CARDIO-ONCOLOGY PRACTICE MANUAL

A COMPANION TO **BRAUNWALD'S HEART DISEASE**

CARDIO-ONCOLOGY PRACTICE MANUAL

A COMPANION TO **BRAUNWALD'S HEART DISEASE**

JOERG **HERRMANN,** MD
Professor of Medicine
Division of Cardiovascular Diseases
Mayo Clinic
Rochester, Minnesota

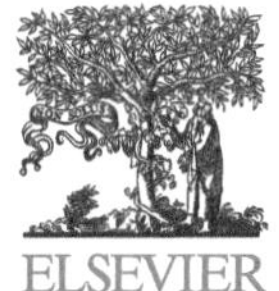

ELSEVIER

Elsevier
1600 John F. Kennedy Blvd.
Ste 1800
Philadelphia, PA 19103-2899

CARDIO-ONCOLOGY PRACTICE MANUAL: A COMPANION TO BRAUNWALD'S HEART DISEASE ISBN: 978-0-323-68135-3

Content Strategist: Robin Carter
Content Development Specialist: Angie Breckon
Content Development Manager: Meghan Andress
Publishing Services Manager: Shereen Jameel
Project Manager: Haritha Dharmarajan
Designer: Renee Duenow

Printed in The United States of America

Last digit is the print number: 9 8 7 6 5 4 3 2 1

To
My family, teachers, and mentors,
and the multitude of patients affected by cancer and cardiovascular disease

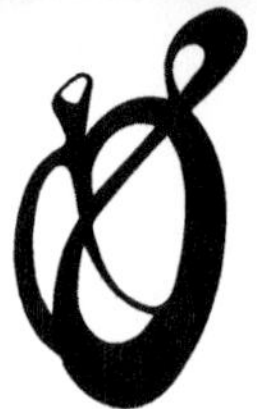

Contributors

Ghosh AK, MBBS, MSc, PhD, FHEA, FACC, FESC, FRCP
University College London
London, UK

Mohamed S. Ali, MD
Fellow, Endocrinology, Diabetes and Metabolism
McGovern Medical School
Houston, Texas, USA

Jose A. Alvarez-Cardona, MD
Instructor
Medicine and Cardiovascular Division
Washington University School of Medicine
Saint Louis, Missouri, USA

Dinu Valentin Balanescu, MD
Beaumont Hospital, Royal Oak
Michigan, USA
Department of Cardiology
The University of Texas MD Anderson Cancer Center
Houston, Texas, USA

Pedro C. Barata, MD, MSc
Tulane Cancer Center
Tulane University School of Medicine
New Orleans, Louisiana, USA

Sara Bouberhan, MD
Program in Gynecologic Medical Oncology
Beth Israel Deaconess Medical Center
Harvard Medical School
Boston, Massachusetts, USA

Ibrahim Büdeyri, MD
Department of General Surgery
University of Muenster
Muenster, Germany

Stephen A. Cannistra, MD
Program in Gynecologic Medical Oncology
Beth Israel Deaconess Medical Center
Harvard Medical School
Boston, Massachusetts, USA

Joseph R. Carver, MD
Abramson Cancer Center of the University of Pennsylvania
Philadelphia, Pennsylvania, USA

Katherine Lee Chuy, MD
John H. Stroger Jr. Hospital of Cook County
Chicago, Illinois, USA

Suparna C. Clasen, MD, MSCE
Department of Medicine
Indiana University School of Medicine
Indianapolis, Indiana, USA

H. M. Connolly, MD
Professor of Medicine
Department of Cardiovascular Medicine
Mayo Clinic
Rochester, Minnesota, USA

Brian A. Costello, MD, MS
Division of Medical Oncology
Mayo Clinic
Rochester, Minnesota, USA

Chen DH, BMED, FRACP
University College London
London, UK

Angela Dispenzieri, MD
Mayo Clinic
Rochester, Minnesota, USA

Stephen J. H. Dobbin, MBChB, MRCP
Institute of Cardiovascular and Medical Sciences
British Heart Foundation Glasgow Cardiovascular Research Centre
University of Glasgow
Glasgow, UK
Department of Internal Medicine
Division of Nephrology and Hypertension
Department of Cardiovascular Diseases
Mayo Clinic
Rochester, Minnesota, USA

Teodora Donisan, MD
Beaumont Hospital, Royal Oak
Michigan, USA
Department of Cardiology
The University of Texas MD Anderson Cancer Center
Houston, Texas, USA

Thomas Eschenhagen, MD
Institute of Experimental Pharmacology and Toxicology
University Medical Center Hamburg-Eppendorf
Hamburg, Germany

William Finch, MD
UCLA Cardio-Oncology Program
Division of Cardiology
Department of Medicine
University of California at Los Angeles
Los Angeles, California, USA

Michael Fradley, MD
Cardio-Oncology Center of Excellence
Division of Cardiology
Perelman School of Medicine at the University of Pennsylvania
Pennsylvania, USA

Sanjeev A. Francis, MD
Assistant Professor
Tufts University School of Medicine
Boston, Massachusetts, USA
Director of Education
Cardiovascular Institute Maine Medical Center
Portland, Maine, USA

Andrea Gallardo-Grajeda, MD
National Institute of Cardiology Ignacio Chavez
Toluca, Mexico

Matthew D. Galsky, MD
Division of Oncology
Mount Sinai Hospital
New York, New York, USA

Alexander Geyer, MD
Pulmonary Service
Division of Subspecialty Medicine
Memorial Sloan Kettering Cancer Center New York, New York, USA

Axel Grothey, MD
Director, GI Cancer Research
Department of Medical Oncology
West Cancer Center and Research Institute
Germantown, Tennessee, USA

Thomas M. Habermann, MD
Division of Hematology
Department of Medicine
Mayo Clinic
Rochester, Minnesota, USA

Robert I. Haddad, MD
Division Chief
Department of Head and Neck Oncology
Dana Farber Cancer Institute
Professor of Medicine
Harvard Medical School
Boston, Massachusetts, USA

Thorvardur R. Halfdanarson, MD
Professor of Oncology
Division of Medical Oncology
Mayo Clinic
Rochester, Minnesota, USA

Christopher L. Hallemeier, MD
Department of Radiation Oncology
Mayo Clinic
Rochester, Minnesota, USA

Joerg Herrmann, MD
Professor of Medicine
Division of Cardiovascular Diseases
Mayo Clinic
Rochester, Minnesota, USA

Sandra M.S. Herrmann, MD
Division of Nephrology and Hypertension
Mayo Clinic
Rochester, Minnesota, USA

William Hogan, MD
Division of Hematology
Mayo Clinic
Rochester, Minnesota, USA

Cezar Iliescu, MD, FACC, FSCAI
Professor Department of Cardiology
Division of Internal Medicine
The University of Texas MD Anderson Cancer Center
Houston, Texas, USA

Robin Jones, MD
Consultant Medical Oncologist
Head of Sarcoma Unit
The Royal Marsden Hospital NHS Foundation Trust
London, UK

Thomas J. Kaley, MD
Beaumont Hospital, Royal Oak
Michigan, USA
Department of Neurology
Memorial Sloan Kettering Cancer Center

Jasvinder Kaur, MBChB
Department of Medical Oncology
University Hospitals Birmingham
Birmingham, Alabama

Alok A. Khorana, MD
Department of Internal Medicine
Western Reserve Health Education/Northeast Ohio Medical University Program
Ohio, USA

Kyle W. Klarich, MD
Vice Chair, Clinical Practice
Department of Cardiology
Mayo Clinic
Rochester, Minnesota, USA

Jörg Kleeff, MD, FACS, FRCS
Department of Visceral, Vascular, and Endocrine Surgery
Halle University Hospital
Martin-Luther-University Halle-Wittenberg
Halle, Germany

Lavanya Kondapalli, DM
Division of Cardiology
University of Colorado School of Medicine
Denver, Colorado, USA

Bonnie Ky, MD, MSCE
Department of Medicine, Division of Cardiology, Perelman School of Medicine at the University of Pennsylvania, Philadelphia, USA
Abramson Cancer Center, Perelman School of Medicine at the University of Pennsylvania, Philadelphia, USA
Department of Biostatistics, Epidemiology & Informatics, Perelman School of Medicine at the University of Pennsylvania, Philadelphia, USA

Ninian N. Lang, BSc (Hons), MBChB, PhD, FRCP
Institute of Cardiovascular and Medical Sciences
British Heart Foundation Glasgow Cardiovascular Research Centre
University of Glasgow
Glasgow, UK

Carolyn M. Larsen, MD
Cardiovascular Medicine
Mayo Clinic
Phoenix, Arizona, USA

Bénédicte Lefebvre, MD, CM
Department of Medicine
Division of Cardiology
Perelman School of Medicine at the University of Pennsylvania
Philadelphia, USA

Daniel J. Lenihan, MD, FACC, FESC
Professor of Medicine
Director, Cardio-Oncology Center of Excellence
Cardiovascular Division
Washington University in Saint Louis
Saint Louis, Missouri, USA

Jennifer E. Liu, MD
Cardiology Service
Memorial Sloan Kettering Cancer Center
New York, New York, USA

S.A. Luis, MBBS, FRACP, FACC, FASE
Co-Director, Pericardial Diseases Clinic
Medical Director, Mayo clinic School of Health Sciences Echocardiography and Advanced Cardiovascular Sonography Programs
Department of Cardiovascular Medicine
Mayo Clinic
Rochester, Minnesota, USA
Senior Lecturer
School of Medicine
The University of Queensland
Brisbane, Australia

Dimitri J. Maamari, MD
American University of Lebanon
Beirut, Lebanon

Priyanka Makkar, MD
Pulmonary Medicine
Memorial Sloan Kettering Cancer Center
New York, New York, USA

Joseph J. Maleszewskic, MD
Professor of Laboratory Medicine and Pathology
Professor of Medicine
Department of Laboratory Medicine and Pathology
Mayo Clinic
Rochester, Minnesota, USA

Robert D. McBane II, MD
Gonda Vascular Center
Department of Cardiovascular Diseases
Mayo Clinic
Rochester, Minnesota, USA

Kristen B. McCullough, PharmD
Department of Pharmacy
Mayo Clinic
Rochester, Minnesota, USA

Christoph W. Michalski, MD
Department of Surgery
Martin Luther University Halle-Wittenberg
Halle, Germany

Yevgeniya Mogilevskaya, DO
Division of pulmonary and critical care medicine
NYU Langone Health
New York, New York, USA

Tomas G. Neilan, MD, MPH
Cardio-Oncology Program
Division of Cardiology
Department of Medicine
Massachusetts General Hospital
Boston, Massachusetts, USA

Vuyisile T. Nkomo, MD, MPH
Division of Structural Heart Disease
Department of Cardiovascular Diseases
Mayo Clinic, Rochester, Minnesota, USA

Jae K. Oh, MD
Division of Structural Heart Disease
Department of Cardiovascular Medicine
Mayo Clinic
Rochester, Minnesota, USA

Mrinal M. Patnaik, MD
Division of Hematology
Department of Internal Medicine
Mayo Clinic
Rochester, Minnesota, USA

P.A. Pellikka, MD
Vice Chair
Department of Cardiovascular Medicine
Betty Knight Scripps Professor of Medicine
Mayo Clinic College of Medicine
Consultant
Department of Cardiovascular Diseases and Internal Medicine
Director
Ultrasound Research Center
Mayo Clinic
Rochester, Minnesota, USA

Shyam K. Poudel, MD
Department of Internal Medicine
Western Reserve Health Education/Northeast Ohio Medical University Program
Ohio, USA

Tienush Rassaf, MD, FESC, FACC
Department of Cardiology and Vascular Medicine
West German Heart and Vascular Center
University Hospital Essen
Essen, Germany

Michael J. Reardon, MD
Allison Family Distinguished Chair of Cardiovascular Research
Department of Cardiovascular Surgery
Professor of Cardiovascular Surgery
Methodist DeBakey Heart and Vascular Center
Houston, Texas, USA

Kathryn J. Ruddy, MD
Division of Medical Oncology
Mayo Clinic Rochester
Rochester, Minnesota, USA

Gagan Sahni, MD, FACC, FACP, FICOS
Associate Professor of Medicine
Cardiovascular Institute
Mount Sinai Hospital
Director, Cardio-Oncology
Mount Sinai Hospital
New York, New York, USA

Jaskanwal Deep Singh Sara, MBChB
Department of Cardiovascular Medicine
Mayo Clinic
Rochester, Minnesota, USA

Oliver Sartor, MD
Tulane Cancer Center
Tulane University School of Medicine
New Orleans, Louisiana, USA

Douglas Sawyer, MD, PhD
Professor of Medicine
Tufts University School of Medicine
Boston, Massachusetts
Chief Academic Office
Division of Cardiovascular Medicine
Maine Medical Center
Portland, Maine, USA

Dirk Schadendorf, MD
Department of Dermatology
University Hospital Essen
Department of Dermatology
Essen, Germany
German Cancer Consortium
Heidelberg, Germany

Wendy Schaffer, MD, PhD
Associate Clinical Member
Memorial Sloan Kettering Cancer Center
New York, New York, USA

Jessica M. Scott, PhD
Memorial Sloan Kettering Cancer Center
Weill Cornell Medical College
New York, New York, USA

Meghan Shea, MD
Program in Gynecologic Medical Oncology
Beth Israel Deaconess Medical Center
Harvard Medical School
Boston, Massachusetts, USA

Mohamed Bassam Sonbol, MD
Assistant Professor of Medicine
Mayo Clinic Cancer Center
Phoenix, Arizona, USA

Aferdita Spahillari, MD
Assistant Professor of Medicine
Massachusetts General Hospital
Boston, Massachusetts, USA

Ray W. Squires, PhD
Department of Cardiovascular Medicine
Division of Preventive Cardiology
Mayo Clinic
Rochester, Minnesota, USA

Jason S. Starr, DO
Assistant Professor of Medicine
Mayo Clinic Florida
Jacksonville, Florida, USA

Richard Steingart, MD
Chief, Cardiology Service
Department of Medicine
Memorial Sloan Kettering Cancer Center
Professor of Medicine
Weill Medical College of Cornell University
New York, New York, USA

A. Keith Stewart, MB, ChB
Director of Mayo Clinic Center for Individualized Medicine
Department of Hematology/Oncology
Mayo Clinic
Phoenix, Arizona, USA

Zoltan Szucs, PhD
Honorary Consultant Medical Oncologist
University College London Hospitals NHS Foundation Trust
London, UK

Rhian M. Touyz, BSc (Hons), MBChB, PhD, FRCP, FRSE, FMedSci
Institute of Cardiovascular and Medical Sciences
British Heart Foundation Glasgow Cardiovascular Research Centre
University of Glasgow
Glasgow, UK

Barry H. Trachtenberg, MD
Assistant Professor of Cardiology
Director of Cardio-Oncology and Cardiac Amyloidosis Program
Methodist DeBakey Heart and Vascular Center
Houston, Texas, USA

Mirela Tuzovic, MD
Division of Cardiovascular Medicine
Department of Medicine
Stanford University Medical center
Stanford, California, USA

Jeena Varghese, MD
Assistant Professor
The University of Texas MD Anderson Cancer Center
Endocrine Neoplasia and Hormonal Disorders
Houston, Texas, USA

Paul V. Viscuse, MD
Department of Medicine
Division of Medical Oncology
Mayo Clinic Rochester
Rochester, Minnesota, USA

Lachelle D. Weeks, MD, PhD
Center for Head and Neck Oncology
Dana Farber Cancer Institute
Harvard Medical School
Boston, Massachusetts, USA

Zhuoer Xie, MD, MS
Department of Medical Oncology
Mayo Clinic
Rochester, Minnesota, USA

Eric H. Yang, MD
Associate Clinical Professor of Medicine
UCLA Cardio-Oncology Program
Division of Cardiology
Department of Medicine
University of California at Los Angeles
Los Angeles, California, USA

Anthony Yu, MD
Assistant Member
Department of Medicine
Memorial Sloan Kettering Cancer Center
New York, New York, USA

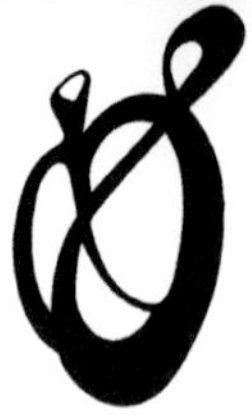

Acknowledgments

Cardio-Oncology Practice Manual: A Companion to Braunwald's Heart Disease is the work and product of many great individuals. First and foremost, I would like to express my deepest gratitude to Dr. Eugene Braunwald for his vision and provision to launch this new title. Furthermore, I would like to thank Elsevier for the wonderful support of the concept taken in the *Cardio-Oncology Practice Manual* and bringing it into production. In particular, I would like to formally acknowledge and thank the following members of the Elsevier team who made this book a reality: Robin Carter, Executive Content Strategist, for the enormous work on this from the very beginning, the relentless positivity and contagious joy; Angie Breckon, Senior Content Development Specialist, for the superb organization, keeping everything together and on track; and Haritha Dharmarajan, Project Manager, for integrating a large volume of material into one coherent production and the excellent final touches. Finally, I would like to give a special thanks to Joanna King from the Mayo Medical Illustration and Animation team for the tremendous work on the art and graphics as well as Mayo Clinic and the Mayo Department of Cardiovascular Medicine for the professional support.

Foreword

FOREWORD TO CARDIO-ONCOLOGY PRACTICE MANUAL

Since the first edition of *Heart Disease: A Textbook of Cardiovascular Medicine* was published in 1980, enormous advances have transformed the management not only of cardiovascular disorders but of cancer as well. Nonetheless, when taken together these two conditions remain responsible for well over half of the deaths in adults in industrially developed nations. Patients with either of these disease states are now living longer and, because both conditions are more common in older patients, with progressive aging of the population their prevalence is rising. Increasingly, survivors of one disease class become at risk for the other. For example, a smoker who develops a large myocardial infarction may survive the acute event owing to modern life-saving care, but faces a heightened future risk of developing lung cancer. Conversely, a patient with a lymphoma that would have been fatal a few years ago who now is cured by the combination of chemotherapy and mediastinal irradiation has enhanced risk of developing cardiomyopathy and coronary artery disease.

Many of the important recent advances in the treatment of cancer entail a variety of cardiovascular toxicities, which can be quite serious and potentially fatal. However, simultaneous advances in cardiology, including the use of non-invasive imaging to monitor cardiac function during cancer therapy, can guide changes in management to minimize or even prevent these complications. This progress has been made possible by the development of a new but important subspecialty, cardio-oncology (or onco-cardiology). An increasing number of caregivers will need training in this challenging, rapidly growing and expanding field.

Dr. Joerg Herrmann, a leader in cardio-oncology, has edited this Practice Manual which could be considered a syllabus for clinicians, cardiologists and oncologists and their trainees alike, as well as for pharmacists, nurses and other professionals on the cardio-oncology team. Dr. Herrmann has selected an excellent cadre of authors and produced a book that we are proud to call a *Companion to Heart Disease: A Textbook of Cardiovascular Medicine*.

Eugene Braunwald, MD
Peter Libby, MD
Robert O. Bonow, MD, MS
Douglas L. Mann, MD
Gordon F Tomaselli, MD
Deepak L. Bhatt, MD, MPH
Scott D. Solomon, MD

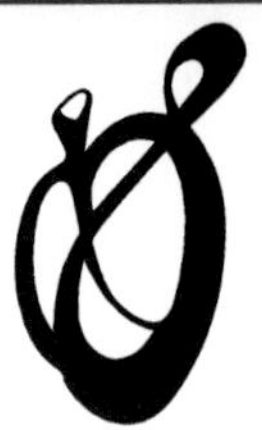

Preface

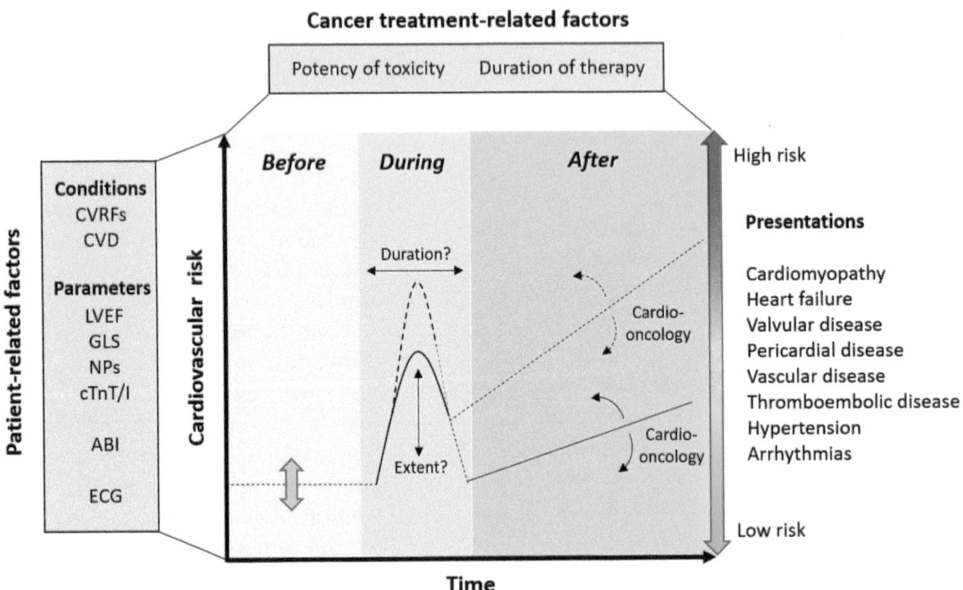

Heart disease and cancer are the two leading causes of death in industrialized countries. Historically seen as separate entities with little to no overlap, this view has changed fundamentally over the last two decades. In particular, with increasing survival rates from malignancies, the acute and long-term complications of cancer therapies have gained more and more prominence. Among these, cardiovascular toxicities are of particular significance given their impact on morbidity and mortality, at times greater than that of the primary malignancy. Attending to the cardiovascular disease aspects of patients with cancer is the essence of the emerging field of cardio-oncology. Furthermore, there has been mounting recognition of a higher risk of malignancies among patients with cardiovascular diseases, which has become known as reverse cardio-oncology.

Although still a relatively new field, cardio-oncology has received a lot of traction with an exponential growth in the initiation of service lines. The momentum of practice initiation has outpaced any evidence base in this area, creating a notable vacuum in terms of knowledge and training. Education, especially self-education in cardio-oncology, has been limited by suitable resources that fit into a busy clinical practice. This aspect, however, is so important, as learning is best received right at the time when the problem arises, and in this case during the clinical encounter. Any resources that aim to be of assistance in this setting need to be readily available, easy to follow, concise, and yet comprehensive.

This book was designed to address these needs and was conceptualized with the busy practitioner in the cardio-oncology clinic in mind. It takes an innovative approach to cover the most common topics in cardio-oncology in a quick and practical manner. Each chapter begins with a Central Illustration and key bullet points that summarize the topic graphically and textually. As appropriate, algorithms are provided that outline the management approach to the presenting problem. The chapter text follows the summary outline, supporting and expanding the key take home points. All chapters are authored by experts in the field who join the reader in their clinical encounter, thereby allowing for a true practice manual experience.

The most common reasons for patients with cancer to be referred to the cardio-oncology clinic are to (1) assess cardiovascular risk, (2) prevent cardiovascular risk, or (3) manage and mitigate cardiovascular complications. The focus of interest shifts slightly before, during, and after cancer treatment. Whereas the emphasis is on risk assessment and prevention before cancer therapy, it is on management and mitigation of complications during cancer therapy and thereafter on long-term disease prevention and management. The content structure follows this continuum of cancer care and thereby allows for the provider to meet the patient in the proper clinical context (see figure on previous page).

Another important aspect this book is addressing is the emerging need for a common understanding of the disease entities and the bidirectional nature of treatment decisions among cardiology, oncology, and hematology providers. Often oncologists/hematologists need to learn more about cardiovascular diseases in patients with cancer and cardiologists need to learn more about malignancies and what to expect in terms of treatment and prognosis. In addition to the coverage of the most important cardiovascular disease entities and cardiovascular comorbidities in patients with cancer, this book henceforth also provides a comprehensive yet concise manual of the most important malignancies.

Last but not least, as cancer therapeutics and their toxicity spectra are so important in everyday cardio-oncology practice, the last part of the book provides a guide to the most commonly used cardiotoxic cancer drugs. The content is made easily accessible in summary tables with further information in text format for the interested reader. This cancer drug guide is also available online with ongoing updates as an invaluable tool of reference.

Taken together, this book is designed to be a one-stop resource for the cardio-oncology practice provider during and outside of clinic hours. Its main intention is to meet the needs of providers so that they can then meet the needs of patients with cancer with or at risk of cardiovascular disease and/or toxicity (from cancer therapy). Never in the history has this patient population been larger than at present with expectations for further growth in the future. To better clinical outcomes, to ease the practice, we hope that this manual will serve patients with cancer and their care team providers well, now and in years to come.

Joerg Herrmann
Professor of Medicine
Division of Cardiovascular Diseases
Mayo Clinic
Rochester, Minnesota

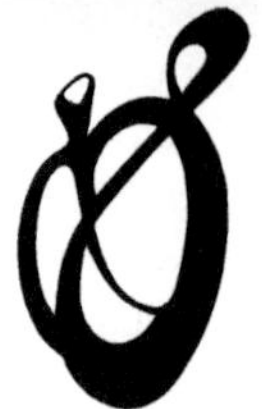

Contents

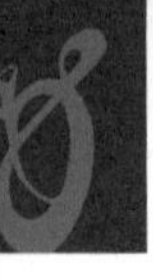

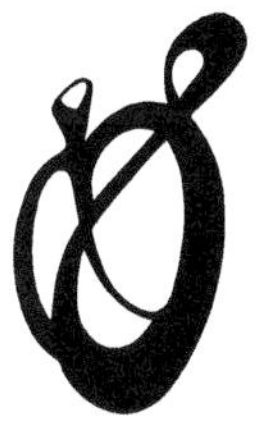

Braunwald's Heart Disease Family of Books

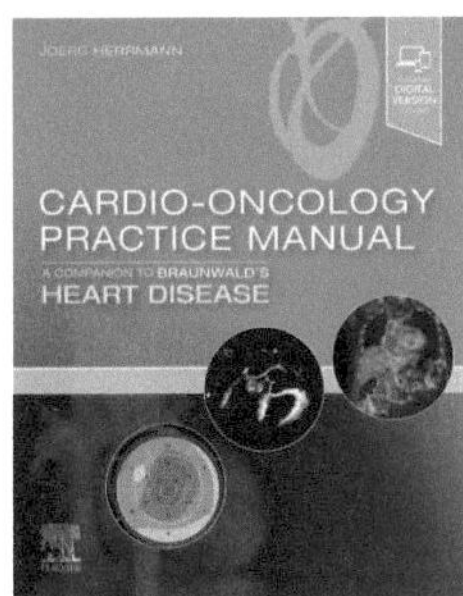

HERRMANN
Cardio-Oncology Practice Manual

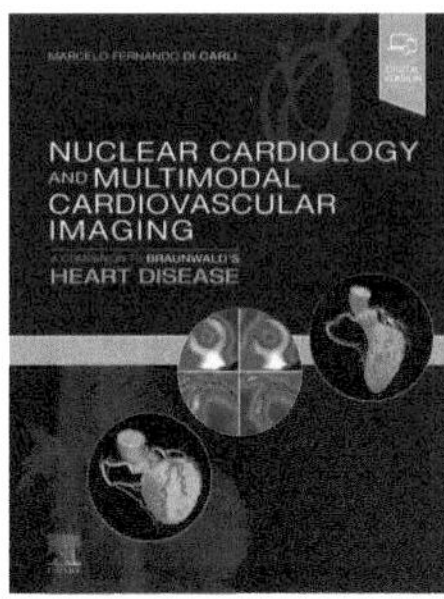

DI CARLI
Nuclear Cardiology and Multimodal Cardiovascular Imaging

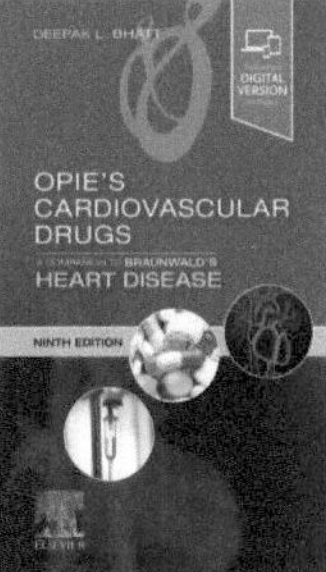

BHATT
Opie's Cardiovascular Drugs

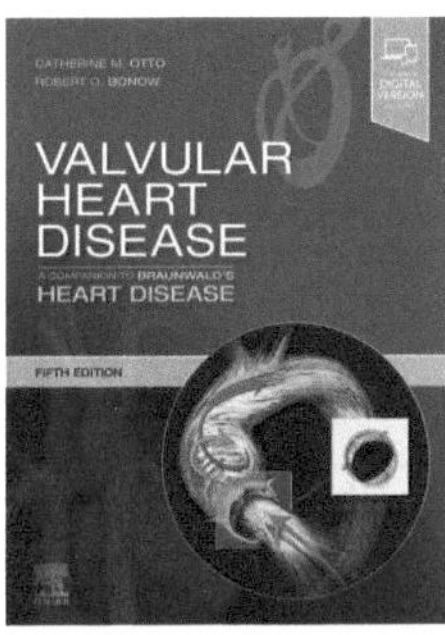

OTTO AND BONOW
Valvular Heart Disease

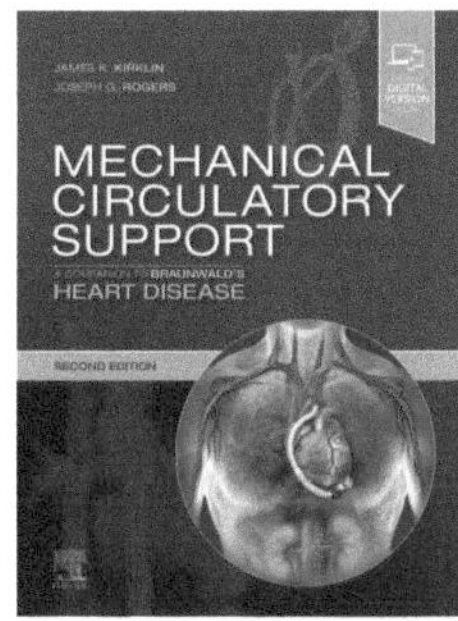

KIRKLIN AND ROGERS
Mechanical Circulatory Support

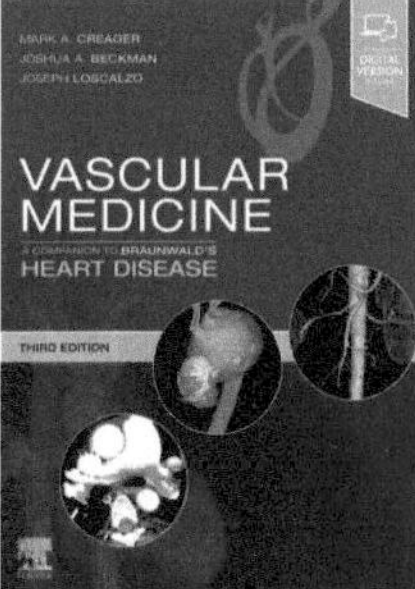

CREAGER
Vascular Medicine

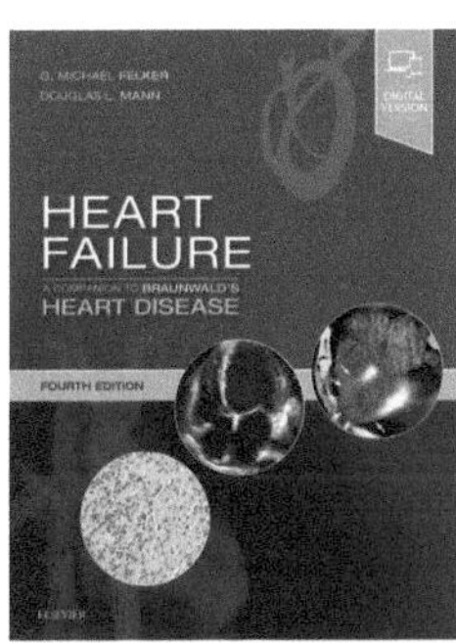

FELKER AND MANN
Heart Failure

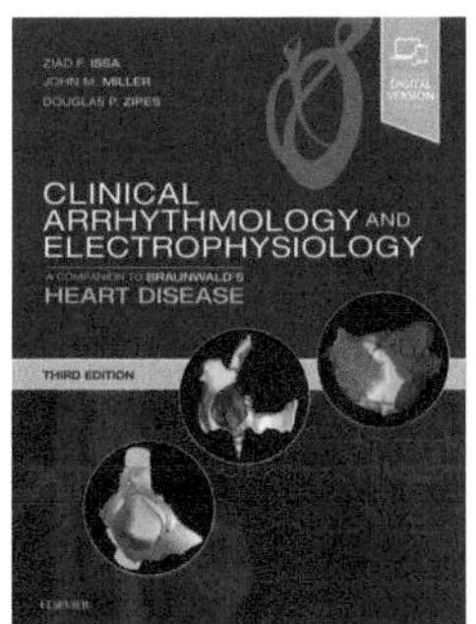

ISSA, MILLER, AND ZIPES
Clinical Arrhythmology and Electrophysiology

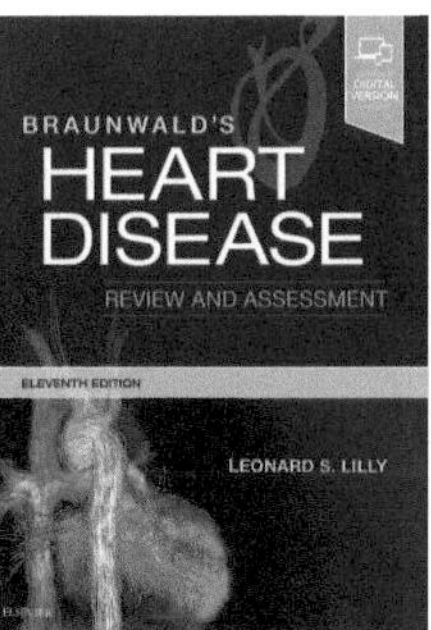

LILLY
Braunwald's Heart Disease

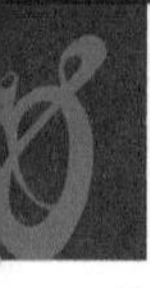

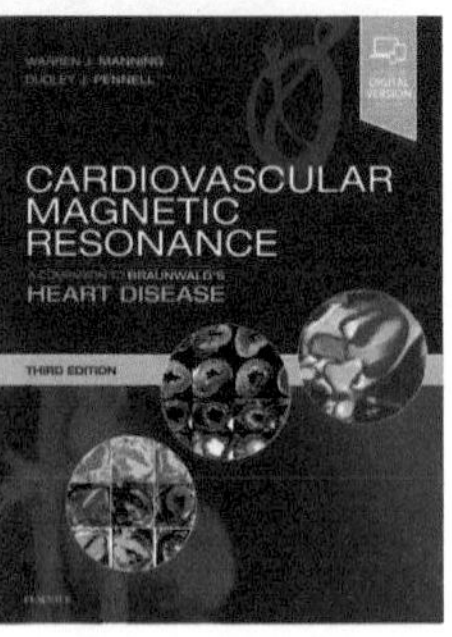

MANNING AND PENNELL
Cardiovascular Magnetic Resonance

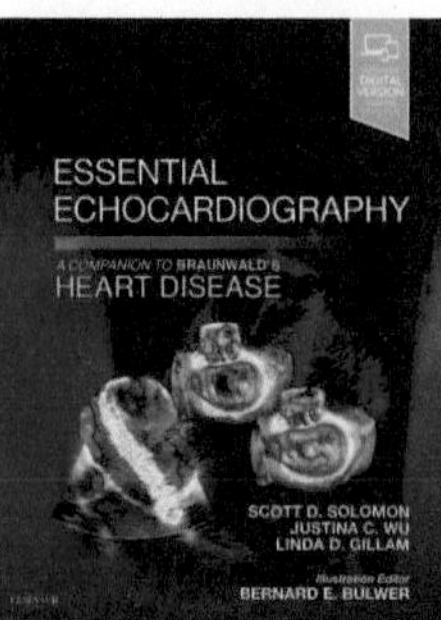

SOLOMON, WU, AND GILLAM
Essential Echocardiography

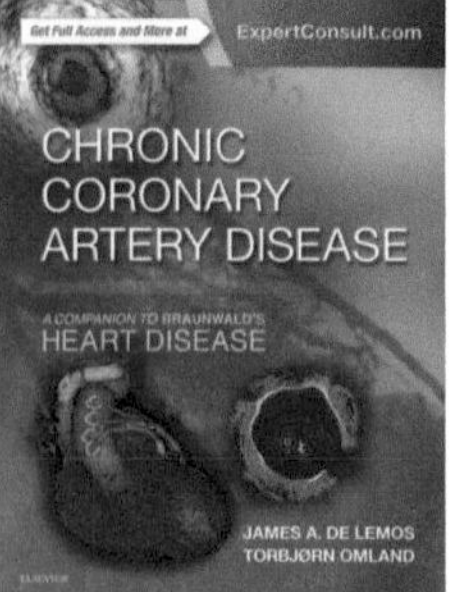

DE LEMOS AND OMLAND
Chronic Coronary Artery Disease

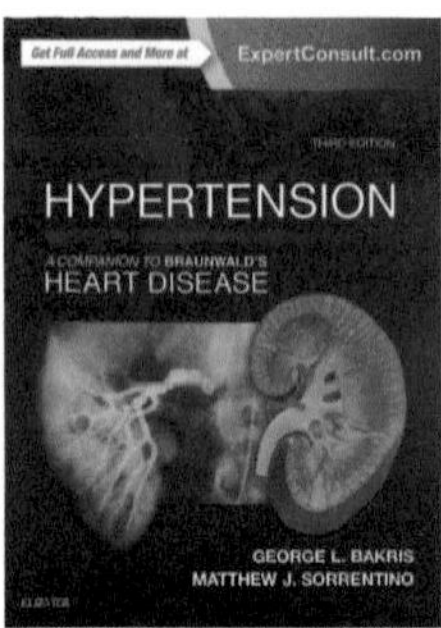

BAKRIS AND SORRENTINO
Hypertension

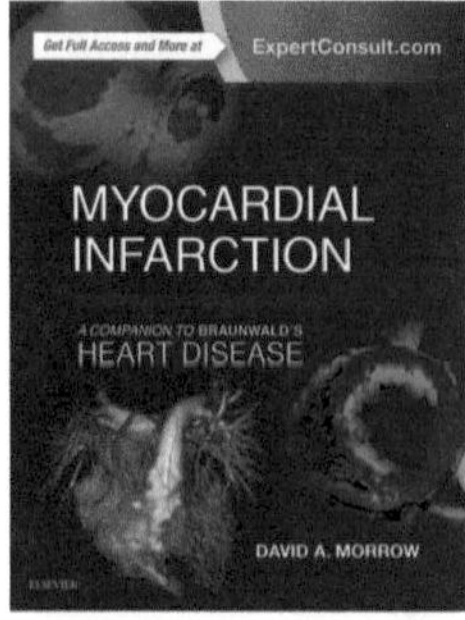

MORROW
Myocardial Infarction

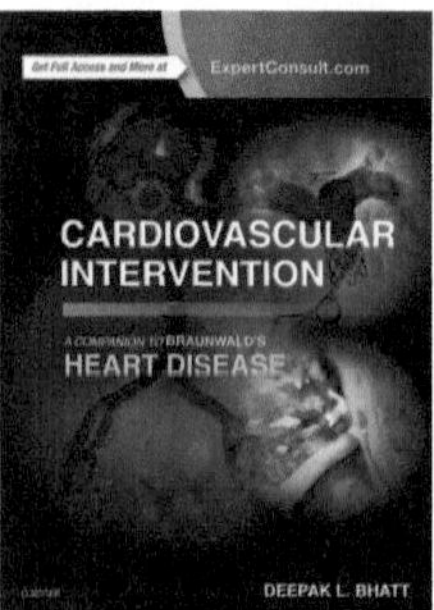

BHATT
Cardiovascular Intervention

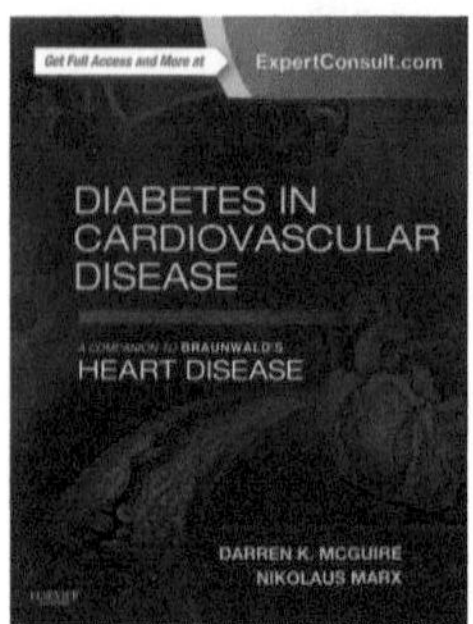

MCGUIRE AND MARX
Diabetes in Cardiovascular Disease

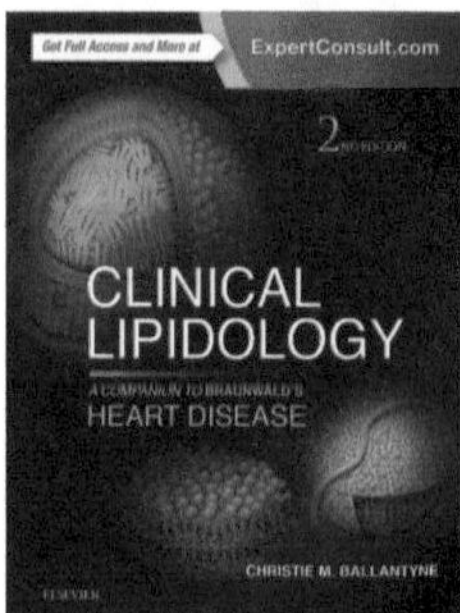

BALLANTYNE
Clinical Lipidology

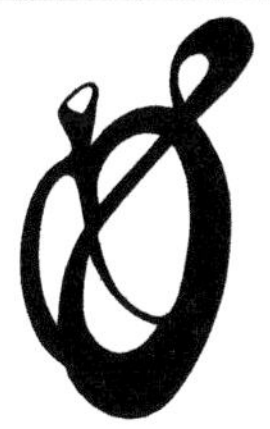

1 The Cardio-Oncology Clinic: Goals, Scope, and Focus of Practice

JOERG HERRMANN

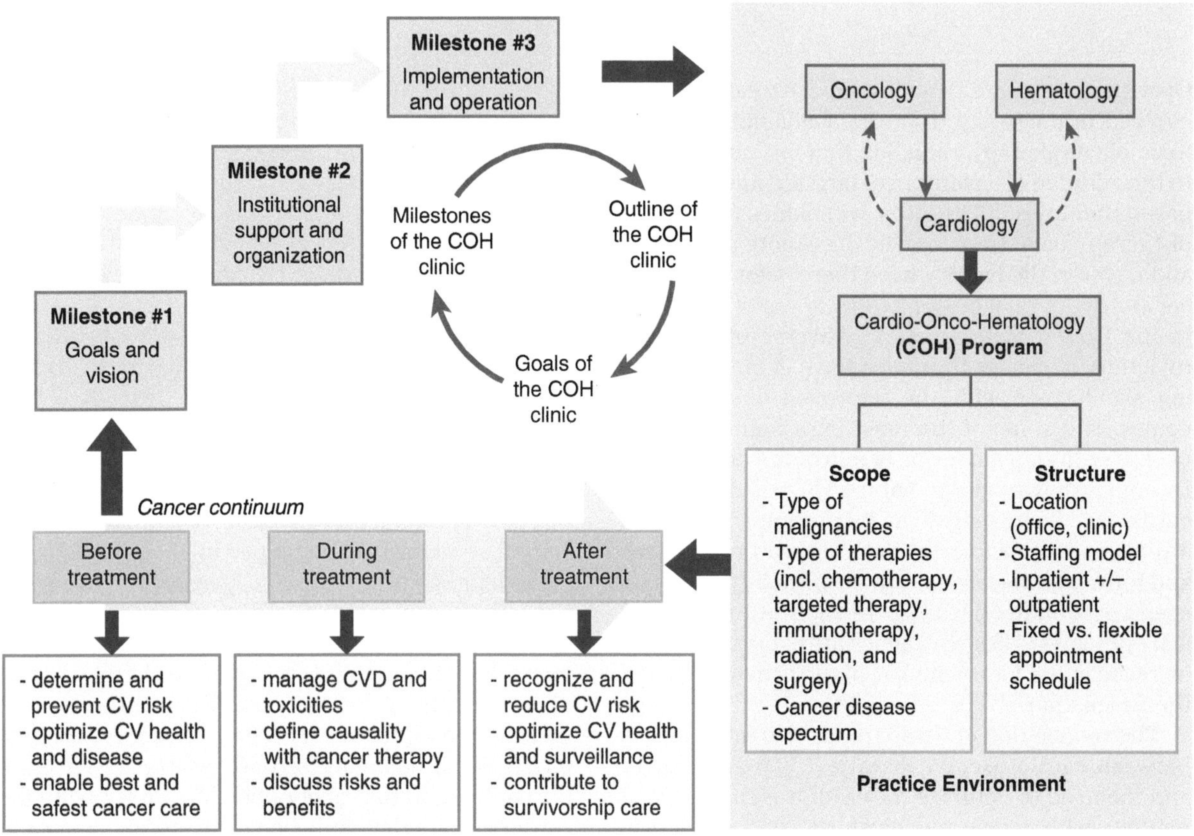

Milestone #3
Implementation and operation

Milestone #2
Institutional support and organization

Milestone #1
Goals and vision

Milestones of the COH clinic

Outline of the COH clinic

Goals of the COH clinic

Cancer continuum

Before treatment
- determine and prevent CV risk
- optimize CV health and disease
- enable best and safest cancer care

During treatment
- manage CVD and toxicities
- define causality with cancer therapy
- discuss risks and benefits

After treatment
- recognize and reduce CV risk
- optimize CV health and surveillance
- contribute to survivorship care

Oncology

Hematology

Cardiology

Cardio-Onco-Hematology **(COH) Program**

Scope
- Type of malignancies
- Type of therapies (incl. chemotherapy, targeted therapy, immunotherapy, radiation, and surgery)
- Cancer disease spectrum

Structure
- Location (office, clinic)
- Staffing model
- Inpatient +/– outpatient
- Fixed vs. flexible appointment schedule

Practice Environment

CHAPTER OUTLINE

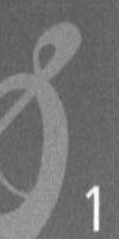

KEY POINTS

- The cardio-oncology clinic covers all cardiovascular aspects of patients with cancer, including tumors that involve the heart and vasculature, cancer therapies that affect the heart and vasculature, and cardiovascular diseases in patients with cancer.
- The key goal of the clinic is to enable patients with cancer to receive the best possible cancer therapy at the lowest possible cardiovascular risk (to uncouple risk and benefit).
- A multidisciplinary team forms the core of the clinic. It is composed of professionals specialized in providing cardiovascular evaluations and treatments for patients across their continuum of cancer care.
- Three milestones can be distinguished toward establishing a cardio-oncology clinic: (1) goals and vision, (2) institutional support and organization, and (3) implementation and operation.
- The structure and scope of the cardio-oncology clinic, which needs to be individualized for the specific practice environment, requires reevaluation and readjustment based on outcome measures and developments in the field.

Over the past three decades cancer treatment has evolved dramatically from the availability of cytotoxic chemotherapy, radiation therapy, and surgery to the addition of a plethora of targeted and immune-based therapies.[1,2] The latter two modes (or pillars) of therapy have transformed the practice radically and never in the history have there been more cancer survivors than presently (in excess of 15 million in the United States alone).[3] Adverse effects and toxicities of cancer therapies have gained increasing significance with the improved survival outcomes, and some of the most important toxicities of cancer therapy in terms of morbidity and mortality are cardiovascular in nature. On the other hand, cardiovascular diseases can be present even before a diagnosis of cancer is made and can complicate and terminate cancer therapy (especially if not managed appropriately) with grave implications for clinical outcomes. These dynamics are expected only to increase in the future in view of the general aging of the population.[4]

The recognition of these trends and interactions between cardiovascular disease (CVD) and cancer and the need to optimize the cardiovascular care of patients with cancer has given rise to a new discipline referred to as "Cardio-Oncology" or "Onco-Cardiology." As the field involves hematology as well, the terminology "Cardio-Onco-Hematology" has also been used at times, but for simplicity and consistency we will use the term "Cardio-Oncology" throughout this book.[5] Clinics providing such services have started to emerge in the mid first decade of the 21st century, and since then, there has been an exponential growth in their number across all continents.[5,6] Milestones and steps toward the successful implementation of a cardio-oncology service line are outlined in prior reviews and the central illustration.[5,6] The very starting point is defined by the needs of the patients, and meeting the needs of the patients defines the success of the cardio-oncology clinic.

MILESTONE #1: GOALS AND VISION

Defining the cardiovascular needs and demands of patients who have cancer at a given practice location will inform about the goals of the cardio-oncology clinic (i.e., what is to be accomplished, which impact one would like to have, which improved outcomes one would like to see). Commonly aspired goals are outlined in Table 1-1.[7,8] A clear vision is absolutely critical and needs to be shaped in cross-disciplinary communications. The perspectives of both, cardiology and oncology/hematology groups, should be taken into account when plans for the clinic are being made, and this should furthermore be in the context of the unique individual practice environment of these groups (private office, group practice, community/regional hospitals, tertiary referral center, cancer center) and the cancer population referred to the cardio-oncology clinic. Based on these foundations, it is possible to summarize and update the vision for the scope and shape of the program:

The cardio-oncology clinic will see ... (type of patients) by ... (cardiologists/oncologists/hematologists) in the .... (heart/cancer center, clinic, hospital). The appointment types might include virtual (e-)consultations as well as in-person, out-patient, and in-patient visits. It should moreover be defined if curbside and on-call options will be made available. Last but not least, based on the defined demand, it can be projected that .... (number of) patients will be seen in the cardio-oncology clinic every month.[5]

TABLE 1.1 **Goals of the Cardio-Onco-Hematology (COH) Clinic**

STAGE IN THE CANCER CONTINUUM	COH CLINIC GOALS
Before	**Recognition and Mitigation of CV Risk**
	• Identification of potential risk factors for cancer therapy-related CV toxicity
	• Optimization of CV health and preexisting CVD (guideline-directed therapies)
	• Discussion of the most efficacious cancer therapy without substantial CV harm
	• Definition of optimal surveillance and preventive efforts for CV complications/toxicities
	• Facilitation of safe administration of anticancer therapies
During	**Early Recognition and Treatment of CVD and CV Toxicities**
	• Implementation of safety measures to avoid cancer therapy interruptions
	• Surveillance, early identification, and treatment of CV complications
	• Defining and prioritizing risks of CVD/CV toxicity vs. cancer therapies
	• Discussions on continuation vs. interruption of cancer therapy
After	**Surveillance and Mitigation of Late CV Complications and CVD**
	• Optimization of preventive strategies
	• Screening for late-onset complications
	• Setup of routine follow-up protocols
	• Enabling health lifestyle measures
	• Referral to cardio-oncology rehabilitation if not done earlier in the continuum

CV, Cardiovascular; *CVD*, cardiovascular diseases.

Although accomplishing these goals is a team effort, a cardio-oncology clinic champion (director) should be identified who will take ownership and will be the main point of contact, integration, and implementation.

MILESTONE #2: INSTITUTIONAL SUPPORT AND ORGANIZATION

For the cardio-oncology clinic to launch, it will need the approval and support of the practice/institution oversight groups.[5,6] From an administrative perspective, a certain volume of patients per week is generally required to build and maintain a practice (Table 1.2). This is important not only as it pertains to investment costs but also for the expertise of the providers. A low volume clinic likely will not develop the necessary experience in this area. Vice versa, an overloaded clinic cannot attend to all the details so important in this field. Various models of defined quantity and quality may therefore be discussed, and the practice environment will dictate the next steps in terms of approval and organization of the cardio-oncology clinic.

Community physicians or private community group practices may have a less complex structure to implement but also to cover all aspects. A strategic partnership with larger regional cardio-oncology service lines are important so that complex cases can be referred for further testing and treatment. Often private practice executive members will make the final decisions in this setting. For any other type of hospital, stakeholders from administration, cardiology and oncology/hematology department leadership will likely form the review group. Individual structures vary as much as the clinic goals and structure, although the outlined principles are the same across the different practice environments.

Once it is decided to proceed, the organization of the clinic can and must take concrete steps. At this stage, allied health staff will need to be centrally involved, and again, the structure will vary depending on practice environment. In private community offices this will include secretaries and desk attendants. In hospitals, the same are to be involved, but also operation managers and staff and appointment coordinators are needed. This is to guarantee that ordering systems are appropriately built, appointment requests are appropriately directed, desk attendants receive instructions on the new type of clinic, and provider schedules are arranged accordingly. Depending on the complexity

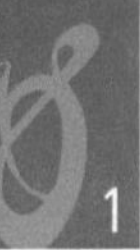

TABLE 1.2 Volume-Based Stratification of Cardio-Onco-Hematology (COH) Programs (Progression/Growth in Service Lines From Left to Right Conceivable)

	LOW-VOLUME COH PROGRAM	MEDIUM-VOLUME COH PROGRAM	LARGE-VOLUME COH PROGRAM	CANCER CENTER
Practice environment	Private office setting Smaller-sized hospitals	Medium-sized hospitals	Larger-sized Hospitals	Specialized High-volume center
Patient volume	<5 per week	5–10 per week	>10 per week	>>10 per week
COH providers	Single COH specialist	Few COH specialists Emerging team	Team of COH specialists; may include nurses, pharmacists, and so forth	Team of focused COH specialists
Cardiology practice	General consultant cardiologists	Consultant cardiologists with specialties	Specialized care in cardiology	General and COH specialized cardiologists In-house staffing or partnership with cardiology center
Oncology/hematology practice	General and focused oncologist/hematologist	General and specialty oncology/hematology	Specialized care in oncology/hematology	Highly specialized care in oncology/hematology
Dedicated outpatient clinic	+ (often on-demand appointments)	+ (half days)	+ (multiple half or full days)	+ (full days)
Inpatient	–	+	+	+
On-call availability	?	+	+	+
Imaging				
Standard echo	+	+	+	+
Advanced echo (strain)	–	+	+	+
CMR, CT, PET	–	+	+	+
Cardiac biomarkers	+	+	+	+
Vascular studies				
ABI	+	+	+	+
Doppler ultrasound	+	+	+	+
Vasoreactivity studies	–	–	+	+
ECG monitoring	+	+	+	+
Procedures Cardiac catheterization, electrophysiology studies, devices, cardiac and vascular surgeries	Upon referral	Routinely	All the time	Variable
Heart transplantation	–	–	+	–
Training program	–	–	+	+
Challenges	Educational experience	In-between stage	Organization and harmonization	Overspecialization

ABI, Ankle-brachial index; *CMR*, cardiac magnetic resonance; *CT*, computed tomography; *ECG*, electrocardiogram; *PET*, positron emission tomography.

of the practice, it may take months for these arrangements to be complete.

Irrespective of the practice environment, the central point for the clinic workflow will be the triage system. Some practices can provide virtual or e-consultations, non-face-to-face and video consultations in addition to in-person, face-to-face consultation (Table 1.3). Whereas the latter is historically the default appointment type, and the preferred route if major treatment decisions are to be made, with decreasing complexity and/or changing environments (e.g., viral pandemics), the other appointment types are valuable. Having these options is also very useful when the volume of consultation requests is high but capacity to see patients in person is limited. The cardio-oncology clinic provider may also be able to guide the oncologist/hematologist with recommendations for drug dosages or tests to order over the

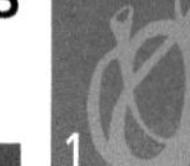

TABLE 1.3 Types and Wait Times for Cardio-Onco-Hematology (COH) Appointment

TYPE OF APPOINTMENT	CHARACTERISTICS, FORMAT, AND INDICATIONS	PROS AND CONS
E-consultation	Virtual chart review of patient's medical records on history, condition, and cardiovascular concerns • Optimization of CV risk factors in asymptomatic patients without CV disease • Advice on drug dosing or drug–drug interactions • Advice on referral for studies, centers, or the COH clinic • Simple follow-up questions of established patients Usually: limited review, no major management decisions, no initiation of new treatments that require in-depth discussion and shared decision making E-messages from the patients may be considered in this category as well (e.g., on symptoms, vital parameters, follow-up tests) Valuable role for a COH clinic nurse is to review incoming requests and messages with responses and triage as appropriate	**Pros:** • Efficient way for requestors to seek specialty opinion • Easy add-on format • Low logistic demand **Cons:** • Disproportional time commitment (and reimbursement)* • Risk of incomplete coverage of the consultation reason*
Non-face-to-face (phone) consultation	As above, but involving a dedicated appointment time for a phone call and direct, real-time communication • Any patient-related questions and concerns • In-depth review of signs and symptoms of disease • In-depth review of test results • Shared decisions on next steps in evaluation or treatment Usually: follow up of established patients or initial review (intake) of new patients for in-person visit planning (streamlining)	**Pros:** • Efficient direct communication • Location flexibility • Low logistic demand **Cons:** • Time commitment and reimbursement* • Limited visual review capacity* • Inability to perform a physical examination
Video consultation	As above, plus ability for video communication • Any patient-related questions and concerns for a more personal review and discussion • Additional visual review of presentation (signs and symptoms) • Additional on-screen review of test results • Additional on-screen education Usually: follow up of established patients or initial review (intake) of new patients with the option of in-person visit planning	**Pros:** • Flexibility for patient and provider location/scheduling • Direct interface **Cons:** • Higher logistic demand (need for setup, often "virtual" check-in desk) • Inability to perform a physical examination
Face-to-face consultation	Standard format for clinic visits • Any of the indication items listed above Usually: any complex clinical scenario, major treatment decisions	**Pros:** • Complete coverage **Cons:** • High demand
Wait Time	**Examples of Clinical Scenarios**	**Location**
Emergent (immediate)	Acute coronary syndrome, flash pulmonary edema, complete heart block, ventricular tachycardia, hypertensive emergency Or initiation of cancer therapy with acutely recognized risk or any of the above outlined presentations	Hospital, ED, rarely outpatient
Urgent (same day)	Initiation of next day cancer therapy in a patient with high CV risk Development of CV complications on cancer therapy with less acuity (e.g., hypertensive urgency, atrial fibrillation with RVR) Logistic reasons	Outpatient, hospital, ED
Semiurgent (within a few days)	Planned cancer therapy in a patient with high CV risk Development of CV complications on cancer therapy with less acuity Uncontrolled, progressive CV conditions, irrespective of therapy	Outpatient
Routine (within a few weeks)	Survivorship visits Post-hospitalization visits Routine follow-up visits	Outpatient

*Especially if complex cases and questions are subjected to e-consultations.
CV, Cardiovascular; *CVD,* cardiovascular diseases; *ED,* emergency department.
Modified from Lenihan, D et al. Cardio-oncology care in the era of the coronavirus disease 2019 (COVID-19) pandemic: an International Cardio-Oncology Society (ICOS) statement. *CA Cancer J Clin*. 2020;70:480–504; Herrmann J, Loprinzi C, Ruddy K. Building a cardio-onco-hematology program. *Curr Oncol Rep*. 2018;20(10):81.

phone. Availability of a triage provider or nurse might help to direct these questions and optimize patient triage and clinic volumes.

Wait times for an appointment differ by appointment type and clinical scenario (see Table 1.3). For patients who need to be started on therapy as soon as possible or have acute cardiovascular complications urgent referrals are usually made and ideally result in a same day appointment. The cardio-oncology program should have enough flexibility and mechanisms in place to accommodate for these cases. Ideally seen as face-to-face consultations, some very urgent cases might also be seen by virtual consultations or telemedicine.

Although coverage of only these very imminent needs might serve as a starting point for a cardio-oncology clinic, this will likely not provide enough volume to develop expertise. As an alternative and to have a more constant flow of patient, one cardio-oncology clinic appointment could be reserved on any given day for any possible (and not only emergent) cardio-oncology consultation. Such slots can be made available for other patients if not taken by those with a cardio-oncology care focus within a defined time interval, providing an administratively attractive model. This also provides for growth, as more and more extra patients will justify having dedicated half-day or full-day clinics. This will then be combined with on-demand capacity to have both a structured standing and flexible clinic model.

Not every group will be able to provide staffing for in-patient services, and may, *de facto*, not need to do so. Providers in the outpatient cardio-oncology clinic may be able to cover questions as they arise, in conjunction with a general inpatient cardiology consultation team. It is to be emphasized that if a cardio-oncology program is present, it should be utilized also as a resource for inpatients. This is becoming more and more important with acute hospitalizations of patients with cancer who present with cardiovascular complications of cancer therapies as their main or concomitant reason for admission.

Once the program structure is established, the availability of the cardio-oncology service line should be communicated. All possible referring providers should be informed, as should local cardiologists so that they can redirect patients with cancer to the new service line if they are subsequently accidentally referred to general or other subspecialty cardiology clinics. The most effective mode of communication is one-on-one. Indeed, the most successful cardio-oncology clinics started based on personal interactions and collaborations between one cardiologist and one oncologist/hematologist.

MILESTONE #3: IMPLEMENTATION AND OPERATION

Although the infrastructure will be tested and major issues declare themselves once the program is in place, it is advisable to follow the first 10 to 20 patients closely to assess for gaps in the scheduling and triage procedure and for lapses in communication. This time period also allows for the development and optimization of algorithms and preorder sets addressing the various reasons for the cardio-oncology consultation (e.g., echocardiogram and cardiac biomarkers for cardiotoxicity, vasoreactivity and ankle-brachial-index studies for vascular toxicity, 24-hour or 48-hour Holter monitoring for arrhythmias prior to the appointment).

The route of communication should be bidirectional. Ideally, the hematology-oncology team will communicate to the cardio-oncology clinic team the context and expectations for the consultation ahead of time. Likewise, cardio-oncology providers should provide a clear report and recommendation to both the patient and the referring provider. A phone call to the referring provider while the patient is in the room is particularly valuable if CVD issues may warrant changes to the cancer treatment plan. This allows for immediate integration of the preferences and wishes of the patient and a joint agreement between all involved parties (shared decision making).[9]

The optimal coordination of care should center on the individual needs of the patient, provided by an integrated multidisciplinary care team.[10] Although this refers primarily to the interaction of the medical disciplines involved, the multidisciplinary team may be much larger and may include a pharmacist, a nurse, and a physician assistant, at times even a nutritionist and an exercise physiologist/therapists. A statement on cardio-oncology rehabilitation was released by the American Heart Association and several programs have adopted this approach.

All members of the multidisciplinary team should be involved in regular 'tumor board-type' meetings to discuss difficult cases, not only from a medical perspective but also the broader context of quality of life and the patient's preferences and goals of care. These sessions or separate all staff multidisciplinary meetings can be utilized to develop local protocols and consensus guidelines for institutional practices and to streamline the communication between professionals involved in the care of patients with cancer.[7] Standardization of clinical processes and care is very important, so that patients receive the same level of care irrespective of the differences in provider staffing of the clinic. It should be emphasized that the overreaching objective is to facilitate oncology treatments, to avoid their interruption, to minimize delays in workup and preparation, and to increase efficiency.

Patient education and enabling patients to be advocates for their own health is an extremely important aspect of cardio-oncology clinics. Patients should have the opportunity to learn more about their disease processes, risk factors that are common to both cancer and CVD, and how these two disease entities and their treatments affect each other. Teaching materials, such as booklets, fact sheets, and educational websites, should be made available. Practices can also consider offering individual and/or group educational sessions as well as community events.

Finally, patient feedback is important as are quality and outcome measures to refine and improve the cardio-oncology program to reach its envisioned goals. Such efforts will also help with any potential moves toward standardization and accreditation of cardio-oncology practices. Cardio-oncology programs will need to remain adaptable, striving continuously to provide the best possible practice.

APPROACH TO THE PATIENT WITH CANCER AT RISK OF OR WITH EVIDENT CARDIOVASCULAR DISEASE

This book is intended to be a companion in the cardio-oncology clinic, a practical guide for the day-by-day encounters and an aid in the approach to patients with cancer who are at risk of or with established CVD. An outline of a cardio-oncology approach is provided in Fig. 1.1. It can be

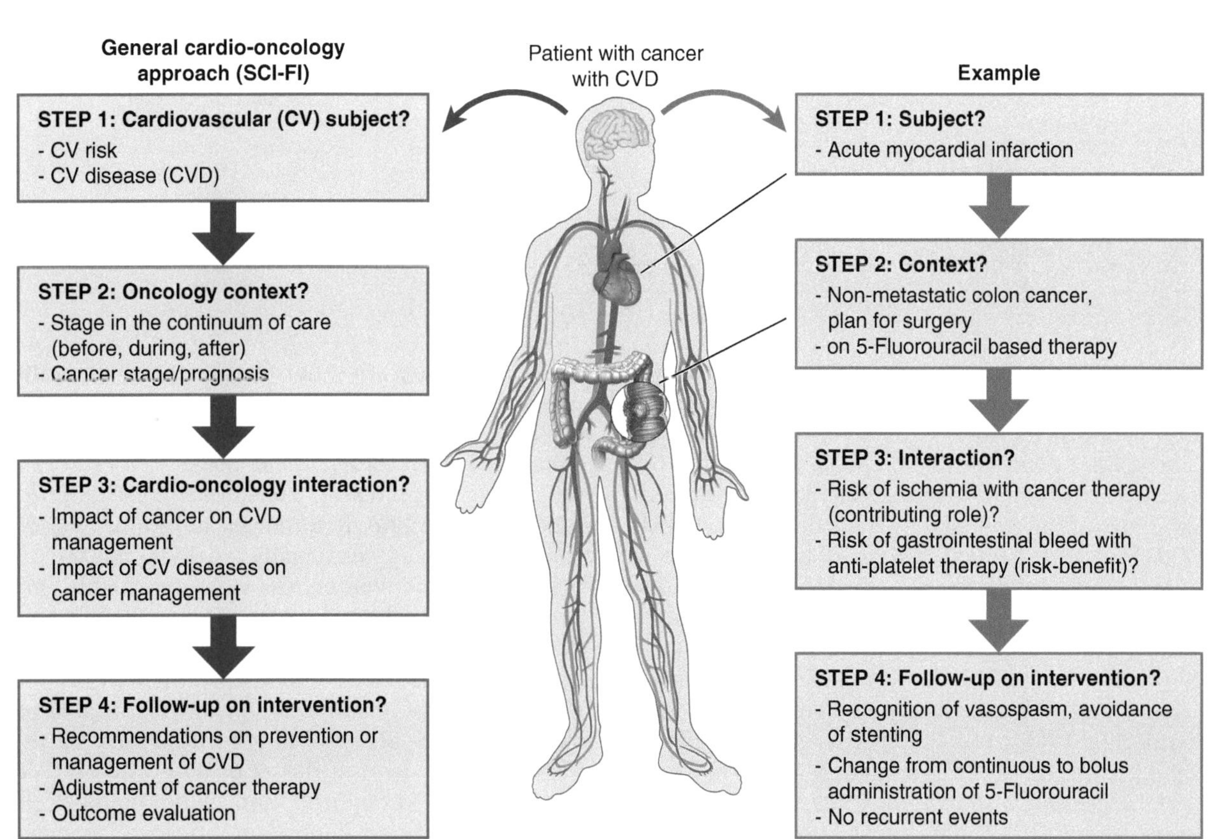

FIG. 1.1 Illustration of a general approach model to patients with cancer who are at risk of or with established cardiovascular diseases.

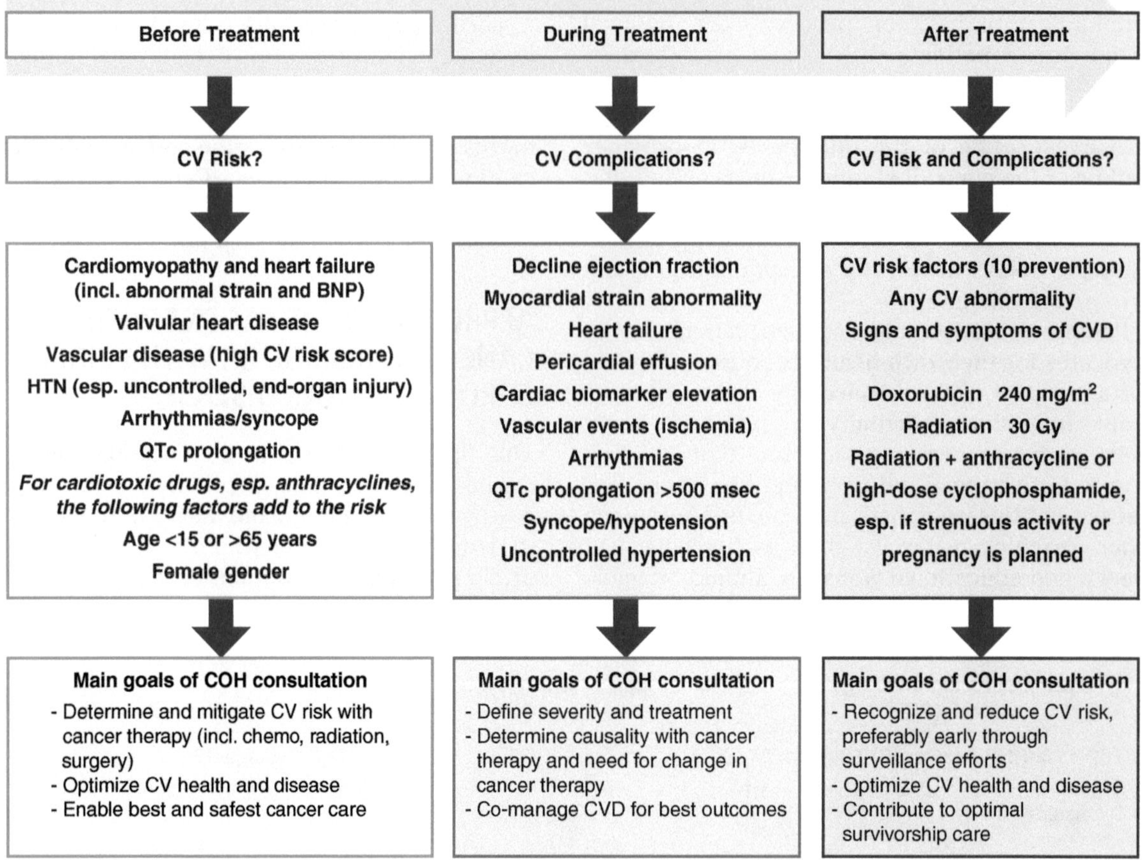

Cancer Continuum
Before Treatment
During Treatment
After Treatment
CV Risk?
CV Complications?
CV Risk and Complications?
Cardiomyopathy and heart failure (incl. abnormal strain and BNP)
Valvular heart disease
Vascular disease (high CV risk score)
HTN (esp. uncontrolled, end-organ injury)
Arrhythmias/syncope
QTc prolongation
For cardiotoxic drugs, esp. anthracyclines, the following factors add to the risk
Age <15 or >65 years
Female gender
Decline ejection fraction
Myocardial strain abnormality
Heart failure
Pericardial effusion
Cardiac biomarker elevation
Vascular events (ischemia)
Arrhythmias
QTc prolongation >500 msec
Syncope/hypotension
Uncontrolled hypertension
CV risk factors (10 prevention)
Any CV abnormality
Signs and symptoms of CVD
Doxorubicin 240 mg/m2
Radiation 30 Gy
Radiation + anthracycline or high-dose cyclophosphamide, esp. if strenuous activity or pregnancy is planned
Main goals of COH consultation
- Determine and mitigate CV risk with cancer therapy (incl. chemo, radiation, surgery)
- Optimize CV health and disease
- Enable best and safest cancer care
Main goals of COH consultation
- Define severity and treatment
- Determine causality with cancer therapy and need for change in cancer therapy
- Co-manage CVD for best outcomes
Main goals of COH consultation
- Recognize and reduce CV risk, preferably early through surveillance efforts
- Optimize CV health and disease
- Contribute to optimal survivorship care

FIG. 1.2 Outline of the cardiovascular care aspects of patients across their continuum of cancer care. *BNP,* brain natriuretic peptide; *COH*, Cardio-onco-hematology; *CV*, cardiovascular; *CVD*, cardiovascular diseases; *HTN,* hypertension.

summarized under the acronym SCI-FI. It begins with the cardiovascular Subject in question, then takes the oncology/hematology Context into consideration and integrates these two elements, the cardio-oncology Interaction. Concrete recommendations and actions are to be provided and their impact should be assessed (e.g., improvement of cardiac function: Follow-up on Intervention). Another proven useful element in the approach to patients with cancer who are at risk of or with evident CVD is to meet them in their continuum of cancer care as cardiovascular care aspects vary accordingly (Fig. 1.2). Before the start of cancer therapy, the question to address is often to define and mitigate the cardiovascular risk and/or optimize preexisting CVD. During cancer therapy, cardiovascular complications often capture the attention or the management of ongoing established CVD. After cancer therapy, the chronic aspects of acute cardiovascular toxicities, late presentations of cardiovascular side effects, and ongoing cardiovascular health issues in cancer survivors are often of greatest interest. The subsequent chapters follow this outline. References and links to additional resources, especially specific consensus statements and guidelines, where available, are provided. On a final note, practice guidelines endorsed by major cardiology societies do generally apply, but with some considerations as exemplified in the supplemental material to two 2020 reviews.[1,2] Thus, at the end, the approach to the patient with cancer at risk of or with evident CVD needs to be thoughtful and individualized, in keeping with good clinical practice and engagement of the patient and multidisciplinary team providers in a shared decision model.

REFERENCES

1. Herrmann J. Adverse cardiac effects of cancer therapies: cardiotoxicity and arrhythmia. *Nat Rev Cardiol.* 2020;17(8):474–502.
2. Herrmann J. Vascular toxic effects of cancer therapies. *Nat Rev Cardiol.* 2020;17(8):503–522.
3. Miller KD, Nogueira L, Mariotto AB, et al. Cancer treatment and survivorship statistics, 2019. *CA Cancer J Clin.* 2019;69(5):363–385.
4. Bluethmann SM, Mariotto AB, Rowland JH. Anticipating the "silver tsunami": prevalence trajectories and comorbidity burden among older cancer survivors in the United States. *Cancer Epidemiol Biomarkers Prev.* 2016;25(7):1029–1036.
5. Herrmann J, Loprinzi C, Ruddy K. Building a cardio-onco-hematology program. *Curr Oncol Rep.* 2018;20(10):81.
6. Snipelisky D, Park JY, Lerman A, et al. How to develop a cardio-oncology clinic. *Heart Fail Clin.* 2017;13(2):347–359.
7. López-Fernández T, Martín García A, Santaballa Beltrán A, et al. Cardio-onco-hematology in clinical practice. Position paper and recommendations. *Rev Esp Cardiol (Engl Ed).* 2017;70(6):474–486.
8. Lancellotti P, Suter TM, López-Fernández T, et al. Cardio-oncology services: rationale, organization, and implementation. *Eur Heart J.* 2019;40(22):1756–1763.
9. Gujral DM, Manisty C, Lloyd G, Bhattacharyya S. Organisation & models of cardio-oncology clinics. *Int J Cardiol.* 2016;214:381–382.
10. Fleissig A, Jenkins V, Catt S, Fallowfield L. Multidisciplinary teams in cancer care: are they effective in the UK? *Lancet Oncol.* 2006;7(11):935–943.

PART I

Cardiovascular Disease Management Before Cancer Treatment

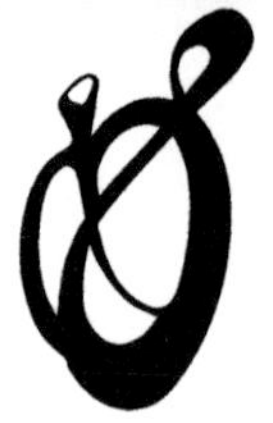

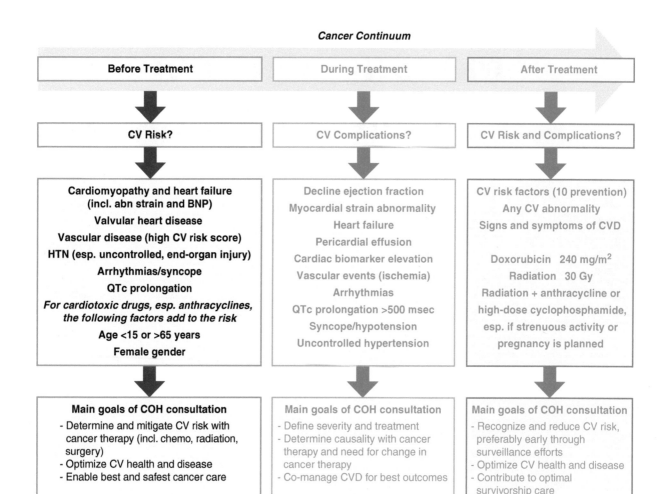

2 Key Points of Cardio-Oncology Evaluation Before Cancer Therapy

JOERG HERRMANN

Cancer Continuum

Before Treatment	During Treatment	After Treatment
CV Risk?	CV Complications?	CV Risk and Complications?
Cardiomyopathy and heart failure (incl. abn strain and BNP) Valvular heart disease Vascular disease (high CV risk score) HTN (esp. uncontrolled, end-organ injury) Arrhythmias/syncope QTc prolongation *For cardiotoxic drugs, esp. anthracyclines, the following factors add to the risk* Age <15 or >65 years Female gender	Decline ejection fraction Myocardial strain abnormality Heart failure Pericardial effusion Cardiac biomarker elevation Vascular events (ischemia) Arrhythmias QTc prolongation >500 msec Syncope/hypotension Uncontrolled hypertension	CV risk factors (10 prevention) Any CV abnormality Signs and symptoms of CVD Doxorubicin 240 mg/m^2 Radiation 30 Gy Radiation + anthracycline or high-dose cyclophosphamide, esp. if strenuous activity or pregnancy is planned
Main goals of COH consultation - Determine and mitigate CV risk with cancer therapy (incl. chemo, radiation, surgery) - Optimize CV health and disease - Enable best and safest cancer care	**Main goals of COH consultation** - Define severity and treatment - Determine causality with cancer therapy and need for change in cancer therapy - Co-manage CVD for best outcomes	**Main goals of COH consultation** - Recognize and reduce CV risk, preferably early through surveillance efforts - Optimize CV health and disease - Contribute to optimal survivorship care

KEY POINTS

- The main objective of the pretherapy evaluation of patients with cancer is to identify cardiovascular (CV) risk, especially as it pertains to the planned cancer therapy and how it could affect its completion and the patient's long-term outcome.
- All cardiovascular disease (CVD) entities should be considered as well as the cluster of CV risk factors because these may decrease the cardiovascular reserve sufficiently to complicate cancer therapy and overall patient clinical outcome.
- Validated risk scores for the various CV toxicities are largely not available and it is challenging to stratify patients as low, intermediate, and high risk.
- Additional studies should be obtained, as needed, to define further risk and preventive strategies.
- Each pretherapy evaluation should conclude with a management plan for surveillance and prevention, even when the risk is deemed low and such efforts are not needed.

The recognition of the profound impact of cardiovascular diseases and toxicities in the lives of those with cancer has led to the discipline of cardio-oncology and should be used to guide its practice. Accordingly, from the very beginning of a patient's journey along the continuum of cancer care, the presence of CVD and the potential for toxicities should be recognized. Unlike many other clinical scenarios in clinical practice, the timing and type of potential injury are known. This knowledge should provide a unique window of opportunity to review, prepare for, and prevent CVDs in patients undergoing cancer therapies.

This section provides an overview of today's main cancer therapies and their cardiovascular risk dimensions, including chemotherapeutics, targeted therapies, radiation therapy, surgery, and bone marrow transplantation. This is followed by an outline of the main CVD entities to consider in patients before the initiation of their cancer therapy, including cardiomyopathy, vascular disease, and arrhythmias. The practical use of this information is in the CV-directed screening and evaluation of every patient with cancer prior to cancer therapy. It provides a framework of what to look for and what to recommend. The management of preexisting CVD and CV risk factors should be optimized before the initiation of therapy. Patients with these conditions are usually at higher risk for complications and should also be set up for (closer) follow up during and after cancer therapy.

The treatment-related CV toxicity risk can be anticipated based on the published literature, although sometimes it is still evolving, especially if treatment is with a new investigational drug.

TABLE 2.1. Baseline Cardio-Oncology Risk Assessment Structure[a]

RISK CATEGORY	DEFINITION
A. Estimate of the cardiovascular toxicity risk with planned cancer therapy based on sum of the risk factors identified (see following tables)	
Low risk	• no risk factors or one one medium-1 point risk factor
Medium risk	• single medium 2-point risk factor or >1 medium-1 point risk factor with points totalling 2–4
High risk	• ≥1 high risk factors or several medium risk factors with points totalling ≥5
Very high risk	• ≥1 very high risk factors
B. Definition of the absolute risk (in terms of likelihood) based on expert consensus as outlined	
Low risk	<2%
Medium risk	2%–9%
High risk	10%–19%
Very high risk	≥20%

[a]Based on the position statement from the cardio-oncology study group of the Heart Failure Association of the European Society of Cardiology in collaboration with the International Cardio-Oncology Society, *Eur J Heart Fail*. 2020;22:1945–1960.

Rigorously validated risk scores for the different CV toxicities are not available; but intuitively, CV toxicity risk is determined by patient- and therapy-related factors. Along these lines, risk proformas have been developed as outlined in Tables 2.1 to 2.7. Also, the cardiovascular reserve concept serves well, as outlined in the exercise chapter 13. In some scenarios, additional tests can help refine risk and direct management, which includes the choice of one type of therapy over another. Some therapies,

TABLE 2.2. Baseline Cardio-Oncology Risk Assessment Before Anthracycline Therapy

RISK FACTOR	RISK FACTOR PRESENT	SCORE	LEVEL OF EVIDENCE
Previous Cardiovascular Disease			
Heart failure or cardiomyopathy		Very High	B
Severe valvular heart disease		High	C
Myocardial infarction or previous CABG		High	C
Stable angina		High	C
Borderline LVEF 50%–54%		Medium-2 points	C
Cardiac Biomarkers (where available)			
Elevated baseline troponin[a]		Medium-1 point	C
Elevated baseline BNP or NT-proBNP[a]		Medium-1 point	C
Demographic and Cardiovascular Risk Factors			
Age ≥80 years		High	B
Age 65–79 years		Medium-2 points	B
Hypertension[b]		Medium-1 point	B
Diabetes mellitus[c]		Medium-1 point	C
Chronic kidney disease[d]		Medium-1 point	C
Previous Cardiotoxic Cancer Treatment			
Previous anthracycline exposure		High	B
Prior radiotherapy to left chest or mediastinum		High	C
Previous non-anthracycline-based chemotherapy		Medium-1 point	C
Lifestyle Risk Factors			
Current smoker		Medium-1 point	C
Obesity (BMI > 30 kg/m^2)		Medium-1 point	C
Risk Level (see Table 2.1A for details)			

[a]Elevated above the upper limit of normal for local laboratory reference range.
[b]Systolic blood pressure (BP) > 140 mm Hg or diastolic BP > 90 mm Hg, or on treatment.
[c]HbA1c > 7.0% or on treatment.
[d]Estimated glomerular filtration rate <60 mL/min/1.73 m^2.
BMI, Body mass index; *BNP*, brain natriuretic peptide; *CABG*, coronary artery bypass graft; *LVEF*, left ventricular ejection fraction; *NT-proBNP*, N-terminal pro-brain natriuretic peptide.

TABLE 2.3 Baseline Cardio-Oncology Risk Assessment Before Trastuzumab Therapy

RISK FACTOR	RISK FACTOR PRESENT	SCORE	LEVEL OF EVIDENCE
Previous Cardiovascular Disease			
Heart failure or cardiomyopathy		Very High	C
Myocardial infarction or CABG		High	B
Stable angina		High	B
Severe valvular heart disease		High	C
Baseline LVEF <50%		High	C
Borderline LVEF 50%–54%		Medium-2 point	B
Arrhythmia[a]		Medium-2 point	C
Cardiac Biomarkers (Where Available)			
Elevated baseline troponin[b]		Medium-2 point	B
Elevated baseline BNP or NT-proBNP[b]		Medium-2 point	C
Demographic and Cardiovascular Risk Factors			
Age ≥80 years		High	B
Age 65–79 years		Medium-2 point	B
Hypertension[c]		Medium-1 point	**B**
Diabetes mellitus[d]		Medium-1 point	C
Chronic kidney disease[e]		Medium-1 point	C
Current Cancer Treatment Regimen			
Anthracycline before HER2-target Tx		Medium-1 point	B
Anthracycline and HER2-Tx concurrently		High	B
Previous Cardiotoxic Cancer Treatment			
Prior trastuzumab cardiotoxicity		Very High	C
Prior (remote) anthracycline exposure[f]		High	B
Prior radiotherapy to left chest or mediastinum		Medium-2 point	C
Lifestyle Risk Factors			
Current smoker or significant smoking hx		Medium-1 point	**C**
Obesity (BMI >30 kg/m^2)		Medium-1 point	C
Risk Level (see Table 2.1A for details)			

[a]Atrial fibrillation, atrial flutter, ventricular tachycardia or ventricular fibrillation
[b]Elevated above the upper limit of normal for local laboratory reference range.
[c]Systolic blood pressure (BP) >140 mm Hg or diastolic BP >90 mm Hg, or on treatment.
[d]HbA1c >7.0% or on treatment.
[e]Estimated glomerular filtration rate <60 mL/min/1.73m^2.
[f]Previous malignancy (not current treatment protocol).
BMI, Body mass index; *BNP*, brain natriuretic peptide; *CABG*, coronary artery bypass graft; *LVEF*, left ventricular ejection fraction; *NT-proBNP*, N-terminal pro-brain natriuretic peptide.

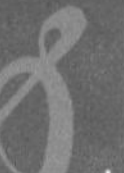

TABLE 2.4. **Baseline Cardio-Oncology Risk Assessment Before vascular growth factor inhibitor (VEGF) Inhibitor Therapy**

RISK FACTOR	RISK FACTOR PRESENT	SCORE	LEVEL OF EVIDENCE
Previous Cardiovascular Disease			
Heart failure or LVSD		Very High	C
Arterial vascular disease (IHD, PCI, CABG, stable angina, TIA, stroke, PVD)		Very High	C
Venous thrombosis (DVT or PE)		High	C
LVEG $< 50\%$		High	C
Borderline LVEF 50%–54%		Medium-2 point	C
QTc $\geq$ 480 ms		High	C
450 ms $\leq$ QTc $<$ 480 ms (men) 460 ms $\leq$ QTc $<$ 480 ms (women)		Medium-2 point	C
Arrhythmia[a]		Medium-2 point	C
Cardiac Biomarkers (Where Available)			
Elevated baseline troponin[b]		Medium-1 point	C
Elevated baseline BNP or NT-proBNP[b]		Medium-1 point	C
Demographic and Cardiovascular Risk Factors			
Age $\geq$75 years		High	C
Age 65–74 years		Medium-1 point	C
Hypertension[c]		High	C
Diabetes mellitus[d]		Medium-1 point	C
Hyperlipidemia[e]		Medium-1 point	C
Chronic kidney disease[f]		Medium-1 point	C
Proteinuria		Medium-1 point	C
Previous Cardiotoxic Cancer Treatment			
Prior anthracycline exposure		High	C
Prior radiotherapy to left chest or mediastinum		Medium-1 point	C
Lifestyle Risk Factors			
Current smoker or significant smoking hx		Medium-1 point	C
Obesity (BMI $>$30 kg/m^2)		Medium-1 point	C
Risk Level (see Table 2.1A for details)			

[a]Atrial fibrillation, atrial flutter, ventricular tachycardia, or ventricular fibrillation.
[b]Elevated above the upper limit of normal for local laboratory reference range.
[c]Systolic blood pressure (BP) $>$140 mm Hg or diastolic BP $>$90mm Hg, or on treatment.
[d]HbA1c $>$7.0% or on treatment.
[e]Total cholesterol level $>$5.2mmol/L.
[f]Estimated glomerular filtration rate $<$60 mL/min/1.73m^2.
BMI, Body mass index; *BNP*, brain natriuretic peptide; *CABG*, coronary artery bypass graft; *DVT*, deep vein thrombosis; *IHD*, ischemic heart disease; *LVEF*, left ventricular ejection fraction; *NT-proBNP*, N-terminal pro-brain natriuretic peptide; *PCI*, percutaneous coronary intervention; *PE*, pulmonary embolism; *QTc*, corrected QT interval; *TIA*, transient ischaemic attack.

TABLE 2.5. Baseline Cardio-Oncology Risk Assessment Before Breakpoint Cluster Region and Abelson (BCR-ABL) Oncogene Fusion Protein

RISK FACTOR	RISK FACTOR PRESENT	SCORE	LEVEL OF EVIDENCE
Previous Cardiovascular Disease			
Arterial vascular disease (IHD, PCI, CABG, stable angina, TIA, stroke, PVD)		Very High	C
Arterial thrombosis with TKI		Very High	C
Heart failure or LVSD		High	C
BCR-ABL TKI-mediated LVSD		High	C
Abnormal ABPI[a]		High	C
Pulmonary arterial hypertension[b]		High	C
Baseline LVEF <50%		High	C
Venous thromboembolism (DVT/PE)		Medium-2 point	C
Arrhythmia[c]		Medium-2 point	C
QTc ≥ 480 ms		High	C
450 ms ≤ QTc < 480 ms (men) 460 ms ≤ QTc < 480 ms (women)		Medium-2 point	C
Demographic and Other CV Risk Factors			
CVD 10-year risk score >20%		High	B
Hypertension[d]		Medium-2 point	B
Diabetes[e]		Medium-1 point	B
Hyperlipidemia[f]		Medium-1 point	B
Age ≥75 years		High	C
Age 65–74 years		Medium-2 point	B
Age ≥60 years		Medium-1 point	B
Chronic kidney disease[g]		Medium-1 point	C
Family history of thrombophilia		Medium-1 point	C
Lifestyle and Other Factors			
Current smoker or significant smoking hx		High	B
Obesity (BMI >30 kg/m^2)		Medium-1 point	C
Risk Level (see Table 2.1A for details)			

[a]Ankle-brachial pressure index ≥1.3.
[b]Peak systolic pulmonary artery pressure at rest ≥35 mm Hg.
[c]Atrial fibrillation, atrial flutter, ventricular tachycardia, or ventricular fibrillation.
[d]Systolic blood pressure (BP) >140 mm Hg or diastolic BP >90mm Hg, or on treatment.
[e]HbA1c >7.0% or on treatment.
[f]Total cholesterol level >5.2 mmol/L.
[g]Estimated glomerular filtration rate <60 mL/min/1.73m^2.
BMI, Body mass index; *CABG*, coronary artery bypass graft; *CVD*, cardiovascular disease *IHD*, ischemic heart disease; *PCI*, percutaneous coronary intervention; *PVD*, peripheral vascular disease; *TIA*, transient ischemic attack; *LVSD*, left ventricular systolic dysfunction.

TABLE 2.6. **Baseline Cardio-Oncology Risk Assessment Before Proteasome Inhibitor and Immunomodulatory Therapy**

RISK FACTOR	RISK FACTOR PRESENT	SCORE	LEVEL OF EVIDENCE
Previous Cardiovascular Disease			
Heart failure or cardiomyopathy		Very High	C
Prior proteasome inhibitor cardiotoxicity		Very High	C
Immunomodulatory drugs cardiotoxicity		High	B
Cardiac amyloidosis		High	C
Arterial vascular disease (IHD, PCI, CABG, stable angina, TIA, stroke, PVD)		High	C
Venous thrombosis (DVT or PE)		High	C
Borderline LVEF 50%–54%		Medium-2 point	C
Arrhythmia[a]		Medium-2 point	C
Left ventricular hypertrophy[b]		Medium-1 point	C
Cardiac Biomarkers (Where Available)			
Elevated baseline troponin[c]		High	B
Elevated baseline BNP or NT-proBNP[c]		High	C
Demographic and CV Risk Factors			
Age ≥75 years		High	C
Age 65–79 years		Medium-1 point	C
Hypertension[d]		Medium-1 point	C
Diabetes mellitus[e]		Medium-1 point	C
Hyperlipidemia[f]		Medium-1 point	C
Chronic kidney disease[g]		Medium-1 point	C
Family history of thrombophilia		Medium-1 point	C
Previous Cardiotoxic Cancer Treatment			
Prior anthracycline exposure		High	C
Prior thoracic spine radiotherapy		Medium-1 point	C
Current Myeloma Treatment			
High-dose dexamethasone >160 mg/month		Medium-1 point	C
Lifestyle Risk Factors			
Current smoker or significant smoking hx		Medium-1 point	C
Obesity (BMI >30 kg/m^2)		Medium-1 point	C
Risk Level (See Table 2.1A for Details)			

[a]Atrial fibrillation, atrial flutter, ventricular tachycardia, or ventricular fibrillation.
[b]Left ventricular wall thickness >1.2 cm.
[c]Elevated above the upper limit of normal for local laboratory reference range.
[d]Systolic blood pressure (BP) >140 mm Hg or diastolic BP >90 mm Hg, or on treatment.
[e]HbA1c >7.0% or on treatment.
[f]Total cholesterol level >5.2 mmol/L.
[g]Estimated glomerular filtration rate <60 mL/min/1.73m^2.
BMI, Body mass index; *BNP*, brain natriuretic peptide; *CABG*, coronary artery bypass graft; *DVT*, deep vein thrombosis; *IHD*, ischemic heart disease; *LVEF*, left ventricular ejection fraction; *NT-proBNP*, N-terminal pro-brain natriuretic peptide; *PCI*, percutaneous coronary intervention; *PE*, pulmonary embolism; *PVD*, peripheral vascular disease; *TIA*, transient ischaemic attack.

TABLE 2.7. Baseline Cardio-Oncology Risk Assessment Before RAF and MEK Inhibitor Combination Therapy

RISK FACTOR	RISK FACTOR PRESENT	SCORE	LEVEL OF EVIDENCE
Previous Cardiovascular Disease			
Heart failure or cardiomyopathy		Very High	C
Myocardial infarction or CABG		High	C
Stable angina		High	C
Severe valvular heart disease		High	C
Borderline LVEF 50%–54%		Medium-2 point	C
Arrhythmia[a]		Medium-1 point	C
Cardiac Biomarkers (Where Available)			
Elevated baseline troponin[b]		Medium-2 point	C
Elevated baseline BNP or NT-proBNP[b]		Medium-2 point	C
Demographic and Cardiovascular Risk Factors			
Age ≥65 years		Medium-1 point	C
Hypertension[c]		Medium-2 point	C
Diabetes mellitus[d]		Medium-1 point	C
Chronic kidney disease[e]		Medium-1 point	C
Previous Cardiotoxic Cancer Treatment			
Prior anthracycline exposure		High	C
Prior radiotherapy to left chest or mediastinum		Medium-2 point	C
Lifestyle Risk Factors			
Current smoker or significant smoking hx		Medium-1 point	C
Obesity (BMI >30 kg/m^2)		Medium-1 point	C
Risk Level (see Table 2.1A for details)			

[a]Atrial fibrillation, atrial flutter, ventricular tachycardia, or ventricular fibrillation.
[b]Elevated above the upper limit of normal for local laboratory reference range.
[c]Systolic blood pressure (BP) > 140 mm Hg or diastolic BP > 90 mm Hg, or on treatment.
[d]HbA1c > 7.0% or on treatment.
[e]Estimated glomerular filtration rate <60 mL/min/1.73 m^2.
[f]Total cholesterol level >5.2 mmol/L.
BMI, Body mass index; *CABG*, coronary artery bypass graft; *CVD*, cardiovascular disease; *IHD*, ischemic heart disease; *LVEF*, left ventricular ejection fraction; *PCI*, percutaneous coronary intervention; *PVD*, peripheral vascular disease; *TIA*, transient ischemic attack; *RAF*, Rapidly accelerated fibrosarcoma; *MEK*, Mitogen-activated protein kinase kinase.

such as anthracyclines and radiation, have a lasting effect, and once therapy is administered, it cannot be undone. Other therapies, such as 5-fluorouracil, have only a transient impact, confined to the time of therapy, which nevertheless can be profound. Various scenarios need to be entertained and, at the end, an individualized management plan should be formulated that pertains to the expected CV toxicities and includes a plan for surveillance and prevention.

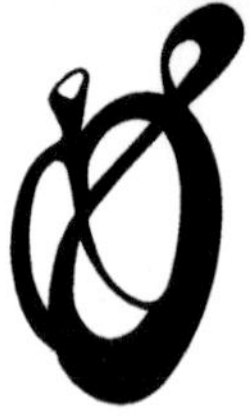

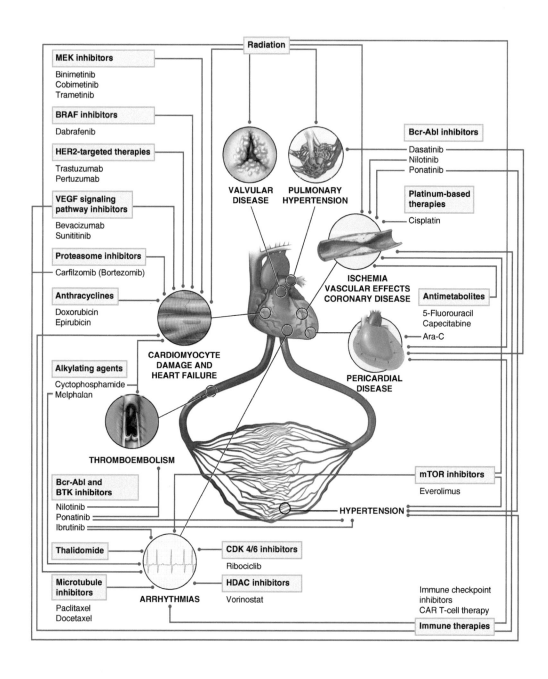

3 Cardiovascular Risks of Chemotherapy

SANJEEV A. FRANCIS AND DOUGLAS SAWYER

Radiation

MEK inhibitors
Binimetinib
Cobimetinib
Trametinib

BRAF inhibitors
Dabrafenib

HER2-targeted therapies
Trastuzumab
Pertuzumab

VEGF signaling pathway inhibitors
Bevacizumab
Sunititinib

Proteasome inhibitors
Carfilzomib (Bortezomib)

Anthracyclines
Doxorubicin
Epirubicin

Alkylating agents
Cyctophosphamide
Melphalan

VALVULAR DISEASE
PULMONARY HYPERTENSION
CARDIOMYOCYTE DAMAGE AND HEART FAILURE
ISCHEMIA VASCULAR EFFECTS CORONARY DISEASE
PERICARDIAL DISEASE
THROMBOEMBOLISM
HYPERTENSION
ARRHYTHMIAS

Bcr-Abl inhibitors
Dasatinib
Nilotinib
Ponatinib

Platinum-based therapies
Cisplatin

Antimetabolites
5-Fluorouracil
Capecitabine
Ara-C

Bcr-Abl and BTK inhibitors
Nilotinib
Ponatinib
Ibrutinib

Thalidomide

Microtubule inhibitors
Paclitaxel
Docetaxel

CDK 4/6 inhibitors
Ribociclib

HDAC inhibitors
Vorinostat

mTOR inhibitors
Everolimus

Immune therapies
Immune checkpoint inhibitors
CAR T-cell therapy

CHAPTER OUTLINE

KEY POINTS

- Cancer therapies can be associated with a broad range of cardiovascular toxicities
- The three most important cardiovascular toxicities in terms of reported incidence and severity are 1) cardiomyopathy and heart failure, 2) vascular toxicities and hypertension, and 3) QTC prolongation and arrhythmias
- The absolute and relative risks of cardiovascular toxicities are drug class specific and will be presented as such in the following
- As evident, one cardiovascular side effect may stand out in particular for one or two agents in any given drug class

Cardio-oncology or onco-cardiology is the discipline at the intersection between cardiovascular disease and cancer, the two leading causes of death in the United States and much of the developed world. A central focus is the cardiovascular risk of cancer therapies. Cardiotoxicity from chemotherapy can be an important source of morbidity and mortality and can limit the use of potentially life-saving cancer therapies. A wide spectrum of cardiovascular toxicities is associated with cancer chemotherapies, including cardiomyopathy, coronary artery disease, atherothrombosis, hypertension, pulmonary hypertension, arrhythmias, conduction system disease, QT prolongation, metabolic effects, peripheral arterial disease, and venous thromboembolism (Table 3.1). These toxicities can result from both on-target and off-target effects; they can occur during treatment or after completion of treatment; and they can contribute to cardiovascular disease long after cancer therapy is completed.

Prompt recognition of cardiovascular toxicity can lead to appropriate mitigation and treatment and optimize health outcomes in patients with cancer. Herein we will discuss the cardiovascular risks of common chemotherapies. The reader is reminded that cardiovascular toxicities of relatively new drugs may not be fully characterized in published clinical trials or initial post-marketing surveillance. Furthermore, long-term cardiovascular risks of currently used therapies require ongoing surveillance and research. This remains a constantly evolving field.

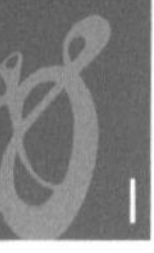

TABLE 3.1 Common Cardiovascular Toxicities With Associated Chemotherapies

Toxicity	Associated Chemotherapies
Cardiomyopathy/ myocyte injury	• Anthracyclines • HER2 inhibitors • VEGF signaling pathway inhibitors • Immune checkpoint inhibitors • Cyclophosphamide (high dose) • Paclitaxel (with anthracycline) • Bcr-Abl inhibitor (Ponatinib) • BRAF + MEK1/2 inhibitor (Vemurafenib + Trametinib) • Proteosome inhibitor (Carfilzomib)
Coronary artery disease/ ischemia	• Antimetabolites (5-Fluorouracil, Capecitabine) • VEGF signaling pathway inhibitors • Bcr-Abl inhibitor (Ponatinib) • Immune modulators (Lenalinomide) • EGFR inhibitor (Erlotinib)
Arrhythmia	• Ibrutinib (atrial fibrillation) • Crizotinib (bradycardia) • Taxanes (bradycardia) • Anthracycline (atrial fibrillation, ventricular ectopy) • Alkylating agents (Ciplatin, Melphalan, Cyclophosphamide) • c-MET inhibitor (Cabozantinib, bradycardia) • HDAC inhibitors (Romidepsin) • Proteosome inhibitor (Carfilozmib) • Immunomodulators (Thalidomide)
QTc prolongation	• Anthracyclines • BRAF inhibitor (Vemurafenib) • EGFR inhibitors (Laptinib, Vandetanib) • c-MET inhibitor (Crizotinib) • HDAC inhibitors (Belinostat)
Peripheral arterial disease	• Bcr-Abl inhibitors (Ponatinib, Nilotinib)
Cerebrovascular accident	• VEGF signaling pathway inhibitors • Bcr-Abl inhibitors (Ponatinib) • EGFR inhibitor (Erlotinib, Vandetanib)
Hypertension	• VEGF signaling pathway inhibitors • Bcr-Abl inhibitor (Ponatinib) • BRAF inhibitor (Vemurafenib) • MEK1/2 inhibitor (Trametinib) • EGFR inhibitor (Vandetanib) • Bruton's tyrosine kinase inhibitor (Ibrutinib) • c-MET inhibitor (Cabozantinib) • Proteosome inhibitor (Carfilzomib)
Pulmonary hypertension	• Bcr-Abl inhibitors (Ponatinib, Dasatinib) • Proteosome inhibitors (Carfilzomib)
Venous thromboembolism	• EGFR inhibitors (Cetuximab, Panitumumab) • Cyclin-dependent kinase inhibitors (Abermaciclib) • c-MET inhibitors (Cabozantinib) • Immunomodulators (Lenalidomide, Thalidomide, Pomalidomide)
Metabolic	• Bcr-Abl inhibitor (Nilotinib) • JAK inhibitor (Tofacitinib) • m-TOR inhibitors

HDAC, Histone deacetylase; *VEGF*, vascular endothelial growth factor.

Chemotherapy for cancer can be divided into two broad categories: standard chemotherapy and targeted therapies, which also includes immunotherapies and anti hormonal therapies (Fig. 3.1). Standard or traditional chemotherapy acts on all dividing cells (cancerous and non cancerous) leading to both therapeutic effects and toxicities. Targeted therapies arose from a greater understanding of the molecular mechanisms of cancers and represent a true revolution in cancer care. Of note, however, "targeted" therapies may have both on-target and off-target effects on non cancerous cells/organs/systems and lead to toxicity.

TRADITIONAL CHEMOTHERAPY

Four classes of traditional chemotherapeutics will be discussed herein: anthracyclines, alkylating agents, anti metabolites, and anti microtubule agents.

Anthracyclines

KEY POINTS

- Main cardiotoxicity is cardiomyopathy with risk factors of cumulative dose, young age at treatment, and traditional cardiovascular risk factors.
- Can have a long latency period from completion of therapy, particularly in childhood cancer survivors.
- Current guidelines recommend screening echocardiography before and 6 to 12 months after completion of treatment in adult and every 1 to 5 years starting 1 to 3 months and up to 5 years after completion of treatment in cases of childhood cancer by various guidelines.[9]

Anthracyclines include doxorubicin, daunorubicin, epirubicin, idarubicin, valrubicin, and mitoxantrone.

The anti cancer therapy effect of anthracyclines relates to topoisomerase II alpha inhibition, which leads to double strand breaks and disarray of the DNA structure in proliferating cells. They are also DNA intercalators, and induction of oxidative stress may further contribute to their cytotoxicity.

Anthracyclines are currently used in the treatment of leukemia, lymphoma, breast cancer, sarcomas, uterine cancer, and gastric cancer.

Cardiomyopathy

Incidence

Anthracycline cardiomyopathy is often broken down into three categories.

Acute: Occurs during active treatment. Estimated incidence is less than 1%.

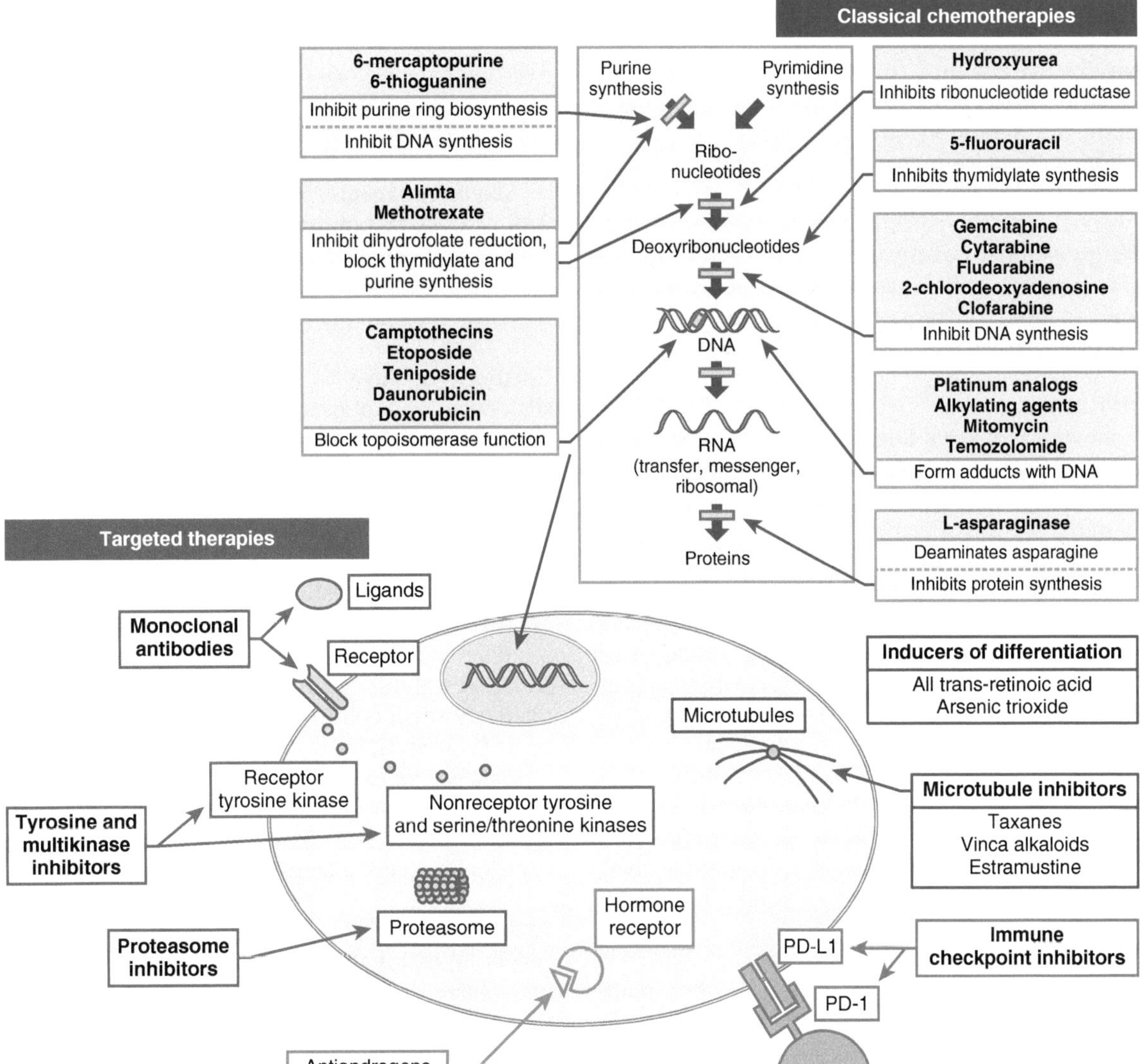

FIG. 3.1 Illustration of the main classes of anti cancer therapeutics and their mode of action on cancer cells.

Early onset: Occurs within 1 year of treatment. Incidence of 9% based on a large prospective series.[1]

Late onset: Occurs after one year of treatment. Incidence varies, depending on series, study cohorts, and definitions used, ranging from 0 to 57%. Most of these are asymptomatic declines in cardiac function. The highest heart failure rates have been projected for childhood patients with cancer exposed to more than 250 mg/m^2 doxorubicin equivalent dose. Chest radiation exposure adds to the risk (as does hypertension, with a more than additive effect in childhood cancer survivors).

Risk Factors

Risk factors include cumulative dose, bolus dosing, extremes of age (very young and old), female gender, concomitant chest radiation, preexisting cardiovascular disease, obesity and genetic factors.[2,3]

Mechanism

The mechanisms of anthracycline-associated cardiomyopathy continue to be the focus of basic and translation research. Central pathways involved include the inhibition of topoisomerase II beta in cardiomyocytes leading to DNA instability and subsequent cell death; oxidative stress manifest by decreases in p53, peroxisome proliferator-activated receptor gamma coactivator-1alpha (PGC-1alpha); and angiogenic imbalance via decreased ErbB/nrg signalling and, subsequently, decreased vascular endothelial growth factor (VEGF) activity.[2]

Arrhythmias

The incidence of atrial fibrillation is estimated at 8% to 10%. It can occur during or immediately after administration of anthracyclines or be a latent effect after months/years. Atrial fibrillation may be a marker for cardiomyopathy and clinical heart failure.[4]

Ventricular arrhythmias have been described during and immediately after administration. In patients qualifying for primary prevention implantable cardioverter defibrillator (ICD) the risk of ventricular arrhythmias in the setting of an anthracycline-associated cardiomyopathy appears to be similar to that seen of patients with ischemic and especially dilated cardiomyopathy.[5]

QTc prolongation has also been described with anthracycline use.[4] In a small study, 12% of patients with acute leukemia developed QTc greater than 450 msec in the setting of anthracycline therapy.[6]

Coronary Artery Disease

Some small studies have demonstrated abnormalities in endothelial dysfunction which might precede the development of atherosclerosis, but that remains speculative.[7] No increase in myocardial infarction was seen in survivors of childhood cancers compared with a healthy sibling cohort.[8]

Alkylating Agents

KEY POINTS

- Cardiomyopathy and hemorrhagic myocarditis can be seen with high-dose cyclophosphamide.
- Atrial fibrillation has been noted with melphalan, and also cisplatin and cyclophosphamide.

Akylating agents include five different categories:

Nitrogen mustards: cyclophosphamide, ifosfamide, bendamustine, chlorambucil, bendamustine, mechlorethamine, melphalan

Nitrosoureas: carmustine, lomustine, streptozocin

Alkyl sulfonates: busulfan

Triazines: dacarbazines, temozolomide

Ethylenimines: altretamine, thiotepa

Metal salts ("platinums"): carboplatin, cisplatin, and oxaliplatin

Alkylating agents promote cell death by induction of DNA instability leading to breakage. These agents, and especially nitrogen mustards and metal salts, are commonly used for a variety of solid and hematologic malignancies.

Cardiomyopathy

High-dose cyclophosphamide can cause a hemorrhagic myocarditis leading to heart failure. This was reported in 1981 using a high dose of 180 mg/kg over 4 days. The incidence of heart failure in this series was 28%.[10] Current, dosing regimens are a fraction of this and consequently the incidence of heart failure is low. In a contemporary study investigating heart failure in the hematopoietic cell transplant (HCT) population no difference was found between patients treated with and without cyclophosphamide.[11] Of note in this relatively small cohort there was a 22% incidence of heart failure post HCT.

Risk factors for cardiotoxicity with high-dose regimens include the following: prior anthracycline treatment, prior chest radiation, obesity, older age, left ventricular ejection factor (LVEF) less than 50%.[12]

Arrhythmias

Cisplatin, melphalan, and high-dose cyclophosphamide have all been associated with atrial fibrillation.[4] Intrapericardial and intrapleural administration of cisplatin is associated with a higher rate of atrial fibrillation. Both acute and late effects have been reported.

Antimetabolites

KEY POINTS

- Most common cardiovascular toxicity with fluorouracil or capecitabine is chest pain, including acute coronary syndrome presentations, which are likely secondary to coronary vasospasm.
- Decline in cardiac function is not common, but can be seen, including Takotsubo cardiomyopathy.
- Ventricular tachycardia (VT) and sudden cardiac death (SCD) have been reported as well, but uncommonly.
- Pericarditis is seen with cytarabine.

Anti-metabolites include 5-fluorouracil (5-FU) fluorouracil, capecitabine, cytarabine, gemcitabine, cladribine, clofarabine, fludarabine, hydroxyurea, mercaptopurine, methotrexate, nelarabine, pemetrexed.

These agents interfere with DNA and RNA synthesis to prevent cell proliferation. Current use includes leukemias, breast, ovary, and gastrointestinal cancers.

Ischemia

5-FU and capecitabine (oral prodrug of fluorouracil) are associated with a syndrome of chest pain, electrocardiographic (ECG) changes, and elevated cardiac biomarkers indicative of myocardial injury. Although not fully understood, the mechanism of cardiotoxicity is often attributed to coronary vasospasm; *in vitro* and animal studies suggest direct endothelial and myocardial injury may be present.[13] The reported incidence ranges from 1% to 19%.

Cardiomyopathy

There are case reports of left ventricular dysfunction and ventricular arrhythmias often associated with the chest pain syndrome described with 5-FU and capecitabine. Based on the available literature this appears to be an uncommon toxicity.[14] Risk factor for "cardiotoxicity" is a history of coronary artery disease.

Antimicrotubule Agents

Anti-microtubule agents taxanes (paclitaxel, docetaxel) and vinca alkaloids (vincristine, vinblastine, vinorelbine).

These agents work by stabilizing microtubules and thus inhibiting cell division, ultimately leading to cell death. Taxanes are commonly used in the treatment of breast cancer, ovarian cancer, and non small-cell lung cancer.

Arrhythmias

Sinus bradycardia during infusion has been reported in up to 30% of patients receiving taxanes.[15] This is largely asymptomatic. ECG changes have been reported, including non specific repolarization abnormalities, sinus bradycardia, and sinus tachycardia in 30% of patients receiving paclitaxel who had normal baseline ECGs. Rarely do these ECG changes have a clinical impact.

Blood Pressure Effects

Hypertension and hypotension have been described as part of the infusion reaction that can be seen with paclitaxel. Serious cardiac events occur infrequently, with an incidence of 1% to 2% according to package insert and these seem to be largely related to events during the infusion period.

Cardiomyopathy

Paclitaxel has been associated with cardiomyopathy in patients treated concomitantly with an anthracycline. Paclitaxel may increase doxorubicin levels contributing to increased risk of cardiomyopathy. There are also case reports of congestive heart failure in the setting of combination therapy with gemcitabine and nab-paclitaxel.

Miscellaneous

The package insert for abraxane reports a 3% incidence of serious cardiac events, possibly related to paclitaxel. These events included cardiac ischemia/infarction, chest pain, cardiac arrest, supraventricular tachycardia, edema, thrombosis, pulmonary thromboembolism, pulmonary emboli, and hypertension.

KEY POINTS

- Most common cardiovascular side effect is sinus bradycardia during infusion.
- Hypotension/hypertension can occur during infusion as well.
- Serious side effects including myocardial infarction (MI) and cardiomyopathy/heart failure are relatively uncommon.

TARGETED THERAPIES

One of the revolutions in medicine has been driven by a better understanding of the molecular mechanisms that drive proliferation and metastasis of cancer cells. The human genome project identified approximately 538 kinases. Dysregulation of these enzymes is seen in many cancers providing an attractive target from a therapeutic perspective. The current landscape of kinase inhibitors includes many different targets. It is important for the reader to understand that this list continues to grow with many new drugs and targets in various stages of development.

HER2 Inhibitors

HER2-inhibitors include trastuzumab, pertuzumab, lapatinib and trastuzumab emtansine (T-DM1)

The discovery that approximately 25% of breast tumors over-express the receptor kinase HER2 set the stage for targeted therapies that have reduced morbidity and mortality for the subset of HER2+ breast patients with cancer. Besides breast cancer, anti-HER2 therapy is used in HER2 expressing gastrointestinal stromal tumors.

Cardiomyopathy

An early clinical trial using the antibody, trastuzumab to target the HER2 receptor in conjunction with anthracyclines noted a 27% incidence of congestive heart failure (New York Heart Association III or IV).[16] Subsequent protocols administered trastuzumab sequentially with an anthracycline and the incidence of clinical heart failure was lowered to 2% to 4% with cardiac dysfunction occurring from 3% to 19%.[17,18] Without concomitant anthracycline therapy the incidence of cardiomyopathy and clinical heart failure with HER2-targeted therapies is even lower.[18] An important caveat is that, in general, clinical trials often enroll patients who are relatively younger and healthier with a lower prevalence of preexisting cardiovascular disease and traditional cardiovascular risk factors compared with the general population. As such, continued vigilance is necessary, as "real world" incidences of cardiotoxicity are often higher. Along the same lines, although clinical trials indicate that cardiac function recovers in the majority of patients with interruption of therapy and that the long-term risk is low clinical registry-based data argue that this is not guaranteed. Mechanistically, the HER2-signaling pathway is an important stress response element in cardiomyocytes with a role in sarcomere structure, cell survival, and metabolism.[19]

The addition of pertuzumab to trastuzumab does not seem to increase the risk of cardiotoxicity at least not in published clinical trials.[19,20] Lapatinib, of note, is associated with a lower risk of cardiotoxicity, possibly related to effects other than HER2 inhibition which could counteract the toxicity risk potential. Intriguingly, T-DM1 is also associated with a lower risk of cardiomyopathy though this agent is a conjugate of trastuzumab and the anti-microtubule agent DM1.

Risk factors for HER2 inhibitor cardiomyopathy include concomitant anthracycline treatment, traditional cardiovascular risk factors (esp. hypertension), and age.

KEY POINTS

- The main cardiovascular toxicity risk with HER2-directed therapy, and mainly trastuzumab, is cardiomyopathy.
- Regular (3-monthly) screening with echocardiography is thus advised as standard of care.
- Beta blockers and angiotensin-converting enzyme inhibitors–angiotensin II receptor blockers (ACEi-ARBs) are indicated in cases of LV dysfunction.
- Most (but not all) patients who develop cardiomyopathy will have full or near full recovery.
- If LVEF improves, HER2 inhibitors can be resumed based on careful risk/benefit discussion.

Bcr-Abl Inhibitors

BCR-Abl inhibitors include imatinib, dasatinib, nilotinib, bosutinib, and ponatinib.

These agents target the molecular fingerprint of Philadelphia chromosome-positive leukemias, which is the Bcr-Abl fusion protein, namely its tyrosine kinase activity. Imatinib was one of the first targeted therapies yielding normal life expectancy in those patients who responded to therapy. However, as not 100% selective, off-target effects can lead to toxicity, including a variety of cardiovascular toxicities.

Risk factors included preexisting coronary artery disease, diabetes mellitus, and hypertension, which increased the risk of cardiotoxicity, particularly with ponatinib.

Cardiomyopathy

Rare event with imatinib and bosutinib cardiovascular events increased with ponatinib, including congestive heart failure, although this may at least be partially related to the increased risk of coronary ischemic events.

Myocardial Infarction

In a trial of ponatinib there was a 10% incidence of myocardial infarction (MI) during a 2+ year follow up.[21]

Pulmonary Hypertension

A 5% incidence of pulmonary hypertension was seen with dasatinib over a 5 year follow-up period in of the DASISION trial.[22] Rarely did the degree of pulmonary hypertension estimated on echocardiography lead to a right heart catheterization, suggesting that this may not be a severe complication. Pleural effusions are also commonly observed, with a reported incidence of 28% with dasatinib, which may be a more frequent etiology of dyspnea.

Metabolic Effects

Nilotinib is associated with hyperglycemia, increased weight, and dyslipidemia.

Peripheral Arterial Disease

Ponatinib and especially nilotinib have been associated with peripheral arterial disease events.

Cerebrovascular Disease

An incidence of cerebrovascular events of 7% has been reported for ponatinib for the 2+ year follow up of the PACE clinical trial.[23]

Hypertension

Consistent with an inhibitory effect on the VEGF signaling pathway a 26% incidence of hypertension has been reported for ponatinib.

QTc Prolongation

Sudden cardiac deaths were noted in early clinical trials with nilotinib, which has led to a "black box" warning and stringent recommendations for QTc interval monitoring. Contrary to the common 500 msec cutoff for grade 3 QTc prolongation (i.e., treatment-relevant toxicity), the cutoff is 480 msec for nilotinib. Overall, the weighted incidence of QTc prolongation is less than 10%, but broad variation can be noted across studies.

Often the spectrum of cardiotoxicity can be linked to the targeted pathways, which have important roles in cardiovascular homeostasis. For example, ponatinib, which has an increased risk of a variety of cardiovascular toxicities, targets vascular endothelial growth factor receptors (VEGFR) 1 to 3, TIE-2, platelet-derived growth factor receptors A and B (PDGFRA/B), and fibroblast growth factor receptors (FGFR) 1 to 4. Basic and translational research can help better understand the mechanism of toxicity and provide insight into the role of particular pathways in cardiovascular function. In a murine model, ponatinib induced a thrombotic microangiopathy and associated left ventricular dysfunction via von Willebrand factor activation of platelets.[24] In a zebra fish model ponatnib inhibits AKT and ERK signaling leading to cardiomyocyte apoptosis.[25]

KEY POINTS

- Ponatinib is associated with an increased risk of a spectrum of cardiovascular toxicities related to its effect on several pathways.
- Dasatinib commonly causes pleural effusions. Pulmonary hypertension is less frequent.
- Nilotinib and ponatinib (less dasatinib) can be associated with progressive atherosclerosis, especially peripheral arterial disease, as well as acute cardiovascular events.
- Nilotinib carries a black box warning for QTc prolongation and risk of sudden cardiac death; concomitant use of QTc-prolonging drugs is to be avoided and ECG should be monitored during treatment.

VEGF Signalling Pathway Inhibitors

VEGF inhibitors include sorafenib, sunitinib, nintedanib, regorafenib, pazopanib, and axitinib.

VEGF is a key angiogenic-signalling protein secreted by cancer cells and, therefore, an attractive target for the inhibition of new blood vessel formation that plays such an important role for tumor growth and metastases. VEGF-signalling pathway inhibitors in the form of monoclonal antibodies, soluble VEGF receptors, and small molecule tyrosine kinase inhibitors are used in the treatment of various cancers, primarily renal cell carcinoma, thyroid cancer, and colorectal cancer.

Cardiomyopathy

Depending on the drug and the definition used the reported incidence of cardiomyopathy with VEGF inhibitors can range from 3% to 28%.[26] Agents that have been linked to cardiomyopathy/heart failure include bevacizumab, sunitinib, sorafenib, pazopanib, vatalanib, axitinib, and regorafenib. Of note, the majority of the publications are retrospective in nature.

Risk factors include older age, preexisting heart failure or coronary artery disease, lower body mass index, and hypertension.

Regarding the mechanisms, mouse models suggest that capillary rarefaction possibly mediated by

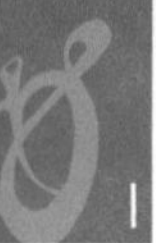

myocardial hypoxia and activation of hypoxia inducible factor.

Hypertension

Hypertension is a common class effect of all VEGF-signalling pathway inhibitors. The incidence ranges from 20% to 50%.[27] The mechanism is related to decreased production of the vasodilators nitric oxide and prostacyclin. The vast majority of hypertension can be managed with standard antihypertensives and either does modification or brief interruptions of VEGF inhibitors. Close monitoring of blood pressure is critical for all patients who are being treated with this class of targeted therapies.

Arterial Thromboembolic Events

Ischemic complications appear to be less frequent, based on the published reports.

Myocardial infarction has been reported with an incidence of 1% to 2%. Stroke has been reported for some VEGF-signalling pathway inhibitors at a rate of 1%.

KEY POINTS

- Given the central role of VEGF signaling in the cardiovascular system, cardiovascular toxicities are common.
- Hypertension is nearly universal and a class effect of VEGF signalling pathway inhibitors.
- Prompt recognition of hypertension and initiation of therapy is important for the majority of patients to continue cancer therapy.
- Cardiomyopathy can be seen with multiple agents. There is no consensus on optimal screening in the absence of symptoms. Consider baseline echocardiogram and a screening echocardiogram in patients with risk factors.

BRAF Inhibitors

B-RAF inhibitors include vemurafenib and dabrafenib.

The Ras-Raf-MAP kinase pathway is the prototype of a growth factor signaling pathway that has been intimately linked to cancer. Ras is the epitome of an oncogene, the one most commonly mutated in human malignancies. Various drugs have been developed that would inhibit kinases activated along the signaling chain of this pathway, and some are even given in combination. Mutations in BRAF gene have been commonly observed in melanoma and papillary thyroid cancer and are present, but less frequently, in a variety of malignancies, including colorectal cancer, non small-cell lung cancer, sarcomas, and breast cancer.

QTc Prolongation

QTc prolongation is reported with vemurafenib. In an open-label multicenter expanded access study of 374 patients, 7% had a QTc increase to greater than 480 msec and 3% had a QTc greater than 500 msec.[28] No clinical arrhythmias were identified during this study. In a second analysis of over 3000 patients, the incidence of QTc prolongation was 10% with 2% experiencing a QTc greater than 500 msec.[29]

The mechanism of QTc prolongation may be via interaction between the BRAF protein and voltage activated K+ channel, hERG, possibly mediated via cAMP. Of note, dabrafenib, when used as a single agent, is not associated with significant cardiotoxicity, including QTc prolongation, arguing against a class effect.

Hypertension

There is a reported incidence of hypertension with vemurafenib of 6% of patients with metastatic melanoma.[29]

Cardiomyopathy

When used in combination with trametinib, cardiomyopathy incidence is 3% per one open-label study.[29]

KEY POINTS

- QTc prolongation can be seen with vemurafenib; concomitant use of QTc prolonging drugs is to be avoided and ECG should be monitored during treatment.
- Hypertension can be seen with vemurafenib.
- Cardiomyopathy can be seen with combination therapy: vemurafenib + trametinib.

MEK1/2 Inhibitors

MEK1/2 inhibitors include Trametinib, cobimetinib, and binimetinib.

These inhibitors are part of the effort to inhibit the Ras-Raf-MAP kinase pathway. They inhibit the downstream target of BRAF. Trametinib is the only FDA-approved agent for monotherapy in BRAF-positive melanoma, the other two are approved in combination therapy with BRAF inhibitors for the same indication.

Cardiomyopathy

The reported incidence of cardiomyopathy ranges from 5% to 11% (7–9% per package insert).[30] Interruption and/or dose reduction can be associated with recovery of LV function. In a trial of cobimetinib plus vemurafenib versus vemurafenib plus placebo, a 26% incidence of cardiomyopathy was seen in the cobimetinib group versus 19% in the vemurafenib alone group. Recovery of LVEF was seen in 61% of patients.[31,32] Bimetinib has also been FDA approved for use in melanoma. In a pivotal trial, left ventricular dysfunction occurred in 8% in the encorafenib plus binimetinib group compared with 2% in the encorafenib alone group. Most of the LV dysfunction was characterized as grade I or II and did not lead to treatment discontinuation.[33]

Hypertension

Trametinib incidence of HTN was 15% compared with 7% in the comparator groups.

KEY POINTS

- Cardiomyopathy is the main cardiovascular toxicity particularly in combination therapy with a BRAF inhibitor.
- Hypertension can be seen with trametinib.

EGFR Inhibitors

EGFR inhibitors include erlotinib, lapatinib, gefitinib, cetuximab, panitumumab, vandetanib, afatinib, and osimertinib.

The EGF receptor is a classic example of a growth factor receptor that signals through the Ras-Raf-MAP kinase pathway into the nucleus. Four subtypes of EGF receptor are known. Beyond HER2, which is an orphan receptor, HER1 is the next best known, commonly referred to as EGFR. EGFR inhibitors are used in a variety of cancers, including such as non small-cell lung, breast, colon, and pancreatic cancers.

Venous Thromboembolism

Venous thromboembolism (VTE) has been reported with cetuximab, and panitumumab. A meta-analysis involving 13 studies and 7611 patients demonstrated a significant increase in the risk of venous thromboembolism.[34] The incidence of VTE with cetuximab was 5.7% compared with 3.9% in the control arms.

QTc Prolongation

QTc prolongation was reported with lapatinib, vandetanib. In a meta-analysis of nine randomized clinical trials involving vandetanib 4813 patients the relative risk of QTc prolongation was 7.9. Baseline and screening ECGs are recommended with interruption and/or dose reduction for a QTc of more than 500 msec.[35] Osimertinib was associated with more than a 60 msec increase in QTc in 2.7% of patients with a 0.2% incidence of QTc greater than 500 msec.

Hypertension

In a meta-analysis the relative risk of HTN compared with a control regimen with vandetanib was 5.6.[35] Vandetanib is also a potent VEGF receptor inhibitor with hypertension a known class effect.

Cardiomyopathy

Lapatinib, which is used to treat breast cancer, has a lower risk of cardiomyopathy than trastuzumab. In a meta-analysis the incidence of decrease in LVEF was 2.2% and the incidence of left ventricular dysfunction was 1.6%. Osimertinib was associated with cardiomyopathy in 1.4% of patients.

Myocardial Infarction

In a trial of erlotinib in patients with pancreatic carcinoma, the incidence of MI was 2.3% compared with 1.6% in the comparator group.

Cerebrovascular accident

In a trial of erlotinib in patients with pancreatic cancer, the incidence of a cerebrovascular accident (CVA) was 2.3% compared with no events in the placebo group. In a trial of medullary thyroid cancer, the incidence of ischemic cerebrovascular events with vandetanib was 1.3% compared with placebo.

KEY POINTS

- Venous thromboembolism is noted with cetuximab and panitumumab
- QTc prolongation is seen with lapatinib and vandetanib
- Arterial thrombotic events (MI, CVA) are noted with erlotinib

Bruton's Tyrosine Kinase (BTK) Inhibitor

BTK inhibitors include ibrutinib, acalabrutinib.

BTK is a component of the B cell receptor signaling pathway. Inhibitors are approved for the treatment of chronic lymphocytic leukemia, mantle cell lymphoma, and Waldenstrom's macroglobulinemia.

Atrial Fibrillation

The incidence of atrial fibrillation has been reported between 3% and 16%.[36] In a pooled meta-analysis of randomized clinical trials the incidence of atrial fibrillation in patients being treated with ibrutinib was 3.3% compared with 0.84% in patients receiving non ibrutinib therapies.[37] Real world retrospective analyses suggest the incidence may be higher, likely reflective of an older population with a higher prevalence of comorbid conditions, such as hypertension.[38] An *in vitro* study using human pluripotent stem cell derived cardiomyocyte suggests that ibrutinib may exert a direct effect on atrial specific cells.[39] A phase II trial of a second generation Bruton's tyrosine kinase inhibitor, alacabruntinib, did not report any episodes of atrial fibrillation.[40] Larger trials with longer follow up will help determine if atrial fibrillation is a class effect.

Hypertension

A pooled meta-analysis of eight studies showed a statistically significant increase in the risk of hypertension with a relative risk of 2.82. The package insert for ibrutinib reports an incidence of hypertension of 12% in clinical trials. The interplay between ibrutinib-associated hypertension and the development of atrial fibrillation requires larger prospective studies.

Cardiomyopathy

There are case reports linking ibrutinib with cardiomyopathy. This appears to be a low frequency event. At present, routine monitoring of LV function is not part of routine surveillance for patients on ibrutinib.

KEY POINTS

- Ibrutinib is associated with an increased risk of atrial fibrillation.
- Hypertension is also seen with ibrutinib use.

Cyclin-Dependent Kinase (CDK) Inhibitors

CDK inhibitors include palbociclib, ribociclib, and abemaciclib.

CDKs are seronine/tyrosine kinases that become active in association with cyclins. They can modify various protein substrates involved in cell cycle progression (e.g., CDK 4/6 promotes the transition from G1 to S phase). CDK4/6 inhibitors are used to interrupt this action and the proliferation of cancer cells. They are used in the treatment of breast cancer.

Venous Thromboembolism

Abermaciclib, in combination with an aromatase inhibitor, was associated with a 5% incidence of venous thromboembolism as compared with 0.6% in the placebo group.

QTc Prolongation

According to the package insert, the incidence of QTc prolongation greater than 60 msec with ribociclib was 6% with only 1% incidence of QTc greater than 500 msec. No cases of torsades de pointes were reported. A baseline and screening ECG is recommended. Use of concomitant drugs the prolong the QTc should be avoided as should strong CYP3A inhibitors which may potentiate the effects of ribociclib.

KEY POINTS

- Venous thromboembolism risk increased with abermaciclib.
- QTc prolongation seen with ribociclib.

c-MET Inhibitors

c-MET inhibitors include cabozantinib (crizotinib, mainly an anaplastic lymphoma kinase [ALK] inhibitor).

c-MET is a receptor tyrosine kinase, which after binding hepatocyte growth factor, its ligand, activates various intracellular signaling pathways involved in proliferation, motility, migration, and invasion. Aberrant activation of c-MET has been documented in many human cancers. Cabozantinib is used in the treatment of hepatocellular carcinoma, renal cell, and thyroid cancer Importantly, cabozantinib blocks a broad range of kinases (MET, VEGFR-1, -2, and -3; AXL; RET; ROS1; TYRO3; MER; KIT; TRKB; FLT-3; and TIE-2). The kinase inhibitory spectrum of crizotinib is not as broad (cMET, ALK, ROS1, RON) and crizotinib is used clinically mainly as an ALK inhibitor in non-small-cell lung cancer.

Arterial Thrombotic Events

The package insert for cabozantinib reports a 2% incidence of arterial thrombotic complications.

Venous Thromboembolic Complications

Similarly, venous thromboembolic complications were reported in 7% of patients treated with cabozantinib.

Hypertension

Cabozantinib is associated with a high incidence of hypertension (36%), including hypertensive crisis, according to the package insert.

Cardiomyopathy

In a small study of 22 patients with metastatic renal cell carcinoma 11% experienced a decline in LVEF of more than 10% during treatment with cabozantinib, with no patients having an LVEF less than 50%.[41] Based on available data, the risk of cardiomyopathy with cabozantinib appears to be minimal.

QTc Prolongation

With crizotinib use, 2% of patients had a QTc greater than 500 msec and 5% had a greater than 60 msec increase in QTc compared with baseline.

Bradycardia

Bradycardia observed with crizotinib: According to the package insert there is a 13% incidence of bradycardia, with syncope in 2.4% compared with 0.6% receiving other therapies.[42] Caution is advised with the concomitant use of beta blocker, calcium channel blockers, and digoxin.

KEY POINTS

- Cabozantinib can be associated with arterial and venous thrombotic events, hypertension, cardiomyopathy likely owing to its effect on multiple pathways.
- Crizotinib can be associated with significant bradycardia and QTc prolongation.

JAK Inhibitors

JAK inhibitors include ruxolitinib and tofacitinib.

JAK is an intracellular, non-receptor tyrosine kinase that regulates gene transcription via the STAT transcription factors. Mutations in JAK are found in many noncr-Abl myeloproliferative disorders, such as essential thrombocythemia, polycythemia vera, and primary myelofibrosis. At present only two JAK inhibitors are approved, with a relatively narrow indication.

Metabolic Changes

Tofacitinib is associated with increases in total cholesterol, low-density lipoprotein and high-density lipoprotein levels, according to the package insert. The clinical relevance of this on cardiovascular outcomes is unclear. Monitoring of lipids 4 to 8 weeks after initiation is recommended.

KEY POINTS

- Tofacitinib can be associated with an increase in serum lipid levels.

Histone Deacylase Inhibitors

Histone deacylase inhibitors include romidepsin, belinostat, vorinostat, and panobinostat.

Histone deacetylases (HDACs) regulate gene expression and their overexpression has been linked to several cancers. Romidepsin, belinostat, and vorinostat are used for the treatment of T-cell lymphomas and panobinostat for multiple myeloma.

In a meta-analysis of 62 studies that included 3268 patients, cardiac effects were noted in 29% of patients.[43] Of note, data on ventricular function were not available in these studies limiting the ability to comment on the impact of HDAC inhibition on ventricular function.

ECG Abnormalities

Non specific ST/T wave abnormalities were reported in 15% in the overall cohort with a higher percentage with romidepsin (25%) and panobinostat (22%) use.

QTc Prolongation

QTc prolongation was seen in 4% of the overall cohort treated with HDAC inhibitors. The highest incidence was observed with belinostat (12%).

Ventricular Tachycardia

Ventricular tachycardia was reported in 2% of patient being treated with romidepsin and 0.2% in patients being treated with panobinostat.

Hypotension

Hypotension was observed in 3% of patients treated with all HDAC inhibitors.

KEY POINTS

- Non specific ECG abnormalities are common.
- QTc prolongation seen with belinostat.
- Ventricular tachycardia reported for romidepsin use.

mTOR Inhibitors

mTOR inhibitors include sirolimus, temsirolimus, everolimus, and ridaforolimus.

The mammalian target of rapamycin, mTOR, plays key roles in metabolism, cell growth, and proliferation, acting at the catalytic subunit of two protein kinase complexes: mTOR 1 and 2. mTORC1 signaling is switched on by several oncogenic signaling pathways. At present mTOR inhibitors have a role in the treatment of renal cell carcinoma, pancreatic neuroendocrine tumors, and advanced breast cancer.

Metabolic Effects

mTOR inhibitors are associated with hyperglycemia and hyperlipidemia. Monitoring before and during therapy is recommended. It is not clear whether this translates to a long-term risk of cardiovascular events.

KEY POINTS

- mTOR inhibitors can be associated with hyperglycemia and hyperlipidemia.

Proteosome Inhibitors

Proteasome inhibitors include bortezomib, carfilzomib, and ixazomib.

The proteasome is the main protein degradation system in eukaryotic cells, operating in conjunction with and independently from the ubiquitin system. Removal of misfolded or otherwise damaged proteins is crucial for cellular health because their accumulation ultimately leads to cytotoxicity. Cells with high protein production (e.g., plasma cells in multiple myeloma) are very sensitive to any compromise of proteasome function. This explains, at least in part, the successful use of proteasome inhibitors primarily in multiple myeloma.

Of the three proteasome inhibitors, bortezomib and ixazomib do not appear to increase the risk of cardiovascular events significantly compared with other treatments. Initial clinical trials with carfilzomib involved patients who were heavily pre treated and had advanced disease. A meta-analysis of clinical trials with carfilzomib reported an incidence of all-grade cardiovascular toxicity of 18%.[44] The mechanisms of carfilzomib-associated cardiotoxicity are not well understood. Of note, patients with multiple myeloma have a high prevalence of cardiac risk factors and co-existing cardiovascular disease. The risk of thrombosis is increased apart from the treatment risks outline below.

Venous Thromboembolism

Bortezomib is often used in conjunction with immunomodulatory agents, such as lenalidomide. Bortezomib is associated with a lower incidence of VTE. Bortezomib does not seem to increase the risk of CV events when compared with control groups in clinical trials and a large meta-analysis.[45] Ixazomib does not seem to be associated with an increased risk based on currently available data.

Hypertension

The incidence of hypertension with carfilozmib is 14% to 25%.[45]

Pulmonary Hypertension

The reported incidence of pulmonary hypertension with carfilzomib is 2%.

Arrhythmia

The reports incidence of arrhythmias with carfilzomib is 13%. Given that it is associated with sudden death, there does appear to be a risk of malignant arrhythmias.

Heart Failure

The incidence of heart failure symptoms with carfilozmib is approximately 5% to 9%.[46] Interestingly, no significant change was noted in EF in carfilzomib compared with control patients, with a low incidence of decline in EF (4%) in each group.

KEY POINTS

- At baseline, cardiovascular risk factors and disease are common in patients with multiple myeloma.
- Bortezomib does not seem to be associated with significant cardiovascular risk.
- Carfilzomib is associated with a spectrum of cardiotoxicities, including hypertension, arrhythmia, heart failure, and sudden death.

Immunomodulatory Drugs

Immunomodulatory drugs include lenalidomide, pomalidomide, thalidomide.

These agents cause selective ubiquitination and degradation of transcription factors that regulate T and B cells. This class of drugs is commonly used in multiple myeloma.

Venous Thromboembolism

The incidence of VTE is greatest when combined with other chemotherapy or dexamethasone. Depending on the drug, study, and whether thromboprophylaxis was used, the incidence ranges from 3% to 75%.[46] High-dose dexamethasone appears to increase the risk significantly and the incidence of VTE is highest in newly diagnosed multiple myeloma, prompting guidelines to recommend thromboprophylaxis in this population. The mechanism is imbalance between pro thrombotic pathways (tissue factor, GPIIb/IIIa, von Willebrand factor) and anti thrombotic factors (endothelial protein C receptor, thrombomodulin).

Arterial Thrombosis

Lenalidomide was associated with an increased risk of MI and stroke of 1.7% and 2.3%, respectively, compared with 0.6% and 0.9% in the control group.

Bradycardia

Bradycardia was seen in 5% of patients on thalidomide.[45]

KEY POINTS

- Venous thromboembolism risk increased, particularly with use of concomitant steroids.
- Thromboprophylaxis recommended, depending on risk factors.
- Arterial thrombosis was less common, but was seen with lenalidomide.

Immune Checkpoint Inhibitors

Includes: PD1 inhibitors—pembrolizumab, nivolumab, cemiplimab; PD-L1 inhibitors—atezolizumab, avelumab, durvalumab; and CTLA-4 inhibitor—ipilimumab

Immune checkpoint proteins PD-L1 and CTLA4 and the receptor PD-1 represent brakes on the immune system that tamp down T-cell-mediated immune responses. Cancer cells express surface proteins that activate these pathways and allow malignant cells to evade the immune system. Immune checkpoint inhibitors release these brakes. Toxicities from this class of medications include autoimmune-mediate phenomena that can affect multiple organ systems: dermatologic, endocrine, gastrointestinal, and muscles. The most feared complication is myocarditis.

Myocarditis

The incidence of myocarditis is estimated to be 0.1% to 1%. A high mortality was published in a series 25% to 50%.[47] Usually presents within the first 6 weeks to 3 months of therapy. Diagnostic tools include ECG, serum biomarkers including troponin, NT-BNP, echocardiography, cardiac MRI, and endomyocardial biopsy. The highest incidence of myocarditis is seen with dual immune checkpoint inhibitor therapy (CTLA-4 and PD1-directed). Treatment generally includes cessation of checkpoint inhibitors and initiation of high-dose steroids. Cases of advanced heart failure and cardiogenic shock (fulminant myocarditis) have been reported. Other immunosuppressive agents, such as antithymocyte globulin (ATG), plasmapheresis, mycophenolate, and intravenous immunoglobulin, have been suggested as well as mechanical circulatory support. Prospective, randomized data are lacking. Other cardiovascular effects that have been reported include pericarditis, arrhythmias, and congestive heart failure.

KEY POINTS

- Myocarditis can be seen in approximately 1% of patients. Risk is highest with dual checkpoint inhibitor treatment.
- Mortality rate with myocarditis is high based on published series.
- Management includes high-dose steroids and consideration of other immunosuppressive agents.

CAR-T Cell Therapy

CAR-T cell therapies include tisagenlecleucel, axicabtagene, lisocabtagene, brexucabtagene (all anti CD19), and idecabtagene (B-cell maturation antigen).

Chimeric antigen receptor (CAR) T-cell therapy involves modifying a patient's own T cells *ex vivo* to express antigen receptors specific to a certain cancer. These modified T cells are then injected back into the patient where they target cancer cells. CAR-T cell therapy is FDA approved for the treatment of refractory acute lymphoblastic leukemia in children (tisagenlecleucel) and refractory diffuse large B-cell lymphoma in adults (axicabtagene and lisocabtagene), refractory mantle cell lymphoma (brexucabtagene), and multiple myeloma (idecabtagene).

Hypotension

Hypotension is attributed to cytokine release syndrome secondary to activation and proliferation of T cells. In a single center study there was a 21%

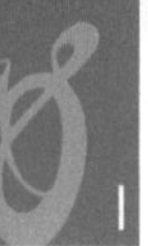

incidence of hypotension requiring inotropic support.[48]

Cardiomyopathy

In a study of pediatric patients with cancer, the vast majority of whom had acute lymphoblastic leukemia, 10% had echocardiographic evidence of new systolic dysfunction. At 6 months of follow up 7% had persistent LV dysfunction with the majority having normal LV function. Preexisting cardiomyopathy or prior anthracycline therapy were not risk factors for development of LV dysfunction in this cohort.

KEY POINTS

- Hypotension can be seen and relates to cytokine release syndrome.
- Cardiomyopathy also seems to relate to cytokine release syndrome and is reversible in the majority of patients
  - arrhythmias may be seen
  - cardiac arrest has been reported.

REFERENCES

1. Cardinale D, Colombo A, Bacchiani G, et al. Early detection of anthracycline cardiotoxicity and improvement with heart failure therapy. *Circulation.* 2015;131(22):1981–1988. doi:10.1161/CIRCULATIONAHA.114.013777.
2. Cowgill JA, Francis SA, Sawyer DB. Anthracycline and peripartum cardiomyopathies. *Circ Res.* 2019;124(11):1633–1646. doi:10.1161/CIRCRESAHA.119.313577.
3. Chang HM, Moudgil R, Scarabelli T, Okwuosa TM, Yeh ETH. Cardiovascular complications of cancer therapy: best practices in diagnosis, prevention, and management: part 1. *J Am Coll Cardiol.* 2017;70(20):2536–2551. doi:10.1016/j.jacc.2017.09.1096.
4. Alexandre J, Moslehi JJ, Bersell KR, Funck-Brentano C, Roden DM, Salem JE. Anticancer drug-induced cardiac rhythm disorders: current knowledge and basic underlying mechanisms. *Pharmacol Ther.* 2018;189:89–103. doi:10.1016/j.pharmthera.2018.04.009.
5. Mazur M, Wang F, Hodge DO, et al. Burden of cardiac arrhythmias in patients with anthracycline-related cardiomyopathy. *JACC Clin Electrophysiol.* 2017;3:139–150. doi:10.1016/j.jacep.2016.08.009.
6. Horacek JM, Jakl M, Horackova J, Pudil R, Jebavy L, Maly J. Assessment of anthracycline-induced cardiotoxicity with electrocardiography. *Exp Oncol.* 2009;31(2):115–117.
7. Wakabayashi I, Groschner K. Vascular actions of anthracycline antibiotics. *Curr Med Chem.* 2003;10:427–436.
8. Mulrooney DA, Yeazel MW, Kawashima T, et al. Cardiac outcomes in a cohort of adult survivors of childhood and adolescent cancer: retrospective analysis of the Childhood Cancer Survivor cohort. *BMJ.* 2009;339:b4606. doi:10.1136/bmj.b4606.
9. Armenian SH, Hudson MM, Mulder RL, et al. Recommendations for cardiomyopathy surveillance for survivors of childhood cancer: a report from the International Late Effects of Childhood Cancer Guideline Harmonization Group. *Lancet Oncol.* 2015;16(3):e123–e136. doi:10.1016/S1470-2045(14)70409-7.
10. Gottdiener JS, Appelbaum FR, Ferrans VJ, Deisseroth A, Ziegler J. Cardiotoxicity associated with high-dose cyclophosphamide therapy. *Arch Intern Med.* 1981;141(6):758–763.
11. Lin CJ, Vader JM, Slade M, DiPersio JF, Westervelt P, Romee R. Cardiomyopathy in patients after posttransplant cyclophosphamide-based hematopoietic cell transplantation. *Cancer.* 2017;123(10):1800–1809. doi:10.1002/cncr.30534.
12. Morandi P, Ruffini PA, Benvenuto GM, Raimondi R, Fosser V. Cardiac toxicity of high-dose chemotherapy. *Bone Marrow Transplant.* 2005;35(4):323–334.
13. Layoun ME, Wickramasinghe CD, Peralta MV, Yang EH. Fluoropyrimidine-induced cardiotoxicity: manifestations, mechanisms, and management. *Curr Oncol Rep.* 2016;18(6):35. doi:10.1007/s11912-016-0521-1.
14. Fradley MG, Barrett CD, Clark JR, Francis SA. Ventricular fibrillation cardiac arrest due to 5-fluorouracil cardiotoxicity. *Tex Heart Inst J.* 2013;40(4):472–476.
15. Rowinsky EK, McGuire WP, Guarnieri T, Fisherman JS, Christian MC, Donehower RC. Cardiac disturbances during the administration of taxol. *J Clin Oncol.* 1991;9(9):1704–1712.
16. Slamon DJ, Leyland-Jones B, Shak S, et al. Use of chemotherapy plus a monoclonal antibody against HER2 for metastatic breast cancer that overexpresses HER2. *N Engl J Med.* 2001;344(11):783–792.
17. Romond EH, Perez EA, Bryant J, et al. Trastuzumab plus adjuvant chemotherapy for operable HER2-positive breast cancer. *N Engl J Med.* 2005;353:1673–1684.
18. Suter TM, Procter M, van Veldhuisen DJ, et al. Trastuzumab-associated cardiac adverse effects in the Herceptin Adjuvant trial. *J Clin Oncol.* 2007;25:3859–3865.
19. Swain SM, Ewer MS, Cortes J, et al. Cardiac tolerability of pertuzumab plus trastuzumab plus docetaxel in patients with HER2-positive metastatic breast cancer in CLEOPATRA: a randomized, double-blind, placebo-controlled phase III study. *Oncologist.* 2013;18:257–264.
20. Baselga J, Cortes J, Kim SB, et al. Pertuzumab plus trastuzumab plus docetaxel for metastatic breast cancer. *N Engl J Med.* 2012;366:109–119.
21. Kantarjian HG, Kim DW, Pinilla-Ibarz J, et al. Ponatinib (PON) in patients (pts) with Philadelphia chromosome-positive (Ph+) leukemias resistant or intolerant to dasatinib or nilotinib, or with the T315I mutation: longer-term follow up of the PACE trial. *J Clin Oncol.* 2014;32(suppl 5):abstr 7081.
22. Cortes JE, Saglio G, Kantarjian HM, et al. Final 5-year study results of DASISION: the Dasatinib Versus Imatinib Study in Treatment-Naïve Chronic Myeloid Leukemia Patients Trial. *J Clin Oncol.* 2016;34(20):2333–2340. doi:10.1200/JCO.2015.64.8899.
23. Cortes JE, Kim D-W, Pinilla-Ibarz J, et al. Ponatinib efficacy and safety in Philadelphia chromosome-positive leukemia: final 5-year results of the phase 2 PACE trial. *Blood.* 2018;132(4):393–404.
24. Latifi Y, Moccetti F, Wu M, et al. Thrombotic microangiopathy as a cause of cardiovascular toxicity from the BCR-ABL1 tyrosine kinase inhibitor ponatinib. *Blood.* 2019;133(14):1597–1606. doi:10.1182/blood-2018-10-881557.
25. Singh AP, Glennon MS, Umbarkar P, et al. Ponatinib-induced cardiotoxicity: delineating the signaling mechanisms and potential rescue strategies. *Cardiovasc Res.* 2019;115(5):966–977. doi:10.1093/cvr/cvz006.
26. Groarke JD, Choueiri TK, Slosky D, Cheng S, Moslehi J. Recognizing and managing left ventricular dysfunction associated with therapeutic inhibition of the vascular endothelial growth factor signaling pathway. *Curr Treat Options Cardiovasc Med.* 2014;16(9):335. doi:10.1007/s11936-014-0335-0.
27. Moslehi JJ. Cardiovascular toxic effects of targeted cancer therapies. *N Engl J Med.* 2016;375:1457–1467. doi:10.1056/NEJMra1100265.
28. Flaherty L, Hamid O, Linette G, et al. A single-arm, open-label, expanded access study of vemurafenib in patients with metastatic melanoma in the United States. *Cancer J.* 2014;20:18–24.
29. Larkin J, Del Vecchio M, Ascierto PA, et al. Vemurafenib in patients with BRAF(V600) mutated metastatic melanoma: an open-label, multicentre, safety study. *Lancet Oncol.* 2014;15:436–444.
30. Shah RR, Morganroth J. Update on cardiovascular safety of tyrosine kinase inhibitors: with a special focus on QT interval, left ventricular dysfunction and overall risk/benefit. *Drug Saf.* 2015;38(8):693–710. doi:10.1007/s40264-015-0300-1.

31. Larkin J, Ascierto PA, Dréno B, et al. Combined vemurafenib and cobimetinib in BRAF-mutated melanoma. *N Engl J Med.* 2014; 371(20):1867–1876. doi:10.1056/NEJMoa1408868.
32. Fiocchi R, Gori M, Taddei F, Trevisani L, Gallo M, Eleftheriou G. Cardiac toxicity of combined vemurafenib and cobimetinib administration. *Int J Clin Pharmacol Ther.* 2019;57(5):259–263. doi:10.5414/CP203379.
33. Dummer R, Ascierto PA, Gogas HJ, et al. Encorafenib plus binimetinib versus vemurafenib or encorafenib in patients with BRAF-mutant melanoma (COLUMBUS): a multicentre, open-label, randomised phase 3 trial. *Lancet Oncol.* 2018;19(5):603–615. doi:10.1016/S1470-2045(18)30142-6.
34. Petrelli F, Cabiddu M, Borgonovo K, Barni S. Risk of venous and arterial thromboembolic events associated with anti-EGFR agents: a meta-analysis of randomized clinical trials. *Ann Oncol.* 2012; 23(7):1672–1679. doi:10.1093/annonc/mdr592.
35. Liu Y, Liu Y, Fan ZW, Li J, Xu GG. Meta-analysis of the risks of hypertension and QTc prolongation in patients with advanced non-small cell lung cancer who were receiving vandetanib. *Eur J Clin Pharmacol.* 2015;71(5):541–547. doi:10.1007/s00228-015-1831-1.
36. Brown JR, Moslehi J, O'Brien S, et al. Characterization of atrial fibrillation adverse events reported in ibrutinib randomized controlled registration trials. *Haematologica.* 2017;102:1796–1805.
37. Leong DP, Caron F, Hillis C, et al. The risk of atrial fibrillation with ibrutinib use: a systematic review and meta-analysis. *Blood.* 2016;128(1):138–140. doi:10.1182/blood-2016–05-712828.
38. Fradley MG, Gliksman M, Emole J, et al. Rates and risk of atrial arrhythmias in patients treated with ibrutinib compared with cytotoxic chemotherapy. *Am J Cardiol.* 2019;124:539–544.
39. Shafaattalab S, Lin E, Christidi E, et al. Ibrutinib displays atrial-specific toxicity in human stem cell-derived cardiomyocytes. *Stem Cell Reports.* 2019;12(5):996–1006. doi:10.1016/j.stemcr.2019.03.011.
40. Wang M, Rule S, Zinzani PL, et al. Acalabrutinib in relapsed or refractory mantle cell lymphoma (ACE-LY-004): a single-arm, multicentre, phase 2 trial. *Lancet.* 2018;391(10121):659–667. doi:10.1016/S0140-6736(17)33108-2.
41. Iacovelli R, Ciccarese C, Fornarini G, et al. Cabozantinib-related cardiotoxicity: a prospective analysis in a real-world cohort of metastatic renal cell carcinoma patients. *Br J Clin Pharmacol.* 2019;85(6):1283–1289. doi:10.1111/bcp.13895.
42. Dikopf A, Wood K, Salgia R. A safety assessment of crizotinib in the treatment of ALK-positive NSCLC patients. *Expert Opin Drug Saf.* 2015;14(3):485–493. doi:10.1517/14740338.2015.1007040.
43. Schiattarella GG, Sannino A, Toscano E, et al. Cardiovascular effects of histone deacetylase inhibitors epigenetic therapies: systematic review of 62 studies and new hypotheses for future research. *Int J Cardiol.* 2016;219:396–403. doi:10.1016/j.ijcard.2016.06.012.
44. Waxman AJ, Clasen S, Hwang WT, et al. Carfilzomib-associated cardiovascular adverse events. A systematic review and meta-analysis. *JAMA Oncol.* 2018;4(3):e174519.
45. Bringhen S, Milan A, Ferri C, et al. Cardiovascular adverse events in modern myeloma therapy - Incidence and risks. A review from the European Myeloma Network (EMN) and Italian Society of Arterial Hypertension (SIIA). European Hematology Association, the European Myeloma Network and the Italian Society of Arterial Hypertension. *Haematologica.* 2018;103(9):1422–1432. doi:10.3324/haematol.2018.191288.
46. Li W, Garcia D, Cornell RF, et al. Cardiovascular and thrombotic complications of novel multiple myeloma therapies: a review. *JAMA Oncol.* 2017;3(7):980–988. doi:10.1001/jamaoncol.2016.3350.
47. Mahmood SS, Fradley MG, Cohen JV, et al. Myocarditis in patients treated with immune checkpoint inhibitors. *J Am Coll Cardiol.* 2018;71(16):1755–1764. doi:10.1016/j.jacc.2018.02.037.
48. Burstein DS, Maude S, Grupp S, Griffis H, Rossano J, Lin K. Cardiac profile of chimeric antigen receptor T cell therapy in children: a single-institution experience. *Biol Blood Marrow Transplant.* 2018;24(8):1590–1595. doi:10.1016/j.bbmt.2018.05.014.

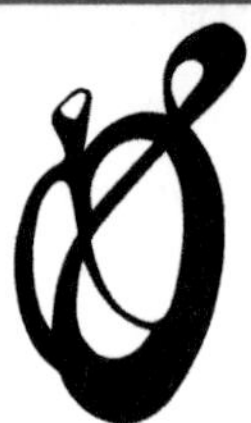

4 Radiation Therapy Cardiovascular Risks

MIRELA TUZOVIC, WILLIAM FINCH, AND ERIC H. YANG

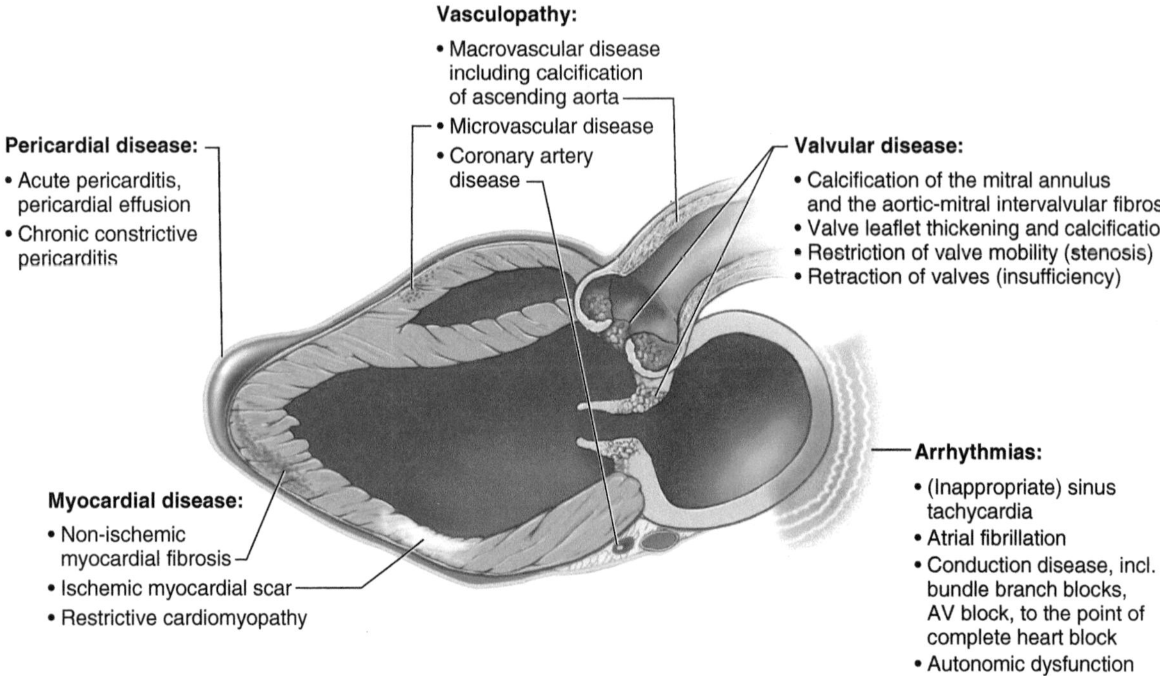
Vasculopathy:
• Macrovascular disease including calcification of ascending aorta
• Microvascular disease
• Coronary artery disease
Pericardial disease:
• Acute pericarditis, pericardial effusion
• Chronic constrictive pericarditis
Valvular disease:
• Calcification of the mitral annulus and the aortic-mitral intervalvular fibrosa
• Valve leaflet thickening and calcification
• Restriction of valve mobility (stenosis)
• Retraction of valves (insufficiency)
Myocardial disease:
• Non-ischemic myocardial fibrosis
• Ischemic myocardial scar
• Restrictive cardiomyopathy
Arrhythmias:
• (Inappropriate) sinus tachycardia
• Atrial fibrillation
• Conduction disease, incl. bundle branch blocks, AV block, to the point of complete heart block
• Autonomic dysfunction

CHAPTER OUTLINE

KEY POINTS

- Radiation therapy can lead to various forms of cardiovascular disease, including cardiomyopathy, heart failure, coronary artery disease, valvular heart disease, pericardial disease, and autonomic dysfunction.
- Dose sparing is the single most important preventive strategy, accomplished by shifting from a large field (e.g., mantle radiation) to an involved field, from photons to protons, and from none to standard use of ancillary techniques such as breath holding and prone positioning.
- Whereas advancements in the delivery of radiation therapy are expected to decrease the long-term risk

KEY POINTS—cont'd

of radiation-induced heart disease, no "safe" radiation dose threshold has been defined and the risk may be rather linear even in the low-dose range spectrum.

- Besides dose, risk factors for radiation-induced heart disease to consider include age at time of radiation exposure (<5 years and >65 years), additional cancer therapies (especially anthracyclines), and the presence of cardiac comorbid conditions (esp., ischemic heart disease and myocardial infarction).
- All risk factors should be considered to direct to the appropriate radiation techniques and patients should be appropriately counseled regarding risks and benefits mitigation strategies.
- Among cardiac surveillance parameters, strain imaging might be the most promising, indicating subclinical cardiac dysfunction during and early after radiation therapy; however, the long-term significance of those changes, including implications for treatment and long-term cardiotoxicity, are unknown.

Radiation therapy (RT) is commonly used to cure, halt, or palliate the manifestations and/or symptoms of many types of cancers (e.g., Hodgkin lymphoma [HL], breast, lung, and esophageal cancer), often in combination with surgical resection and/or chemotherapy. Although RT can provide significant benefit for the treatment of cancer, it is important to recognize that RT carries significant risks to healthy tissue that may inadvertently be exposed. RT causes tissue injury primarily through the generation of oxidative stress; inflammation is seen acutely and fibrosis over time.[1]

Radiation-induced heart disease (RIHD) is typically noted in patients who receive high doses of radiation for thoracic malignancies where the cardiac silhouette overlaps with the radiation field. RIHD can manifest in a variety of disease states, including cardiomyopathy, coronary artery disease, valvular dysfunction, and pericardial disease (see Central Illustration). The risk of RIHD is influenced by multiple factors, including the radiation dose and technique, concomitant administration of cardiotoxic chemotherapy such as with anthracycline agents, age at the time of exposure, time interval since exposure, and patient-specific cardiovascular risk factors (Table 4.1). It is critical for providers to consider the risk, appropriately counsel patients, and to participate in discussions with care team providers regarding the best modes of therapies and risk mitigation strategies before radiation therapy is applied. The specific disease elements of RIHD, including screening and management, will be discussed in Chapter 26.

RADIATION DOSE AND TECHNIQUE

Modern RT for the treatment of HL, breast, lung, and esophageal cancer is performed using medical linear accelerators to produce megavoltage x-ray beams, with the beam being tailored to the tumor using collimators and blocks.[2] Radiation dose is commonly described in terms of gray (Gy), the International System (SI) unit for absorbed radiation dose (Table 4.2). Therapeutic doses of radiation for common malignancies range from 30 to 60 Gy delivered to the tumor. They are fractionated into multiple doses separated temporally (Table 4.3). Dose-sparing is the single most important preventive strategy; a list of techniques used to reduce radiation exposure to the heart is provided in Table 4.4.

Historically, large areas (e.g., mantle field radiation) and high doses of radiation (40 to 45 Gy) were

TABLE 4.1 Types of Radiation-Induced Heart Disease and Relevant Risk Factors

RADIATION-INDUCED HEART DISEASE	RISK FACTORS
Pericarditis	Radiation dose
Ischemic heart disease	History of coronary artery disease, cardiovacular risk factors, younger age at time of exposure
Cardiomyopathy/congestive heart failure	Anthracycline use, cardiovacular risk factors
Valve disease	Radiation dose, anthracycline use

TABLE 4.2 Units of Radiation Exposure

UNIT	TYPE OF UNIT	CONVERSION FACTOR
Rad[a]	Absorbed radiation dose	1 rad = 0.01 Gy
Gray (Gy)[a]	Absorbed radiation dose; SI unit	1J/kg = 1 Gy = 100 rad
Rem[b]	Dose equivalent	1 rem = 0.01 Sv; 1 rem = 1 rad[c]
Sievert (Sv)[b]	Dose equivalent; SI unit	1 Sv = 100 rem; 1 Sv = 1 Gy[c]

[a]Rad and grays are units of energy per mass.
[b]Rem and sieverts are units of energy per mass adjusted by a dimensionless factor to account for a potential for biological damage.
[c]Rem and rad are equivalent and sieverts and grays are equivalent for radiograph and gamma radiation.

TABLE 4.3 Malignancies Whose Treatment May Include Radiation Therapy at the Outlined Doses and Generation of a Radiation Risk to the Heart

MALIGNANCY	DOSE (Gy)
Hodgkin lymphoma	30–36
Breast cancer	45–50
Gastric carcinoma	45–50
Esophageal carcinoma	45–50
Lung cancer	50–60
Thymoma	60

Adapted from Finch W, Lee MS, Yang EH. Radiation-induced heart disease: long-term manifestations, diagnosis, and management. In: Herrmann J, ed. *Clinical Cardio-oncology*. 1st ed. Philadelphia: Elsevier, 2016.

TABLE 4.4 Cardiac-Sparing Mechanisms

TECHNIQUE	CARDIAC-SPARING MECHANISM
Breath hold	With inspiration, distance from chest wall to the heart increases
Prone position	Breast falls away from chest wall Increases distance from the heart to radiation therapy (RT) beam
Intensity modulated RT	Computerized leaves and dose planning algorithms allow for shaping of radiation field to limit cardiac dose
Proton beam irradiation	Utilizes difference in properties of protons compared with photons to allow for reduced dose fall off
Accelerated partial breast irradiation	Smaller target volume allows for possible decreased dose to the heart
Intraoperative RT	Smaller target volume and, in some cases. lower energy reduced dose to the heart

Adapted from Shah C, Badiyan S, Berry S, et al. Cardiac dose sparing and avoidance techniques in breast cancer radiotherapy. *Radiother Oncol*. 2014;112(1):9–16.

used for the treatment of HL. Of note, doses of 30 Gy or higher have been associated with the greatest proportion of morbidity and mortality caused by RIHD.[3] With the aforementioned dose-sparing techniques, such as radiation blocks (shielding), smaller dose fractions, and involved-node radiation therapy (in which only the involved nodes are irradiated),[4,5] the relative cardiovascular mortality risk could be reduced from 5.3 to 1.4.[5] Acute manifestations, such as pericarditis, are nearly eliminated nowadays.[6]

The cardioprotective benefit of dose fractionation is supported by experimental studies.[4,7,8] For patients, the ideal fractionation regimen to reduce RIHD is not known, but hypofractionated whole breast irradiation (42.56 Gy/16 fractions) resulted in a lower rate of acute toxicity compared with conventional radiation (50 Gy/25 fractions).[9] Otherwise there are no indications of inferior outcomes at 10 years when hypofractionated RT is compared with conventional RT.[9–11] Evidence of obstructive coronary artery disease and abnormalities on myocardial perfusion scans correlate with the left ventricular volume included in the radiation therapy field.[12] Newer radiation techniques with smaller radiation fields help to minimize the radiation volume. Intensity-modulated radiation therapy (IMRT), for example, can improve dose distribution with the ultimate goal of delivering homogeneous radiation to target tissue and minimizing doses absorbed by critical structures[13] (Fig. 4.1A). IMRT may be particularly beneficial in patients undergoing repeat RT for relapsed disease or for patients with very large tumor burden.[14]

In addition to fractionation and minimizing the delivered dose, RT planning and custom radiation blocks can reduce the dose absorbed by the heart. In the case of breast cancer, RIHD is primarily a concern with RT of the left breast, which results in at least twice the radiation dose to the heart compared with that to the right breast, and a higher risk for accelerated atherosclerosis.[15,16] No safe threshold of cardiac radiation dose exists: for every gray of absorbed dose there is an approximate 7% increased risk of coronary artery disease (CAD), with a higher risk observed in patients with conventional CAD risk factors.[17] The lowest dose that has been found to be associated with CAD is 2.8 Gy.[18] This being said, no "safe" radiation dose threshold has been defined and the risk may be rather linear even in the low-dose range spectrum (Fig. 4.2).

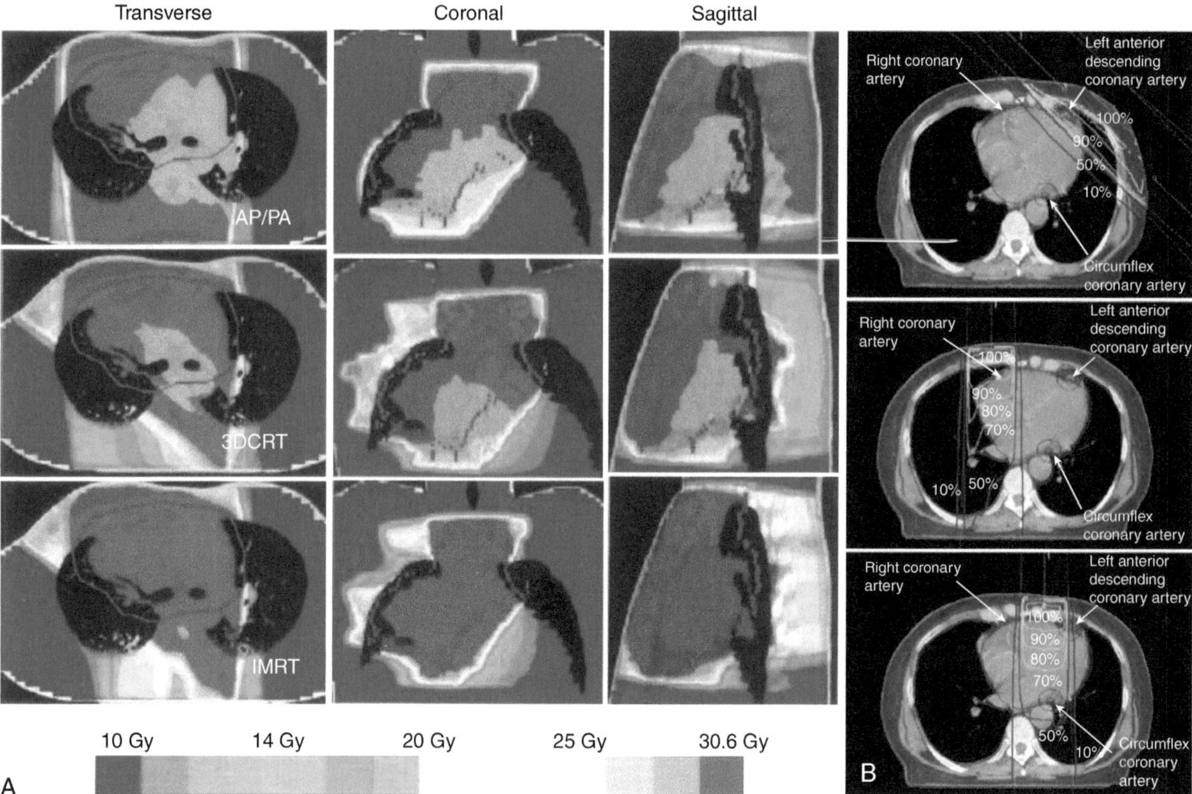

FIG. 4.1 **A,** Comparison of dose distribution of conventional parallel opposed (*AP/PA*) versus three-dimensional conformal radiation therapy (3-*DCRT*) versus intensity-modulated radiation therapy (*IMRT*) plans. (a) Example 1: large volume. (b) Example 2: repeat radiation therapy (RT). **B.** Axial computed tomography sections showing dose distributions from right and left 6-MV direct anterior internal mammary fields and left ^{60}Co pair radiotherapy. *Isodose lines* correspond to percentages of given dose. Three main coronary arteries are outlined, with 1-cm margin added to each. (**A,** From Goodman KA, Toner S, Hunt M, Wu EJ, Yahalom J. Intensity-modulated radiotherapy for lymphoma involving the mediastinum. *Int J Radiol Oncology Biol Phys*. 2005;62:198–206. **B,** From Taylor CW, Nisbet A, McGale P, Darby SC. Cardiac exposures in breast cancer radiotherapy: 1950–1990s. *Int J Radiation Oncology Biol Phys*. 2007;69(5):1484–1495.)

Strategies to reduce cardiac dose during left breast RT include computed tomography planning to ensure the heart is not within the radiation field (see Fig. 4.1B), tangential (as opposed to anterior) radiation beams, and cardiac radiation protection blocks.[19–21] Historically the myocardium involving the left anterior descending coronary artery would receive higher doses, but with contemporary RT CAD is no longer lateralized, depending on which breast is treated.[22,23] Furthermore, the recent Danish Breast Cancer Cooperative Group trials, which randomized patients to RT and surgery or surgery alone, found no increase in atherosclerotic cardiovascular disease with RT.[21,22] These more recent studies suggest that modern cardiac dose reduction strategies are proving effective at minimizing RIHD. RT of the internal mammary chain of lymph nodes is also utilized. Internal mammary node RT, which is often delivered using anterior fields, increases the absorbed dose of the heart and techniques between 1979 and 1986 continued to be associated with an elevated risk of heart failure.[24] With modern techniques the overall cardiac toxicity of internal mammary RT appears to be low at least on short-term follow up.[25] Internal mammary RT has not been found to result in increased RIHD-related mortality at 10-year follow up and it reduces the risk of breast cancer recurrence.[26,27]

AGE AT TIME OF EXPOSURE

Children are more vulnerable to serious radiation-related complications compared with adults, both

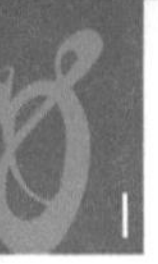

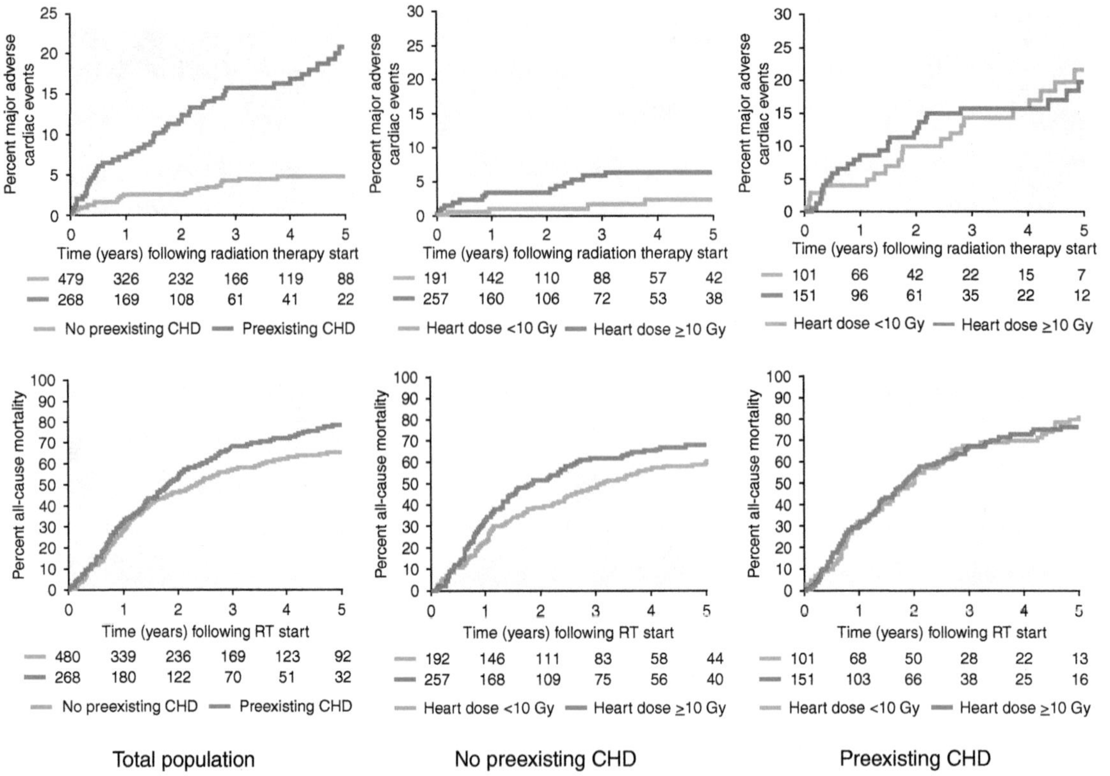

FIG. 4.2. Cardiac radiation dose, cardiac disease, and mortality in patients with lung cancer. *Upper panels*: Cumulative incidence of major adverse cardiac events (MACE) stratified by preexisting coronary heart disease (*CHD*) (Gray's $P < .001$) or MHD in patients without preexisting CHD (Gray's $P = .025$) and patients with preexisting CHD (Gray's $P = .98$). *Lower panels:* All-cause mortality estimates stratified by preexisting CHD (log-rank $P = .003$) or mean heart dose (MHD) in patients without preexisting CHD (log-rank $P = .014$), and patients with preexisting CHD (log-rank $P = .66$). (From Atkins KM, Rawal B, Chaunzwa TL, et al. Cardiac Radiation Dose, Cardiac Dose, and Mortality in Patients with Lung Cancer. *J Am Coll Cardiol*. 2019:73:2976–987.)

owing to growing and developing organs and to a longer life expectancy with more time to develop complications.[28,29] Adult childhood cancer survivors from the Childhood Cardiac Registry in the Netherlands had a 27% prevalence of cardiac dysfunction based on screening with echocardiography. Multivariate regression analysis showed that younger age at diagnosis (age 0 to 5 had an odds ratio [OR] of 2.94 compared with age >15 years), time since diagnosis (>25 years following diagnosis had an OR of 0.11 compared with 5 to 10 years following treatment), anthracycline dose (cumulative doses of 151 to 300 mg/m^2 had an OR of 3.98, whereas cumulative doses of >450 mg/m^2 had an OR of 10.58 when compared with 1 to 150 mg/m^2), and thoracic radiotherapy were all predictive of left ventricular dysfunction. It is worth noting that two-thirds of the patients had also received chemotherapy with anthracyclines, which are known to cause cardiomyopathy.[30] Children and adolescents with HL treated with radiation and/or chemotherapy at Stanford Hospital between 1961 and 1991 had high risks of death from heart disease (relative risk [RR], 29.6), death from acute myocardial infarction (MI; RR, 41.5), and death from other cardiac disease (RR, 21.2).[31] Patients who died had received between 42 and 45 Gy of radiation to the mediastinum between the ages of 9 and 20 years.[32] A second analysis on a broader spectrum of 2232 patients with HL treated with radiation therapy (72% mantle field) at Stanford Hospital between 1960 and 1990 confirmed a 45 times higher risk of death owing to acute MI with radiation exposure before age 19.[5]

TIME INTERVAL AFTER RADIATION THERAPY

As alluded to above, the risk of RIHD and cardiac mortality increases with a longer duration after radiation therapy. In the Stanford study noted above, the risk of cardiac death increased substantially with increasing duration of follow up: the relative risk of death caused by an acute MI was 2 for patients within 5 years of treatment compared with a relative risk of 5.6 at 20 years following radiation.[5] A retrospective cohort study of the medical records of 2524 Dutch patients with HL treated between 1965 and 1995 evaluated more types of cardiac disease, which showed a significant increase in the risk of ischemic heart disease, as well as cardiomyopathy/congestive heart failure (HF) and valvular heart disease even 35 years or more after treatment. The highest risk of cardiac disease was noted in patients treated before age 25 and in those who were 20 to 47 years posttreatment (when compared with those patients treated 5 to 10 years ago).[30] Similar results have been shown for patients with breast cancer where the excess risk of cardiac death may not be apparent until up to 20 years following treatment in patients with left-sided disease compared with right-sided disease.[33] In a large, long-term follow-up study of 7425 patients with breast cancer, longer follow-up time was associated with increasing risk of cardiovascular death: HR 1.0 at $\leq$10 years, HR 1.5 at 10 to 20 years, and HR 2.9 $>$20 years.[34] A review of 19 published reports on patients with breast cancer is likewise in agreement with the conclusion that extended follow-up duration is associated with excess risk of cardiac mortality.[35]

ANTHRACYCLINE EXPOSURE

Anthracyclines, which are commonly used to treat various hematologic and solid cancers, represent the classic cardiotoxin.[36] Although there is likely no "safe" dose of anthracyclines, the risk of cardiotoxicity seems to be significantly increased with cumulative doses $>$240 mg/m^2. Although anthracyclines and RT independently increase the risk for cardiotoxicity, they may also have a synergistic effect on cardiac toxicity. In a study of 1474 patients with HL, RT and anthracycline treatment was found to increase the risk of congestive HF (HR, 7.37 and 2.44, respectively). Combination treatment with RT and anthracyclines further increased this risk for congestive HF and valve disease (HR, 2.81 for congestive HF and 2.10 for valve disorders compared with RT alone), but not for MI or angina.[37] A prospective study of 299 patients with breast cancer undergoing either 5 or 10 cycles of chemotherapy with cyclophosphamide and doxorubicin showed that patients treated with 10 cycles have an increased risk of cardiac events compared with those in the Framingham population, whereas those treated with 5 cycles do not. Treatment with RT in addition to chemotherapy, which accounted for 41% of patients, was associated with an increased risk of events, particularly in those patients receiving moderate to high doses of radiation.[38]

COMORBID CONDITIONS

Most data suggest that the presence of cardiovascular comorbidities, especially preexisting coronary artery disease increases the risk of RIHD (Figs. 4.2 and 4.3). A history of cardiac problems, including MI, arrhythmias, valvular dysfunction, right atrial hypertrophy, and ventricular septum defects, indicated they were important modifiers of ischemic heart disease risk following radiation.[39] Likewise, the incidence of fatal and nonfatal ischemic cardiac disease was higher than expected (based on age, gender, and calendar period) for patients treated with mediastinal radiation for HL (between 30 and 45 Gy) who had cardiovascular risk factors such as hypertension, smoking, obesity, hypercholesterolemia, diabetes mellitus, or a history of ischemic cardiac disease (RR, 2.36).[40] Although it is clear that patients treated with radiation during childhood are particularly vulnerable to RIHD, as patients approach middle age, the relative rate of ischemic cardiac events decreases when compared with the rate of expected events, even though the absolute rate increases.[5]

How much optimal risk factor control reduces the risk remains to be determined.[24,33]

RISKS DURING OR EARLY AFTER RT

Whereas RIHD typically manifests years to decades following treatment, acute pericarditis can develop during treatment. Acute pericarditis usually occurs

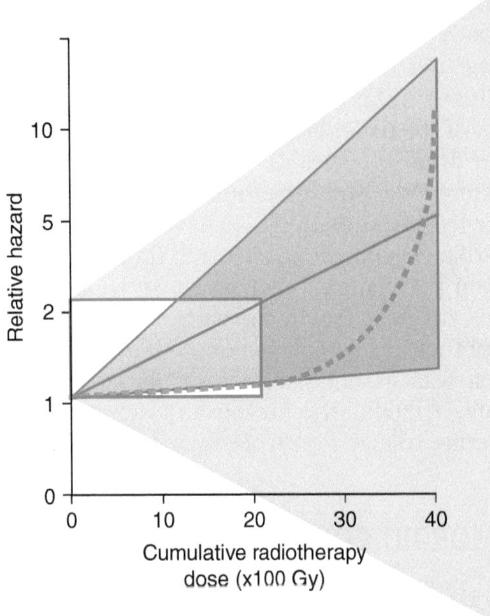

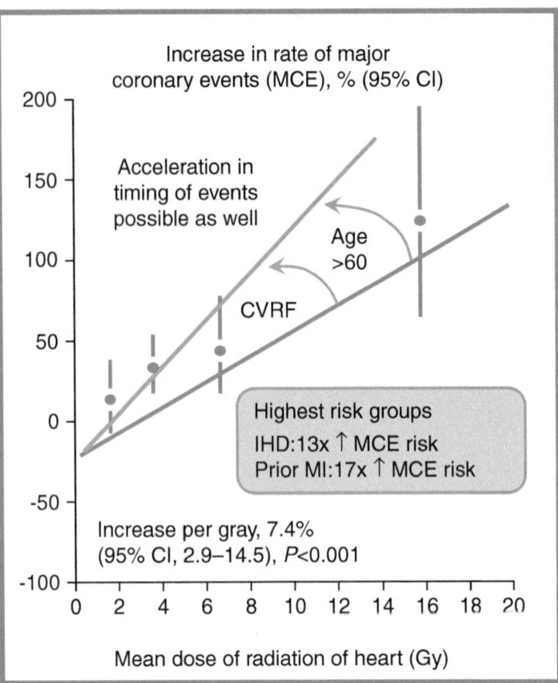

FIG. 4.3. *Left panel:* Rate of major coronary events according to mean radiation dose to the heart in a conceptual exponential (cut-off) or linear model based on dose estimates in patients (major coronary events includes myocardial infarction, coronary revascularization, and death from ischemic heart disease). *Right panel:* The values for the *solid line* were calculated with the use of dose estimates for individual women. The *circles* show values for groups of women, classified according to dose categories; the associated *vertical lines* represent 95% confidence intervals. All estimates were calculated after stratification for country and for age at breast-cancer diagnosis, year of breast-cancer diagnosis, interval between breast-cancer diagnosis and first major coronary event for case patients or index date for controls (all in 5-year categories), and presence or absence of a cardiac risk factor. The radiation categories were less than 2, 2 to 4, 5 to 9, and 10 Gy or more, and the overall averages of the mean doses to the heart of women in these categories were 1.4, 3.4, 6.5, and 15.8 Gy, respectively). *CVRF*, Cardiovascular risk factors. (Modified from Darby SC, Ewertz M, McGale P. Risk of ischemic heart disease in women after radiotherapy for breast cancer. *N Engl J Med.* 2013;368(11):987–998.)

in patients with large mediastinal tumors.[41] It is thought to develop owing to inflammation from tumor necrosis as opposed to direct radiation injury to the pericardium.[41] Acute pericarditis, which is less common than chronic pericarditis, typically presents with chest pain, fever, tachycardia, and a pericardial rub. Typical electrocardiographic (ECG) features include diffuse ST elevations with PR depressions. An effusion may or may not be present; however, if present, development of a pericardial effusion may be a risk factor for chronic pericarditis.[42]

Radiation therapy on its own does not appear to cause any significant changes on ECG acutely.[40,43] In one study of 16 patients aged 15 to 33 years who received >3500 rads to the heart, ECG abnormalities included nonspecific ST segment or T-wave changes, low voltage, or complete right bundle branch block.[44] However, the exact timing of the electrocardiogram with respect to completion of radiation therapy was not specified; therefore, some of the ECG changes may be owing to progressive RIHD as opposed to acute radiation injury.

CARDIAC BIOMARKERS

Radiation therapy alone does not commonly increase the levels of typical cardiac biomarkers, and in general, abnormal biomarkers warrant further evaluation for the etiology and should not be routinely attributed to radiation-induced injury. In patients with breast cancer undergoing ~45 Gy of whole-breast radiation treatment, no changes in troponin levels were seen before and after treatment.[45] Similarly, in patients with thoracic malignancies, biomarkers including troponin, NT-proBNP, and CK-MB were not significantly elevated during or after completion of radiation treatment.[46] Only one study showed troponins did increase following radiation in patients with left-sided breast cancer compared with those with right-sided disease; however, the increased values were still within the normal range.[47] NT-proBNP levels may be more affected by RT compared with troponin levels. NT-proBNP was elevated in patients with breast cancer after RT compared with the control group that consisted of patients with breast cancer who were radiation naïve.[14] Increase in NT-proBNP correlated with receiving high doses in a small volume of the heart and ventricles.[14] Consistent with the other studies, troponin levels remained normal in both groups.[14]

STRAIN IMAGING

Deformation imaging with strain is a sensitive way to detect myocardial dysfunction and is widely used in the assessment of oncology patients, particularly those undergoing treatment with anthracyclines.[48] Evidence indicates that strain is abnormal in patients with cancer exposed to radiation and regional changes in strain correspond to the RT fields used during therapy.[49] Regional strain changes can present immediately and up to 14 months following RT in patients with left-sided breast cancer, but are not seen in patients with right-sided breast cancer.[47,50] The long-term significance of these early changes in strain imaging after RT are unclear.

FUTURE AVENUES

Cardiovascular risk assessment remains a challenging task owing to the heterogeneous modalities of RT, accompanying chemotherapy and targeted therapy regimens, preexisting cardiovascular risk factors, and other multifactorial variables. An individualized assessment for each cancer case is essential, which includes a risk-to-benefit discussion of potential short- and long-term consequences of RT in the absence of large-scale evidence. Aggressive management of cardiovascular comorbidities should be pursued to the degree that is tolerated during and after cancer treatments, particularly with malignancies that confer favorable, long-term prognosis.

In regard to society guidelines reflective of cardiovascular risk assessment with RT, the American Society of Clinical Oncology Clinical Practice Guidelines in 2017 stated that patients with cancer who experienced high dose RT ($\geq$30 Gy) in the area of the heart, or lower doses in combination with anthracycline chemotherapy were considered at increased risk for developing cardiac dysfunction—regardless of prior risk factors. However, suggested preventative strategies were limited in scope owing to an overall lack of robust evidence of efficacy of interventions, with the recommendation of performing a comprehensive assessment of screening for cardiovascular risk factors and avoiding or minimizing the use of potentially cardiotoxic therapies if established alternatives exist that would not compromise cancer outcomes. In regard to RT techniques, it was recommended that clinicians select lower radiation doses when clinically appropriate, use more precise or tailored radiation fields (excluding as much of the heart as possible), include deep-inspiration breath holding for patients with mediastinal tumors or breast cancer, and use intensity-modulated RT that varies the delivery of radiation energy to precisely contour the desired radiation distribution and minimize involving normal tissue.[49]

In closing, wide-scale efforts are needed to capture the dynamic epidemiology of the effects of RT in a diverse spectrum of cancer states and survivors. Such research efforts may involve tracking outcomes in national/international registries, as well as evaluating the effects of cardiovascular interventions and imaging surveillance for cardiotoxicity in prospective, randomized trials. As many effects of RT may not manifest for decades, such registries are crucial toward our understanding of the natural history of RIHD, which has yet to be defined accurately.

REFERENCES

1. Straub JM, New J, Hamilton CD, Lominska C, Shnayder Y, Thomas SM. Radiation-induced fibrosis: mechanisms and implications for therapy. *J Cancer Res Clin Oncol.* 2015;141(11):1985–1994.
2. Podgorsak EB. Treatment machines for external beam radiotherapy. In: Podgorsak EB, ed. *Radiation Oncology Physics: A Handbook for Teachers and Students.* Vienna: International Atomic Energy Agency, 2005.

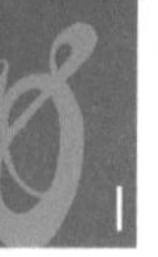

3. Finch W, Lee MS. Radiation-induced heart disease: long-term manifestations, diagnosis, and management. In: Herrmann J, ed. *Clinical Cardio-Oncology*. Philadelphia: Elsevier, 2016.
4. Lauk S, Rüth S, Trott KR. The effects of dose-fractionation on radiation-induced heart disease in rats. *Radiother Oncol*. 1987;8(4):363–367.
5. Hancock SL, Tucker MA, Hoppe RT. Factors affecting late mortality from heart disease after treatment of Hodgkin's disease. *JAMA*. 1993;270(16):1949–1955.
6. Carmel RJ, Kaplan HS. Mantle irradiation in Hodgkin's disease. An analysis of technique, tumor eradication, and complications. *Cancer*. 1976;37(6):2813–2825.
7. Gagliardi G, Constine LS, Moiseenko V, et al. Radiation dose-volume effects in the heart. *Int J Radiat Oncol Biol Phys*. 2010;76 (suppl 3):S77–S85.
8. Gillette SM, Gillette EL, Shida T, Boon J, Miller CW, Powers BE. Late adiation response of canine mediastinal tissues. *Radiother Oncol*. 1992;23(1):41–52.
9. Shaitelman SF, Schlembach PJ, Arzu I, et al. Acute and short-term toxic effects of conventionally fractionated vs hypofractionated whole-breast irradiation: a randomized clinical trial. *JAMA Oncol*. 2015;1(7):931–941.
10. Appelt AL, Vogelius IR, Bentzen SM. Modern hypofractionation schedules for tangential whole breast irradiation decrease the fraction size-corrected dose to the heart. *Clin Oncol*. 2013;25(3):147–152.
11. Whelan TJ, Pignol JP, Levine MN, et al. Long-term results of hypofractionated radiation therapy for breast cancer. *N Engl J Med*. 2010;362(6):513–520.
12. Marks LB, Yu X, Prosnitz RG, et al. The incidence and functional consequences of RT-associated cardiac perfusion defects. *Int J Radiat Oncol Biol Phys*. 2005;63(1):214–223.
13. Yeoh KW, Mikhaeel NG. Role of radiotherapy in modern treatment of Hodgkin's lymphoma. *Adv Hematol*. 2011;2011:258797.
14. D'Errico MP, Grimaldi L, Petruzzelli MF, et al. N-terminal pro-B-type natriuretic peptide plasma levels as a potential biomarker for cardiac damage after radiotherapy in patients with left-sided breast cancer. *Int J Radiat Oncol Biol Phys*. 2012;82(2):e239–e246.
15. Darby SC, McGale P, Taylor CW, Peto R. Long-term mortality from heart disease and lung cancer after radiotherapy for early breast cancer: prospective cohort study of about 300 000 women in US SEER cancer registries. *Lancet Oncol*. 2005;6(8):557–565.
16. Taylor CW, Nisbet A, McGale P, Darby SC. Cardiac exposures in breast cancer radiotherapy: 1950s–1990s. *Int J Radiat Oncol Biol Phys*. 2007;69(5):1484–1495.
17. Darby SC, Ewertz M, McGale P, et al. Risk of ischemic heart disease in women after radiotherapy for breast cancer. *N Engl J Med*. 2013;368(11):987–998.
18. Carr ZA, Land CE, Kleinerman RA, et al. Coronary heart disease after radiotherapy for peptic ulcer disease. *Int J Radiat Oncol Biol Phys*. 2005;61(3):842–850.
19. Topolnjak R, Borst GR, Nijkamp J, Sonke JJ. Image-guided radiotherapy for left-sided breast patients with cancer: geometrical uncertainty of the heart. *Int J Radiat Oncol Biol Phys*. 2012;82(4):e647–e655.
20. Rutqvist LE, Lax I, Fornander T, Johansson H. Cardiovascular mortality in a randomized trial of adjuvant radiation therapy versus surgery alone in primary breast cancer. *Int J Radiat Oncol Biol Phys*. 1992;22(5):887–896.
21. Højris I, Overgaard M, Christensen JJ, Overgaard J. Morbidity and mortality of ischaemic heart disease in highrisk breast-patients with cancer after adjuvant postmastectomy systemic treatment with or without radiotherapy: analysis of DBCG 82b and 82c randomised trials. Radiotherapy Committee of the Danish Brea. *Lancet*. 1999;354(9188):1425–1430.
22. Høst H, Brennhovd IO, Loeb M. Postoperative radiotherapy in breast cancer—long-term results from the Oslo study. *Int J Radiat Oncol Biol Phys*. 1986;12(5):727–732.
23. Giordano SH, Kuo YF, Freeman JL, Buchholz TA, Hortobagyi GN, Goodwin JS. Risk of cardiac death after adjuvant radiotherapy for breast cancer. *J Natl Cancer Inst*. 2005;97(6):419–424.
24. Hooning MJ, Botma A, Aleman BM, et al. Long-term risk of cardiovascular disease in 10-year survivors of breast cancer. *J Natl Cancer Inst*. 2007;99(5):365–375.
25. Verma V, Vicini F, Tendulkar RD, et al. Role of internal mammary node radiation as a part of modern breast cancer radiation therapy: a systematic review. *Int J Radiat Oncol Biol Phys*. 2016;95(2):617–631.
26. Whelan TJ, Olivotto IA, Parulekar WR, et al. Regional nodal irradiation in early-stage breast cancer. *N Engl J Med*. 2015;373(4):307–316.
27. Poortmans PM, Collette S, Kirkove C, et al. Internal mammary and medial supraclavicular irradiation in breast cancer. *N Engl J Med*. 2015;373(4):317–327.
28. Kleinerman RA. Cancer risks following diagnostic and therapeutic radiation exposure in children. *Pediatr Radiol*. 2006;36(suppl 2):121–125.
29. Adams MJ, Hardenbergh PH, Constine LS, Lipshultz SE. Radiation-associated cardiovascular disease. *Crit Rev Oncol Hematol*. 2003;45(1):55–75.
30. van Nimwegen FA, Schaapveld M, Janus CP, et al. Cardiovascular disease after Hodgkin lymphoma treatment: 40-year disease risk. *JAMA Intern Med*. 2015;175(6):1007–1017.
31. Hancock SL, Donaldson SS, Hoppe RT. Cardiac disease following treatment of Hodgkin's disease in children and adolescents. *J Clin Oncol*. 1993;11(7):1208–1215.
32. van der Pal HJ, van Dalen EC, Hauptmann M, et al. Cardiac function in 5-year survivors of childhood cancer: a long-term follow-up study. *Arch Intern Med*. 2010;170(14):1247–1255.
33. Harris EE, Correa C, Hwang WT, et al. Late cardiac mortality and morbidity in early-stage breast patients with cancer after breast-conservation treatment. *J Clin Oncol*. 2006;24(25):4100–4106.
34. Hooning MJ, Aleman BM, van Rosmalen AJ, Kuenen MA, Klijn JG, van Leeuwen F. Cause-specific mortality in long-term survivors of breast cancer: a 25-year follow-up study. *Int J Radiat Oncol Biol Phys*. 2006;64(4):1081–1091.
35. Demirci S, Nam J, Hubbs JL, Nguyen T, Marks LB. Radiation-induced cardiac toxicity after therapy for breast cancer: interaction between treatment era and follow-up duration. *Int J Radiat Oncol Biol Phys*. 2009;73(4):980–987.
36. Von Hoff DD, Layard MW, Basa P, et al. Risk factors for doxorubicin-induced congestive heart failure. *Ann Intern Med*. 1979;91(5):710–717.
37. Aleman BM, van den Belt-Dusebout AW, De Bruin ML, et al. Late cardiotoxicity after treatment for Hodgkin lymphoma. *Blood*. 2007;109(5):1878–1886.
38. Shapiro CL, Hardenbergh PH, Gelman R, et al. Cardiac effects of adjuvant doxorubicin and radiation therapy in breast patients with cancer. *J Clin Oncol*. 1998;16(11):3493–3501.
39. Reinders JG, Heijmen BJ, Olofsen-van Acht MJ, van Putten WL, Levendag PC. Ischemic heart disease after mantlefield irradiation for Hodgkin's disease in long-term follow-up. *Radiother Oncol*. 1999;51(1):35–42.
40. Glanzmann C, Kaufmann P, Jenni R, Hess OM, Huguenin P. Cardiac risk after mediastinal irradiation for Hodgkin's disease. *Radiother Oncol*. 1998;46(1):51–62.
41. Stewart JR, Fajardo LF. Radiation-induced heart disease: an update. *Prog Cardiovasc Dis*. 1984;27(3):173–194.
42. Heidenreich PA, Kapoor JR. Radiation induced heart disease: systemic disorders in heart disease. *Heart*. 2009;95:252–258.
43. Green DM, Gingell RL, Pearce J, Panahon AM, Ghoorah J. The effect of mediastinal irradiation on cardiac function of patients treated during childhood and adolescence for Hodgkin's disease. *J Clin Oncol*. 1987;5(2):239–245.
44. Brosius FC III, Waller BF, Roberts WC. Radiation heart disease. Analysis of 16 young (aged 15 to 33 years) necropsy patients who received over 3,500 rads to the heart. *Am J Med*. 1981;70(3):519–530.
45. Hughes-Davies L, Sacks D, Rescigno J, Howard S, Harris J. Serum cardiac troponin T levels during treatment of early-stage breast cancer. *J Clin Oncol*. 1995;13(10):2582–2584.
46. Kozak KR, Hong TS, Sluss PM, et al. Cardiac blood biomarkers in patients receiving thoracic (chemo)radiation. *Lung Cancer*. 2008;62(3):351–355.

47. Erven K, Florian A, Slagmolen P, et al. Subclinical cardiotoxicity detected by strain rate imaging up to 14 months after breast radiation therapy. *Int J Radiat Oncol Biol Phys*. 2013;85(5): 1172–1178.
48. Plana JC, Galderisi M, Barac A, et al. Expert consensus for multimodality imaging evaluation of adult patients during and after cancer therapy: a report from the American Society of Echocardiography and the European Association of Cardiovascular Imaging. *Eur Heart J Cardiovasc Imaging*. 2014;15(10):1063–1093.
49. Tuohinen SS, Skyttä T, Poutanen T, et al. Radiotherapy-induced global and regional differences in early-stage left-sided versus right-sided breast patients with cancer: speckle tracking echocardiography study. *Int J Cardiovasc Imaging*. 2017;33(4):463–472.
50. Erven K, Jurcut R, Weltens C, et al. Acute radiation effects on cardiac function detected by strain rate imaging in breast patients with cancer. *Int J Radiat Oncol Biol Phys*. 2011;79(5):1444–1451.

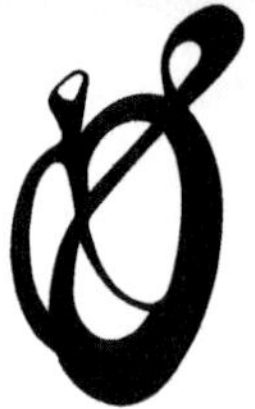

5 Bone Marrow Transplantation Risks

WILLIAM HOGAN

Autologous Stem Cell Transplantation

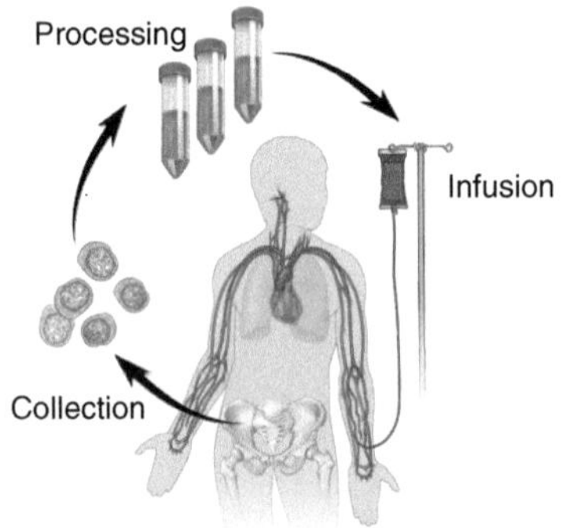

Indications:

- Multiple myeloma
- Non-Hodgkin lymphoma
- Hodgkin lymphoma
- Acute myeloid leukemia
- Neuroblastoma
- Germ cell tumors
- Autoimmune disorders

Early complications (<100 days):

CV
- Arrhythmias
- Pericarditis
- Heart failure/pulmonary edema
- Thromboembolic disease

Non-CV
- Myelosuppression
- Infection
- Bleeding
- Diffuse alveolar hemorrhage
- Mucositis
- Engraftment syndrome
- Graft failure
- Chemotherapy toxicity

Late complications (>100 days):

CV
- Atherosclerotic cardiovascular disease (ASVCD)
- Heart failure
- Thromboembolic disease

Non-CV
- Relapse
- Infection
- Gonadal failure
- Secondary malignancy

Allogeneic Stem Cell Transplantation

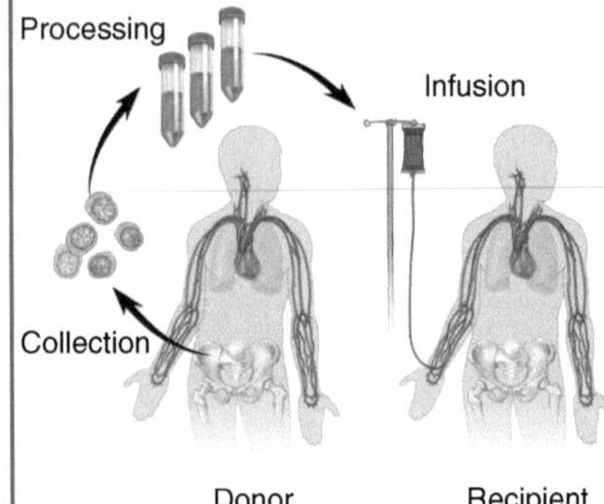

Indications:

- Acute myeloid leukemia
- Acute lymphoblastic leukemia
- Chronic myeloid leukemia
- Chronic lymphoblastic leukemia
- Myeloproliferative disorders
- Myelodysplastic syndromes
- Multiple myeloma
- Non-Hodgkin lymphoma
- Hodgkin lymphoma
- Aplastic anemia

Early complications (<100 days):

CV
- Arrhythmias
- Pericarditis
- Heart failure/pulmonary edema
- Thrombotic microangiopathy
- Sinusoidal obstruction (liver)
- Thromboembolic disease

Non-CV
- Myelosuppression
- Infection
- Bleeding
- Mucositis
- Interstitial pneumonia syndrome
- Acute graft versus host disease
- Graft failure
- Chemotherapy toxicity
- Radiation toxicity

Late complications (>100 days):

CV
- ASCVD
- Heart failure
- Thromboembolic disease

Non-CV
- Chronic graft versus host disease
- Infection
- Relapse
- Gonadal failure
- Cataracts
- Secondary malignancy
- Chemotherapy toxicity
- Radiation toxicity

CHAPTER OUTLINE

KEY POINTS

- Hematopoietic stem cell transplantation (HSCT) involves the infusion of multipotent hematopoietic stem cells, usually derived from the bone marrow, peripheral blood, or umbilical cord, and using cells from either the patient him-/herself (autologous), a donor (allogeneic), or an identical twin (syngeneic).
- A preparative or conditioning regimen is a critical element in HSCT for two reasons: to eradicate the underlying disease for which HSCT is given and to provide adequate immunosuppression to prevent rejection of the transplanted graft.
- Conditioning has traditionally been achieved by delivering maximally tolerated doses of combination chemotherapy with non-overlapping toxicities plus or minus total body radiation; non-myeloablative regimens have been developed as novel approaches to allow older patients or those with comorbid conditions to undergo HSCT.
- Following HSCT two periods are distinguished: early (within the first 100 days) and late (>100 days); arrhythmias, especially SVT and atrial fibrillation/flutter dominate cardiovascular complications early on, whereas cardiometabolic risk factors, atherosclerotic cardiovascular disease (ASCVD), and heart failure typically present later.
- The traditional comprehensive history and physical examination by an experienced clinician remains the most critical component of pretransplant screening, supplemented by the HCT comorbidity index.
- For long-term follow-up, optimal cardiovascular (CV) risk factor control and screening for evolving cardiovascular disease (CVD) is crucial, especially in patients identified as high risk for CVD.

HEMATOPOIETIC STEM CELL TRANSPLANTATION AND CONDITIONING REGIMENS

In the past referred to as bone marrow transplantation (BMT) but now termed hematopoietic (stem) cell transplantation (H(S)CT) because of the utilization of stem cell resources other than the bone marrow, HSCT constitutes a life-saving or life prolonging intervention for many patients with hematologic malignancies and occasionally for patients with benign hematologic and non-hematologic disorders. The indications for HSCT have been rapidly evolving; innovations in HSCT, in combination with new targeted therapies for malignancies, allow older and more medically tenuous patients to be considered for transplantation. These developments have had a significant impact on pretransplant screening and posttransplant monitoring for cardiovascular diseases (CVD) in HSCT recipients.

Two types of HSCT can be distinguished: autologous and allogeneic. Autologous HSCT entails the use of the patient's own stem cells for reconstitution of the bone marrow. These cells, which are collected in advance, allow for higher dose chemotherapy to be given, which is frequently employed for diseases such as recurrent non-Hodgkin lymphoma, Hodgkin lymphoma, and multiple myeloma. Allogeneic HSCT entails the use of stem cells from a donor to reconstitute the bone marrow. Early studies focused on the use of escalating doses of chemo- and radiation therapy to achieve the dual goals of more effective eradication of chemoresistant malignant cells and preventing immunologic graft rejection by paralyzing the recipient immune system. Chemotherapy doses can be escalated by about three-fold when healthy stem cells from a donor are used after chemotherapy exposure to repopulate the marrow. This strategy is effective because hematopoietic cells are much more sensitive to lethal toxicity compared with other organs, permitting escalation to a dose that is sublethal to other organs, especially the lungs, liver, kidneys, and heart. To permit such high doses of chemotherapy and radiation, patients who were considered appropriate candidates were highly selected to be young (typically <35 years) with excellent organ function.

Subsequent experience clearly indicated that high-dose chemoradiation was only partially responsible for eradication of malignant clone and that immunologic targeting by the donor's immune system contributed significantly. In fact, this graft-versus-tumor effect was relatively more important in certain diseases, such as chronic lymphocytic leukemia, and relatively less so in other diseases, such as multiple myeloma (MM). It was also associated with potentially severe or life-threatening toxicity when the donor immune system targeted normal recipient tissues and organs resulting in graft-versus-host disease (GVHD) with potentially lethal injury to organs, such as the colon. This can result in bacterial translocation and sepsis, and in the context of immunologic dysregulation a high mortality rate.

Certain diseases that rely predominantly on chemotherapy dose escalation, such as dysproteinemic disorders and lymphomas, typically have much better outcomes when the recipient's own stem cells are collected in advance of the high-dose conditioning regimen and reinfused afterward (autologous transplantation). This strategy works well when the stem cells are unaffected and the likelihood of transmitting malignant cells with the autologous stem cells is low. The toxicity of this approach is much lower because it avoids immunosuppressive drugs after the stem cell infusion and typically avoids the risk of GVHD. However, for other diseases, such as myeloid disorders, acute leukemias, and bone marrow failure syndromes, a donor-derived (allogeneic) graft is essential for disease control and bone marrow reconstitution, this approach is associated with much greater risk.

Increasing recognition that graft-versus-tumor activity could replace some of the benefit of high-dose chemoradiation for malignant cell eradication led to the possibility of less-intense chemotherapy regimens (Table 5.1 and Fig. 5.1). Progress was accelerated with the development of the purine analogs (e.g., fludarabine and cladribine), which prevent graft rejection with less toxicity. These reduced-intensity or non-myeloablative

TABLE 5.1 Preconditioning Regimens for Hematopoietic Cell Transplantation

REGIMEN	COMPONENTS	CARDIOVASCULAR TOXICITIES
Myeloablative Regimens		
Attempts to eliminate all hematopoietic cells in the bone marrow, resulting in profound pancytopenia within 1–3 weeks, which is prolonged, usually irreversible, and often fatal, unless rescued by infusion of hematopoietic stem cells.		
BEAM	BCNU (carmustine, 300 mg/m^2) over 1 day Etoposide (400–800 mg/m^2) over 4 days cytosine Arabinoside (800 mg/m^2) over 4 days, and Melphalan (140 mg/m^2) over 1 day (most common regimen for patients with non-Hodgkin or Hodgkin lymphoma)	Carmustine: Chest pain, arterial occlusive disease, tachycardia Etoposide: Hypotension (with rapid infusion) cytosine Arabinoside: Chest pain, pericarditis Melphalan: Atrial fibrillation, peripheral edema
Cy/TBI TBI/Cy	The Cy/TBI regimen combines cyclophosphamide 120 mg/kg total dose over 2 days Total body irradiation (TBI, 12–13.2 Gy) over 3 days TBI is given first, followed by cyclophosphamide. (may include etoposide (60 mg/kg) instead of cyclophosphamide or in addition to cyclophosphamide for patients with advanced disease not in remission)	Cyclophosphamide: Arrhythmias Hemorrhagic myocarditis Pericarditis, pericardial effusion, even tamponade Myocardial infarction Arterial and venous thrombosis Radiation-induced heart and vascular disease
Bu4/Cy	Busulfan 12.8 mg/kg total dose over 4 days Cyclophosphamide 120 mg/kg over 2 days	Busulfan: Arrhythmia, including atrial fibrillation, premature contractions, (complete) atrioventricular block, Peripheral edema Hypertension and hypotension Thrombosis Chest pain Cardiomyopathy (endocardial fibrosis)

TABLE 5.1 **Preconditioning Regimens for Hematopoietic Cell Transplantation—cont'd**

REGIMEN	COMPONENTS	CARDIOVASCULAR TOXICITIES
Flu/Bu4	Fludarabine 120–180 mg/m^2 Busulfan 12.8 mg/kg total dose, each over 4 days	Fludarabine: Edema Arrhythmia, esp. supraventricular tachycardia Heart failure Angina pectoris Myocardial infarction Cerebrovascular accident Transient ischemic attacks (≤1%) Deep vein thrombosis Phlebitis Aneurysm
High dose melphalan	Melphalan (200 mg/m^2) (common prior to autologous HCT for multiple myeloma; lower dose to be used patient >70 years, with renal dysfunction, or multiple comorbidities.)	See above
Reduced Intensity Regimens		
Causes cytopenia, which may be prolonged and can result in significant morbidity and mortality, thus requiring hematopoietic stem cell support.		
Flu/Mel	Fludarabine (125–150 mg/m^2 total dose) over 5 days Melphalan (140 mg/m^2) administered over 2 days	See above
Flu/Bu2 and Flu/Bu3	Fludarabine (150–160 mg/m^2 total dose) over 4–5 days Busulfan (8–10 mg/kg) over 2–3 days	See above
Flu/Cy	Fludarabine (150–180 mg/m^2 total dose) over 5–6 days Cyclophosphamide (120–140 mg/kg) administered over 2 days	See above
Flu/Bu3/TT	Fludarabine 150 mg/m^2 total dose over 3 days Busulfan (8 mg/kg) over 3 days Thiotepa (5–10 mg/m^2) over 1–2 days	See above
Nonmyeloablative Regimens		
Causes minimal cytopenia (but significant lymphopenia), not requiring stem cell support; however, usually becomes myeloablative because the engrafting donor T cells will eventually eliminate host hematopoietic cells, allowing the establishment of donor hematopoiesis.		
Flu/TBI	Fludarabine 90 mg/m^2 total dose over 3 days Low dose total body irradiation (TBI, 2 Gy) on the day of graft infusion	See above
TLI/ATG	Total lymphoid irradiation (TLI, 8–12 cGy) over 11 days Antithymocyte globulin (ATG; 1.25 mg/kg) over 5 days	ATG: Hypertension and hypotension Peripheral edema Tachycardia Chest pain

regimens permitted older patients (into the 7th and 8th decade of life) and more fragile patients to be considered for allogeneic transplantation and thereby the advantage of potentially curative therapy. As a result, the comorbidity and risk spectrum for HCT has increased greatly in the current era.

PRETRANSPLANT SCREENING

From a cardiac perspective the goals of the pretransplant evaluation are to determine whether:

1. The patient has modifiable cardiovascular risk factors that can be improved prior to proceeding, and

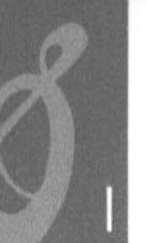

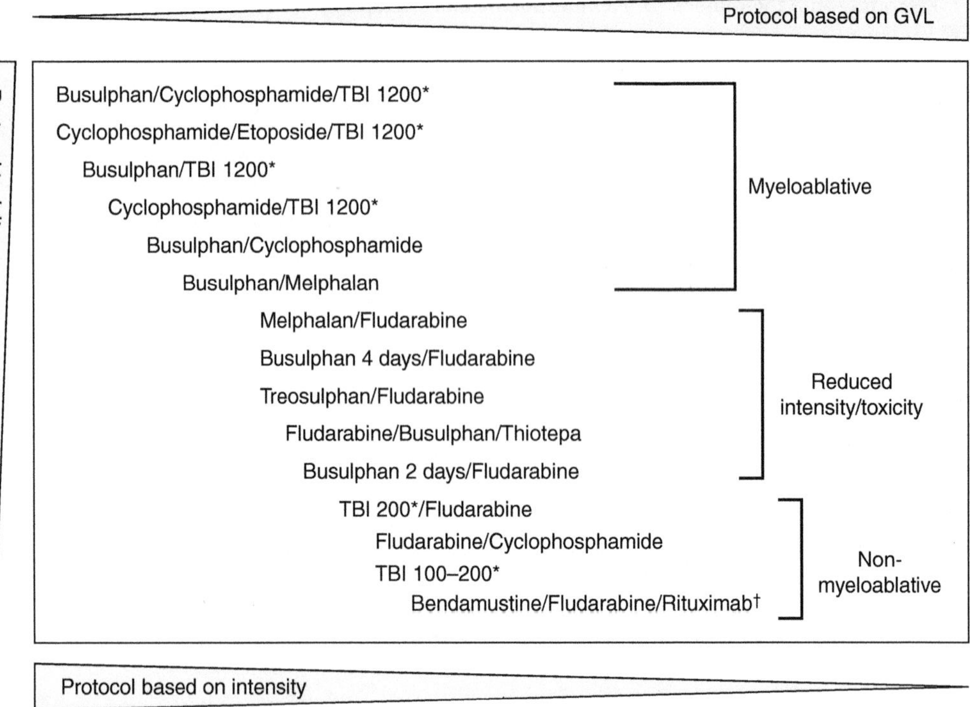

FIG. 5.1 Illustration of the three main conditioning approaches. The more intense (myeloablative) the protocol, the more toxic it is and typically less reliant on early graft-versus-leukemia (GVL) effect for disease control. Reduced-intensity regimens are less toxic and rely more on an immunotherapeutic GVL effect to prevent relapse. Conditioning may include also the use of antithymocyte globulin in matched unrelated donor (MUD) hematopoietic stem cell transplantation (HSCT). TBI, total body irradiation. *The number represents the radiation dose in rads. †New conditioning in phase II trial for chronic lymphocytic leukemia patients. (From Henig I, Zuckerman T. Hematopoietic stem cell transplantation—50 years of evolution and future perspectives. *Rambam Maimonides Med J.* 2014;5 (4):e0028. doi:10.5041/RMMJ.10162.)

2. If the patient will have an acceptable risk-to-benefit ratio (after appropriate intervention), factoring into the equation the relevant comorbid conditions and the potential benefit of transplant in controlling the underlying hematologic disorder.

The HCT comorbidity index (HCT-CI)[1] provides an objective way to determine the impact of multiorgan comorbidity prior to transplant. Symptomatic valvular disease, reduced left ventricular zejection fraction, or a history of arrhythmia all contribute points to the calculation of the HCT-CI, predicting nonrelapse mortality. A score greater than 4, (indicative of multiple comorbid conditions, such as cardiac, pulmonary, liver, renal, or psychiatric dysfunction, or a history of nonhematologic malignancy) predicts a non-relapse mortality of 40% or greater. With the increasing age of potential recipients, comorbid conditions, such as hypertension, coronary artery disease, atrial fibrillation, and diabetes, are much more common and must be considered in conjunction with the traditional cardiac challenges of prior anthracycline exposure, mediastinal radiation, and the effects of hematologic disease-related complications, such as amyloid deposition, leukemic infiltration of the cardiovascular system, or pericarditis. Further complicating the situation is the explosion of new antimicrobials and molecularly targeted therapies, which bring new concerns ranging from direct cardiac toxicities to pharmacologic interactions that predispose to potentially lethal arrhythmias. This has led to a refined approach with an initial risk assessment of patients prior to transplant, altered monitoring of patients during the peritransplant period, and new considerations for surveillance of long-term survivors.

Despite the availability of an extensive array of sophisticated tools to assess cardiac function, the most critical component of pretransplant screening remains the traditional comprehensive history and physical examination by an experienced clinician. Relevant cardiovascular risk factors to assess include age, smoking, hypertension, diabetes, family history of coronary artery disease, and obesity. In addition, knowledge of the underlying hematologic disorder, the specific treatment administered, the presence of unrelated cardiovascular risks, and the potential cardiotoxicity of the proposed conditioning and GVHD prophylaxis regimen are important. A retrospective study from Loyola, for instance, suggested that age (>60 years), graft source, and a history of atrial fibrillation were predictive of a very high cardiac risk with HCT.[2] For patients with cardiac amyloidosis, significant hypotension, elevated troponin, and multiorgan involvement have been strongly associated with increased peritransplant mortality. Pretransplant screening with serum troponin in addition to echocardiography performed by an experienced echocardiographer looking for classic signs of advanced cardiac amyloidosis with intraventricular hypertrophy and left ventricular strain can be very helpful in determining whether HSCT is likely to provide durable benefit or to be associated with excessive risk. Appropriate patient selection and subsequent close attention to fluid and arrhythmia management have been instrumental in reducing the peritransplant mortality for patients with primary systemic amyloidosis which ultimately led the Centers for Medicare & Medicaid Services to determine that autologous transplant was an appropriate treatment option for patients with fewer than three organs involved and an ejection fraction of at least 45%. Whereas assessment of pretransplant troponin and left ventricular strain are invaluable tools for risk stratification of patients with cardiac amyloidosis, these components of evaluation have a less proven role for other pretransplant scenarios.

The potential for cardiac decompensation related to neutropenic fever, bacteremia, and sepsis needs to be considered during the pretransplant evaluation. The use of contemporary antifungals, such as posaconazole and voriconazole, has had a major impact on the risk of death from fungal infection during HSCT. However, these agents have a significant impact on the metabolism of many drugs such as calcineurin inhibitors. These interactions can lead to renal toxicity, accelerated hypertension, and subsequent cardiovascular events and need to be preempted with appropriate dose modifications. The interaction of the azole antifungal agents with sirolimus is particularly potent and is frequently contraindicated. Additionally, drug interactions with quinolones, especially when combined with tyrosine kinase inhibitors or novel targeted agents such as FLT3 (fms like tyrosine kinase 3) inhibitors, can lead to clinically relevant QTc prolongation and the risk for life-threatening arrhythmia, especially in the context of electrolyte derangement. Electrolyte abnormalities, including hypokalemia/hyperkalemia and hypomagnesemia, are a ubiquitous finding in patients on therapeutic doses of calcineurin inhibitors. These risks also need to be proactively anticipated and managed as part of the pretransplant planning process when determining eligibility and risk management strategies. Collaboration between the transplant physician and cardio-oncology specialist can be very valuable in assessing such complex patients and averting predictable adverse events.

Finally, the extent of anthracycline exposure can be a significant factor in determining transplant eligibility, including whether a patient is a potential candidate for a myeloablative conditioning regimen, because these patients may be more vulnerable to cardiotoxicity even with relatively satisfactory pretransplant testing. Cardiac rhythm should be assessed, typically with an electrocardiogram (ECG), and systolic function should be assessed typically by echocardiography, cardiac magnetic resonance imaging, or multiple gated acquisition scan. For patients with documented anthracycline-induced cardiomyopathy, beta blockade, and angiotensin-converting enzyme inhibition is to be initiated.

PERITRANSPLANT MANAGEMENT

For patients who have been cleared for transplant, close monitoring during the conditioning regimen and subsequent hematopoietic nadir is critical because this is a high-risk period. The specific considerations are highly context dependent. For all patients the high-dose conditioning regimen is expected to result in profound pancytopenia; however, the implications of this may vary, depending on the specific regimen. For instance, myeloablative regimens are more likely to cause injury to the gastrointestinal tract with a greater risk of gram-negative bacterial translocation and subsequent sepsis. Certain populations, such as

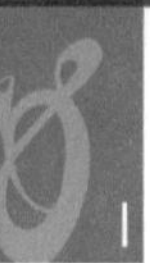

those with gastrointestinal amyloidosis, are particularly susceptible to gastrointestinal injury resulting in bleeding and sepsis. This can be particularly devastating in the patient with advanced cardiac amyloidosis with a stiff, noncompliant heart and dramatically impaired ability to compensate for the demands of bleeding or sepsis.

Typical antimicrobial treatment during the anticipated nadir includes fluoroquinolone antibacterial and azole antifungal prophylaxis. The introduction of these antimicrobial strategies has dramatically reduced mortality from infection. However, these drugs can contribute to lethal arrhythmias by significantly prolonging the QTc. In the allogeneic setting the frequent presence of electrolyte derangement, especially hypomagnesemia as a result of renal tubular magnesium loss caused by calcineurin inhibitors enhances the risk as does any concomitantly used QTc prolonging drug or genetic predisposition. An ECG 2 to 5 days after the introduction of these agents or any new drug anticipated to prolong the QTc should be obtained to ensure that the QTc is maintained at an acceptable level, typically < 500 msec.

The recent expansion of the use of haploidentical (half matched) transplantation has had a major impact on the availability of acceptable donors for many patients who previously did not have a well-matched family member or unrelated volunteer donor. Lack of acceptable donor availability is a particular challenge for ethnic minorities as a result of both the greater HLA antigen diversity of the population and the relative lack of diversity of donors in the "Be the Match" registry. Haploidentical transplantation has allowed a half-matched sibling, parent, or child (or occasionally a second-degree relative) to be considered as a donor. This innovation became mainstream only with the development of safer and more effective GVHD prophylaxis regimens that include posttransplant cyclophosphamide.

Cyclophosphamide is a nitrogen mustard alkylating agent with antineoplastic and immunosuppressive properties, which can have an impact on both, cell-mediated and humoral immunity. This drug plays a critical role in BMT as both, an effective component of many conditioning regimens and more recently as an effective posttransplant GVHD prophylactic agent for haploidentical transplantation, with an emerging role even for matched donors. Cyclophosphamide is a prodrug that requires activation in the liver, therefore drug-drug interactions at the level of the hepatic microsome cytochrome p450 level may be pertinent.[3] Cyclophosphamide has well-described cardiotoxicity. Determining which patients are at highest risk is challenging, although anecdotal evidence suggests that young women may be particularly vulnerable. Interestingly, previous studies have suggested that a reduced ejection fraction of < 50% or previous modest anthracycline exposure does not necessarily confer an elevated risk of cyclophosphamide-induced cardiac toxicity. This might fit with the possibility that this complication is more pharmacogenomically driven. Clinically a high degree of suspicion is required to diagnose cyclophosphamide-induced cardiomyopathy rapidly. Onset typically is within 2 days of exposure, but may occur up to 7 to 10 days afterward. Treatment is supportive, based on the presentation, which can include arrhythmias, hypotension, and heart failure. Although there are anecdotal reports of a possible benefit with theophylline and ascorbic acid, no consistent evidence supports such an approach. For patients with advanced heart failure in cardiogenic shock, management in the intensive care unit with circulatory support and use of extracorporeal membrane oxygenation and mechanical circulatory support may provide a window of opportunity to allow for recovery.

EARLY POSTTRANSPLANT MANAGEMENT (UNTIL DAY 100)

Life-threatening cardiac events are relatively common after allogeneic transplant; they have been reported in 5% to 12.5% of patients. This risk is much higher in patients over the age of 60 or those over the age of 40 with peripheral vascular disease or diabetes who were reported to have a risk of post-HCT cardiac events of up to 33%. Not surprisingly, there is an increased mortality risk at day 100 and at 1 year for patients who experience cardiovascular events after transplant. Management of cardiac complications is frequently challenged by the unique needs of this patient population. In general, however, no good evidence appears to suggest that management of cardiac complications occurring in the immediate posttransplant interval should vary significantly from standard management in keeping with the American Heart Association and American College of Cardiology guidelines. The main additional considerations are related to the frequent concomitant use of drugs, which may have significant potential for drug-drug interactions. The presence of liver function test abnormalities results in challenges with the use of statins. Furthermore, the frequent use of antineoplastic or supportive care medications generates the potential for significant and potentially life-threatening drug interactions. A particular challenge can be an acute coronary event occurring in the context of severe thrombocytopenia. This complicates the decision-making process regarding medical management versus coronary intervention with stenting. The likely duration of severe thrombocytopenia and the potential serious bleeding risk associated with potent antiplatelet therapy are important considerations in making the choice regarding coronary intervention using a bare metal stent, drug-eluting stent, or alternatively choosing a noninterventional approach with medical therapy. These situations are typically most successfully managed with multidisciplinary input from experienced transplant and cardiology physicians working in real time. Given the paucity of randomized clinical trial data in this subset of patients, many management recommendations are extrapolated from noncancer populations. Expertise in cardio-oncology is invaluable here.

LATE POSTTRANSPLANT MANAGEMENT (AFTER DAY 100)

Late cardiac complications are well described in patients with hematologic malignancies and after both autologous and allogeneic HSCT. For patients cured of their underlying disease or hematologic malignancy the 15-year cumulative incidence of severe or life-threatening chronic health conditions exceeds 40% and results in premature mortality with CVD as a primary cause[4] (Fig. 5.2). The insidious onset of late complications mandates lifelong monitoring and pristine control of CV risk factors. Indeed, the impact of CV risk factors is

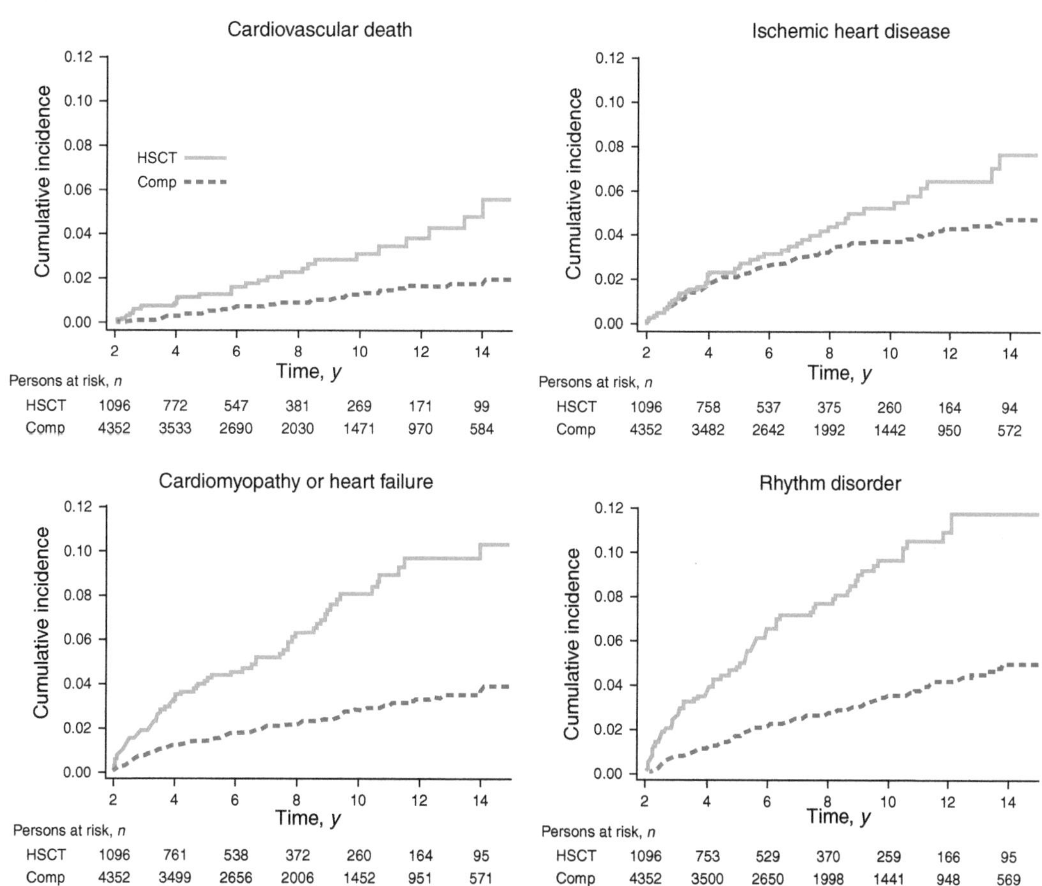

FIG. 5.2 Cumulative incidences of cardiovascular outcomes (including cardiovascular mortality, ischemic heart disease, cardiomyopathy, and arrhythmias) in 1096 hematopoietic stem cell transplant (HSCT) recipients, matched to a comparison group (comp) of 4352 individuals from the general population (log-rank <0.01 for all outcomes). (From *Ann Intern Med*. 2011;155(1):21–32. doi:10.7326/0003-4819-155-1-201107050-00004.)

profound, especially in those with additional cardiotoxic therapy exposure (Fig. 5.3). Prediction models have been developed that aid with risk prediction (Fig. 5.4).

In this context it is very relevant that up to 30% of those who survive cancer smoke, particularly those of younger age. This can be particularly devastating for recipients of allogeneic transplant given the risk of secondary cancers, advanced lung injury in the context of GVHD and accelerated CVD. Effective nicotine cessation efforts are critical, but often challenging to achieve. The use of alternatives to smoking, such as vaping, is more prevalent in younger populations and has not yet been systematically studied in regards to the risk of cardiotoxicity in this group. The additional challenges brought by exposure to medications, such as corticosteroids, calcineurin inhibitors, sirolimus, and tyrosine kinase inhibitors, substantially increase the cardiovascular risk for this population. Standard recommendations regarding diet, exercise, and weight should be included as part of the recommended counseling. This includes at least 150 minutes of moderate exercise per week regardless of age or treatment during transplant; however, this clearly needs to be adjusted to the functional status of the recipient. In apparently healthy survivors, however, this is an appropriate recommendation.

In addition to smoking, metabolic syndrome is extremely common; the 10-year cumulative incidence of diabetes alone exceeds 18%. A fasting plasma glucose screen has been recommended at least every 3 years after the age of 45 or earlier if there is hypertension (>135/80 mm Hg). The risk of metabolic syndrome is even greater in children and therefore the Children's Oncology Group recommends a fasting glucose every 2 years after transplant, particularly if radiation was included as part of the preparative regimen.

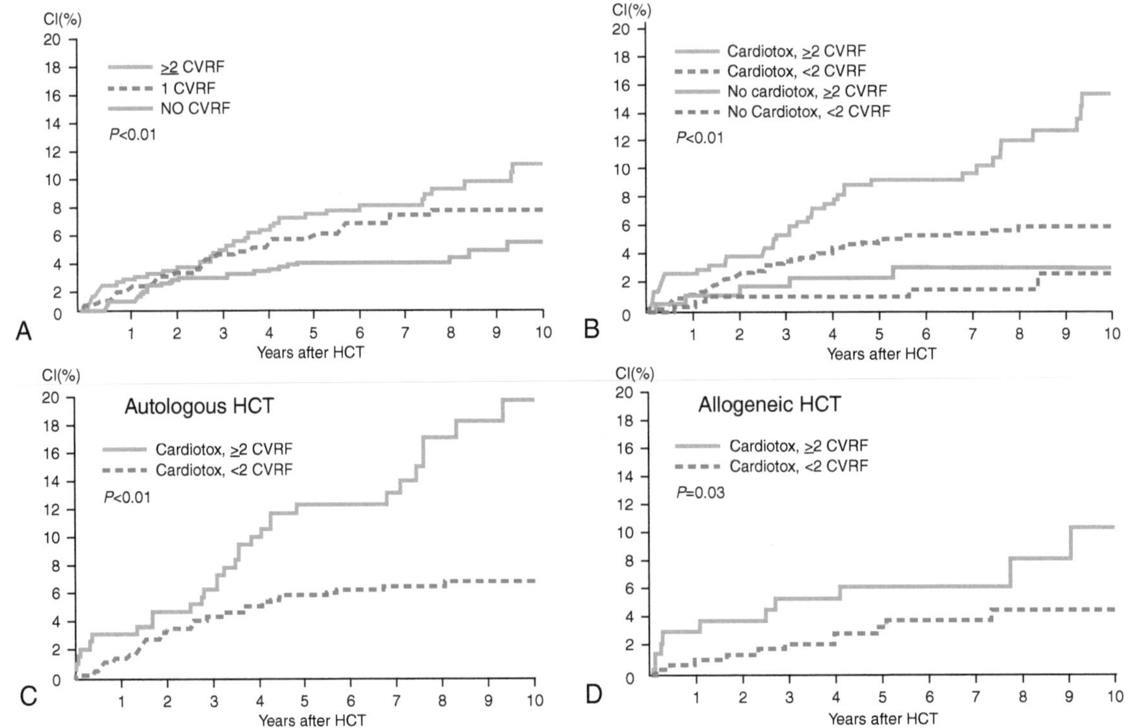

FIG. 5.3 Cumulative incidence of cardiovascular events after hematopoietic cell transplantation (HCT) by number of cardiovascular risk factors (CVRFs; **A**), by number of CVRFs and pre-HCT cardiotoxic exposure (**B**), by autologous HCT survivors with pre-HCT cardiotoxic exposure (**C**), and by allogeneic HCT survivors with pre-HCT cardiotoxic exposure (**D**). Cardiotoxic exposure refers to anthracycline or chest radiation. (From Armenian SH, Sun CL, Vase T, et al. Cardiovascular risk factors in hematopoietic cell transplantation survivors: role in development of subsequent cardiovascular disease. *Blood*. 2012;120(23):4505– 4512. doi:10.1182/blood-2012-06-437178. Epub 2012 Oct 3. PubMed PMID: 23034279; PubMed Central PMCID: PMC3512230.)

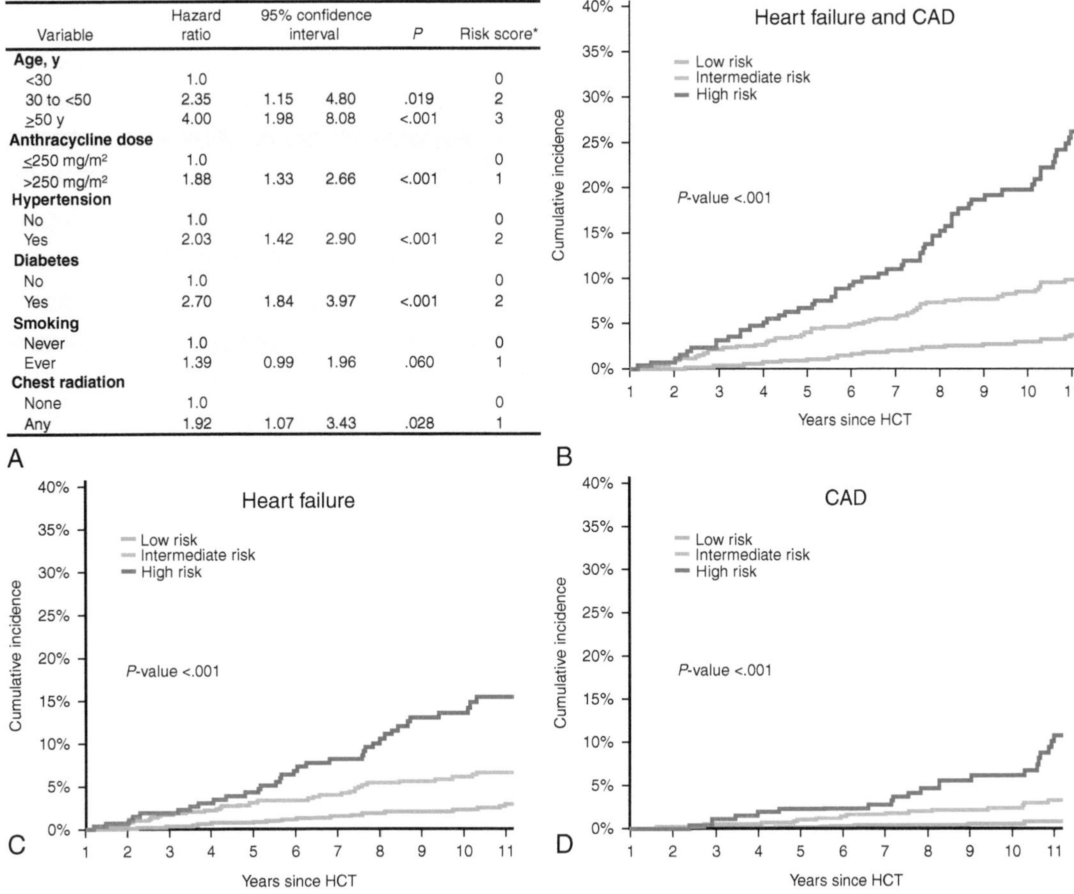

Variable	Hazard ratio	95% confidence interval		*P*	Risk score*
Age, y					
<30	1.0				0
30 to <50	2.35	1.15	4.80	.019	2
≥50 y	4.00	1.98	8.08	<.001	3
Anthracycline dose					
≤250 mg/m²	1.0				0
>250 mg/m²	1.88	1.33	2.66	<.001	1
Hypertension					
No	1.0				0
Yes	2.03	1.42	2.90	<.001	2
Diabetes					
No	1.0				0
Yes	2.70	1.84	3.97	<.001	2
Smoking					
Never	1.0				0
Ever	1.39	0.99	1.96	.060	1
Chest radiation					
None	1.0				0
Any	1.92	1.07	3.43	.028	1

FIG. 5.4 Ten-year cumulative incidence of cardiovascular disease by integer risk score (**A**) and by risk groups (**B**). Cumulative incidence of heart failure (**C**) and coronary artery disease (**D**) by risk groups. Curves start at index date (1 year from hematopoietic cell transplantation). (From Armenian SH, et al. *Blood Adv.* 2018;2:1756–1764.)

Hyperlipidemia is noted in nearly half or more transplant survivors and is compounded by the fact that many survivors have multiple cardiac risk factors. For patients without other cardiovascular risk factors fasting lipids should be checked every 5 years beginning at age 35 for men and at age 45 for women. For those with other cardiovascular risk factors, screening is recommended to begin at age 20 for adult recipients and beginning 2 years after transplant for children, particularly those who have had exposure to radiation.

The role of electrocardiogram screening is less standardized, but it could potentially be useful in those with known cardiovascular disease, significant risk factors, or at risk of QTc prolongation. Cardiac imaging is not generally recommended for asymptomatic adults without cardiac risk factors posttransplant. In individuals with significant risk factors, including traditional cardiac risk factors, mediastinal radiation, or cardiac amyloidosis, echocardiography or stress echocardiography may have a role. There are specific recommendations for pediatric transplant survivors made by the Children's Oncology Group with regard to imaging. Some evidence suggests that aggressive screening to monitor for left ventricular dysfunction with subsequent early pharmacologic intervention may be cost effective. The exact interval has not been well defined. Similarly, routine use of screening for peripheral arterial disease is not generally recommended, but it may have a role for specific populations, including those treated with radiation to the neck or pediatric populations. Those treated with nilotinib or ponatinib, tyrosine kinase inhibitors well known to result in a greater risk of serious coronary artery or peripheral vascular disease, may also be considered for screening in the absence of robust data at this time.

Screening recommendations for survivors of BMT have been developed jointly by the European Group for Blood and Marrow Transplantation (EBMT) and the American Society of Blood and Marrow Transplant (ASBMT)/Center for International Blood and Marrow Transplantation (CIBMTR).[5] In addition, the Children's Oncology Group and the CIBMTR have developed guidelines for the treatment of cardiovascular risk factors in pediatric survivors of transplant.[6,7] Of note, the guidelines differ from those recommended for the general population and are generally consensus based rather than evidence based, given that the long latency and relatively small numbers pose significant challenges to performing well-designed, randomized clinical trials in this context. Survivorship programs should include these recommendations and an overview for the cardio-oncologist is provided in Tables 5.2 to 5.4.

In survivors of autologous bone marrow transplant a cumulative anthracycline dose of greater

TABLE 5.2 Multisociety Recommendations for Long-Term Survivors After Hematopoietic Cell Transplantation

LATE COMPLICATIONS	GENERAL RISK FACTORS	MONITORING TESTS	MONITORING TESTS AND PREVENTIVE
• Cardiomyopathy • Congestive heart failure • Arrhythmias • Valvular anomaly • Coronary artery disease • Cerebrovascular disease • Peripheral arterial disease	• Anthracycline exposure • TBI/radiation exposure to neck or chest • Older age at HCT • Allogeneic HCT • Cardiovascular risk factors before/after HCT • Chronic kidney disease • Metabolic syndrome	• Cumulative dose of anthracyclines • Echocardiogram with ventricular function, ECG in patients at risk and in symptomatic patients • Fasting lipid profile (including HDL-C, LDL-C, and triglycerides) • Fasting blood sugar	• Routine clinical assessment of cardiovascular risk factors as per general health maintenance at 1 year and at least yearly thereafter • Education and counseling on "heart" healthy lifestyle (regular exercise, healthy weight, no smoking, dietary counseling) • Early treatment of cardiovascular risk factors, such as diabetes, hypertension and dyslipidemia • Administration of antibiotics for endocarditis prophylaxis according to American Heart Association guidelines

ECG, Electrocardiogram; [*HCT*, hematopoietic cell transplantation; *HDL*, high-density lipoprotein; *LDL*, low-density lipoprotein; *TBI*, total body irradiation.
From Majhail et al. *Bone Marrow Transplant*. 2012;47(3):337–341.

TABLE 5.3 Screening Guidelines for Metabolic Syndrome and Cardiovascular Risk Factors for Adult and Pediatric Patients Among the General Population and HCT Survivors

	ADULT LONG-TERM HCT SURVIVORS (MAJHAIL, ET AL. 2012)	PEDIATRIC LONG-TERM HCT SURVIVORS (PULSIPHER. ET AL. 2012)	CIBMTR/EBMT MetS COLLABORATION (DE FILIPP, ET AL. 2017)
Weight, Height, BMI	No specific recommendations	Weight, height, and BMI assessment yearly	Weight, height, and BMI assessment at every clinic visit (at least yearly) Waist circumference measurement yearly Consider DXA to assess sarcopenia
Dyslipidemia	Lipid profile assessment every 5 years in males aged ≥35 years and females aged ≥45 years. Screening should start at age 20 for anyone at increased risk (smokers, DM, HTN, BMI ≥30 kg/m^2, family history of heart disease before age 50 for male relatives or before age 60 for female relatives).	Lipid profile at least every 5 years; if abnormal, screen annually.	For all allo-HCT recipients, initial lipid profile 3 months after HCT. For high-risk patients with ongoing risk factors (including those on sirolimus, calcineurin inhibitors, corticosteroids), repeat evaluation every 3–6 months. For standard-risk patients, lipid profile assessment every 5 years in males aged ≥35 years and females aged ≥45 years. The interval for screening should be shorter for people who have lipid levels close to those warranting therapy.

TABLE 5.3 Screening Guidelines for Metabolic Syndrome and Cardiovascular Risk Factors for Adult and Pediatric Patients Among the General Population and HCT Survivors—cont'd

	ADULT LONG-TERM HCT SURVIVORS (MAJHAIL, ET AL. 2012)	PEDIATRIC LONG-TERM HCT SURVIVORS (PULSIPHER. ET AL. 2012)	CIBMTR/EBMT MetS COLLABORATION (DE FILIPP, ET AL. 2017)
Blood Pressure	Blood pressure assessment at least every 2 years	Blood pressure assessment at each visit and at least annually	Blood pressure assessment at every clinic visit (at least yearly)
Hyperglycemia	Screening for type 2 DM every 3 years in adults aged ≥45 years or in those with sustained higher blood pressure (>135/80 mm Hg).	Fasting glucose at least every 5 years; if abnormal, screen annually.	For high-risk patients with ongoing risk factors (including those on systemic corticosteroids), screen for abnormal blood glucose (HbA1C or fasting plasma glucose) 3 months after HCT with repeat evaluation every 3–6 months. Consider oral glucose tolerance test to evaluate abnormal screening results. For standard-risk adult patients, screening for abnormal blood glucose every 3 years in adults aged ≥45 years or in those with sustained higher blood pressure (>135/80 mm Hg). For standard-risk pediatric patients, fasting glucose at least every 5 years; if abnormal, screen annually.
			Risk factors to consider when screening for components of metabolic syndrome in transplant recipients: Personal history Family history Type of transplant (allogeneic or autologous) TBI as part of pretransplant conditioning Development of acute or chronic GVHD Ongoing therapy with corticosteroids Ongoing therapy with calcineurin inhibitors Ongoing therapy with sirolimus Presence of additional metabolic syndrome components

BMI, Body mass index; *CIBMTR*, Center for International Blood and Marrow Transplant Research; *DM*, diabetes mellitus; *DXA*, dual X-ray absorptiometry; *EBMT*, European Group for Blood and Marrow Transplantation; *GVHD*, graft-versus-host disease; *HbA1C*, hemoglobin A1C; *HCT*, hematopoietic cell transplantation; HTN, hypertension; TBI, total body irradiation.

From De Filipp Z, et al. *Bone Marrow Transplant*. 2017;52(2):173–182; Majhail NS, et al. *Biol Blood Marrow Transplant*. 2012;18(3):348–371; Pulsipher MA, et al. *Biol Blood Marrow Transplant*. 2012;18(3):334-347.

than 250 mg/m^2 is associated with a 10-fold increased risk of congestive heart failure. The additional impact of hypertension is more than additive, increasing the risk of congestive heart failure more than 35-fold.[8] The risk of congestive heart failure is also similarly increased with the combination of anthracycline exposure and diabetes (27-fold increased risk),[9] and total body radiation increases the risk for dyslipidemia and diabetes.[10] As in the general population, data indicate that a healthier lifestyle can attenuate the risk of CVD in patients after transplant, particularly with regard to the risk of hypertension, diabetes, and dyslipidemia. It is possible, however, that the pathophysiology of CVD in HCT recipients differs significantly from that in the general population. For this reason it may not be possible to extrapolate directly recommendations from those of the general population. In the absence of well-designed studies this nevertheless may be a reasonable approach.

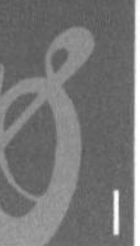

TABLE 5.4 Preventive Practice Recommendations for Metabolic Syndrome and Cardiovascular Risk Factors for Adult and Pediatric Patients Among the General Population and HCT Survivors

	ADULT LONG-TERM HCT SURVIVORS (MAJHAIL, ET AL. 2012)	CIBMTR/EBMT MetS COLLABORATION (DE FILIPP, ET AL. 2017)
Weight control	Recommend education and counseling on "heart" healthy lifestyle (regular exercise, healthy weight, no smoking, dietary counseling).	Provide advice regarding intensive, multicomponent behavioral interventions focused on achieving and maintaining healthy weight by reducing caloric intake and increasing physical activity.
Dyslipidemia control	Recommend education and counseling on "heart" healthy lifestyle (regular exercise, healthy weight, no smoking, dietary counseling). Treatment goals are based on overall risk of heart disease (e.g., >10% chance of coronary heart disease in 10 years). Overall risk assessment will include the following risk factors: age, sex, diabetes, clinical atherosclerotic disease, hypertension, family history, low HDL (<40 mg/dL or 1.0 mmol/L), and smoking.	Lifestyle modifications and lipid-lowering therapies to achieve risk-adapted target for LDL is primary goal. The decision to initiate lipid-lowering therapy should include assessment of overall risk of heart disease (http://cvdrisk.nhlbi.nih.gov). If TG >500 mg/dL (5.65 mmol/L), initiate fibrate or nicotinic acid.
Blood pressure control	Nonpharmacologic treatments may also be tried for mild hypertension; they include moderate dietary sodium restriction, weight reduction in the obese, avoidance of excess alcohol intake, and regular aerobic exercise. Treatment is indicated for readings >140/90 in adults on two separate visits at least 1 week apart, unless hypertension is mild or can be attributed to a temporary condition or medication (e.g., cyclosporine).	Nonpharmacologic treatments may also be tried for mild hypertension; they include moderate dietary sodium restriction, weight reduction in the obese, avoidance of excess alcohol intake, and regular aerobic exercise. Treatment is indicated for readings >140/90 in adults on two separate visits at least 1 week apart, unless hypertension is mild or can be attributed to a temporary condition or medication (e.g., cyclosporine).
Glycemic control	Recommend education and counseling on "heart" healthy lifestyle (regular exercise, healthy weight, no smoking, dietary counseling).	For IFG, encourage weight reduction and increased physical activity. For type 2 DM, lifestyle therapy, and pharmacotherapy, if necessary, should be used to achieve near-normal HbA1C (<7%).

BP, Blood pressure; *CIBMTR*, Center for International Blood and Marrow Transplant Research; *CHILD-1*, Cardiovascular Health Integrated Lifestyle Diet; *DM*, diabetes mellitus; *EBMT*, European Group for Blood and Marrow Transplantation; *HbA1C*, hemoglobin A1C; *HCT*, hematopoietic cell transplantation; *HDL*, high-density lipoprotein cholesterol; *HTN*, hypertension; *IFG*, impaired fasting glucose; *LDL*, low-density lipoprotein; *TG*, triglyceride.

From De Filipp Z, et al. *Bone Marrow Transplant.* 2017;52(2):173–182) ; Majhail NS, et al. *Biol Blood Marrow Transplant.* 2012;18(3):348–371.

REFERENCES

1. Sorror ML. How I assess comorbidities before hematopoietic cell transplantation. *Blood.* 2013;121(15):2854–2863.
2. Henry M, Guo R, Parthasarathy M, Lopez J, Stiff P. Cardiac complications following allogeneic bone marrow transplantation: evaluation of risk factors, outcomes and enhanced screening for at risk populations. *Blood.* 2012;120:3070.
3. Black JL, Litzow MR, Hogan WJ, et al. Correlation of CYP2B6, CYP2C19, ABCC4 and SOD2 genotype with outcomes in allogeneic blood and marrow transplant patients. *Leuk Res.* 2012;36(1):59–66. doi:10.1016/j.leukres.2011.06.020.
4. Armenian SH, Chow EJ. Cardiovascular disease in survivors of hematopoietic cell transplantation. *Cancer.* 2014;120(4):469–479.
5. Majhail NS, Rizzo JD, Lee SJ, et al. Recommended screening and preventive practices for long-term survivors after hematopoietic stem cell transplantation. *Bone Marrow Transplant.* 2012;47(3):337–341.
6. Shankar SM, Marina N, Hudson MM, et al. Monitoring for cardiovascular disease in survivors of childhood cancer: report from the cardiovascular disease task force of the Children's Oncology Group. *Pediatrics.* 2008;121:e387–e396.
7. Chow EJ, Anderson L, Baker KS, et al. Late effects surveillance recommendations among survivors of childhood hematopoietic cell transplantation: a Children's Oncology Group report. *Biol Blood Marrow Transplant.* 2016;22(5):782–795.
8. Armenian SH, Sun CL, Shannon T, et al. Incidence and predictors of congestive heart failure after autologous hematopoietic cell transplantation. *Blood.* 2011;118(23):6023–6029.
9. Chow EJ, Baker KS, Lee SJ, et al. Influence of conventional cardiovascular risk factors and lifestyle characteristics and cardiovascular disease after hematopoietic cell transplantation. *J Clin Oncol.* 2014;32(3); 191–198.
10. Armenian SH, Sun CL, Vase T, et al. Cardiovascular risk factors in hematopoietic cell transplantation survivors: role in development of subsequent cardiovascular disease. *Blood.* 2012;120 (23):4505–4512.

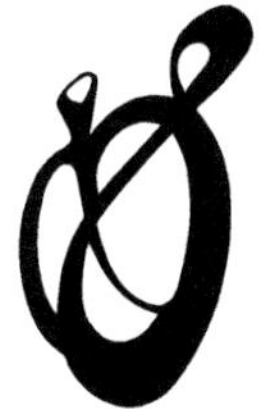

6 Surgical Risks

BARRY H. TRACHTENBERG AND MICHAEL J. REARDON

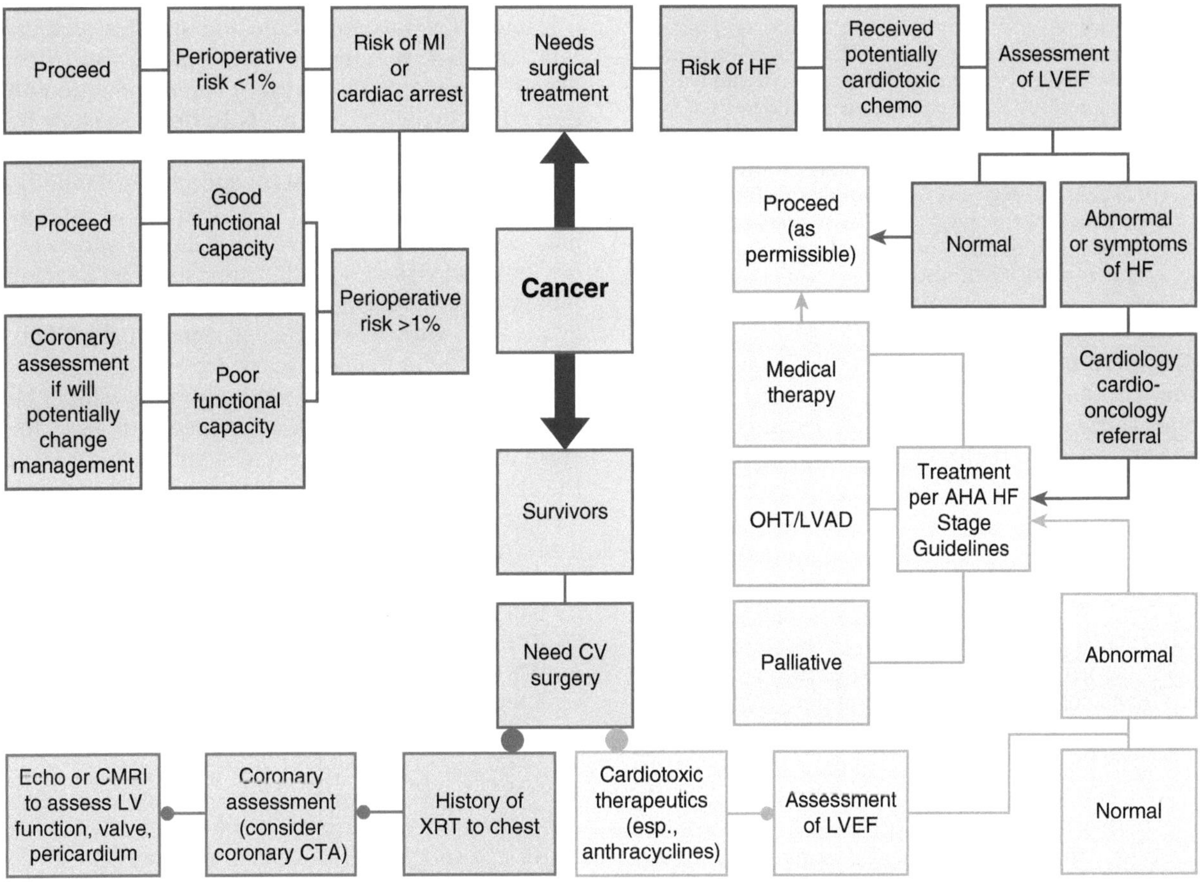

Proceed

Perioperative risk <1%

Risk of MI or cardiac arrest

Needs surgical treatment

Risk of HF

Received potentially cardiotoxic chemo

Assessment of LVEF

Proceed

Good functional capacity

Coronary assessment if will potentially change management

Poor functional capacity

Perioperative risk >1%

Cancer

Proceed (as permissible)

Normal

Abnormal or symptoms of HF

Medical therapy

Cardiology cardio-oncology referral

OHT/LVAD

Treatment per AHA HF Stage Guidelines

Survivors

Palliative

Abnormal

Need CV surgery

Echo or CMRI to assess LV function, valve, pericardium

Coronary assessment (consider coronary CTA)

History of XRT to chest

Cardiotoxic therapeutics (esp., anthracyclines)

Assessment of LVEF

Normal

CHAPTER OUTLINE

KEY POINTS

- Cardiovascular risks depend on traditional risk factors, cancer type, and type of surgical procedures.
- Assessment of left ventricular (LV) function should be performed preoperatively in patients who have received potentially cardiotoxic chemotherapies, including but not limited to anthracyclines and her-2 receptor antagonists.
- Preoperative coronary ischemia assessment should be reserved for symptomatic patients *or* patients with coronary artery disease (CAD) risk factors, poor functional capacity, and perioperative risk of myocardial infarction (MI) or cardiac arrest above 1%.
- Cancer survivors who undergo subsequent cardiac surgery (i.e., coronary artery bypass; valve, left ventricular assist device [LVAD] transplant) have unique considerations that need to be considered, particularly in the context of prior mediastinal radiation exposure and/or treatment with cardiotoxic chemotherapies.

There are currently more than 15.5 million cancer survivors in the United States, nearly half of whom have survived ten or more years.[1] Patients with cancer not only commonly undergo surgery as part of their cancer treatment, but owing to increased long-term survival they also frequently undergo cardiac surgeries that may or may not be a consequence of their cancer treatment. Many unique aspects of cancer and cancer treatment confer additional cardiovascular risks to patients who undergo cardiovascular surgery. Among long-term cancer survivors, cardiovascular mortality is a common cause of death, especially among patients with lung and bladder cancers.[2] In this chapter, we (1) review cardiovascular risk assessment in general, (2) outline individual cardiovascular concerns for a few specific cancers that are both common and frequently require surgery, and (3) address unique issues for patients who have cardiovascular complications from cancer treatment that require surgery. A risk assessment specific for each individual cancer type is beyond the scope of this chapter.

PREOPERATIVE CARDIOVASCULAR RISK ASSESSMENT

RISK OF MYOCARDIAL INFARCTION (MI)

From a perioperative cardiac complication standpoint, the risk of myocardial infarction and cardiac arrest (MICA) is of greatest concern. The risk is obviously highest in the setting of an acute coronary syndrome, and revascularization should be performed in appropriate patients followed by delay in any nonemergent surgery. Timing of cancer surgery would depend on the temporal urgency of resection to decrease local and metastatic spread coupled with appropriate timing for consideration of interrupting dual antiplatelet therapy (impacted by factors such as stent type and size, lesion location, number of stents). The general guidance, based predominantly on the recommended length of dual antiplatelet therapy, is to delay surgery by 14 days after balloon angioplasty (rarely indicated), 30 days after bare metal stent and ideally 6 months after drug-eluting stent (DES), although 3 months may be acceptable if the risk of delaying surgery is greater than risk of stent thrombosis.[3] The specific timelines are changing with updated data gathered in patients with newer DES designs. For patients who have undergone coronary artery bypass grafting (CABG), timing of noncardiac surgery should be delayed for a minimum of 4 to 6 weeks to allow for sternal healing. For patients who have had an MI in the absence of intervention, the current 2014 American College of Cardiology/American Heart Association (ACC/AHA) guidelines recommend to delay noncardiac surgery until the risk of MI and mortality has exponentially decreased, commonly at least 60 days.[4] Patients who undergo revascularization for MI fare better (50% lower risk); however, antiplatelet therapy considerations pertain to percutaneous coronary intervention (PCI) and the above outlined aspects to bypass surgery.

Patients who have a higher perioperative risk (e.g., surgery type with >1% risk of major adverse cardiac events or based on risk scores such as the revised cardiac risk index or RCRI[5]) with good functional capacity should proceed to surgery. If functional capacity is poor or unknown, noninvasive coronary assessment (e.g., stress echocardiography, radionuclide stress myocardial perfusion imaging, computed topography coronary angiography) should be performed if it will change perioperative management (Fig. 6.1).[6] Indeed, it is a major message of the ACC/AHA guidelines on perioperative risk assessment to consider noninvasive evaluation for coronary arterial disease only if the results would change management.[4] In addition to the RCRI score, newer risk scores include the National Surgical Quality Improvement Program (NSQIP) Surgical

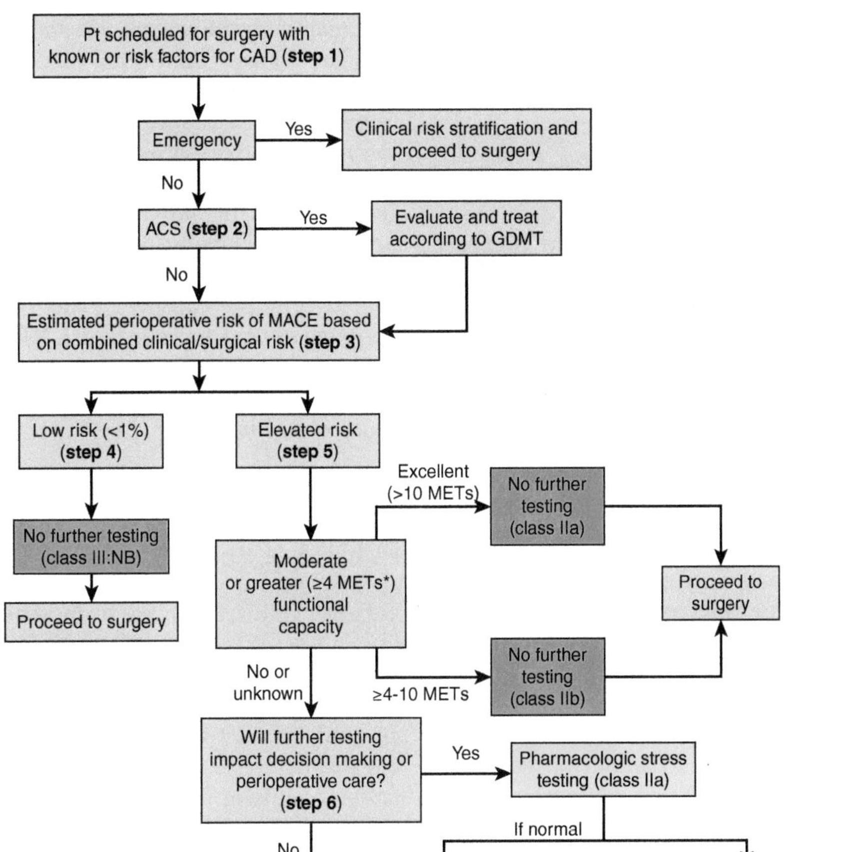

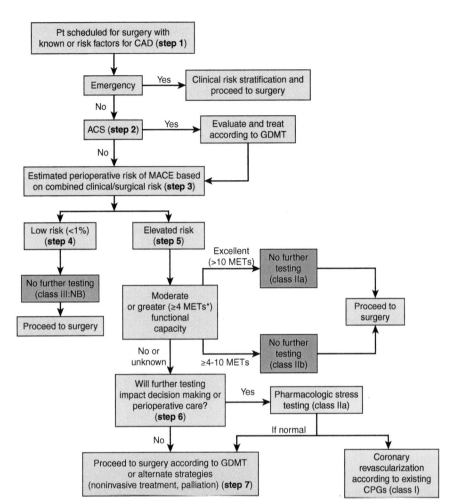

FIG. 6.1 Stepwise approach to perioperative cardiac assessment for CAD. **Step 1:** In patients scheduled for surgery with risk factors for or known CAD, determine the urgency of surgery. If an emergency, then determine the clinical risk factors that may influence perioperative management and proceed to surgery with appropriate monitoring and management strategies based on the clinical assessment. **Step 2:** If the surgery is urgent or elective, determine if the patient has an ACS. If yes, then refer patient for cardiology evaluation and management according to GDMT according to the UA/NSTEMI and STEMI CPGs (18,20). **Step 3:** If the patient has risk factors for stable CAD, then estimate the perioperative risk of MACE based on the combined clinical/surgical risk. This estimate can use the American College of Surgeons NSQIP risk calculator (http://www.surgicalriskcalculator.com) or incorporate the RCRI (131) with an estimation of surgical risk. For example, a patient undergoing very low-risk surgery (e.g., ophthalmologic surgery), even with multiple risk factors, would have a low risk of MACE, whereas a patient undergoing major vascular surgery with few risk factors would have an elevated risk of MACE. **Step 4:** If the patient has a low risk of MACE (<1%), then no further testing is needed, and the patient may proceed to surgery. **Step 5:** If the patient is at elevated risk of MACE, then determine functional capacity with an objective measure or scale, such as the DASI (133). If the patient has moderate, good, or excellent functional capacity (≥4 METs), then proceed to surgery without further evaluation. **Step 6:** If the patient has poor (<4 METs) or unknown functional capacity, then the clinician should consult with the patient and perioperative team to determine whether further testing will have an impact on patient decision making (e.g., decision to perform original surgery or willingness to undergo CABG or PCI, depending on the results of the test) or perioperative care. If yes, then pharmacologic stress testing is appropriate. In those patients with unknown functional capacity, exercise stress testing may be reasonable to perform. If the stress test is abnormal, consider coronary angiography and revascularization depending on the extent of the abnormal test. The patient can then proceed to surgery with GDMT or consider alternative strategies, such as noninvasive treatment of the indication for surgery (e.g., radiation therapy for cancer) or palliation. If the test is normal, proceed to surgery according to GDMT. **Step 7:** If testing will not have an impact on decision making or care, then proceed to surgery according to GDMT or consider alternative strategies, such as noninvasive treatment of the indication for surgery (e.g., radiation therapy for cancer) or palliation. *ACS,* Acute coronary syndrome; *CABG,* coronary artery bypass graft; *CAD,* coronary artery disease; *CPG,* clinical practice guideline; *DASI,* Duke Activity Status Index; *GDMT,* guideline-directed medical therapy; *MACE,* major adverse cardiac event; *MET,* metabolic equivalent; *NB,* No Benefit; *NSQIP,* National Surgical Quality Improvement Program; *PCI,* percutaneous coronary intervention; *RCRI,* Revised Cardiac Risk Index; *STEMI,* ST-elevation myocardial infarction; *UA/NSTEMI,* unstable angina/non–ST-elevation myocardial infarction.

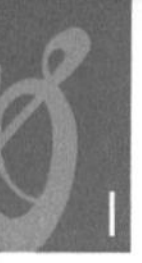

Risk calculator and the NSQIP MICA risk calculator (Table 6.1).[7,8]

RISK OF HEART FAILURE DECOMPENSATION

Whereas symptomatic heart failure has the highest cardiovascular risk for patients undergoing surgery in general, asymptomatic left ventricular (LV) dysfunction also carries an increased risk of cardiovascular morbidity and mortality compared with patients without heart failure or abnormal LV function.[9] In a large retrospective study of mostly male veterans undergoing a variety of surgical procedures, for example, 90-day mortality was 1.2%, 4.8%, and 10.1% for patients without heart failure, asymptomatic systolic dysfunction, or symptomatic heart failure, respectively.[10] Patients with symptomatic heart failure (with preserved or reduced ejection fraction [EF]) and patients with asymptomatic LV dysfunction should be assessed by a cardiologist prior to surgery for evaluation and medical optimization with guideline-directed therapies. Assessment of LV function prior to surgery should be performed particularly in any patient who has been exposed to potentially cardiotoxic therapies including (but not limited to) anthracyclines, human epidermal growth factor receptor (her-2) antagonists, certain vascular endothelial growth factor inhibitors and tyrosine kinase inhibitors, and immunotherapies (see Central Illustration). While strain parameters (e.g., derived by speckle tracking echocardiography) have been shown to predict cardiotoxicity with cancer therapeutics,[11] their value to assess surgical risks of patients with cancer has not yet been defined. Finally, biomarkers such as brain natriuretic peptide (BNP) and NT-proBNP can also help stratify the cardiovascular risk of patients undergoing noncardiac surgery. A NT-BNP greater than 300 ng/L or a BNP greater than 92 mg/L is associated with a four-fold increase in the postoperative risk of death or nonfatal MI.[12]

RISK OF CEREBROVASCULAR EVENTS (CVE)

Patients with cancer are at increased risk of atrial fibrillation (AF) and this risk increases with surgery.[13] Owing in part to the increased hypercoaguable state, patients with many types of cancer are also at increased risk for CVE independent of AF. AF occurs in approximately 12.6% of patients with cancer who are undergoing lung resection and it is also common in patients with cancer undergoing colectomy or esophageal resection. Elevated perioperative NT-BNP is associated with an increased risk of AF after lung

TABLE 6.1 Comparison of the Three Major Risk Scores

	RCRI	NSQIP MICA	NSQIP SURGICAL RISK
Criteria	1 point for each • [a]High-risk surgery • Hx ischemic heart disease • Hx CHF • Hx CVA • Preoperative trt with insulin • Preoperative Cr >2 mg/dL	Risk calculator based on following variables: • Type of surgery • Dependent functional status • Abnormal Cr • Increased age • American Society of Anesthesiologists Class	[b]20 variable calculator based on type of surgery and various patient variables
	Outcome parameters: MI, cardiac arrest, ventricular fibrillation, complete heart block, pulmonary edema for RCRI for the other two: MI and cardiac death Low risk: score of 0-1	Outcome parameters: MI or cardiac arrest Low risk: risk <1%	Outcome parameters: MI, cardiac arrest, heart failure Low risk: <1%
Pros	Simple and easy to use	Accuracy higher than RCRI Large derivation and validation cohort	Highest mortality accuracy (c-statistic 0.944)
Cons	Newer models perform better	Requires online calculator	Not externally validated More complex

[a]Defined by intraperitoneal, intrathoracic, or suprainguinal vascular surgery.
[b]See riskcalculator.facs.org/riskcalculator/index.jsp.
CHF, Congestive heart failure; *Cr,* serum creatinine; *CVA,* cerebrovascular accident; *MICA,* Myocardial infarction and cardiac arrest; *NSQIP,* National Surgical Quality Improvement Program; *RCRI,* Revised Cardiac Risk Index; *trt,* treatment.

cancer resection.[14] Although AF confers a five-fold increased risk of CVE in the general population, the risk of CVE in those with cancer with post operative AF is not well studied nor is the optimal treatment approach. No evidence supports the use of routine preoperative carotid imaging prior to surgery.

RISK OF VENOUS THROMBOEMBOLIC EVENTS (VTE)

The risk of venous thromboembolism is markedly elevated in patients with cancer. Those undergoing surgery have two times higher rates of postoperative VTE than do patients without cancer.[15] In addition to patient characteristics, such as advanced age, morbid obesity, and prolonged hospitalization, cancer type is a major risk factor for VTE in those patients undergoing surgery. For example, the 30-day incidence of VTE after breast cancer surgery is very low (~0.30%); however, the VTE incidence for patients undergoing esophagectomy, cystectomy, and pancreatectomy is very high (~7.3%, 4.9%, and 3.4%, respectively).[16] Patients should have prophylaxis for VTE administered postoperatively as soon as feasible, from a postoperative bleeding perspective.

UNIQUE RISK ASSESSMENT IN SPECIFIC CANCERS

BREAST CANCER

The lifetime risk of developing breast cancer for women in the United States is approximately 1 in 8. Most patients with stages I to III breast cancer will undergo a surgical intervention as part of their treatment plan, whether it is breast-conserving surgery (BCS; i.e., lumpectomy or partial mastectomy) or complete mastectomy.[17] Among women with stage I or II breast cancer, 61% have BCS and 36% have mastectomy, whereas among those with stage III breast cancer 21% undergo BCS and 72% undergo mastectomy. In addition, more than half of patients without metastatic disease who had mastectomies opt to have reconstructive surgery.[18] Preexisting cardiovascular risk factors (e.g., obesity, diabetes) are highly associated with the risk of complications after breast surgery.[19] Most of these complications are wound-related; the risk of major cardiovascular events perioperatively overall is quite low (<1%).[20] Given the relatively low risk of perioperative MI, preoperative ischemic assessment should be reserved for those who would warrant evaluation independent of surgical consideration (e.g., symptomatic ischemic heart disease) in line with societal guidelines.[4]

Those patients with breast cancer who have received potentially cardiotoxic chemotherapies, particularly anthracyclines or her-2 antagonists, are at risk for heart failure or asymptomatic LV dysfunction. An echocardiogram should be obtained in patients who have received these therapies prior to surgery.

LUNG CANCER

Surgical treatment is common for patients with lung cancer. For example, 69% of patients with stage I or II non–small-cell carcinoma undergo surgery as part of their treatment. Cardiac morbidity is high among patients with lung cancer, in part owing to age and the commonality of cigarette smoking and thus concomitant cardiovascular disease in this population. In fact, one in three patients undergoing lung resection from the European Society of Thoracic Surgery registry had cardiac comorbidities, including hypertension (23.4%), coronary artery disease (5.8%), and arrhythmias (2.6%).[21] The presence of at least one cardiac comorbidity increased the risk of mortality from 2.3% to 3.2%. Other factors leading to worse survival in this registry included age (i.e., >75 years), type of surgery (i.e., open vs. video-assisted thoracoscopic surgery; pneumonectomy worse than bilobectomy), and predicted postoperative forced expiratory volume (i.e., <70%). Other studies have shown a similar incidence of major cardiac events within 30 days of lung surgery, ranging between 1.7% and 4.3%.[22] An adaptation of the Revised Cardiac Risk Index (RCRI) called the Thoracic Revised Cardiac Risk Index (ThRCRI) has been used to predict perioperative cardiac outcomes in patients undergoing lung resection. The ThRCRI incorporates the following variables: the presence of ischemic heart disease, preoperative serum creatinine above 2.0 mg/dL, cerebrovascular disease, and pneumonectomy.[22] The use of this risk score has been shown to be predictive of the risk of major CV events in this patient population, with those with a ThRCRI score 2 or greater having a rate of major cardiac complications three times higher than those with a score of 0 (4.8% vs. 1.3%). Those who had major cardiac complications had a 40-fold increase in 30-day mortality. This database reported a 9% prevalence of ischemic heart disease; however, it should be emphasized that the presence of coronary artery disease is likely underestimated in this and other database studies.[23]

Although data are limited in sample size, the outcomes of patients who undergo simultaneous cardiac surgery and resection of isolated solitary lung nodules appear to be highly dependent on histology, with a 5-year survival of 86% in patients with benign lesions versus 44% in those with malignant solitary nodules.[24] Finally, patients who undergo left upper lobe lobectomy for lung cancer have an increased risk of CVE owing to the risk of thrombosis in the left upper pulmonary vein stump site.[25]

COLORECTAL CANCER

Approximately 1.4 million Americans have colorectal cancer; 85% of those patients are over the age of 60.[18] Surgery is indicated for patients without stage IV disease. The risk of MI in patients after colorectal surgery (including for noncancerous indications) is approximately 1% to 2%, with mortality greatly increased in these patients.[26] The strongest risk factors associated with mortality include advanced age, history of heart failure, chronic kidney disease, and hypoalbuminemia.[26] Patients who undergo surgery for cancer (vs. other colorectal surgeries) and those undergoing emergency surgeries also have decreased survival. Patients with heart failure who have preoperative ascites are at particularly increased risk, with a nearly two-fold increase in mortality compared with those patients with heart failure without ascites.[27] Randomized studies have shown that laparoscopic surgery has similar survival outcomes compared with open surgery. Other studies have shown a decreased mortality rate with a laparoscopic approach, particularly in elderly patients.[28] Additional factors that have been suggested to mitigate risk, although not studied in a prospective fashion, is limiting the need for blood transfusions and using board-certified anesthesiologists for high-risk cases such as those with American Society of Anesthesiology classification 3 or greater.[29]

CARDIAC TUMORS

Complete resection is the optimal treatment for most cardiac tumors. Benign tumors, such as papillary fibroelastomas (PFEs) and myxomas, should be considered for resection owing to the risk of embolization. For PFEs, tumor size does not consistently predict outcomes but the mobility of the mass and prior history of embolization are important factors in consideration of resection. We advocate for resection of all left-sided PFE in patients who are appropriate surgical candidates. Patient with myxomas can develop obstructive symptoms and sudden cardiac death, thus rendering the need for surgery more urgent. Perioperative mortality for patients undergoing myxoma resection is generally less than 5%. Common postoperative risks include AF and atrioventricular conduction defects.[30] Although the risk of recurrence is low (i.e., <5%) for completely resected myxoma, long-term surveillance is recommended.[31] For left-sided malignant tumors as well as some complex benign left atrial tumors, cardiac auto-transplantation (cardiac explant followed by *ex vivo* resection of tumor and reimplantation) is feasible and safe.[32] The need for pneumonectomy during the procedure, however, is associated with decreased survival and is a contraindication. Patients who have complete surgical resection for cardiac sarcomas have an increased survival compared with those who have incomplete resection or those with unresectable masses.[33] For primary right-sided heart sarcomas, which tend to be bulky and difficult to treat, neoadjuvant chemotherapy prior to surgical resection leads to improved survival compared with resection alone.[34] However, long-term survival of patients with cardiac sarcoma is still quite poor despite current treatment options. Right-sided masses should always be biopsied prior to treatment to differentiate primary cardiac lymphomas from sarcomas and other types of malignancies.

MALIGNANT PERICARDIAL EFFUSIONS

In the cancer population, pericardial effusions may arise from metastatic cancers (especially lung, breast, and Hodgkin lymphoma), cancer treatment such as checkpoint inhibitors, graft-versus-host disease after stem cell transplant, and other etiologies. Echocardiography is the diagnostic modality of choice to assess size of effusion and hemodynamic significance, and to evaluate for the presence of constrictive physiology. Cardiac magnetic resonance imaging may be considered if the effusion size is difficult to ascertain on echocardiogram and/or with a concern for underlying pericarditis that cannot be determined clinically. The median survival of patients with malignant effusions is poor[31]; thus, decision making for treatment options should be carefully discussed with both the patient and the oncologist.

Pericardiocentesis can be considered for the acute management; recurrence rate is high (36% to 60%) with isolated drainage but can be reduced with prolonged catheter drainage.[35,36] Surgical options include the creation of a pericardial "window" into the pleural cavity or balloon pericardiotomy, in which a deflated single or double balloon catheter is inserted into the pericardial space. These options are associated with a lower recurrence rate (<20%) compared with pericardiocentesis, although data are limited to retrospective series and systematic reviews.[37] A window may be performed via open surgery (subxiphoid or minithoracotomy) or using video-assisted thoracoscopy.

UNIQUE CONSIDERATIONS FOR CANCER SURVIVORS UNDERGOING CARDIAC SURGERY

CARDIOPULMONARY BYPASS (CPB)

A theoretic concern exists that CPB can weaken the immune system and thus promote conditions that increase the risk of cancer. For example, CPB is known to increase cytokines, such as IL-10, transforming growth factor-beta, tumor necrosis factor, and others. Data on whether CPB is associated with an increased risk of cancer has been mixed. One of the largest studies, albeit retrospective, failed to show an overall statistically significant increased risk of cancer, but did observe an increased risk of melanoma and lung cancer among patients who underwent CPB compared with "off-pump" cardiac surgery. However, this has not been replicated and currently insufficient data exist to identify CPB as being associated with an increased risk of malignancy.

Additional data suggest that those undergoing cardiac surgery with CPB who have cancer that was recently diagnosed or currently under treatment have decreased survival compared with patients in remission and those without cancer. The decreased survival was largely attributed to cancer recurrence.[38]

VALVE SURGERY

Patients with neuroendocrine tumors, such as carcinoid disease who have severe valve disease as a result, should be considered for valve surgery. Long-term outcomes are highly dependent on response to somatostatin analogues and this should factor into decisions regarding the type of valve (i.e., bioprosthetic vs. mechanical) and surgical candidacy, although palliative surgeries can be considered in select patients. There is a high incidence of valve deterioration postoperatively and, thus, mechanical valves should be considered in these patients despite the risk of anticoagulation. In carefully selected patients, 30-day mortality ranges from 11% to 18%.[39,40] Postoperative mortality most often is attributed to progression of carcinoid disease.

Patients with cancer requiring surgical treatment who have concomitant valvular disease may consider catheter-based approaches. Transaortic valve replacement (TAVR), for example, is now available for patients with severe symptomatic aortic stenosis who are at intermediate or high risk for surgery and may allow earlier definitive cancer surgery for them compared with patients who undergo surgical AVR.[41]

ADVANCED HEART FAILURE THERAPIES IN CANCER SURVIVORS

Many cancer survivors develop heart failure so advanced that they need end-organ interventions, such as mechanical circulatory support (MCS) devices or heart transplantation (HT). Analysis of heart transplant and MCS databases informs much of what we know about outcomes, although these are largely limited to patients with heart failure who received anthracycline-based chemotherapy. Although the incidence of stage D (refractory) heart failure owing to chemotherapy is estimated to be approximately 2% to 4%, various reports from transplant registries show that the incidence is increasing.[42]

Unique considerations for the eligibility of MCS and HT in this population include the impact of mediastinal radiation therapy (discussed above). In addition, because of the concern for recurrence of malignancy (esp., in the setting of systemic immunosuppression), many centers have a requirement for a 5-year cancer-free interval prior to acceptance for heart transplantation (HT).

Analysis of the Interagency Registry for Mechanically Assisted Circulatory Support (INTERMACS) registry from 2006 to 2011 shows that 2% of patients who had a left ventricular assist device (LVAD) placed had a history of chemotherapy-induced cardiomyopathy (CCMP). Patients with CCMP were more likely to receive the LVAD with a strategy of destination therapy compared with other LVAD recipients. Importantly, patients were twice as likely to require a right ventricular assist device (19% vs. 9%) than those without a history of cancer, likely owing to the global cardiac dysfunction caused by the chemotherapy.[43] Thus, careful consideration should be given to alternative strategies, such as total artificial heart or HT, in eligible patients who are determined to have a high risk of right ventricular (RV) failure. Despite the increased risk of RV failure, patients with CCMP had similar survival compared with all other patients. The increased risks may have been mitigated by the facts that patients with CCMP had fewer comorbid conditions and were younger.

In addition, an analysis from the International Society for Heart and Lung Transplantation registry from 2000 to 2008 compared patients with CCMP and dilated nonischemic cardiomyopathy. No difference was seen in overall survival between the two groups. There was a higher incidence of malignancies in the CCMP group within one year of HT (5% vs. 2% in the control group), although five of nine cancers were skin cancers. No increased risk of death owing to recurrent cancers was seen, a finding that was also replicated in analysis of the United Network of Organ Sharing (UNOS) database.[42]

These databases are not only limited by lack of information on specific chemotherapy regimens and dosages, but they may be subject to misclassification of patients with CCMP under more generic terms, such as "nonischemic" or "idiopathic" cardiomyopathy. In our single center study analyzing outcomes of patients with CCMP referred for advanced therapies, we found that we had indeed failed to properly designate 60% and 40% of those patients appropriately to the UNOS and INTERMACS registries, respectively.[44]

Finally, our knowledge on the outcomes of advanced therapies is mainly confined to anthracycline-based chemotherapy. As the use of targeted therapies, such as tyrosine kinase inhibitors and vascular endothelial growth factor inhibitors, as well as immunotherapies continues to expand considerably, the implications for those who develop stage D heart failure from these therapies remain wholly unknown. More data are needed on patients with cardiomyopathies owing to novel chemotherapies and immunotherapies in terms of their candidacy, unique complications, and outcomes for consideration of heart transplant and LVAD placement.

RISKS IN PATIENTS WITH PRIOR MEDIASTINAL RADIATION

In addition to the unique risks for patients with cancer mentioned above, those who have undergone radiation therapy to the mediastinum or chest face an increased the risk of developing heart disease. These complications can include coronary artery and valvular disease, pericardial constriction, restrictive myocardial disease, and conduction defects. The risk of mortality from heart disease, for example, is 27% higher where patients have had their breast cancer irradiated compared with those who had not, although newer techniques have been developed to minimize heart field radiation exposure.[45] Patients who undergo surgery for a specific element of radiation-induced heart disease should also be evaluated for the concomitant presence of additional sequelae from radiation (e.g., concomitant CAD in patients undergoing valve surgery).

The impact of radiation on surgical outcomes is substantial. Patients with a history of radiation-induced heart disease undergoing cardiovascular surgery have significantly worse outcomes compared with age and gender matched controls.[46] Risk scores, such as the EuroScore or Society of Thoracic Surgeons score underestimate surgical risks when used for patients with radiation-induced heart disease. Patients with radiation-associated heart disease who have constrictive pericarditis are at a particularly high risk for increased early mortality.[47] Patients with severe aortic stenosis caused by radiation who undergo surgical valve replacement have worse long-term outcomes compared with age- and gender-matched controls, although good outcomes are reported for those who are candidates for TAVR.[48]

Additionally, heart transplant outcomes according to analysis from the UNOS database were compared with patients with other forms of restrictive cardiomyopathy and all other patients who have had a HT. Patients with radiation-CMP were younger, more likely female, and were more likely to have previous cardiac surgeries. Compared with the other groups, patients with cardiomyopathy caused by radiation had lower 1- and 5-year survival.[49]

Whereas risk scores underperform in this population, known additive risks in these populations include amount of radiation exposure and concomitant surgeries. Also, it has been noted increased thickness of the aorto-mitral curtain as measured by echocardiography is an independent predictor of risk,[60] but further studies should validate this finding before used routinely in clinical practice.

CONCLUSION

Despite advances in cancer treatments, surgery is still commonly indicated in the treatment of various malignancies. The type of cancer, the treatments, and comorbid conditions contribute to unique considerations that must be considered when evaluating cardiac risk and determining the need for additional testing and treatment. In addition, as survivorship continues to improve, there is a need for increased awareness of the unique risks in this population as patients undergo standard cardiac surgeries owing to aging, cancer treatment, or their underlying comorbid diseases.

REFERENCES

1. American Cancer Society. *Cancer Treatment and Survivorship Facts and Figures 2016–2017*. Atlanta: American Cancer Society; 2019.
2. Abdel-Rahman O. Risk of cardiac death among cancer survivors in the United States: a SEER database analysis. *Expert Rev Anticancer Ther*. 2017;17(9):873–878. doi:10.1080/14737140.2017.1344099.
3. Levine GN, Bates ER, Bittl JA, et al. 2016 ACC/AHA guideline focused update on duration of dual antiplatelet therapy in patients with coronary artery disease: a report of the American College of Cardiology/American Heart Association Task Force on clinical practice guidelines. *J Am Coll Cardiol*. 2016;68(10):1082–1115. doi:10.1016/j.jacc.2016.03.513.
4. Fleisher LA, Fleischmann KE, Auerbach AD, et al. 2014 ACC/AHA guideline on perioperative cardiovascular evaluation and management of patients undergoing noncardiac surgery: a report of the American College of Cardiology/American Heart Association Task Force on practice guidelines. *J Am Coll Cardiol*. 2014;64(22):e77–e137. doi:10.1016/j.jacc.2014.07.944.
5. Lee TH, Marcantonio ER, Mangione CM, et al. Derivation and prospective validation of a simple index for prediction of cardiac risk of major noncardiac surgery. *Circulation*. 1999;100(10):1043–1049. doi:10.1161/01.cir.100.10.1043.
6. Patel AY, Eagle KA, Vaishnava P. Cardiac risk of noncardiac surgery. *J Am Coll Cardiol*. 2015;66(19):2140–2148. doi:10.1016/j.jacc.2015.09.026.
7. Bilimoria KY, Liu Y, Paruch JL, et al. Development and evaluation of the universal ACS NSQIP surgical risk calculator: a decision aid and informed consent tool for patients and surgeons. *J Am Coll Surg*. 2013;217(5):833–842.e1–e3. doi:10.1016/j.jamcollsurg.2013.07.385.
8. Gupta PK, Gupta H, Sundaram A, et al. Development and validation of a risk calculator for prediction of cardiac risk after surgery. *Circulation*. 2011;124(4):381–387. doi:10.1161/CIRCULATIONAHA.110.015701.
9. Flu WJ, van Kuijk JP, Hoeks SE, et al. Prognostic implications of asymptomatic left ventricular dysfunction in patients undergoing vascular surgery. *Anesthesiology*. 2010;112(6):1316–1324. doi:10.1097/ALN.0b013e3181da89ca.
10. Lerman BJ, Popat RA, Assimes TL, Heidenreich PA, Wren SM. Association of left ventricular ejection fraction and symptoms with mortality after elective noncardiac surgery among patients with heart failure. *JAMA*. 2019;321(6):572–579. doi:10.1001/jama.2019.0156.
11. Thavendiranathan P, Poulin F, Lim KD, Plana JC, Woo A, Marwick TH. Use of myocardial strain imaging by echocardiography for the early detection of cardiotoxicity in patients during and after cancer chemotherapy: a systematic review. *J Am Coll Cardiol*. 2014;63(25 Pt A):2751–2768. doi:10.1016/j.jacc.2014.01.073.
12. Duceppe E, Parlow J, MacDonald P, et al. Canadian Cardiovascular Society guidelines on perioperative cardiac risk assessment and management for patients who undergo noncardiac surgery. *Can J Cardiol*. 2017;33(1):17–32. doi:10.1016/j.cjca.2016.09.008.
13. Farmakis D, Parissis J, Filippatos G. Insights into onco-cardiology: atrial fibrillation in cancer. *J Am Coll Cardiol*. 2014;63(10):945–953. doi:10.1016/j.jacc.2013.11.026.
14. Cardinale D, Colombo A, Sandri MT, et al. Increased perioperative N-terminal pro-B-type natriuretic peptide levels predict atrial fibrillation after thoracic surgery for lung cancer. *Circulation*. 2007; 115(11):1339–1344. doi:10.1161/CIRCULATIONAHA.106.647008.
15. Timp JF, Braekkan SK, Versteeg HH, Cannegieter SC. Epidemiology of cancer-associated venous thrombosis. *Blood*. 2013;122(10):1712–1723. doi:10.1182/blood-2013-04-460121.
16. De Martino RR, Goodney PP, Spangler EL, et al. Variation in thromboembolic complications among patients undergoing commonly performed cancer operations. *J Vasc Surg*. 2012;55(4):1035–1040.e4. doi:10.1016/j.jvs.2011.10.129.
17. American Cancer Society. *Breast Cancer Facts and Figures 2017–2018*. Atlanta: American Cancer Society; 2017.
18. Miller KD, Siegel RL, Lin CC, et al. Cancer treatment and survivorship statistics, 2016. *CA Cancer J Clin*. 2016;66(4):271–289. doi:10.3322/caac.21349.
19. Huang BZ, Camp MS. Burden of preoperative cardiovascular disease risk factors on breast cancer surgery outcomes. *J Surg Oncol*. 2016;114(2):144–149. doi:10.1002/jso.24298.
20. de Blacam C, Ogunleye AA, Momoh AO, et al. High body mass index and smoking predict morbidity in breast cancer surgery: a multivariate analysis of 26,988 patients from the national surgical quality improvement program database. *Ann Surg*. 2012;255(3):551–555. doi:10.1097/SLA.0b013e318246c294.
21. Salati M, Brunelli A, Decaluwe H, et al. Report from the European Society of Thoracic Surgeons Database 2017: patterns of care and perioperative outcomes of surgery for malignant lung neoplasm. *Eur J Cardiothorac Surg*. 2017;52(6):1041–1048. doi:10.1093/ejcts/ezx272.
22. Thomas DC, Blasberg JD, Arnold BN, et al. Validating the Thoracic Revised Cardiac Risk Index following lung resection. *Ann Thorac Surg*. 2017;104(2):389–394. doi:10.1016/j.athoracsur.2017.02.006.
23. Ferguson MK, Saha-Chaudhuri P, Mitchell JD, Varela G, Brunelli A. Prediction of major cardiovascular events after lung resection using a modified scoring system. *Ann Thorac Surg*. 2014;97(4):1135–1140. doi:10.1016/j.athoracsur.2013.12.032.
24. Zhang R, Wiegmann B, Fischer S, et al. Simultaneous cardiac and lung surgery for incidental solitary pulmonary nodule: learning from the past. *Thorac Cardiovasc Surg*. 2012;60(2):150–155. doi:10.1055/s-0030-1271147.
25. Yamamoto T, Suzuki H, Nagato K, et al. Is left upper lobectomy for lung cancer a risk factor for cerebral infarction? *Surg Today*. 2016;46(7):780–784. doi:10.1007/s00595-015-1233-0.
26. Moghadamyeghaneh Z, Mills SD, Carmichael JC, Pigazzi A, Stamos MJ. Risk factors of postoperative myocardial infarction after colorectal surgeries. *Am Surg*. 2015;81(4):358–364.
27. Moghadamyeghaneh Z, Carmichael JC, Mills SD, Pigazzi A, Stamos MJ. Effects of ascites on outcomes of colorectal surgery in congestive heart failure patients. *Am J Surg*. 2015;209(6):1020–1027. doi:10.1016/j.amjsurg.2014.08.021.

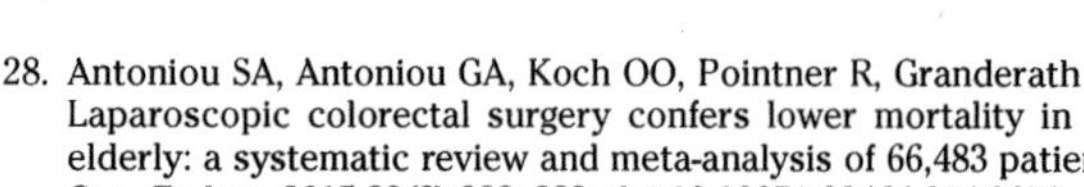

28. Antoniou SA, Antoniou GA, Koch OO, Pointner R, Granderath FA. Laparoscopic colorectal surgery confers lower mortality in the elderly: a systematic review and meta-analysis of 66,483 patients. *Surg Endosc*. 2015;29(2):322–333. doi:10.1007/s00464-014-3672-x.
29. Bottger TC, Hermeneit S, Muller M, et al. Modifiable surgical and anesthesiologic risk factors for the development of cardiac and pulmonary complications after laparoscopic colorectal surgery. *Surg Endosc*. 2009;23(9):2016–2025. doi:10.1007/s00464-008-9916-x.
30. Pinede L, Duhaut P, Loire R. Clinical presentation of left atrial cardiac myxoma. A series of 112 consecutive cases. *Medicine (Baltimore)*. 2001;80(3):159–172.
31. Lee KS, Kim GS, Jung Y, et al. Surgical resection of cardiac myxoma—a 30-year single institutional experience. *J Cardiothorac Surg*. 2017;12(1):18. doi:10.1186/s13019-017-0583-7.
32. Ramlawi B, Al-Jabbari O, Blau LN, et al. Autotransplantation for the resection of complex left heart tumors. *Ann Thorac Surg*. 2014;98(3):863–968. doi:10.1016/j.athoracsur.2014.04.125.
33. Truong PT, Jones SO, Martens B, et al. Treatment and outcomes in adult patients with primary cardiac sarcoma: the British Columbia Cancer Agency experience. *Ann Surg Oncol*. 2009;16(12):3358–3365. doi:10.1245/s10434-009-0734-8.
34. Abu Saleh WK, Ramlawi B, Shapira OM, et al. Improved outcomes with the evolution of a neoadjuvant chemotherapy approach to right heart sarcoma. *Ann Thorac Surg*. 2017;104(1):90–96. doi:10.1016/j.athoracsur.2016.10.054.
35. Laham RJ, Cohen DJ, Kuntz RE, Baim DS, Lorell BH, Simons M. Pericardial effusion in patients with cancer: outcome with contemporary management strategies. *Heart*. 1996;75(1):67–71. doi:10.1136/hrt.75.1.67.
36. Tsang TS, Seward JB, Barnes ME, et al. Outcomes of primary and secondary treatment of pericardial effusion in patients with malignancy. *Mayo Clin Proc*. 2000;75(3):248–253. doi:10.4065/75.3.248.
37. DeCamp MM Jr, Mentzer SJ, Swanson SJ, Sugarbaker DJ. Malignant effusive disease of the pleura and pericardium. *Chest*. 1997;112(suppl 4):291S–295S. doi:10.1378/chest.112.4_supplement.291s.
38. Carrascal Y, Gualis J, Arevalo A, et al. Cardiac surgery with extracorporeal circulation in patients with cancer: influence on surgical morbidity and mortality and on survival. *Rev Esp Cardiol*. 2008;61(4):369–375.
39. Bhattacharyya S, Raja SG, Toumpanakis C, Caplin ME, Dreyfus GD, Davar J. Outcomes, risks and complications of cardiac surgery for carcinoid heart disease. *Eur J Cardiothorac Surg*. 2011;40(1):168–172. doi:10.1016/j.ejcts.2010.10.035.
40. Manoly I, McAnelly SL, Sriskandarajah S, McLaughlin KE. Prognosis of patients with carcinoid heart disease after valvular surgery. *Interact Cardiovasc Thorac Surg*. 2014;19(2):302–305. doi:10.1093/icvts/ivu146.
41. Reardon MJ, Van Mieghem NM, Popma JJ, et al. Surgical or transcatheter aortic-valve replacement in intermediate-risk patients. *N Engl J Med*. 2017;376(14):1321–1331. doi:10.1056/NEJMoa1700456.
42. Oliveira GH, Hardaway BW, Kucheryavaya AY, Stehlik J, Edwards LB, Taylor DO. Characteristics and survival of patients with chemotherapy-induced cardiomyopathy undergoing heart transplantation. *J Heart Lung Transplant*. 2012;31(8):805–810. doi:10.1016/j.healun.2012.03.018.
43. Oliveira GH, Dupont M, Naftel D, et al. Increased need for right ventricular support in patients with chemotherapy-induced cardiomyopathy undergoing mechanical circulatory support: outcomes from the INTERMACS Registry (Interagency Registry for Mechanically Assisted Circulatory Support). *J Am Coll Cardiol*. 2014;63(3):240–248. doi:10.1016/j.jacc.2013.09.040.
44. Araujo-Gutierrez R, Ibarra-Coretz S, Estep JD, et al. Incidence and outcomes of cacer treatment-related cardiomyopathy among referrals for advanced heart failure. *Cardiooncology*. 2018;4:3.
45. Clarke M, Collins R, Darby S, et al. Effects of radiotherapy and of differences in the extent of surgery for early breast cancer on local recurrence and 15-year survival: an overview of the randomised trials. *Lancet*. 2005;366(9503):2087–2106. doi:10.1016/S0140-6736(05)67887-7.
46. Wu W, Masri A, Popovic ZB, et al. Long-term survival of patients with radiation heart disease undergoing cardiac surgery: a cohort study. *Circulation*. 2013;127(14):1476–1484. doi:10.1161/CIRCULATIONAHA.113.001435.
47. Handa N, McGregor CG, Danielson GK, et al. Valvular heart operation in patients with previous mediastinal radiation therapy. *Ann Thorac Surg*. 2001;71(6):1880–1884.
48. Dijos M, Reynaud A, Leroux L, et al. Efficacy and follow-up of transcatheter aortic valve implantation in patients with radiation-induced aortic stenosis. *Open Heart*. 2015;2(1):e000252. doi:10.1136/openhrt-2015-000252.
49. Al-Kindi SG, Oliveira GH. Heart transplantation outcomes in radiation-induced restrictive cardiomyopathy. *J Card Fail*. 2016;22(6):475–478. doi:10.1016/j.cardfail.2016.03.014.
50. Desai MY, Wu W, Masri A, et al. Increased aorto-mitral curtain thickness independently predicts mortality in patients with radiation-associated cardiac disease undergoing cardiac surgery. *Ann Thorac Surg*. 2014;97(4):1348–1355. doi:10.1016/j.athoracsur.2013.12.029.

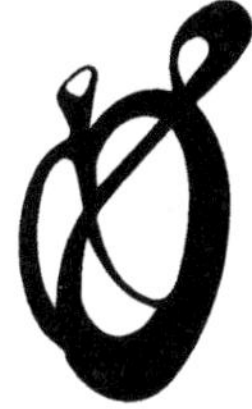

7 Prevention of Heart Failure and Cardiomyopathy in Patients With Cancer

JOSE A. ALVAREZ-CARDONA AND DANIEL J. LENIHAN

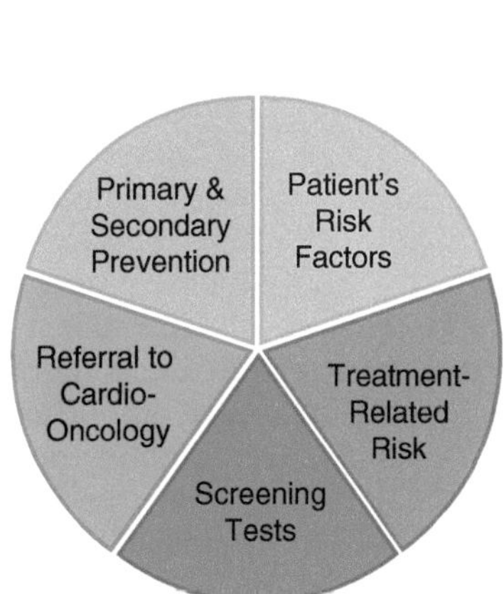

Patient's Risk Factors	Treatment Related Risk	Screening Tests	Referral to Cardio-Oncology	Primary & Secondary Prevention

• Age <15 or >65 years
• Obesity
• Cardiomyopathy
• Valvular heart disease
• Arrhythmias
• Coronary artery disease
• Peripheral vascular disease
• Diabetes mellitus
• Hypertension
• Hyperlipidemia
• Chronic kidney disease
• Prior anthracycline therapy
• Prior chest radiation
• Tobacco use
	• High-dose anthracycline monotherapy or in combination with other cardiotoxic agents
	• High-dose cyclophosphamide
	• Trastuzumab
	• 5-Fluorouracil, capecitabine
	• Carfilzomib
	• Combined MEK/BRAF inhibitors
	• Immune checkpoint inhibitors
	• Concurrent chest radiation
		• Baseline ventricular function
		  • 2D or 3D echo with strain imaging
		  • Cardiac MRI with gadolinium
		• ECG
		• Chest imaging
		  • X-ray
		  • CT scan
		• Cardiac biomarkers
		  • Troponin I or T
		  • NT-proBNP or BNP
		• High-sensitivity C-reactive protein
		• Lipid panel
			• Preexisting cardiomyopathy or HF
			• High CV risk
			• High risk therapy
			• Symptomatic CV disease: CAD, HF, PAD
			• Abnormal screening CV test
				• Risk factor modification
				• Optimize medical therapy
				• Screen for symptomatic CV disease: CAD, HF, PAD
				• Exercise

CHAPTER OUTLINE

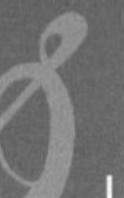

KEY POINTS

- All patients should undergo screening for preexisting/concomitant cardiovascular (CV) risk factors, cancer-specific risks for cardiomyopathy, and previous cancer therapy-related risk factors for cardiomyopathy before initiation of cancer treatment.
- Cardiomyopathy or heart failure (CM/HF) can emerge early during cancer therapy, shortly after completion, or many years later.
- The goal of the pretherapy assessment is to identify the presence or risks of CV disease and consequently CM/HF, and to define a screening, prevention, and treatment plan.
- These efforts should enable patients to complete the best possible cancer therapy without the deterioration or development of CM/HF or have premature discontinuation of planned cancer therapy resulting from cardiotoxicity.

A wide array of risk factors has been linked to the development of cardiovascular (CV) disease. Some of these CV risk factors overlap with known risk factors for the development of cancer and create a complex interplay resulting in disease progression of both of these two leading causes of death. As a result, an interdisciplinary approach is necessary for the cardiovascular care of the oncology patient before, during, and after treatment. Prevention of CV disease in such patients should focus on these five interventions: (1) establishing patient- and (2) treatment-related risk, (3) screening for asymptomatic and symptomatic CV disease, (4) appropriate use of screening tools, and (5) prompt referral to a cardio-oncologist for further evaluation and management when necessary (Central Illustration).

ESTABLISHING A PATIENT'S CARDIOVASCULAR RISK

The American College of Cardiology's Atherosclerotic Cardiovascular Disease (ASCVD) Risk Estimator Plus allows clinicians to calculate a patient's 10-year risk for ASCVD (primary prevention only). It considers a patient's age, race, gender, blood pressure, cholesterol (total cholesterol and high-density lipoprotein), history of diabetes mellitus and hypertension, history of tobacco use, and aspirin use. Based on the calculated 10-year risk for ASCVD, the patient's risk is classified as low (<5%), borderline (5% to 7.4%), intermediate (7.5% to 19.9%), and high (≥20%). Depending on the patient's risk, preventative strategies, such as initiating statin therapy, are recommended. It is important to emphasize that none of these risk assessment calculators has been validated in the cancer population, especially those who have had prior cancer therapy.

Certain cancers (e.g., lung cancer, multiple myeloma) have an inherently higher risk of CV complications, and this is frequently coupled with treatment-related CV adverse effects (e.g., radiation-induced heart disease, drug-related cardiac dysfunction).

Patients with known CV disease, such as coronary artery disease and peripheral vascular disease should be screened for symptoms, and medical optimization should be pursued when possible. Knowing the extent of their CV disease and prior cancer treatment plays a key role when providing recommendations about the patient's risk with certain cancer therapies (e.g., a tyrosine kinase inhibitor, such as nilotinib) that are associated with increased risk for vascular toxicity (e.g., development of atherosclerosis, endothelial dysfunction, thrombosis, or vasospasm). Additionally, certain cancer therapies (e.g., high-dose cytarabine) have important hematologic complications (e.g., thrombocytopenia) that could preclude guideline-based therapy. Anticipating these issues becomes critically important—for example, the use of dual antiplatelet agents in patients with recent percutaneous coronary intervention who are undergoing treatment for a hematologic malignancy.

The differential diagnosis of heart failure (HF) in the oncology population is essentially the same as for the general population, except for the complications that may arise from cancer itself or its therapy. Table 7.1 provides a list of possible causes of HF in this population. In general, cardiomyopathy or (CM) or HF can result from any combination of direct cardiotoxic effects from the cancer itself (e.g., multiple myeloma, amyloidosis), cardiotoxic treatments (e.g., anthracyclines), or as an exacerbation of a preexisting CV disease or a systemic condition (e.g., sepsis).

Treatment of patients with congenital heart disease is particularly challenging, because, in many cases, there are residual structural abnormalities even if surgically corrected. Hemodynamic compromise may result during cancer treatment because of fluid changes, such as with dehydration and anemia.

TABLE 7.1 Differential Diagnosis of Heart Failure (HF) and Management Considerations in Patients With Cancer

Cancer therapy-related cardiomyopathy	• Anthracyclines: doxorubicin, epirubicin, idarubicin • HER2-targed therapies: trastuzumab, pertuzumab • Proteasome inhibitors: carfilzomib • BRAF/MEK inhibitors
Primary or secondary cardiac tumors	• Hemodynamic effects of obstructive lesions: LVOT, RVOT, valvular • Tumor migration and invasion from SVC/IVC or pulmonary veins
Myocarditis	• Immune checkpoint inhibitors (ICIs): ipilimumab, pembrolizumab, nivolumab • Viral myocarditis
Ischemic cardiomyopathy	• Severity and extent of coronary artery disease • Residual disease at risk for ischemia or infarction • Need for dual antiplatelet therapy based on prior revascularization
Valvular heart disease	• Clinical significance (at least moderate regurgitation and/or stenosis), etiology, mechanism • Hemodynamic complications owing to cancer-related issues: dehydration, renal failure, anasarca, anemia • Eligibility for valvular repair or replacement before, during, or after cancer treatment
Pericardial disease	• Constrictive pericarditis owing to radiation exposure • Cardiac tamponade • Metastatic pericardial disease • Chemotherapy or immunotherapy associated with pericardial effusion: high-dose cyclophosphamide, ICIs
Arrhythmias and conduction disease	• Supraventricular tachycardias: AVNRT • Atrial fibrillation or flutter • Chemotherapy or immunotherapy associated with arrhythmias: taxanes, arsenic trioxide, ibrutinib • Benefits and risks of antiarrhythmic therapy and catheter-based ablation
Vascular disease	• Pulmonary arterial hypertension (e.g., dasatinib), Eisenmenger syndrome, pulmonary venoocclusive disease • Pulmonary embolism and right HF

AVNRT, Atrioventricular nodal reentry tachycardia; *IVC*, inferior vena cava; *LVOT*, left ventricular outflow tract; *RVOT*, right ventricular outflow tract; *SVC*, superior vena cava.

TREATMENT-RELATED RISK

Understanding the risk of left ventricular (LV) dysfunction and HF associated with different chemotherapy agents is necessary when planning a safe and personalized treatment regimen.

Risk factors specific to patients with cancer include prior anthracycline therapy and chest or mediastinal radiation.

It is well recognized that anthracycline cardiotoxicity is dose-dependent and there is no safe dose. Knowing the cumulative dose allows clinicians to consider different protective strategies, such as anthracycline dose reduction, continuous versus bolus infusion to avoid peak levels,[1,2] liposomal doxorubicin,[3,4] and dexrazoxane.[5,6] This is especially crucial in cases where the benefits of anthracycline therapy outweigh its risks.

Unlike anthracyclines, the decline in ejection fraction is classically seen at the time of therapy for trastuzumab and recovers in most cases upon cessation of therapy, although irreversible declines and persistent reduction in cardiac function have been described as well; patients receiving trastuzumab after anthracycline therapy are considered to represent the highest risk group.

The 2016 American Society of Clinical Oncology (ASCO) practice guidelines consider those patients with cancer at high risk for cardiotoxicity if they are receiving a cumulative doxorubicin dose 250 mg/m^2 or greater, chest radiation 30 Gy or greater with the heart in the radiation field, combination of these two even at lower dose cutoffs, anthracycline at any dose, trastuzumab in combination with with either anthracycline or radiation therapy, or CV risk factors or CVD (Table 7.2).

Efforts have been pursed to express the overall cardiotoxicity risk as an integral score based on patient and treatment-related risk factors, but these are conceptual models in need of validation.[7] At present not sufficient data support either a universal cardiotoxicity risk prediction model (either for all patients and therapies or for one therapy and all possible cardiovascular toxicities), given the heterogeneity of variables involved. Identifying patients at risk for cardiotoxicity from cancer treatment remains a challenge in clinical practice, even when focus is only on one drug and one patient

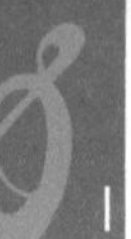

TABLE 7.2 2016 American Society of Clinical Oncology (ASCO) Clinical Practice Guideline on the Prevention and Monitoring of Cardiac Dysfunction in Survivors of Adult Cancers

1. Which patients with cancer are at increased risk for developing cardiac dysfunction?

Recommendation 1.1. It is recommended that patients with cancer who meet any of the following criteria should be considered at increased risk for developing cardiac dysfunction. (Evidence based; benefits outweigh harms; Evidence quality: intermediate; Strength of recommendation: moderate)

Treatment that includes any of the following:

- High-dose anthracycline (e.g., doxorubicin ≥250 mg/m^2, epirubicin ≥600 mg/m^2)
- High-dose radiotherapy (RT; ≥30 Gy) where the heart is in the treatment field
- Lower-dose anthracycline (e.g., doxorubicin <250 mg/m^2, epirubicin <600 mg/m^2) in combination with lower-dose RT (<30 Gy) where the heart is in the treatment field

Treatment with lower-dose anthracycline (e.g., doxorubicin <250 mg/m^2, epirubicin <600 mg/m^2) or trastuzumab alone, and presence of any of the following risk factors:

- Multiple cardiovascular risk factors (≥2 risk factors), including smoking, hypertension, diabetes, dyslipidemia, and obesity, during or after completion of therapy
- Older age (≥60 years) at cancer treatment
- Compromised cardiac function (e.g., borderline low left ventricular ejection fraction (50%–55%), history of myocardial infarction, ≥moderate valvular heart disease) at any time before or during treatment

Treatment with lower-dose anthracycline (e.g., doxorubicin <250 mg/m^2, epirubicin <600 mg/m^2) followed by trastuzumab (sequential therapy)

Recommendation 1.2. No recommendation can be made on the risk of cardiac dysfunction in patients with cancer with any of the following treatment exposures (Evidence based; Evidence quality: low):

- Lower-dose anthracycline (e.g., doxorubicin <250 mg/m^2, epirubicin <600 mg/m^2) or trastuzumab alone and no additional risk factors (as defined in Recommendation 1.1)
- Lower-dose RT (<30 Gy) where the heart is in the treatment field and no additional cardiotoxic therapeutic exposures or risk factors (as defined in Recommendation 1.1)
- Kinase inhibitors

2. Which preventative strategies minimize risk before initiation of therapy?

Recommendation 2.1. Avoid or minimize the use of potentially cardiotoxic therapies if established alternatives exist that would not compromise cancer-specific outcomes. (Consensus based; benefits outweigh harms; Strength of recommendation: strong)

Recommendation 2.2. Clinicians should perform a comprehensive assessment in patients with cancer that includes a history and physical examination, screening for cardiovascular disease risk factors (hypertension, diabetes, dyslipidemia, obesity, smoking), and an echocardiogram before initiation of potentially cardiotoxic therapies. (Evidence and consensus based; benefits outweigh harms; Evidence quality: high; Strength of recommendation: strong)

3. Which preventive strategies are effective in minimizing risk during the administration of potentially cardiotoxic cancer therapy?

Recommendation 3.1. Clinicians should screen for and actively manage modifiable cardiovascular risk factors (smoking, hypertension, diabetes, dyslipidemia, obesity) in all patients receiving potentially cardiotoxic treatments. (Informal consensus and evidence based; benefits outweigh harms; Evidence quality: insufficient; Strength of recommendation: moderate)

Recommendation 3.2. Clinicians may incorporate a number of strategies, including use of the cardioprotectant dexrazoxane, continuous infusion, or liposomal formulation of doxorubicin, for prevention of cardiotoxicity in patients planning to receive high-dose anthracyclines (e.g., doxorubicin ≥250 mg/m^2, epirubicin ≥600 mg/m^2). (Evidence based; benefits outweigh harms; Evidence quality: intermediate; Strength of recommendation: moderate)

Recommendation 3.3. For patients who require mediastinal RT that might impact cardiac function, clinicians should select lower radiation doses when clinically appropriate and use more precise or tailored radiation fields with exclusion of as much of the heart as possible. These goals can be accomplished through use of advanced techniques including the following. (Evidence based and informal consensus; benefits outweigh harms; Evidence quality: intermediate; Strength of recommendation: strong):

- Deep-inspiration breath holding for patients with mediastinal tumors or breast cancer in which the heart might be exposed
- Intensity-modulated RT that varies the radiation energy while treatment is delivered to precisely contour the desired radiation distribution and avoid normal tissues

4. What are the preferred surveillance and monitoring approaches during treatment in patients at risk for cardiac dysfunction?

Recommendation 4.1. Clinicians should complete a careful history and physical examination in patients who are receiving potentially cardiotoxic treatments. (Informal consensus; benefits outweigh harms; Evidence quality: insufficient; Strength of recommendation: strong)

TABLE 7.2 2016 American Society of Clinical Oncology (ASCO) Clinical Practice Guideline on the Prevention and Monitoring of Cardiac Dysfunction in Survivors of Adult Cancers—cont'd

Recommendation 4.2. In individuals with clinical signs or symptoms concerning for cardiac dysfunction during routine clinical assessment, the following strategy is recommended:

- Echocardiogram for diagnostic workup. (Evidence based; benefits outweigh harms; Evidence quality: intermediate; Strength of recommendation: strong)
- Cardiac magnetic resonance imaging (MRI) or multigated acquisition (MUGA) scan if echocardiogram is not available or technically feasible (e.g., poor image quality), with preference given to cardiac MRI. (Evidence based; benefits outweigh harms; Evidence quality: intermediate; Strength of recommendation: moderate)
- Serum cardiac biomarkers (troponins, natriuretic peptides) or echocardiography-derived strain imaging in conjunction with routine diagnostic imaging. (Evidence based; benefits outweigh harms; Evidence quality: intermediate; Strength of recommendation: moderate)
- Referral to a cardiologist based on findings. (Informal consensus; benefits outweigh harms; Evidence quality: insufficient; Strength of recommendation: strong)

Recommendation 4.3. Routine surveillance imaging may be offered during treatment in asymptomatic patients considered to be at increased risk (Recommendation 1.1) of developing cardiac dysfunction. In these individuals, echocardiography is the surveillance imaging modality of choice that should be offered. Frequency of surveillance should be determined by health care providers based on clinical judgment and patient circumstances. (Evidence based; benefits outweigh harms; Evidence quality: intermediate; Strength of recommendation: moderate)

Recommendation 4.4. No recommendations can be made regarding continuation or discontinuation of cancer therapy in individuals with evidence of cardiac dysfunction. This decision, made by the oncologist, should be informed by close collaboration with a cardiologist, fully evaluating the clinical circumstances and considering the risks and benefits of continuation of therapy responsible for the cardiac dysfunction. (Informal consensus; benefits outweigh harms; Evidence quality: insufficient)

Recommendation 4.5. Clinicians may use routine echocardiographic surveillance in patients with metastatic breast cancer continuing to receive trastuzumab indefinitely. The frequency of cardiac imaging for each patient should be determined by health care providers based on clinical judgment and patient circumstances. (Evidence based and informal consensus; benefits outweigh harms; Evidence quality: low; Strength of recommendation: moderate)

5. What are the preferred surveillance and monitoring approaches after treatment in patients at risk for cardiac dysfunction?

Recommendation 5.1. Clinicians should complete a careful history and physical examination in survivors of cancer previously treated with potentially cardiotoxic therapies. (Informal consensus; benefits outweigh harms; Evidence quality: insufficient; Strength of recommendation: strong)

Recommendation 5.1.1. In individuals with clinical signs or symptoms concerning for cardiac dysfunction, the following approaches should be offered as part of recommended care:

Echocardiogram for diagnostic workup. (Evidence based; benefits outweigh harms; Evidence quality: intermediate; Strength of recommendation: strong)

Cardiac MRI or MUGA if echocardiogram is not available or technically feasible (e.g., poor image quality), with preference given to cardiac MRI. (Evidence based; benefits outweigh harms; Evidence quality: intermediate; Strength of recommendation: moderate)

Serum cardiac biomarkers (troponins, natriuretic peptides). (Evidence based; benefits outweigh harms; Evidence quality: intermediate; Strength of recommendation: moderate)

Referral to a cardiologist based on findings. (Informal consensus; benefits outweigh harms; Evidence quality: insufficient; Strength of recommendation: strong)

Recommendation 5.2. An echocardiogram may be performed between 6 and 12 months after completion of cancer-directed therapy in asymptomatic patients considered to be at increased risk. (Recommendation 1.1 of cardiac dysfunction.) (Evidence based; benefits outweigh harms; Evidence quality: intermediate; Strength of recommendation: moderate)

Recommendation 5.2.1. Cardiac MRI or MUGA may be offered for surveillance in asymptomatic individuals if an echocardiogram is not available or technically feasible (e.g., poor image quality), with preference given to cardiac MRI. (Evidence based; benefits outweigh harms; Evidence quality: intermediate; Strength of recommendation: moderate)

Recommendation 5.3. Patients identified to have asymptomatic cardiac dysfunction during routine surveillance should be referred to a cardiologist or a health care provider with Cardio-Oncology expertise for further assessment and management. (Informal consensus; benefits outweigh harms; Evidence quality: insufficient; Strength of recommendation: strong)

Recommendation 5.4. No recommendations can be made regarding the frequency and duration of surveillance in patients at increased risk (Recommendation 1.1) who are asymptomatic and have no evidence of cardiac dysfunction on their 6- to 12-month posttreatment echocardiogram. (Informal consensus; relative balance of benefits and harms; Evidence quality: insufficient)

Recommendation 5.5. Clinicians should regularly evaluate and manage cardiovascular risk factors such as smoking, hypertension, diabetes, dyslipidemia, and obesity in patients previously treated with cardiotoxic cancer therapies. A heart-healthy lifestyle, including the role of diet and exercise, should be discussed as part of long-term follow-up care. (Evidence based and consensus; benefits outweigh harms; Evidence quality: intermediate; Strength of recommendation: moderate) population such as trastuzumab in patients with breast cancer.[8]

Radiation-induced heart disease (RIHD) consists of a series of events that ultimately lead to myocardial dysfunction and HF. It involves direct and indirect vascular damage and upregulation of inflammatory markers that can result in ischemia, thrombosis, and stenosis of the major vessels (e.g., coronary artery disease, superior vena cava syndrome).[9–11] It also has a detrimental effect on cardiac valves, which may result in calcification leading to significant regurgitation and/or stenosis.

Pericardial disease can manifest as constrictive pericarditis in patients with prior chest radiation or as pericardial effusion and/or tamponade caused by inflammation, medications (e.g., high-dose cyclophosphamide), or malignant involvement.

Immune checkpoint inhibitors are associated with rare, but sometimes fatal, cardiovascular immune-related adverse events, particularly myocarditis.[12] Nonetheless, other manifestations include pericardial disease,[13,14] vasculitis,[14] Takotsubo cardiomyopathy,[15] conduction abnormalities,[16] and destabilization of atherosclerotic lesions.[17]

PRIMARY AND SECONDARY PREVENTATIVE STRATEGIES

Patients at risk for CM/HF prior to undergoing cancer treatment should be screened and managed according to the American College of Cardiology and American Heart Association guidelines (Fig. 7.1).

SCREENING AND MONITORING

Patients without prior CV disease should be screened for traditional CV risk factors: family history, obesity, hypertension, diabetes, hyperlipidemia, and tobacco use. This includes reviewing prior computed tomography scan(s) or positron emission tomography scan(s) that could reveal evidence of atherosclerosis.

Baseline ventricular function assessment is recommended for all patients receiving cancer treatment who are at risk for LV dysfunction. This can be obtained by means of 2D or 3D echocardiography or cardiac magnetic resonance imaging, and should

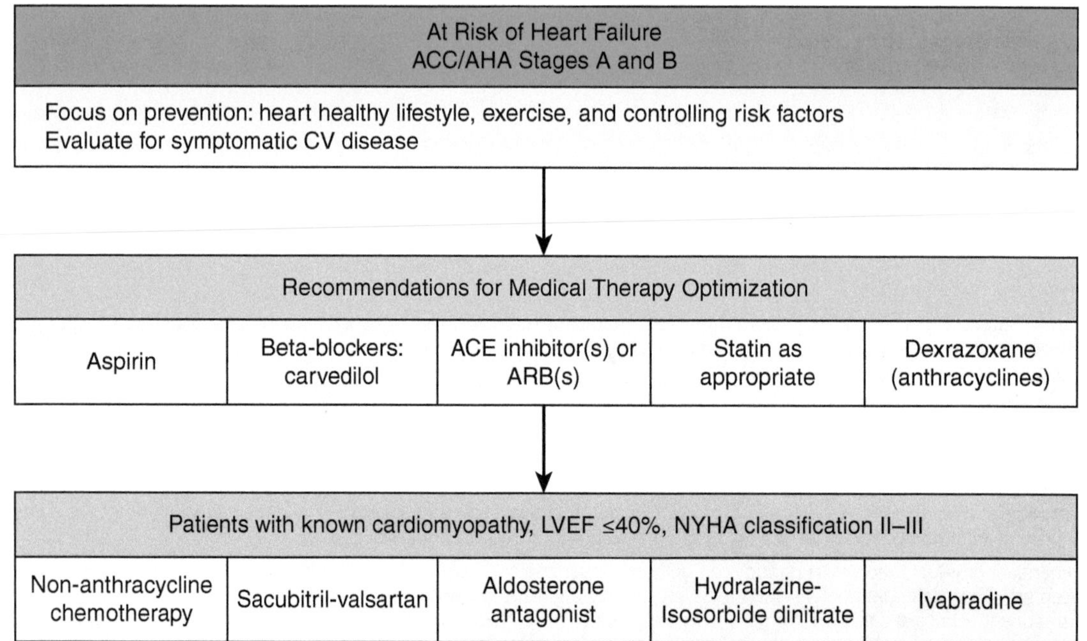

FIG. 7.1 Preventative approach to patients at risk for cardiomyopathy or heart failure (CM/HF) who are scheduled to receive cancer treatment.[5,6,18,19–23] *ACE*, Angiotensin-converting enzyme; *ARB*, angiotensin receptor blocker; *CV*, cardiovascular; *LEVF*, left ventricular ejection fraction.

include assessment of myocardial strain, when clinically feasible.

Assessment of NT-proBNP is recommended in patients at risk of developing HF and in those presenting with dyspnea, and to establish prognosis or disease severity in chronic HF.[18,24,25]

Obtaining a baseline troponin I (or T) level is reasonable in patients at risk of myocardial injury from cancer treatment (e.g., myocarditis, leukostasis). In fact, the ASCO guideline recommendations are for a baseline electrocardiogram (ECG) and troponin level prior to immune checkpoint inhibitor therapy.[26]

INFLAMMATORY MARKERS, SUCH AS HIGH-SENSITIVITY C-REACTIVE PROTEIN (HS-CRP), MAY BE USEFUL IN GUIDING CLINICAL DECISION MAKING WHEN MYOCARDITIS IS SUSPECTED.

A combination of serial biomarker and imaging assessments is strongly recommended, especially in those patients undergoing high-risk cancer therapy. Abnormal biomarkers may precede LV dysfunction and this can help guide medical therapy and the frequency of reassessments in any given patient.

REFERRAL TO CARDIO-ONCOLOGY

Patients with high-risk features should be evaluated by a cardiologist or cardio-oncologist prior to initiation of cancer treatment.

Patients with abnormal screening tests should be referred to a cardio-oncologist, if possible, to direct further evaluation. This can include ischemic risk stratification or optimization of HF therapy in preparation for cancer treatment.

Patients with significant valvular heart disease should be referred to a valve center or a cardio-oncologist experienced in the management of complex valve disease. Decision about pursuing valve repair or replacement will depend on the patient's symptoms and functional status as well as the overall prognosis from a cancer standpoint. Percutaneous interventions (e.g., transcatheter valve replacement) are now available and should be considered in this particular population.

The cardio-oncologist will work closely with the oncologist/hematologist to determine if the patient's presentation is thought to be related to cancer therapy and establish a surveillance and treatment plan. This should include specific recommendations regarding the timing of therapy continuation, need for cancer treatment modification, frequency and modality for cardiac surveillance, and addition or adjustment of cardioprotective medications.

Summaries of the 2016 ASCO Clinical Practice Guideline on the Prevention and Monitoring of Cardiac Dysfunction in Survivors of Adult Cancers[27] and the 2020 European Society of Medicine Oncology (ESMO) Consensus recommendations for the management of cardiac disease in patients with cancer throughout the continuum of cancer[28] care are provided in Tables 7.2 and 7.3.

TABLE 7.3 2020 European Society of Medicine Oncology Consensus Recommendations for the Management of Cardiac Disease in Patients With Cancer Throughout Oncologic Treatment

SECTION	RECOMMENDATIONS
1. General principles	1.1 Screening for known cardiovascular (CV) risk factors in patients with cancer is recommended; treatment of identified CV risk factors according to current guidelines is recommended (LOE: I, GOR: A). 1.2 Many types of cancer therapy, especially mediastinal and left-sided chest radiation and certain chemotherapy and targeted agents can substantially affect the heart and vascular system and it is recommended that CV safety be monitored (LOE: I, GOR: A). 1.3 Close and early collaboration between cardiologists, oncologists, hematologists, and radiation oncologists is recommended to ensure lifelong CV health and to avoid unnecessary discontinuation of cancer therapy (LOE: III, GOR: C).
2. Before cancer treatment: Screening	2.1 Routine use of cardiac biomarkers (cardiac troponins [TnI or TnT], B-type natriuretic peptide or N-terminal pro-brain natriuretic peptide [BNP or NT-proBNP]) for patients undergoing potentially cardiotoxic chemotherapy is not well established. However, for patients at high risk (with preexisting significant cardiovascular disease) and those receiving high doses of cardiotoxic chemotherapy, such as anthracycline, baseline measurement of such cardiac biomarkers should be considered (LOE: III, GOR: A).

Continued

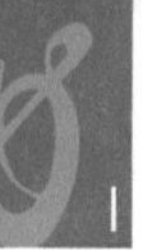

TABLE 7.3 2020 European Society of Medicine Oncology Consensus Recommendations for the Management of Cardiac Disease in Patients With Cancer Throughout Oncologic Treatment—Cont'd

SECTION	RECOMMENDATIONS
	2.2 For patients with a cancer diagnosis that requires treatment with a potentially cardiotoxic treatment, a baseline electrocardiogram (ECG), including measurement of a heart-rate corrected QT interval (QTc), is recommended (LOE: I, GOR: A). *QTc should be calculated by either of the two most standardized methods—Bazett's or Fridericia's—and the comparative measurements during treatment should all be done using the same method.* 2.3 In patients scheduled to undergo cancer therapy associated with heart failure (HF) or left ventricular dysfunction (LVD), baseline evaluation of left ventricular ejection fraction (LVEF), with strain imaging, when possible, and diastolic function according to accepted comprehensive imaging practice is recommended (LOE: I, GOR: A).
3. Before cancer treatment: Primary prevention therapy	3.1 In patients with a normal LVEF scheduled to undergo cancer therapy with known cardiotoxic agents and risk factors for cardiac toxicity, prophylactic use of angiotensin-converting enzyme inhibitors (ACE-I) or alternatively, angiotensin receptor blocker (ARB), and/or selected beta-blockers (BB) may be considered to reduce the risk of cardiotoxicity (LOE: II, GOR: B). • Dexrazoxane has been validated as a cardio-protectant in selected populations who are receiving anthracycline-based chemotherapy (LOE: II, GOR: C). • In patients with pre existing cardiomyopathy, who require anthracycline-based chemotherapy (ChT), concomitant administration of dexrazoxane from the beginning of anthracycline therapy can be considered regardless of the type of cancer (LOE: III, GOR: C). 3.2 Patients with evidence of hyperlipidemia may benefit from treatment during active cancer therapy, especially cardiotoxic chemotherapy (LOE: II, GOR: C).
4. During cancer treatment: Cardiac safety surveillance	4.1 The following general principles are recommended for medical imaging in patients with cancer at risk for cardiac complications particularly for the periodic assessment of LV systolic function: • Highly reproducible, quantitative volumetric, nonirradiating imaging with quality control is recommended (quantitative 2-dimensional [2D] and 3-dimensional [3D] echocardiography, and cardiac magnetic resonance imaging [MRI]) (LOE: I, GOR: A). • For each patient, the same imaging modality at the same facility is highly recommended for serial testing (LOE: I, GOR: A). • LV global longitudinal strain (GLS) imaging may be considered, when available, for baseline and serial LV systolic function monitoring (LOE: III, GOR: C). 4.2 Asymptomatic patients receiving anthracycline-based chemotherapy with no cardiac biomarker or imaging abnormalities should undergo surveillance for risk stratification and the early detection of cardiac toxicity: • Periodic (every 3–6 weeks or prior to each cycle) measurement of TnI or TnT and BNP or NT-proBNP using the same institutional laboratory with an acceptable 99% upper limit of normal reference range being the threshold for abnormal (LOE: III, GOR: C). • Reassessment of LVEF and GLS (when possible) following the general imaging principles is recommended after a cumulative dose of 250 mg/m^2 of doxorubicin or its equivalent anthracycline, after approximately each additional 100 mg/m^2 (or ~200 mg/m^2 of epirubicin) beyond 250 mg/m^2, and at the end of therapy even if the cumulative dose is less than 400 mg/m^2 (LOE: I, GOR: A). 4.3 Aligned to the current recommendations by the US Food and Drug Administration (FDA) for patients who are asymptomatic and nonmetastatic undergoing adjuvant trastuzumab treatment, routine surveillance consisting of cardiac imaging every 3 months should be considered for the early detection of cardiac toxicity. However, the effectiveness of this strategy in patients at low CV risk with no evidence of early LV dysfunction has not been demonstrated (LOE: II, GOR: B). 4.4 Cardiac biomarker assessment may be considered as a valuable tool for cardiac safety surveillance in patients receiving adjuvant anti-HER2-based treatment (LOE: III, GOR: C). 4.5 Asymptomatic patients receiving anti-HER2-based treatment (trastuzumab, pertuzumab, T-DM1) for metastatic disease should have general surveillance for cardiac toxicity that may consist of periodic physical examination, cardiac biomarkers, and/or cardiac imaging (LOE: I, GOR: B). 4.6 In patients receiving cancer therapeutics associated with risk of systemic hypertension, especially anti–vascular endothelial growth factor (anti-VEGF) based therapy, establishment of a baseline blood pressure (BP) measurement and serial BP monitoring is recommended along with surveillance for the early detection of CV toxicity that may consist of periodic cardiac examination, cardiac biomarkers, and/or cardiac imaging (LOE: I, GOR: A).

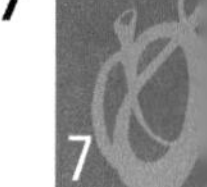

TABLE 7.3 2020 European Society of Medicine Oncology Consensus Recommendations for the Management of Cardiac Disease in Patients With Cancer Throughout Oncologic Treatment—Cont'd

SECTION	RECOMMENDATIONS
5. During cancer treatment: Asymptomatic, new laboratory abnormalities (or preclinical toxicity)	5.1 In asymptomatic patients receiving treatment with anthracyclines, an LVEF decrease of ≥10% from baseline to below 50%, or decrease in LVEF to ≥40% but <50%, the following evaluations are recommended (LOE: III, GOR: A): • Cardiology consultation (preferably a Cardio-Oncology specialist). • Consider initiation of cardio-protective treatment (Angiotensin-converting enzyme inhibitor [ACE-I] or angiotensin receptor blocker [ARB] ± beta blocker [BB] and perhaps a statin), if not already prescribed. • Consider measuring cardiac biomarkers (TnI or TnT and BNP or NT-proBNP) and perform a cardiac focused physical examination after each dose of anthracycline. • Repeat LVEF ± GLS measurement after every other dose of anthracycline-based chemotherapy. • If further anthracycline therapy is planned, the benefit risk assessment of continued anthracycline-based therapy as well as options of nonanthracycline regimens should be discussed, with consideration for the use of dexrazoxane and/or liposomal doxorubicin. 5.2 In asymptomatic patients receiving treatment with trastuzumab, an LVEF decrease of ≥10% from baseline to below 50%, or a decrease in LVEF to ≥40% but <50%, the following evaluations are recommended (LOE: III, GOR: A): • Cardiology consultation (preferably a Cardio-Oncology specialist). • Consider initiation of cardio-protective treatment (ACE-I or ARB ± BB), if not already prescribed. • Consider measuring cardiac biomarkers (TnI or TnT and BNP or NT-proBNP) at a suggested interval of every 4–6 weeks and a periodic cardiac-focused physical examination for ongoing monitoring of cardiac toxicity. • Repeat LVEF ± GLS measurement within 3–6 weeks after holding trastuzumab, and if LVEF ± GLS has normalized, trastuzumab therapy can be resumed. 5.3 In asymptomatic patients receiving treatment with any cardiotoxic cancer therapy with normal LVEF, but a decrease in average GLS from baseline assessment (≥12% relative decrease or ≥5% absolute decrease), the following evaluation and treatment should be considered (LOE: III, GOR: B): • Consider initiation of cardio-protective treatment (ACE-I or ARB ± BB), if not already prescribed. • Repeat LVEF ± GLS measurement every 3 months, or sooner, if cardiac symptoms develop • Life-saving cancer treatment should not be altered solely based on changes in LV strain. 5.4 In asymptomatic patients undergoing treatment with cardiotoxic anticancer therapy and an elevation in cardiac troponin, the following measures should be considered (LOE: III, GOR: C): • Cardiology consultation, preferably a Cardio-Oncology specialist. • Consider LVEF and GLS assessment with echocardiography. • Appropriate evaluation to exclude ischemic heart disease as a comorbidity. • Consider initiation of cardioprotective treatments (ACEIs, ARBs, and/or BBs), if not already prescribed. • Consider initiation of dexrazoxane in patients undergoing anthracycline-based ChT. • It is possible that anticancer therapy may be continued without interruption if only mild elevations in cardiac biomarkers occur without significant LVD.
6. During cancer treatment: Clinical cardiac dysfunction	6.1 In patients with an abnormal LVEF <50% but ≥40%, medical therapy with an ACE-I (or ARB) and/or BB is recommended prior to starting potential cardiotoxic treatment (LOE: I, GOR: A). 6.2 For those with an LVEF <40%, anthracycline therapy, in particular, is not recommended unless no other effective alternative cancer treatment option is available (LOE: IV, GOR: A). 6.3 For a patient receiving treatment with any cardiotoxic agent presenting with potentially cardiac-related but unexplained signs and symptoms such as (but not limited to) sinus tachycardia, rapid weight gain, dyspnea, peripheral edema or ascites, it is recommended to obtain a Cardio-Oncology consultation, reassess LVEF ± GLS, and potentially measuring cardiac biomarkers (LOE: III, GOR: A). 6.4 For a patient receiving treatment with trastuzumab (or any HER2 targeted molecular therapy) with signs and symptoms of heart failure, or an asymptomatic patient with an LVEF <40%, the same assessments as those for an LVEF ≥40% are recommended. In addition, trastuzumab (or any HER2 targeted molecular therapy) should be held until the cardiac status has stabilized and a discussion regarding the risk/benefits of continuation should be held with the multidisciplinary team and the patient (LOE: I, GOR: A).

Continued

TABLE 7.3 2020 European Society of Medicine Oncology Consensus Recommendations for the Management of Cardiac Disease in Patients With Cancer Throughout Oncologic Treatment—Cont'd

SECTION	RECOMMENDATIONS
	6.5 For a patient in whom trastuzumab (or any HER2 targeted molecular therapy) has been interrupted, whose LVEF has increased to ≥40% and/or whose signs and symptoms of heart failure have resolved, resumption of trastuzumab (or any HER2 targeted molecular therapy) should be considered, along with the following recommendations (LOE: III, GOR: B): • Continued medical therapy for heart failure and ongoing cardiology care • Periodic cardiac biomarker (BNP or NT-proBNP) assessment • Periodic LVEF assessments during ongoing treatment 6.6 For a patient in whom trastuzumab (or any HER2 targeted molecular therapy) has been interrupted, whose signs and symptoms of heart failure do not resolve, cardiac biomarker does not normalize, and/or LVEF remains <40%, resumption of trastuzumab may be considered if no alternative therapeutic options exist. The risk-benefit assessment of prognosis from cancer versus heart failure should be discussed with the multidisciplinary team and the patient (LOE: IV, GOR: C). 6.7 For a patient receiving treatment with sunitinib (or any other anti-VEGF based therapy) with signs and symptoms of heart failure, assessment of BP control is recommended and measurement of LVEF and/or cardiac biomarkers should be considered. In addition, sunitinib (or any other anti-VEGF based therapies) should be interrupted until the appropriateness of reinstituting this therapy has been fully assessed (LOE: III, GOR: A).
7. After cancer treatment	7.1 For asymptomatic patients who have been treated with cardiotoxic agents and have normal cardiac function, periodic screening for the development of new asymptomatic LV dysfunction with cardiac biomarkers and potentially cardiac imaging should be considered at 1- and 2-years after treatment, and consideration for reassessment periodically thereafter (LOE: III, GOR: B). 7.2 For patients who developed asymptomatic LV dysfunction or heart failure owing to trastuzumab (or any other HER2 targeted molecular therapy), anthracycline, or other cancer therapy, CV care including medical treatment with ACE-I (or ARB) and/or BB, and regular CV evaluation (e.g., annually, if asymptomatic) should be continued indefinitely, regardless of improvement in LVEF or symptoms. Any decision to withdraw guideline-based medical therapy should only be done after a period of stability, no active cardiac risk factors, and no further active cancer therapy (LOE: III, GOR: B). 7.3 For patients with a history of mediastinal or chest radiation, evaluation for coronary artery disease and myocardial ischemia as well as valvular heart disease is recommended, even if asymptomatic, starting at 5 years posttreatment and then at least every 3–5 years thereafter (LOE: I, GOR: A).
8. Immune checkpoint inhibitor-associated CV toxicity	8.1 For patients who develop new CV symptoms or are incidentally noted to have any arrhythmia, conduction abnormality on ECG or LVSD on echocardiogram, while undergoing (or after recent completion) of ICI therapy, further appropriate work-up (ECG, troponin, BNP or NT-pro BNP, C-reactive protein, viral titer, echocardiogram with GLS, cardiac MRI) for immune checkpoint inhibitor (ICI)-associated CV toxicity, particularly myocarditis and other common differential diagnoses should be carried out promptly (LOE: IV, GOR: C). 8.2 Endomyocardial biopsy for diagnosis should be considered if the diagnosis is highly suspected with otherwise negative work-up (LOE:IV, GOR:C). 8.3 With either suspicion or confirmation of ICI-associated myocarditis, further therapy with ICIs should be withheld and high-dose corticosteroids (methylprednisolone 1000 mg/day followed by oral prednisone 1 mg/kg/day) should be initiated promptly. Corticosteroids should be continued until resolution of symptoms and normalization of troponin, LV systolic function and conduction abnormalities (LOE: IV, GOR: C). 8.4 For steroid-refractory or high-grade myocarditis with hemodynamic instability, other immunosuppressive therapies such as antithymocyte globulin, infliximab (except in patients with HF), mycophenolate mofetil or abatacept should be considered (LOE: IV, GOR: C). 8.5 For patients with cardiomyopathy and/or HF, appropriate guideline-directed medical therapy and hemodynamic support should be provided as indicated (LOE: IV, GOR: C). 8.6 For patients with atrial or ventricular tachyarrhythmia or heart block, appropriate medical and supportive care should be provided, as indicated (LOE: IV, GOR: C). 8.7 ICI therapy should be permanently discontinued with any clinical myocarditis. The decision regarding restarting ICI therapy in the absence of alternative available antineoplastic therapy needs to be individualized with multidisciplinary discussion considering the cancer status, response to prior therapy, severity of cardiotoxicity, regression of toxicity with immunosuppressive therapy, and patient preference after weighing the risks and benefits. If ICI therapy needs to be restarted, monotherapy with an antiprogrammed cell death protein 1 (anti-PD-1) agent might be considered with very close surveillance for cardiotoxicity development (LOE: V, GOR: C).

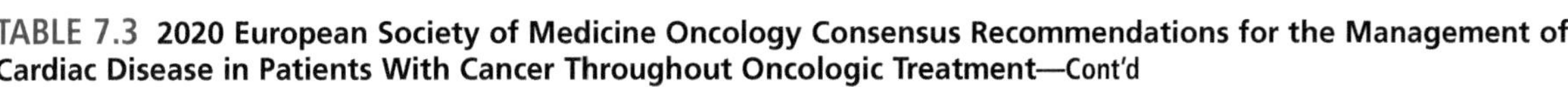

TABLE 7.3 **2020 European Society of Medicine Oncology Consensus Recommendations for the Management of Cardiac Disease in Patients With Cancer Throughout Oncologic Treatment—Cont'd**

SECTION	RECOMMENDATIONS
Level of evidence (LOE)	I. Evidence from at least one large randomized, controlled trial of good methodologic quality (low potential for bias) or meta-analyses of well-conducted randomized trials without heterogeneity II. Small randomized trials or large randomized trials with a suspicion of bias (lower methodologic quality) or meta-analyses of such trials or of trials with demonstrated heterogeneity III. Prospective cohort studies IV. Retrospective cohort studies or case-control studies V. Studies without control group, case reports, expert opinions
Grading of recommendation (GOR)	A. Strong evidence for efficacy with a substantial clinical benefit, strongly recommended B. Strong or moderate evidence for efficacy, but with a limited clinical benefit, generally recommended C. Insufficient evidence for efficacy or benefit does not outweigh the risk or the disadvantages (adverse events, costs, and so forth), optional D. Moderate evidence against efficacy or for adverse outcome, generally not recommended E. Strong evidence against efficacy or for adverse outcome, never recommended

REFERENCES

1. Legha SS, Benjamin RS, Mackay B, et al. Adriamycin therapy by continuous intravenous infusion in patients with metastatic breast cancer. *Cancer*. 1982;49:1762–1766.
2. Lipshultz SE, Miller TL, Lipsitz SR, et al. Continuous versus bolus infusion of doxorubicin in children with ALL: long-term cardiac outcomes. *Pediatrics*. 2012;130:1003–1011.
3. van Dalen EC, van der Pal HJ, Caron HN, Kremer LC. Different dosage schedules for reducing cardiotoxicity in patients with cancer receiving anthracycline chemotherapy. *Cochrane Database Syst Rev*. 2009;(4):CD005008.
4. van Dalen EC, van der Pal HJ, Kremer LC. Different dosage schedules for reducing cardiotoxicity in people with cancer receiving anthracycline chemotherapy. *Cochrane Database Syst Rev*. 2016; 3:CD005008.
5. Swain SM, Whaley FS, Gerber MC, Ewer MS, Bianchine JR, Gams RA. Delayed administration of dexrazoxane provides cardioprotection for patients with advanced breast cancer treated with doxorubicin-containing therapy. *J Clin Oncol*. 1997;15:1333–1340.
6. Swain SM, Whaley FS, Gerber MC, et al. Cardioprotection with dexrazoxane for doxorubicin-containing therapy in advanced breast cancer. *J Clin Oncol* 1997;15:1318-1332.
7. Herrmann J, Lerman A, Sandhu NP, Villarraga HR, Mulvagh SL, Kohli M. Evaluation and management of patients with heart disease and cancer: cardio-oncology. *Mayo Clin Proc*. 2014;89:1287–1306.
8. Ezaz G, Long JB, Gross CP, Chen J. Risk prediction model for heart failure and cardiomyopathy after adjuvant trastuzumab therapy for breast cancer. *J Am Heart Assoc*. 2014;3:e000472.
9. Darby SC, Ewertz M, McGale P, et al. Risk of ischemic heart disease in women after radiotherapy for breast cancer. *N Engl J Med*. 2013;368:987–998.
10. Zhang D, Guo W, Al-Hijji MA, et al. Outcomes of patients with severe symptomatic aortic valve stenosis after chest radiation: transcatheter versus surgical aortic valve replacement. *J Am Heart Assoc*. 2019;8:e012110.
11. Liu LK, Ouyang W, Zhao X, et al. Pathogenesis and prevention of radiation-induced myocardial fibrosis. *Asian Pac J Cancer Prev*. 2017;18:583-587.
12. Mahmood SS, Fradley MG, Cohen JV, et al. Myocarditis in patients treated with immune checkpoint inhibitors. *J Am Coll Cardiol*. 2018;71:1755–1764.
13. Altan M, Toki MI, Gettinger SN, et al. Immune checkpoint inhibitor-associated pericarditis. *J Thorac Oncol*. 2019;14:1102, et al1108.
14. Salem JE, Manouchehri A, Moey M, et al. Cardiovascular toxicities associated with immune checkpoint inhibitors: an observational, retrospective, pharmacovigilance study. *Lancet Oncol*. 2018;19: 1579–1589.
15. Anderson RD, Brooks M. Apical takotsubo syndrome in a patient with metastatic breast carcinoma on novel immunotherapy. *Int J Cardiol*. 2016;222:760–761.
16. Reddy N, Moudgil R, Lopez-Mattei JC, et al. Progressive and reversible conduction disease with checkpoint inhibitors. *Can J Cardiol*. 2017;33:1335.e13–1335.e15.
17. Tomita Y, Sueta D, Kakiuchi Y, et al. Acute coronary syndrome as a possible immune-related adverse event in a lung patient with cancer achieving a complete response to anti-PD-1 immune checkpoint antibody. *Ann Oncol*. 2017;28:2893–2895.
18. Yancy CW, Jessup M, Bozkurt B, et al. 2017 ACC/AHA/HFSA Focused Update of the 2013 ACCF/AHA Guideline for the Management of Heart Failure: a report of the American College of Cardiology/American Heart Association Task Force on Clinical Practice Guidelines and the Heart Failure Society of America. *Circulation*. 2017;136:e137–e161.
19. Bosch X, Rovira M, Sitges M, et al. Enalapril and carvedilol for preventing chemotherapy-induced left ventricular systolic dysfunction in patients with malignant hemopathies: the OVERCOME trial (preventiOn of left Ventricular dysfunction with Enalapril and caRvedilol in patients submitted to intensive ChemOtherapy for the treatment of Malignant hEmopathies). *J Am Coll Cardiol*. 2013;61:2355–2362.
20. Gulati G, Heck SL, Ree AH, et al. Prevention of cardiac dysfunction during adjuvant breast cancer therapy (PRADA): a 2 × 2 factorial, randomized, placebo-controlled, double-blind clinical trial of candesartan and metoprolol. *Eur Heart J*. 2016;37:1671–1680.
21. Acar Z, Kale A, Turgut M, et al. Efficiency of atorvastatin in the protection of anthracycline-induced cardiomyopathy. *J Am Coll Cardiol*. 2011;58:988–989.
22. Avila MS, Ayub-Ferreira SM, de Barros Wanderley Jr MR, et al. Carvedilol for prevention of chemotherapy-related cardiotoxicity: the CECCY trial. *J Am Coll Cardiol*. 2018;71:2281–2290.
23. Yancy CW, Jessup M, Bozkurt B, et al. 2013 ACCF/AHA guideline for the management of heart failure: executive summary: a report of the American College of Cardiology Foundation/American Heart Association Task Force on practice guidelines. *Circulation*. 2013;128:1810–1852.
24. Ledwidge M, Gallagher J, Conlon C, et al. Natriuretic peptide-based screening and collaborative care for heart failure: the STOP-HF randomized trial. *JAMA*. 2013;310:66–74.
25. Huelsmann M, Neuhold S, Resl M, et al. PONTIAC (NT-proBNP selected prevention of cardiac events in a population of diabetic patients without a history of cardiac disease): a prospective randomized controlled trial. *J Am Coll Cardiol*. 2013;62:1365–1372.
26. Brahmer JR, Lacchetti C, Thompson JA, et al. Management of immune–related adverse events in patients treated with immune checkpoint inhibitor therapy: American Society of Clinical Oncology Clinical Practice Guideline Summary. *J Oncol Pract*. 2018;14:247–249.
27. Armenian SH, Lacchetti C, Barac A, et al. Prevention and monitoring of cardiac dysfunction in survivors of adult cancers: American Society of Clinical Oncology Clinical Practice Guideline. *J Clin Oncol*. 2017;35:893–911
28. Curigliano C, Lenihan D, Fradley M, et al. Management of cardiac disease in patients with cancer throughout oncological treatment: ESMO Consensus Recommendations. *Ann Oncol*.2020;31:171–190.

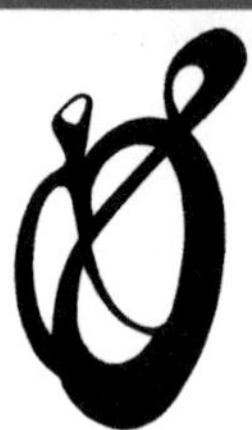

8 Vascular Disease Prevention: Before Cancer Therapy

JOERG HERRMANN

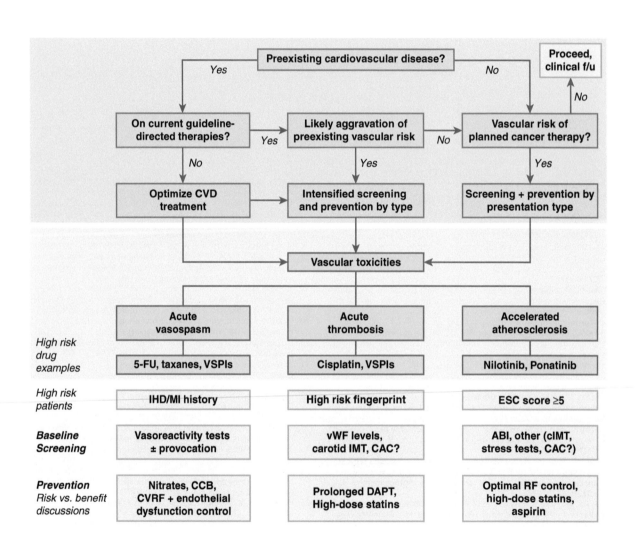

Preexisting cardiovascular disease?

Yes / No

On current guideline-directed therapies?

Yes → Likely aggravation of preexisting vascular risk

No → Vascular risk of planned cancer therapy?

No → Proceed, clinical f/u

No → Optimize CVD treatment → Intensified screening and prevention by type

Yes → Intensified screening and prevention by type

Yes → Screening + prevention by presentation type

Vascular toxicities

	Acute vasospasm	Acute thrombosis	Accelerated atherosclerosis
High risk drug examples	5-FU, taxanes, VSPIs	Cisplatin, VSPIs	Nilotinib, Ponatinib
High risk patients	IHD/MI history	High risk fingerprint	ESC score ≥5
Baseline Screening	Vasoreactivity tests ± provocation	vWF levels, carotid IMT, CAC?	ABI, other (cIMT, stress tests, CAC?)
Prevention *Risk vs. benefit discussions*	Nitrates, CCB, CVRF + endothelial dysfunction control	Prolonged DAPT, High-dose statins	Optimal RF control, high-dose statins, aspirin

CHAPTER OUTLINE

KEY POINTS

- The goal of the pretherapy vascular assessment is to define the likelihood that vascular events will develop during cancer therapy, complicating the clinical course
- Vascular risk is defined by the patient's underlying vascular disease status, the vascular toxicity potential of the cancer therapy, and the interaction potential of these
- Screening tests for vascular health, such as endothelial function/vasoreactivity test, von Willebrand factor levels, and carotid intima-media thickness, may be useful
- Preventive strategies for those at high risk are tailored to the specific subtype of arterial vascular complications/toxicity risk: acute vasospasm, acute thrombosis, and accelerated atherosclerosis
- Correlating with the vascular toxicity potential, patients should receive a thorough discussion of the cardiovascular risks and benefits of the planned cancer therapy

Historically, thromboembolism has been the main, if not the only, concern in terms of vascular complications in patients with cancer.[1] In recent years, however, arterial vascular complications have been increasingly recognized.[2] A number of cancer therapies, including classical chemotherapeutics (Table 8.1), targeted therapies (Table 8.2), immunotherapies, and radiation therapy, have the potential to cause a variety of vasotoxicities.[3] These entail typical and atypical chest pain episodes, myocardial infarction, transient ischemic attack, stroke, claudication, critical limb ischemia, Raynaud's as well as deep venous thrombosis, and pulmonary embolism (Fig. 8.1).[3] Thromboembolic disease will be discussed elsewhere (see **Chapter 8**). This chapter will focus on arterial toxicities, specifically the assessment before cancer therapy. Chapters covering the management of arterial toxicities during and after cancer therapy follow (see Chapters 17 and 29).

VASCULAR RISKS AND IDENTIFYING THE PATIENT AT HIGH RISK

The goal of the pretherapy assessment is to define the cardiovascular risk of the individual patient in general and in the context of the planned cancer therapy. To do so requires familiarity with the drugs that can cause cardiovascular toxicities, the malignancies for which they are used, and their success rates. This is important for risk-benefit discussions, which should take place with the patient and the oncologist/hematologist as needed.

Importantly, although the vascular toxicity spectrum is broad, three principal types of presentations can be defined: acute vasospasm, acute thrombosis, and accelerated atherosclerosis (Table 8.3). It is valuable to think in these categories because risk evaluation and prevention differ for these presentations types (Fig. 8.2). A fourth type to consider is vasculitis, which can contribute to all three previously mentioned disease processes. Also, certain drugs are associated with the risk of more than one, possibly with all of these vascular toxicity presentations (e.g., cisplatin and especially vascular endothelial growth factor [VEGF] signaling pathway inhibitors). This needs to be taken into account.

Acute vasospasm can involve various and sometimes even multiple different vascular territories, the most common being the peripheral vasculature (Raynaud's) and the coronary vasculature (ischemic heart disease [IHD]).[4–6] Of these two, most attention has been given to coronary vasospasm given its potential for fatal implications.[7,8] This being said, Raynaud's can lead to debilitating symptoms and even losses of digits.[9,10] For some, for example, patients undergoing therapy with bleomycin, Raynaud's can precede manifestations of IHDs arguing for a systemic effect. Other cancer therapeutics known to cause vasospasm include 5-FU, capecitabine, paclitaxel, cisplatin, bleomycin, VEGF inhibitors such as sorafenib, and Bcr-Abl inhibitors such as dasatinib.

The cardiovascular toxicity presentations with 5-FU treatment can span from myocardial ischemia to unstable angina, VT, cardiac function decline, and even sudden cardiac death.[11–14] Cardiovascular disease (CVD) and especially IHD is a prominent risk factor (eight-fold higher risk).[15] In fact, assessing for a history of myocardial infarction (MI) seems to suffice to identify the high risk individual (see Fig. 8.1).[15] Thus, a thorough history should be obtained in each patient, and those with a history of IHD/MI should be appropriately "flagged." Based on the outlined observations, screening for subclinical IHD does not seem to be needed and may not translate into a tangible difference. Furthermore, it would remain a matter for debate if a functional (noninvasive cardiac stress test) or an

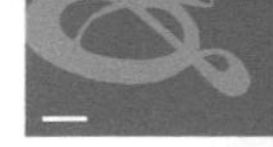

TABLE 8.1 Spectrum of Vascular Toxicities of Conventional Chemotherapies[1]

THERAPY	CANCER THERAPY INDICATIONS (LABEL AND OFF-LABEL)	TOXICITY HTN	ANGINA	AMI	RAYNAUD SYNDROME	STROKE	PAD	PULMONARY HTN	DVT/PE
Alkylating Agents									
Cisplatin	Bladder cancer, breast cancer, cervical cancer, endometrial carcinoma, esophageal and gastric cancer, head and neck cancer, HL, malignant pleural mesothelioma, multiple myeloma, NHL, osteosarcoma, ovarian cancer, penile cancer, SCLC, testicular cancer	–	++	++	+	+	+	–	–
Cyclophosphamide	ALL, breast cancer, CLL, Ewing sarcoma, HL, multiple myeloma, NHL, SCLC, stem-cell transplant condition	–	+	+	–	–	–	+	–
Antimetabolites									
5-Fluorouracil	Anal carcinoma, bladder cancer, breast cancer, cervical cancer, colorectal cancer, esophageal cancer, gastric cancer, hepatobiliary cancer, pancreatic cancer, squamous cell carcinomas	–	ND	ND	ND	ND	–	–	–
Capecitabine	Anal carcinoma, breast cancer, colorectal cancer, esophageal cancer, gastric cancer, hepatobiliary cancer, ovarian, fallopian peritoneal cancer, pancreatic cancer, cancer of unknown primary	+	++	++	+	+	–	–	+
Gemcitabine	Breast cancer, NSCLC, ovarian cancer, pancreatic cancer, bladder cancer, cervical cancer, head and neck cancer, hepatobiliary cancer, HL, malignant pleural mesothelioma, non-NHL, sarcomas, SCLC, testicular cancer, adenocarcinoma of unknown primary, uterine cancer	–	+	+	+	–	–	–	–
Microtubule-Binding Agents									
Paclitaxel	Breast cancer, NSCLC, ovarian cancer, Kaposi sarcoma, bladder cancer, cervical cancer, esophageal and gastric cancer, head and neck cancers, penile cancer, SCLC, soft tissue sarcoma, testicular germ cell tumors, thymoma, adenocarcinoma of unknown primary	+	+	+	–	–	–	–	+
Antitumor Antibiotics									
Bleomycin	HL, testicular cancer, ovarian germ cell cancer	–	+	+	+	+		+	–
Vinca Alkaloids									
Vincristine	ALL, central nervous system tumors, HL, NHL, Ewing sarcoma, gestational trophoblastic tumors, multiple myeloma, ovarian cancer, primary CNS lymphoma, SCLC, thymoma	ND	ND	ND	ND	–	–	–	–
Immunomodulatory Drugs									
IFNa2B	Hairy cell leukemia, lymphoma, malignant melanoma, Kaposi sarcoma	++	+++	++	++	++	++	++	++

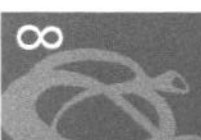

TABLE 8.1 Spectrum of Vascular Toxicities of Conventional Chemotherapies[1]—cont'd

THERAPY	CANCER THERAPY INDICATIONS (LABEL AND OFF-LABEL)	TOXICITY HTN	ANGINA	AMI	RAYNAUD SYNDROME	STROKE	PAD	PULMONARY HTN	DVT/PE
Thalidomide	Multiple myeloma, systemic light chain amyloidosis, Waldenstrom macroglobulinemia	–	–	–	–	–	–	–	+++
Lenalidomide	CLL, diffuse large B-cell lymphoma, mantle cell lymphoma, multiple myeloma, myelodysplastic syndrome	++	++	++	–	++	–	–	+++

Based on data from IBM Micromedex (IBM, NY, USA) and Lexicomp (Wolters Kluwer, Netherlands).
–, not reported; +, uncommon (<1%), ++, common (1–10%), +++, very common (>10%).
ALL, Acute lymphoblastic leukemia; *AMI,* acute myocardial infarction; *CLL,* chronic lymphocytic leukemia; *CML,* chronic myeloid leukemia; *CNS,* central nervous system; *DVT,* deep vein thrombosis; *GIST,* gastrointestinal stromal tumors; *HL,* Hodgkin lymphoma; *HTN,* hypertension; *ND,* frequency not defined; *NHL,* non-Hodgkin lymphoma; *NSCLC,* non–small-cell lung cancer; *PAD,* peripheral artery disease; *PE,* pulmonary embolism; *SCLC,* small-cell lung cancer.

TABLE 8.2 Spectrum of Vascular Toxicities of Targeted Cancer Therapies[1]

THERAPY	CANCER THERAPY INDICATIONS (LABEL AND OFF-LABEL)	TOXICITY HTN	ANGINA	AMI	RAYNAUD SYNDROME	STROKE	PAD	PULMONARY HTN	DVT/PE
Proteasome Inhibitors									
Bortezomib	Multiple myeloma, mantle cell lymphoma, T-cell lymphoma, follicular lymphoma, systemic light chain amyloidosis, Waldenstrom macroglobulinemia	+	–	ND	–	ND	–	ND	ND
Carfilzomib	Multiple myeloma, Waldenstrom macroglobulinemia	+++	+++	+++	–	–	–	++	–
mTOR Inhibitors									
Everolimus	Breast cancer, neuroendocrine tumors, RCC	+++	++	+	–	–	–	–	++
Temsirolimus	RCC	++	+++	–	–	–	–	–	++
Monoclonal Antibodies (Target)									
Rituximab (anti-CD20)	Burkitt lymphoma, CLL, CNS lymphoma, HL, NHL, Waldenstrom macroglobulinemia	+++	+	+	–	–	–	–	–
Bevacizumab (anti-VEGF–VEGFR2)	Glioblastoma, persistent/recurrent/metastatic cervical cancer, metastatic colorectal cancer, non–small (nonsquamous)-cell lung cancer	+++	++	++	–	++	–	–	+++
Ramucirumab (anti-VEGF–VEGFR2)	Metastatic NSCLC, metastatic gastric, metastatic colorectal cancer	+++	–	++	–	++	–	–	–

Continued

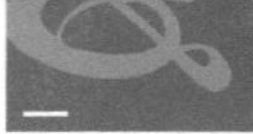

TABLE 8.2 **Spectrum of Vascular Toxicitiesof Targeted Cancer Therapies[1]—cont'd**

THERAPY	CANCER THERAPY INDICATIONS (LABEL AND OFF-LABEL)	TOXICITY							
		HTN	ANGINA	AMI	RAYNAUD SYNDROME	STROKE	PAD	PULMONARY HTN	DVT/PE
VEGFR Fusion Molecules									
Aflibercept	Metastatic colorectal cancer	+++	–	++	–	++	–	–	++
Multi-Targeted Kinase Inhibitors (Primary Target)									
Axitinib (VEGFR1–3)	RCC, thyroid cancer	+++	+	++	–	+	–	–	++
Cabozantinib (VEGFR2)	RCC, thyroid cancer, hepatocellular carcinoma	+++	–	++	–	++	–	–	++
Lenvatinib (VEGFR1–3)	RCC, thyroid cancer, hepatocellular carcinoma	+++	–	++	–	–	–	–	++
Regorafenib (VEGFR2)	Colorectal cancer, GIST, hepatocellular carcinoma	+++	+	+	–	–	–	–	++
Sorafenib (VEGFR1–3)	Hepatocellular cancer, RCC, thyroid cancer, angiosarcoma, GIST	+++	+	++	–	+	–	–	+
Sunitinib (VEGFR1–3)	GIST, pancreatic neuroendocrine tumors, RCC, soft tissue sarcoma, thyroid cancer	+++	+++	+	–	+	–	–	++
Pazopanib (VEGFR1–3)	RCC, soft tissue carcinoma, thyroid cancer	+++	+++	++	–	+	–	–	++
Vandetanib (VEGFR)	Thyroid cancer	+++	–	–	–	+	–	–	++
Dasatinib (BCR–ABL1)	Philadelphia chromosome-positive ALL and CML, GIST		++	–	–	–	–	++	<1%
Nilotinib (BCR–ABL1)	Philadelphia chromosome-positive ALL and CML, GIST	++	++	+	–	++	+++	–	ND
Ponatinib (BCR–ABL1)	Philadelphia chromosome-positive ALL and CML	+++	+++	+++		++	++		++
Alectinib (ALK)	NSCLC	–	–	–	–	–	–	–	+
Crizotinib (ALK)	NSCLC	–	–	–	–	–	–	–	++

TABLE 8.2 Spectrum of Vascular Toxicities of Targeted Cancer Therapies[1]—cont'd

THERAPY	CANCER THERAPY INDICATIONS (LABEL AND OFF-LABEL)	TOXICITY HTN	ANGINA	AMI	RAYNAUD SYNDROME	STROKE	PAD	PULMONARY HTN	DVT/PE
Dacomitinib (EGFR)	NSCLC	–	++	–	–	–	–	–	
Erlotinib (EGFR)	NSCLC, pancreatic cancer	–	+++	++[a]	–	++[a]	–	–	+++[a]
Dabrafenib (BRAF)	Melanoma, NSCLC, thyroid cancer	+++	–	–	–	–	–	–	+
Cabozantinib (MET)	Hepatocellular carcinoma, RCC, thyroid cancer	+++	–	+	–	+	–	–	++
Crizotinib (MET)	NSCLC		–	–	–	–	–	–	++
Binimetinib (MEK)	Melanoma	++	–	–	–	–	–	–	++[b]
Trametinib (MEK)	Melanoma, NSCLC, thyroid cancer	+++	–	–	–	–	–	–	++[b]

Based on data from IBM Micromedex (IBM, NY, USA) and Lexicomp (Wolters Kluwer, Netherlands).

+, uncommon (<1%); ++, common (1–10%); +++, very common (>10%).

ALL, Acute lymphoblastic leukemia; *AMI,* acute myocardial infarction; *CLL,* chronic lymphocytic leukemia; *CML,* chronic myeloid leukemia; *CNS,* central nervous system; *DVT,* deep vein thrombosis; *GIST,* gastrointestinal stromal tumors; *HL,* Hodgkin lymphoma; *HTN,* hypertension; *mTOR,* mechanistic target of rapamycin; *ND,* frequency not defined; *NHL,* non-Hodgkin lymphoma; *NSCLC,* non–small-cell lung cancer; *PAD,* peripheral artery disease; *PE,* pulmonary embolism; *RCC,* renal cell carcinoma; *SCLC,* small-cell lung cancer; *VEGF,* vascular endothelial growth factor; *VEGFR,* vascular endothelial growth factor receptor.

[a]In combination with gemcitabine.

[b]In combination with a BRAF inhibitor.

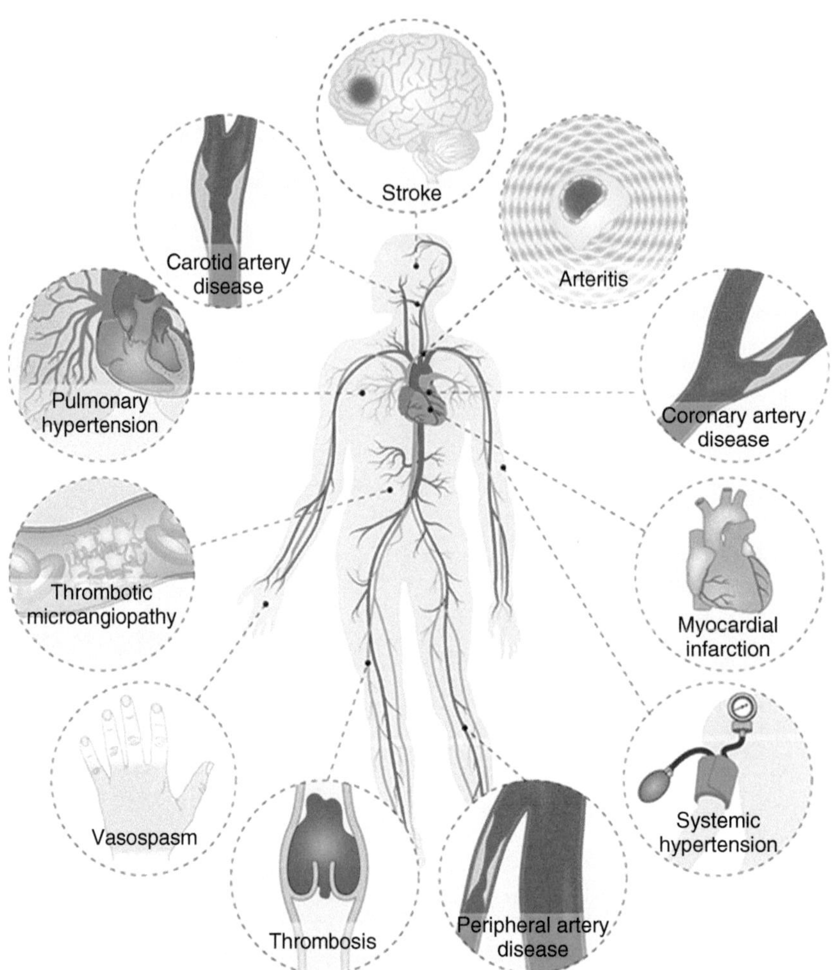

FIG. 8.1 Outline of the spectrum of vascular toxicities with cancer therapies. (From Herrmann J. Vascular toxic effects of cancer therapies. *Nat Rev Cardiol*. 2020;17(8):503–522. doi:10.1038/s41569-020-0347-2.)

anatomic test (coronary computed tomography angiography) would provide better information. The latter would outline the overall burden of coronary artery disease (CAD). Decisions on coronary angiography are to be made in the context of the findings, the comorbidities, the planned cancer therapies, and the patient's wishes. Most certainly they should not routinely be made, and as outlined, simple history taking may suffice.

Risk factors for peripheral vasospasm in patients with cancer are not defined in this cohort of patients, but very likely smoking is a significant factor.[16] Other cardiovascular risk factors are likely of significance as well, especially in combination. They can impair endothelial function and thereby play a facilitating role for vasospastic presentations.[17] Peripheral arterial vasoreactivity studies with provocation maneuvers can be used to test baseline predisposition. The Endo-PAT evaluates both endothelium-dependent and-independent vasoreactivity of the forearm and hand circulation.[18] On the contrary, flow-mediated dilatation of the brachial artery is more specific for site and function (endothelium-dependent vasoreactivity). It is often also more difficult to do, whereas the Endo-PAT can be easily done without much training and operator dependence.[19]

Cancer drugs associated with *acute thrombosis* include cisplatin and VSP inhibitors.[20,21] Among patients undergoing treatment with the VSP inhibitor bevacizumab, patients at highest risk of arterioembolic events (ATE) are those >65 years of age with a

TABLE 8.3 **Overview of the Three Principal Presentations of Arterial Vascular Toxicity With Cancer Therapy**[1]

	MAIN PRESENTATION		
CHARACTERISTICS	ACUTE VASOSPASM	ACUTE THROMBOSIS	ACCELERATED ATHEROSCLEROSIS
Onset after start of cancer therapy	Days to weeks	Weeks to years	Months to decades
Reversibility	Very likely	Likely	Very unlikely
Primary culprit	Vascular smooth muscle cells	Endothelial cells	Endothelial cells
Secondary culprit	Endothelial cells	Platelets	Bone-marrow derived cells, proinflammatory cells
High levels of circulating endothelial cells	+	++	+
Low levels of endothelial progenitor cells	+	+	+
Procoagulant microvesicles	–	+	–
Examples of cancer therapeutics	5-Fluorouracil, capecitabine, platinum drugs, VEGF inhibitors	Platinum drugs, bleomycin, vinca alkaloids, VEGF inhibitors, ICIs	Nilotinib, ponatinib, cisplatin, VEGF inhibitors
Treatment	Nitrates, calcium-channel blocker (CCB)	Thrombectomy with/without PTCA, stent; DAPT, statin therapy	Revascularization, aspirin, statins, amlodipine, ACE inhibitor, exercise
On-therapy screening	Signs and symptoms	Signs and symptoms	Signs and symptoms
	Vasoreactivity studies, ECG (ST-segment elevation) monitoring	vWF levels, circulating endothelial cell and/or endothelial progenitor cell levels	Ankle–brachial index, cardiac stress test, coronary CT angiography
Pretherapy screening and prevention	Prophylactic therapy with nitrates and CCB	DAPT, statin therapy	Strict risk factor control, especially lipids (anti-IL-1β), aspirin, statin and/or other therapies
	CVD risk stratification: risk factors and/or disease, testing for subclinical ASCVD and/or abnormal vasoreactivity, including endothelial dysfunction	CVD risk stratification: risk factors, testing for subclinical ASCVD, endothelial dysfunction, vWF levels	CVD risk stratification: risk factors, testing for subclinical ASCVD

ACE, Angiotensin-converting enzyme; *ASCVD,* atherosclerotic cardiovascular disease; *CVD,* cardiovascular disease; *DAPT,* dual antiplatelet therapy; *ECG,* electrocardiogram; *ICI,* immune checkpoint inhibitor; *PTCA,* percutaneous transluminal coronary angioplasty, *VEGF,* vascular endothelial growth factor; *vWF,* von Willebrand factor.

prior ATE.[22] For patients with cancer undergoing cisplatin-based therapy a clinical high risk fingerprint has been identified, defined by the presence of at least 3 risk factors (BMI >25 kg/m^2, current smoking, BP >140/90 mm Hg [or treated], hyperlipidemia [or treated], elevated fasting plasma glucose).[23] Of further note, carotid intima-media-thickness (IMT) is higher in these patients arguing for the use of new cardiovascular risk markers in these patients. C-reactive protein levels, however, are likely confounded by the malignant process and whether coronary calcium screening or CCTA is of value and cost-effective is not known. This being said, von Willebrand factor (vWF) has recently emerged as a possible marker of high risk. Levels of vWF are higher at baseline and show a clear rise and fall pattern in patients with testicular cancer cisplatin-based chemotherapy who develop ATEs (see Fig. 8.2).[23,24]

Accelerated atherosclerosis is the third presentation and has become known as *progressive arterial occlusive disease* with the use of Bcr-Abl inhibitors such as nilotinib and ponatinib.[25–30] It may also be seen with VEGF inhibitors and cisplatin.[31–36] Most commonly it had been associated with radiation therapy in the past, which remains of concern though recent changes in radiation therapy have substantially reduced the

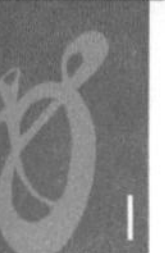

Vasospasm Example 5-FU	Arterial Thrombosis Example Cisplatin	Accelerated Atherosclerosis Example Nilotinib
At risk groups: Ischemic heart disease history, specifically history of prior myocardial infarction (MI)	High risk fingerprint (≥3 of the following): • BMI >25 kg/m² • Current smoking • BP >140/90 mm Hg (or treated) • Hyperlipidemia (or treated) • Elevated FPG	ESC Score (varies by high/low risk country): • Age • Current smoking • Systolic blood pressure • Total cholesterol level • Gender

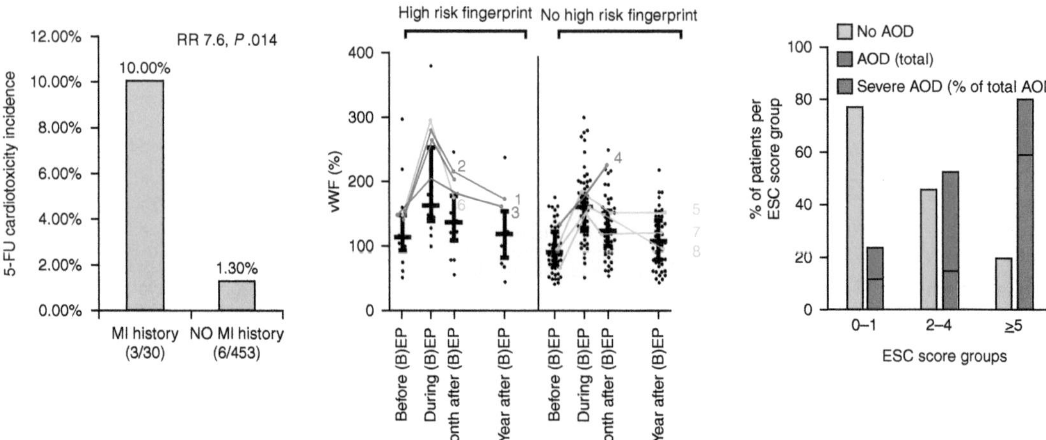

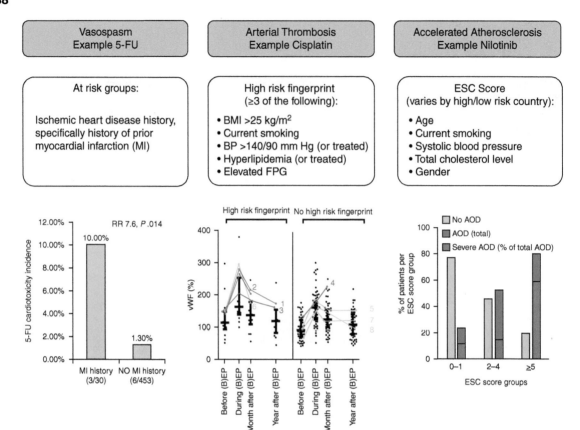

FIG. 8.2 Overview of defined risk factors for high risk groups in the three vascular toxicity presentation categories.

risk.[37–39] The manifestations with radiation therapy are territorial, that is, arterial disease matches radiation exposure in location and intensity/severity. With nilotinib, the lower extremity circulation is predisposed, but involvement of coronary and cerebral vasculature is seen as well. The distribution pattern of vascular disease with ponatinib is more diverse but also involves the peripheral vasculature in a substantial number of patients. For VEGF inhibitors and cisplatin no predilection sites have been defined.

Based on the distribution patterns, the ankle-brachial index might be a very suitable test for patients on Bcr-Abl inhibitors.[40] This test can be performed in the office and is an ideal tool for serial follow-up. An evaluation for preexisting disease prior to initiation of therapy is important for establishing a baseline (similar to cardiac function with therapies that can cause cardiotoxicity). Patients with preexisting disease likely have a reduced reserve and may show more rapid progression. This concept is confirmed by the observation that an ESC score cutoff of 5 seems to differentiate very clearly between those who do not and those who do develop severe arterial occlusive disease (see Fig. 8.2).[41] This being said, even a small percentage of patients without preexisting atherosclerosis and a low risk score can develop accelerated and severe atherosclerosis.

Arteriosclerotic cardiovascular disease (ASCVD) or ESC risk scores will likely also help to define the at risk patients undergoing VEGF inhibitor and cisplatin therapy as well as those undergoing radiation therapy. For patients with breast cancer it has been shown that those who undergo left-sided radiation treatment, the risk of an acute coronary event is highest among those with a clinical history of IHD and especially MI.[42] Whether screening for silent CAD is useful is unknown at this point.

PREVENTION

Ideally patients at high risk for any of the outlined potential arterial vascular toxicities would be identified before initiation of therapy and subjected to effective primary preventive therapies. At present only limited recommendations can be provided as the current evidence base does not allow for official practice guidelines.

Regarding primary prevention efforts of *vasospasm*, for example, for patients undergoing 5-FU therapy, those identified as high risk based on a history of IHD should be provided sublingual nitroglycerin and possibly even long-acting nitrates. In fact, such patients are often already on nitrates and calcium channel blockers (CCBs) and remain at higher risk.[15] An important aspect is that vascular function/reactivity dynamics do not correlate one-to-one with the anatomic atherosclerotic plaque burden. The luminal margin, however, is reduced at stenosis sites, and the combination of functional and anatomic luminal reduction can quickly exhaust the reserve. Intervening on stenoses might thus have a beneficial impact locally but would not address the globally dysfunctional endothelium in these patients. If side effects are minor one could argue for starting any patients with CAD on vasodilator therapy. It has to be mentioned as well though that vasodilator therapy does not always prevent 5-FU cardiotoxicity, in keeping with the view that mechanisms other than vasospasm contribute to it.[11]

Defining patients at risk for peripheral vasospasm might be more difficult unless they have a history of Raynaud's. Baseline assessment of vasoreactivity ± provocation maneuvers might be useful in this subgroup. One easy-to-use modality is the Endo-PAT, and this testing modality could also be used to follow patients in their response to vasodilator therapy and cancer therapy. Peripheral and coronary vasoreactivity correlate to some degree.[43] Thus, this modality, or flow-mediated dilation of the brachial artery could serve as a general vascular assessment. The duration of assessment would continue until exposure to potentially harmful agents is complete. For some agents like cisplatin this may not be possible as circulating levels can remain elevated for years.

For *acute thrombosis*, preventive efforts should be directed toward improving endothelial health, which will likely reduce the risk of all three vascular toxicities. These interventions include optimal control of cardiovascular risk factors, statins and angiotensin-converting enzyme (ACE) inhibitors, and exercise. Patients at highest ATE risk while undergoing treatment with bevacizumab (and possibly any other type of VEGF inhibitor therapy) should be started on aspirin. These are patients ≥65 years with a prior ATE.[22] Based on their medical history they qualify for secondary prevention antiplatelet therapy regardless. In line with recent data on primary prevention with aspirin, age alone does not qualify and neither is there any other convincing subgroup in view of the increased risk of bleeding any such intervention need to be balanced with. This holds true as well when considering dual antiplatelet therapy (DAPT). For patients with cancer on cisplatin, an argument can be made to initiate or continue antiplatelet therapy in those deemed at high risk, for example, those with a high-risk fingerprint as outlined above or higher baseline vWF levels (>120%). Importantly, vWF stimulates platelet aggregation via a different signaling cascade than aspirin and P2Y inhibitors are designed to target; thus it may not be as potent and may unnecessarily expose patients to bleeding risk.[44] Overall, the bleeding risk may be highest with VEGF inhibitors.[45–48] Whether a patient develops thrombosis or bleeding may, however, not only be a function of platelet activity and inhibition but rather the consequence of the effects of VEGF receptor signaling inhibition on endothelial viability and vascular integrity within the context of the specific environment. Along these lines, capillary networks are more prone to collapse with the complications being either thrombosis with ischemia or rupture with bleeding.[49]

Patients, who are flagged as at high risk for *accelerated atherosclerosis* during therapy with the Bcr-Abl inhibitor nilotinib based on an ESC score ≥ 5, should be on high-dose statins, even if not hyperlipidemic, and on ACE inhibitor and/or amlodipine if hypertensive. Superb cardiovascular risk factor control is key, facilitated by optimal diet, weight, and exercise efforts. Lifestyle changes are the most difficult to implement. However, even modest changes can be impactful; for example, for exercise even only 150 minutes of moderate intensity exercise per week is sufficient. Smoking cessation is a must and includes all types of exposures. These patients should be instructed on signs and symptoms of vascular disease and the merit of serial ABIs.

For patients on VEGF inhibitor therapy or those undergoing radiation therapy optimal cardiovascular risk factor management is key and those with high ASCVD or ESC scores should follow the same management scheme outlined above.[50] For radiation, the effect is regionally more defined and follow-up can be directed accordingly to recognize and intervene on trends of progression early on. For VEGF inhibitors, this is more diffuse and follow-up evaluations need to be individualized.

In summary, the goal of the pre-therapy evaluation is to identify patients at high risk for vascular disease/events/toxicity not to categorically exclude from cancer therapy but to enable as many preemptive, preventive efforts as possible so that these patients can proceed with best possible cancer therapy adequately monitored and managed.

REFERENCES

1. Herrmann J. Vascular toxic effects of cancer therapies. *Nat Rev Cardiol.* 2020;17(8):503–522. doi:10.1038/s41569-020-0347-2.
2. Khorana AA, Francis CW, Culakova E, Kuderer NM, Lyman GH. Thromboembolism is a leading cause of death in patients with cancer receiving outpatient chemotherapy. *J Thromb Haemost.* 2007;5(3): 632–634.
3. Herrmann J, Yang EH, Iliescu CA, et al. Vascular toxicities of cancer therapies: the old and the new—an evolving avenue. *Circulation.* 2016;133(13):1272–1289.
4. Vogelzang NJ, Bosl GJ, Johnson K, Kennedy BJ. Raynaud's phenomenon: a common toxicity after combination chemotherapy for testicular cancer. *Ann Inter Med.* 1981;95(3):288–292.
5. Burger AJ, Mannino S. 5-Fluorouracil-induced coronary vasospasm. *Am Heart J.* 1987;114(2):433–436.
6. Schnetzler B, Popova N, Collao Lamb C, Sappino AP. Coronary spasm induced by capecitabine. *Ann Oncol.* 2001;12(5):723–724.
7. Fradley MG, Barrett CD, Clark JR, Francis SA. Ventricular fibrillation cardiac arrest due to 5-fluorouracil cardiotoxicity. *Tex Heart Inst J.* 2013;40(4):472–476.
8. Hayasaka K, Takigawa M, Takahashi A, et al. A case of ventricular fibrillation as a consequence of capecitabine-induced secondary QT prolongation: a case report. *J Cardiol Cases.* 2017;16(1):26–29.
9. Elomaa I, Pajunen M, Virkkunen P. Raynaud's phenomenon progressing to gangrene after vincristine and bleomycin therapy. *Acta Med Scand.* 1984;216(3):323–326.
10. Kopterides P, Tsavaris N, Tzioufas A, Pikazis D, Lazaris A. Digital gangrene and Raynaud's phenomenon as complications of lung adenocarcinoma. *Lancet Oncol.* 2004;5(9):549.
11. Sara JD, Kaur J, Khodadadi R, et al. 5-Fluorouracil and cardiotoxicity: a review. *Ther Adv Med Oncol.* 2018;10:1758835918780140.
12. Cerny J, Hassan A, Smith C, Piperdi B. Coronary vasospasm with myocardial stunning in a patient with colon cancer receiving adjuvant chemotherapy with FOLFOX regimen. *Clin Colorectal Cancer.* 2009;8(1):55–58.
13. Kobayashi N, Hata N, Yokoyama S, Shinada T, Shirakabe A, Mizuno K. A case of Takotsubo cardiomyopathy during 5-fluorouracil treatment for rectal adenocarcinoma. *J Nippon Med Sch.* 2009; 76(1):27–33.
14. Y-Hassan S, Tornvall P, Törnerud M, Henareh L. Capecitabine caused cardiogenic shock through induction of global Takotsubo syndrome. *Cardiovasc Revasc Med.* 2013;14(1):57–61.
15. Meyer CC, Calis KA, Burke LB, Walawander CA, Grasela TH. Symptomatic cardiotoxicity associated with 5-fluorouracil. *Pharmacotherapy.* 1997;17(4):729–736.
16. Wigley FM, Flavahan NA. Raynaud's phenomenon. *N Engl J Med.* 2016;375(6):556–565.
17. Lanza GA, Careri G, Crea F. Mechanisms of coronary artery spasm. *Circulation.* 2011;124(16):1774–1782.
18. Nohria A, Gerhard-Herman M, Creager MA, Hurley S, Mitra D, Ganz P. Role of nitric oxide in the regulation of digital pulse volume amplitude in humans. *J Appl Physiol (1985).* 2006;101(2):545–548.
19. Arrebola-Moreno AL, Laclaustra M, Kaski JC. Noninvasive assessment of endothelial function in clinical practice. *Rev Esp Cardiol (Engl Ed).* 2012;65(1):80–90.
20. Ito D, Shiraishi J, Nakamura T, et al. Primary percutaneous coronary intervention and intravascular ultrasound imaging for coronary thrombosis after cisplatin-based chemotherapy. *Heart Vessels.* 2012;27(6):634–638.
21. Moore RA, Adel N, Riedel E, et al. High incidence of thromboembolic events in patients treated with cisplatin-based chemotherapy: a large retrospective analysis. *J Clin Oncol.* 2011;29(25):3466–3473.
22. Scappaticci FA, Skillings JR, Holden SN, et al. Arterial thromboembolic events in patients with metastatic carcinoma treated with chemotherapy and bevacizumab. *J Natl Cancer Inst.* 2007;99(16): 1232–1239.
23. Lubberts S, Boer H, Altena R, et al. Vascular fingerprint and vascular damage markers associated with vascular events in testicular patients with cancer during and after chemotherapy. *Eur J Cancer.* 2016;63:180–188.
24. Dieckmann KP, Struss WJ, Budde U. Evidence for acute vascular toxicity of cisplatin-based chemotherapy in patients with germ cell tumour. *Anticancer Res.* 2011;31(12):4501-4505.
25. Aichberger KJ, Herndlhofer S, Schernthaner GH, et al. Progressive peripheral arterial occlusive disease and other vascular events during nilotinib therapy in CML. *Am J Hematol.* 2011;86(7):533–539.
26. Le Coutre P, Rea D, Abruzzese E, et al. Severe peripheral arterial disease during nilotinib therapy. *J Natl Cancer Inst.* 2011;103(17): 1347–1348.
27. Giles FJ, Mauro MJ, Hong F, et al. Rates of peripheral arterial occlusive disease in patients with chronic myeloid leukemia in the chronic phase treated with imatinib, nilotinib, or non-tyrosine kinase therapy: a retrospective cohort analysis. *Leukemia.* 2013;27(6):1310–1315.
28. Kim TD, Rea D, Schwarz M, et al. Peripheral artery occlusive disease in chronic phase chronic myeloid leukemia patients treated with nilotinib or imatinib. *Leukemia.* 2013;27(6):1316–1321.
29. Breccia M, Molica M, Zacheo I, Serrao A, Alimena G. Application of systematic coronary risk evaluation chart to identify chronic myeloid leukemia patients at risk of cardiovascular diseases during nilotinib treatment. *Ann Hematol.* 2015;94(3):393–397.
30. Valent P, Hadzijusufovic E, Schernthaner GH, Wolf D, Rea D, le Coutre P. Vascular safety issues in CML patients treated with BCR/ABL1 kinase inhibitors. *Blood.* 2015;125(6):901–906.
31. Winnik S, Lohmann C, Siciliani G, et al. Systemic VEGF inhibition accelerates experimental atherosclerosis and disrupts endothelial homeostasis—implications for cardiovascular safety. *Int J Cardiol.* 2013;168(3):2453–2461.
32. Meinardi MT, Gietema JA, van der Graaf WT, et al. Cardiovascular morbidity in long-term survivors of metastatic testicular cancer. *J Clin Oncol.* 2000;18(8):1725–1732.
33. van den Belt-Dusebout AW, Nuver J, de Wit R, et al. Long-term risk of cardiovascular disease in 5-year survivors of testicular cancer. *J Clin Oncol.* 2006;24(3):467–475.
34. van den Belt-Dusebout AW, de Wit R, Gietema JA, et al. Treatment-specific risks of second malignancies and cardiovascular disease in 5-year survivors of testicular cancer. *J Clin Oncol.* 2007; 25(28):4370–4378.
35. Haugnes HS, Wethal T, Aass N, et al. Cardiovascular risk factors and morbidity in long-term survivors of testicular cancer: a 20-year follow-up study. *J Clin Oncol.* 2010;28(30):4649–4657.
36. Huddart RA, Norman A, Shahidi M, et al. Cardiovascular disease as a long-term complication of treatment for testicular cancer. *J Clin Oncol.* 2003;21(8):1513–1523.
37. Brosius FC III, Waller BF, Roberts WC. Radiation heart disease. Analysis of 16 young (aged 15 to 33 years) necropsy patients who received over 3,500 rads to the heart. *Am J Med.* 1981;70(3):519–530.
38. Veinot JP, Edwards WD. Pathology of radiation-induced heart disease: a surgical and autopsy study of 27 cases. *Hum Pathol.* 1996;27(8):766–773.
39. Virmani R, Farb A, Carter AJ, Jones RM. Pathology of radiation-induced coronary artery disease in human and pig. *Cardiovasc Radiat Med.* 1999;1(1):98–101.

40. Moslehi JJ, Deininger M. Tyrosine kinase inhibitor-associated cardiovascular toxicity in chronic myeloid leukemia. *J Clin Oncol.* 2015;33(35):4210–4218.
41. Hadzijusufovic E, Albrecht-Schgoer K, Huber K, et al. Nilotinib-induced vasculopathy: identification of vascular endothelial cells as a primary target site. *Leukemia.* 2017;31(11):2388–2397.
42. Darby SC, Ewertz M, McGale P, et al. Risk of ischemic heart disease in women after radiotherapy for breast cancer. *N Engl J Med.* 2013;368(11):987–998.
43. Bonetti PO, Pumper GM, Higano ST, Holmes DR Jr, Kuvin JT, Lerman A. Noninvasive identification of patients with early coronary atherosclerosis by assessment of digital reactive hyperemia. *J Am Coll Cardiol.* 2004;44(11):2137–2141.
44. Shatzel JJ, Olson SR, Tao DL, McCarty OJT, Danilov AV, DeLoughery TG. Ibrutinib-associated bleeding: pathogenesis, management and risk reduction strategies. *J Thromb Haemost.* 2017;15(5):835–847.
45. Qi WX, Tang LN, Sun YJ, et al. Incidence and risk of hemorrhagic events with vascular endothelial growth factor receptor tyrosine-kinase inhibitors: an up-to-date meta-analysis of 27 randomized controlled trials. *Ann Oncol.* 2013;24(12):2943–2952.
46. Hang XF, Xu WS, Wang JX, et al. Risk of high-grade bleeding in patients with cancer treated with bevacizumab: a meta-analysis of randomized controlled trials. *Eur J Clin Pharmacol.* 2011;67(6):613–623.
47. Hapani S, Sher A, Chu D, Wu S. Increased risk of serious hemorrhage with bevacizumab in patients with cancer: a meta-analysis. *Oncology.* 2010;79(1-2):27–38.
48. Je Y, Schutz FA, Choueiri TK. Risk of bleeding with vascular endothelial growth factor receptor tyrosine-kinase inhibitors sunitinib and sorafenib: a systematic review and meta-analysis of clinical trials. *Lancet Oncol.* 2009;10(10):967–974.
49. Lee S, Chen TT, Barber CL, et al. Autocrine VEGF signaling is required for vascular homeostasis. *Cell.* 2007;130(4):691–703.
50. Touyz RM, Herrmann SMS, Herrmann J. Vascular toxicities with VEGF inhibitor therapies-focus on hypertension and arterial thrombotic events. *J Am Soc Hypertens.* 2018;12(6):409–425.

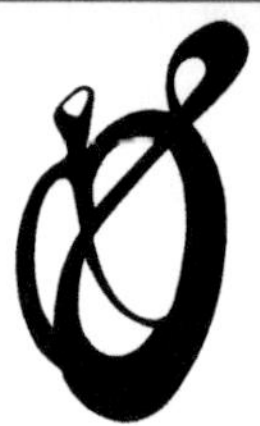

9 Thromboembolic Disease Prevention Before Cancer Therapy

SHYAM K. POUDEL AND ALOK A. KHORANA

Risk factors for VTE

Patient-related
(e.g., advanced age, anemia, infection, obesity, immobility)

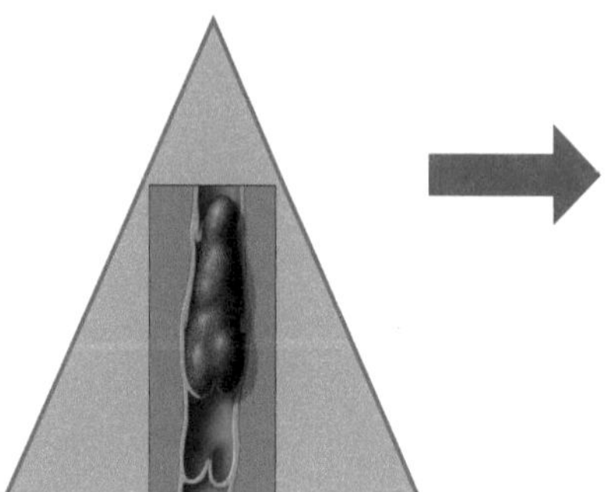

Cancer-related
(cancer type and stage, e.g., multiple myeloma, brain, pancreas, gastric, lung cancer, stage III/IV)

Therapy-related
(e.g., systemic chemotherapy, central catheters)

Khorana Prediction Score

Patient characteristic	Risk score
Site of cancer	
Very high risk (stomach, pancreas)	2
High risk (lung, lymphoma, gyn., bladder, testicular)	1
Pre-chemotherapy platelet count ≥350 × 10^9/L	1
Hb level <10.0 g/L or use of red cell growth factors	1
Pre-chemotherapy leukocyte count ≥11 × 10^9/L	1
BMI 35 kg/m^2 or more	1
0 = Low risk **1–2 = Intermediate risk** **3 = High risk**	

VTE prophylaxis recommended

- Multiple myeloma patients on thalidomide- or lenalidomide-based regimens with chemotherapy and/or dexamethasone should be offered thromboprophylaxis with either aspirin or LMWH for low-risk patients and LMWH for higher-risk patients (ASCO)
- Hospitalized patients with active cancer who have an acute medical illness or reduced mobility and no contraindications (most commonly LMWH)

VTE prophylaxis suggested

- DOACs (clinical trial evidence for apixaban and rivaroxaban) as primary thrombo-prophylaxis in ambulatory patients with cancer starting chemotherapy with a Khorana score ≥2 in patients with no drug-drug interactions and not at high risk for bleeding (unlike patients with gastroesophageal cancers)
- Final treatment decision should be made after considering the risk of both VTE and bleeding, as well as patients' preference and values.
- If DOACs are used, administer for up to 6 months after the initiation of chemotherapy, monitor platelet counts and risk of bleeding

CHAPTER OUTLINE

KEY POINTS

- Patients with cancer account for more than 20% of all newly diagnosed cases of venous thromboembolic events (VTEs); they are six times more likely to develop VTEs
- Risk factors for VTE in patients with cancer are patient-, cancer-, and treatment-related
- As one single risk factor does not reliably predict risk, risk assessment models have been developed, such as the Khorana Risk Score
- Patients with cancer who have a Khorana Risk Score of 3 or greater who are undergoing low-molecular-weight heparin (LMWH) therapy or 2 or greater undergoing direct oral anticoagulant (DOAC) experience a 60% reduction in VTE and/or VTE-related deaths
- American Society of Clinical Oncology (ASCO), International Society on Thrombosis and Hemostasis (ISTH), and International Initiative on Thrombosis and Cancer (ITAC) guidelines suggest the use of DOACs as primary thromboprophylaxis in ambulatory patients with cancer starting chemotherapy with a Khorana score of 2 or greater, in patients with no drug-drug interactions and not at high risk for bleeding
- LMWH remains an option for outpatient thromboprophylaxis in patients at high risk
- Patients with multiple myeloma receiving immunomodulatory drugs (IMiD)-based combination therapy, current guidelines recommend aspirin 81 to 325 mg daily if none or only one individual/myeloma risk factor, otherwise LMWH equivalent to 40 mg enoxaparin daily or full-dose warfarin
- In hospitalized patients with major surgery or acute medical illness, thromboprophylaxis with heparin or LMWH is recommended per standard recommendations with consideration for 4 weeks extension postoperatively in patients at high risk in the setting of abdominal and pelvic surgery for malignancy

Thromboembolic events can manifest either synchronously or metachronously in the course of a malignancy and can involve both the venous and arterial systems. Venous thromboembolism (VTE) includes deep-vein thrombosis (DVT), visceral vein thrombosis, and pulmonary embolism (PE), and is much more prevalent. Compared with the general population, patients with cancer are six times more likely to develop VTE and they account for more than 20% of all newly diagnosed cases of VTE.[1] Arterial events, such as stroke and myocardial infarction, are also more common in patients with cancer than in the general population (as reviewed in Chapter 8).

Thrombosis is often associated with detrimental effects in patients with cancer. VTE can complicate postoperative recovery, medical hospitalization, and systemic chemotherapy and increase the cost of cancer treatments and hospitalizations.[2] A strong association exists of VTE with short- and long-term mortality, and thromboembolism is the second-leading cause of death among outpatients with cancer after cancer itself.[3] Therapeutic anticoagulation carries a substantial risk for both serious bleeding complications and recurrence of VTE in patients with cancer.[4] Indeed, one in four patients with cancer-associated VTE require readmission owing to bleeding or VTE recurrence.[5] Therefore, appropriate prevention of thrombosis is important to reduce its impact on patients on patients with cancer and on the health system in general. This chapter provides an overview of risk stratification approaches and prevention of VTE in patients with cancer. **Chapters 18 and 30** will cover the management of incident and recurrent VTE.

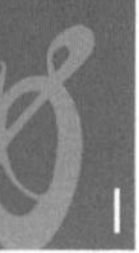

Risk Factors for Cancer-Associated VTE

Risk factors for VTE in patients with cancer can be considered in three main categories: patient, cancer, and treatment-related (Table 9.1).

- **Patient-related risk factors** include advanced age, black race, and associated comorbidities such as obesity, infection, anemia, and renal and pulmonary disease.
- **Cancer-related risk factors:** The risk for VTE also varies according to the primary site and histologic subtype of the cancer. Patients with advanced malignancies and primary brain tumors, pancreatic, stomach, and lung cancers have the highest risk (Fig. 9.1). In hematologic malignancies, patients with lymphoma are also at increased risk for VTE. The natural history of the cancer itself is another risk factor, in which, the greatest risk for VTE has been shown in the first 3 months of initial diagnosis.
- **Treatment-related risk factors:** Risk for cancer-associated thrombosis increases with the use of systemic chemotherapy, usually by two- to six-fold.[6] Long-term use of central catheters has also been found to increase the risk for VTE in patients with cancer. Antiangiogenic agents, such as bevacizumab, increase the risk for both arterial and venous events.[6] Thalidomide and lenalidomide also increase the risk for VTE in patients with multiple myeloma when combined with dexamethasone.[6] In addition to systemic chemotherapy, other supportive therapies, including the use of erythropoiesis stimulating agents, red blood cell and platelet transfusions, further increase the risk for VTE.[6]

TABLE 9.1 Risk Factors for Venous Thromboembolism in Patients With Cancer

VARIABLES	RISK FACTORS
Patient-related	Advanced age Ethnicity (higher in Blacks) Comorbidities (obesity, infection, anemia, renal, and pulmonary disease)
Cancer-related	Primary site of cancer Histologic subtype Natural history of cancer
Treatment-related	Indwelling catheters Systemic chemotherapy Supportive therapies (e.g., erythropoiesis-stimulating agents; red blood cell and platelet transfusion)

VTE, Venous thromboembolism.

CANCER-ASSOCIATED ARTERIAL THROMBOEMBOLISM

Patients with cancer also face an increased short-term risk of arterial thromboembolic events, including myocardial infarction and stroke. In a recent study, compared with patients without cancer,

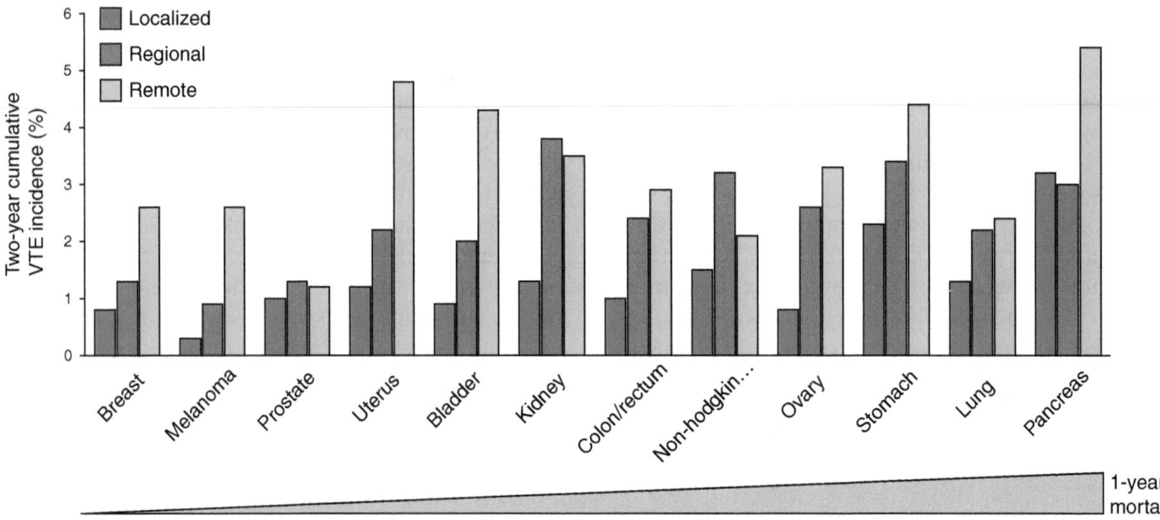

FIG. 9.1 Two-year cumulative incidence (%) of venous thromboembolism (VTE) per type and stage of cancer. Types of cancer were ordered by their respective 1-year mortality rates. (From Timp JF, Braekkan SK, Versteeg HH, Cannegieter SC. Epidemiology of cancer-associated venous thrombosis. *Blood*. 2013;122:1712–1713.)

the 6-month cumulative incidence of arterial thromboembolism (4.7% vs. 2.2%), myocardial infarction (2% vs. 0.7%), and ischemic stroke (3% vs. 1.6%) was significantly higher in patients with cancer.[7] Arterial events are frequently occurring complications during cancer therapies, mainly attributed to the toxicity profiles of vascular endothelial growth factor (VEGF) antagonists, such as bevacizumab, sunitinib, and sorafenib.[8] Such agents can induce endothelial dysfunction with a decrease in the levels of nitric oxide and prostacyclin, thereby leading to platelet activation.[9] These mechanisms might stir up a downstream cascade of events in patients with preexisting coronary and cerebral artery diseases to promote thrombosis. As mentioned previously, an increased risk of arterial thromboembolic events also exists in patients with multiple myeloma who are treated with lenalidomide.

Compared with VTE, there is a paucity of information regarding risk factors and prevention of cancer-associated arterial thromboembolism. Further discussion in this chapter is primarily focused on the prevention of venous events, prevention of arterial events is covered in Chapter 8.

RISK ASSESSMENT

Given that VTE in cancer is multifactorial and that any given single risk factor does not reliably predict risk, risk-assessment models have been developed. Among these, the Khorana score (see Central Illustration) has been validated in multiple large cohorts of patients with cancer who have a variety of malignancies.[10] The Khorana score is calculated by assigning points to clinical variables, such as site of cancer, hematologic parameters, and body mass index, that can be easily obtained in most of these patients. The score was derived from a development cohort of 2701 patients and subsequently validated in an independent cohort of 1365 patients.

The utility of risk assessment lies in its role in education, screening, and prophylaxis.

- **Education:** In one prospective, observational study, investigators incorporated the Khorana score into the electronic medical record.[11] Patients stratified into intermediate- or high-risk had a message sent to their providers to include a discussion of warning signs and symptoms of cancer-associated thrombosis. During the follow-up period, 11% of patients in the intermediate- to high-risk group developed VTE.
- **Screening:** Single- and multi-institutional studies have demonstrated high rates of subclinical DVT detected on screening.[12–14] Rates range from 9% to 12% for patients with Khorana score 3 or greater and approximately 4.5% for a Khorana score 2 or greater.
- **Prophylaxis:** The utility of risk score to identify patients suitable for thromboprophylaxis has been shown in studies where absolute risk of VTE was substantially lower with low-molecular-weight heparin (LMWH) in the high-risk (Khorana score ≥3) patient subgroups.[15–17] In a pooled analysis of these three reported studies (Prophylaxis of Thromboembolism during Chemotherapy (PROTECHT), Evaluation of AVE5026 in the Prevention of Venous Thromboembolism in Patients with Cancer Undergoing Chemotherapy (SAVE-ONCO), and A Study of Dalteparin Prophylaxis in High-Risk Ambulatory Patients with Cancer (PHACS)) of thromboprophylaxis in patients with a Khorana score 3 or greater, the pooled relative risk for VTE with thromboprophylaxis was 0.41 (95% confidence interval [CI], 0.22 to 0.78; P = .006).[17] Two recent studies (A Study to Evaluate the Efficacy and Safety of Rivaroxaban Venous Thromboembolism Prophylaxis in Ambulatory Cancer Participants Receiving Chemotherapy (CASSINI) and Apixaban for the Prevention of Venous Thromboembolism in Patients with Cancer (AVERT)) used direct oral anticoagulants (DOACs) and focused on a population of patients with a lower cutoff of the risk score (i.e., ≥2) and demonstrated substantial reduction in VTE, with a number needed to treat (NNT) of 17 (based on symptomatic rates in AVERT).[14,18]

OVERVIEW OF PROPHYLAXIS GUIDELINES

Thromboprophylaxis in Surgical Patients With Cancer

Venous thromboembolism is more frequent during the perioperative period in patients with cancer. In one clinical outcome study, persistent risk of VTE after the perioperative period was seen with a 40% VTE event rate three weeks after surgery.[19] Indeed, an increased risk of VTE after abdominopelvic cancer surgery and the duration of anticoagulation with

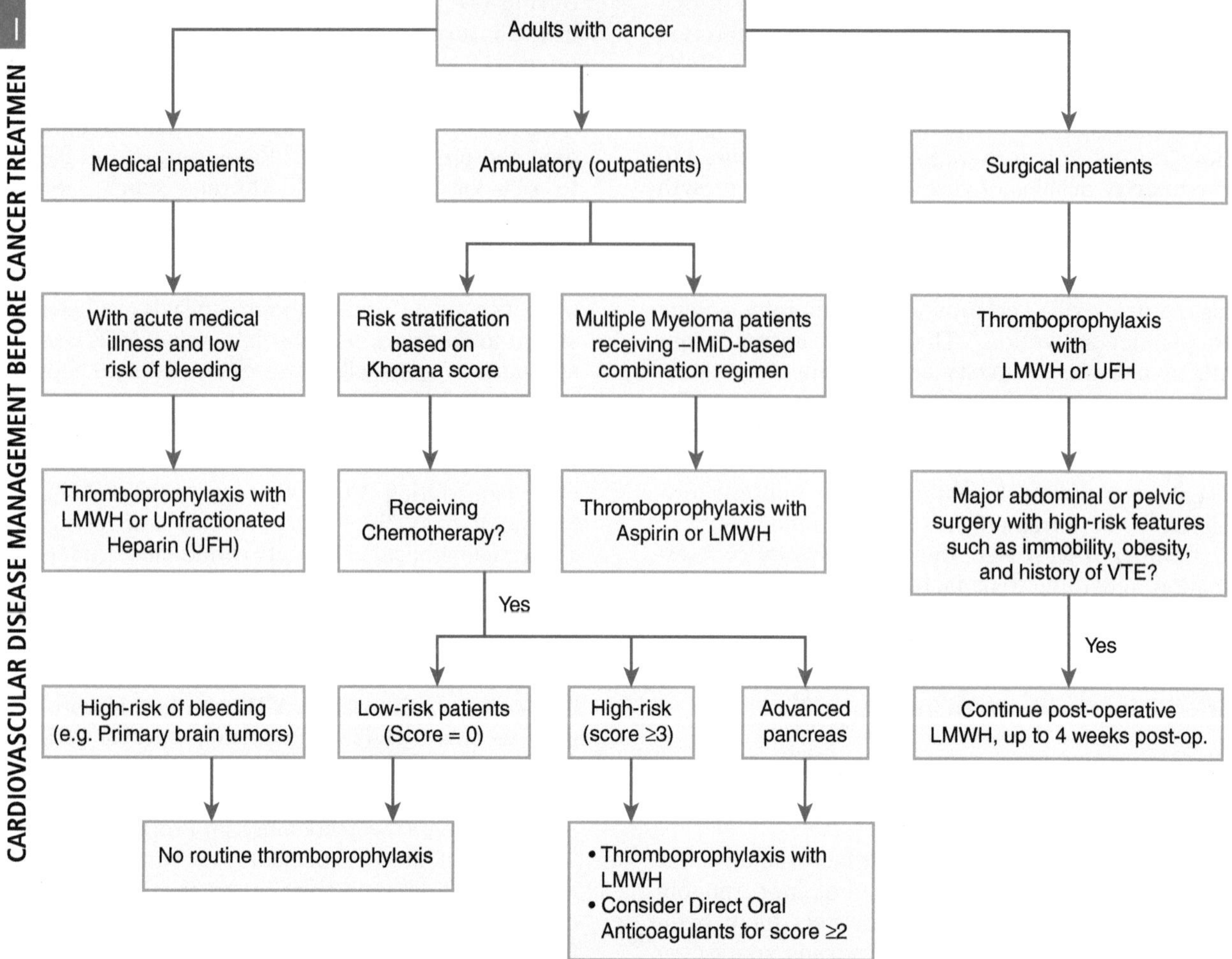

(**Figure CENTRAL ILLUSTRATION ON VTE PROPHYLAXIS IN ADULT PATIENTS WITH CANCER. ABBREVIATIONS:** *IMiD*, immunomodulator drugs; *LMWH*, low molecular weight heparin; *VTE*, venous thromboembolism; *UFH*, unfractionated heparin)

LMWH remained highly heterogeneous in the past. In a recent meta-analysis, investigators compared extended duration of thromboprophylaxis (2 to 6 weeks) with a conventional approach (≤2 weeks) in the postoperative period in patients with cancer who had abdominopelvic surgery. From seven randomized and prospective studies pooled into the analysis, extended thromboprophylaxis was associated with a significantly reduced incidence of all VTEs (2.6% vs. 5.6%; relative risk [RR], 0.44; 95% CI, 0.28 to 0.70; NNT, 39) and proximal DVT (1.4% vs. 2.8%; RR, 0.46; 95% CI, 0.23 to 0.91; NNT, 71) when compared with conventional duration of prophylaxis.[20] No differences were found in the incidence of symptomatic pulmonary embolism, major bleeding, and 3-month mortality. Current recommendation is to consider extended thromboprophylaxis in the setting of abdominal and pelvic surgery for those patients with cancer at high risk.[21]

Mechanical devices have also been explored for thromboprophylaxis in patients with cancer. Despite the lack of evidence, these devices still provide an option for thromboprophylaxis in patients at high risk of hemorrhagic complications, and as an adjunct to pharmacologic thromboprophylaxis.[22]

Thromboprophylaxis in Hospitalized Patients With Cancer

Patients with cancer who are hospitalized with an acute medical illness are at high risk of developing VTE. However, relative contraindications, such as thrombocytopenia, high risk for hemorrhage, and active hemorrhage, frequently limit the use of anticoagulants in this patient population. A recent multicenter study demonstrated that nearly one third of hospitalized patients with cancer had a relative contraindication to thromboprophylaxis, mainly thrombocytopenia (65.2%) and active hemorrhage (17.4%).[23]

Studies looking exclusively at thromboprophylaxis in cancer-specific cohorts are lacking. Indeed, most of the data have been derived from randomized trials that were not specifically conducted for patients with cancer. In a recent subgroup analysis of three placebo-controlled, randomized trials comparing the rates of VTE events in hospitalized patients with cancer, no significant benefit of thromboprophylaxis was seen (RR, 0.91; 95% CI, 0.21 to 4.0; I=68%).[24]

However, given the known high risk of VTE in hospitalized patients with cancer, current recommendation is to provide routine thromboprophylaxis for hospitalized patients with active cancer who have acute medical illness or reduced mobility, in the absence of coraindications, Prophylaxis should not be offered to patients admitted for the sole purpose of minor procedures or chemotherapy infusion, nor to patients undergoing stem-cell/bone marrow transplantation.[21]

Thromboprophylaxis in Ambulatory Patients With Cancer

Patients receiving anticancer therapy in the outpatient setting are at high risk for VTE. Recent trials have compared LMWHs and DOACs versus placebo for VTE prophylaxis in this setting. In multiple randomized trials outlined below, a lower incidence of VTE was noted in patients who received thromboprophylaxis.

- PROTECHT randomly assigned 1150 patients with metastatic or locally advanced solid tumors to receive once daily subcutaneous nadroparin (3800 U) or placebo, up to a maximum of four months.[25] Compared with placebo, patients in the nadroparin arm had (1) a lower incidence of thromboembolic event (2% vs. 3.9%) and (2) similar incidence of major bleeding events (0.7% vs. 0%), minor bleeding events (7.4% vs. 7.9%), overall adverse events (15.7% vs. 17.6%), and serious adverse events related to the investigational drug alone (1.2% vs. 1.6%).
- SAVE-ONCO randomly assigned 3212 patients with metastatic or locally advanced solid tumors commencing chemotherapy to receive either the ultra-LMWH semuloparin or placebo for a median duration of 3.5 months. Patients in the semuloparin arm had (1) a lower incidence of VTE (1.2% vs. 3.4%) and (2) similar incidences of major bleeding events (1.2% vs. 1.1%) and clinically relevant nonmajor bleeding events (1.6% vs. 0.9%).
- CASSINI randomly assigned 841 patients with various solid tumors or lymphomas initiating a new systemic regimen and at increased risk for VTE (Khorana score ≥2) to receive either oral rivaroxaban (10 mg once daily) or placebo, for up to 180 days.[14] Compared with placebo, patients receiving rivaroxaban had (1) nonsignificantly reduced VTE events and VTE-related deaths in the up-to-day 180 observation period owing to high rates of discontinuation (hazard ratio[HR], 0.66; 95% CI, 0.40 to 1.09; P = .101; NNT, 35), (2) significantly reduced VTE and VTE-related deaths during the intervention period (HR, 0.40; 95% CI, 0.20 to 0.80; NNT, 26), (3) nonsignificantly increased major bleeding (HR, 1.96; 95% CI, 0.59 to 6.49; P = .265; number needed to harm [NNH], 101), and (4) nonsignificantly increased clinically relevant nonmajor bleeding (HR, 1.34; 95% CI, 0.54 to 3.32; P = .53; NNH, 135).
- In AVERT, 563 patients with various malignancies and at increased risk of VTE (Khorana Risk Score ≥2) were randomized to oral apixaban (2.5 mg twice daily) or placebo over a follow-up period of 180 days.[18] Patients receiving apixaban had (1) reduced VTE events (4.2% vs. 10.2%; HR, 0.41; 95% CI, 0.26 to 0.65; P <.001; NNT, 17) and (2) higher rate of major bleeding (3.5% vs. 1.8%; HR, 2.00; 95% CI, 1.01 to 3.95; NNH, 59).

Randomized trials in patients with pancreatic cancer have also shown greater benefits with anticoagulation compared with those with other solid tumors. In FRAGEM and PROSPECT-CONKO 004 trials, patients with locally advanced and metastatic pancreatic cancers who received thromboprophylaxis with LMWH during chemotherapy had a substantially reduced rate of VTE during subsequent follow up.[26,27]

In patients with multiple myeloma, immunomodulatory drugs (IMiD)-based combination regimens are associated with an increased risk for VTE. In a recent study in previously untreated patients with multiple myeloma who were receiving lenalidomide, aspirin and LMWH demonstrated similar benefit in reducing the incidence of VTE.[28]

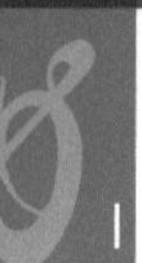

Current established guidelines recommend routine thromboprophylaxis with LMWH in high-risk outpatients receiving systemic chemotherapy for solid tumors.[21] New guidelines and guidance statements from American Society of Clinical Oncology (ASCO), International Society on Thrombosis and Hemostasis (ISTH), and International Initiative on Thrombosis and Cancer (ITAC) suggest or recommend the use of DOACs (rivaroxaban or apixaban) as primary thromboprophylaxis in ambulatory patients with cancer starting chemotherapy with Khorana score 2 or greater, in patients with no drug-drug interactions and not at high risk for bleeding (Table 9.2). In patients with multiple myeloma receiving IMiD-based combination regimens, thromboprophylaxis with aspirin or LMWH in low-risk cases and LMWH in high-risk cases are recommended.[21]

EVOLVING ROLE OF DIRECT ORAL ANTICOAGULANTS AND THE CHANGING LANDSCAPE

Direct oral anticoagulants include the direct factor IIa inhibitor dabigatran and the factor Xa inhibitors apixaban, rivaroxaban, edoxaban, and betrixaban, currently approved for VTE prevention in multiple countries. Results from CASSINI and AVERT trials are encouraging and support the potential benefit of rivaroxaban and apixaban in primary prevention of cancer-associated thrombosis. Recent guidelines and guidance statements from ASCO, ISTH, and ITAC suggest the changing landscape in thromboprophylaxis in ambulatory patients with cancer in which the roles of DOACs have been sufficiently highlighted (see Table 9.2).

TABLE 9.2 Society Recommendations for Thromboprophylaxis in Primary Prevention of VTE in Ambulatory Patients With Cancer

ORGANIZATION	RECOMMENDATIONS
ASCO[21]	• Routine pharmacologic thromboprophylaxis should not be offered to all outpatients with cancer. • High-risk outpatients with cancer (Khorana score of ≥2 prior to starting a new systemic chemotherapy regimen) may be offered thromboprophylaxis with apixaban, rivaroxaban, or LMWH provided there are no significant risk factors for bleeding and no drug interactions. Considerations of such therapy should be accompanied by a discussion with the patient about the relative benefits and harms, drug cost, and duration of prophylaxis in this setting. • Patients with multiple myeloma receiving thalidomide- or lenalidomide-based regimens with chemotherapy and/or dexamethasone should be offered pharmacologic thromboprophylaxis with either aspirin or LMWH for low-risk patients and LMWH for higher-risk patients.
ISTH[29]	• ISTH suggests the use of DOACs as primary thromboprophylaxis in patients with cancer who are ambulatory starting chemotherapy with Khorana score ≥2 in patients with no drug-drug interactions and not at high risk for bleeding (such as patients with gastroesophageal cancers). Currently, apixaban and rivaroxaban are the only DOACs with evidence from randomized clinical trials. A final treatment decision should be made after considering the risk of both VTE and bleeding, as well as patients' preference and values. • ISTH suggests that if DOACs were to be used for primary thromboprophylaxis in ambulatory patients with cancer, it is administered for up to 6 months after the initiation of chemotherapy. ISTH recommends monitoring of platelet counts and risk of bleeding complications while on anticoagulation.
ITAC[30]	• Primary pharmacologic thromboprophylaxis with LMWH is indicated in ambulatory patients with locally advanced or metastatic pancreatic cancer treated with systemic anticancer therapy and who have a low risk of bleeding. However, it is not recommended outside of a clinical trial for patients with locally advanced or metastatic lung cancer treated with systemic anticancer therapy, including patients who have a low risk of bleeding. • Primary prophylaxis with DOAC (rivaroxaban or apixaban) is recommended in ambulatory patients who are receiving systemic anticancer therapy at intermediate-to-high risk of VTE, identified by cancer type (i.e., pancreatic) or by a validated risk assessment model (i.e., a Khorana score ≥2), and not actively bleeding or not at a high risk of bleeding.

ASCO, American Society of Clinical Oncology; *DOAC*, direct oral anticoagulant; *ISTH*, International Society on Thrombosis and Hemostasis; *ITAC*, International Initiative on Thrombosis and Cancer; *LMWH*, low-molecular-weight heparin; *VTE*, venous thromboembolism.

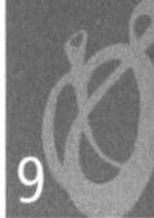

REFERENCES

1. Geerts WH, Bergqvist D, Pineo GF, et al. Prevention of venous thromboembolism: American College of Chest Physicians Evidence-Based Clinical Practice Guidelines (8th Edition). *Chest.* 2008;133: 381S–453S.
2. Khorana AA, Dalal MR, Lin J,Connolly GC. Health care costs associated with venous thromboembolism in selected high-risk ambulatory patients with solid tumors undergoing chemotherapy in the United States. *Clinicoecon Outcomes Res.* 2013;5:101–108.
3. Khorana AA, Francis CW, Culakova E, Kuderer NM, Lyman GH. Thromboembolism is a leading cause of death in patients with cancer receiving outpatient chemotherapy. *J Thromb Haemost.* 2007;5:632–634.
4. Prandoni P, Lensing AW, Piccioli A, et al. Recurrent venous thromboembolism and bleeding complications during anticoagulant treatment in patients with cancer and venous thrombosis. *Blood.* 2002;100:3484–3488.
5. Bullano MF, Willey V, Hauch O, Wygant G, Spyropoulos AC, Hoffman L. Longitudinal evaluation of health plan cost per venous thromboembolism or bleed event in patients with a prior venous thromboembolism event during hospitalization. *J Manag Care Pharm.* 2005;11:663–673.
6. Donnellan E, Khorana AA. Cancer and venous yhromboembolic disease: a review. *Oncologist.* 2017;22:199–207.
7. Navi BB, Reiner AS, Kamel H, et al. Risk of arterial thromboembolism in patients with cancer. *J Am Coll Cardiol.* 2017;70:926-938.
8. Choueiri TK, Schutz FA, Je Y, Rosenberg JE, Bellmunt J. Risk of arterial thromboembolic events with sunitinib and sorafenib: a systematic review and meta-analysis of clinical trials. *J Clin Oncol.* 2010;28: 2280–2285.
9. Herrmann J, Yang EH, Iliescu CA, et al. Vascular toxicities of cancer therapies: the old and the new—an evolving avenue. *Circulation.* 2016;133:1272–1289.
10. Khorana AA, Kuderer NM, Culakova E, Lyman GH, Francis CW. Development and validation of a predictive model for chemotherapy-associated thrombosis. *Blood.* 2008;111:4902–4907.
11. Lustig DB, Rodriguez R, Wells PS. Implementation and validation of a risk stratification method at The Ottawa Hospital to guide thromboprophylaxis in ambulatory patients with cancer at intermediate-high risk for venous thrombosis. *Thromb Res.* 2015;136:1099–1102.
12. Khorana AA, Rubens D, Francis CW. Screening high-risk patients with cancer for VTE: a prospective observational study. *Thromb Res.* 2014;134:1205–1207.
13. Kunapareddy G, Switzer B, Jain P, et al. Implementation of an electronic medical record tool for early detection of deep vein thrombosis in the ambulatory oncology setting. *Res Pract Thromb Haemost.* 2019;3:226–233.
14. Khorana AA, Soff GA, Kakkar AK, et al. Rivaroxaban for thromboprophylaxis in high-risk ambulatory patients with cancer. *N Engl J Med.* 2019;380:720–728.
15. Verso M, Agnelli G, Barni S, Gasparini G, LaBlanca R. A modified Khorana risk assessment score for venous thromboembolism in patients with cancer receiving chemotherapy: the Protecht score. *Intern Emerg Med.* 2012;7:291–292.
16. George D, Agnelli G, Fisher W, et al. Venous thromboembolism (VTE) prevention with semuloparin in patients with cancer initiating chemotherapy: benefit-risk assessment by VTE risk in SAVE-ONCO. *Blood.* 2011;118:206.
17. Khorana AA, Francis CW, Kuderer NM, et al. Dalteparin thromboprophylaxis in patients with cancer at high risk for venous thromboembolism: a randomized trial. *Thromb Res.* 2017;151:89–95.
18. Carrier M, Abou-Nassar K, Mallick R, et al. Apixaban to prevent venous thromboembolism in patients with cancer. *N Engl J Med.* 2019;380:711–719.
19. Agnelli G, Bolis G, Lorenzo C, et al. A clinical outcome-based prospective study on venous thromboembolism after cancer surgery: the @RISTOS project. *Ann Surg.* 2006;243: 89–95.
20. Fagarasanu A, Alotaibi GS, Hrimiuc R, Lee AY, Wu C. Role of extended thromboprophylaxis after abdominal and pelvic surgery in patients with cancer: a systematic review and meta-analysis. *Ann Surg Oncol.* 2016;23:1422–1430.
21. Key NS, Khorana AA, Kuderer NM, et al. Venous thromboembolism prophylaxis and treatment in patients with cancer: ASCO Clinical Practice Guideline Update. *J Clin Oncol.* 2020;38:496–520.
22. Stanley A, Young A. Primary prevention of venous thromboembolism in medical and surgical oncology patients. *Br J Cancer.* 2010; 102(suppl 1):S10–S16.
23. Zwicker JI, Rojan A, Campigotto F, et al. Pattern of frequent but nontargeted pharmacologic thromboprophylaxis for hospitalized patients with cancer at academic medical centers: a prospective, cross-sectional, multicenter study. *J Clin Oncol.* 2014;32:1792–1796.
24. Carrier M, Khorana AA, Moretto P, Le Gal G, Karp R, Zwicker JI. Lack of evidence to support thromboprophylaxis in hospitalized medical patients with cancer. *Am J Med.* 2014;127:82–86.e1.
25. Agnelli G, Gussoni G, Bianchini C, et al. Nadroparin for the prevention of thromboembolic events in ambulatory patients with metastatic or locally advanced solid cancer receiving chemotherapy: a randomised, placebo-controlled, double-blind study. *Lancet Oncol.* 2009;10:943–949.
26. Maraveyas A, Waters J, Roy R, et al. Gemcitabine versus gemcitabine plus dalteparin thromboprophylaxis in pancreatic cancer. *Eur J Cancer.* 2012;48:1283–1292.
27. Riess H, Pelzer U, Hilbig A, et al. Rationale and design of PROSPECT-CONKO 004: a prospective, randomized trial of simultaneous pancreatic cancer treatment with enoxaparin and chemotherapy). *BMC Cancer.* 2008;8:361.
28. Larocca A, Cavallo F, Bringhen S, et al. Aspirin or enoxaparin thromboprophylaxis for patients with newly diagnosed multiple myeloma treated with lenalidomide. *Blood.* 2012;119:933–939, quiz 1093.
29. Wang TF, Zwicker JI, Ay C, et al. The use of direct oral anticoagulants for primary thromboprophylaxis in ambulatory patients with cancer: guidance from the SSC of the ISTH. *J Thromb Haemost.* 2019;17:1772–1778.
30. Farge D, Frere C, Connors JM, et al. 2019 international clinical practice guidelines for the treatment and prophylaxis of venous thromboembolism in patients with cancer. *Lancet Oncol.* 2019; 20:e566–e581.

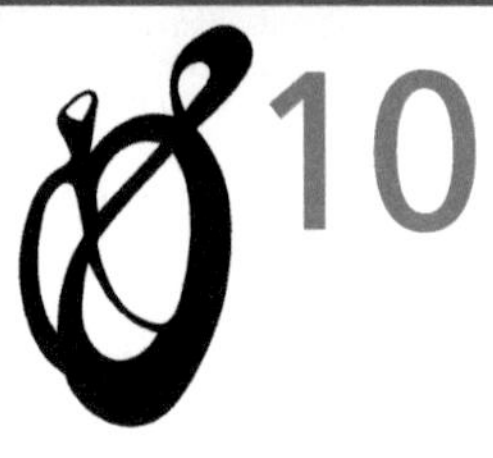

10 Arrhythmia Prevention and Device Management: Before Cancer Therapy

MICHAEL FRADLEY

Patient with cancer

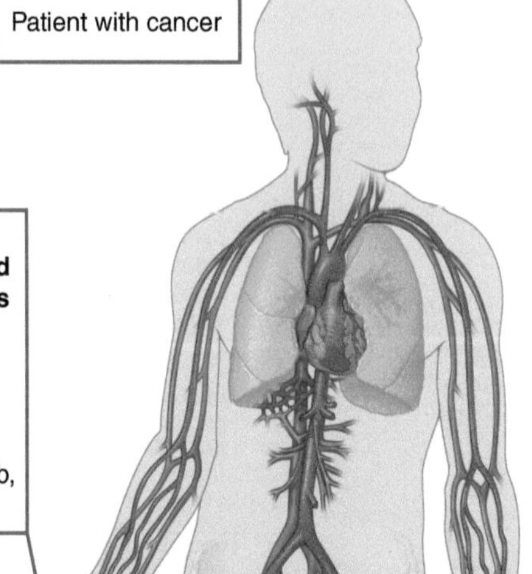

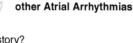

Atrial Fibrillation (AF) and other Atrial Arrhythmias

- Prior history?
- AF risk factors?
- At risk population (e.g., CLL)?
- At risk cancer therapies (e.g. ibrutinib, melphalan, immune therapies)?

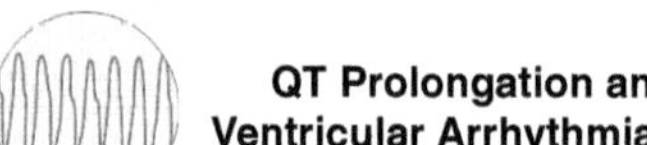

QT Prolongation and Ventricular Arrhythmias

- LQ or VT history?
- Cardiomyopathy?
- Electrolyte abnormalities?
- Exposure to cancer therapies with associated risk (ribocuclib, TKIs)?
- Drug-drug interactions?

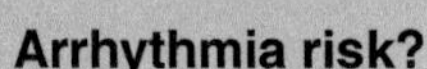

Arrhythmia risk?

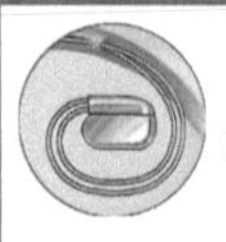

Cardiac Implantable Devices (pacemaker, ICD)

- Device status?
- Pacemaker dependence?
- Thoracic/cardiac surgery?
- Any radiation therapy to the chest or high energy radiation with potential chest exposure?

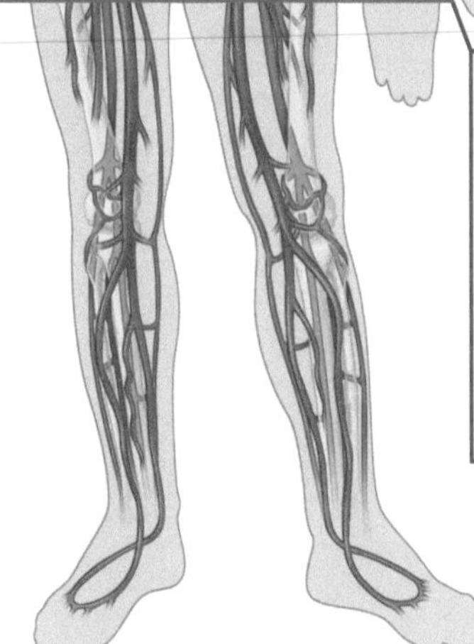

Bradyarrhythmias and Autonomic Dysfunction

- Prior history, incl. syncope of any form?
- Sinus tachycardia?
- Abnormal heart rate recovery?
- Any prior or planned radiation therapy to the neck or chest?

CHAPTER OUTLINE

KEY POINTS

- All patients with cancer should be evaluated for the presence and risk of developing arrhythmias because these can significantly complicate treatments and outcomes
- The intake should include preexisting atrial fibrillation, QTc prolongation, and cardiac device status
- In patients with cancer who have atrial fibrillation, rhythm control strategies to maintain sinus rhythm can be challenging and drug-drug interactions must be anticipated even when a rate-controlling approach is used (beta-blocker often first-line therapy)
- Anticoagulation decisions in patients with cancer who have atrial fibrillation must be considered in the context of planned cancer therapeutics, comorbid conditions, including cytopenias, and drug-drug interactions
- It is essential to minimize the potential for QT prolongation and risk of torsades prior to the initiation of cancer therapy; this includes monitoring of electrolyte abnormalities and drug interactions
- Cardiac implantable device status should be assessed in all cancer cases and managed proactively in patients undergoing chest surgery with (electro-) cauterization or chest radiation therapy
- Whereas cardiac device malfunction is rare and repositioning prior to cancer therapy is rarely necessary, routine device interrogation before and after is recommended
- Cardiac device reprogramming into a "safe mode" should be considered in those patients who are expected to be at higher risk of developing device malfunction (i.e., mainly those who receive a higher absorbed dose of radiation and higher energy photons)

With the aging population, a significant number of patients with newly diagnosed cancer will also have coexisting cardiovascular (CV) diseases. Additionally, many different cancer therapeutics from traditional cytotoxic chemotherapies to the newer targeted and immunotherapies can themselves be cardiotoxic. As such, optimizing patients from a CV standpoint prior to the initiation of cancer treatment can help to prevent serious complications or treatment disruption. Although preventative strategies have often focused on heart failure and left ventricular dysfunction, patients with underlying arrhythmias may also benefit from aggressive pretreatment evaluation and management. The broad scope of arrhythmias that have been reported with cancer therapeutics is outlined in Table 10.1.[1]

ATRIAL FIBRILLATION AND OTHER ATRIAL ARRHYTHMIAS

Atrial fibrillation (AF) is an especially common arrhythmia in older individuals. In fact, the lifetime risk of developing AF after age 40 for individuals of European descent is 26% for men and 23% for women.[2] In addition to age, risk factors for developing AF include hypertension, obesity, obstructive sleep apnea, thyroid disease, alcohol use, and underlying cardiovascular disease.[2] In addition, patients with cancer are at increased risk for developing AF, and some cancer therapeutics are particularly arrhythmogenic. These scenarios are well illustrated in patients with chronic lymphocytic leukemia (CLL), who are at a two-fold higher risk of AF, further increased at least three-fold in patients on ibrutinib (Fig. 10.1).[3,4] AF risk prediction models were developed for patients with CLL and remain applicable for patients on ibrutinib (see Fig. 10.1). Given that many patients with newly diagnosed cancer will have preexisting AF, it is especially important to optimize their treatment prior to the initiation of therapy in order to minimize potential complications. Both, preexisting and newly developing AF are prognostic implications for thromboembolism, heart failure (esp., newly developing) and mortality (esp., preexisting AF; Fig. 10.2).

Management of AF in patients with newly diagnosed cancer should follow the same algorithms as the general population (Fig. 10.3). For asymptomatic individuals, a rate control strategy is most appropriate, with a goal resting heart rate of less than 110 beats per minute (bpm).[2] In general, patients with

TABLE 10.1 Types of Arrhythmia Reported With the Use of Cancer Therapeutics

THERAPY CLASS	AGENT NAME (TARGET)	AF	SVT	BRADYCARDIA	AV BLOCK	QTch	TdP	VT/VF	SCD
Miscellaneous	Arsenic trioxide	++	++	–	+	+++	++	–	+
Alkylating agents	Anthracyclines (acute)	x	–	x	x	x	–	x	
	Busulfan	x	x	–	x	–	–	–	x
	Cyclophosphamide	x	–	–	x	x	–	x	–
	Ifosfamide	x	–	x	–	–	–	x	x
	Melphalan	x	x	–	–	–	–	x	
Antimetabolites	5-Fluorouracil	x		x	x	x	–	x	x
	Capecitabine	++	–	++	–	+	–	–	+
	Clofarabine	x	x	x	–	–	–	–	–
	Cytarabine	x		x	–	–	–	–	–
	Gemcitabine	+	+	–	–	–	–	–	–
Microtubule-binding agents	Paclitaxel	+	+	++	+	–	–	+	–
Platinum drugs	Cisplatin	+	+	+	+	–	–	+	–
Immunomodulatory drugs	Thalidomide	+		+	–	–	–	–	–
	Lenalidomide	x	x	x	–	–	–	–	–
Proteasome inhibitors	Bortezomib	x	–	x	x	x	x	x	x
	Carfilzomib	x	x	x	x	–	–	–	x
HDAC inhibitors	Romidepsin	+	++	–	–	++	+	++	+
	Vorinostat	–	–	–	–	++	–	–	–
	Panobinostat	–	–	–	–	++	–	–	–
CDK4/CDK6 inhibitors	Ribociclib	–	–	–	–	++	–	–	–
mTOR inhibitors	Everolimus	++	–	–	–	–	–	–	–
Monoclonal antibodies	Alemtuzumab (anti-CD52)	++	–	++	–	–	–	+	+
	Cetuximab (anti-EGFR/HER1)	+		+	–	–	–	+	+
	Necitumumab (anti-EGFR/HER1)	–	+	–	–	–	–	–	++
	Pertuzumab (anti-EGFR/HER1)	+	+	+	–	–	–	+	+
	Rituximab (anti-CD20)	+	+	+	+	+	+	+	+
	Trastuzumab (anti-HER2/ ERBB2)	++	++	+	–	–	–	+	–

TABLE 10.1 Types of Arrhythmia Reported With the Use of Cancer Therapeutics—cont'd

THERAPY CLASS	AGENT NAME (TARGET)	AF	SVT	BRADYCARDIA	AV BLOCK	QTch	TdP	VT/VF	SCD
Multi-targeted kinase Inhibitors	Lenvatinib (VEGFR)	–	–	–	–	++	–	–	–
	Sunitinib (VEGFR)	–	–	+	–	+	+	–	–
	Sorafenib (VEGFR)	+	–	+	+	+	+	–	–
	Pazopanib (VEGFR)	–	–	+++	–	++	–	–	–
	Vandetanib (VEGFR)	–	–	–	–	+++	–	+	+
	Lapatinib (HER2/ ERBB2)	+	+	–	–	+	–	–	–
	Bosutinib (BCR–ABL1)	–	–	+	–	++	–	–	–
	Dasatinib (BCR–ABL1)	+	+	–	–	+	–	+	+
	Imatinib (BCR–ABL1)	+	+	–	–	–	–	–	–
	Nilotinib (BCR–ABL1)	++		++	++	++	–	–	+
	Ponatinib (BCR–ABL1)	++	+	+	+	+	–	+	
	Ibrutinib (BTK)	+++	–	–	–	–	–	+	+
	Alectinib (ALK)	–	–	+++	–	+	–	–	–
	Ceritinib (ALK)	–	–	+	–	++	–	–	–
	Crizotinib (ALK)	–	–	+++	–	+	–	–	–
	Brigatinib (ALK)	–	–	++	–	–	–	–	–
	Lorlatinib (ALK)	–	–	–	+	–	–	–	–
	Osimertinib (EGFR/HER1)	–	–	–	–	++	–	–	–
	Encorafenib (BRAF)	–	–	–	–	+	–	–	–
	Vemurafenib (BRAF)	++		+	–	+++	+	–	–
	Gilteritinib (FTL3)	–	–	–	–	++	–	–	–
	Trametinib (MEK)	–	–	++	–	++	–	–	–
	Ruxolitinib (JAK)	–	–	+	–	+	–	–	–
Immune checkpoint inhibitors	Ipilimumab (anti-CTLA4)	+	–	+	+	–	–	+	+
	Nivolumab (anti-PD1)	+	–	+	+	–	–	+	+
	Pembrolizumab (anti-PD1)	+	–	+	+	–	–	+	+

Frequency not always defined for the individual entities, but when available: +, uncommon (<1%); ++, common (1% to 10%); +++, very common (>10%); x, frequency not defined.

AF, Atrial fibrillation; *CTLA4*, cytotoxic T lymphocyte antigen 4; *HDAC*, histone deacetylase; *JAK*, Janus kinase; mTOR, mechanistic target of rapamycin; *NA*, not applicable; *PD1*, programmed cell death protein 1; *SCD*, sudden cardiac death; *SVT*, supraventricular tachycardia; TdP, torsades de pointes, *VEGF*, vascular endothelial growth factor; *VEGFR*, vascular endothelial growth factor receptor; *VF*, ventricular fibrillation; *VT*, ventricular tachycardia.

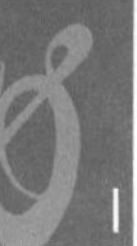

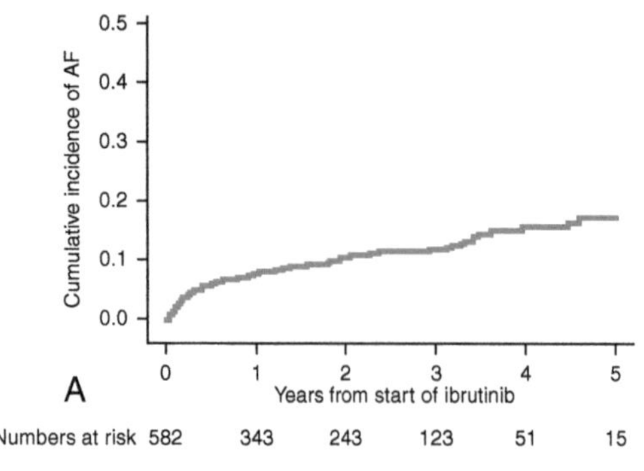

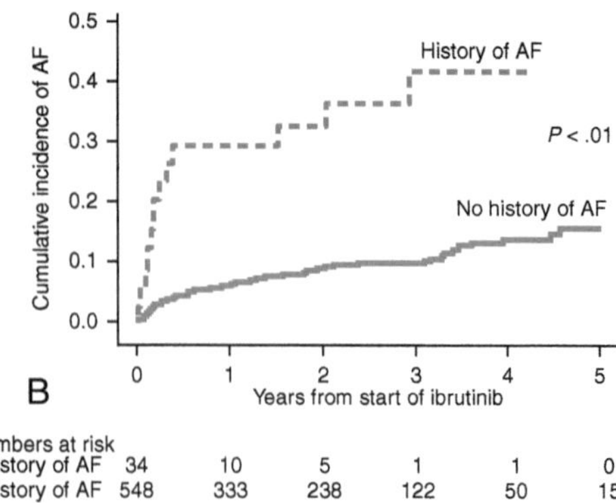

Characteristic	Adverse factor	Risk value[a]
Age	<65	0
	65–74	2
	75+	3
Sex	Female	0
	Male	1
Valvular heart disease	Absent	0
	Present	2
Hypertension	Absent	0
	Present	1

Overall AF risk score[a]	Patients N (%)	HR (95% CI)
0–1	904 (39.4%)	Ref
2–3	789 (34.4%)	2.4 (1.5–3.9)
4	414 (18.1%)	4.3 (2.6–7.2)
≥5[b]	185 (8.1%)	8.3 (4.9–14.3)

C

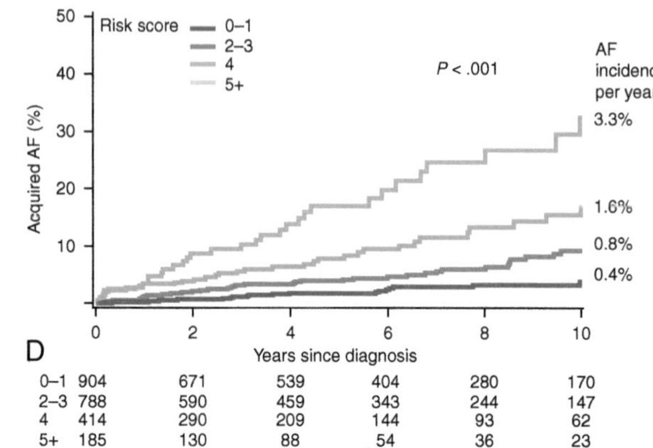

FIG. 10.1 Atrial fibrillation (*AF*) incidence in patients with chronic lymphocytic leukemia (CLL) on ibrutinib over time (**A**) and stratified by history of atrial fibrillation (**B**). Mayo atrial fibrillation risk prediction score for patients with CLL (**C**) and accordingly stratified incidence of atrial fibrillation (**D**;overall incidence for this population 1%/year). (**A** and **B**, From Shanafelt TD, Parikh SA, Noseworthy PA, et al. Atrial fibrillation in patients with chronic lymphocytic leukemia (CLL). *Leuk Lymphoma.* 2017;58 (7):1630–1639; **C** and **D**, From Wiczer TE, Levine LB, Brumbaugh J, et al. Cumulative incidence, risk factors, and management of atrial fibrillation in patients receiving ibrutinib. *Blood Adv.* 2017;1(20):1739–1748.)

cancer are more likely to develop tachycardia as a manifestation of autonomic dysfunction. Conversely, it is also important to recognize that some cancer therapeutics may lead to heart rate slowing—particularly crizotinib, an anaplastic lymphoma kinase inhibitor used for non-small-cell lung cancer, as well as taxanes, a class of chemotherapies with broad applicability.[5] Additionally, certain cancer therapeutics may affect the metabolism of nodal blocking agents. For example, non-dihydropyridine calcium channel blockers should be avoided with treatments that affect the cytochrome P450 system, including vascular endothelial growth factor (VEGF) inhibitors and the antiandrogen, abiraterone, can increase levels of certain beta blockers.[5] As such, cardio-oncologists should be prepared to adjust pharmacologic therapy if necessary.

In symptomatic patients a rhythm control strategy may be necessary; however, patients with cancer pose unique management challenges. Although cardioversion can lead to a rapid resolution of an atrial arrhythmia, it often fails to have long-term durability, particularly if the primary stressor is still present, as is the case in patients with active cancer undergoing treatment. Antiarrhythmic medications must be used with caution in patients with cancer, given frequent drug-drug interactions, which can lead to serious issues, including QT prolongation and ventricular arrhythmias. As such they often require dose adjustment or cessation. Catheter ablation may be an option for more durable rhythm control for select patients.[6] Success rates for AF ablation ranges from 60% to 80% in the general population. It should be noted that patients must be able to tolerate anticoagulation for a minimum of 3 months after ablation regardless of CHA_2DS_2-VASc score (see Fig. 31.1). Therefore, patients who are expected to develop a contraindication to anticoagulation in the first three

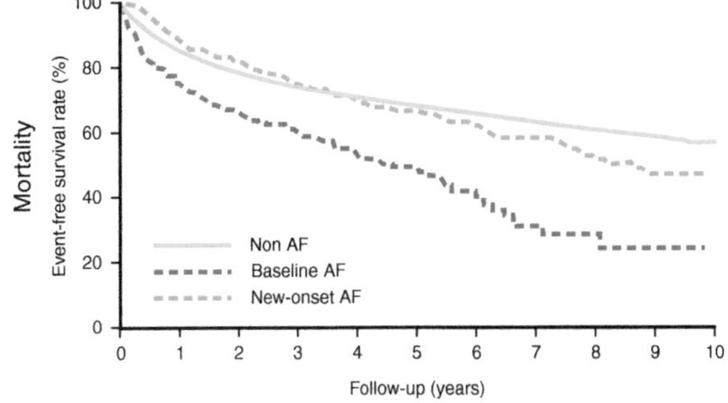

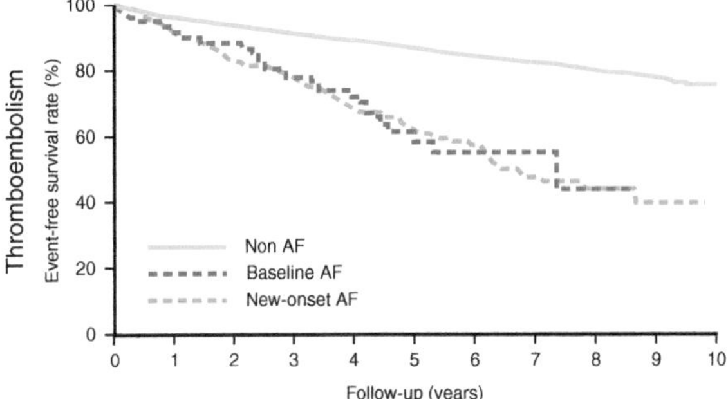

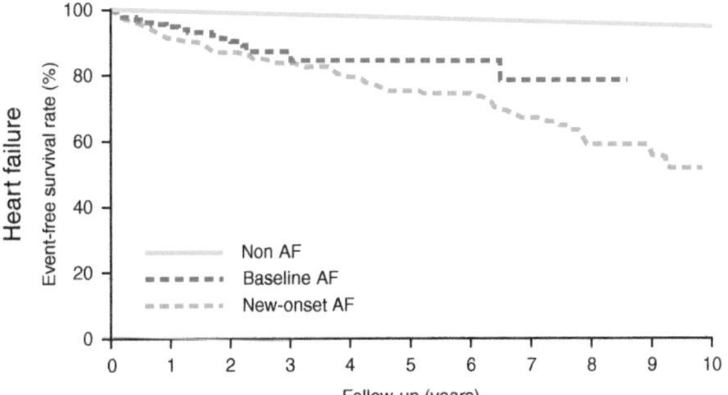

FIG. 10.2 Overall survival (**A**), survival free of thromboembolism (**B**), and survival free of heart failure in patients with cancer with no baseline or new-onset atrial fibrillation (AF). Mortality was higher in patients with baseline AF ($P < .001$ vs. the other two groups); both new-onset and baseline AF were associated with higher incidence of thromboembolism and a higher incidence of heart failure ($P < .0001$ vs. non-AF group for all). (From Hu Y-f, Liu C-j, Chang P M-h, et al. Incident thromboembolism and heart failure associated with new-onset atrial fibrillation in patients with cancer. *Int J Cardiol.* 2013;165(2):355–357.)

months after an ablation should not be referred for this procedure.[2] Moreover, it should be noted that catheter ablation is not considered protective against stroke and decision for long-term anticoagulation should be determined based on the patient's CHA_2DS_2-VASc score. Finally, catheter ablation has not been specifically studied in patients with cancer. The success of ablation in patients with active cancer or in those receiving arrhythmogenic cancer therapies is not established.

Both AF and atrial flutter are known to increase the risk of stroke and systemic thromboembolism. Anticoagulation is the mainstay of therapy to minimize this risk. In the general population, the CHA_2DS_2-VASc score is a validated system to help guide anticoagulation decisions. Recent guidelines suggest utilization of direct oral anticoagulants (DOACs) in men with a CHA_2DS_2-VASc of 2 or greater or in women with a CHA_2DS_2-VASc of 3 or greater to reduce the risk of thromboembolism in the absence of significant contraindications.[7] It is not clear, however, if the CHA_2DS_2-VASc score is truly predictive of adverse events in patients with cancer based on data from several large studies.[8,9] Furthermore, it is advisable to weigh the benefits of anticoagulation against the risk of bleeding. This is commonly done by utilizing the HAS-BLED (Hypertension, Abnormal renal and liver function, Stroke, Bleeding, Labile INR, Elderly, Drugs or alcohol) score (see Chapter 31, Fig. 31.1), but this score model is also not validated in patients with cancer.[7] Recommendations on anticoagulation in patients with cancer with atrial fibrillation thus remain conceptual (see Fig. 31.2).

Although DOACs are preferred in most scenarios in patients without cancer, the choice of anticoagulant in patients with cancer remains challenging (see Fig. 31.3). Warfarin is often avoided owing to drug-drug interactions and difficulties maintaining a therapeutic window; however, it may be necessary if patients also possess mechanical prosthetic valves. Low-molecular-weight heparin (LMWH) has traditionally been the anticoagulant of choice for patients with cancer who have venous thromboembolism (VTE), given the results from the CLOT (Randomized Comparison of Low-Molecular-Weight Heparin Versus Oral Anticoagulant Therapy for the Prevention of Recurrent Venous Thromboembolism in Patients With Cancer) trial[10]; however, the mechanism of thrombus formation in AF is different and the superiority of LMWH for this disease process is not established. This being said, LMWH may be preferred when drug-drug interactions and cytopenias are of concern and/or unpredictable. Recently several studies have demonstrated the efficacy and safety of DOACs in the treatment of cancer-associated VTE[11,12]; however, dedicated studies evaluating DOACs to prevent atrial thrombus formation in patients with AF

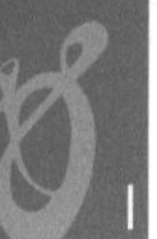

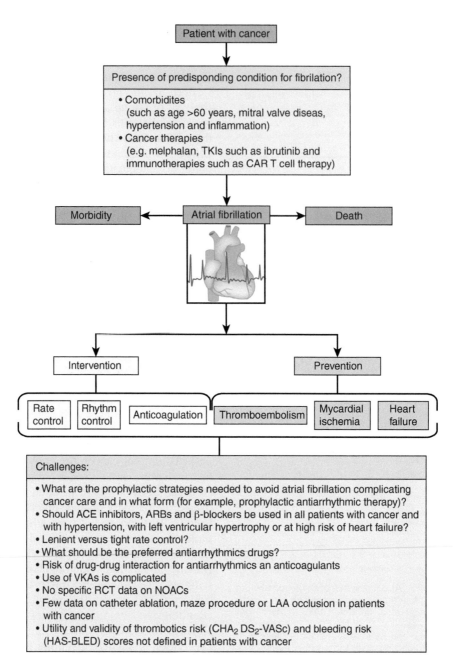

Patient with cancer

Presence of predisponding condition for fibrilation?

- Comorbidites
  (such as age >60 years, mitral valve diseas, hypertension and inflammation)
- Cancer therapies
  (e.g. melphalan, TKIs such as ibrutinib and immunotherapies such as CAR T cell therapy)

Morbidity ← Atrial fibrillation → Death

Intervention
- Rate control
- Rhythm control
- Anticoagulation

Prevention
- Thromboembolism
- Mycardial ischemia
- Heart failure

Challenges:

- What are the prophylactic strategies needed to avoid atrial fibrillation complicating cancer care and in what form (for example, prophylactic antiarrhythmic therapy)?
- Should ACE inhibitors, ARBs and β-blockers be used in all patients with cancer and with hypertension, with left ventricular hypertrophy or at high risk of heart failure?
- Lenient versus tight rate control?
- What should be the preferred antiarrhythmics drugs?
- Risk of drug-drug interaction for antiarrhythmics an anticoagulants
- Use of VKAs is complicated
- No specific RCT data on NOACs
- Few data on catheter ablation, maze procedure or LAA occlusion in patients with cancer
- Utility and validity of thrombotics risk (CHA_2 DS_2-VASc) and bleeding risk (HAS-BLED) scores not defined in patients with cancer

FIG. 10.3 Main elements in the treatment of patients with cancer and atrial fibrillation. *ACE*, Angiotensin-converting enzyme; *ARB*, angiotensin-receptor blocker; *HAS-BLED*, Hypertension, Abnormal renal and liver function, Stroke, Bleeding, Labile INR, Elderly, Drugs or alcohol; *LAA*, left atrial appendage; *NOAC*, non-vitamin K antagonist oral anticoagulant; *RCT*, randomized clinical trials; *TKI*, tyrosine kinase inhibitor; *VKA*, vitamin K antagonist. (From Herrmann, J. Adverse cardiac effects of cancer therapies: cardiotoxicity and arrhythmia. *Nat Rev Cardiol* 17, 474–502 (2020). https://doi.org/10.1038/s41569-020-0348-1.)

and cancer is lacking because patients with cancer have generally been excluded or underrepresented in the seminal DOAC trials. Nevertheless, a subanalysis of the ARISTOTLE (Apixaban for Reduction in Stroke and Other Thromboembolic Events in Atrial Fibrillation) trial demonstrated greater protection from thromboembolism with apixaban than warfarin in patients with active cancer when compared with patients without cancer.[13] Similar findings were reported in a sub study of the ENGAGE AF-TIMI 48 (Effective Anticoagulation with Factor Xa Next Generation in Atrial Fibrillation–Thrombolysis in Myocardial Infarction 48) trial with edoxaban.[14] A retrospective analysis of more than 16,000 patients with cancer suggested similar reduction in ischemic stroke with the different DOACs, and lower rates of bleeding with apixaban.[15]

Multiple issues ranging from limited life expectancy to increased bleeding from hematologic abnormalities or intracerebral metastases may prevent long-term anticoagulant use in patients receiving cancer therapy. Furthermore, the benefits of thromboembolism reduction must be balanced with the potential for bleeding complications. For example, ibrutinib is associated with increased bleeding owing to the effects on the glycogen VI collagen activation pathway.[16] Studies have demonstrated increased rates of intracerebral bleeds with the concomitant use of ibrutinib and vitamin K antagonists.[17] As a result warfarin is generally avoided with this drug, although DOACs appear to be relatively safe. Moreover, multiple cancer therapeutics can interact with anticoagulants, especially warfarin and the DOACs, leading to increased bleeding and/or decreased efficacy. Dabigatran is particularly susceptible to interactions with p-glycoprotein, whereas apixaban and rivaroxaban are both metabolized via the cytochrome P450 3A4 system. As such, their efficacy is affected by both inducers and inhibitors of this system. For example, enzalutamide, a non-steroidal antiandrogen used for prostate cancer can increase levels of apixaban and rivaroxaban and therefore the concomitant use of these DOACs should be avoided.[5,6]

In patients who are at very high risk for stroke but in whom anticoagulation is likely to be contraindicated, left atrial appendage occlusion devices may be an option, however they have not been specifically evaluated in patients with cancer. It is also important to note that current recommendations require short-term anticoagulation with warfarin followed by long-term treatment with antiplatelets. For patients who are not candidates for short-term oral anticoagulation, the ASAP-TOO trial is currently enrolling patients to determine the safety and efficacy of the Watchman left atrial appendage closure device without postprocedural anticoagulation.[18] If the device arm demonstrates favorable results, this could become an important option to protect newly diagnosed cancer cases in patients with AF who may not be candidates for anticoagulation.

QT INTERVAL ASSESSMENT

Significant attention is paid to the QT prolonging potential of many different cancer therapeutics. The QT interval is the electrocardiographic manifestation of ventricular myocardial depolarization and repolarization. At the cellular level the process of depolarization and repolarization is known as the action potential and is controlled by the influx and efflux of sodium, calcium, and potassium ions. The action potential of the ventricular myocardium is divided into five phases: phase 0—depolarization, primarily driven by the rapid opening of sodium channels; phase 1—early repolarization, owing to the rapid transient outflow of potassium ions; phase 2—plateau phase, resulting from the balance of inward calcium and outward potassium flow; phase 3—rapid depolarization, controlled by the opening of outward potassium channels; phase 4—return to baseline resting membrane potential.[19]

Normal QT intervals for men are generally between 350 and 450 milliseconds and for women between 360 and 470 milliseconds. Anything greater than the 99th percentile (>470 milliseconds for men and 480 milliseconds for women) should be considered abnormal. Significant prolongation (>500 milliseconds regardless of gender) confers an increased risk of the potentially life-threatening ventricular arrhythmia, *torsades de points* (TdP).[20] Accurate assessment of the QT interval can be challenging, especially when U waves, AF, bundle branch blocks, or pacing are present. Key points for accurate QT interval measurement are listed in Table 10.2.

It is well established that the QT interval varies with heart rate such that at faster heart rates the QT interval is shorter and at slower heart rates the

TABLE 10.2 Key Points for Accurate QT Measurement

1. Measure longest QT interval
2. Manually verify electronic QT measurements
3. Average measurement over multiple beats
4. Use tangent method to determine the end of the T wave
5. Avoid measuring U waves in most circumstances
6. During atrial fibrillation, average the QT interval more than 10 beats
7. Utilize correction formulae in the setting of bundle branch blocks or ventricular pacing

From Fradley MG, Moslehi J. QT prolongation and oncology drug development. *Card Electrophysiol Clin*. 2015;7(2):341–355.

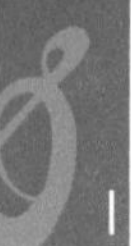

TABLE 10.3 QT Correction Formulae

	BAZETT	FRIDERICIA	FRAMINGHAM	HODGES
Mathematical formulae	$QTc = QT/(RR)^{1/2}$	$QTc = QT/(RR)^{1/3}$	$QTc = QT + 0.154 \times (1 - RR)$	$QTc = QT + 1.75 \times (\text{Heart rate} - 60)$
Advantages	Simple calculation	More accurate at slower heart rates; simple calculation	Accuracy at faster and slower heart rates	Accuracy at faster and slower heart rates
Disadvantages	Overcorrects at fast heart rates and undercorrects at slow heart rates	Overcorrects at fast heart rates	Complicated calculation. Unclear validity outside of original study population.	Complicated calculation.

Adapted from Chandrasekhar S, Fradley MG. QT interval prolongation associated with cytotoxic and targeted cancer therapeutics. *Curr Treat Options Oncol.* 2019;20(7):55.

TABLE 10.4 Cancer Therapeutics With a High Risk of QTc Prolongation, Ventricular Tachycardia (VT) or Fibrillation (VF), Torsades de Pointes (TdP), and Sudden Cardiac Death (SCD)

THERAPY CLASS	AGENT NAME (TARGET)	QTc PROLONGATION	TdP	VT/VF	SCD
HDAC inhibitors	Arsenic trioxide	+++	++	–	+
	Romidepsin	++	+	++	+
	Vorinostat	++	–	–	–
	Panobinostat	++	–	–	–
CDK4/CDK6 inhibitors	Ribociclib	++	–	–	–
Multi-targeted kinase inhibitors	Lenvatinib (VEGFR)	++	–	–	–
	Pazopanib (VEGFR)	++	–	–	–
	Vandetanib (VEGFR)	+++	–	+	+
	Bosutinib (BCR–ABL1)	++	–	–	–
	Nilotinib (BCR–ABL1)	++	–	–	+
	Ceritinib (ALK)	++	–	–	–
	Osimertinib (EGFR/HER1)	++	–	–	–
	Vemurafenib (BRAF)	+++	+	–	–
	Gilteritinib (FTL3)	++	–	–	–
	Trametinib (MEK)	++	–	–	–

HDAC, Histone deacetylase; *VEGFR*, vascular endothelial growth factor receptor.

QT interval is longer. Different mathematic correctional formulae have been developed to standardize the QT interval across the range of heart rates (Table 10.3). The Bazett formula is relatively easy to calculate and it is the most frequent algorithm utilized on electronic electrocardiographic equipment; however, it associated with the most error, overcorrecting at faster heart rates and undercorrecting at slower heart rates when TdP is most likely to occur. The Fridericia formula is also easy to calculate manually and is considered a more accurate assessment than the Bazett formula in most circumstances. In general, the Fridericia formula is the preferred correction for patients with patients. Prior to the initiation of cancer treatments that are known to prolong the QT interval, it is recommended to obtain a baseline electrocardiogram to assess the QT interval. The QT interval should be manually measured and the Fridericia formula should be utilized to correct for heart rate.[21]

There are many reasons for QT prolongation in patients with cancer. Multiple cancer therapeutics are known to prolong the QT interval (Table 10.4), however, patients with patients are also frequently treated with other medications that are also known to prolong the QT interval, such as antiemetics, psychiatric medications, and antibiotics. Moreover, cancer treatment complications including electrolyte abnormalities and renal dysfunction can contribute to abnormal QT interval measurements. Finally, patient characteristics, including gender and baseline CV disease can prolong the QT interval. Prior to the initiation of cancer therapeutics, cardio-oncologists must treat any modifiable risk factors. For example, electrolytes must be aggressively repleted and, if possible, the use of concomitant QT prolonging medications should be avoided, with alternative therapeutics considered.[21]

CARDIAC IMPLANTABLE ELECTRONIC DEVICE EVALUATION

The number of patients with cardiac implantable electronic devices (CIEDs) with newly diagnosed cancer has been increasing significantly over the last several decades as has the proportion of these undergoing radiation therapy. CIEDs include pacemakers, implantable cardioverter defibrillators, and cardiac resynchronization therapy pacemakers/defibrillators. External beam radiation may interact with CIEDs, especially when used to treat thoracic lymphomas, breast, lung, and esophageal cancers, although subdiaphragmatic malignancies may also pose a concern if high-energy radiation therapy is used.[22]

Although most modern CIEDs are designed to withstand diagnostic radiation, therapeutic ionizing radiation can pose a risk to device function. Nevertheless, the vast majority of patients tolerate radiation therapy without any issues or damage to their devices. Most problems occur when the total absorbed dose of radiation by the device exceeds 10 grays (Gy) or the radiation energy is high enough to produce neutrons (generally >10 mV), which are more damaging to the boron and lithium components of devices.[23] The most common device malfunctions are soft errors that damage device software. Most of these are minor and only recorded in the data log of the device. In addition, device resets may occur, which can occasionally require device reprogramming. Hard errors that damage the device hardware are exceedingly rare.[24]

Prior to the initiation of radiation therapy, cardiology and/or electrophysiology should be consulted to interrogate the device and determine pacemaker dependency. In addition, a radiation physicist should estimate the radiation dose to the device. In general, pacemaker-dependent patients and those expected to receive a cumulative dose of greater than 10 Gy to the device require closer evaluation and monitoring. In addition, patients exposed to high energy photons (>10 mV) should also be considered at elevated risk for device damage even if the radiation is directed further from the device, such as below the diaphragm. In patients deemed high risk, device evaluations should occur prior to and after each fraction of radiation.[23,24]

Whereas device relocation is often considered when the absorbed dose is expected to be high, few data to support this practice. In a study of 21 patients who had their device relocated prior to radiation, 4 of them still had evidence of malfunction. If relocation had been protective, the odds ratio (OR) should have been less than 1; however, in this study the OR was actually 2.65.[25] Device repositioning should only be considered if the tumor is directly posterior to the CIED and radiation cannot effectively be delivered to the malignancy because of the device location.

REFERENCES

1. Herrmann J. Adverse cardiac effects of cancer therapies: cardiotoxicity and arrhythmia. *Nat Rev Cardiol.* 2020;17:474–502. doi:10.1038/s41569-020-0348-1.
2. January CT, Wann LS, Alpert JS, et al. 2014 AHA/ACC/HRS guideline for the management of patients with atrial fibrillation: a report of the American College of Cardiology/American Heart Association Task Force on practice guidelines and the Heart Rhythm Society. *Circulation.* 2014;130(23):e199–e267. doi:10.1161/CIR.0000000000000041.
3. Shanafelt TD, Parikh SA, Noseworthy PA, et al. Atrial fibrillation in patients with chronic lymphocytic leukemia (CLL). *Leuk Lymphoma.* 2017;58(7):1630–1639. doi:10.1080/10428194.2016.1257795.
4. Wiczer TE, Levine LB, Brumbaugh J, et al. Cumulative incidence, risk factors, and management of atrial fibrillation in patients receiving ibrutinib. *Blood Adv.* 2017;1(20):1739–1748. doi:10.1182/bloodadvances.2017009720.
5. Rhea I, Burgos PH, Fradley MG. Arrhythmogenic anticancer drugs in cardio-oncology. *Cardiol Clin.* 2019;37(4):459–468. doi:10.1016/j.ccl.2019.07.011.
6. Rhea IB, Lyon AR, Fradley MG. Anticoagulation of cardiovascular conditions in the patient with cancer: review of old and new therapies. *Curr Oncol Rep.* 2019;21(5):45. doi:10.1007/s11912-019-0797-z.
7. January CT, Wann LS, Calkins H, et al. 2019 AHA/ACC/HRS focused update of the 2014 AHA/ACC/HRS Guideline for the Management of Patients with Atrial Fibrillation: a report of the American College of Cardiology/American Heart Association Task Force on Clinical Practice Guidelines and the Heart Rhythm Society in collaboration with the Society of Thoracic Surgeons. *Circulation.* 2019;140(2):e125–e151. doi:10.1161/CIR.0000000000000665.
8. D'Souza M, Carlson N, Fosbøl E, et al. CHA_2 DS_2-VASc score and risk of thromboembolism and bleeding in patients with atrial fibrillation and recent cancer. *Eur J Prev Cardiol.* 2018;25(6):651–658. doi:10.1177/2047487318759858.
9. Patell R, Gutierrez A, Rybicki L, Khorana AA. Usefulness of CHADS2 and CHA_2DS_2-VASc scores for stroke prediction in patients with cancer and atrial fibrillation. *Am J Cardiol.* 2017;120(12):2182–2186. doi:10.1016/j.amjcard.2017.08.038.
10. Lee AY, Rickles FR, Julian JA, et al. Randomized comparison of low molecular weight heparin and coumarin derivatives on the survival of patients with cancer and venous thromboembolism. *J Clin Oncol.* 2005;23(10):2123–2129. doi:10.1200/JCO.2005.03.133.

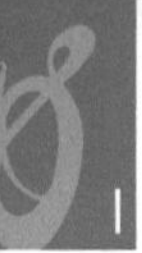

11. Raskob GE, van Es N, Verhamme P, et al. Edoxaban for the treatment of cancer-associated venous thromboembolism. *N Engl J Med.* 2018;378(7):615–624. doi:10.1056/NEJMoa1711948.
12. Young AM, Marshall A, Thirlwall J, et al. Comparison of an oral factor Xa inhibitor with low molecular weight heparin in patients with cancer with venous thromboembolism: results of a randomized trial (SELECT-D). *J Clin Oncol.* 2018;36(20):2017–2023. doi:10.1200/JCO.2018.78.8034.
13. Melloni C, Dunning A, Granger CB, et al. Efficacy and safety of apixaban versus warfarin in patients with atrial fibrillation and a history of cancer: insights from the ARISTOTLE trial. *Am J Med.* 2017;130(12):1440–1448.e1. doi:10.1016/j.amjmed.2017.06.026.
14. Fanola CL, Ruff CT, Murphy SA, et al. Efficacy and safety of edoxaban in patients with active malignancy and atrial fibrillation: analysis of the ENGAGE AF - TIMI 48 trial. *J Am Heart Assoc.* 2018;7(16):e008987. doi:10.1161/JAHA.118.008987.
15. Shah S, Norby FL, Datta YH, et al. Comparative effectiveness of direct oral anticoagulants and warfarin in patients with cancer and atrial fibrillation. *Blood Adv.* 2018;2(3):200–209. doi:10.1182/bloodadvances.2017010694.
16. Levade M, David E, Garcia C, et al. Ibrutinib treatment affects collagen and von Willebrand factor-dependent platelet functions. *Blood.* 2014;124(26):3991–3995. doi:10.1182/blood-2014-06-583294.
17. Wang ML, Rule S, Martin P, et al. Targeting BTK with ibrutinib in relapsed or refractory mantle-cell lymphoma. *N Engl J Med.* 2013;369(6):507–516. doi:10.1056/NEJMoa1306220.
18. Holmes DR, Reddy VY, Buchbinder M, et al. The assessment of the Watchman device in patients unsuitable for oral anticoagulation (ASAP-TOO) trial. *Am Heart J.* 2017;189:68–74. doi:10.1016/j.ahj.2017.03.007.
19. Chandrasekhar S, Fradley MG. QT Interval prolongation associated with cytotoxic and targeted cancer therapeutics. *Curr Treat Options Oncol.* 2019;20(7):55. doi:10.1007/s11864-019-0657-y.
20. Drew BJ, Ackerman MJ, Funk M, et al. Prevention of torsade de pointes in hospital settings: a scientific statement from the American Heart Association and the American College of Cardiology Foundation. *J Am Coll Cardiol.* 2010;55(9):934–947. doi:10.1016/j.jacc.2010.01.001.
21. Fradley MG, Moslehi J. QT prolongation and oncology drug development. *Card Electrophysiol Clin.* 2015;7(2):341–355. doi:10.1016/j.ccep.2015.03.013.
22. Zaremba T, Jakobsen AR, Sogaard M, et al. Risk of device malfunction in patients with cancer with implantable cardiac device undergoing radiotherapy: a population-based cohort study. *Pacing Clin Electrophysiol.* 2015;38(3):343–356. doi:10.1111/pace.12572.
23. Zecchin M, Severgnini M, Fiorentino A, et al. Management of patients with cardiac implantable electronic devices (CIED) undergoing radiotherapy: a consensus document from Associazione Italiana Aritmologia e Cardiostimolazione (AIAC), Associazione Italiana Radioterapia Oncologica (AIRO), Associazione Italiana Fisica Medica (AIFM). *Int J Cardiol.* 2018;255:175–183. doi:10.1016/j.ijcard.2017.12.061.
24. Viganego F, Singh R, Fradley MG. Arrhythmias and other electrophysiology issues in patients with cancer receiving chemotherapy or radiation. *Curr Cardiol Rep.* 2016;18(6):52. doi:10.1007/s11886-016-0730-0.
25. Bagur R, Chamula M, Brouillard E, et al. Radiotherapy-induced cardiac implantable electronic device dysfunction in patients with cancer. *Am J Cardiol.* 2017;119(2):284–289. doi:10.1016/j.amjcard.2016.09.036.

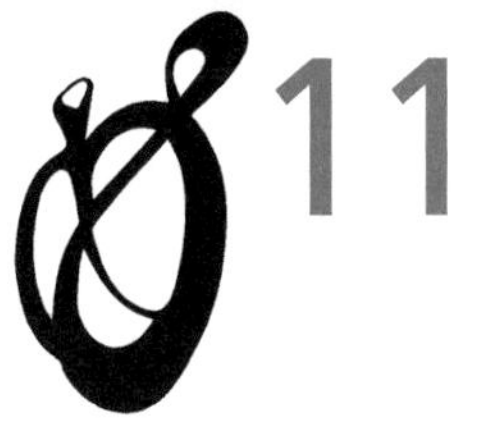

11 Hypertension and Renal Disease Prevention Before Cancer Therapy

STEPHEN J.H. DOBBIN, SANDRA M.S. HERRMANN, NINIAN N. LANG, JOERG HERRMANN, AND RHIAN M. TOUYZ

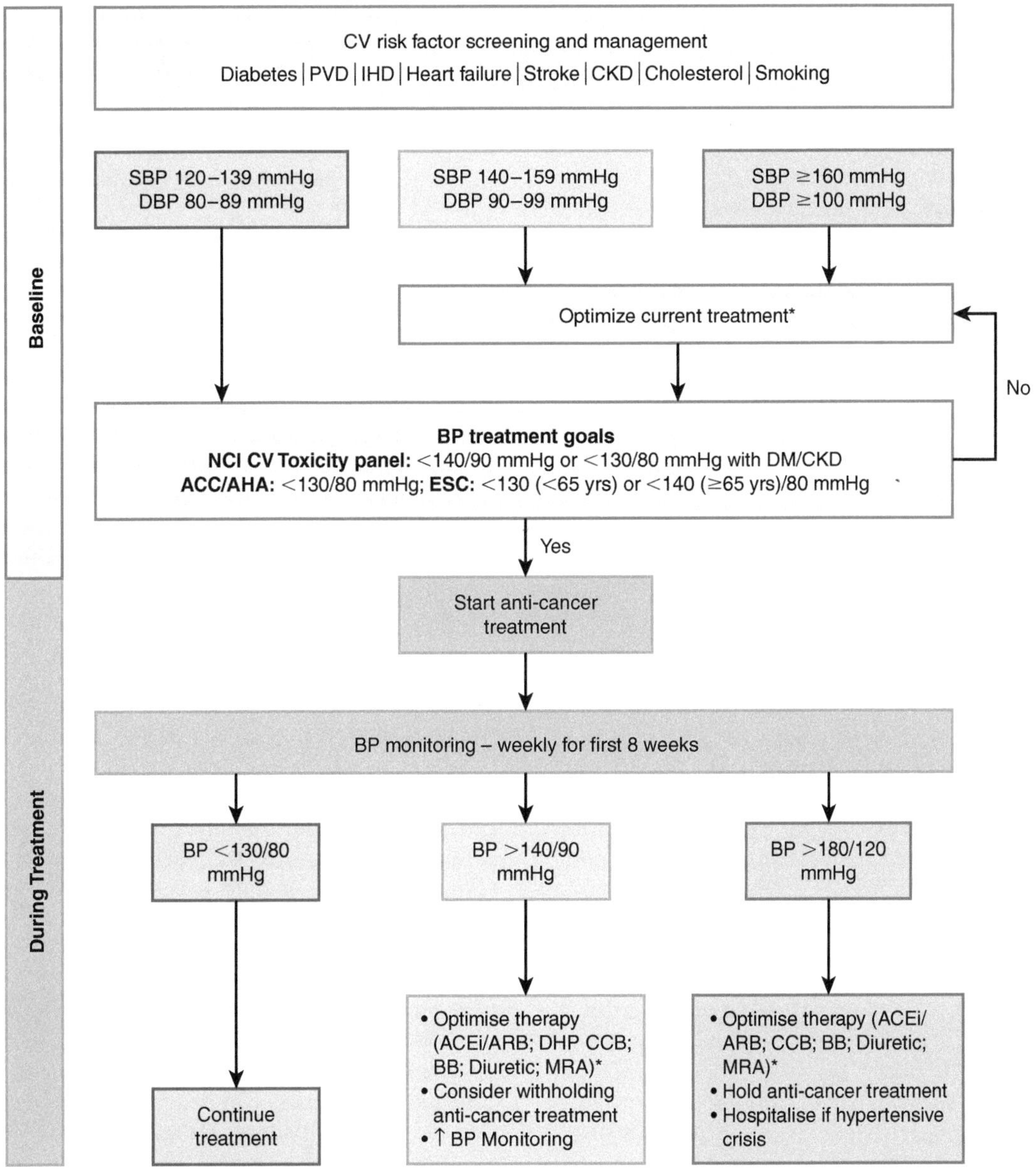

Baseline

CV risk factor screening and management
Diabetes | PVD | IHD | Heart failure | Stroke | CKD | Cholesterol | Smoking

SBP 120–139 mmHg
DBP 80–89 mmHg

SBP 140–159 mmHg
DBP 90–99 mmHg

SBP ≥160 mmHg
DBP ≥100 mmHg

Optimize current treatment*

BP treatment goals
NCI CV Toxicity panel: <140/90 mmHg or <130/80 mmHg with DM/CKD
ACC/AHA: <130/80 mmHg; **ESC:** <130 (<65 yrs) or <140 (≥65 yrs)/80 mmHg

No

Yes

During Treatment

Start anti-cancer treatment

BP monitoring – weekly for first 8 weeks

BP <130/80 mmHg

BP >140/90 mmHg

BP >180/120 mmHg

Continue treatment

- Optimise therapy (ACEi/ARB; DHP CCB; BB; Diuretic; MRA)*
- Consider withholding anti-cancer treatment
- ↑ BP Monitoring

- Optimise therapy (ACEi/ARB; CCB; BB; Diuretic; MRA)*
- Hold anti-cancer treatment
- Hospitalise if hypertensive crisis

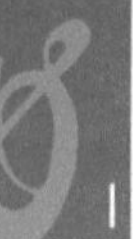

CHAPTER OUTLINE

KEY POINTS

- Hypertension and renal disease, which are common in patients with cancer, can have a significant impact on outcomes, including induction and aggravation of cardiotoxicity
- Baseline risk factors for hypertension and renal disease/toxicity should be recognized and addressed as much as possible before starting anticancer therapy
- Vascular endothelial growth factor (VEGF) inhibitors, in particular, are associated with both hypertension and the risk of renal toxicity and this risk is to be considered in patients to be started on these drugs
- Antihypertensive therapy should be optimized before commencing cancer treatment and the patient should be provided with a blood pressure monitoring and management plan
- Preventive efforts to reduce the risk of acute kidney injury and progression of chronic kidney disease should be implemented and continued throughout cancer therapy
- Correct estimation of renal function is key for dose calculations of cancer therapies

Hypertension is a well-established cardiovascular effect of anticancer therapy, particularly with vascular endothelial growth factor inhibitors (VEGFI),[1] and is associated with adverse outcomes.[2,3] Hypertension is the most common comrbidity in patients diagnosed with cancer.[4] In order to minimize the risk of end-organ effects, it is important that blood pressure (BP) management is optimised prior to commencing cancer therapy wherever possible. Particular attention should be paid to up-front BP management in patients who are to be exposed to potentially cardiotoxic chemotherapeutic agents as well as in patients to be treated with drugs associated with acute hypertensive effects, such as VEGFI or mammalian target of rapamycin (mTOR) inhibitors, platinum-based compounds, and proteasome inhibitors (see Chapter 20). Renal side effects, including acute kidney injury, also have been reported with VEGFI, but are also associated with many other anticancer therapies that have a broad range of potentially harmful effects on the kidneys. Chronic kidney disease may be a consequence of long-standing hypertension and renal disease can lead to hypertension. Thus, there is a bidrectional component in the pathogenesis and progression of both hypertension and renal disease. Importantly, hypertension is one of the most common risk factors reported for cardiotoxicity and decreasing renal function can profoundly limit treatment options. For these reasons, careful attention needs to be paid to these related comorbidites in the cardio-oncology clinic.

RISK STRATIFICATION AND SCREENING FOR HYPERTENSION AND RENAL DYSFUNCTION

Assessment for preexisting cardiovascular disease and cardiovascular risk factors should be made in all patients prior to starting VEGFI therapy (Table 11.1). This should be performed by the oncology team in the first instanceand should include a detailed history, physical examination, and focused investigations to screen for risk factors and preexisting end-organ damage.[5–7] It is important to identify any history of preexisting hypertension or established cardiovascular disease, including ischemic heart disease, cerebrovascular disease, peripheral arterial disease, retinal disease, and heart

TABLE 11.1 Diagnostic Workup Before Cancer Therapies That Increase the Risk of Hypertension

Baseline assessment of cardiovascular risk factors (performed by oncologist):	Detailed history and clinical examination Blood pressure measurement Electrocardiography and echocardiography Blood analysis—electrolytes and renal function Cholesterol and glucose/Hb_{A1C} measurement Lifestyle factors: smoking, alcohol consumption, exercise, weight reduction
Risk factor modification and optimization of cardiovascular status takes place prior to starting cancer treatment	
Referral to cardiovascular-oncologist for optimization of cardiovascular status in patients at high risk	
Collaboration with oncology and cardiovascular-oncology specialist on timing of introduction of anticancer therapy	
Aim to commence cancer therapy once satisfactory risk factor control achieved, or sooner depending on clinical mandate.	
In patients with hypertension, ensure good blood pressure control with standard antihypertensive drugs based on hypertension guidelines.	

failure. Additional cardiovascular risk factors, including smoking and family history of premature cardiovascular disease, should be identified. Renal function should be assessed at baseline via serum creatinine and estimated glomerular filtration rate (GFR) measurement. Preexisting proteinuria should also be assessed, at a minimum by use of urinary dispstick, and preferably by laboratory measurement of protein-to-creatine ratio.[8] Where possible, ambulatory BP monitoring should be used to identify preexisting hypertension and office BP should always be measured prior to commencing therapy.[9,10] Lipid profile andfasting plasma glucose should be measured in all patients. A baseline electrocardiogram and echocardiogram should be obtained.[11]

The over-arching aim of these assessments is not to exclude patients from treatment with a VEGFI, but to provide a systematic means of identifying and addressing modifiable risk factors to reduce the risk of developing acute cardiovascular complications during and after treatment. By addressing these issues proactively, it is intended that patients should be able to receive the optimal cancer therapy, at the optimal dose, and for the optimal time to allow maximum anticancer effects to be achieved without interruption or cessation because of concerns about cardiovascular toxicity. It is very important to note that the treatment of VEGFI-associated hypertension does not impair the VEGFI anticancer effect.[12]

Given that almost every patient commenced on VEGFI therapy will have a treatment-associated rise in blood pressure (outlined in detail in Chapter 20),[5,13] it is important to identify those at greatest risk. It is clear that there would be clinical value in a risk prediction tool for VEGFI-associated hypertension and end-organ effects from hypertension. This could be used to facilitate more intensive BP monitoring and early intervention, particularly in those most vulnerable. However, the currently available data are insufficient to inform such a tool and the use of circulating and urinary biomarkers to identify such patients is limited at present. In the absence of validated risk-stratification tools, clinical assessment should focus on conventional cardiovascular risk factors.

In patients proposed to receive other treatments with cardiotoxicity potential similar attention should be paid to the assessment and treatment of blood pressures. Whereas the primary cardiotoxic effect of many of these drugs is on the myocardium, the consequences of myocardial toxicity are further potentiated by coexisting hypertension.[14]

CORRECTING MODIFIABLE RISK FACTORS

It is accepted that strict control of cardiovascular risk factors to minimize the risk of the development of toxicity is an important part of the treatment of patients. Adequate BP control should be accomplished before starting treatment, and intensive monitoring of BP and up-titration of antihypertensive therapy may be required to minimize any delay in starting cancer treatment.[15] Lifestyle modifications should be instituted, including reduced alcohol consumption, smoking cessation and, where possible, physical exercise. Management of diabetes should also be optimized, with input from diabetologists where appropriate.

The risks of delaying anticancer therapy for optimization of the cardiovascular status always need to be balanced with the hazards of incomplete control or suboptimal management of cardiovascular disease and risks.

DIAGNOSIS AND MONITORING OF HYPERTENSION BEFORE TREATMENT

The criteria for the diagnosis of hypertension vary across international guidelines and this variation is primarily a reflection of a differing interpretation of data from the Systolic Blood Pressure Intervention Trial (SPRINT) trial.[16] SPRINT demonstrated that cardiovascular outcomes in patients at high risk were improved by intensive blood pressure reduction.[16] This trial was conducted in a noncancer population and extrapolation of the results to those with cancer and particularly those to be treated with VEGFI requires careful consideration. Patients with cancer may be at greater risk of iatrogenic hypotension, particularly in the context of intercurrent infection or hemorrhage. Additionally, the balance of competing cardiovascular and oncologic risk needs careful assessment. The Cardiovascular Toxicities Panel, Convened by the Angiogenesis Task Force of the National Cancer Institute Investigational Drug Steering Committee recommended a goal of blood pressure less than 140/90 mm Hg for patients on VEGFI therapy and a goal of less than 130/80 mm Hg for those with diabetes and/or chronic kidney disease.[10] More recent American College of Cardiology/American Heart Association guidelines recommend more stringent BP control, with antihypertensive therapy being commenced in patients with blood pressure greater than 130/80 mm Hg and with high cardiovascular risk, defined as individuals with existing cardiovascular disease, a calculated 10-year cardiovascular risk of more than 10%, or those who have other risk factors (e.g., kidney disease or diabetes).[15] Conversely, current European Society of Cardiology guidelines and its position paper on cardiovascular toxicity of anticancer therapy recommend treatment initiation at blood pressures above 140/90 mm Hg.[17,18] Taking these variations in recommendations and the increased risk of the rapid and potentially severe rise in BP seen with almost all patients receiving VEGFI therapy into consideration, we recommend a target BP of below 130/80 mm Hg prior to starting treatment. However, the start of anticancer treatment should not be delayed in order to achieve strict blood pressure control, and we agree with the National Cancer Institute Investigational Drug Steering Committee's recommendation that blood pressure should be below 140/90 mm Hg before initiating VEGFI therapy as an absolute minimum. Decisions on antihypertensive therapy, BP control, and timing of initiation of VEGFI therapy should be made following input from both oncology and cardiovascular specialists to ensure timely optimal cardiovascular status is achieved prior to commencing VEGFI therapy.

For those patients with preexisting hypertension already receiving antihypertensive treatment, it is important to ensure adherence to therapy, the optimal choice of agent, and the dosing regimen. It may be necessary to change to an alternative agent, up-titrate the current dosing regimen or to add an additional agent. In most cases the choice of antihypertensive drug(s) should follow clinical guidelines for the general, noncancer, population, but particular preference for the use of ACEi/ARB (angiogensin-converting enzyme inhibitor/angiotensin receptor blocker) in patients with hypertension scheduled to receive drugs with a known cardiotoxic profile, particularly anthracyclines and/or trastuzumab. Non-dihydropyridine calcium channel blockers should be avoided in patients due to be treated with VEGFI. Other pertinent aspects for the choice of antihypertensive therapy in patients with cancer are outlined elsewhere (see Chapter 20, Table 20.2). Referral to a hypertension specialist or cardiovascular-oncologist may be appropriate if there is any difficulty with achieving target blood pressure.[19]

RENAL DISEASE IN PATIENTS WITH CANCER

Evaluation of kidney function is a critical element in the assessment of the patient with cancer before initiating cancer therapy for several reasons.[20] First, determination of renal function is essential for the calculation of the correct dose of cancer therapeutics. Second, preexisting chronic kidney disease (CKD) is a risk factor for acute kidney injury during cancer therapy. Third, CKD identifies a patient population with worse clinical outcomes.

The Insuffisance Rénale et Médicaments Anticancéreux studies were the first to report on the prevalence of CKD in patients with cancer.[21] With 90 mL/min/1.72 m^2 as the cutoff for CKD, at least half of the patients with solid tumors had reduced renal function and CKD stage III and IV were seen in 12% each.[21] These numbers are particularly high in patients with renal cell carcinoma (RCC), with nearly 90% having some reduction in glomerular function rate GFR to less than 90 mL/min/1.72 m^2 and 26% having CKD Stage III or IV.[22] Among patients who undergo nephrectomy for localized RCC, approximately 25% to 30% have CKD prior to surgery. This high prevalence may reflect the presence of risk factors that are common to both RCC and CKD, such as older age, male sex, smoking, obesity, diabetes, and hypertension. Assessment of the nonneoplastic tissue obtained from tumor nephrectomy specimens may provide important information about the cause of CKD and the risk of disease progression in these patients. In one study, kidney disease (most frequently, diabetic nephropathy and hypertensive nephropathy) was identified in 15% of tumor nephrectomy specimens; 74% of these cases also showed evidence of severe arteriolosclerosis.[23] Patients with a GFR less than 60 mL/min/1.72 m^2 have a worse cancer-related survival prognosis of 4 to 9 months, and some studies suggest an 18% increase in cancer-related mortality for every 10 mL/min/1.72 m^2 drop in GFR.[21]

ESTIMATION OF RENAL FUNCTION IN PATIENTS WITH CANCER

When estimating renal function in patients with cancer, the Chronic Kidney Disease Epidemiology Collaboration formula is the method of choice currently. However, the Modification of the Diet in Renal Disease and Janowitz equations may be used as alternatives.[24] In patients with presumed low muscle mass, including those with advanced disease and debility, creatinine-based formulas can be misleading and calculations based on cystatin C are advisable.

RENAL DYSFUNCTION AND IMPLICATIONS FOR MANAGEMENT

A critical element of the precancer therapy evaluation is the recognition of the risk of renal failure (Table 11.2).[20] A number of clinical conditions predispose, and special attention needs to be paid to, nephrotoxic cancer therapeutics (Table 11.3).[25] These mandate viliglance and surveillance, and preventive measures as available. When a patient has an estimated GFR of less than 60 mL/min/1.73 m^2, whenever possible nephrotoxic drugs should be avoided and the least nephrotoxic drugs should be used, if otherwise of equal efficiency (i.e., oxaliplatin > carboplatin > cisplatin). Preventive measures include minimizing the use of any additional nephrotoxins such as contrast agents and ACEi/ ARBs.

The management of the complications related to CKD (e.g., hypertension, anemia, mineral bone disease) in patients with cancer is broadly similar to that in patients without cancer with some nuances. For instance, erythropoiesis-stimulating agents should only be prescribed with caution because of concerns for hypertension, higher rates of thromboembolism, and faster progression of malignancy.

CANCER-ASSOCIATED RENAL DISEASE

Several malignacies are associated with renal (glomerular) disease. In distinction from the renal toxicities above, these improve with cancer therapy.[20]

Among cancer-associated glomerular diseases, membranous nephropathy (MN) and minimal change disease (MCD) are the most common. MN is more often associated with solid tumors (e.g., carcinomas of the lung, prostate, or gastrointestinal tract) and less commonly with hematologic malignancies (e.g., chronic lymphocytic leukemia [CLL]). Treatment of the cancer is often associated with improvement in renal function. Indeed, patients diagnosed with MN should undergo routine cancer screening. MCD, is associated in particular with hematologic maliganices, especially Hodgkin lymphoma and, less commonly, with lymphoproliferative disorders and solid tumors. Lymphoma-associated MCD is frequently resistant to treatment with glucocorticoids and cyclosporine. Therefore, a poor response to the treatment of MCD with these agents should prompt an investigation for an underlying malignancy. In some, but not all, patients with lymphoma-associated MCD, the course of MCD correlates with that of the lymphoma. An association with malignancy has also been described with membranoproliferative glomerulonephritis, immunoglobulin A (IgA) nephropathy, IgA vasculitis (Henoch-Schönlein purpura), and amyloid A amyloidosis.

Proteinuria and the nephrotic syndrome are common presenting features of disorders associated with multiple myeloma or other monoclonal gammopathies. These include amyloidosis (see Chapter 51). Light chain (AL) amyloidosis is the most common variant of primary amyloidosis, and Ig-associated amyloidosis typically presents with proteinuria, nephrotic syndrome, and renal failure. Monoclonal immunoglobulin deposition disease (MIDD) is pathogenetically similar to Ig-associated amyloidosis except that the light (or heavy) chain fragments deposited within the membranes do not form fibrils and do not stain Congo red positive. Based on the composition of the deposits, three types of MIDD can be differentiated: light chain deposition disease, heavy chain deposition disease, and light and heavy chain deposition disease. MIDD is most frequently seen in patients with multiple myeloma, but also in those with Waldenström macroglobulinemia, CLL, and nodal marginal zone lymphoma. Proteinuria, renal impairment, and hypertension are the typical triad of presenting features of MIDD.

Other monoclonal gammopathy-associated disorders that can cause proteinuria and nephrotic syndrome include monoclonal cryoglobulinemia, membranoproliferative glomerulonephritis, crystalline podocytopathy, fibrillary glomerulonephritis and immunotactoid glomerulopathy, and membranous-like

TABLE 11.2 **Factors to Evaluate for Acute and Chronic Renal Insufficiency Before, During, and After Cancer Therapy**

	BEFORE	DURING	AFTER
AKI			
RIFLE Criteria Risk Increased serum Cr ≥ 1.5-fold the normal value, or GFR decrease [25% normal value] Or UO < 0.5 mL/kg/h for 6 h Injury Increased serum Cr ≥ 2-fold the normal value, or GFR decrease [50% normal value] UO < 0.5 mL/kg/h for 12 h Failure Increased serum Cr ≥ 3-fold the normal value, GFR decrease [75% normal value] or serum Cr C 4 mg/dL with acute rise C 0.5 mg/dL Or UO < 0.3 mL/kg/h for 24 h, or anuria for 12 h Loss Need for renal replacement therapy for 4 weeks ESRD Need for renal replacement therapy for 4 weeks	**Goals** Identify and reduce risk of renal function decline	**Goals** Screen for, reduce and treat renal complications and function decline	**Goals** Screen for, reduce, and treat renal complications and function decline

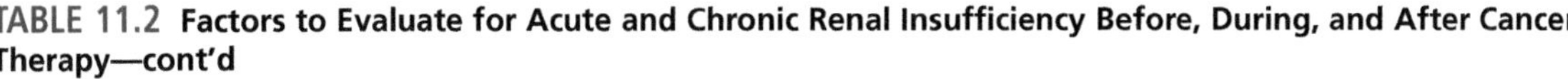

TABLE 11.2 Factors to Evaluate for Acute and Chronic Renal Insufficiency Before, During, and After Cancer Therapy—cont'd

	BEFORE	DURING	AFTER
AKIN Classification			

Stage I
Increase in serum Cr ≥ 1.5–2-fold from baseline or C 0.3 mg/dL
OR UO < 0.5 mL/kg/h for more than 6 h
Stage II
Increase in serum Cr ≥ 2–3-fold from baseline
OR UO < 0.5 mL/kg/h for more than 12 h
Stage III
Increase in serum Cr > 3-fold from baseline, or serum Cr ≥ 4 mg/dL with acute increase ≥ 0.5 mg/dL
OR UO < 0.3 mL/kg/h for 24 h, or anuria for 12 h
	Prerenal causes
	• Volume depletion
	• Infection
	• Hypercalcemia
	• Hyperuricemia
	• Reduced cardiac output
	• Medications
	  • ACE inhibitors or ARBs
	  • Diuretics
	  • NSAIDs
	  • Iodinated contrast
	Intrarenal causes
	• Additional risk factors for acute interstitial nephritis (e.g., concomitant medications)
	• Additional risk factors for acute tubular necrosis (e.g., hypotension)
	• Tumor infiltration of the kidney
	• Risk factors for tumor lysis syndrome
	Postrenal causes
	• Obstruction
	• Retroperitoneal fibrosis
	Other risk factors for AKI:
	• Advanced cancer stage
	• Older age
	• CKD
	• Diabetes
	• Concomitant use of diuretics, ACE inhibitors or ARBs
	• Immune response genes (increased allergic reactions to drugs)
	• Pharmacogenomics in favor of toxicity (gene mutations in metabolizing enzymes and transport proteins)
	• Renal drug handling, high blood delivery rate to the kidney, high uptake and metabolic rate, relatively hypoxic renal environment
		Prerenal causes
		• Volume depletion
		• Decreased oral intake
		• Gastrointestinal losses
		• Reduced cardiac output
		• Sepsis
		• Hypercalcemia
		• Medications
		  • ACE inhibitors or angiotensin receptor blockers
		  • Diuretics
		  • Iodinated contrast
		  • NSAIDs
		• Sinusoidal obstruction syndrome (veno-occlusive disease)
		Intrarenal causes
		Glomerular disease
		• Monoclonal gammopathy-associated proliferative glomerulonephritis
		• Rapidly progressive glomerulonephritis
		Tubulointerstitial
		• Acute interstitial nephritis
		• Acute tubular necrosis
		• Light chain cast nephropathy
		• Lysozymuria
		• Nephrotoxic anticancer agents
		• High-dose and prolonged exposure to therapy
		• Tumor infiltration of the kidney
		• Tumor lysis syndrome
		Vascular
		• Thrombotic microangiopathy
		Nephrectomy
		Postrenal causes
		Intratubular obstruction
		Uric acid nephropathy
		Methotrexate
		Case nephropathy (MM)
		Extrarenal obstruction
		Bladder outlet or urethral obstruction
		GU > GI malignancies retroperitoneal fibrosis
			Early after HCT
			Prerenal causes
			• HRS
			• Hypovolemia
			• Calcineurin inhibitors
			• Amphotericin B
			Intrarenal causes
			• ATN
			• Methotrexate
			Postrenal causes
			• Hemorrhagic cystitis
			• Fungal infection
			Late after HCT
			• TMA
			• Calcineurin inhibitors
			• AKI after nephrectomy
			Highest risk period first 90 days after systemic therapy
			None HCT
			Pre-, intra-, and post-renal causes as seen in the general population

Continued

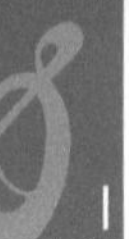

TABLE 11.2 **Factors to Evaluate for Acute and Chronic Renal Insufficiency Before, During, and After Cancer Therapy—cont'd**

	BEFORE	DURING	AFTER
CKD			
CKD Stages	**Goals** Assessment of renal function prior to cancer therapy	**Goals** Screen for and identify decline of renal function and responsible factors	**Goals** Screen for and identify decline of renal function and responsible factors
Stage I: Normal GFR > 90 mL/min **Stage II: Mild CKD** GFR = 60–89 mL/min **Stage IIIA: Mild-moderate CKD** GFR = 45–59 mL/min **Stage IIIB: Moderate CKD** GFR = 30–44 mL/min **Stage IV: Severe CKD** GFR = 15–29 mL/min **Stage V End-stage CKD** GFR < 15 mL/min	• Recognize preexisting CKD (e.g., due to diabetes or hypertension, or chronic obstructive nephropathy) • If renal function is reduced, avoid nephrotoxic drugs whenever possible, if this is not possible, implement strategies to prevent renal toxicity • Adjust dosing of all medications, including all cancer drugs properly based on estimated renal clearance (see recommended formulas)	Dynamics could be due to • Worsening preexisting CKD • Non-recovery from AKI • Chronic obstructive nephropathy • Nephrotoxicity of anticancer agents	Dynamics could be due to • Worsening preexisting CKD • Non-recovery from AKI • Chronic obstructive nephropathy • Nephrotoxicity of anticancer agents • Reduction in renal mass following nephrectomy for renal cell (RCC) or urothelial cancers • Kidney irradiation • Chronic TMA after HCT

ACE, Angiotensin-converting enzyme; *AKI*, acute kidney injury; *AKIN*, acute kidney injury network; *ARBs*, angiotensin receptor blockers; *ATN*, acute tubular necrosis; *CKD*, chronic kidney disease; *ESRD*, end-stage renal disease; *GFR*, glomerular filtration rate; *HCT*, hematopoietic cell transplantation; *HRS*, hepatorenal syndrome; *MM*, multiple myeloma; *NSAIDs*, nonsteroidal anti-inflammatory drugs; *RIFLE*, risk, injury, failure, loss of kidney function, and end-stage kidney disease; *TMA*, thrombotic microangiopathy; UO, urine output.

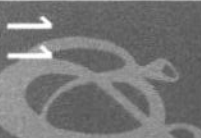

TABLE 11.3 Drug-Based Approach to Nephrotoxicity of Cancer Therapeutics

	CLINICAL PRESENTATIONS									HISTOPATHOLOGY									PREVENTION[a]
	HTN	AKI	PROT.	HEM.	FANCONI	NDI	NA↓	MG↓	TLS	TMA	ATI	AIN	CIN	IF	CRYST.	FSG	GN	MCD	
Chemotherapeutics																			
Anthracyclines		√	√							√						√		√	
Cyclophos-phamide				√[b]			√[c]												IV fluid, Mesna
Gemcitabine	√	√	√	√						√									
Ifosfamide		√			√	√					√								IV fluids, dose ↓
Melphalan																			
Methotrexate		√					√[c]				√				√				IV fluids, urine alkalization
Mitomycin C	√	√	√	√						√									
Nitrosorurea		√[d]											√						IV fluids
Pemetrexed		√			√	√					√			√					IV fluids
Platinum drugs		√			√	√	√[e]	√			√								IV fluids, IV Mg, dose ↓
Proteasome inhibitor (carfilzomib)	√	√	√							√	√								
Vinca alkaloids							√[c]												
Targeted Therapeutics																			
ALK TKI		√						√[f]			√	√							
Bcl-2 inhibitors									√										
BRAF TKI		√						√[f]			√	√							
BCR-Abl TKI (imatinib)		√[d]									√								
BTK TKI (ibrutinib)	√	√																	
EGFR inhibitors								√											
FGFR inhibitors		√									√								
Rituximab		√							√		√				√				IV fluids, hypourecemics
VEGF inhibitors	√	√	√							√	√	√				√			

Continued

TABLE 11.3 Drug-Based Approach to Nephrotoxicity of Cancer Therapeutics—cont'd

	CLINICAL PRESENTATIONS									HISTOPATHOLOGY									PREVENTION[a]
	HTN	AKI	PROT.	HEM.	FANCONI	NDI	NA↓	MG↓	TLS	TMA	ATI	AIN	CIN	IF	CRYST.	FSG	GN	MCD	
Immunotherapeutics																			
CAR-T cells		√[g]						√[f]	√										Steroids
CTLA-4 inhibitors		√	√									√					√	√	
Interferons		√	√							√						√			
Interleukin-2		√[g]																	IV fluids
ICI (PD-1 inhibitors)		√										√							

[a]In addition to minimizing exposure to other nephrotoxins.
[b]Hemorrhagic cystitis.
[c]Syndrome of inappropriate antidiuretic hormone.
[d]Chronic kidney disease predisposition.
[e]Salt wasting.
[f]Electrolyte disorders (in addition, e.g., calcium, phosphate).
[g]Capillary leak syndrome with AKI.

AIN, Acute interstitial nephritis; *AKI*, acute kidney injury; *ALK*, anaplastic lymphoma kinase; *ATI*, acute tubular injury; *Bcl-2*, B cell lymphoma-2; *BTK*, Bruton tyrosine kinase; *CIN*, chronic interstitial nephritis; *CTLA-4*, cytotoxic T-lymphocyte-associated protein 4; *Cryst.*, crystalline nephropathy; *EGFR*, epidermal growth factor receptor; *FGFR*, fibroblast growth factor receptor; *FSG*, focal segmental glomerulosclerosis; GN, glomerulonephritis; Hem., hematuria; HTN, hypertension; *ICI*, immune checkpoint inhibitors; *IF*, interstitial fibrosis; *MCD*, minimal change disease; *Mg↓*, hypomagnesemia; *Na↓*, hyponatremia; *NDI*, nephrogenic diabetes insipidus; *PD-1*, programmed death 1; *Prot.*, proteinuria; *TKI*, tyrosine kinase inhibitor; *TLS*, tumor lysis syndrome; *TMA*, thrombotic microangiopathy; *VEGF*, vascular endothelial growth factor nephropathy with masked immunoglobulin G (IgG)-kappa.

CANCER THERAPY-INDUCED RENAL DISEASE

Proteinuria and nephrotic syndrome (as well as renal failure and hypertension) can also be a consequence of glomerular disease induced by cancer therapies. This occurs, in particular, in patients treated with VEGFI. Proteinuria occurs as a dose-dependent side effect in up to 60% of patients (on average in 10% to 15% of patients) treated with bevacizumab (a monocolonal antibody directed against VEGF). Although the majority of cases are not severe, grade 3 or 4 proteinuria occurs in up to 6% of treated patients.[26,27] Small molecule tyrosine kinase inhibitors of VEGF are associated with a similarly high incidence of developing grade 2 or higher proteinuria.[28] Low levels of proteinuria are often accepted during VEGFI treatment, but should be closely monitored.[29] The development of nephrotic syndrome and renal impairment with VEGFI therapy will require further evalautions. However, even in 35% of those with small amounts of proteinuria and no evidence of renal function impairment, renal thrombotic microangiopathy (TMA) has been noted.[30] Although proteinuria is most often reversible upon interruption of treatment, severe cases may require cessation of VEGFI therapy, espeically if renal disease is noted.[31] An increase in serum creatinine has been reported with sunitinib therapy in up to 70% of patients, but severe renal dysfunction (grade 3 and 4 events) occurs in less than 1%.[32,33] Unlike patients with proteinuria alone, it has been observed that in those who develop renal dysfunction in association with VEGFI, only a minority (16.6%) have an improvement in kidney function following VEGFI withdrawal.[34] Other reports though do indicate improvement in renal function in patients with biopsy proven VEGFI-induced renal impairment with the introduction of antihypertensive therapy and discontinuation of VEGFI therapy.[35] The role of kidney biopsy is unclear given the bleeding risk associated with the procedure; however, it may be indicated in some patients to exclude paraneoplastic MN.[29] Minimal change nephrotic syndrome, which can evolve to focal segmental glomerulosclerosis (FSGS), and TMA are the two main renal toxicity phenotypes of VEGF inhibitor therapy. Risk factors for the development of VEGFI-induced proteinuria and renal disease have not been extensively studied. However, one analysis of 1392 patients treated with sunitinib and pazopanib showed that Asian ethnicity, diabetes, preexisting hypertension, and prior grade 1 proteinuria were risk factors for the development of any grade proteinuria with hazard ratios of 4.12, 1.45, 1.14, and 1.65 respectively.[36] TMA is mainly seen with bevacizumab (and VEGF-Trap), whereas minimal change nephrotic syndrome/FSGS-like presentation seem to relate to VEGF-TKI therapy.[37]

Chronic therapy with interferons can cause FSGS and MCD. The onset of proteinuria and/or nephrotic syndrome may occur days to years after the initiation of interferon treatment. Discontinuation of interferon generally leads to complete remission of nephrotic syndrome in patients with MCD; however, remission is less consistent in those with FSGS.

Other therapies include the mTOR inhibitors, in particular sirolimus causing collapsing FSGS. In addition, rare cases of membranoproliferative glomerulonephritis, MN, and IgA nephropathy have reported with sirolimus.

Immune checkpoint inhibitors can cause antibody-induced lupus nephritis and acute kidney injury (AKI; most commonly, from acute tubulointerstitial nephritis). Last but not least one needs to be aware of the possibility of pseudo-AKI, that is, an asymptomatic rise in serum creatinine, which spontaneously returns to baseline upon discontinuation of the offending drug. This has been seen, for instance, with capmatinib.[38]

ACKNOWLEDGMENTS

RMT is supported by grants from the British Heart Foundation (BHF) (CH/12/429762; RE/18/6/34217) and SD is funded through the BHF Research Excellence Award (RE/13/5/30177).

REFERENCES

1. Małyszko J, Małyszko M, Kozlowski L, Kozlowska K, Małyszko J. Hypertension in malignancy—an underappreciated problem. *Oncotarget*. 2018;9:20855–20871. doi:10.18632/oncotarget.25024.
2. Armstrong GT, Oeffinger KC, Chen Y, et al. Modifiable risk factors and major cardiac events among adult survivors of childhood cancer. *J Clin Oncol*. 2016;31(29):3673–3680. doi:10.1200/JCO.2013.49.3205.

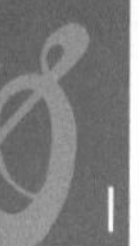

3. Armenian SH, Xu L, Ky B, et al. Cardiovascular disease among survivors of adult-onset cancer: a community-based retrospective cohort study. *J Clin Oncol.* 2016;34(10):1122–1130. doi:10.1200/JCO.2015.64.0409.
4. Piccirillo JF, Tierney RM, Costas I, Grove L, Spitznagel EL. Prognostic importance of comorbidity in a hospital-based cancer registry. *J Am Med Assoc.* 2004;291(20):2441–2447. doi:10.1001/jama.291.20.2441.
5. Small HY, Montezano AC, Rios FJ, Savoia C, Touyz RM. Hypertension due to antiangiogenic cancer therapy with vascular endothelial growth factor inhibitors: understanding and managing a new syndrome. *Can J Cardiol.* 2014;30(5):534–543. doi:10.1016/j.cjca.2014.02.011.
6. Cameron AC, Touyz RM, Lang NN. Vascular complications of cancer chemotherapy. *Can J Cardiol.* 2016;32(7):852–862. doi:10.1016/j.cjca.2015.12.023.
7. Dobbin SJH, Cameron AC, Petrie MC, Jones RJ, Touyz RM, Lang NN. Toxicity of cancer therapy: what the cardiologist needs to know about angiogenesis inhibitors. *Heart.* 2018;104(24):1995–2002. doi:10.1136/heartjnl-2018–313726.
8. Tesařová P, Tesař V. Proteinuria and hypertension in patients treated with inhibitors of the VEGF signalling pathway—incidence, mechanisms and management. *Folia Biol (Praha).* 2013;59(1):15–25.
9. Maitland ML, Kasza KE, Karrison T, et al. Ambulatory monitoring detects sorafenib-induced blood pressure elevations on the first day of treatment. *Clin Cancer Res.* 2009;15(19):6250–6257. doi:10.1158/1078–0432.CCR-09–0058.
10. Maitland ML, Bakris GL, Black HR, et al. Initial assessment, surveillance, and management of blood pressure in patients receiving vascular endothelial growth factor signaling pathway inhibitors. *J Natl Cancer Inst.* 2010;102(9):596–604. doi:10.1093/jnci/djq091.
11. James PA. Evidence-based guideline for the management of high blood pressure in adults. *JAMA.* 2014;311(5):507–520. doi:10.1001/jama.2013.284427.
12. Rini BI, Cohen DP, Lu DR, et al. Hypertension as a biomarker of efficacy in patients with metastatic renal cell carcinoma treated with sunitinib. *J Natl Cancer Inst.* 2011;103(9):763–773. doi:10.1093/jnci/djr128.
13. Abdel-Qadir H, Ethier J-L, Lee DS, Thavendiranathan P, Amir E. Cardiovascular toxicity of angiogenesis inhibitors in treatment of malignancy: a systematic review and meta-analysis. *Cancer Treat Rev.* 2017;53:120–127. doi:10.1016/j.ctrv.2016.12.002.
14. Szmit S, Jurczak W, Zaucha JM, et al. Pre-existing arterial hypertension as a risk factor for early left ventricular systolic dysfunction following (R)-CHOP chemotherapy in patients with lymphoma. *J Am Soc Hypertens.* 2014;8(11):791–799. doi:10.1016/j.jash.2014.08.009.
15. Whelton PK, Carey RM, Aronow WS, et al. 2017 ACC/AHA/AAPA/ABC/ACPM/AGS/APhA/ASH/ASPC/NMA/PCNA Guideline for the prevention, detection, evaluation, and management of high blood pressure in adults: executive summary. *J Am Soc Hypertens.* 2018;71(6):1269–1324. doi:10.1016/j.jash.2018.06.010.
16. SPRINT Research Group. A randomized trial of intensive versus standard blood-pressure control. *N Engl J Med.* 2015;373(22):2103–2116. doi:10.1097/HCR.0000000000000175.
17. Williams B, Mancia G, Spiering W, et al. 2018 Practice guidelines for the management of arterial hypertension of the European Society of Hypertension (ESH) and the European Society of Cardiology (ESC). *Blood Press.* 2018;27(6):314–340. doi:10.1080/08037051.2018.1527177.
18. Zamorano JL, Lancellotti P, Muñoz DR, et al. 2016 ESC position paper on cancer treatments and cardiovascular toxicity developed under the auspices of the ESC committee for practice guidelines: the task force for cancer treatments and cardiovascular toxicity of the European Society Of Cardiology (ESC). *Russ J Cardiol.* 2017;143(3):105–139. doi:10.15829/1560–4071-2017-3-105-139.
19. Rizzoni D, De Ciuceis C, Porteri E, Agabiti-Rosei C, Agabiti-Rosei E. Use of antihypertensive drugs in neoplastic patients. *High Blood Press Cardiovasc Prev.* 2017;24(2):127–132. doi:10.1007/s40292-017-0198-z.
20. Rosner MH, Perazella MA, Magee CC. Overview of kidney disease in the patient with cancer. *UpToDate.* 2020.
21. Launay-Vacher V, Janus N, Deray G. Renal insufficiency and cancer treatments. *ESMO Open.* 2016;1(4):e000091. doi:10.1136/esmoopen-2016–000091.
22. Huang WC, Levey AS, Serio AM, et al. Chronic kidney disease after nephrectomy in patients with renal cortical tumours: a retrospective cohort study. *Lancet Oncol.* 2006;7(9):735–740. doi:10.1016/S1470-2045(06)70803–8.
23. Salvatore SP, Cha EK, Rosoff JS, Seshan SV. Nonneoplastic renal cortical scarring at tumor nephrectomy predicts decline in kidney function. *Arch Pathol Lab Med.* 2013;137(4):531–540. doi:10.5858/arpa.2012-0070-OA.
24. Capasso A, Benigni A, Capitanio U, et al. Summary of the International Conference on Onco-Nephrology: an emerging field in medicine. *Kidney Int.* 2019;96(3):555–567. doi:10.1016/j.kint.2019.04.043.
25. Perazella MA. Onco-nephrology: renal toxicities of chemotherapeutic agents. *Clin J Am Soc Nephrol.* 2012;7(10):1713–1721. doi:10.2215/CJN.02780312.
26. Kappers MHW, Van Esch JHM, Sleijfer S, Danser AJ, Van Den Meiracker AH. Cardiovascular and renal toxicity during angiogenesis inhibition: Clinical and mechanistic aspects. *J Hypertens.* 2009;27(12):2297–2309. doi:10.1097/HJH.0b013e3283309b59.
27. Wu S, Kim C, Baer L, Zhu X. Bevacizumab increases risk for severe proteinuria in patients with cancer. *J Am Soc Nephrol.* 2010;21(8):1381–1389. doi:10.1681/asn.2010020167.
28. Rixe O, Bukowski RM, Michaelson MD, et al. Axitinib treatment in patients with cytokine-refractory metastatic renal-cell cancer: a phase II study. *Lancet Oncol.* 2007;8(11):975–984. doi:10.1016/S1470-2045(07)70285–1.
29. Izzedine H. Anti-VEGF cancer therapy in nephrology practice. *Int J Nephrol.* 2014;2014:143426. doi:10.1155/2014/143426.
30. Izzedine H, Soria JC, Escudier B. Proteinuria and VEGF-targeted therapies: an underestimated toxicity? *J Nephrol.* 2013;26(5):807–810. doi:10.5301/jn.5000307.
31. Land JD, Chen AH, Atkinson BJ, Cauley DH, Tannir NM. Proteinuria with first-line therapy of metastatic renal cell cancer. *J Oncol Pharm Pract.* 2016;22(2):235–241. doi:10.1177/1078155214563153.
32. Motzer RJ, Hutson TE, Tomczak P, et al. Overall survival and updated results for sunitinib compared with interferon alfa in patients with metastatic renal cell carcinoma. *J Clin Oncol.* 2009;27(22):3584–3590. doi:10.1200/JCO.2008.20.1293.
33. Zhu X, Stergiopoulos K, Wu S. Risk of hypertension and renal dysfunction with an angiogenesis inhibitor sunitinib: systematic review and meta-analysis. *Acta Oncol (Madr).* 2009;48(1):9–17. doi:10.1080/02841860802314720.
34. Baek SH, Kim H, Lee J, et al. Renal adverse effects of sunitinib and its clinical significance: a single-center experience in Korea. *Korean J Intern Med.* 2014;29(1):40–48. doi:10.3904/kjim.2014.29.1.40.
35. Izzedine H, Escudier B, Lhomme C, et al. Kidney diseases associated with anti-vascular endothelial growth factor (VEGF): an 8-year observational study at a single center. *Med (United States).* 2014;93(24):333–339. doi:10.1097/MD.0000000000000207.
36. Sorich MJ, Rowland A, Kichenadasse G, Woodman RJ, Mangoni AA. Risk factors of proteinuria in renal cell carcinoma patients treated with VEGF inhibitors: a secondary analysis of pooled clinical trial data. *Br J Cancer.* 2016;114(12):1313–1317. doi:10.1038/bjc.2016.147.
37. Izzedine H, Escudier B, Lhomme C, et al. Kidney diseases associated with anti-vascular endothelial growth factor (VEGF): an 8-year observational study at a single center [published correction appears in *Medicine (Baltimore).* 2014;93(24):414]. *Medicine (Baltimore).* 2014;93(24):333–339. doi:10.1097/MD.0000000000000207.
38. Mohan A, Herrmann SM. Capmatinib-induced pseudo-acute kidney injury: a case report. *Am J Kidney Dis.* 2021;S0272-6386(21)00640-5. doi:10.1053/j.ajkd.2021.04.009.

12 Prevention and Management of Pulmonary Conditions in Patients With Cancer Before Therapy

ALEXANDER GEYER

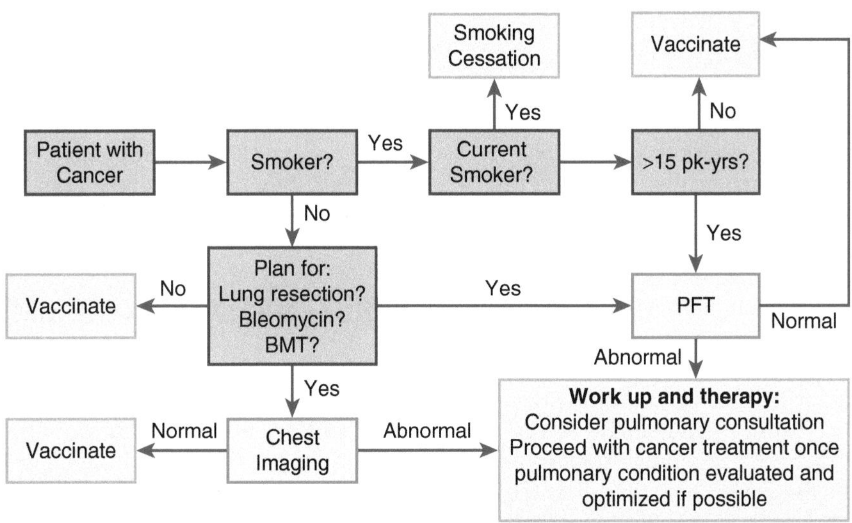

CHAPTER OUTLINE

KEY POINTS

- Current and former heavy smokers and patients with respiratory symptoms should be screened for the presence of pulmonary disease at the time of cancer diagnosis
- Smoking cessation improves treatment outcomes in patients with cancer
- All patients with cancer should receive inactivated influenza vaccination (yearly) and either have documentation of or receive appropriate pneumococcal vaccination
- Physiologic evaluation (pulmonary function test [PFT], quantitative V/Q scan, cardiopulmonary exercise test [CPET]) helps risk stratify patients being considered for lung resection surgery
- Preoperative optimization of pulmonary function in patients with asthma and chronic obstructive pulmonary disease (COPD) and preoperative pulmonary rehabilitation in patients with COPD can reduce the risk of postoperative pulmonary complications
- Conducting PFT before bleomycin therapy or stem cell transplantation is recommended

Smoking is a major risk factor for many types of cancer, including colorectal, head and neck, esophagus, lung, and others.[1] It is also the most important risk factor for chronic obstructive pulmonary disease (COPD).[2] As a result, lung disease and cancer often coexist. Moreover, pulmonary disorders develop frequently in patients with cancer, either as a manifestation of their malignancy or a complication of treatment. It is therefore important to identify patients at risk for these complications and mitigate the risks when possible.

GENERAL RECOMMENDATIONS

Although US Preventive Services Task Force recommends against screening for COPD in the general population,[3] identification of COPD or other pulmonary disorders, such as asthma or pulmonary fibrosis, may be beneficial when planning potentially pneumotoxic therapies. A somewhat arbitrary cutoff of 15 years of smoking history or presence of respiratory symptoms (e.g., chronic cough or dyspnea) regardless of smoking history is suggested as an indication for pulmonary function testing (PFT) or chest imaging in newly diagnosed cases of cancer. If either is abnormal, a consultation with a pulmonologist may be useful. The benefits of smoking cessation in the general smoking population are well established.[1] Smoking cessation after cancer diagnosis is associated with improved treatment outcomes.[4] It is therefore important to screen for tobacco use and encourage smoking cessation in patients with cancer.

Adults with cancer should receive yearly inactivated influenza vaccination.[5] Even though immune response to the inactivated vaccines is likely reduced in patients receiving chemotherapy, the risk of influenza-related morbidity and mortality is high and vaccination seems prudent. An exception is patients receiving anti-B cell antibodies. Because immunogenicity is so poor in these patients, influenza vaccination should be delayed for at least six months.[5] Intranasally administered live attenuated influenza vaccine should not be given to immunocompromised individuals, including those with cancer. Individuals 65 years of age or older should receive *high-dose* inactivated influenza vaccine regardless of whether cancer is present.

Pneumococcal infections are an important cause of morbidity and mortality in patients with cancer. Pneumococcal vaccine should be administered to all patients with cancer, preferably before initiating chemotherapy because immunogenicity to the polysaccharide vaccine is significantly diminished afterward. The Infectious Diseases Society of America and the United States Advisory Committee on Immunization Practices recommend that both a pneumococcal polysaccharide vaccine (e.g., PPSV23, Pneumovax) and a pneumococcal conjugate vaccine (PCV13, Prevnar 13) be administered.[5] Pneumococcal vaccine naïve patients should receive a single dose of PCV13 followed by a dose of PPSV12 at least 8 weeks later. Patients who have previously received one or more doses of PPSV23, a single dose of PCV13 should be given at least one year after the last PPSV23. A repeat dose of PPSV23, if needed, should be administered no sooner than 8 weeks after PCV13 and at least 5 years after the most recent PPSV23. Specific pneumococcal vaccines vary by country and patients should be vaccinated according to their national guidelines.

SURGERY-RELATED RECOMMENDATIONS

Physiologic evaluation, including PFT and, when indicated, quantitative ventilation perfusion scanning and/or integrated cardiopulmonary exercise testing, of patients with lung cancer being considered for resectional surgery is useful in preoperative assessment and the corresponding guidelines have been published by the American College of Chest Physicians[6] and the European Respiratory Society.[7] Evaluation of the perioperative risk of pulmonary complications plays an important role in any surgery, with cancer surgery being no exception. Patient-related risk factors (e.g., history of COPD, functional status, recent respiratory tract infection) and surgery-related risk factors (i.e., proximity of the surgical site to the chest and duration of general anesthesia) can be used to estimate the risks of perioperative pulmonary complications, including pneumonia and respiratory failure. Several prediction equations, such as the ARISCAT Risk Index[8] and Gupta calculators for postoperative respiratory failure[9] and postoperative pneumonia,[10] have been published and are available online.

Several strategies exist to prevent pulmonary complications after cancer surgery. Smoking cessation prior to elective surgery appears to reduce the incidence of postoperative pulmonary complications and improve wound healing.[11] Longer (e.g., >8 weeks) periods of smoking cessation are more effective than shorter ones; despite the earlier concerns about an increased risk of pulmonary complications in patients who quit fewer than 2 months before surgery,[12] subsequent systematic reviews and meta-analyses have not supported this finding.[13] Patients with known and well-controlled asthma or COPD should continue to receive therapy according to the previously published and routinely updated guidelines (www.ginasthma.org and www.goldcopd.org). If symptoms of an exacerbation are present, surgery should be delayed, and the exacerbation treated before proceeding with surgery. Those who have received more than 20 mg of daily prednisone or its equivalent for more than three weeks during the previous six months should receive perioperative empiric stress dose steroids. Preoperative exercise and pulmonary rehabilitation may improve postoperative outcomes after lung or abdominal surgery.[14,15]

CHEMOTHERAPY-RELATED RECOMMENDATIONS

Owing to the high incidence of potentially life-threatening pneumonitis, pretreatment PFT is recommended in patients with germ cell tumors and older adults with Hodgkin lymphoma planned to receive a bleomycin-containing chemotherapy regimen.[16] Pretreatment PFT serves as a baseline for future comparison. Low diffusing capacity for carbon monoxide (DLCO) may identify patients at a higher risk of symptomatic pulmonary toxicity with even a small degree of bleomycin injury, but pretreatment DLCO alone should not be used to exclude patients from this therapy because no prospective data validate this approach.

Pretransplant PFT (particularly DLCO) plays a role in determining eligibility for allogeneic hematopoietic cell transplantation with patients whose pretransplant DLCO is below 60% of predicted traditionally excluded from transplantation. More recently it has been shown that a subset of patients with DLCO less than 60% predicted can receive transplant safely.[17] Nevertheless, low diffusing capacity is associated with increased posttransplant mortality and avoidance of known pneumotoxic conditioning agents, such as bleomycin, is recommended in patients with DLCO.

REFERENCES

1. Samet JM. Health benefits of smoking cessation. *Clin Chest Med.* 1991;12(4):669–679.
2. Bhatt SP, Kim YI, Harrington KF, et al. Smoking duration alone provides stronger risk estimates of chronic obstructive pulmonary disease than pack-years. *Thorax.* 2018;73(5):414–421.
3. US Preventive Services Task Force (USPSTF), Bibbins-Domingo K, Grossman DC, et al. Screening for chronic obstructive pulmonary disease: US Preventive Services Task Force Recommendation Statement. *JAMA.* 2016;315(13):1372–1377.
4. Warren GW. Mitigating the adverse health effects and costs associated with smoking after a cancer diagnosis. *Transl Lung Cancer Res.* 2019;8(suppl 1):S59–S66.
5. Rubin LG, Levin MJ, Ljungman P, et al. 2013 IDSA clinical practice guideline for vaccination of the immunocompromised host. *Clin Infect Dis.* 2014;58(3):309–318.
6. Brunelli A, Kim AW, Berger KI, Addrizzo-Harris DJ. Physiologic evaluation of the patient with lung cancer being considered for resectional surgery: diagnosis and management of lung cancer, 3rd ed: American College of Chest Physicians evidence-based clinical practice guidelines. *Chest.* 2013;143(suppl 5):e166S–e190S.
7. Brunelli A, Charloux A, Bolliger CT, et al. ERS/ESTS clinical guidelines on fitness for radical therapy in lung patients with cancer (surgery and chemo-radiotherapy). *Eur Respir J.* 2009;34(1):17–41.
8. Canet J, Gallart L, Gomar C, et al. Prediction of postoperative pulmonary complications in a population-based surgical cohort. *Anesthesiology.* 2010;113(6):1338–1350.
9. Gupta H, Gupta PK, Fang X, et al. Development and validation of a risk calculator predicting postoperative respiratory failure. *Chest.* 2011;140(5):1207–1215.
10. Gupta H, Gupta PK, Schuller D, et al. Development and validation of a risk calculator for predicting postoperative pneumonia. *Mayo Clin Proc.* 2013;88(11):1241–1249.
11. Mastracci TM, Carli F, Finley RJ, et al. Effect of preoperative smoking cessation interventions on postoperative complications. *J Am Coll Surg.* 2011;212(6):1094–1096.
12. Warner MA, Offord KP, Warner ME, Lennon RL, Conover MA, Jansson-Schumacher U. Role of preoperative cessation of smoking and other factors in postoperative pulmonary complications: a blinded prospective study of coronary artery bypass patients. *Mayo Clin Proc.* 1989;64(6):609–616.
13. Mills E, Eyawo O, Lockhart I, Kelly S, Wu P, Ebbert JO. Smoking cessation reduces postoperative complications: a systematic review and meta-analysis. *Am J Med.* 2011;124(2):144–154.e8.
14. Pouwels S, Fiddelaers J, Teijink JA, Woorst JF, Siebenga J, Smeenk FW. Preoperative exercise therapy in lung surgery patients: a systematic review. *Respir Med.* 2015;109(12):1495–1504.
15. Valkenet K, van de Port IG, Dronkers JJ, de Vries WR, Lindeman E, Backx FJ. The effects of preoperative exercise therapy on postoperative outcome: a systematic review. *Clin Rehabil.* 2011;25(2):99–111.
16. Watson RA, De La Peña H, Tsakok MT, et al. Development of a best-practice clinical guideline for the use of bleomycin in the treatment of germ cell tumours in the UK. *Br J Cancer.* 2018;119(9):1044–1051.
17. Chien JW, Sullivan KM. Carbon monoxide diffusion capacity: how low can you go for hematopoietic cell transplantation eligibility? *Biol Blood Marrow Transplant.* 2009;15(4):447–453.

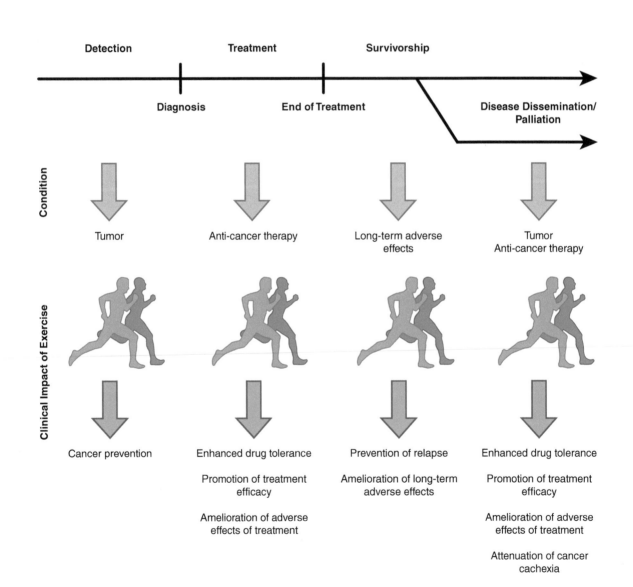

13 Cardiopulmonary Exercise for Management of Cardiovascular Toxicity

JESSICA M. SCOTT

CHAPTER OUTLINE

KEY POINTS

- Exercise therapy is a pleiotropic intervention with the potential to prevent/reverse therapy-related cardiotoxicity across the cancer continuum
- Patients at high cardiovascular risk according to American Society of Clinical Oncology (ASCO) guidelines may need clearance from a cardiologist prior to initiating an exercise program
- Preexercise screening should include assessment of current physical activity levels and/or cardiopulmonary exercise test for exercise safety or to determine cardiorespiratory fitness
- Patients can be stratified into not meeting American College of Sports Medicine (ACSM) exercise guidelines/low cardiorespiratory fitness versus meeting these exercise guidelines or normal to high cardiorespiratory fitness to guide exercise prescriptions
- Exercise prescriptions should follow frequency, intensity, time, type, and sequence (i.e., F.I.T.T.S) guidelines

EXERCISE TO MODULATE CARDIOVASCULAR TOXICITY: OVERVIEW OF THE EVIDENCE

The direct and secondary adverse consequences of anticancer treatment have an impact on both cardiac function and the entire cardiovascular-skeletal muscle axis (i.e., whole-organism cardiovascular toxicity).[1] This multisystem toxicity creates a strong rationale for pleiotropic treatment strategies. Exercise is one such therapy that has been shown to augment cardiovascular function leading to substantial improvements in the prevention and treatment of cardiovascular disease (CVD) in nononcology clinical populations (Fig. 13.1).[2] However, exercise is not considered a standard of care therapy in patients with cancer. In this chapter, the evidence base for the efficacy of exercise therapy on cardiovascular toxicity across the continuum of cancer treatment is outlined, and strategies for patient stratification and implementation of exercise in patients with a history of cancer are provided.

EXERCISE ACROSS THE CANCER CONTINUUM

The cancer continuum encompasses several distinct phases, typically beginning with the diagnosis of the primary disease and surgical management, continuing with adjuvant (drug or radiation) therapy (but this treatment can also be before surgery, i.e., neoadjuvant therapy), followed by postcancer therapy surveillance (often referred to as survivorship). The fourth phase, palliation or end-of-life with diagnosis of distant disease recurrence (metastasis) is beyond the scope of the current chapter. An organizing framework outlining the potential role and application of exercise across the first three phases of the cancer continuum is presented in Figure 13.2.[3] The impact of exercise on treatment-related cardiovascular toxicities (e.g., CVD, CVD risk factors, cardiorespiratory fitness [CRF)] from definitive (phase 3) clinical trials, observational cohorts, and smaller randomized controlled trials (RCT) is outlined in each phase.

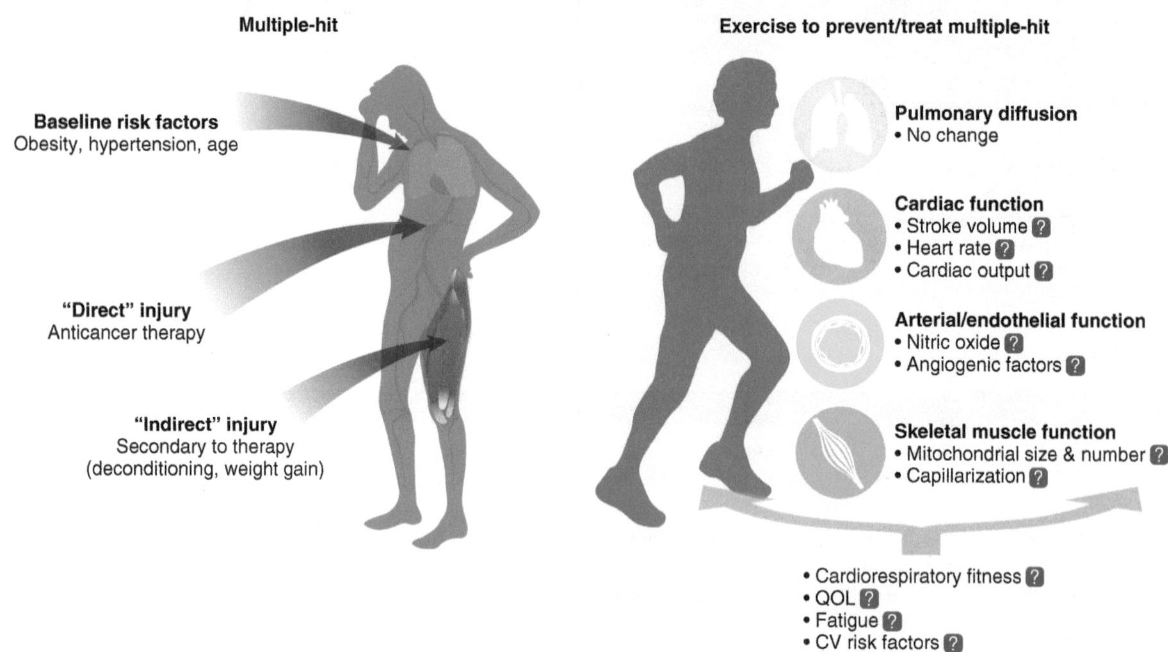

FIG. 13.1 Potential benefits that exercise training may confer to patients with cancer at a heightened risk for cardiovascular disease. CV, Cardiovascular; *QOL*, quality of life. (Reprinted with permission from Gilchrist SC, Barac A, Ades PA, et al. Cardio-oncology rehabilitation to manage cardiovascular outcomes in patients with cancer and survivors: a scientific statement from the American Heart Association. *Circulation*. 2019;139:e997–e1012; © 2019 American Heart Association, Inc.)

Presurgery/Therapy

The presurgery or therapy setting is broadly defined as investigating the impact of exercise in the period between primary diagnosis and surgical intervention. This setting is typically characterized as (1) a period of one to six weeks without administration of any anticancer therapy or (2) a period of several months with administration of chemotherapy with or without radiation (i.e., chemoradiation) or endocrine therapy until surgical resection (known as induction or neoadjuvant therapy). In the most common presurgery clinical scenario (i.e., no concurrent treatment administration), the primary question of interest is whether short-term exercise training can augment cardiovascular (physiologic) function (e.g., CRF) to, in turn, lower complications/recovery or even impact surgical eligibility. In a meta-analysis of 14 RCTs, single arm trials, and retrospective cohort studies investigating the effects of preoperative exercise in patients with lung cancer, Garcia and colleagues[4] reported that, in comparison to usual care, exercise decreased hospital stay (mean difference, −4.83 days; 95% CI, −5.9 to −3.76) and significantly reduced postoperative complications risk (risk ratios [RR], 0.45; 95% CI, 0.28–0.74]). The two RCTs, which assessed postoperative outcomes in cancer types other than lung, had conflicting results. Dronkers and colleagues[5] evaluated the efficacy of two to four weeks of preoperative aerobic training (2 days/week supervised, 4 days/week unsupervised 60 minutes/session at 55% to 75% peak heart rate) in 42 patients scheduled for abdominal surgery for colorectal cancer; no differences in postoperative complications or length of hospital stay were observed between groups. In contrast, Dunne and colleagues[6] reported that four weeks of exercise (3 days/week, 30 minutes/session alternating between 90% and 60% of CRF) led to a four-day decrease in hospital stay compared with usual care in 38 patients undergoing liver resection for colorectal liver metastasis. In studies on CRF, Stefanelli and colleagues[7] randomized 40 patients with non-small-cell lung cancer and chronic obstructive pulmonary disease to aerobic exercise (5 days/week, 30 minutes/

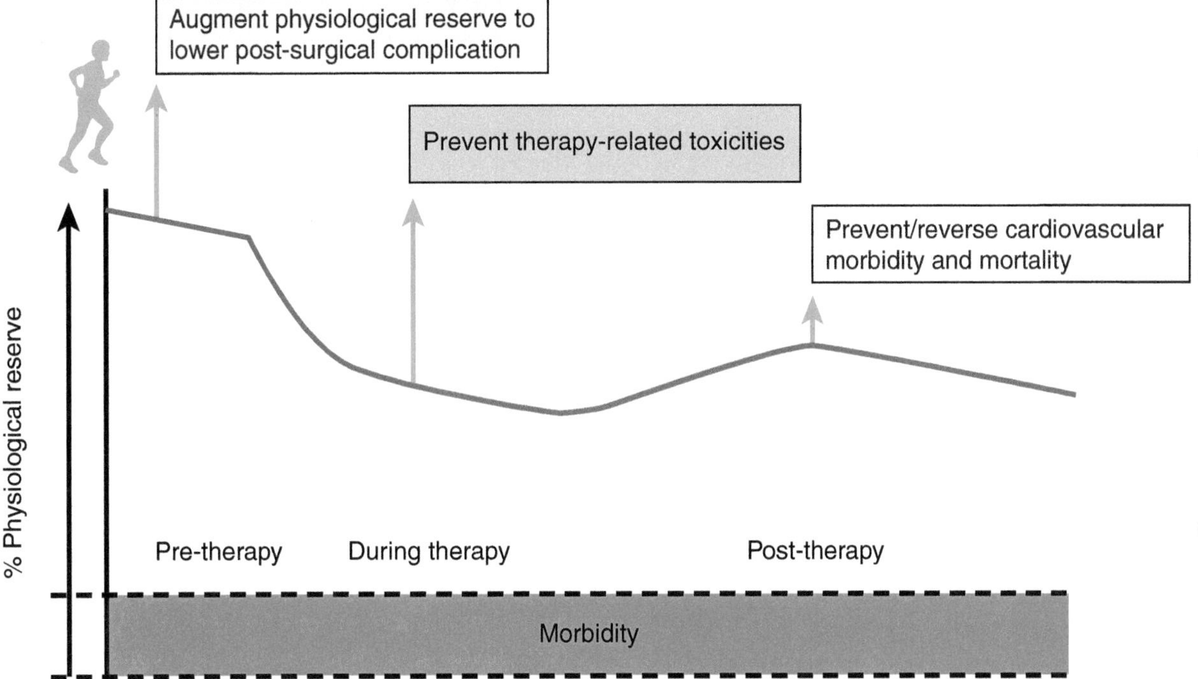

FIG. 13.2 Trajectory decline in physiologic reserve across the cancer continuum. The postulated trajectories of decline in patients with early-stage cancer (*pink line*) compared with age-matched decline in individuals without a history of cancer (*blue line*). As reserve depletes below a critical threshold, asymptomatic maladaptation occurs, which, without intervention, leads to overt clinical dysfunction (e.g., heart failure, myocardial infarction) and ultimately chronic morbidity and premature mortality. Exercise (*yellow dotted lines*) may augment reserve prior to therapy, mitigate decline during therapy, and reverse decline after therapy. (Modified from Scott JM, Dolan LB, Norton L, Charles JB, Jones LW. Multisystem toxicity in cancer: lessons from NASA's countermeasures program. *Cell*. 2019;179(5);1003–1009.)

session at 70% of CRF), or usual care control for three weeks. Exercise training led to, 17% in CRF compared with no change in usual care. Collectively, extant evidence indicates that presurgical exercise therapy is an effective intervention to augment CRF and reduce postoperative complications.

During Adjuvant Therapy

The adjuvant therapy setting is defined as investigation of exercise during any form of primary adjuvant therapy (i.e., chemotherapy, radiation, or molecularly targeted therapy, except hormone deprivation therapy) following curative-intent. Key questions in this setting relate to whether exercise can prevent and/or mitigate common toxicities (e.g., cardiovascular dysfunction, anemia). Data from at least one observational cohort study support the initial contention that exposure to exercise during or around the period of adjuvant therapy may alter chronic therapy-related outcomes. In a study of 4015 patients with primary breast cancer, exercise exposure of, 18 metabolic equivalent hours per week (MET-h/week) was associated with an adjusted 37% (95% CI, 0.43 to 0.80) lower risk of any CVD event compared with less than 2 MET-h/week after 12.7 years of follow-up.[8] Exercise is also associated with improvements in CRF in this setting. In a meta-analysis of RCTs evaluating the effects of exercise training on CRF in patients with adult-onset cancer, Scott and colleagues[9] reported that among 14 studies conducted during therapy, exercise training improved CRF compared with usual care (weighted mean differences [WMD], +1.37 mL O_2/kg/min favoring exercise training; 95% CI,0.58 to 2.16).

Few studies have assessed the effects of exercise on cardiovascular outcomes other than CRF.

In a single-arm study investigating the effects of 16 weeks of supervised linear aerobic training (3 days/week, 30 to 60 minutes/session at 60% to 0% peak heart rate) on CRF and cardiac function in 17 women previously treated with anthracycline-containing chemotherapy and currently receiving trastuzumab for human epidermal growth factor receptor 2 (HER2) positive early breast cancer, Haykowsky and colleagues[10] found no significant change in CRF, that resting and peak end diastolic and end systolic left ventricle volumes significantly increased, and that resting and peak left ventricle ejection fraction significantly decreased.[1] In sum, short-term (12 to 26 weeks) anticancer therapy markedly decreases CRF. Structured exercise training during this period may abrogate this marked decline; however, limited evidence exists regarding the effects of exercise on other CVD risk factors, and whether an exercise-induced attenuation in CRF decline is clinically meaningful is not known.

After Adjuvant Therapy (Survivorship)

This setting is defined as investigation of exercise after the cessation of any form of primary adjuvant therapy, where exercise is applied to prevent and/or reverse CVD-related morbidity and mortality. Three epidemiologic studies have investigated whether exposure to exercise after primary treatment cessation lowers long-term risk of cause-specific late mortality. Jones and colleagues examined the association between exercise exposure and risk of major CVD events among adult survivors of childhood Hodgkin lymphoma (n = 1187; median age, 31.2 years; median follow up, 11.9 years)[11] and women with primary breast cancer (n = 2973; mean age, 57 years; median follow up, 8.6 years).[12] Adherence to national exercise guidelines was associated with an adjusted 23% (breast cancer)[12] and 51% (Hodgkin lymphoma)[11] lowered risk of CVD events, in comparison with not meeting guidelines. In extension of this work, Scott and colleagues[13] reported that 3 or more MET-h/wk was associated with a 19% ($P = .026$), 39% ($P = .026$), and 11% ($P = .17$) reduction in all-cause, recurrence/progression and health-related deaths, respectively, in 15,450 adult survivors of childhood cancer after median follow up of 10 years. Increase in exercise exposure (+7.9 ± 4.4 MET-h/week) over an 8-year period was associated with a 40% reduction in all-cause mortality rate compared with maintenance of low exercise exposure (RR, 0.60; 95% CI, 0.44 to 0.82).[13] In a meta-analysis evaluating the effects of exercise training on CRF in RCTs (outlined above), Scott and colleagues[9] reported that among 27 studies conducted after therapy, exercise was associated with a significant increase in CRF compared with usual care (WMD, +2.45 mL O_2/kg/min; 95% CI, 1.71 to 3.19).

Several studies have assessed the effects of exercise on cardiovascular outcomes other than CRF. For instance, Jones and colleagues[14] investigated the efficacy of supervised nonlinear aerobic training (5 days/week [3 supervised, 2 home-based]; 30 to 60 minutes/session at 55% to 100% of CRF for 24 weeks) compared with usual care in 50 patients with prostate cancer and found that exercise improved endothelial function (as measured by flow-mediated dilatation of brachial artery), but there were no changes in body composition (as assessed by dual-energy x-ray absorptiometry), cardiac function (resting left ventricular ejection fraction), or biochemical CVD markers (e.g., lipids, glucose).[14] Adams and colleagues[15] reported that, compared with usual care, 12 weeks of exercise (3 days/week, 35 minutes/session at 75% to 95% VO_{2peak}) improved vascular function (adjusted mean group differences of −0.6 mm, 1.54 10^{-3}/kPa, and −2.02 m/s for carotid intima-media thickness, carotid distensibility, arterial stiffness, respectively), and Framingham risk score (adjusted mean group difference −0.6%) in 63 patients with testicular cancer.

Finally, in an unplanned, ancillary retrospective analysis of the Heart Failure: A Controlled Trial Investigating Outcomes of Exercise Training (HF-ACTION) trial, Jones and colleagues[16] reported that among 90 patients with cancer and with heart failure, the incidence of cardiovascular mortality or cardiovascular hospitalization was significantly higher in the exercise group compared with the usual care group (67% vs. 41%; HR, 1.94; 95% CI, 1.12 to 3.16). In summary, most studies support the conclusion that exercise training after therapy augments CRF and improves CVD risk factors; only one small retrospective analysis has investigated the effects of exercise on clinical end points in patients with overt CVD (e.g., cardiovascular death, all-cause mortality).

In totality, meta-analyses and systematic reviews of the extant data conclude that exercise, and particularly supervised exercise, improves CRF in a broad array of patients with cancer before, during, and after treatment.[17–19] Emerging data suggest that exercise during these periods may lower the risk of death from CVD and all causes following diagnosis, although confirmatory data from RCTs are not yet available.

IMPLEMENTATION OF EXERCISE IN PATIENTS WITH A HISTORY OF CANCER

The development of exercise prescriptions requires an initial evaluation of clinical and/or medical parameters that permits stratification of patients into more homogeneous subgroups.[20] In this context a patient stratification approach to guide exercise prescriptions is outlined below and in Figure 13.3.

IDENTIFICATION OF PATIENTS WITH HIGH CARDIOVASCULAR RISK

Several models are available that predict individual patient risk of late-occurring CVD following a cancer diagnosis and assist in the stratification of patients on the basis of available clinical information, such as gender and radiation or chemotherapy exposures.[21] For instance, the Childhood Cancer Survivor Study developed and validated risk prediction models for heart failure,[22] ischemic heart disease, and stroke,[23] and the American Society of Clinical Oncology (ASCO) guidelines[24] identified various patient subgroups considered "high" risk of cardiac dysfunction or heart failure.[24] It is likely that patients considered "high risk" should receive cardiology clearance prior to initiating an exercise program; however, this has

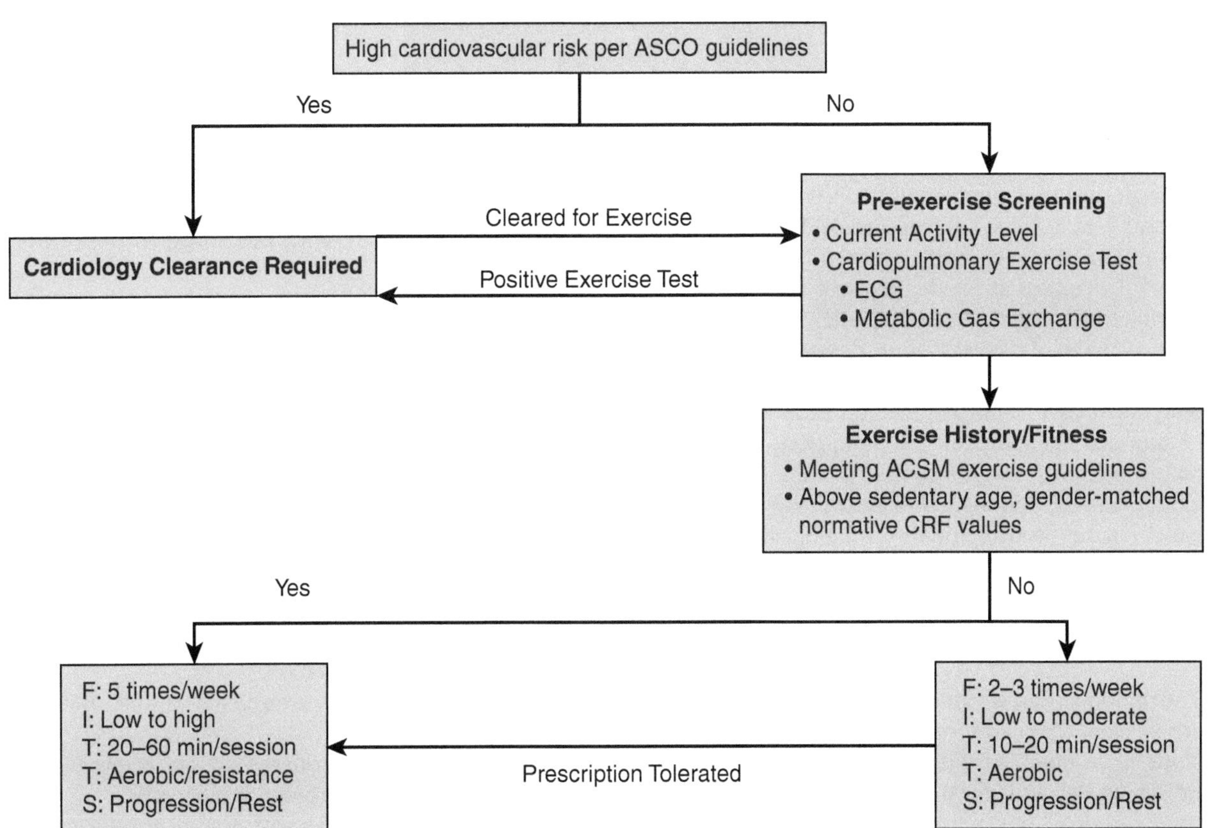

FIG. 13.3 Algorithm for risk stratification and exercise based on current guidelines. *ASCO*, American Society of Clinical Oncology; *ECG*, electrocardiogram; *CRF*, cardiorespiratory fitness; *F.I.T.T.S*, frequency, intensity, time, type, sequence.

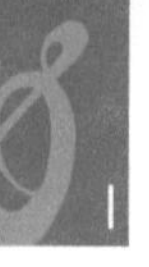

not been systematically addressed to date. Of note, ASCO guidelines do not include all cancer therapies implicated in overall CVD risk (e.g., immunotherapy,[25] androgen-deprivation therapy[26]).

Preexercise Screening

Available risk stratification models specify important information regarding potential CVD risk; however, they provide limited guidance on exercise safety or how to design exercise prescriptions. Accordingly, additional exercise testing and/or physical activity assessments are valuable tools for further stratification.

Exercise Testing

Exercise testing is an ideal tool both to provide safety screening (to identify contraindications to exercise) and to guide the design of exercise prescriptions.[27] A detailed description of exercise testing guidelines is provided by the American Heart Association and the ACSM guidelines.[28] In brief, a standard 12-lead electrocardiogram (ECG) should be obtained before and during exercise and compared with previously obtained ECGs to determine if changes have occurred over time. Resting blood pressure and oxygen saturation (SpO_2) should also be monitored for abnormalities.[29] Patients with abnormal test results will require additional medical evaluation and clearance prior to initiating exercise.[30,31] Maximal stress testing can also be used to estimate CRF[27] and measured peak heart rate can be used to facilitate prescription design.[27] In addition, measurement of ventilatory gas exchange is preferable because it can provide an objective assessment of submaximal and peak CRF (i.e., peak oxygen consumption, VO_2peak), as well as guide individualized exercise prescriptions.[28] Normative VO_2peak values can then be used to identify patients below, at, or above age and gender-matched individuals.[32]

PHYSICAL ACTIVITY

The national exercise guidelines for patients with cancer suggest that endurance (aerobic) exercise, either alone or in combination with resistance training, be prescribed at a moderate-intensity (50% to 75% of a predetermined physiologic parameter, typically age-predicted heart rate maximum or reserve), achieved in two to five sessions per week, for 10 to 60 minutes per session, with the ultimate objective of achieving at least 150 minutes of moderate-intensity or at least 75 minutes of vigorous-intensity exercise per week.[17,18] Thus patients can be stratified into meeting or not meeting these guidelines based on self-reported physical activity,[33] or more objective physical activity data obtained from commonly used digital devices (e.g., Fitbit).[34]

Exercise Prescriptions

Major components of any exercise prescription include several key features: *frequency* (sessions/week), *intensity* (percentage of a predetermined physiologic parameter, such as maximum heart rate obtained from baseline cardiopulmonary exercise test), *type* (exercise modality – cycle ergometry, treadmill, resistance training), *time* (session duration), and *sequence* (progressive overload, and rest/recovery).[35] Based on preexercise screening, these major components can be manipulated to provide more personalized exercise prescriptions.

Exercise Frequency

Prolonged periods of inactivity are associated with negative physiologic changes,[36] as such, exercise is recommended at least two times per week for patients with low CRF/physical activity, and five times per week for patients with moderate to high CRF/physical activity.

Exercise Intensity

Intensity is one of the most important considerations for exercise. Exercise intensities that are too low may not provide physiologic challenge to patients with high fitness, whereas exercise intensities that are too high may not be safe or feasible.[1] According to the National Comprehensive Cancer Network,[37] exercise intensity can be described as follows:

- Low-intensity exercise: No noticeable change in breathing pattern.
- Moderate-intensity exercise: Can talk, but not sing.
- High-intensity exercise: Can say a few words without stopping to catch a breath.

Intensity should begin with low to moderate intensity for patients with low CRF/physical activity, and include low to high intensity for patients with higher fitness.

Exercise Time

For patients not currently exercising, exercise duration can be broken down into more manageable time (e.g., three 5-minute sessions) throughout the day with the aim of achieving a total 20 minutes per session. For patients with higher fitness, exercise time can range from 20 to 60 minutes per session.

Exercise Type

The two primary types of exercise that may help prevent and treat cancer-related cardiovascular toxicity are aerobic exercise training (i.e., sustained exercise that increases heart rate or breathing rate)[38] and resistance exercise training (i.e., voluntary muscle contractions against a resistance greater than that normally encountered in activities of daily living).[38] Patients with limited exercise experience should begin with aerobic exercise; patients with higher fitness can incorporate both aerobic and resistance exercise.

Exercise Sequence

Repetitive exposure to a training load above habitual levels promotes adaptation[39,40]; thus subsequent increases in training load (i.e., progressive overload) are required for continued adaptation.[35,41] However, progressive overload only confers physiologic adaptation with adequate rest and recovery to maximize the adaptive response.[35,41,42] Chronically overloading a system without adequate rest and recovery can lead to fatigue, maladaptation, and illness (overtraining).[39,43] This could stimulate worsening symptoms or inferior clinical outcomes in certain clinical populations.[1] Collectively, an exercise sequence should include sessions with higher intensity or duration followed by rest or recovery sessions that are at a lower intensity or duration.[35]

Additional Considerations for Exercise

A "one size, fits all" approach clearly cannot address the complex safety, tolerability, and efficacy needs of all individuals with a history of cancer.[1] Stratifying patients according to CVD risk is one step; however, many additional individual patient factors (e.g., ostomy, lymphedema) should be considered for exercise program design. The ACSM has a specialized certification training course for exercise professionals working with patients/survivors of cancer; patients interested in beginning a structured exercise program can be referred to these professionals (e.g., LIVESTRONG at the YMCA).[44]

SUMMARY

Exercise is a multisystem intervention that is likely to become an important strategy in cardiovascular toxicity prevention and control in patients with a history of cancer. Appropriate stratification to identify patients at high risk of cardiovascular toxicity and patients with limited exercise history is needed to optimize the safety and efficacy of exercise across the cancer continuum.

REFERENCES

1. Scott JM, Nilsen TS, Gupta D, et al. Exercise therapy and cardiovascular toxicity in cancer. *Circulation,* 2018;137:1176–1191.
2. Lavie CJ, Thomas RJ, Squires RW, et al. Exercise training and cardiac rehabilitation in primary and secondary prevention of coronary heart disease. *Mayo Clin Proc*. 2009;84:373–383.
3. Courneya KS, Friedenreich CM. Framework PEACE: an organizational model for examining physical exercise across the cancer experience. *Ann Beh Med*. 2001;23:263–272.
4. Garcia RS, Brage MIY, Moolhuyzen EG, et al. Functional and postoperative outcomes after preoperative exercise training in patients with lung cancer: a systematic review and meta-analysis. *Interact Cardiovasc Thorac Surg*. 2016;23:486–497.
5. Dronkers JJ, Lamberts H, Reutelingsperger IM, et al. Preoperative therapeutic programme for elderly patients scheduled for elective abdominal oncological surgery: a randomized controlled pilot study. 2010;24:614–622.
6. Dunne DF, Jack S, Jones RP, et al. Randomized clinical trial of prehabilitation before planned liver resection. *Br J Surg*. 2016;103:504–512.
7. Stefanelli F, Meoli I, Cobuccio R, et al. High-intensity training and cardiopulmonary exercise testing in patients with chronic obstructive pulmonary disease and non-small-cell lung cancer undergoing lobectomy. *Eur J Cardiothorac Surg*. 2013;44:e260–e265.
8. Okwuosa TM, Roberta RM, Palomo A, et al. Pre-diagnosis exercise and cardiovascular events in primary breast cancer women's health initiative. *JACC: CardioOncology*. 2019;1:41–50.
9. Scott JM, Zabor EC, Schwitzer E, et al. Efficacy of exercise therapy on cardiorespiratory fitness in patients with cancer: a systematic review and meta-analysis. *J Clin Oncol*. 2018;36:2297–2305.
10. Haykowsky MJ, Mackey JR, Thompson RB, et al. Adjuvant trastuzumab induces ventricular remodeling despite aerobic exercise training. *Clin Cancer Res*. 2009;15:4963–4967.
11. Jones LW, Liu Q, Armstrong GT, et al. Exercise and risk of major cardiovascular events in adult survivors of childhood hodgkin lymphoma: a report from the childhood cancer survivor study. *J Clin Oncol*. 2014;32:3643–3650.
12. Jones LW, Habel LA, Weltzien E, et al. Exercise and risk of cardiovascular events in women with nonmetastatic breast cancer. *J Clin Oncol*. 22016;34:2743–2749.
13. Scott JM, Li N, Liu Q, et al. Association of exercise with mortality in adult survivors of childhood cancer.*JAMA Oncol*. 2018;4:1352–1358.
14. Jones LW, Hornsby WE, Freedland SJ, et al. Effects of nonlinear aerobic training on erectile dysfunction and cardiovascular function following radical prostatectomy for clinically localized prostate cancer. *Eur Urol*. 2014;65:852–855.

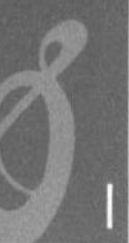

15. Adams SC, DeLorey DS, Davenport MH, et al. Effects of high-intensity aerobic interval training on cardiovascular disease risk in testicular cancer survivors: a phase 2 randomized controlled trial. *Cancer.* 2017;123:4057–4065.
16. Jones LW, Douglas PS, Khouri MG, et al. Safety and efficacy of aerobic training in patients with cancer who have heart failure: an analysis of the HF-ACTION randomized trial. *J Clin Oncol.* 2014;32:2496–502.
17. Schmitz KH, Courneya KS, Matthews C, et al. American College of Sports Medicine roundtable on exercise guidelines for cancer survivors. *Med Sci Sports Exerc.* 2010;42:1409–14.
18. Rock CL, Doyle C, Demark-Wahnefried W, et al. Nutrition and physical activity guidelines for cancer survivors. *CA Cancer J Clin.* 2012;62:243–274.
19. Buffart LM, Kalter J, Sweegers MG, et al. Effects and moderators of exercise on quality of life and physical function in patients with cancer: an individual patient data meta-analysis of 34 RCTs. *Cancer Treat Rev.* 2017;52:91–104.
20. Collins FS, Varmus H. A new initiative on precision medicine. *N Engl J Med.* 2015;372:793– 795.
21. Chow EJ, Chen Y, Hudson MM, et al. Prediction of ischemic heart disease and stroke in survivors of childhood cancer. *J Clin Oncol.*2018;36:44–52.
22. Chow EJ, Chen Y, Kremer LC, et al. Individual prediction of heart failure among childhood cancer survivors. *J Clin Oncol.* 2015;33:394–402.
23. Chow EJ, Chen Y, Hudson MM, et al. Prediction of ischemic heart disease and stroke in survivors of childhood cancer. *J Clin Oncol.* 2018;36:44–52.
24. Armenian SH, Lacchetti C, Barac A, et al. Prevention and monitoring of cardiac dysfunction in survivors of adult cancers: American Society of Clinical Oncology Clinical Practice Guideline. *J Clin Oncol.* 217;35:893–911.
25. Moslehi JJ. Cardiovascular toxic effects of targeted cancer therapies. *N Engl J Med.* 2016;375:1457–1467.
26. Moslehi J. The cardiovascular perils of cancer survivorship. *N Engl J Med.* 2013;368:1055–1056.
27. Ross R, Blair SN, Arena R, et al. Importance of assessing cardiorespiratory fitness in clinical practice: a case for fitness as a clinical vital sign: a scientific statement from the American Heart Association. *Circulation.* 2016;134:e653–e699.
28. American Thoracic Society; American College of Chest Physicians. ATS/ACCP statement on cardiopulmonary exercise testing. *Am J Respir Crit Care Med.* 2003;167:211–277.
29. American College of Sports Medicine. *ACSM's Guidelines for Exercise Testing and Prescription*, ed 9. Philadelphia, PA: Lippincott Williams & Wilkins, 2013.
30. Gibbons RJ, Balady GJ, Beasley JW, et al. ACC/AHA guidelines for exercise testing: a report of the American College of Cardiology/American Heart Association task force on practice guidelines (committee on exercise testing). *J Am Coll Cardiol.* 1997;30:260–311.
31. Thomas SG, Goodman JM, Burr JF. Evidence-based risk assessment and recommendations for physical activity clearance: established cardiovascular disease. *Appl Physiol Nutr Metab.* 2011;36(suppl 1): S190–S213.
32. Fitzgerald MD, Tanaka H, Tran ZV, et al. Age-related declines in maximal aerobic capacity in regularly exercising vs. sedentary women: a meta-analysis. *JJ Appl Physiol (1985).* 1997;83(1):160–165.
33. Godin G, Jobin J, Bouillon J. Assessment of leisure time exercise behavior by self-report: a concurrent validity study. *Can J Public Health.* 1986;77:359–362.
34. Sushames A, Edwards A, Thompson F, et al. Validity and reliability of Fitbit Flex for step count, mModerate to vigorous physical activity and activity energy expenditure. *PLoS One.* 2016;11:e0161224.
35. Sasso JP, Eves ND, Christensen JF, et al. A framework for prescription in exercise-oncology research. *J Cachexia Sarcopenia Muscle.* 2015;6:115–124.
36. Scott JM, Martin D, Ploutz-Snyder R, et al. Efficacy of exercise and testosterone to mitigate atrophic cardiovascular remodeling. *Med Sci Sports Exerc.* 2018;50:1940–1949.
37. Denlinger CS, Sanft T, Baker KS, et al. Survivorship, Version 2.2017, NCCN clinical practice guidelines in oncology. *J Natl Compr Canc Netw.* 2017;15:1140–1163.
38. Garber CE, Blissmer B, Deschenes MR, et al. American College of Sports Medicine position stand. Quantity and quality of exercise for developing and maintaining cardiorespiratory, musculoskeletal, and neuromotor fitness in apparently healthy adults: guidance for prescribing exercise. *Med Sci Sports Exerc.* 2011;43:1334–1359.
39. McEwen BS. Stressed or stressed out: what is the difference? *J Psychiatry Neurosci.* 2005;30:315–318.
40. McEwen BS, Wingfield JC. The concept of allostasis in biology and biomedicine. *Horm Behav.* 2003;43:2–15.
41. Kraemer WJ, Adams K, Cafarelli E, et al. American College of Sports Medicine position stand. Progression models in resistance training for healthy adults. *Med Sci Sports Exerc.* 2002;34:364–380.
42. Hickson RC, Hagberg JM, Ehsani AA, et al. Time course of the adaptive responses of aerobic power and heart rate to training. *Med Sci Sports Exerc.* 1981;13:17–20.
43. Kreher JB, Schwartz JB. Overtraining syndrome: a practical guide. *Sports Health.* 2012;4:128–138.
44. Irwin ML, Cartmel B, Harrigan M, et al. Effect of the LIVESTRONG at the YMCA exercise program on physical activity, fitness, quality of life, and fatigue in cancer survivors. *Cancer.* 2017;123: 1249–1258.
45. Gilchrist SC, Barac A, Ades PA, et al. Cardio-oncology rehabilitation to manage cardiovascular outcomes in patients with cancer and survivors: a scientific statement from the American Heart Association. *Circulation.* 2019;139:e997–e1012.
46. Scott JM, Dolan LB, Norton L, Charles JB, Jones LW. Multisystem toxicity in cancer: lessons from NASA's countermeasures program. *Cell.* 2019;179(5);1003–1009.

PART II

Cardiovascular Disease Management During Cancer Treatment

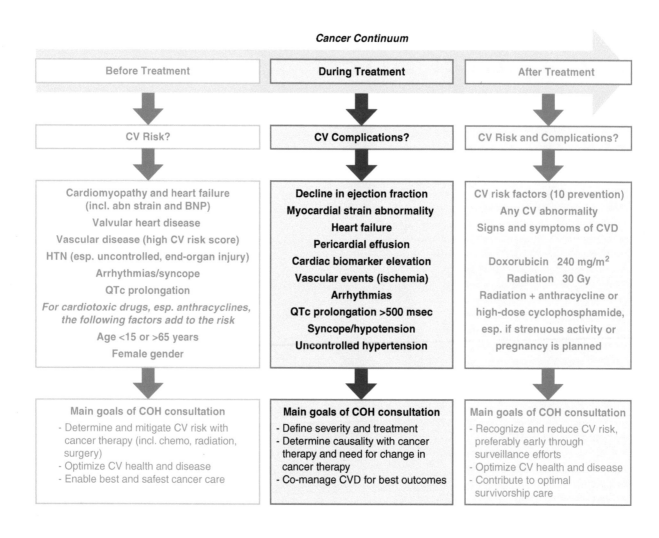

14 Key Points of Cardio-Oncology Evaluation During Cancer Therapy

JOERG HERRMANN

Cancer Continuum

Before Treatment

CV Risk?

Cardiomyopathy and heart failure (incl. abn strain and BNP)
Valvular heart disease
Vascular disease (high CV risk score)
HTN (esp. uncontrolled, end-organ injury)
Arrhythmias/syncope
QTc prolongation
For cardiotoxic drugs, esp. anthracyclines, the following factors add to the risk
Age <15 or >65 years
Female gender

Main goals of COH consultation
- Determine and mitigate CV risk with cancer therapy (incl. chemo, radiation, surgery)
- Optimize CV health and disease
- Enable best and safest cancer care

During Treatment

CV Complications?

Decline in ejection fraction
Myocardial strain abnormality
Heart failure
Pericardial effusion
Cardiac biomarker elevation
Vascular events (ischemia)
Arrhythmias
QTc prolongation >500 msec
Syncope/hypotension
Uncontrolled hypertension

Main goals of COH consultation
- Define severity and treatment
- Determine causality with cancer therapy and need for change in cancer therapy
- Co-manage CVD for best outcomes

After Treatment

CV Risk and Complications?

CV risk factors (10 prevention)
Any CV abnormality
Signs and symptoms of CVD

Doxorubicin 240 mg/m^2
Radiation 30 Gy
Radiation + anthracycline or high-dose cyclophosphamide, esp. if strenuous activity or pregnancy is planned

Main goals of COH consultation
- Recognize and reduce CV risk, preferably early through surveillance efforts
- Optimize CV health and disease
- Contribute to optimal survivorship care

KEY POINTS

- The main objective of the on-therapy evaluation of patients with cancer is to identify cardiovascular (CV) complications, especially as it pertains to the cancer therapy the patient is receiving
- The spectrum of cardiovascular diseases (CVD) is broad; it encompasses all of cardiology and ranges from asymptomatic changes within the CV system to life-threatening clinical scenarios
- Fulminant myocarditis, ventricular tachycardia/fibrillation, complete heart block, cardiac tamponade, cardiogenic shock, as well as ST-segment myocardial infarction and stroke are true emergencies that can occur in patients with cancer as a consequence of their therapy
- Defining the severity, trajectory, and treatment of the clinical presentation is essential
- Equally important is the definition of causality with the administered cancer therapy and addressing the question if the CV presentation is prohibitive to any further therapy, or if changes could be implemented that would allow for safe continuation of cancer therapy
- Multidisciplinary risk-benefit discussions and management decisions should be sought

Cardiovascular (CV) complications and toxicities are at the heart of cardio-oncology. The first to be recognized were cardiotoxicities and these still are the most common reason for referral to the cardio-oncology clinic. However, other CV toxicities have been increasingly encountered in recent years, somewhat paradoxically as the newer targeted therapies were envisioned to be safer as more directed toward the molecular finger print of the malignant disease process.

This section covers the main CV toxicities as they arise during cancer therapy, including cardiac, vascular, valvular, pericardial, and rhythm abnormalities as well as hypertension, and renal and pulmonary diseases. As broad as the spectrum of disease entities, so is their clinical presentation, ranging from asymptomatic to life-threatening. This applies to all the outlined disease entities in this section. Rapidly identifying any potentially fatal case scenarios is extremely important for obvious reasons. Further along these lines, some patients will need to be seen and followed in the hospital setting and even the intensive care unit. Treating patients with active cancer who develop cardiovascular disease (CVD) is often the most challenging situation because the unique characteristics and comorbidities of this patient population require a broader knowledge and experience of their trajectory. Standard practice guidelines written for the general population may therefore need to be modified, although for the most part these should be followed and translate into better clinical outcomes. Pertinent societal recommendations and considerations for patients with cancer who present with CVD are covered elsewhere (https://static-content.springer.com/esm/art%3A10.1038%2Fs41569-020-0348-1/MediaObjects/41569_2020_348_MOESM1_ESM.pdf and https://static-content.springer.com/esm/art%3A10.1038%2Fs41569-020-0347-2/MediaObjects/41569_2020_347_MOESM1_ESM.pdf).

Each time CVD or CV toxicity is noted in a patient with cancer who is on active cancer therapy, a key objective should be to define causality (i.e., to answer the question if the cancer therapy administered is causally responsible for the CV presentation). For obvious reasons, this has profound implications for the continuation of cancer therapy. Thoughtful risk-benefit decisions are to be made, which requires expert insight into both, the CVD and cancer aspects, and is therefore most ideally to be vetted in a multidisciplinary manner.

15 Diagnosis and Management of Cardiomyopathy and Heart Failure During Cancer Treatment

JOSE A. ALVAREZ-CARDONA AND DANIEL J. LENIHAN

Baseline CV Health

- Known CV risk factors
- Established cardiomyopathy or structural heart disease

Type of HF

- Heart failure with reduced ejection fraction (HFrEF)
- Heart failure with preserved ejection fraction (HFpEF)

Onset of Symptoms

- During cancer treatment
- After cancer treatment

Diagnosis

- Biomarkers: troponin, NT-proBNP, BNP, lipid profile, high-sensitive C-reactive protein
- Imaging: 2D/3D echo with strain, cardiac MRI, stress test
- Cardiac catheterization, coronary CTA

Potential Causes

- Cancer treatment-related: chemotherapy, immunotherapy, radiation therapy
- Coronary artery disease: acute coronary syndrome, chronic coronary artery disease
- Valvular heart disease
- Arrhythmias
- Stress-induced (Takotsubo) cardiomyopathy

Impact on Cancer Treatment

- Provide an accurate assessment of the risks and benefits of continuing cancer treatment

CHAPTER OUTLINE

KEY POINTS

- The management of cardiomyopathy or heart failure (CM/HF) in patients during cancer therapy ideally should be a continuation of pretherapy efforts (i.e., these patients should have been identified as high risk before any cancer therapy was given); only in the minority of patients should CM come as a surprise and HF should not be the first presentation
- Common universal classifications should be used, including asymptomatic decline in left ventricular ejection fraction (EF; i.e., ACC/AHA Stage B HF, and symptomatic HF with preserved or reduced EF ([HFpEF or HFrEF], American College of Cardiology/American Heart Association (ACC/AHA) stage C HF
- No universal definition of cardiotoxicity exists. The most common definition of cardiotoxicity, based on oncology clinical trials, is a greater than 10% reduction in left ventricular ejection fraction (LVEF) from baseline to less than or equal to 50%. Alternatively, cancer therapy-related cardiac dysfunction has been defined as a drop in LVEF by more than 10% to less than 53% by the American Society of Echocardiography)
- For any patient with a new presentation of CM/HF, all potential etiologies need to be entertained and treatment needs to be directed accordingly
- Whenever CM/HF is identified during cancer treatment, the risks and benefits of continued cancer therapy need to be carefully weighed on an individual basis, taking into account any potential long-term impact

The approach to heart failure (HF) during cancer treatment requires understanding the patient's current condition, including diagnosis and therapy. Common conditions are found in patients with cancer and should be evaluated accordingly.

Key points to consider include the following:

- Type of HF: heart failure with reduced ejection fraction (HFrEF) or heart failure with preserved ejection fraction (HFpEF)
- Chronicity of HF: acute or chronic
- Patient's hemodynamic status: warm and dry, warm and wet, cold and wet, or cold and dry
- Potential causes: acute coronary syndrome, arrhythmias, valvular heart disease, acute pulmonary embolism, or cancer therapy-related
- Sufficient evidence to recommend temporary or permanent discontinuation of cancer therapy after discussion with the oncology team

A proposed algorithm for monitoring and treating patients undergoing potentially cardiotoxic anticancer therapy is detailed below (Figs. 15.1 and 15.2). It highlights the importance of combining different screening tools, including imaging, electrocardiogram (ECG), and cardiac and inflammatory markers. These are complementary to the patient's symptoms and clinical findings, allowing clinicians to determine the severity of the patient's condition and need for specific treatment. The frequency of monitoring should be individualized, based on the severity of the patient's condition and current cancer therapy. In certain circumstances, if potentially cardiotoxic therapy is the only viable option for cancer treatment, the continuation of life-saving cancer therapy can be considered after close collaboration with a cardio-oncologist.

STRESS-INDUCED (TAKOTSUBO) CARDIOMYOPATHY IN PATIENTS WITH CANCER

Stress-induced (Takotsubo) cardiomyopathy is an acute presentation of HFrEF in the setting of significant physical or psychologic stress. Although most cases have been reported in women older than 55 years, men and younger patients are also affected.[1–3] Patients with cancer are intrinsically considered to have significant physical and emotional stress. A recent analysis from the International Takotsubo Registry found that about one in six patients with Takotsubo syndrome has a malignancy, with an overall prevalence of 18.2% in the Takotsubo cohort and 11.1% in those with acute coronary syndrome. Certain clinical characteristics in the malignancy group, including older age, were discovered, more commonly experiencing a physical rather than an emotional trigger, having dyspnea more frequently than chest pain, a lower LVEF, and having higher high-sensitivity C-reactive protein baseline and peak levels.[4] In addition, specific chemotherapy and immunotherapy agents have been associated with Takotsubo syndrome: 5-fluorouracil, capecitabine, axitinib, sunitinib, bevacizumab, ibrutinib, trastuzumab, rituximab, nivolumab, and ipilimumab.[5–16]

Table 15.1 summarizes the most widely used diagnostic criteria for Takotsubo syndrome. Its diagnosis may be challenging, but can definitively be

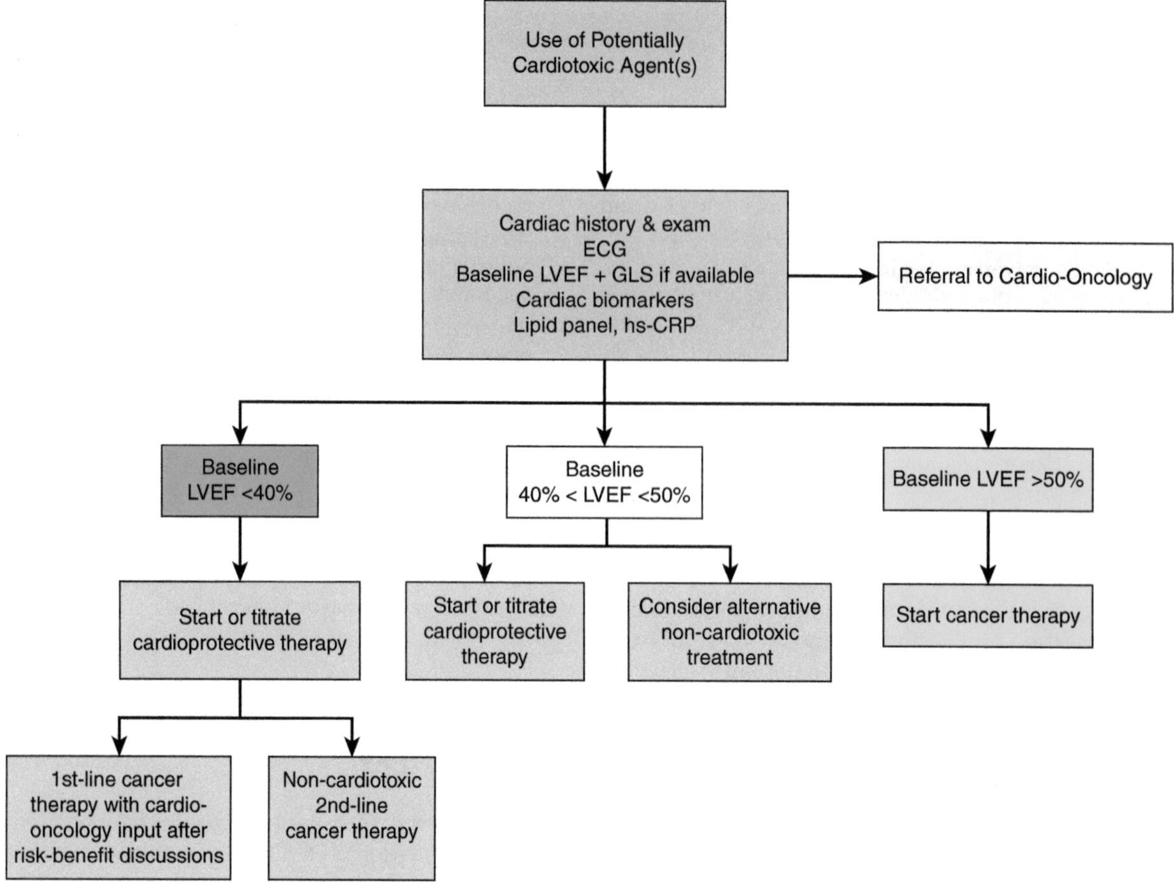

*Cardioprotective therapy includes angiotensin-converting enzyme inhibitor, angiotensin receptor blocker, carvedilol, mineralocorticoid receptor antagonist, statin, and dexrazoxane (applies to anthracycline-based chemotherapy)

FIG. 15.1 Proposed monitoring and management approach for patients undergoing potentially cardiotoxic anticancer therapy (Part 1). *ECG*, Electrocardiogram; *GLS*, global longitudinal strain; *LVEF*, left ventricular ejection fraction.

established once acute coronary syndrome has been excluded and its reversible nature has been demonstrated (Fig. 15.3). During the initial presentation a probable diagnosis can be made, especially when very specific clinical features are present, such as a regional wall motion abnormality that extends beyond a single vascular distribution. The InterTAK International Registry Group developed a diagnostic score that includes five clinical variables; depending on the score, a diagnosis of Takotsubo can be made with a specificity of 95% (Table 15.2).[17]

The management of Takotsubo syndrome depends on the patient's hemodynamic status and the presence or absence of LV outflow tract obstruction, usually caused by hypercontractility of basal segments. The management of cardiogenic shock owing to Takotsubo syndrome is beyond the scope of this chapter, but the reader is directed to thoughtful algorithms.[18–22] For patients who have a reduced LV systolic function but are otherwise hemodynamically stable and without LV outflow tract obstruction, treatment is the same as that published for patients with HFrEF.[23,24] In general, treatment of patients with cancer and heart failure should follow the ACC/AHA/HFSA Heart Failure Guidelines.

IMMUNE CHECKPOINT INHIBITORS AND CARDIAC IMMUNE-RELATED ADVERSE EVENTS

Immune checkpoint inhibitors (ICI) represent a new class of cancer therapy that directs the immune system to recognize and target cancer cells (see

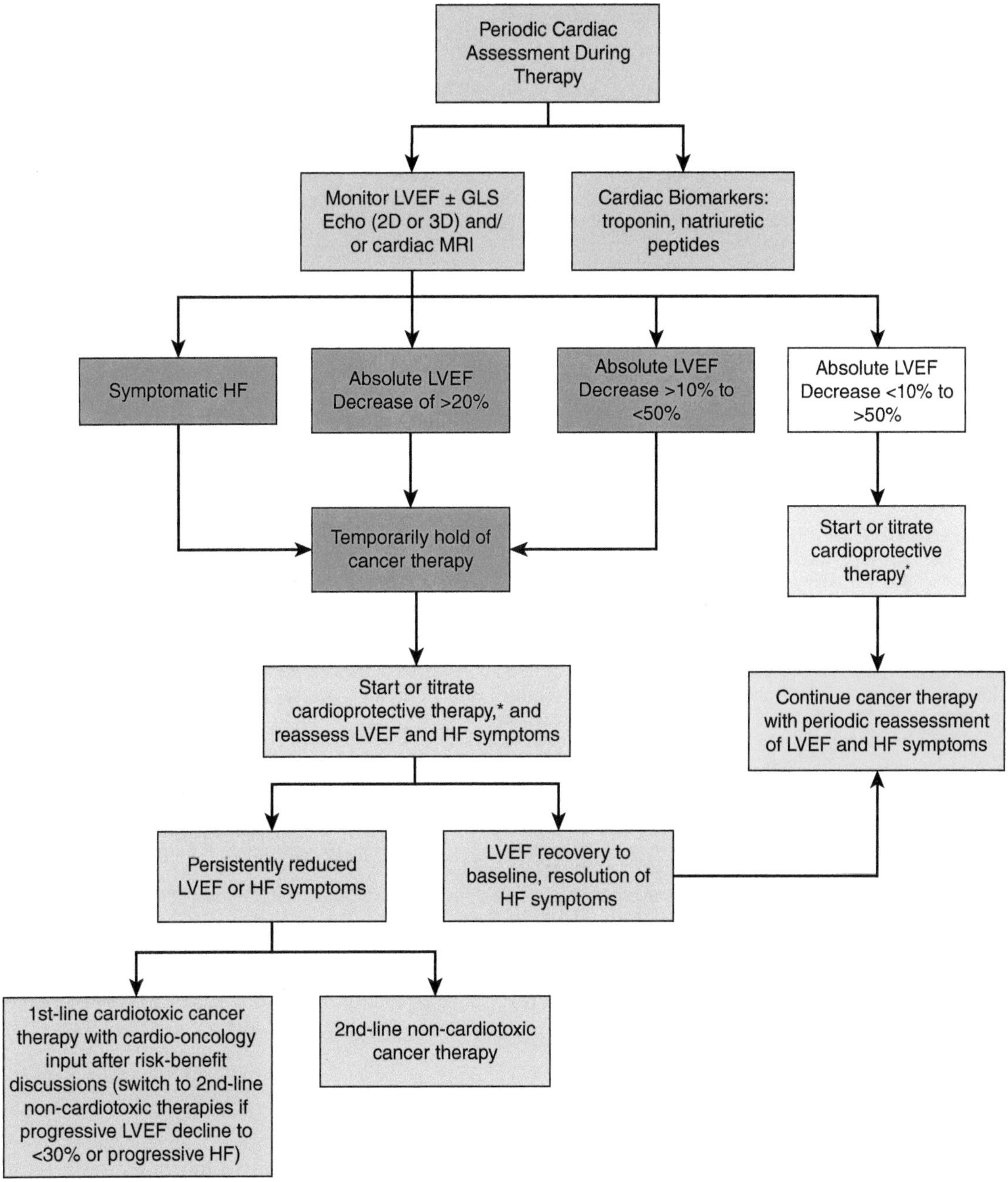

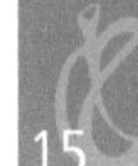

Periodic Cardiac Assessment During Therapy

Monitor LVEF ± GLS Echo (2D or 3D) and/or cardiac MRI

Cardiac Biomarkers: troponin, natriuretic peptides

Symptomatic HF

Absolute LVEF Decrease of >20%

Absolute LVEF Decrease >10% to <50%

Absolute LVEF Decrease <10% to >50%

Temporarily hold of cancer therapy

Start or titrate cardioprotective therapy*

Start or titrate cardioprotective therapy,* and reassess LVEF and HF symptoms

Continue cancer therapy with periodic reassessment of LVEF and HF symptoms

Persistently reduced LVEF or HF symptoms

LVEF recovery to baseline, resolution of HF symptoms

1st-line cardiotoxic cancer therapy with cardio-oncology input after risk-benefit discussions (switch to 2nd-line non-cardiotoxic therapies if progressive LVEF decline to <30% or progressive HF)

2nd-line non-cardiotoxic cancer therapy

*Cardioprotective therapy includes angiotensin-converting enzyme inhibitor, angiotensin receptor blocker, carvedilol, mineralocorticoid receptor antagonist, statin, and dexrazoxane (applies to anthracycline-based chemotherapy).

FIG. 15.2 Proposed monitoring and management approach for patients undergoing potentially cardiotoxic anticancer therapy (Part 2). *GLS*, Global longitudinal strain; *LVEF*, left ventricular ejection fraction; *MRI*, magnetic resonance image.

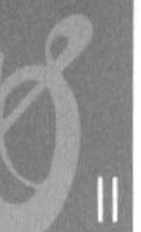

TABLE 15.1 **Diagnostic Criteria for Takotsubo Syndrome**

International Takotsubo Diagnostic Criteria (InterTAK Diagnostic Criteria)[18]
1. Patients show transient LV dysfunction (hypokinesia, akinesia, or dyskinesia) presenting as apical ballooning or midventricular, basal, or focal wall motion abnormalities. RV involvement can be present. Besides these regional wall motion patterns, transitions between all types can exist. The regional wall motion abnormality usually extends beyond a single epicardial vascular distribution; however, rare cases can exist where the regional wall motion abnormality is present in the subtended myocardial territory of a single coronary artery (focal Takotsubo cardiomyopathy). 2. An emotional, physical, or combined trigger can precede the Takotsubo syndrome event, but this is not obligatory. 3. Neurologic disorders (e.g., subarachnoid hemorrhage, stroke/TIA, or seizures) as well as pheochromocytoma may serve as triggers for Takotsubo syndrome. 4. New ECG abnormalities are present (ST-segment elevation, ST-segment depression, T-wave inversion, and QTc prolongation); however, rare cases exist without any ECG changes. 5. Levels of cardiac biomarkers (troponin and creatinine kinase) are moderately elevated in most cases; significant elevation of brain natriuretic peptide is common. 6. Significant coronary artery disease is not a contraindication in Takotsubo syndrome. 7. Patients have no evidence of infectious myocarditis. 8. Postmenopausal women are predominantly affected.
Heart Failure Association of the European Society of Cardiology[19]
1. Transient regional wall motion abnormalities of LV or RV myocardium which are frequently, but not always, preceded by a stressful trigger (emotional or physical). 2. The regional wall motion abnormalities usually extend beyond a single epicardial vascular distribution, and often result in circumferential dysfunction of the ventricular segments involved. 3. The absence of culprit atherosclerotic coronary artery disease including acute plaque rupture, thrombus formation, and coronary dissection or other pathological conditions to explain the pattern of temporary LV dysfunction observed (e.g., hypertrophic cardiomyopathy, viral myocarditis). 4. New and reversible ECG abnormalities (ST-segment elevation, ST depression, LBBB, T-wave inversion, and/or QTc prolongation) during the acute phase (3 months). 5. Significant elevated serum natriuretic peptide (BNP or NT-proBNP) during the acute phase. 6. Positive but relatively small elevation in cardiac troponin measured with a conventional assay (i.e., disparity between the troponin level and the amount of dysfunctional myocardium present). 7. Recovery of ventricular systolic function on cardiac imaging at follow-up (3–6 months).
Revised Mayo Clinic Criteria[20,21]—All 4 Criteria Must be Met
1. Transient hypokinesis, akinesis, or dyskinesis of the LV mid segments with or without apical involvement; the regional wall motion abnormalities extend beyond a single epicardial vascular distribution; a stressful trigger is often, but not always present. There are rare exceptions to these criteria such as those patients in whom the regional wall motion abnormality is limited to a single coronary territory. 2. Absence of obstructive coronary disease or angiographic evidence of acute plaque rupture. It is possible that a patient with obstructive coronary atherosclerosis may also develop Takotsubo syndrome. 3. New ECG abnormalities (either ST-segment elevation and/or T-wave inversion) or modest elevation in cardiac troponin. 4. Absence of pheochromocytoma and myocarditis.

BNP, Brain natriuretic peptide; *ECG*, electrocardiogram; *LBBB*, left bundle branch block; *LV*, left ventricle; *NT-proBNP*, N-terminal pro-brain natriuretic peptide; *RV*, right ventricle; *TIA*, transient ischemic attack.

Chapter 54). Upregulation of the immune system sometimes results in immune-related adverse events, which can affect different multiple organ systems. Cardiac immune-related adverse events are now increasingly recognized (Fig. 15.4), in particular, myocarditis. A recent study by Mahmood et al.[25] found that myocarditis usually occurs early during treatment (median time of 34 days after starting) and was more common with combination ICI, even though 66% of cases were seen with monotherapy. The rate of mortality remains unacceptably high, estimated at 50% of confirmed cases of myocarditis. In addition, a depressed LVEF was not a requirement for serious adverse CV events, but the degree of troponin elevation was a predictor of such events. Treatment with steroids, particularly at high doses, was associated with lower adverse cardiac events.[25] These findings illustrate the importance of surveillance and prompt diagnosis in patients treated with ICI.

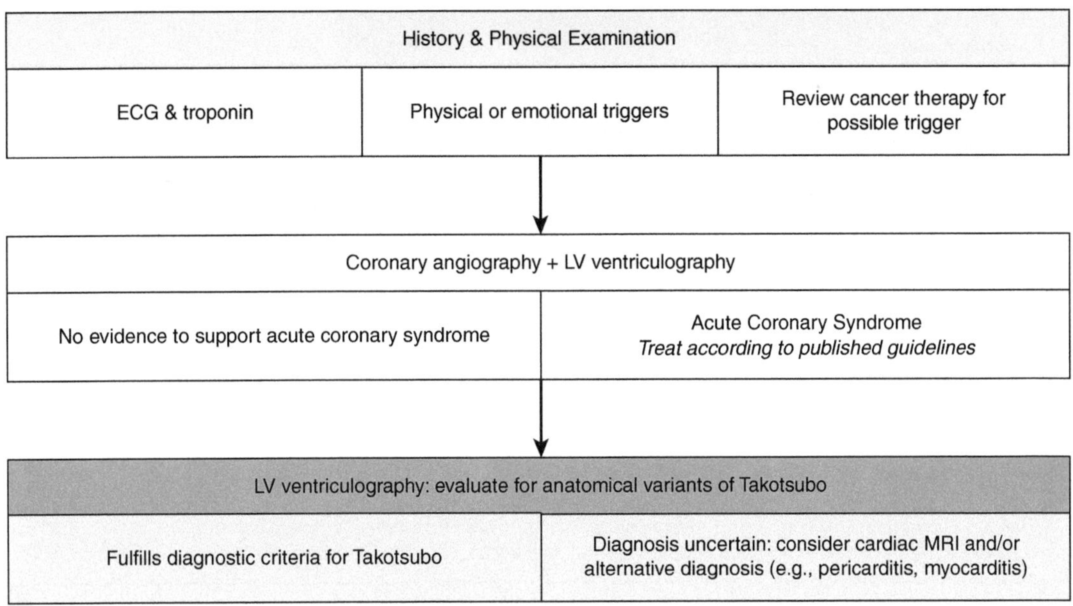

FIG. 15.3 General diagnostic approach to Takotsubo syndrome in patients receiving cancer therapy. *ECG*, Electrocardiogram; *LV*, left ventricle; *MRI*, magnetic resonance image.

TABLE 15.2 InterTAK Diagnostic Score: Takotsubo Versus Acute Coronary Syndrome[17]

CRITERIA	POINTS
Female	25
Emotional trigger	24
Physical trigger	13
Absence of ST-segment depression (except in lead aVR)	12
Psychiatric disorders	11
Neurologic disorders	9
QTc prolongation	6
Diagnosis (cutoff value, range 0–100)	
Takotsubo syndrome	≥50 (specificity 95%)
Acute coronary syndrome	≤31 (specificity 95%)

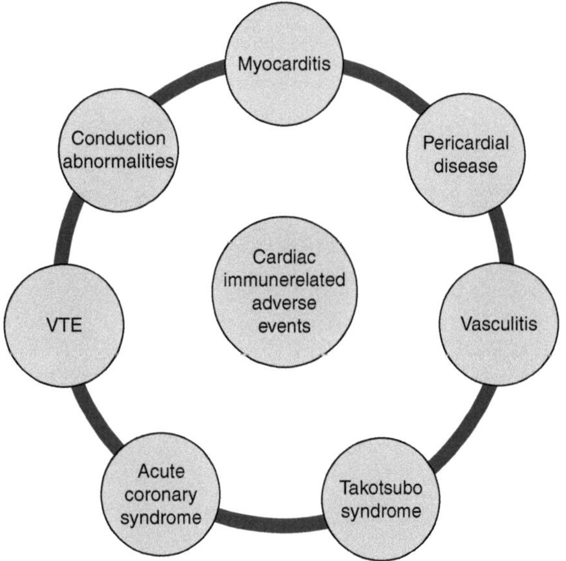

FIG. 15.4 Potential cardiac immune-related adverse events in patients treated with immune checkpoint inhibitor therapy. *VTE*, Venous thromboembolism.[25,–31]

In summary:

- Cardiac immune-related adverse events appear to be more frequent with cytotoxic T-lymphocyte-associated antigen 4 (CTLA-4) antagonists compared with programmed death 1 (PD-1) inhibitors, and the risk increases with combination therapy.[26,32–34]
- Cardiac immune-related adverse events usually happen early during treatment.
- These adverse events usually respond well to high-dose steroids.
- More research is warranted to determine if comorbid conditions and/or concurrent therapy with other agents and/or radiation therapy

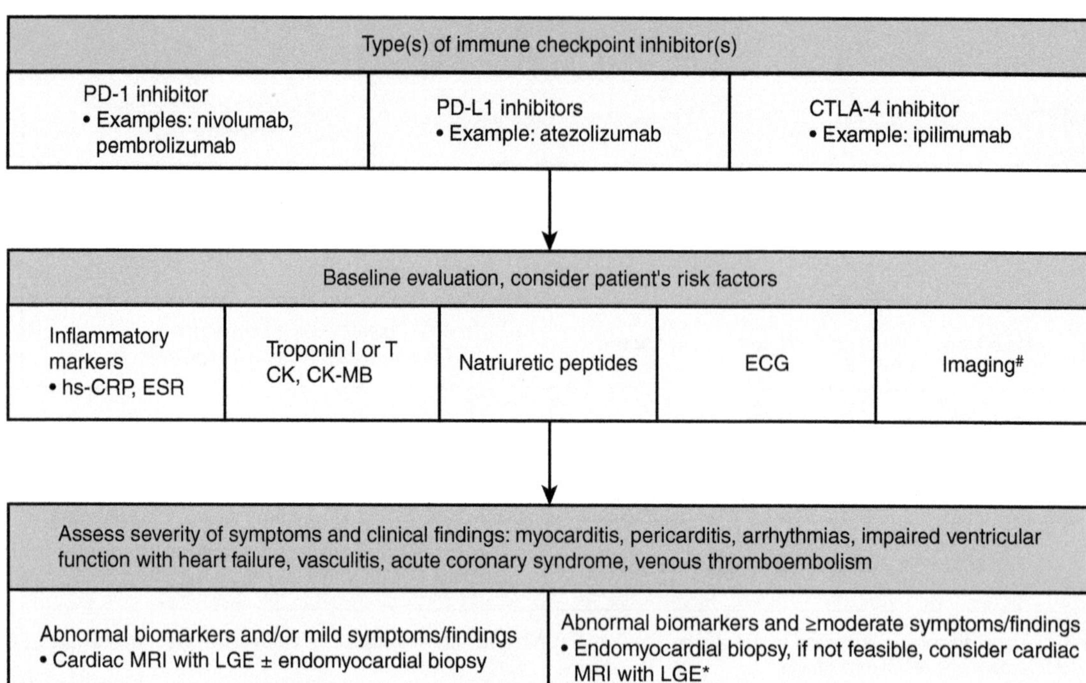

*Treatment initiation should not be delayed.
#Imaging includes chest XR, 2D or 3D echo, cardiac MRI, cardiac catheterization, stress test
CK = creatinine kinase; CK-MB = creatinine kinase muscle/brain; ECG = electrocardiogram; ESR = erythrocyte sedimentation rate; CTLA-4 = cytotoxic T-lymphocyte-associated-4; LGE = late gadolinium enhancement; PD-1 = programmed cell death protein 1; PD-L1 = programmed death-ligand 1

FIG. 15.5 Approach to the patient receiving immune checkpoint inhibitor therapy.

TABLE 15.3 Management of Cardiac Immune-Related Adverse Events as Recommended by ASCO[35]

GRADING	MANAGEMENT

Grade 1: Abnormal cardiac biomarker testing, including abnormal ECG
Grade 2: Abnormal screening tests with mild symptoms
Grade 3: Moderately abnormal testing or symptoms with mild activity
Grade 4: Moderate to severe decompensation, intravenous medication or intervention required, life-threatening conditions
	• All grade warrant work-up and intervention given potential for cardiac compromise
	• Consider the following:
	  • Hold ICPi and permanently discontinue after G1
	  • High-dose corticosteroid (1–2 mg/kg of prednisone) initiated rapidly (oral or IV depending on symptoms)
	  • Admit patient, cardiology consultation
	  • Management of cardiac symptoms according to ACC/AHA guidelines and with guidance from cardiology
	  • Immediate transfer to a coronary care unit for patients with elevated troponin or conduction abnormalities
	• In patients without an immediate response to high-dose corticosteroids, consider early institution of cardiac transplant rejection doses of corticosteroids (methylprednisolone 1 g every day) and the addition of mycophenolate mofetil, infliximab, or antithymocyte globulin

ACC, American College of Cardiology; *AHA*, American Heart Association; *ASCO*, American Society of Clinical Oncology; *ECG*, electrocardiogram; *ICPi*, immune checkpoint inhibitor; *IV*, intravenous.

impact the likelihood of cardiac immune-related adverse events.

- Owing to potentially fatal toxicity, an aggressive and emergent approach to diagnosis and treatment is recommended (Fig. 15.5 and Table 15.3).

REFERENCES

1. Roshanzamir S, Showkathali R. Takotsubo cardiomyopathy a short review. *Curr Cardiol Rev.* 2013;9:191–196.
2. Schneider B, Athanasiadis A, Stollberger C, et al. Gender differences in the manifestation of tako-tsubo cardiomyopathy. *Int J Cardiol.* 2013;166:584–588.

3. Templin C, Ghadri JR, Diekmann J, et al. Clinical features and outcomes of Takotsubo (stress) cardiomyopathy. *N Engl J Med.* 2015;373:929–938.
4. Cammann VL, Sarcon A, Ding KJ, et al. Clinical features and outcomes of patients with malignancy and Takotsubo syndrome: observations from the International Takotsubo Registry. *J Am Heart Assoc.* 2019;8:e010881.
5. Basselin C, Fontanges T, Descotes J, et al. 5-Fluorouracil-induced tako-tsubo-like syndrome. *Pharmacotherapy.* 2011;31:226.
6. Ederhy S, Cautela J, Ancedy Y, Escudier M, Thuny F, Cohen A. Takotsubo-like syndrome in patients with cancer treated with immune checkpoint inhibitors. *JACC Cardiovasc Imaging.* 2018;11:1187–1190.
7. Franco TH, Khan A, Joshi V, Thomas B. Takotsubo cardiomyopathy in two men receiving bevacizumab for metastatic cancer. *Ther Clin Risk Manag.* 2008;4:1367–1370.
8. Geisler BP, Raad RA, Esaian D, Sharon E, Schwartz DR. Apical ballooning and cardiomyopathy in a melanoma patient treated with ipilimumab: a case of takotsubo-like syndrome. *J Immunother Cancer.* 2015;3:4.
9. Grunwald MR, Howie L, Diaz Jr LA. Takotsubo cardiomyopathy and fluorouracil: case report and review of the literature. *J Clin Oncol.* 2012;30:e11–e14.
10. Khanji M, Nolan S, Gwynne S, Pudney D, Ionescu A. Tako-Tsubo syndrome after trastuzumab—an unusual complication of chemotherapy for breast cancer. *Clin Oncol (R Coll Radiol).* 2013;25:329.
11. Knott K, Starling N, Rasheed S, et al. A case of Takotsubo syndrome following 5-fluorouracil chemotherapy. *Int J Cardiol.* 2014;177:e65–e67.
12. Kobayashi N, Hata N, Yokoyama S, Shinada T, Shirakabe A, Mizuno K. A case of Takotsubo cardiomyopathy during 5-fluorouracil treatment for rectal adenocarcinoma. *J Nippon Med Sch.* 2009;76:27–33.
13. Ng KH, Dearden C, Gruber P. Rituximab-induced Takotsubo syndrome: more cardiotoxic than it appears? *BMJ Case Rep.* 2015;2015: bcr2014208203. doi:10.1136/bcr-2014-208203.
14. Numico G, Sicuro M, Silvestris N, et al. Takotsubo syndrome in a patient treated with sunitinib for renal cancer. *J Clin Oncol,* 2012;30:e218–e220.
15. Ovadia D, Esquenazi Y, Bucay M, Bachier CR. Association between takotsubo cardiomyopathy and axitinib: case report and review of the literature. *J Clin Oncol.* 2015;33:e1–e3.
16. Ozturk MA, Ozveren O, Cinar V, Erdik B, Oyan B. Takotsubo syndrome: an underdiagnosed complication of 5-fluorouracil mimicking acute myocardial infarction. *Blood Coagul Fibrinolysis.* 2013;24:90–94.
17. Ghadri JR, Cammann VL, Jurisic S, et al. A novel clinical score (InterTAK Diagnostic Score) to differentiate takotsubo syndrome from acute coronary syndrome: results from the International Takotsubo Registry. *Eur J Heart Fail.* 2017;19:1036–1042.
18. Ghadri JR, Wittstein IS, Prasad A, et al. International expert consensus document on takotsubo syndrome (Part I): clinical characteristics, diagnostic criteria, and pathophysiology. *Eur Heart J.* 2018;39:2032–2046.
19. Lyon AR, Bossone E, Schneider B, et al. Current state of knowledge on Takotsubo syndrome: a position statement from the Taskforce on Takotsubo Syndrome of the Heart Failure Association of the European Society of Cardiology. *Eur J Heart Fail.* 2016;18:8–27.
20. Bybee KA, Kara T, Prasad A, et al. Systematic review: transient left ventricular apical ballooning: a syndrome that mimics ST-segment elevation myocardial infarction. *Ann Intern Med.* 2004;141:858–865.
21. Prasad A, Lerman A, Rihal CS. Apical ballooning syndrome (Tako-Tsubo or stress cardiomyopathy): a mimic of acute myocardial infarction. *Am Heart J.* 2008;155:408–417.
22. de Chazal HM, Del Buono MG, Keyser-Marcus L, et al. Stress cardiomyopathy diagnosis and treatment: JACC state-of-the-art review. *J Am Coll Cardiol.* 2018;72:1955–1971.
23. Yancy CW, Jessup M, Bozkurt B, et al. 2017 ACC/AHA/HFSA focused update of the 2013 ACCF/AHA guideline for the management of heart failure: a report of the American College of Cardiology/ American Heart Association Task Force on clinical practice guidelines and the Heart Failure Society of America. *Circulation.* 2017;136:e137–e161.
24. Yancy CW, Jessup M, Bozkurt B, et al. 2013 ACCF/AHA guideline for the management of heart failure: executive summary: a report of the American College of Cardiology Foundation/American Heart Association Task Force on practice guidelines. *Circulation.* 2013; 128:1810–1852.
25. Mahmood SS, Fradley MG, Cohen JV, et al. Myocarditis in patients treated with immune checkpoint inhibitors. *J Am Coll Cardiol.* 2018;71:1755–1764.
26. Johnson DB, Balko JM, Compton ML, et al. Fulminant myocarditis with combination immune checkpoint blockade. *N Engl J Med.* 2016; 375:1749–1755.
27. Reddy N, Moudgil R, Lopez-Mattei JC, et al. Progressive and reversible conduction disease with checkpoint inhibitors. *Can J Cardiol.* 2017;33:1335.e13–1335.e15.
28. Salem JE, Manouchehri A, Moey M, et al. Cardiovascular toxicities associated with immune checkpoint inhibitors: an observational, retrospective, pharmacovigilance study. *Lancet Oncol.* 2018;19: 1579–1589.
29. Altan M, Toki MI, Gettinger SN, et al. Immune checkpoint inhibitor-associated pericarditis. *J Thorac Oncol.* 2019;14:1102–1108.
30. Anderson RD, Brooks M. Apical takotsubo syndrome in a patient with metastatic breast carcinoma on novel immunotherapy. *Int J Cardiol,* 2016;222:760–761.
31. Tomita Y, Sueta D, Kakiuchi Y, et al. Acute coronary syndrome as a possible immune-related adverse event in a lung patient with cancer achieving a complete response to anti-PD-1 immune checkpoint antibody. *Ann Oncol.* 2017;28:2893–2895.
32. Larkin J, Chiarion-Sileni V, Gonzalez R, et al. Combined nivolumab and ipilimumab or monotherapy in untreated melanoma. *N Engl J Med.* 2015;373:23–34.
33. Tawbi HA, Forsyth PA, Algazi A, et al. Combined nivolumab and ipilimumab in melanoma metastatic to the birain. *N Engl J Med.* 2018;379:722–730.
34. Topalian SL, Hodi FS, Brahmer JR, et al. Safety, activity, and immune correlates of anti-PD-1 antibody in cancer. *N Engl J Med.* 2012;366:2443–2454.
35. Brahmer JR, Lacchetti C, Thompson JA. Management of immune-related adverse events in patients treated with immune checkpoint inhibitor therapy: American Society of Clinical Oncology clinical practice guideline summary. *J Oncol Pract.* 2018;14:247–249.

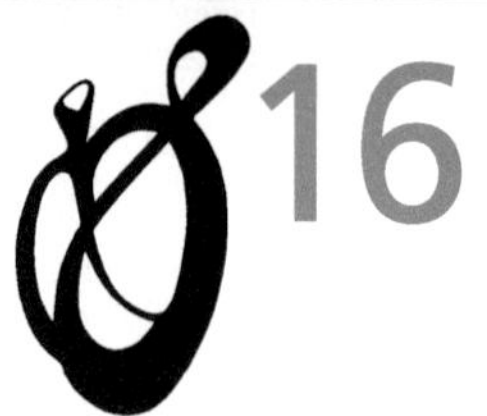

16 Structural Heart Disease Management During Cancer Treatment

VUYISILE T. NKOMO, DIMITRI J. MAAMARI, AND JAE K. OH

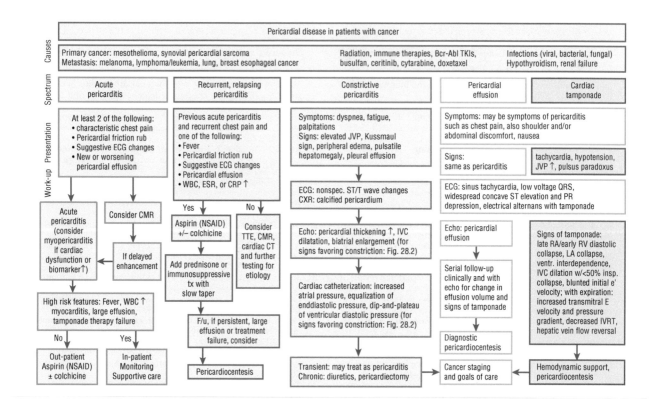

Pericardial disease in patients with cancer

Causes

Primary cancer: mesothelioma, synovial pericardial sarcoma
Metastasis: melanoma, lymphoma/leukemia, lung, breast esophageal cancer

Radiation, immune therapies, Bcr-Abl TKIs, busulfan, ceritinib, cytarabine, doxetaxel

Infections (viral, bacterial, fungal)
Hypothyroidism, renal failure

Spectrum

Acute pericarditis | Recurrent, relapsing pericarditis | Constrictive pericarditis | Pericardial effusion | Cardiac tamponade

Work-up Presentation

Acute pericarditis

At least 2 of the following:
- characteristic chest pain
- Pericardial friction rub
- Suggestive ECG changes
- New or worsening pericardial effusion

→ Acute pericarditis (consider myopericarditis if cardiac dysfunction or biomarker↑)

→ Consider CMR → If delayed enhancement → Acute pericarditis (consider myopericarditis if cardiac dysfunction or biomarker↑)

→ High risk features: Fever, WBC ↑ myocarditis, large effusion, tamponade therapy failure

No → Out-patient Aspirin (NSAID) ± colchicine

Yes → In-patient Monitoring Supportive care

Recurrent, relapsing pericarditis

Previous acute pericarditis and recurrent chest pain and one of the following:
- Fever
- Pericardial friction rub
- Suggestive ECG changes
- Pericardial effusion
- WBC, ESR, or CRP ↑

Yes → Aspirin (NSAID) +/− colchicine → Add prednisone or immunosuppressive tx with slow taper → F/u, if persistent, large effusion or treatment failure, consider → Pericardiocentesis

No → Consider TTE, CMR, cardiac CT and further testing for etiology

Constrictive pericarditis

Symptoms: dyspnea, fatigue, palpitations
Signs: elevated JVP, Kussmaul sign, peripheral edema, pulsatile hepatomegaly, pleural effusion

→ ECG: nonspec. ST/T wave changes
CXR: calcified pericardium

→ Echo: pericardial thickening ↑, IVC dilatation, biatrial enlargement (for signs favoring constriction: Fig. 28.2)

→ Cardiac catheterization: increased atrial pressure, equalization of enddiastolic pressure, dip-and-plateau of ventricular diastolic pressure (for signs favoring constriction: Fig. 28.2)

→ Transient: may treat as pericarditis
Chronic: diuretics, pericardiectomy → Cancer staging and goals of care

Pericardial effusion / Cardiac tamponade

Symptoms: may be symptoms of pericarditis such as chest pain, also shoulder and/or abdominal discomfort, nausea

Signs (pericardial effusion): same as pericarditis
Signs (cardiac tamponade): tachycardia, hypotension, JVP ↑, pulsus paradoxus

ECG: sinus tachycardia, low voltage QRS, widespread concave ST elevation and PR depression, electrical alternans with tamponade

Pericardial effusion: Echo: pericardial effusion → Serial follow-up clinically and with echo for change in effusion volume and signs of tamponade → Diagnostic pericardiocentesis → Cancer staging and goals of care

Cardiac tamponade: Signs of tamponade: late RA/early RV diastolic collapse, LA collapse, ventr. interdependence, IVC dilation w/<50% insp. collapse, blunted initial e' velocity; with expiration: increased transmitral E velocity and pressure gradient, decreased IVRT, hepatic vein flow reversal → Hemodynamic support, pericardiocentesis → Cancer staging and goals of care

CHAPTER OUTLINE

KEY POINTS

- Baseline transthoracic echocardiogram is important for the assessment of heart structure and function, and the determination of the presence or absence of pericardial or valvular heart disease prior to initiation of cancer treatment.
- On autopsy, pericardial involvement is noted in 1% to 20% of patients with cancer, most commonly lung cancer, but also breast and esophageal cancer, melanoma, lymphoma, and leukemia.
- Pericardial disease in patients with cancer can manifest as pericarditis, pericardial effusion, cardiac tamponade, or constrictive pericarditis.
- Pericarditis during cancer treatment typically responds to anti-inflammatory therapy, but can pose a risk for tamponade acutely and for recurrent pericarditis later on.
- Patients with cancer are at an increased risk of infective endocarditis; nonbacterial thrombotic endocarditis may be an associated complication of cancer.
- Preexisting valvular heart disease can complicate cancer therapy owing to increased pressure and/or volume load and predispose to heart failure presentations.
- Valve repair or replacement is recommended for severe valve disease, especially with the advances in percutaneous techniques and when cardiotoxic cancer therapy is unavoidable.
- Guidelines recommend valve intervention if life expectancy is more than 12 months.

PERICARDIAL DISEASE

Incidence

- Malignancy is newly diagnosed in 5% to 10% of patients presenting with pericarditis, and chances are higher (20% to 30%) in those presenting with a large pericardial effusion, cardiac tamponade, and lack of response to anti-inflammatory therapy or recurrent/persistent pericarditis.
- Around 50% of pericardial effusions are malignancy-related (including patients with known cancer), and pericardial effusion can complicate 5% to 15% of late-stage cancers.[1]
- Pericardial disease can be seen in 6% to 30% of patients with cancer undergoing radiation therapy, but pericardial constriction is usually a late (20 to 30 years) complication seen in survivors (see Chapter 28).

Risk Factors

Risk factors include types of cancer, chemotherapy drugs, radiation, and infection related to a compromised state.

Causes

Drugs

- Anthracyclines, cyclophosphamide, cytarabine, (pericarditis ± myocarditis)
- Tyrosine kinase inhibitors (imatinib, dasatinib, bosutinib, and ceritinib (pericarditis ± pleural effusion)
- Interferon-α (for melanoma)
- Retinoic acid (retinoic acid syndrome = fever, systemic hypotension, acute renal failure, pleural effusion, pericardial effusion)
- Busulfan (late pericardial and myocardial fibrosis)
- Methotrexate, arsenic trioxide, 5-fluorouracil, and docetaxel
- High-dose chemotherapy (circulating tumor cell [CTC] regimen consisting of four courses daily of fluorouracil, epirubicin, cyclophosphamide every three weeks, followed by high-dose chemotherapy with cyclophosphamide, carboplatin, and thiotepa divided over four days is the reported cause of constrictive pericarditis that began as an effusion two months after chemotherapy and 2 weeks later had no effusion, but needed pericardiectomy for constrictive pericarditis)
- Immune checkpoint inhibitors, such as anti-PD1 (e.g., nivolumab, pembrolizumab) and anti-PDL1 agents (e.g., atezolizumab)

Radiation

- 6% to 30% of patients receiving radiation therapy[2–6]

Direct or Metastatic Tumor Invasion/Extension

- Primary involvement of the pericardium is seen with pericardial mesothelioma and pericardial fibrosarcoma or angiosarcoma.
- Direct local extension into the pericardium is seen with lung, breast, or esophageal cancer.
- Hematogenous and/or lymphangitic spread is seen with leukemia, lymphoma, and melanoma.

Infectious Causes

- Infections related to the immunocompromised state of patients
- Infections following thoracic or cardiac surgery

Obstruction of Mediastinal Lymphatic Drainage

- Compression by mediastinal tumor mass
- Mediastinal lymph node removal
- Radiation therapy

Diagnosis

Pericarditis

Symptoms suggesting pericarditis include positional sharp chest pain, dyspnea, and palpitations. Physical examination and detection of a pericardial friction rub is important in the assessment of patients suspected of having pericarditis because pericarditis may or may not be accompanied by a pericardial effusion. Electrocardiogram changes can be seen in pericarditis, such as tachycardia, PR depression or ST-segment elevation.

Cardiac magnetic resonance imaging or computed tomography show enhancement or thickening of the pericardium in acute pericarditis.

Pericardial Effusion

Pericardial effusion could result in hemodynamic compromise based on the size and rapidity of accumulation of pericardial fluid.[7,8] A pericardial effusion should be suspected when there is an enlarging cardiac silhouette. Cardiomegaly on chest X-ray does not manifest until the pericardial fluid reaches at least 200 mL.[8] Some patients report fatigue, dyspnea, and chest heaviness. Transthoracic echocardiography is the diagnostic tool of choice for the evaluation of presence, size, and hemodynamic sequelae of a pericardial effusion. It is not uncommon for the pericardial effusion to be detected first by computed tomography or cardiac magnetic resonance imaging during chest imaging prior to echocardiography. Electrocardiographic findings of pericardial effusion include tachycardia, low voltage, and electrical alternans. Pericardial fluid should be sent for testing to investigate the cause of pericardial effusion including cytology, aerobic and anaerobic cultures, protein, glucose, and lactate dehydrogenase, pH, specific gravity, and hemoglobin if the effusion is bloody.

Cardiac Tamponade

Cardiac tamponade is a medical emergency that culminates in cardiogenic shock hemodynamics (hypotension and tachycardia). Physical examination findings include jugular venous distention and its paradoxical rise with inspiration (Kussmaul sign); a pulsus paradoxus (drop in systolic blood pressure by $>$10 mm Hg with inspiration) may also be seen.

Cardiac tamponade dynamics are seen with large or rapidly accumulating pericardial effusions. The diagnostic tool of choice is the transthoracic echocardiography. Echocardiographic features of tamponade include a swinging heart, mitral inflow respiratory variability of greater than 25%, right-sided cardiac chamber diastolic compression, and inferior vena cava changes, such as a dilated, minimally collapsing, or not collapsing inferior vena cava.

Myopericarditis

Pericarditis, with or without a pericardial effusion, may be associated with varying degrees of myocardial involvement (myopericarditis). Myopericarditis may manifest as global reduction in left ventricular ejection fraction or as regional wall motion abnormalities that do not necessarily follow a coronary distribution. Sometimes, myocardial involvement is minor and is not associated with any myocardial structural changes; but elevations in cardiac biomarkers such as cardiac troponins are indicative in this setting. Cardiac magnetic resonance imaging is helpful in detecting myocarditis associated with pericarditis,[9–11] as well as the extent to which the pericardium or myocardium is involved. Coronary angiogram may be necessary to exclude coronary artery disease and myocardial infarction, especially when cardiac troponin elevation is present and clinical (chest pain) presentation and echocardiographic findings are not conclusive.

Prognosis

Patients with acute pericarditis are at risk of developing chronic pericarditis.[12]

Malignant pericardial effusion portends worse prognosis than nonmalignant pericardial effusion in patients with lung cancer. However, this has not been seen in patients with breast cancer.[13] The prognosis in general is more favorable in hematologic than in solid malignancies and relates to the ability to provide effective cancer-directed therapies.

Prevention

If possible, cancer drugs not associated with pericardial effusion should be chosen. New radiation techniques, such as proton beam therapy, have shown lower rates of cardiotoxicity in certain cancer populations.[14,15]

Treatment Overview

Acute Pericarditis

Acute pericarditis is treated with anti-inflammatory drugs. Colchicine is recommended as first-line therapy, in addition to a nonsteroidal anti-inflammatory drug (NSAID) or high-dose aspirin. It usually takes three months of the medications to heal the pericardial inflammation. Corticosteroids are used as second-line therapy, in cases of nonresponsiveness to the previous medications, or in patients with contraindication to NSAIDs or aspirin, to avoid corticosteroid-dependence.[16] If a specific cause is identified (e.g., infection), therapy should be directed accordingly.

Although dose adjustment can be considered, there is no indication to interrupt radiation therapy because pericarditis responds well to anti-inflammatory drug therapy.[17]

Constrictive hemodynamics can be present transiently with acute pericarditis, but should be able to be managed by medical therapy (see Chapter 28).

Pericardial Effusion and Cardiac Tamponade

In case of pericardial effusions with underlying pericarditis, pharmacotherapy is similar to that of acute pericarditis, especially when the effusion is neither large nor associated with tamponade physiology. If pharmacotherapy fails to reduce the effusion, pericardiocentesis should be considered.[16]

In cases of isolated pericardial effusion, without signs of ongoing inflammation, pericardiocentesis should be considered if the effusion is associated with either cardiac tamponade[16] or systemic venous congestion. Pericardiocentesis should also be of consideration in case of general anesthesia (e.g., in the setting of surgery) to avoid hemodynamic instability and cardiovascular collapse during induction.

Echocardiogram-guided pericardiocentesis has been shown to be effective and safe with very low complication rates in multiple studies.[18,19]

After successful drainage, pericardial fluid should be sent for testing (see Diagnosis of Pericardial Effusion). For residual fluid draining, it is recommended to withdraw the introducer sheath and to keep a pigtail catheter in the pericardial space for intermittent drainage. Then, 10 mL 1% xylocaine are injected in the pericardial space for chest pain prophylaxis and treatment. Proper pericardial care should include flushing 3 to 5 mL of sterile saline, aspiration of all available fluid with recording of the retrieved amount followed by injection of 3 to 5 mL of sterile saline, every 4 to 6 hours.[20,21] Contemporary practice at Mayo Clinic is to leave the pericardial catheter until the net drainage is less than 50 mL over 24 hours.[20,21] On average, the time to minimal catheter output is three days. Compared with pericardiocentesis alone, the combination of pericardiocentesis with extended catheter drainage decreases the risk of recurrence by approximately two-thirds. A pericardiotomy (pericardial window) is the other alternative for management of pericardial effusions and reduction of their recurrence. The reported recurrence rates vary considerably and are as high as 60%. Furthermore, about 20% of the patients who undergo pericardiocentesis develop effusive-constrictive pericarditis, which can be detected by persistent elevation of jugular venous pressure and constrictive features on echocardiography. They need to be treated with NSAID and colchicine for 3 months.[22] Most patients with "constrictive pericarditis" fall in this category.

Myopericarditis

Anti-inflammatory medications such as NSAIDs or high-dose aspirin should be considered for management of chest pain in myopericarditis. Corticosteroids can also be prescribed as second-line agents when NSAIDs or aspirin are not effective, contraindicated, or not tolerated by the patient.[16] Some studies have shown increased mortality in animal models when myopericarditis is treated with NSAIDs,[16] leading some to recommend using the lowest possible dose of anti-inflammatory medications. The approach also needs to be modified, depending on cancer therapy exposure. For instance, myopericarditis in the setting of immune checkpoint inhibitors should be treated with high-dose steroid therapy with a slow gradual taper. Acute myopericarditis with cyclophosphamide can likewise progress to a medical emergency requiring mechanical support.

VALVE DISEASE

Incidence

Risk of endocarditis is higher in patients with cancer compared with patients without cancer even when matched by other comorbidities.[23]

Risk Factors

Aging, prior cardiovascular risk factors,[24,25] prior rheumatic fever,[26] previous radiation with median time from radiation to onset of 12 years and adjuvant chemotherapy at time of radiation,[5,27,28] and active cancer[23,29] are the major risk factors.

Causes

Causes of valve diseases may be primary valve disease (e.g., congenital or degenerative valve disease or endocarditis) or secondary valve disease (e.g., cardiomyopathies or indwelling catheters, such as defibrillators/pacemakers).

Diagnosis

Valve disease is typically diagnosed when a heart murmur is detected during physical examination. Valve disease is also frequently diagnosed for the first time during echocardiography examination in patients referred for indications other than valve disease. Echocardiography is the diagnostic tool of choice for the evaluation and management of cancer cases and a cardio-oncology echocardiogram is recommended by the guidelines.[30] Grading severity of valve disease and determining timing of intervention should follow guidelines.[31,32]

Prognosis

Chronic regurgitant valve lesions are typically better tolerated than stenotic lesions, but both are associated with poor prognosis when severe and left untreated. The main indications for valve intervention are stages C and D of valve disease (Tables 16.1 to 16.5).[31]

Treatment

Valve repair or replacement is the mainstay treatment for severe valve diseases. Surgery is more urgent when valve disease is acute and severe, when symptoms are present, or when associated with reduced left ventricular ejection fraction.[31,33] Choice of valve repair versus replacement or surgery versus transcatheter therapies is based on, among other things, nature of valve lesion, acuity, surgical risk, life expectancy, and availability of percutaneous options. Special consideration is given to asymptomatic, severe valve disease with preserved left ventricular systolic function in patients needing cancer therapy. In these patients, valve repair or

TABLE 16.1 Stages of Aortic Valve Stenosis and Concomitant Parameters Independently Indicating Valve Repair or Replacement

	AORTIC STENOSIS				
	STAGE C		STAGE D		
	Stage C1	Stage C2	Stage D1	Stage D2[a]	Stage D3[b]
Symptoms	No	No	Yes	Yes	Yes
Aortic valve area	≤1 cm^2	≤1 cm^2	≤1 cm^2	≤1 cm^2	≤1 cm^2
Peak velocity	≥4 m/sec	≥4 m/sec	≥4 m/sec	<4 m/sec	<4 m/sec
Mean gradient	≥40 mm Hg	≥40 mm Hg	≥40 mm Hg	<40 mm H g	<40 mm Hg
LVEF	≥50%	<50%	≥50%	<50%	≥50%
SVi				<35 mL/m^2	<35 mL/m^2

[a]Stage D2: Dobutamine hemodynamic study or aortic valve computed tomography calcium score recommended.
[b]Stage D3: Aortic valve computed tomography calcium score recommended.
LVEF, Left ventricular ejection fraction; *SVi*, stroke volume index.

TABLE 16.2 **Stages of Aortic Valve Regurgitation and Concomitant Parameters Independently Indicating Valve Repair or Replacement**

	AORTIC REGURGITATION		
	Stage C1	Stage C2	Stage D
Symptoms	No	No	Yes
ERO	≥0.3 cm^2	≥0.3 cm^2	≥0.3 cm^2
Rvol	≥60 mL	≥60 mL	≥60 mL
Vena contracta	>0.6 cm	>0.6 cm	>0.6 cm
Angiographic	>3+	>3+	>3+
LVEF	50%	<50%	Any

ERO, Effective regurgitant orifice; *LVEF*, left ventricular ejection fraction; *Rvol*, regurgitant volume.

TABLE 16.3 **Stages of Mitral Valve Stenosis and Concomitant Parameters Independently Indicating Valve Repair or Replacement**

	MITRAL STENOSIS	
	Stage C	Stage D
Symptoms	No	Yes
Mitral valve area	≤1.5 cm^2	≤1.5 cm^2

TABLE 16.4 **Stages of Mitral Valve Regurgitation and Concomitant Parameters Independently Indicating Valve Repair or Replacement**

	MITRAL REGURGITATION		
	Stage C1	Stage C2	Stage D
Symptoms	No	No	Yes
ERO	≥0.4 cm^2	≥0.4 cm^2	≥0.4 cm^2
Rvol	≥60 mL	≥60 mL	≥60 mL
Vena contracta	≥0.7 cm	≥0.7 cm	≥0.7 cm
Angiographic	>3+	>3+	>3+
LVEF	≥60%	<60%	Any

ERO, Effective regurgitant orifice; *LVEF*, left ventricular ejection fraction; *Rvol*, regurgitant volume.

replacement should be undertaken if it will not result in unacceptable delay in cancer treatment while allowing for recuperation from valve intervention, typically 4 to 6 weeks following open heart surgery versus 2 to 4 weeks following percutaneous therapies (the latter often preferred for this reason). Guidelines recommend valve intervention if expected life expectancy is more than 12 months.[31] The prognosis of the malignancy therefore has to be taken into account as well as the impact any

TABLE 16.5 **Stages of Tricuspid Valve Regurgitation and Concomitant Parameters Independently Indicating Valve Repair or Replacement**

	TRICUSPID REGURGITATION	
	Stage C	Stage D
Symptoms	No	Yes
ERO	≥0.4 cm^2	≥0.4 cm^2
Rvol	≥45 mL	≥45 mL
Vena contracta	>0.7 cm	>0.7 cm
Angiographic	>3+	>3+

ERO, Effective regurgitant orifice.

holding of cancer therapy for the purpose of surgery might have versus its continuation on surgical complications and outcomes. Vice versa, the prognosis of the valve disease needs to be balanced against the risk of intervention in these patients.[34]

Risk of endocarditis is higher in patients diagnosed with cancer[23,35] and the decision to intervene before or during cancer treatment has to weigh risk of valve disease versus holding or continuing cancer treatment and prognosis related to cancer.[34] Endocarditis prophylaxis guidelines should be followed.[36,37] Careful attention should be paid to unique predisposing factors and the microbiology of infective endocarditis in patients with cancer.[34,38,39] At a minimum Infectious Disease, Cardiology, and Cardiovascular Surgery services should be consulted on all cases of endocarditis to help guide investigations, choice of antibiotic therapy, and indications and timing of valve surgery.

Aortic Valve Stenosis

Aortic Valve Stenosis Severity

Surgical or transcatheter aortic valve replacement is indicated when aortic valve stenosis is severe and symptomatic or associated with a left ventricular ejection fraction (LVEF) below 50%. Recent data suggest that the patients with severe aortic stenosis and a LVEF of 50% to 60% are at increased risk of mortality, and aortic valve replacement may be considered in that situation.[40] In the setting of low gradient aortic valve stenosis (mean gradient <40 mm Hg and peak velocity <4 m/sec in the setting of aortic valve area ≤1 cm^2), guidelines recommend additional hemodynamic assessment of severity of aortic stenosis via dobutamine echocardiography, dobutamine cardiac catheterization, or evaluation of anatomic severity of aortic stenosis with computed

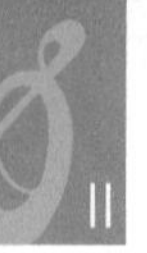

tomography calcium score to confirm severe aortic stenosis.

Mitral Valve Stenosis

Mitral Valve Stenosis Severity

Guidelines consider severe mitral valve stenosis to be present when the mitral valve area is 1.5 cm^2 or less and very severe when the mitral valve area is less than 1 cm^2. When mitral valve stenosis is related to rheumatic valve disease, mitral balloon valvuloplasty is the mainstay of treatment in suitable anatomy without significant calcification, especially of the commissures. However, radiation-induced valve disease is unlike rheumatic heart disease and mitral stenosis is typically related to calcification of the mitral annulus and mitral valve leaflets with sparing of the mitral valve tips and commissures. Mitral annulus calcification complicates mitral valve surgery and balloon valvuloplasty may not be suitable, limiting options for intervention. Alternative transcatheter mitral valve replacement procedures are possible for severe mitral annulus calcification, although these procedures carry additional risk[41–43] and careful preprocedural planning is important to address the risk of periprosthetic regurgitation, iatrogenic left ventricular outflow tract obstruction, or transcatheter heart valve embolization (see Chapter 28).

Mitral Valve Regurgitation

Mitral Valve Regurgitation Severity

Guidelines classify mitral valve regurgitation as primary or secondary. Surgical mitral valve repair is the procedure of choice for primary mitral valve regurgitation needing intervention; otherwise, an alternative is transcatheter mitral valve repair with MitraClip in patients who are at increased surgical risk. The most common cause of primary mitral valve regurgitation is mitral valve prolapse or flail leaflet. Secondary or functional mitral valve regurgitation is caused by left ventricular remodeling with apical displacement of the mitral valve apparatus and tethering of the leaflets. This may improve with optimal guideline-directed heart failure medical therapy and surgical mitral valve repair for does not offer any survival benefit in this setting. A recent trial, however, did show benefit for the MitraClip in patients with severe functional mitral valve regurgitation refractory to guideline-directed medical therapy, including cardiac resynchronization therapy where indicated.[44]

Mitral regurgitation may also be caused by mitral valve and annulus calcification from previous radiation (see Mitral Stenosis and Chapter 28).

Aortic Valve Regurgitation

Aortic Valve Regurgitation Severity

Surgical aortic valve replacement is the mainstay for treatment of severe valve regurgitation needing intervention. Aortic valve repair is feasible and a good alternative in patients with a repairable valve, such as leaflet prolapse or focal leaflet perforation.[45] The aortic valve can be spared in some cases during aortic surgery when aortic valve regurgitation is caused by aortic root dilatation. Currently, no approved percutaneous therapies exist for aortic valve regurgitation.

Tricuspid Valve Regurgitation

Tricuspid Valve Regurgitation Severity

Tricuspid valve regurgitation is usually well tolerated and the patient responds well to diuretic therapy. Tricuspid valve repair is indicated when there is refractory right-sided heart failure or moderate right ventricular enlargement or moderate decrease in right ventricular systolic function. Percutaneous therapies for tricuspid valve repair are in development, although severe tricuspid regurgitation in selected patients has been treated successfully with MitraClip.[46]

Prosthetic Valve Failure

In patient with bioprosthetic valve failure requiring replacement, surgical management has been the conventional approach. In patients at high risk, such as those with heart failure and New York Heart Association class III or IV or prior coronary artery bypass graft, transcatheter valve replacement can be preferred over the surgical approach.[47]

Paravalvular leak is another complication that is seen in either bioprosthetic or mechanical valves. Percutaneous paravalvular regurgitation leak closure has been shown to be successful in decreasing symptoms of heart failure or hemolysis and increase survival in patients.[48]

REFERENCES

1. Gornik HL, Gerhard-Herman M, Beckman JA. Abnormal cytology predicts poor prognosis in patients with cancer with pericardial effusion. *J Clin Oncol*. 2005;23(22):5211–5216.
2. Gaya AM, Ashford RF. Cardiac complications of radiation therapy. *Clin Oncol (R Coll Radiol)*. 2005;17(3):153–159.
3. Morton DL, Glancy DL, Joseph WL, Adkins PC. Management of patients with radiation-induced pericarditis with effusion: a note on the development of aortic regurgitation in two of them. *Chest*. 1973;64(3):291–297.
4. Filopei J, Frishman W. Radiation-induced heart disease. *Cardiol Rev*. 2012;20(4):184–188.
5. Heidenreich PA, Hancock SL, Lee BK, Mariscal CS, Schnittger I. Asymptomatic cardiac disease following mediastinal irradiation. *J Am Coll Cardiol*. 2003;42(4):743–749.
6. Jaworski C, Mariani JA, Wheeler G, Kaye DM. Cardiac complications of thoracic irradiation. *J Am Coll Cardiol*. 2013;61(23):2319–2328.
7. Spodick DH. Acute cardiac tamponade. *N Engl J Med*. 2003;349(7): 684–690.
8. Swami A, Spodick DH. Pulsus paradoxus in cardiac tamponade: a pathophysiologic continuum. *Clin Cardiol*. 2003;26(5):215–217.
9. Friedrich MG, Sechtem U, Schulz-Menger J, et al. Cardiovascular magnetic resonance in myocarditis: a JACC white paper. *J Am Coll Cardiol*. 2009;53(17):1475–1487.
10. Wassmuth R, Schulz-Menger J. Cardiovascular magnetic resonance imaging of myocardial inflammation. *Expert Rev Cardiovasc Ther*. 2011;9(9):1193–1201.
11. Ball S, Ghosh RK, Wongsaengsak S, et al. Cardiovascular toxicities of immune checkpoint inhibitors: JACC review topic of the week. *J Am Coll Cardiol*. 2019;74(13):1714–1727.
12. Arsenian MA. Cardiovascular sequelae of therapeutic thoracic radiation. *Prog Cardiovasc Dis*. 1991;33(5):299–311.
13. El Haddad D, Iliescu C, Yusuf SW, et al. Outcomes of patients with cancer undergoing percutaneous pericardiocentesis for pericardial effusion. *J Am Coll Cardiol*. 2015;66(10):1119–1128.
14. Verma V, Shah C, Mehta MP. Clinical outcomes and toxicity of proton radiotherapy for breast cancer. *Clin Breast Cancer*. 2016;16(3):145–154.
15. Chang HM, Okwuosa TM, Scarabelli T, Moudgil R, Yeh ETH. Cardiovascular complications of cancer therapy: best practices in diagnosis, prevention, and management: part 2. *J Am Coll Cardiol*. 2017;70(20):2552–2565.
16. Adler Y, Charron P. The 2015 ESC guidelines on the diagnosis and management of pericardial diseases. *Eur Heart J*. 2015;36(42):2873–2874.
17. Hancock SL, Donaldson SS, Hoppe RT. Cardiac disease following treatment of Hodgkin's disease in children and adolescents. *J Clin Oncol*. 1993;11(7):1208–1215.
18. Tsang TS, Freeman WK, Sinak LJ, Seward JB. Echocardiographically guided pericardiocentesis: evolution and state-of-the-art technique. *Mayo Clin Proc*. 1998;73(7):647–652.
19. Akyuz S, Zengin A, Arugaslan E, et al. Echo-guided pericardiocentesis in patients with clinically significant pericardial effusion. Outcomes over a 10-year period. *Herz*. 2015;40(suppl 2):153–159.
20. Fenstad ER, Le RJ, Sinak LJ, et al. Pericardial effusions in pulmonary arterial hypertension: characteristics, prognosis, and role of drainage. *Chest*. 2013;144(5):1530–1538.
21. Lekhakul A, Fenstad ER, Assawakawintip C, et al. Incidence and management of hemopericardium: impact of changing trends in invasive cardiology. *Mayo Clin Proc*. 2018;93(8):1086–1095.
22. Kim KH, Miranda WR, Sinak LJ, et al. Effusive-constrictive pericarditis after pericardiocentesis: incidence, associated findings, and natural history. *JACC Cardiovasc Imaging*. 2018;11(4):534–541.
23. García-Albéniz X, Hsu J, Lipsitch M, Logan RW, Hernández-Díaz S, Hernán MA. Infective endocarditis and cancer in the elderly. *Eur J Epidemiol*. 2016;31(1):41–49.
24. Stewart BF, Siscovick D, Lind BK, et al. Clinical factors associated with calcific aortic valve disease. Cardiovascular health study. *J Am Coll Cardiol*. 1997;29(3):630–634.
25. Pawade TA, Newby DE, Dweck MR. Calcification in aortic stenosis: the skeleton key. *J Am Coll Cardiol*. 2015;66(5):561–577.
26. Watkins DA, Johnson CO, Colquhoun SM, et al. Global, regional, and national burden of rheumatic heart disease, 1990–2015. *N Engl J Med*. 2017;377(8):713–722.
27. Carlson RG, Mayfield WR, Normann S, Alexander JA. Radiation-associated valvular disease. *Chest*. 1991;99(3):538–545.
28. Wethal T, Lund MB, Edvardsen T, et al. Valvular dysfunction and left ventricular changes in Hodgkin's lymphoma survivors. A longitudinal study. *Br J Cancer*. 2009;101(4):575–581.
29. Edoute Y, Haim N, Rinkevich D, Brenner B, Reisner SA. Cardiac valvular vegetations in patients with cancer: a prospective echocardiographic study of 200 patients. *Am J Med*. 1997;102(3):252–258.
30. Plana JC, Galderisi M, Barac A, et al. Expert consensus for multimodality imaging evaluation of adult patients during and after cancer therapy: a report from the American Society of Echocardiography and the European Association of Cardiovascular Imaging. *J Am Soc Echocardiogr*. 2014;27(9):911–939.
31. Nishimura RA, Otto CM, Bonow RO, et al. 2014 AHA/ACC guideline for the management of patients with valvular heart disease: a report of the American College of Cardiology/American Heart Association Task Force on practice guidelines. *J Am Coll Cardiol*. 2014;63(22):e57–e185.
32. Nishimura RA, Otto CM, Bonow RO, et al. 2017 AHA/ACC focused update of the 2014 AHA/ACC guideline for the management of patients with valvular heart disease: a report of the American College of Cardiology/American Heart Association Task Force on clinical practice guidelines. *J Am Coll Cardiol*. 2017;70(2):252–289.
33. Yancy CW, Jessup M, Bozkurt B, et al. 2017 ACC/AHA/HFSA focused update of the 2013 ACCF/AHA guideline for the management of heart failure: a report of the American College of Cardiology/American Heart Association Task Force on clinical practice guidelines and the Heart Failure Society of America. *J Am Coll Cardiol*. 2017;70(6): 776–803.
34. Kim K, Kim D, Lee SE, et al. Infective endocarditis in patients with cancer—causative organisms, predisposing procedures, and prognosis differ from infective endocarditis in on-patients with cancer. *Circ J*. 2019;83(2):452–460.
35. Cahill TJ, Prendergast BD. Infective endocarditis. *Lancet*. 2016; 387(10021):882–893.
36. Wilson W, Taubert KA, Gewitz M, et al. Prevention of infective endocarditis: guidelines from the American Heart Association: a guideline from the American Heart Association Rheumatic Fever, Endocarditis, and Kawasaki Disease Committee, Council on Cardiovascular Disease in the Young, and the Council on Clinical Cardiology, Council on Cardiovascular Surgery and Anesthesia, and the Quality of Care and Outcomes Research Interdisciplinary Working Group. *Circulation*. 2007;116(15):1736–1754.
37. Habib G, Hoen B, Tornos P, et al. Guidelines on the prevention, diagnosis, and treatment of infective endocarditis (new version 2009): the Task Force on the Prevention, Diagnosis, and Treatment of Infective Endocarditis of the European Society of Cardiology (ESC). Endorsed by the European Society of Clinical Microbiology and Infectious Diseases (ESCMID) and the International Society of Chemotherapy (ISC) for Infection and Cancer. *Eur Heart J*. 2009;30(19):2369–2413.
38. Janszky I, Gémes K, Ahnve S, Asgeirsson H, Möller J. Invasive procedures associated with the development of infective endocarditis. *J Am Coll Cardiol*. 2018;71(24):2744–2752.
39. Wisplinghoff H, Bischoff T, Tallent SM, Seifert H, Wenzel RP, Edmond MB. Nosocomial bloodstream infections in US hospitals: analysis of 24,179 cases from a prospective nationwide surveillance study. *Clin Infect Dis*. 2004;39(3):309–317.
40. Ito S, Miranda WR, Nkomo VT, et al. Reduced left ventricular ejection fraction in patients with aortic stenosis. *J Am Coll Cardiol*. 2018;71(12):1313–1321.
41. Guerrero M, Urena M, Himbert D, et al. 1-Year outcomes of transcatheter mitral valve replacement in patients with severe mitral annular calcification. *J Am Coll Cardiol*. 2018;71(17): 1841–1853.
42. Russell HM, Guerrero ME, Salinger MH, et al. Open atrial transcatheter mitral valve replacement in patients with mitral annular calcification. *J Am Coll Cardiol*. 2018;72(13):1437–1448.
43. Guerrero M, Eleid M, Foley T, Said S, Rihal C. Transseptal transcatheter mitral valve replacement in severe mitral annular calcification (transseptal valve-in-MAC). *Ann Cardiothorac Surg*. 2018;7(6): 830–833.

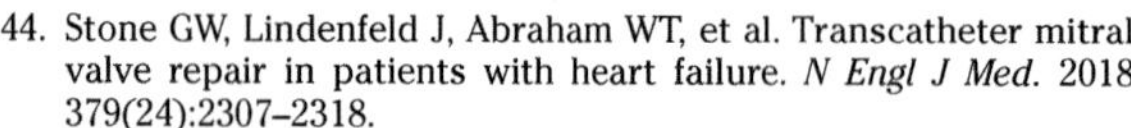

44. Stone GW, Lindenfeld J, Abraham WT, et al. Transcatheter mitral-valve repair in patients with heart failure. *N Engl J Med.* 2018; 379(24):2307–2318.
45. Minakata K, Schaff HV, Zehr KJ, et al. Is repair of aortic valve regurgitation a safe alternative to valve replacement? *J Thorac Cardiovasc Surg.* 2004;127(3):645–653.
46. Sorajja P, Cavalcante JL, Gossl M, Bae R. Transcatheter repair of tricuspid regurgitation with MitraClip. *Prog Cardiovasc Dis.* 2019; 62(6):488–492.
47. Stulak JM, Tchantchaleishvili V, Daly RC, et al. Conventional redo biological valve replacement over 20 years: surgical benchmarks should guide patient selection for transcatheter valve-in-valve therapy. *J Thorac Cardiovasc Surg.* 2018;156(4): 1380–1390.e1.
48. El Sabbagh A, Eleid MF, Matsumoto JM, et al. Three-dimensional prototyping for procedural simulation of transcatheter mitral valve replacement in patients with mitral annular calcification. *Catheter Cardiovasc Interv.* 2018;92(7):E537–E549.

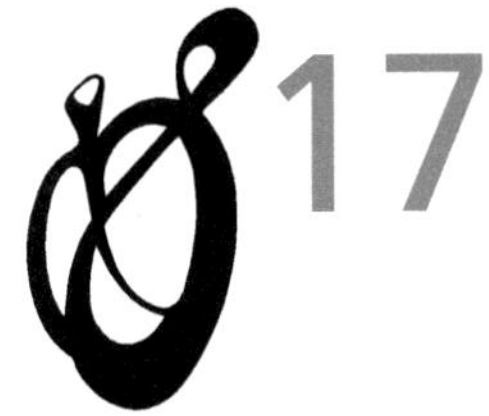

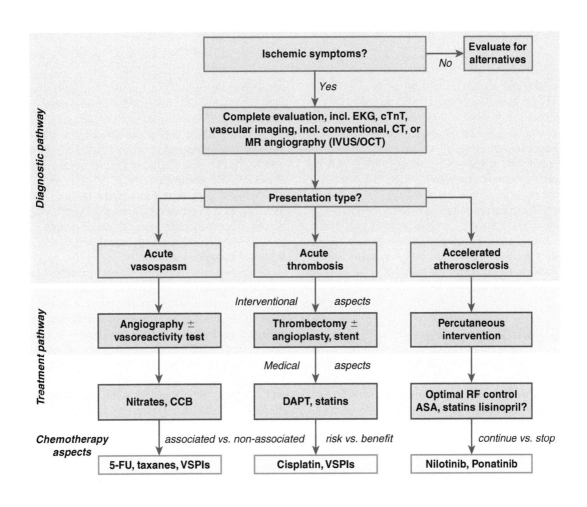

17 Vascular Disease During Cancer Therapy

JOERG HERRMANN

Diagnostic pathway

Ischemic symptoms?

No → Evaluate for alternatives

Yes ↓

Complete evaluation, incl. EKG, cTnT, vascular imaging, incl. conventional, CT, or MR angiography (IVUS/OCT)

Presentation type?

Acute vasospasm | Acute thrombosis | Accelerated atherosclerosis

Treatment pathway

Interventional aspects

Angiography ± vasoreactivity test | Thrombectomy ± angioplasty, stent | Percutaneous intervention

Medical aspects

Nitrates, CCB | DAPT, statins | Optimal RF control ASA, statins lisinopril?

Chemotherapy aspects

associated vs. non-associated → 5-FU, taxanes, VSPIs

risk vs. benefit → Cisplatin, VSPIs

continue vs. stop → Nilotinib, Ponatinib

CHAPTER OUTLINE

PRESENTATIONS
DIAGNOSIS
TREATMENT
IMPLICATIONS FOR CANCER THERAPY AND SECONDARY PREVENTION

KEY POINTS

- Patients who have cancer are at risk of developing vascular complications during cancer therapy owing to preexisting cardiovascular disease and/or risk factors and the toxicity potential of cancer therapeutics
- Three principal presentations of arterial vascular complications/toxicity can be distinguished: acute vasospasm, acute thrombosis, and accelerated atherosclerosis
- The diagnostic evaluation needs to keep both a broad differential and to define the most likely presentation category as the basis for further treatment
- Treatment is composed of invasive and medical therapy based on presentation
- Finally, presentation and treatment evaluations allow for a critical review of the potentially contributing role of cancer therapeutics and risk/benefit discussions of the continuation of these drugs with close clinical follow up

Various vascular toxicities can be seen in patients with cancer including typical and atypical chest pain episodes, myocardial infarction, transient ischemic attack, stroke, claudication, critical limb ischemia, Raynaud, in addition to the classic venous thromboembolic disease spectrum, which will be discussed elsewhere (see Chapter 18). This chapter will focus on arterial toxicities during active cancer treatment (pre- and postcare are discussed in Chapters 8 and 29). Although the spectrum of manifestations is broad as is the number of cancer therapies potentially associated with it, key scenarios with a few key therapies account for most of what is seen in clinical practice and will be covered herein.

PRESENTATIONS

Three principal presentations of arterial vascular toxicities can be differentiated: acute vasospasm, acute thrombosis, and accelerated atherosclerosis (Fig. 17.1). A summary of the pertinent aspects is provided in Chapter 8, Table 8.3.

Acute vasospasm is one of the most classic presentations, as it emerged with one of the drugs first associated with vascular toxicities: 5-FU.[1–3] Several reports have outlined chest pain episodes with ST segment elevation that resolve with vasodilator therapy. Alteration of coronary vasoreactivity, predisposing to coronary vasospasm has been shown in invasive provocation studies and relates mechanistically to changes in protein kinase C signaling and calcium handling in vascular smooth muscle cells (hypercontractility).[4] Sympathetic innervation (catecholamines), molecular vasoconstrictors, and endothelial dysfunction play a contributing role.[5] Severe complications that can evolve as a consequence of profound and prolonged coronary vasospasm include myocardial infarction, arrhythmias such as ventricular tachycardia and ventricular fibrillation to the point of sudden cardiac death, and cardiac dysfunction, even Takotsubo cardiomyopathy, with presentations of heart failure and even shock ("5-FU cardiotoxicity").[6–9] Other drugs that can induce coronary vasospasm include the oral prodrug of 5-FU capecitabine, paclitaxel, cisplatin, bleomycin, vascular endothelial growth factor (VEGF) inhibitors, such as sorafenib, and Bcr-Abl inhibitors, such as dasatinib.

Acute thrombosis is the second principal presentation of vascular toxicity in those with cancer. Almost intuitively these patients have been considered to be at a higher thrombotic risk relating to a procoagulant state. Indeed, evidence is emerging that supports a higher risk not only of venous but also of arterial thromboembolic events.[10] The risk is seemingly highest just around the time of diagnosis and abates over two years, most profoundly within the first 12 months.[11] The risk is highest with advanced (stage III and IV) cancers and those of the gastrointestinal tract and the lung, similar to venous thromboembolism.[11] Intriguingly, for instance, gastric adenocarcinomas (especially undifferentiated and advanced stages) have been shown to express von Willebrand factor (vWF), thereby adding to platelet activation.[12] Cancer cells can also express a number of other platelet agonists, such as adenosine diphosphate and thromboxane A2, and platelets can contribute to cancer growth and spread ("platelet-cancer loops").[10] One of the classic examples of a chemotherapeutic associated with thrombosis is cisplatin. vWF and circulating endothelial cells increase in patients undergoing cisplatin-based therapy, reflecting endothelial injury and apoptosis.[13,14]

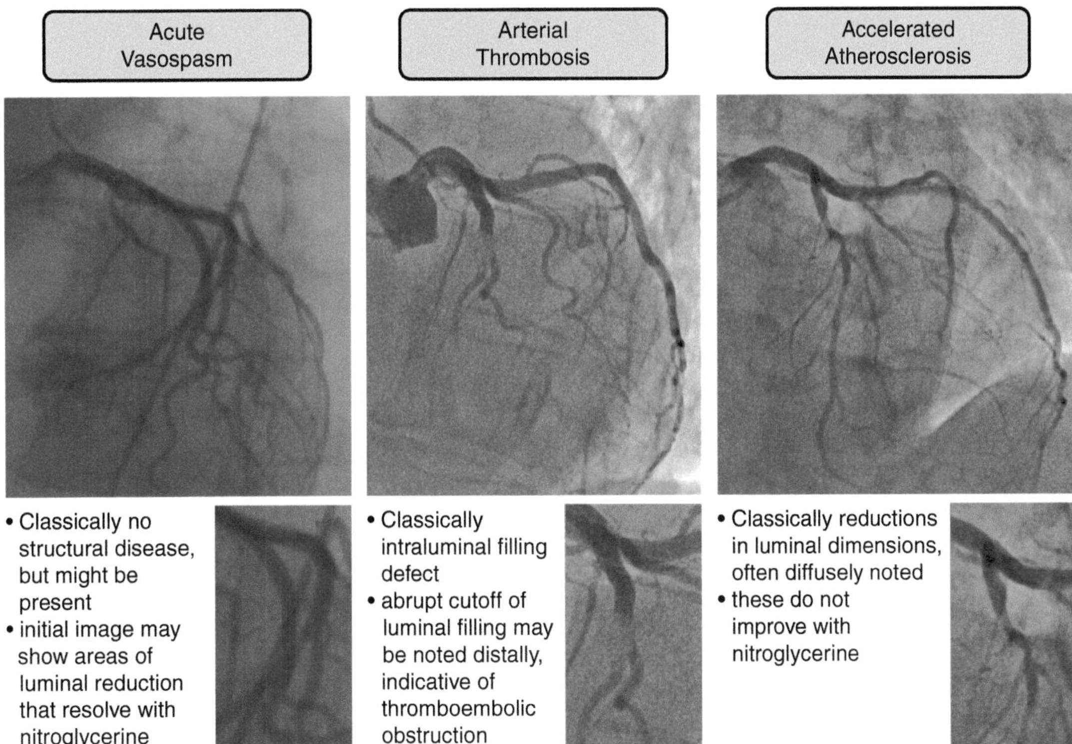

Acute Vasospasm
Arterial Thrombosis
Accelerated Atherosclerosis
• Classically no structural disease, but might be present
• initial image may show areas of luminal reduction that resolve with nitroglycerine
• Classically intraluminal filling defect
• abrupt cutoff of luminal filling may be noted distally, indicative of thromboembolic obstruction
• Classically reductions in luminal dimensions, often diffusely noted
• these do not improve with nitroglycerine

FIG. 17.1 Coronary angiograms displaying the characteristically different presentations of patients with acute vasospasm, acute thrombosis, and accelerated atherosclerosis.

A number of agents, such as cisplatin, also suppress local (in-growth of surrounding endothelial cells) and remote (endothelial progenitor cells) regenerative capacity.[15] This generates the unfortunate constellation of induction of endothelial injury and reduction of endothelial repair capacity. The fact that no underlying plaques and thus no potential for plaque rupture was noted in patients developing acute coronary thrombosis on cisplatin supports the view that erosions account for *in situ* thrombosis.[16] These patients are also at risk for systemic thrombotic complications as thrombus burden can be high. Other drugs associated with acute thrombosis include mainly VEGF inhibitors.

Accelerated atherosclerosis in patients with cancer used to be thought of only in the context of radiation therapy. Radiation is a potent injurious stimulus that can induce and enhance the atherosclerotic disease process as outlined in Chapter 26. A central element is injury to the endothelium (though radiation also injures the vascular smooth muscle layer of media and induces inflammation in the media).[17–19] Drug therapies that have recently emerged to be potentially contributing to vascular disease include immune checkpoint inhibitors. These have been shown, at least experimentally, to reactivate giant cell arteritis, which is an adventitial inflammation that affects the entire arterial wall and can even lead to complete luminal obstruction.[20] The most aggressive forms of arterial disease with any cancer therapeutics have been reported with nilotinib and ponatinib as progressive arterial occlusive disease with acute ischemic events of the peripheral lower extremity, the visceral, the cerebral, and the coronary circulation.[21–32] Standard atherosclerotic cardiovascular disease risk prediction models support the view that these two drugs, indeed, accelerate atherosclerosis rather than leading to alternative forms of accelerated arterial disease such as vasculitis.[32,33] Endothelial injury is thought to be a key element underlying the pathophysiology of progressive arterial occlusive disease.[33,34] Both drugs inhibit the VEGF signaling pathway, as well as the Abl signaling pathway in endothelial cells, and it may be this combination that yields the detrimental momentum. Pan-VEGF receptor inhibition does lead to accelerated (but not necessarily unstable/vulnerable) atherosclerosis in a rodent model, but there have not been many clinical reports of events.[35] Finally, patients undergoing cisplatin-based therapy may not only be vulnerable to acute thrombotic events and abnormal vascular reactivity but also to more accelerated atherosclerosis, especially if they underwent concomitant radiation therapy as seen in those with testicular patients.[36-40]

DIAGNOSIS

Based on careful history taking and signs and symptoms an initial differential diagnosis is to be made. Awareness and background knowledge of the side effect potential of cancer therapeutics is key to define the clinical presentation as precisely as possible, which will then guide further testing and management.

For *vasospasm*, it is the typical constellation of ischemic manifestations that characterize Raynaud's for the periphery and the constellation of typical angina or angina-like chest pain (atypical features being night-time presentations, provocation by mental stress and cold exposure), and concomitant ST segment elevation on electrocardiogram (ECG), all resolving promptly with vasodilator therapy. Angiography typically does not show structural disease (stenosis), but it might, in which case even smaller degrees of vasoconstriction can provoke hemodynamically relevant lumen reductions and ischemia. In case of 5-FU, the presentation can be so typical that treatment with vasodilator therapy is all that is needed. Cardiac biomarkers, ECG, and echocardiogram, however, should be obtained to assess for myocardial injury/infarction, arrhythmias, and cardiac dysfunction in this setting. Furthermore, especially in patients with risk factors for atherosclerosis and especially those with a family history of premature coronary artery disease (CAD), should undergo testing for CAD. Coronary computed tomography angiography (CCTA) might be valuable to screen for underlying structural disease, which can be underestimated by functional stress tests. The knowledge of the presence and extent of CAD is important for long-term prognosis and to guide adequate additional measures, such as statins, optimal blood pressure, and glucose control.

For *acute thrombosis*, the first step to diagnosis is the recognition of signs and symptoms of acute ischemia that vary based on the vascular territory. It can range from unstable angina to myocardial infarction with and without arrhythmias (polymorphic VT or heart block) in the coronary circulation, from transient ischemic attack to stroke in the carotid/cerebral circulation, and bowl ischemia, acute renal failure, and critical limb ischemia in the peripheral circulation. The precise diagnosis is made by vascular imaging, in most cases angiography. An intraluminal filling defect is the classic angiographic sign. This may not be present in case of spontaneous resolution or embolization of the thrombus. A careful assessment of the distal vasculature is very important in this setting and in general. Truncation of side branches and the distal segments is diagnostic as is slow flow, which is indicative of microcirculatory impairment.

For *accelerated atherosclerosis* signs and symptoms of ischemia in the various vascular territories as outlined above are seen, but are not as acute unless there is superimposed vasospasm or thrombus. The former is more common and both can be present once platelet activation ensues. Typically accelerated atherosclerosis presents with and should be suspected in cases of symptoms of end-organ ischemia that is becoming more noticeable, including stable chronic angina, transient neurologic deficits, postprandial ischemia, and claudication.

Overall, the diagnostic pathway is similar to that in patients without cancer and in keeping with societal guidelines.

TREATMENT

Treatment is directed to the underlying pathophysiology and thus, as outlined above, a precise definition of the disease process is key.

For patients experiencing *acute vasospasm* on 5-FU, paclitaxel, cisplatin, VEGF inhibitors, or other cancer therapeutics, vasodilators, such as nitrates and calcium channel blockers (CCBs), are mainstay therapy. CCBs are more effective in cases of microcirculatory involvement (microvascular angina). They are also usually first-line therapy for patients with Raynaud's. Importantly, beta-blockers should be used with caution in these patients. If any need to be used, carvedilol as a combined alpha-/beta-blocker is the preferred choice. The other aspect is to define any additional provoking and contributing factors. For instance, one may advise on avoidance of cold exposure, mental stress management, and absolute cessation of nicotine exposure (first- and second-hand). Patients with structural vascular disease will need optimal treatment of atherosclerosis as well.

For the treatment of *acute thrombosis* the following general interventions are to be entertained: anticoagulation, fibrinolysis, antiplatelet therapy, revascularization, and treatment of the underlying cause. This includes treatment of the underlying malignancy and the prothrombotic state it generates. If plaque rupture was noted on angiography plus or minus advanced intravascular imaging (intravascular ultrasound [IVUS] and optical coherence tomography [OCT]), revascularization strategies are pursued, mainly stenting. Manual thrombectomy is no longer universally recommended in view of higher stroke rates and no decisive coronary/myocardial ischemic benefit. However, it can be performed in individual cases. Surgery is to be considered if the location and extent of disease are unfavorable for a percutaneous approach. Erosions are not revascularized in the absence of significant plaque burden compromising luminal dimensions. However, dual antiplatelet therapy (DAPT) should be recommended. Based on current American College of Cardiology and American Heart Association guideline, DAPT should be continued for one year in patients with acute coronary syndrome, thereafter guided by risk calculators. These, however, do not take malignancy into consideration. Similar to venous thromboembolic event recommendations, one might argue for the continuation of DAPT as long as active cancer is present. However, there are no clinical trial data for such recommendation even though a recent study has outlined an increased (stent) thrombosis risk in patients with cancer after percutaneous coronary intervention (PCI), especially in those patients with cancer with a high DAPT score.[41] The higher bleeding risk of patients with cancer needs to be taken into consideration. In this context thrombocytopenia is an important factor to consider and the Society for Cardiovascular Angiography and Interventions (SCAI) recommendations for platelet cutoffs are as following: for surgical interventions platelet counts greater than 50 k, for PCI with DAPT platelet counts greater than 30 k, and for angiography platelet counts greater than 10 k.[42]

Patients with cancer who experience *accelerated atherosclerosis* should be treated in keeping with societal guidelines. Optimal guideline-directed medical therapy is the very foundation. It is directed at optimal cardiovascular risk factor control, stabilization of atherosclerotic plaques, and the reduction of further growth of stenoses. Defining the dynamic of disease progression by serial evaluation is especially important with nilotinib and ponatinib. Percutaneous or surgical intervention, in general, mainly serves the purpose of symptom control and quality-of-life improvement. However, in the setting of a large burden of myocardial ischemia, revascularization can be of prognostic benefit as well. Further, progressive luminal obstruction, unhalted by other efforts, is likely to require intervention to maintain patency and perfusion. Again, this is illustrated in the accelerated nature of peripheral arterial disease in patients on nilotinib and ponatinib, which can lead to limb ischemia and limb loss. Accordingly, a more proactive approach may be needed to help avoid severe complications in these patients and, very importantly, to enable continuation of cancer therapy.

IMPLICATIONS FOR CANCER THERAPY AND SECONDARY PREVENTION

Ideally patients at high risk for any of the outlined potential arterial vascular toxicities would be identified before initiation of therapy and subjected to effective primary preventive therapies (see Chapter 8). Once signs and symptoms have evolved, the focus shifts to secondary prevention efforts and the assessment of the risk of resuming or continuing any cancer therapy in relation to the cardiovascular presentations. For all manifestations, the key questions are (1) is the current cardiovascular presentation associated or not associated with the current cancer therapy, (2) what is the associated risk of the current cancer therapy versus its benefit, (3) is the risk-to-benefit ratio in favor of continuing or stopping the current cancer therapy?

For patients who developed cardiovascular toxicities with 5-FU, reexposure is of 5-FU is of particular concern and it was previously not recommended in case of myocardial infarction or cardiac dysfunction in the setting of 5-FU therapy. However, the sensitivity for myocardial infarction has increased with the implementation of highly sensitive cardiac troponin assays. Furthermore, there has been experience now with careful reexposure of 5-FU using a bolus regimen and coverage with vasodilator therapy just before, throughout, and for a short time after the treatment course. Such strategy, however, is not always successful, arguing for other pathomechanisms to be involved, at least for 5-FU cardiotoxicity. Patients being reexposed to 5-FU after experiencing cardiotoxicity should have ECG monitoring to detect ischemic changes and arrhythmias. These patients should also have a repeat ECG after reexposure even if the patient is completely asymptomatic.

For other patients who develop clinically significant *vasospasm* with drugs other than 5-FU, the question is how severe the vasospasm and how amendable to vasodilator therapy. Thus, the episode on therapy defines the ability to continue therapy with vasodilator coverage with long-acting nitrates and CCBs. Monitoring should be in line with the initial presentation, usually chest pain symptoms or Raynaud's. The value of vascular reactivity studies is not defined and providers need to evaluate how baseline and on therapy vascular reactivity compare. Importantly, one would like to know how these dynamics were in those patients who did and those patients who did not develop symptomatic vasospasm. ECG-Holter monitoring to track ST segment changes is another testing modality.

The risk of *acute thrombosis* is difficult to define in the individual patient. However, certain at-risk populations, such as patients with testicular cancer undergoing cisplatin-based therapy display a "high-risk fingerprint," defined as three or more of the following: body mass index above 25 kg/m^2, current smoking, blood pressure greater than 140/90 mm Hg (or treated), hypcrlipidemia (or treated), elevated fasting plasma glucose (FPG).[40,42] These patients have a higher intima-media thickness and higher baselined vWF levels.[40,42] On therapy, these but not non-high-risk fingerprint patients show a significant rise in circulating levels of vWF.[40,42] Whether any of these parameters apply to patients on cisplatin therapy for other malignancies is unknown. Gastrointestinal malignancies and advanced (stage III and IV) and undifferentiated cancers also pose a higher risk group. Currently no randomized controlled trial or other collateral evidence supports a recommendation for preemptive DAPT. However, this would be the intuitive implication. A main concern is the bleeding risk and a careful consideration of risk and benefit is required.

For patients who develop *accelerated atherosclerosis* while on cancer therapy associated with such toxicity, it often becomes a very difficult risk-benefit discussion. A key question is if anything is modifiable. In some cases patients might have continued to smoke and other cardiovascular risk factor might not be as tightly controlled either. Modification of dose or type of therapy is another important question. For instance, patients on nilotinib might be able to transition to another Bcr-Abl inhibitor such as bosutinib. If this is not possible, the dose of nilotinib possibly could be reduced. All these considerations need to take place in discussions with the hematologist. Revascularization approaches address emerging needs, but the risk remains of restenosis and progression of disease in other vascular areas. Overall, general societal treatment recommendations apply for patients with cancer presenting with vascular toxicities, but with some considerations (https://www.nature.com/articles/s41569-020-0347-2#Sec24).[43]

REFERENCES

1. Kleiman NS, Lehane DE, Geyer CE Jr, Pratt CM, Young JB. Prinzmetal's angina during 5-fluorouracil chemotherapy. *Am J Med.* 1987;82(3):566–568.
2. Collins C, Weiden PL. Cardiotoxicity of 5-fluorouracil. *Cancer Treat Rep.* 1987;71(7–8):733–736.
3. Schnetzler B, Popova N, Lamb CC, Sappino AP. Coronary spasm induced by capecitabine. *Ann Oncol.* 2001;12(5):723–724.
4. Mosseri M, Fingert HJ, Varticovski L, Chokshi S, Isner JM. In vitro evidence that myocardial ischemia resulting from 5-fluorouracil chemotherapy is due to protein kinase C-mediated vasoconstriction of vascular smooth muscle. *Cancer Res.* 1993;53(13):3028–3033.
5. Lanza GA, Careri G, Crea F. Mechanisms of coronary artery spasm. *Circulation.* 2011;124(16):1774–1782.
6. Sara JD, Kaur J, Khodadadi R, et al. 5-Fluorouracil and cardiotoxicity: a review. *Ther Adv Med Oncol.* 2018,10:1758835918780140.
7. Cerny J, Hassan A, Smith C, Piperdi B. Coronary vasospasm with myocardial stunning in a patient with colon cancer receiving adjuvant chemotherapy with FOLFOX regimen. *Clin Colorectal Cancer.* 2009;8(1):55–58.
8. Kobayashi N, Hata N, Yokoyama S, Shinada T, Shirakabe A, Mizuno K. A case of Takotsubo cardiomyopathy during 5-fluorouracil treatment for rectal adenocarcinoma. *J Nippon Med Sch.* 2009;76(1):27–33.
9. Y-Hassan S, Tornvall P, Törnerud M, Henareh L. Capecitabine caused cardiogenic shock through induction of global Takotsubo syndrome. *Cardiovasc Revasc Med.* 2013;14(1):57–61.
10. Oren O, Herrmann J. Arterial events in patients with cancer—the case of acute coronary thrombosis. *J Thorac Dis.* 2018;10(suppl 35):S4367–S4385.
11. Navi BB, Reiner AS, Kamel H, et al. Risk of arterial thromboembolism in patients with cancer. *J Am Coll Cardiol.* 2017;70(8):926–938.
12. Yang AJ, Wang M, Wang Y, et al. Cancer cell-derived von Willebrand factor enhanced metastasis of gastric adenocarcinoma. *Oncogenesis.* 2018;7(1):12.
13. Dieckmann KP, Struss WJ, Budde U. Evidence for acute vascular toxicity of cisplatin-based chemotherapy in patients with germ cell tumour. *Anticancer Res.* 2011;31(12):4501–4505.

14. Lubberts S, Boer H, Altena R, et al. Vascular fingerprint and vascular damage markers associated with vascular events in testicular patients with cancer during and after chemotherapy. *Eur J Cancer.* 2016;63:180–188.
15. Soultati A, Mountzios G, Avgerinou C, et al. Endothelial vascular toxicity from chemotherapeutic agents: preclinical evidence and clinical implications. *Cancer Treat Rev.* 2012;38(5):473–483.
16. Ito D, Shiraishi J, Nakamura T, et al. Primary percutaneous coronary intervention and intravascular ultrasound imaging for coronary thrombosis after cisplatin-based chemotherapy. *Heart Vessels.* 2012; 27(6):634–638.
17. Brosius FC III, Waller BF, Roberts WC. Radiation heart disease. Analysis of 16 young (aged 15 to 33 years) necropsy patients who received over 3,500 rads to the heart. *Am J Med.* 1981;70(3):519–530.
18. Veinot JP, Edwards WD. Pathology of radiation-induced heart disease: a surgical and autopsy study of 27 cases. *Hum Pathol.* 1996; 27(8):766–773.
19. Virmani R, Farb A, Carter AJ, Jones RM. Pathology of radiation-induced coronary artery disease in human and pig. *Cardiovasc Radiat Med.* 1999;1(1):98–101.
20. Weyand CM, Berry GJ, Goronzy JJ. The immunoinhibitory PD-1/PD-L1 pathway in inflammatory blood vessel disease. *J Leukoc Biol.* 2018;103(3):565–575.
21. Aichberger KJ, Herndlhofer S, Schernthaner GH, et al. Progressive peripheral arterial occlusive disease and other vascular events during nilotinib therapy in CML. *Am J Hematol.* 2011;86(7): 533–539.
22. Le Coutre P, Rea D, Abruzzese E, et al. Severe peripheral arterial disease during nilotinib therapy. *J Natl Cancer Inst.* 2011;103(17): 1347–1348.
23. Tefferi A, Letendre L. Nilotinib treatment-associated peripheral artery disease and sudden death: yet another reason to stick to imatinib as front-line therapy for chronic myelogenous leukemia. *Am J Hematol.* 2011;86(7):610–611.
24. Breccia M, Efficace F, Alimena G. Progressive arterial occlusive disease (PAOD) and pulmonary arterial hypertension (PAH) as new adverse events of second generation TKIs in CML treatment: who's afraid of the big bad wolf? *Leuk Res.* 2012;36(7):813–814.
25. Giles FJ, Mauro MJ, Hong F, et al. Rates of peripheral arterial occlusive disease in patients with chronic myeloid leukemia in the chronic phase treated with imatinib, nilotinib, or non-tyrosine kinase therapy: a retrospective cohort analysis. *Leukemia.* 2013; 27(6):1310–1315.
26. Kim TD, Rea D, Schwarz M, et al. Peripheral artery occlusive disease in chronic phase chronic myeloid leukemia patients treated with nilotinib or imatinib. *Leukemia.* 2013;27(6):1316–1321.
27. Levato L, Cantaffa R, Kropp MG, Magro D, Piro E, Molica S. Progressive peripheral arterial occlusive disease and other vascular events during nilotinib therapy in chronic myeloid leukemia: a single institution study. *Eur J Haematol.* 2013;90(6):531–532.
28. Tefferi A. Nilotinib treatment-associated accelerated atherosclerosis: when is the risk justified? *Leukemia.* 2013;27(9):1939–1940.
29. Maurizot A, Beressi JP, Manéglier B, et al. Rapid clinical improvement of peripheral artery occlusive disease symptoms after nilotinib discontinuation despite persisting vascular occlusion. *Blood Cancer J.* 2014;4:e247.
30. Breccia M, Molica M, Zacheo I, Serrao A, Alimena G. Application of systematic coronary risk evaluation chart to identify chronic myeloid leukemia patients at risk of cardiovascular diseases during nilotinib treatment. *Ann Hematol.* 2015;94(3):393–397.
31. Mirault T, Rea D, Azarine A, Messas E. Rapid onset of peripheral artery disease in a chronic myeloid leukemia patient without prior arterial disorder: direct relationship with nilotinib exposure and clinical outcome. *Eur J Haematol.* 2015;94(4):363–367.
32. Valent P, Hadzijusufovic E, Schernthaner GH, Wolf D, Rea D, le Coutre P. Vascular safety issues in CML patients treated with BCR/ABL1 kinase inhibitors. *Blood.* 2015;125(6):901–906.
33. Hadzijusufovic E, Albrecht-Schgoer K, Huber K, et al. Nilotinib-induced vasculopathy: identification of vascular endothelial cells as a primary target site. *Leukemia.* 2017;31(11):2388–2397.
34. Gover-Proaktor A, Granot G, Shapira S, et al. Ponatinib reduces viability, migration, and functionality of human endothelial cells. *Leuk Lymphoma.* 2017;58(6):1455–1467.
35. Winnik S, Lohmann C, Siciliani G, et al. Systemic VEGF inhibition accelerates experimental atherosclerosis and disrupts endothelial homeostasis—implications for cardiovascular safety. *Int J Cardiol.* 2013;168(3):2453–2461.
36. Meinardi MT, Gietema JA, van der Graaf WT, et al. Cardiovascular morbidity in long-term survivors of metastatic testicular cancer. *J Clin Oncol.* 2000;18(8):1725–1732.
37. van den Belt-Dusebout AW, Nuver J, de Wit R, et al. Long-term risk of cardiovascular disease in 5-year survivors of testicular cancer. *J Clin Oncol.* 2006;24(3):467–475.
38. van den Belt-Dusebout, AW, de Wit R, Gietema JA, et al. Treatment-specific risks of second malignancies and cardiovascular disease in 5-year survivors of testicular cancer. *J Clin Oncol.* 2007;25(28): 4370–4378.
39. Haugnes HS, Wethal T, Aass N, et al. Cardiovascular risk factors and morbidity in long-term survivors of testicular cancer: a 20-year follow-up study. *J Clin Oncol.* 2010;28(30):4649–4657.
40. Huddart RA, Norman A, Shahidi M, et al. Cardiovascular disease as a long-term complication of treatment for testicular cancer. *J Clin Oncol.* 2003;21(8):1513–1523.
41. Guo W, Fan X, Lewis BR, et al. Patients with cancer have a higher risk of thrombotic and ischemic events after percutaneous coronary intervention. *JACC Cardiovasc Interv.* 2021;14(10):1094–1105.
42. Iliescu CA, Grines CL, Herrmann J, et al. SCAI expert consensus statement: evaluation, management, and special considerations of cardio-oncology patients in the cardiac catheterization laboratory (endorsed by the Cardiological Society of India, and Sociedad Latino Americana de Cardiologia intervencionista). *Catheter Cardiovasc Interv.* 2016;87(5):E202–E223.
43. Herrmann J. Vascular toxic effects of cancer therapies. *Nat Rev Cardiol.* 2020;17(8):503–522. doi:10.1038/s41569-020-0347-2.

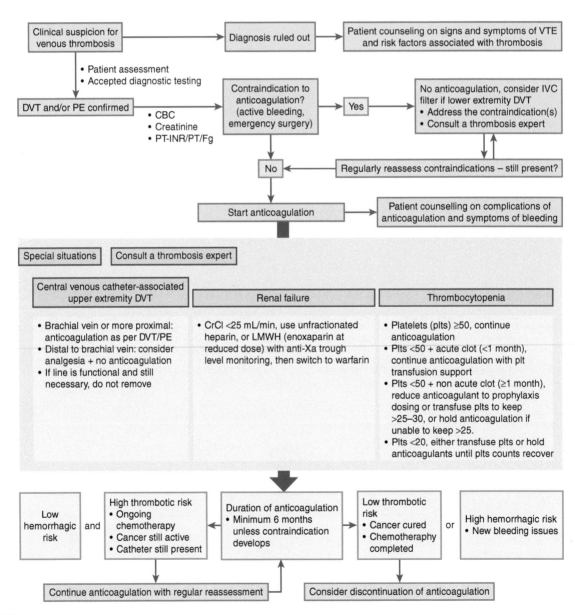

18 Thromboembolic Disease Treatment During Cancer Therapy

ROBERT D. MCBANE II

- Clinical suspicion for venous thrombosis → Diagnosis ruled out → Patient counseling on signs and symptoms of VTE and risk factors associated with thrombosis
- Clinical suspicion for venous thrombosis → (• Patient assessment • Accepted diagnostic testing) → DVT and/or PE confirmed
- DVT and/or PE confirmed → (• CBC • Creatinine • PT-INR/PT/Fg) → Contraindication to anticoagulation? (active bleeding, emergency surgery)
- Yes → No anticoagulation, consider IVC filter if lower extremity DVT
  - Address the contraindication(s)
  - Consult a thrombosis expert
- ↔ Regularly reassess contraindications – still present? → No
- No → Start anticoagulation → Patient counselling on complications of anticoagulation and symptoms of bleeding

Special situations | Consult a thrombosis expert

Central venous catheter-associated upper extremity DVT	Renal failure	Thrombocytopenia
• Brachial vein or more proximal: anticoagulation as per DVT/PE • Distal to brachial vein: consider analgesia + no anticoagulation • If line is functional and still necessary, do not remove	• CrCl <25 mL/min, use unfractionated heparin, or LMWH (enoxaparin at reduced dose) with anti-Xa trough level monitoring, then switch to warfarin	• Platelets (plts) ≥50, continue anticoagulation • Plts <50 + acute clot (<1 month), continue anticoagulation with plt transfusion support • Plts <50 + non acute clot (≥1 month), reduce anticoagulant to prophylaxis dosing or transfuse plts to keep >25–30, or hold anticoagulation if unable to keep >25. • Plts <20, either transfuse plts or hold anticoagulants until plts counts recover

Duration of anticoagulation
- Minimum 6 months unless contraindication develops

Low hemorrhagic risk and High thrombotic risk
- Ongoing chemotherapy
- Cancer still active
- Catheter still present

→ Continue anticoagulation with regular reassessment → (back to Duration of anticoagulation)

Low thrombotic risk
- Cancer cured
- Chemotheraphy completed

or High hemorrhagic risk
- New bleeding issues

→ Consider discontinuation of anticoagulation

CHAPTER OUTLINE

KEY POINTS

- Active cancer increases the risk of venous thromboembolism (VTE) by four-fold without chemotherapy and seven-fold with chemotherapy
- The likelihood of developing VTE is highest during the first 3 months after the cancer diagnosis and the majority of thrombotic events occur within the first year
- Management of cancer-associated VTE is challenging because these patients are at risk of both thrombotic and bleeding events
- Risk of anticoagulation failure (i.e., VTE recurrence despite anticoagulation) is highest with warfarin at 2.5% per month or 16% at 6 months
- Low-molecular-weight heparin (LMWH, dalteparin) has been shown to have superior efficacy compared with warfarin with similar major bleeding rates
- Compared with LMWH (dalteparin), the direct oral anticoagulants (DOACs) have similar (edoxaban) or improved (rivaroxaban, apixaban) efficacy rates. Major bleeding and clinically relevant nonmajor bleeding remain important considerations for DOAC therapy
- Treatment should continue for as long as the cancer disease process is deemed active, a minimum 6 months

As outlined in Chapter 9, patients with cancer face an increased risk of venous thromboembolism (VTE), which is attributable to a combination of cancer-specific prothrombotic activity, complications of cancer-directed therapy (e.g., hormonal therapy, chemotherapy, targeted agents or radiotherapy, surgery, or hospital confinement), or the use of chronic indwelling central venous catheters for chemotherapy administration.[1–3] The risk is highest in the first months to a year after diagnosis (Fig. 18.1). Once diagnosed, the management of VTE in patients with active cancer can be challenging given their increased

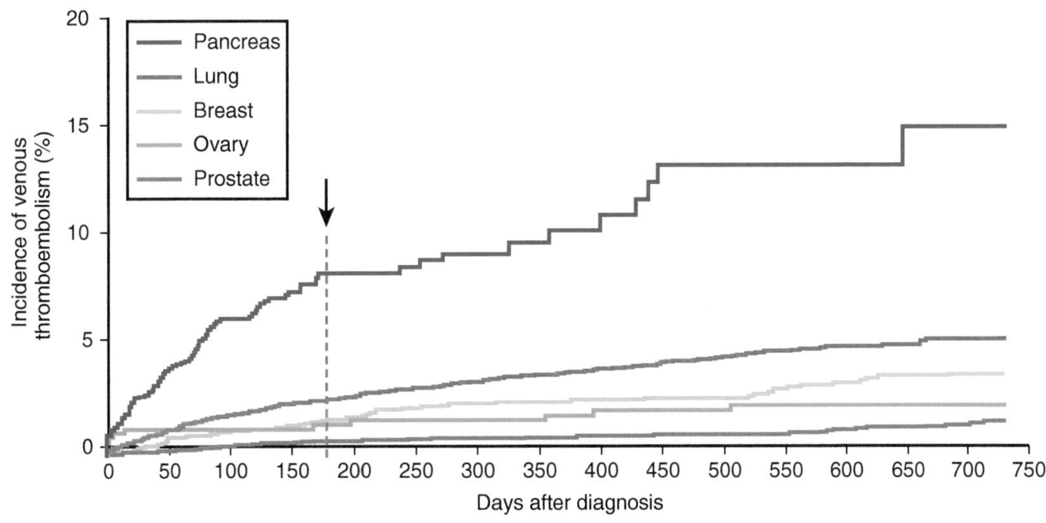

FIG 18.1 Cancer Associated Venous Thromboembolism Management. (From Chew HK, Wun T, Harvey D, Zhou H, White RH. Incidence of venous thromboembolism and its effect on survival among patients with common cancers. *Arch Intern Med.* 2006;166(4):458–464.)

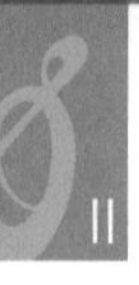

propensity for both recurrent VTEs as well as major bleeding.[1–4] The risk of recurrence relates to the persistence of risk factors, at least in part (Chapter 30). An increased risk of anticoagulant-associated major bleeding may result from hepatic dysfunction (primary liver cancer, liver metastasis, hepatic injury owing to chemotherapy), kidney injury, thrombocytopenia, tumor friability, or supratherapeutic international normalized ratio (INR) while on a vitamin K antagonist owing to malnutrition, vomiting, or medication-interactions.[1–4] Balancing efficacy and safety can be challenging and adds complexity to the treatment of these patients.

TREATMENT TRIALS

A number of important treatment trials of cancer-associated VTE have been conducted (Table 18.1).[5–15] The initial trials compared warfarin with low-molecular- weight heparin (LMWH). The Comparison of Low-Molecular-Weight Heparin versus Oral Anticoagulant Therapy for the Prevention of Recurrent Venous Thromboembolism in Patients with Cancer (CLOT) trial remains the landmark cancer VTE treatment trial, which formed the basis for current treatment guidelines and against which all contemporary trials are compared.[5,7] Subsequent trials

TABLE 18.1 Trials for VTE Treatment in Patients With Cancer

TRIAL	SIZE	DESIGN	DRUG	COMPARATOR	FOLLOW-UP DURATION	PRIMARY OUTCOMES
CLOT[5]	672	Randomized, open label	Dalteparin 200 IU/kg/day × 30 day then 150 IU/kg/day	Dalteparin-coumarin	6 months	• Dalteparin resulted in lower recurrent VTE rates (9% vs. 17%) • Similar major bleeding (6% vs. 4%) • Similar mortality (39% vs. 41%)
French Cooperate Group[8]	146	Randomized, open label	Enoxaparin 1.5 mg/kg/day	Enoxaparin-warfarin	3 months	• Trial terminated prematurely owing to slow enrollment • Similar recurrent VTE and major bleeding composite endpoint (10.5% vs. 21.1%) • Similar major bleeding (7% vs. 16%) • Similar mortality (11.3% vs. 22.7%)
ONCENOX[9]	122	Randomized, open label	**Group 1a** Enoxaparin 1.0 mg/kg twice daily for 5 days then 1.0 mg/kg once daily **Group 1b** Enoxaparin 1.0 mg/kg twice daily for 5 days then 1.5 mg/kg once daily	Enoxaparin-warfarin	6 months	• VTE recurrence was similar across three groups: Group 1a (6.9%), Group 1b (6.3%), warfarin (10%) • Major bleeding rates were similar: Group 1a (6.5%), Group 1b (11.1%), warfarin (2.9%) • Mortality rates were similar: Group 1a (22.6%), Group 1b (41.7%), warfarin (32.4%) • Statistical differences between groups were limited by small sample sizes.
LITE[10]	200	Randomized, open label	Tinzaparin 175 IU/kg/day continued for 3 months	Unfractionated heparin/ warfarin continued for 3 months	Treatment: 3 months Surveillance: 12 months	• At 3 months, VTE recurrence rates were similar (6% vs. 10%). • At 12 months, fewer patients on LMWH had a VTE recurrence (7% vs. 16%) • Similar major bleeding (7% vs. 7%) • Similar mortality at 3 months (20% vs. 19%) and at 12 months (47% vs. 47%)

TABLE 18.1 **Trials for VTE Treatment in Patients with Cancer—cont'd**

TRIAL	SIZE	DESIGN	DRUG	COMPARATOR	FOLLOW-UP DURATION	PRIMARY OUTCOMES
CATCH[11]	900	Randomized, open label	Tinzaparin 175 IU/kg/day	Tinzaparin-warfarin	6 months	• VTE recurrence was borderline lower in tinzaparin arm (7.2% vs. 10.5%). • Symptomatic DVT were less frequent with tinzaparin (2.7% vs. 5.3%). • PE rates were similar (4.5% vs. 4.5%). • Major bleeding rates were similar (2.7% vs. 2.4%). • Similar mortality rates (23.4% vs. 20.6%)
Hokusai VTE Cancer[12]	1050	Randomized, open label	LMWH × 5 days then edoxaban 60 mg daily	Dalteparin 200 IU/kg/day × 30 days then 150 IU/kg/day	6–12 months	• Composite of VTE recurrence or major bleeding at 12 months was noninferior (12.8% vs. 13.5%). • Recurrent VTE was similar (7.9% vs. 11.3%). • Major bleeding was higher for edoxaban arm (6.9% vs. 4.0%). • Death rates were similar (39.5% vs. 36.6%).
SELECT-D[13]	406	Randomized, open label	Rivaroxaban 15 mg twice daily for 21 days then 20 mg daily	Dalteparin 200 IU/kg/day × 30 days then 150 IU/kg/day	6 months	• Recurrent VTE was lower for rivaroxaban (4% vs. 11%). • Major bleeding was similar (6% vs. 4%). • Death rates were similar (25% vs. 30%).
ADAM VTE[14]	300	Randomized, open label	Apixaban 10 mg twice daily for 7 days then 5 mg twice daily	Dalteparin 200 IU/kg/day × 30 days then 150 IU/kg/day	6 months	• Major bleeding was similar between arms (0% vs. 1.4%). • Recurrent VTE was lower for the apixaban arm (0.7% vs. 6.3%). • Death rates were similar (16% vs. 11%).
CARAVAGGIO[15]	1155	Randomized, open label	Apixaban 10 mg twice daily for 7 days then 5 mg twice daily	Dalteparin 200 IU/kg/day × 30 days then 150 IU/kg/day	6 months	• Recurrent VTE was noninferior for apixaban arm (5.6% vs. 7.9%). • Major bleeding was similar between arms (3.8% vs. 4.0%). • Death rates were similar (24.3% vs. 26.4%).
Vedovati[16]	595	Meta-analysis of DOAC VTE trials limited to patients with cancer	Apixaban (n = 81)	Heparin/warfarin	6 months	• VTE rates were similar (3.7% vs. 6.4%). • Major bleeding rates were similar (2.3% vs. 5.0%).
			Dabigatran (n = 173)			• VTE rates were similar (5.7% vs. 7.4%). • Major bleeding rates were similar (3.8% vs. 4.6%).
			Edoxaban (n = 109)			• VTE rates were similar (3.7% vs. 7.0%). • Major bleeding rates were similar (4.6% vs. 3.0%).
			Rivaroxaban (n = 232)			• VTE rates were similar (2.6% vs. 4.0%). • Major bleeding rates were similar (2.6% vs. 4.1%).

DVT, Deep venous thrombosis; *LMWH*, Low-molecular-weight heparin; *PE*, pulmonary embolism; *VTE*, venous thromboembolism.

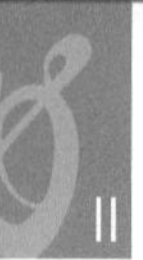

have compared the direct oral anticoagulants (DOACs) with LMWH and will be discussed separately.

Low-Molecular-Weight Heparin Compared With Warfarin

The CLOT trial randomized 672 patients with active cancer and acute proximal deep vein thrombosis (popliteal or more proximal), pulmonary embolism, or both to receive either LMWH (dalteparin 200 IU/kg/day for 1 month followed by 150 IU/kg/day for 5 months) or dalteparin transitioned to adjusted dose warfarin.[5] *Active cancer was defined as cancer diagnosed within 6 months of enrollment, any cancer treatment within the past 6 months, or recurrent or metastatic disease.* After a trial duration of 6 months, symptomatic recurrent venous thromboembolism occurred in 9% in the dalteparin group compared with 17% in the warfarin group (hazard ratio [HR], 0.48; 95% confidence interval [CI], 0.30 to 0.77; *P* = .002). No differences were found in major bleeding rates (dalteparin 6% vs. warfarin 4%) or overall mortality (dalteparin 39% vs. warfarin 41%; *P* = .53). A subsequent *post hoc* analysis[6] revealed a survival benefit at 12 months among patients with cancer without metastasis receiving dalteparin compared with warfarin (mortality: dalteparin 20% vs. warfarin 36%; HR, 0.50; 95% CI, 0.27 to 0.95; *P* = .03). The survival benefit was not apparent for those patients with metastatic disease (dalteparin 72% vs. warfarin 69%; HR, 1.1; 95% CI, 0.87 to 1.4; *P* = .46).

The CATCH trial randomized 900 patients with cancer who had acute symptomatic leg deep venous thrombosis (DVT) or pulmonary embolism (PE) to receive either tinzaparin (175 IU/kg once daily) or tinzaparin transitioned to warfarin[11] for 6 months. The primary composite endpoint was symptomatic DVT recurrence, PE, or incidental VTE. Of the recruited patients, 55% had known metastasis and 42% were receiving active systemic therapy. During the 6 months of treatment, VTE recurrence was similar in the tinzaparin (7.2%) compared with the warfarin group (10.5%; HR, 0.65, *P* = .07). Major bleeding did not differ between treatment groups (tinzaparin 2.7% vs. warfarin 2.4%; HR, 0.89; *P* = .77). Clinically relevant nonmajor bleeding rates favored tinzaparin therapy (10.9% vs. 15.3%; *P* = .004). Mortality rates were similar for both treatment arms (tinzaparin 34.7% vs. warfarin 32.2%). The most frequent cause of death was cancer progression. Fatal pulmonary embolism occurred in 3.8% of each group and fatal bleeding in one warfarin treated patient.

Apart from these two trials, a number of smaller negative trials have compared LMWH with warfarin, including a French Cooperate Group,[8] the ONCENOX pilot,[9] and the Long-term Innovations in TreatmEnt (LITE) trial[10] (see Table 18.1)

Based primarily on the CLOT trial, treatment guidelines had recommended a preference for LMWH, both for initial therapy during the first three months (grade 2B) and for extended therapy beyond three months (grade 2C) regardless of bleeding risk.[7] Anticoagulants are continued until no evidence exists of active malignancy, defined as any evidence of cancer on cross-sectional imaging or any cancer-related treatment (surgery, radiation, or chemotherapy) within the preceding six months.

Low-Molecular-Weight Heparin Limitations

Chronic subcutaneous LMWH therapy has several disadvantages. First, these injections may be painful and cause considerable local ecchymoses and hematomas. Second, for individuals without insurance, the cost may be prohibitive, particularly given the extended nature of treatment. Third, thrombocytopenia, which may frequently accompany cancer or cancer treatment, may limit its use. Thrombocytopenia in the setting of heparin therapy may also raise concerns for heparin-induced thrombocytopenia. A history of heparin-induced thrombocytopenia precludes the use of this medication. Fourth, protamine is an imperfect antidote for LMWH therapy if the patient develops major bleeding complications. Fifth, renal impairment, which is not infrequent among patients with cancer, may limit the use of LMWH. For these combined reasons, an alternative anticoagulation therapy for patients with cancer associated VTE would be extremely attractive.

Direct Oral Anticoagulants Compared With Low-Molecular-Weight Heparin

DOACs offer an attractive alternative to either LMWH or warfarin for the treatment of acute venous thrombosis in patients with cancer. To date, there have been four treatment trials in this setting and one important meta-analysis comparing dalteparin with the direct factor Xa inhibitors, edoxaban, rivaroxaban, and apixaban.[12–16]

TABLE 18.2 Guidelines for Treatment of Cancer Associated Venous Thromboembolism

	2019 ITAC[48]	2019 ASCO[49]	2020 NCCN[50]
Initial treatment	LMWH if creatinine clearance ≥30 mL/min preferred over VKA. Rivaroxaban or edoxaban if risk of GI/GU bleeding is low and creatinine clearance ≥30 mL/min.[a] Fondaparinux or UFH as alternative	Initial anticoagulation may include LMWH, UFH, fondaparinux, or rivaroxaban. LMWH, edoxaban, or rivaroxaban are preferred over VKA. VKA may be used where LMWH or DOACs are not accessible.	DOACs (apixaban, edoxaban, rivaroxaban) preferred in the absence of GI lesions. LMWH preferred for patients with GI lesions. Dabigatran, fondaparinux, or warfarin as alternatives (initial therapy with LMWH or UFH for at least 5 days if edoxaban or dabigatran, start of warfarin concurrently with LMWH, UFH, or fondaparinux until INR 2–3)
Duration of initial treatment	Treatment duration is for a minimum of 6 months (minimum of 3 months for catheter-related)	Treatment duration is for a minimum of 6 months	Treatment duration is at least 3 months
Long-term secondary prevention	After 6 months, continued anticoagulation should be individualized based on risk-to-benefit ratio, tolerability, drug availability, patient preference, and cancer activity.	After 6 months, continued anticoagulation should be offered to select patients with active cancer, metastatic cancer, or active chemotherapy. Decision-making should be individualized based on a continued favorable risk-benefit profile.	Continue as long as cancer is active, under treatment, or risk factors for recurrence persist, or as long as catheter is in place.
Special considerations/ absolute contraindications	Special considerations: Brain tumor: LWMH or DOACs CrCl <30 mL/min: UFH followed by warfarin or LMWH adjusted to anti-Xa levels Platelet count <50,000: case-based with caution Platelet count >50,000: no adjustment Obesity: higher doses of LMWH Pregnancy: LWMH	Absolute contraindications: active, serious, or potentially life-threatening bleeding not reversible with intervention Severe, uncontrolled malignant hypertension Severe, uncompensated coagulopathy Severe platelet dysfunction of inherited bleeding disorder Persistent, severe thrombocytopenia (<20,000/μL) High-risk invasive procedure in a critical site Concurrent use of potent P-glycoprotein or CYP3A4 inhibitors or inducers (DOACs)	Absolute contraindications: active bleeding (major), indwelling neuraxial catheters, neuraxial anesthesia/lumbar puncture, interventional spine and pain procedure For LWMH and UFH: recent/ acute HIT For fondaparinux: CrCl <30 mL/min For DOACs: CrCl <30 mL/min (except for apixban <25 mL/min), ASI/AST >3 × ULN (except for apixaban or edoxaban >2 × ULN), or strong inducers/inhibitors of CYP3A4 and P-glycoprotein (latter for dabigatran and edoxaban, both for apixaban and rivaroxaban)
Anticoagulation failure (recurrence while on anticoagulation)	LMWH: increase LMWH by 20%–25% or switch to DOACs DOACs: switch to LMWH Warfarin: switch to LMWH or DOACs	LWMH: increase the dose, or switch to an alternative regimen. All other: switch to alternative agent	LMWH: switch to twice daily, increase dose by 25%–25%, or switch to fondaparinux or DOAC DOACs: switch to LMWH or fondaparinux Fondaparinux: switch to UFH, LMWH, or DOAC Warfarin: all other options

[a]Guidelines published prior to ADAM VTE and CARAVAGGIO trials with apixaban.

DOAC, Direct oral anticoagulant; *GI*, gastrointestinal; *GU*, genitourinary; *INR*, international normalized ratio; *LMWH*, low-molecular-weight heparin; *UFH*, unfractionated heparin; *VKA*, vitamin K antagonist (warfarin).

Edoxaban

The Hokusai VTE Cancer trial investigators compared a strategy of LMWH for 5 days followed by oral edoxaban (60 mg daily) with dalteparin (200 IU/kg/day × 30 days then 150 IU/kg daily) for at least 6 months and up to 12 months for the treatment of acute symptomatic or incidentally detected proximal leg DVT or pulmonary embolism.[12] Patients had to have active cancer or a diagnosis of cancer within the prior 2 years. During the recruitment period, 1050 patients were enrolled, of whom 53% had metastatic disease and 72% were receiving active cancer treatment. The median duration of antithrombotic treatment was 211 days for the edoxaban arm and 184 days for the dalteparin arm. The primary composite outcome included recurrent VTE or major bleeding, which occurred in 12.8% of the edoxaban-treated patients and 13.5% of the dalteparin-treated patients (P = .006 for noninferiority; HR, 0.97; 95% CI, 0.70 to 1.36). Recurrent VTE rates were similar (edoxaban 7.9% vs. dalteparin 11.3%; P = .09). Major bleeding rates were 2.9% higher for the edoxaban group (6.9% vs. 4.0%; HR, 1.77; 95% CI, 1.03 to 3.04; P = .04). Of the major bleeding events in the edoxaban group, most did not represent a clinical emergency (66.7%). In a subgroup analysis of patients with gastrointestinal malignancy, major bleeding rates favored dalteparin therapy (edoxaban 13.2% vs. dalteparin 2.4%; P = .0169). No fatal bleeding events occurred in the edoxaban arm and only one fatal bleed occurred in the dalteparin arm. All-cause mortality rates were similar for both arms (39.5% vs. 36.6%).

Rivaroxaban

The SELECT-D trial compared rivaroxaban (15 mg twice daily for 3 weeks, then 20 mg once daily for a total of 6 months) with dalteparin (200 IU/kg daily during month 1, then 150 IU/kg daily for months 2 to 6) for treatment of acute symptomatic leg DVT, symptomatic or incidental PE in patients with active cancer.[13] To qualify for the trial, patients had to have an ECOG performance score of 2 or less. The primary outcome was VTE recurrence. Secondary outcomes were major and clinically relevant nonmajor bleeding. During the recruitment period, 406 patients were randomized. Of these, 70% were actively receiving cancer therapy and 58% had metastatic disease. Nearly half of qualifying thrombi (48%) were symptomatic and 52% were found incidentally. VTE recurrence rates at 6 months were 4% for the rivaroxaban arm and 11% for the dalteparin arm (HR, 0.43; 95% CI, 0.19 to 0.99). There were two patients with symptomatic PE and one fatal PE in each treatment arm.

The site of the primary tumor influenced VTE recurrence rates. Patient with stomach or pancreas cancer had more than a five-fold greater risk of recurrence (HR, 5.55; 95% CI, 1.97 to 15.66), whereas those with lung, lymphoma, gynecologic, or bladder cancer had more than a two-fold increased risk (HR, 2.69; 95% CI, 1.11 to 6.53). Patients presenting with symptomatic VTE as a qualifying event also had more than a two-fold increased risk of recurrence compared with those with an incidental PE (HR, 2.78; 95% CI, 1.20 to 6.41).

Major bleeding rates were 6% for rivaroxaban and 4% for dalteparin (HR, 1.83; 95% CI, 0.68 to 4.96). Most major bleeding events involved the gastrointestinal (GI) tract. Patients with upper GI cancer were more likely to experience a major bleed with rivaroxaban. Clinically relevant nonmajor bleeding was also more frequent with rivaroxaban (13% vs. 4%; HR, 3.76; 95% CI, 1.63 to 8.69) and primarily involved GI or genitourinary (GU) sources. There were no intracranial bleeds. Overall survival at 6 months was similar for both arms (rivaroxaban 75% vs. dalteparin 70%).

Apixaban

The Apixaban versus Dalteparin in Active Malignancy associated VTE (ADAM VTE) trial randomized 300 patients with cancer to receive either apixaban (10 mg twice daily for 7 days followed by 5 mg twice daily) for 6 months or subcutaneous dalteparin (200 IU/kg for 1 month followed by 150 IU/kg once daily).[14] The primary outcome was major bleeding. Major bleeding up to 6 months occurred in 0% assigned to apixaban and in 1.4% assigned to dalteparin (P = .138; HR and 95% CI not estimable owing to 0 bleeding events in the apixaban arm). The major bleeding events in the dalteparin arm included one retroperitoneal and one intracranial bleed. Secondary outcomes included VTE recurrence and a composite of major plus clinically relevant nonmajor bleeding. Recurrent VTE occurred in 0.7% in the apixaban group and 6.3% in the dalteparin group (HR, 0.099; 95% CI, 0.013 to 0.780; P = .0281). Quality-of-life surveys were obtained monthly to assess satisfaction with anticoagulant delivery. By the first month cycle, survey results favored apixaban for most measures: bruising, stress, irritation, burden of delivery, and overall satisfaction with anticoagulant therapy ($P <$ .05). A monthly bruise survey also favored apixaban.

The CARAVAGGIO trial randomized 1155 patients with cancer with a newly diagnosed symptomatic or incidental leg DVT or PE to receive apixaban (10 mg twice daily for 7 days followed by 5 mg twice daily for 6 months) or therapeutic dalterparin.[15] Patients with active cancer or a history of cancer within 2 years of enrollment were eligible for participation. The primary efficacy outcome, recurrent VTE, was confirmed in 5.6% of patients assigned to apixaban compared with 7.9% receiving dalteparin (HR, 0.63; 95% CI, 0.37 to 1.07), reaching noninferiority ($P <$ .001), but not superiority (P = .09). Rates of major bleeding, GI bleeding and non-GI bleeding were similar for both arms. There was no fatal bleeding in the apixaban group and two fatal bleeding events in the dalteparin group. All-cause mortality rates were similar across treatment groups.

A meta-analysis analyzing the outcomes of patients with cancer participating in six DOAC trials for venous thromboembolism treatment were included in the analysis for a total of 1132 patients.[16] In general, outcomes were favorable for DOAC therapy.

When taken together, DOAC therapy was found to be a reasonable treatment alternative to LMWH for acute VTE in patients with active cancer and now have guideline endorsement (Table 18.2)[48–50]. This conclusion is supported by a meta-analysis of the six major DOAC trials for VTE treatment compared with conventional therapy with warfarin in a total of 1132 patients[16]; both VTE recurrence rates (DOAC 3.9% vs. warfarin 6.0%) and major bleeding rates (DOAC 3.2% vs. warfarin 4.2%) were not significantly lower in patients treated with DOAC. DOACs are as effective or at least not inferior to LMWH in the setting of cancer. The benefit of oral delivery over parenteral injections is clear and may serve to improve patient adherence to therapy. An obstacle to DOAC therapy remains anticoagulant-related bleeding. Most bleeding episodes are from gastrointestinal sources. Both intracranial bleeding and fatal bleeding are infrequent. Some investigators have suggested avoiding DOAC use in patients with gastrointestinal, particularly upper GI tract cancers.

Duration of Anticoagulation

In patients with cancer-associated thrombosis, the optimal duration of anticoagulation therapy has not been established. Owing to the perceived high risk of VTE recurrence in this patient population, it is generally recommended to continue extended anticoagulant therapy as long as there is evidence of active cancer or the patient is receiving cancer-directed therapies.[7,16] Active cancer carries a risk of recurrent VTE two- to nine-fold higher compared with patients without cancer.[17–24] VTE recurrence increases the risk of death three-fold, particularly with recurrent pulmonary embolism.[24] Guideline recommendations are to continue anticoagulation therapy until the cancer is no longer evident.[7] These recommendations are limited to expert opinion given the lack of randomized controlled data (grade 2C).[7] Patients with cancer also have an increased risk of anticoagulant-associated major bleeding and balancing these competing risks can be challenging.[19,22,24,25] Prolonged anticoagulant therapy may not be beneficial for all patients with cancer.

Limited data exist to inform decision-making for treatment duration in patients with cancer (Table 18.3). The LITE investigators randomized 200 patients with cancer to receive warfarin or LMWH, tinzaparin, for 3 months for the acute treatment of VTE.[10] Thereafter, patients were treated "per usual care" by their primary provider. Patients were then assessed for an additional 9 months. At 3 months, 6% of those patients randomized to tinzaparin compared with 10% on warfarin suffered an acute VTE recurrence which did not differ significantly between treatment allocations. At 12 months, an additional 7% of patients in the tinzaparin group (total of 13%) compared with an additional 16% in the warfarin arm (total of 26%) suffered VTE recurrence (P = .044; RR, 0.44; absolute difference, 9.0%; 95% CI, −21.7% to −0.7%). Major bleeding events were 7% for both groups at 3 months. Death occurred in 20% for both groups at 3 months and 47% of both groups at 12 months.

The Cancer-DACUS trial assessed patients with cancer with the first episode of DVT who had been treated with LMWH for 6 months.[26] After 6 months, patients underwent duplex ultrasound imaging to assess residual DVT. Those with residual thrombus were then randomly assigned to continue LMWH for an additional 6 months or to discontinue therapy. For those patients with thrombus resolution (no residual thrombus), anticoagulation was discontinued. They enrolled 347 patients of whom 242 patients had residual DVT. Of these, 22 of the 119 patients (18%) with continued LMWH had VTE recurrence compared with 27 of 123 patients (22%)

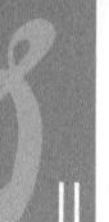

TABLE 18.3 Secondary Prevention Trials

TRIAL	SIZE	DESIGN	DRUG	FOLLOW-UP DURATION	PRIMARY OUTCOMES
LITE[10]	200	Randomized, open label	Tinzaparin 175 IU/kg/ day for 3 months UFH/warfarin for 3 months	12 months	• Subjects were treated for 3 months and then followed for an additional 9 months. • At 12 months, fewer LMWH patients had a VTE recurrence (7% vs. 16%). • Similar major bleeding (7% vs. 7%). • Similar mortality (47% vs. 47%).
DACUS[27]	347	Randomized, open label LMWH for 6 months followed by ultrasound for residual DVT	If no residual DVT: then no further therapy (group B1) If residual DVT, then either: nadroparin 97 IU/kg twice daily (group A1) No therapy (group A2)	12 months	• VTE recurrence was lowest in patients with no residual DVT on follow-up ultrasound (2.9%). • For patients with residual DVT on ultrasound, VTE recurrence rates were not lower for those who continued LMWH (A1, 18%) compared with those who stopped treatment (A2, 22%). • Major bleeding rates were similar between groups. (A1, 5.8%; A2, 1.2%; B1, 1.9%). • Mortality rates were similar between groups (A1, 10.1%; A2, 15.4%; B1, 10.5%).
DALTECAN[28]	334	Multicenter, open label, single arm	Dalteparin 200 IU/kg/ day for 1 month, then 150 IU/kg/day for 11 months	12 months	• VTE recurrence was 11.1%. • Major bleeding was 10.2% • Mortality rate was 33.8%

DVT, Deep venous thrombosis; *LMWH*, low-molecular-weight heparin; *UFH*, unfractionated heparin; *VTE*, venous thromboembolism.

who stopped therapy. For those patients without residual thrombus, the recurrence rate was low at 2.9% (3 of 105 patients). This study suggests that continued anticoagulant therapy beyond 6 months based on ultrasound evidence of residual thrombus provides only a modest reduction in recurrent venous thromboembolism. Decisions based on the presence of residual thrombus after acute therapy has not been deemed sufficiently well validated to receive guideline endorsement.[7]

DALTECAN was a multicenter open-label, single-arm study of dalteparin therapy for cancer-associated VTE.[27] Patients (n = 334) received dalteparin 200 IU/kg daily for 4 weeks with a maximal daily dose of 18,000 IU. Thereafter, patients received a dose reduction that amounted to 150 IU/kg daily for months 2 through 12. Major bleeding occurred in 34 patients (10.2%) and was highest during the first month of therapy (3.6%). Thirty-seven patients (11%) had recurrent VTE, which was also highest during the first month (5.7%). There were 116 deaths (33.8%) primarily owing to cancer progression. Four patients died from recurrent pulmonary embolism and 2 patients died from major bleeding.

In summary, decision-making for continued therapy after 6 months of anticoagulation can be challenging (see Chapter 30). Balancing the risk of recurrent thrombosis, the risk of major bleeding and patient-specific preferences is most appropriate.

Anticoagulation Failures

One of the difficulties of anticoagulation management in patients with cancer is the problem of its failure.[1–4] These are patients who develop recurrent thrombotic events despite anticoagulation therapy. Unfortunately, treatment failures are not infrequent. In recent clinical trials of patients with cancer with acute VTE, the frequency of anticoagulation failure for DOACs was 4% at 6 months and up to 8% at 12 months (Table 18.4). For those treated with warfarin, the rate was approximately 2.5% per month or up to 16% at 6 months. For patients receiving LMWH, the rates were 10% at 6 months and up to 14% at 12 months. The treatment failures appeared to be more frequent with biologically aggressive tumors. For example, in the SELECT-D trial, the likelihood of anticoagulant failure was more

TABLE 18.4 Anticoagulation Failures in Patients With Cancer by Type of Anticoagulation Therapy

AGENT	TRIAL	TRIAL DURATION (DAYS)	TREATMENT FAILURES (%)
Parenteral Agents			
Dalteparin	CLOT[1]	180	9
	DALTECAN[28]	180 365	9 14
	Hokusai Cancer VTE[8]	365	13.5
	SELECT-D[9]	180	11
	ADAM VTE[10]	180	6.3
Tinzaparin	CATCH[7]	160	7.2
Oral Agents			
Warfarin	CLOT[1]	180	16
	CATCH[7]	160	10.5
Edoxaban	Hokusai Cancer VTE[8]	365	7.9
Rivaroxaban	SELECT-D[7]	180	4
Apixaban	ADAM VTE[10]	180	0.7

than five-fold higher for patients with stomach or pancreatic cancer compared with other tumors (HR, 5.55; 95% CI, 1.97 to 15.66).[13] For subjects with lymphoma, lung, GYN or bladder cancer, the risk was more than two-fold higher (HR, 2.69; 95% CI, 1.11 to 6.53). Symptomatic VTE at presentation carried a higher risk of anticoagulant failure compared with incidentally identified thrombi.

Determining the best treatment for such patients can be challenging and requires a systematic approach:

1. It is important to confirm anticoagulant failure through careful imaging review with side-by-side comparisons whenever feasible. To be classified as a recurrent event, there must be a new filling defect evident on the second study not appreciated on the original images or an interval study that had clearly documented interim thrombus resolution. As the problem of anticoagulant failure is of such importance and not infrequent among cancer cases, it is imperative to obtain a complete assessment of thrombus burden at the time of the initial thrombosis diagnosis. This allows for a complete and thorough comparison should the issue of anticoagulation failure arise in the future.
2. It is important to determine whether drug metabolism is occurring as anticipated for the patient. This includes confirmation that the patient is taking the correct dose. Where available, it is helpful to assess drug levels. Ideally this would be accomplished prior to discontinuing or altering the anticoagulation strategy for the patient. For young individuals with excellent renal function, "hyper-clearance" of the drug may be occurring. This is particularly true for anticoagulants such as LMHW, dabigatran, and edoxaban.[28,29] Significant drug interactions, such as the concomitant use of severe CYP 3A4 inducers and direct factor Xa inhibitors, should be excluded. Proper drug administration should be confirmed, particularly for patients taking rivaroxaban, which requires a fatty meal to improve drug absorption.[30] Anatomic confounders, such as altered GI motility, gastric bypass, or intestinal resection may impair drug absorption.[31,32]
3. It is important to ensure that the patient has been compliant with the medications prescribed. Many reasons exist for noncompliance, including patient-related factors, such as health literacy, cognitive function, and disease-related knowledge. Drug-related factors include polypharmacy and both real and perceived adverse effects. Then, logistic factors may relate to barriers obtaining medications, such as financial constraints and physical impairment sufficient to limit pharmacy access. Real-world experience has shown that medical adherence to anticoagulants is only slightly better than 50% at the end of the first year of therapy.[33,34] Furthermore, DOAC adherence has not been shown to be superior to warfarin adherence. Although DOAC and LMWH therapy avoids the necessity of regular clinic visits for INR monitoring and drug adjustments, guideline recommendations include active participation by the management health care team to promote compliance with assessment of drug levels, pill counts, pharmacy reviews, and DOAC management agreement cards.[35]
4. Temporary anticoagulant interruptions for invasive procedures may promote thrombosis for several reasons (see next section). The invasive procedure itself may augment the propensity for thrombosis.[36–39] Blood product transfusions for bleeding associated with surgery further increases this risk. Central venous lines, common to large surgical procedures will also increase the thrombotic risk. The temporary interruption of anticoagulants will expose the underlying substrate that prompted the original thrombotic event.

5. Drug-specific complications may augmented the thrombotic risk. This specifically relates to heparin-induced thrombocytopenia, which may complicate LMWH delivery.
6. The thrombus propagation may not be owing to bland thrombus, but rather to tumor thrombus. Key tumors for which this type of complication may occur include renal cell carcinoma, sarcoma, Wilm's tumor, adrenal cortical carcinoma, and hepatocellular carcinoma.[40] Contrast-enhanced computed tomography, magnetic resonance imaging, and positron emission tomography imaging may help differentiate tumor thrombus from bland thrombus is such cases.[41–44]

Thus, if anticoagulation failure occurs despite therapeutic levels and confirmed compliance, guidance recommendations favor transitioning the patient to therapeutic LMWH.[7] This should include twice daily dosing with careful monitoring to ensure adequate delivery and metabolism. If the recurrence occurs while receiving LMWH, the recommendation is to increase the current dosing by 25% to 33%.[7] Given the results of recent DOAC trials in this context, it would not be unreasonable to switch to one of these agents in the setting of LMWH failure. In general, inferior vena cava (IVC) filter placement should be avoided unless anticoagulation is contraindicated (e.g., active bleeding). In this situation, a retrievable filter should be considered with prompt reinitiation of anticoagulants as soon as clinically feasible.

Temporary Anticoagulation Cessation for Invasive Procedures

It is anticipated that patients with active cancer will require invasive procedures throughout their clinical course. For patients without cancer on anticoagulation therapy, approximately 15% will require an invasive procedure each year.[36–39] By comparison, patients with cancer undergo much more frequent invasive procedures requiring temporary anticoagulant cessation. In one trial, nearly 30% of those with cancer required an invasive procedure over 6 months of follow up.[47] During this period, careful anticoagulation management is crucial to avoid periprocedural major hemorrhage or thromboembolic complications. For elective procedures, a step-wise systematic approach should be adopted and carefully followed:

1. The date and type of procedure should to be confirmed and recorded.[36] A growing number of minor procedures may be performed without anticoagulant cessation; consultation with the team performing the anticipated procedure can be informative. It is also helpful to document renal function, liver function, and platelet counts during this decision-making visit.
2. The timing of anticoagulation discontinuation will be agent specific. It is important to allow sufficient time for drug metabolism to occur such that minimal circulating drug is present at the time of the procedure. The interval between drug discontinuation and procedure also depends on the anticipated bleeding risk of the procedure.
3. On the morning of the procedure, it is often helpful to obtain drug levels when feasible to ensure that complete or near complete metabolism has occurred. Postprocedure, patients should receive prophylactic dose anticoagulants; the first prophylactic dose is to be given 24 hours after the procedure. Therapeutic anticoagulants should be withheld for at least 48 hours after the procedure and not initiated until adequate hemostasis is confirmed.

This approach was followed for 83 patients participating in the ADAM VTE trial.[14] Of these interventions, 43% would be considered major procedures from a bleeding perspective. Within the 30-day interval following the procedures, no VTE or major bleeding events occurred.

SUMMARY

Treatment of patients with cancer-associated VTE is complicated and must take into account the risk of thrombosis recurrence and major bleeding. This includes decision-making for anticoagulant choice and duration as well as the evaluation and treatment of anticoagulant failures. In contrast to patients without cancer, a high percentage of those with cancer will require an invasive procedure. Successful treatment of these patients requires a thoughtful plan to avoid periprocedural bleeding or thromboembolism. Lastly, further work is needed to improve the overall survival of patients with cancer who have had a thrombotic event.

REFERENCES:

1. Chee CE, Ashrani AA, Marks RS, et al. Predictors of venous thromboembolism recurrence and bleeding among active patients with cancer: a population-based cohort study. *Blood*. 2014;123:3972–3978.

2. Prandoni P, Trujillo-Santos J, Surico T, et al. Recurrent thromboembolism and major bleeding during oral anticoagulant therapy in patients with solid cancer: findings from the RIETE registry. *Haematologica*. 2008;93:1432–1434.
3. Monreal M, Falgá C, Valdés M, et al. Fatal pulmonary embolism and fatal bleeding in patients with cancer with venous thromboembolism: findings from the RIETE registry. *J Thromb Haemost*. 2006;4:1950–1956.
4. Trujillo-Santos J, Nieto JA, Ruíz-Gamietea A, et al. Bleeding complications associated with anticoagulant therapy in patients with cancer. *Thromb Res*. 2010;125(suppl 2):S58–S61.
5. Lee AYY, Levine MN, Baker RI, et al. Low-molecular-weight heparin versus a coumarin for the prevention of recurrent venous thromboembolism in patients with cancer. *N Engl J Med*. 2003;349:146–153.
6. Lee AY, Rickles FR, Julian JA, et al. Randomized comparison of low molecular weight heparin and coumarin derivatives on the survival of patients with cancer and venous thromboembolism. *J Clin Oncol*. 2005;23:2123–2129.
7. Kearon C, Akl EA, Ornelas J, et al. Antithrombotic therapy for VTE disease: CHEST guideline and expert panel report. *Chest*. 2016;149: 315–352.
8. Meyer G, Marjanovic Z, Valcke J, et al. Comparison of low-molecular-weight heparin and warfarin for the secondary prevention of venous thromboembolism in patients with cancer: a randomized controlled study. *Arch Intern Med*. 2002;162:1729–1735.
9. Deitcher SR, Kessler CM, Merli G, et al. Secondary prevention of venous thromboembolic events in patients with active cancer: enoxaparin alone versus initial enoxaparin followed by warfarin for a 180-day period. *Clin Appl Thromb Hemost*. 2006;12:389–396.
10. Hull RD, Pineo GF, Brant RF, et al. Long-term low-molecular-weight heparin versus usual care in proximal-vein thrombosis patients with cancer. *Am J Med*. 2006;119:1062–1072.
11. Lee AY, Kamphuisen PW, Meyer G, et al. Tinzaparin vs warfarin for treatment of acute venous thromboembolism in patients with active cancer: a randomized clinical trial. *JAMA*. 2015;314:677–686.
12. Raskob GE, van Es N, Verhamme P, et al. Edoxaban for the treatment of cancer-associated venous thromboembolism. *N Engl J Med*. 2018;378:615–624.
13. Young AM, Marshall A, Thirlwall J, et al. Comparison of an oral factor Xa inhibitor with low molecular weight heparin in patients with cancer with venous thromboembolism: results of a randomized trial (SELECT-D). *J Clin Oncol*. 2018;36:2017–2023.
14. McBane RD, Wysokinski WE, Le-Rademacher JG, et al. Apixaban and dalteparin in active malignancy-associated venous thromboembolism: the ADAM VTE trial. *J Thromb Haemost*. 2020;18(2):411–421.
15. Agnelli G, Becattini C, Meyer G, et al. Caravaggio investigators. Apixaban for the treatment of venous thromboembolism associated with cancer. *N Engl J Med*. 2020;382(17):1599–1607
16. Vedovati MC, Germini F, Agnelli G, Becattini C. Direct oral anticoagulants in patients with VTE and cancer: a systematic review and meta-analysis. *Chest*. 2015;147:475–483.
17. Khorana AA, Carrier M, Garcia DA, Lee AY. Guidance for the prevention and treatment of cancer-associated venous thromboembolism. *J Thromb Thrombolysis*. 2016;41:81–91.
18. Heit JA, Mohr DN, Silverstein MD, Petterson TM, O'Fallon WM, Melton LJ III. Predictors of recurrence after deep vein thrombosis and pulmonary embolism: a population-based cohort study. *Arch Intern Med*. 2000;160:761–768.
19. Hutten BA, Prins MH, Gent M, Ginsberg J, Tijssen JG, Buller HR. Incidence of recurrent thromboembolic and bleeding complications among patients with venous thromboembolism in relation to both malignancy and achieved international normalized ratio: a retrospective analysis. *J Clin Oncol*. 2000;18:3078–3083.
20. Hansson PO, Sorbo J, Eriksson H. Recurrent venous thromboembolism after deep vein thrombosis: incidence and risk factors. *Arch Intern Med*. 2000;160(6):769–774.
21. Douketis JD, Foster GA, Crowther MA, Prins MH, Ginsberg JS. Clinical risk factors and timing of recurrent venous thromboembolism during the initial 3 months of anticoagulant therapy. *Arch Intern Med*. 2000;160:3431–3436.
22. Prandoni P, Lensing AW, Piccioli A, et al. Recurrent venous thromboembolism and bleeding complications during anticoagulant treatment in patients with cancer and venous thrombosis. *Blood*. 2002;100:3484–3488.
22. Descourt R, Le Gal G, Couturaud F, et al. Recurrent venous thromboembolism under anticoagulant therapy: a high risk in adenocarcinoma? *Thromb Haemost*. 2006;95:912–913.
23. Heit JA, Lahr BD, Petterson TM, Bailey KR, Ashrani AA, Melton LJ III. Heparin and warfarin anticoagulation intensity as predictors of recurrence after deep vein thrombosis or pulmonary embolism: a population-based cohort study. *Blood*. 2011;118(18):4992–4999.
24. Trujillo-Santos J, Ruiz-Gamietea A, Luque JM, et al. Predicting recurrences or major bleeding in women with cancer and venous thromboembolism. Findings from the RIETE Registry. *Thromb Res*. 2009;123(suppl 2):S10–S15.
25. Palareti G, Legnani C, Lee A, et al. A comparison of the safety and efficacy of oral anticoagulation for the treatment of venous thromboembolic disease in patients with or without malignancy. *Thromb Haemost*. 2000;84:805–810.
26. Napolitano M, Saccullo G, Malato A, et al. Optimal duration of low molecular weight heparin for the treatment of cancer-related deep vein thrombosis: the cancer-DACUS study. *J Clin Oncol*. 2014;32:3607–3612.
27. Francis CW, Kessler CM, Goldhaber SZ, et al. Treatment of venous thromboembolism in patients with cancer with dalteparin for up to 12 months: the DALTECAN study. *J Thromb Haemost*. 2015;13:1028–1035.
28. Yu HT, Yang PS, Kim TH, et al. Impact of renal function on outcomes with edoxaban in real-world patients with atrial fibrillation. *Stroke*. 2018;49:2421–2429.
29. Del-Carpio Munoz F, Yao X, Abraham NS, et al. Dabigatran versus warfarin in relation to renal function in patients with atrial fibrillation. *J Am Coll Cardiol*. 2016;68:129–131.
30. Stampfuss J, Kubitza D, Becka M, Mueck W. The effect of food on the absorption and pharmacokinetics of rivaroxaban. *Int J Clin Pharmacol Ther*. 2013;51:549–561.
31. Rottenstreich A, Barkai A, Arad A, Raccah BH, Kalish Y. The effect of bariatric surgery on direct-acting oral anticoagulant drug levels. *Thromb Res*. 2018;163:190–195.
32. Martin KA, Lee CR, Farrell TM, Moll S. Oral anticoagulant use after bariatric surgery: a literature review and clinical guidance. *Am J Med*. 2017;130:517–524.
33. Castellucci LA, Shaw J, van der Salm K, et al. Self-reported adherence to anticoagulation and its determinants using the Morisky medication adherence scale. *Thromb Res*. 2015;136:727–731.
34. Miyazaki M, Nakashima A, Nakamura Y, et al. Association between medication adherence and illness perceptions in atrial fibrillation patients treated with direct oral anticoagulants: an observational cross-sectional pilot study. *PLoS One*. 2018;13:e0204814.
35. Steffel J, Verhamme P, Potpara TS, et al. The 2018 European Heart Rhythm Association Practical Guide on the use of non-vitamin K antagonist oral anticoagulants in patients with atrial fibrillation. *Eur Heart J*. 2018;39:1330–1393.
36. Baron TH, Kamath PS, McBane RD. Antithrombotic therapy and invasive procedures. *N Engl J Med*. 2013;369(11):1079–1080.
37. Tafur AJ, Wysokinski WE, McBane RD, et al. Cancer effect on periprocedural thromboembolism and bleeding in anticoagulated patients. *Ann Oncol*. 2012;23:1998–2005.
38. Tafur AJ, McBane R II, Wysokinski WE, et al. Predictors of major bleeding in peri-procedural anticoagulation management. *J Thromb Haemost*. 2012;10:261–267.
39. McBane RD, Wysokinski WE, Daniels PR, et al. Periprocedural anticoagulation management of patients with venous thromboembolism. *Arterioscler Thromb Vasc Biol*. 2010;30:442–448.
40. Quencer KB, Friedman T, Sheth R, Oklu R. Tumor thrombus: incidence, imaging, prognosis and treatment. *Cardiovasc Diagn Ther*. 2017;7:S165–S177.
41. Catalano OA, Choy G, Zhu A, Hahn PF, Sahani DV. Differentiation of malignant thrombus from bland thrombus of the portal vein in patients with hepatocellular carcinoma: application of diffusion-weighted MR imaging. *Radiology*. 2010;254:154–162.
42. Rohatgi S, Howard SA, Tirumani SH, Ramaiya NH, Krajewski KM. Multimodality Imaging of tumour thrombus. *Can Assoc Radiol J*. 2015;66:121–129.

43. Ravina M, Hess S, Chauhan MS, Jacob MJ, Alavi A. Tumor thrombus: ancillary findings on FDG PET/CT in an oncologic population. *Clin Nucl Med*. 2014;39:767–771.
44. Elting LS, Escalante CP, Cooksley C, et al. Outcomes and cost of deep venous thrombosis among patients with cancer. *Arch Intern Med*. 2004;164:1653–1661.
45. Douketis JD, Spyropoulos AC, Spencer FA, et al. Perioperative management of antithrombotic therapy: antithrombotic therapy and prevention of thrombosis, 9th ed: American College of Chest Physicians Evidence-Based Clinical Practice Guidelines. *Chest*. 2012;141:e326S–e350S.
46. Garcia D, Alexander JH, Wallentin L, et al. Management and clinical outcomes in patients treated with apixaban vs warfarin undergoing procedures. *Blood*. 2014;124:3692–3698.
47. Healey JS, Eikelboom J, Douketis J, et al. Periprocedural bleeding and thromboembolic events with dabigatran compared with warfarin: results from the randomized evaluation of long-term anticoagulation therapy (RE-LY) randomized trial. *Circulation*. 2012;126:343–348.
48. Farge D, Frere C, Connors JM, et al., International Initiative on Thrombosis and Cancer (ITAC) advisory panel. 2019 international clinical practice guidelines for the treatment and prophylaxis of venous thromboembolism in patients with cancer.. *Lancet Oncol*. 2019;20(10):e566–e581.
49. Key NS, Khorana AA, Kuderer NM, et al. Venous thromboembolism prophylaxis and treatment in patients with cancer: ASCO clinical practice guideline update. *J Clin Oncol*. 2020;38(5): 496–520.
50. NCCN Clinical Practice Guidelines in Oncology. Cancer-Associated Venous Thromboembolic Disease. Version 1.2020. https://www.nccn.org/professionals/physician_gls/pdf/vte.pdf.

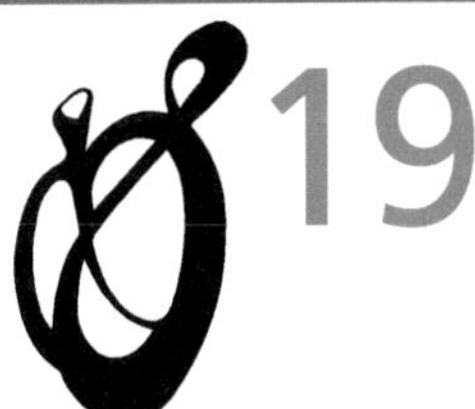

19 Arrhythmia and Device Assessment During Cancer Treatments

MICHAEL FRADLEY

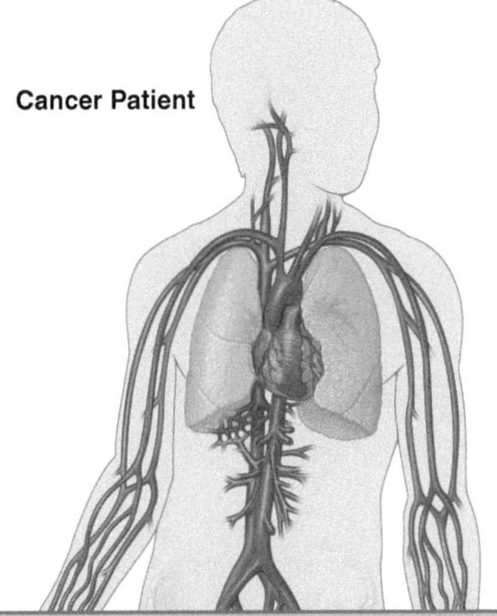

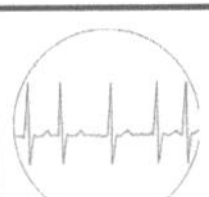

Atrial Fibrillation and Other Atrial Arrhythmias

- Symptoms or complications?
- Need for additional studies?
- Rate versus rhythm control?
- Anticoagulation decisions?
  (CHADS2-VASC/HAS-BLED score unverified)
- Relationship with cancer therapy?
- Drug-drug interactions?

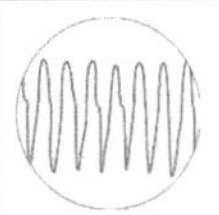

QT Prolongation and Ventricular Arrhythmias

- Underlying cardiovascular disease?
- Need for additional studies?
- Arrhythmic +/– device therapy?
- Renal function/e'lyte abnormality?
- Relationship with cancer therapies?
- Drug-drug interactions?

Arrhythmias during cancer therapy

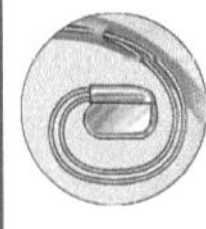

Cardiac Implantable Devices (pacemaker, ICD)

- Adjustment to programming based on therapy (radiation) and clinical presentation
- ICD, CRT-D, pacemaker indication?
  (survival prognosis and code status?)
- Device infection?

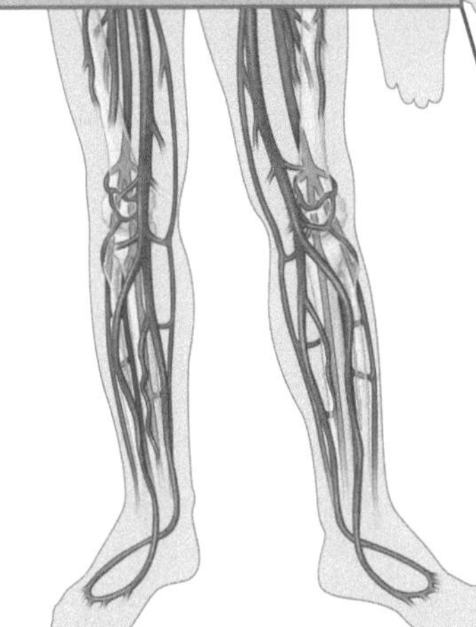

Bradyarrhythmlas and Autonomic Dysfunction

- Symptoms, incl. palpitations, lightheadedness, syncope?
- Need for additional studies?
- Need for medical or device therapy?
- Any modifiable cause or factor?
- Relationship with cancer therapies?

CHAPTER OUTLINE

KEY POINTS

- Atrial fibrillation and other atrial arrhythmias are common complications of many different cancer therapeutics.
- The CHA_2DS_2-VASc and the HAS-BLED scores may not be appropriate to determine thromboembolic and bleeding risk in patients with cancer receiving active therapy.
- Ventricular arrhythmias are an infrequent, but potentially life-threatening, complication of various cancer therapeutics, most often related to QT prolongation or secondary to other toxicities, such as ischemia or left ventricular dysfunction.
- Bradyarrhythmias are frequently asymptomatic and rarely require intervention.
- Heart block may be the first manifestation of checkpoint inhibitor myocarditis.
- Autonomic dysfunction is commonly observed in patients after head, neck, and chest radiation.
- The majority of patients with cardiac implantable devices can safely receive radiation therapy.
- Additional monitoring precautions should be offered to pacemaker-dependent patients and those with devices who are exposed to high beam energy and/or cumulative absorbed dose.

The landscape of cancer therapeutics has significantly changed over the last decade owing to an improved understanding of cancer biology. Patients are now living longer and, in many cases, surviving their disease. Unfortunately, cardiovascular (CV) toxicities are an increasingly important and often treatment-limiting problem. Whereas much of the focus has been on left ventricular dysfunction and heart failure, many cancer treatments are known to be arrhythmogenic and can have a significant impact on patient morbidity and mortality (see Chapter 10, Table 10.1, concise overview provided in Table 19.1). Although atrial fibrillation and other supraventricular arrhythmias are more commonly encountered, ventricular arrhythmias and QT prolongation can also occur during cancer treatment (see Chapter 10, Tables 10.1 and 10.4). Management of electrophysiology issues poses unique challenges in patients with cancer and requires a collaborative effort between cardio-oncologists and the rest of the treatment team.

ATRIAL FIBRILLATION AND OTHER SUPRAVENTRICULAR ARRHYTHMIAS

Atrial arrhythmias, especially atrial fibrillation (AF) are frequently observed in patients undergoing cancer therapy. The "REasons for Geographic and Racial Differences in Stroke" (REGARDS) cohort of more than 15,000 patients reported a 20% higher adjusted risk of AF in patients with cancer, especially within the first year of diagnosis.[1] This can be for multiple reasons, ranging from the malignancy itself and the associated inflammatory state (breast, colorectal, and hematologic malignancies are all associated with higher rates of AF), to specific cancer treatments, including chemo- and targeted therapies. Additionally, patients with cancer and AF have worse outcomes with a two-fold higher risk for thromboembolic complications, a 6-fold higher adjusted risk for heart failure, and a 10-fold higher risk of adjusted 30-day mortality compared with patients not having cancer.[2] It is essential to identify and manage

TABLE 19.1 **Arrhythmias Associated With Anticancer Agents**

DRUG CLASS	EXAMPLE	ASSOCIATED ARRHYTHMIAS	POTENTIAL MECHANISM
Alkylating agents	Melphalan	Atrial arrhythmias	Unknown
Anthracyclines	Doxorubicin	Atrial arrhythmias	Free radical/toxin accumulation; direct myocardial damage/ cardiomyopathy
		Ventricular arrhythmia	Direct myocardial damage/cardiomyopathy; increased ventricular repolarization indices
Arsenic		QT prolongation	Potassium channel inhibition
Cyclin-dependent kinase 4/6 inhibitors	Ribociclib	QT prolongation	Unknown
Fluoropyrimidines	5-Fluorouracil	Ventricular arrhythmias	Secondary to coronary vasospasm/ myocardial ischemia
Immunotherapies	Checkpoint inhibitors (e.g., pembrolizumab)	Atrial arrhythmias Ventricular arrhythmias Bradyarrhythmias	Myocarditis/inflammatory Myocarditis/inflammatory Myocarditis/inflammatory
Proteasome inhibitors	Carfilzomib	Atrial arrhythmias	Unknown: possibly owing to accumulation of abnormal intracellular proteins
Taxanes	Paclitaxel	Bradyarrhythmais	Effects on histamine receptor
Tyrosine kinase inhibitors	Ibrutinib (frequent) Ponatinib, Bosutinib, Sorafenib (infrequent)	Atrial arrhythmias	PI3K pathway inhibition; impaired sarcoplasmic reticulum calcium handling; left atrial fibrosis
	Nilotinib, Sunitinib, Vemurafenib, Vandetanib	QT prolongation	Impaired intracellular signaling leading to enhanced late sodium and decreased potassium currents
	Ibrutinib	Ventricular arrhythmias	Unknown
	ALK inhibitors	Bradyarrhythmias	Decrease I_f (funny channel) currents in sinoatrial nodal cells

ALK, Anaplastic lymphoma kinase.

aggressively those patients with cancer with AF, whereas providing appropriate treatment can be challenging and often requires a nuanced, multidisciplinary approach in order for patients to have the best oncologic and CV outcomes.

ANTHRACYCLINES

Although heart failure and left ventricular dysfunction are the most common cardiotoxicities of doxorubicin and other anthracyclines, arrythmias are also frequently encountered. For example, rates of AF with doxorubicin infusion are reported between 6% and 10% in the absence of other cardiovascular pathology.[3,4] Moreover, also found are increased rates of AF in the setting of anthracycline-mediated cardiomyopathy, with a prevalence of more than 50%, which is similar to other nonischemic cardiomyopathy etiologies.[5,6] The arrhythmic mechanism is not clear, but is likely caused by impaired intracellular signaling, damage from free radicals and other toxins, and/or direct myocardial injury.[7]

ALKYLATING AGENTS AND STEM CELL TRANSPLANTATION

Alkylating agents, including melphalan and cyclophosphamide, are a class of cytotoxic chemotherapeutics that disrupt the DNA double helix and are used in the treatment of various solid and hematologic malignancies. Moreover, melphalan is a common agent used in stem cell transplant (SCT) preconditioning regimens. In one study, 11% of patients who received melphalan prior to

SCT developed atrial arrhythmias, including AF, which was significantly higher than in patients who received other treatment regimens.[8] Moreover, SCT itself increases the likelihood of developing AF, with rates as high as 27%.[9] Risk factors for the development of AF after transplant include renal failure, hypertension, and exposure to melphalan. Moreover, the development of AF during transplant portends a worse prognosis, with elevated rates of intensive care unit admissions as well as 30-day and 1-year mortality compared with those patients without arrhythmias.[10]

TYROSINE KINASE INHIBITORS

Tyrosine kinase inhibitors (TKI) affect intracellular pathways that regulate cell growth. A variety of cardiotoxicities are observed with these agents, including AF and other arrhythmias. In one study, the incidence of AF with the TKI sorafenib was reported at 5%.[11] Similarly, arrhythmias can be seen with TKIs used to treat chronic myeloid leukemia that target the BCR-ABL protein. Although vascular toxicities, raging from stroke to myocardial infarction, are most often associated with these TKIs, arrhythmias can also occur. For example, in the EPIC study, the incidence of AF associated with ponatinib use was reported at 3%, compared with 0% for the imatinib treated group.[12] Similarly, rates of AF are around 2% with bosutinib.[13] Whereas the mechanism of arrhythmia remains unclear, it may be related to off-target effects on the phosphoinositide 3-kinase (PI3K) pathway .

Ibrutinib is the TKI most associated with the development of AF. This is a small molecule inhibitor of the Bruton's tyrosine kinase, used to treat various B-cell malignancies, including chronic lymphocytic leukemia (CLL), mantle cell lymphoma, and Waldenstrom's macroglobulinemia, as well as chronic graft-versus-host disease. Rates of AF have been reported between 10% and 15%, with ibrutinib itself identified as an independent risk factor for the development of AF.[14] Other risk factors include a prior history of AF, left atrial enlargement, and an elevated Framingham Heart Study AF risk score.[15] As other Bruton's tyrosine kinase inhibitors, such as acalabrutinib, are associated with a significantly lower incidence of AF, off-target effects of ibrutinib have been postulated, among these. Inhibition of the PI3K pathway, enhanced left atrial fibrosis, and/or impaired sarcoplasmic reticulum calcium handling.

PROTEASOME INHIBITORS

Proteasomes are essential in the elimination of the majority of intracellular proteins, including those modified by oxidative stress and tagged for degradation by the ubiquitin system. Proteasome inhibitors (PIs) block the proteolytic activity of the proteasome complex, leading to protein accumulation, even aggregation, and the activation of apoptotic pathways and cell death. PIs are used primarily in the treatment of multiple myeloma and AL amyloidosis. AF is quite common in patients with multiple myeloma, with a prevalence of 14.6%.[16] This is caused, in part, to PI exposure, particularly to carfilzomib, in which the associated incidence of AF/atrial flutter (AFL) is between 3% and 4%.[17]

IMMUNOTHERAPY

Immunotherapies are an increasingly important class of therapeutics in the treatment of various cancers. They range from immunomodulatory drugs and interleukin-2, to immune checkpoint inhibitors and chimeric antigen receptor therapy. Among the immunomodulatory drugs, atrial arrhythmias are most commonly seen with lenalidomide, occurring in 4% to 7% of patients, especially in combination with a PI.[18] Interleukin-2 therapy is less common and is now used primarily in adoptive cell therapy protocols; however, rates of AF have been reported to exceed 14%.[19] The majority of AF/AFL episodes with ICIs occur in the setting of myocarditis,[20] whereas arrhythmias associated with chimeric antigen receptor therapy often occur as a result of cytokine release syndrome.[21]

MANAGEMENT OF ATRIAL FIBRILLATION AND ATRIAL ARRHYTHMIAS

Whereas the management recommendations for AF in the setting of cancer are similar to the general population, patients with active malignancy undergoing treatment can pose several unique challenges. It is well known that an increased risk of thromboembolism (TE) exists in the setting of AF and atrial

CHA_2DS_2-VASc	Score	HAS-BLED	Score
Congestive heart failure/LV dysfunction	1	Hypertension i.e., uncontrolled BP	1
Hypertension	1	Abnormal renal/liver function	1 or 2
Aged ≥75 years	2	Stroke	1
Diabetes mellitus	1	Bleeding tendency or predisposition	1
Stroke/TIA/TE	2	Lebile INR	1
Vascular disease (prior MI, PAD, or aortic plaque)	1	Age (e.g., >65)	1
Aged 65–74 years	1	Drugs (e.g., concomitant aspirin or NSAIDSs) or alcohol	1
Sex category (i.e., female gender)	1		
Maximum score	**9**		**9**

FIG. 19.1 Overview of the elements of the CHA_2DS_2-VASc score and the HAS-BLED score.

flutter, and this risk may be even higher in patients with cancer. The CHADS-VASc score is the primary determinant of a patient's risk of stroke or TE in the setting of AF or flutter (Fig. 19.1). The mainstay for minimizing this risk is anticoagulation, with current guidelines recommending initiation of anticoagulation in men with a CHADS-VASc of 2 or greater, and in women with a score of 3 or greater.[22] Nevertheless, the CHADS-VASc score has not been validated in patients with cancer and several large epidemiologic studies have highlighted its limitations in this population. For example, a study by D'Souza and colleagues[23] reported higher rates of TE in patients with cancer who had a CHADS-VASc of 1 compared with patients without cancer, but lower rates at higher CHADS-VASc scores.[23] Similarly, a study from Taiwan suggested the risk of ischemic stroke was attenuated with higher CHADS-VASc score in patients with cancer, with an area under the curve suggesting poor predictive ability of this model in those patients.[24] Likewise, there is no validation of the HAS-BLED score, used to assess the patient's risk of bleeding, important for risk-benefit discussions and net benefit determinations and decisions (see Fig. 19.1). As such, risk scores specific to the population of patients with cancer must be developed to help guide appropriate clinical decision-making (Fig. 19.2).

Whereas use of a direct oral anticoagulant (DOAC) is preferred in most situations to reduce the risk of AF-associated stroke and TE, no prospective clinical trials have evaluated the safety and efficacy of these agents in the setting of active malignancies. Nonetheless, an increasing body of retrospective literature supports the use of DOACs in patients with cancer with AF. The results from a substudy of the ARISTOTLE trial with apixaban,[25] and the ENGAGE-AF with edoxaban were promising, suggesting both safety and efficacy.[26] A Marketscan database analysis of over 16,000 patients with cancer and AF reported lower rates of bleeding with apixaban compared with warfarin with similar reductions in stroke and thromboembolism with each of the DOACs and warfarin.[27]

Anticoagulation can be challenging in patients with cancer for various reasons, ranging from drug-drug interactions to increased bleeding complications. Many patients with cancer have hematologic abnormalities, including anemia and thrombocytopenia, as a result of the cancer itself or associated therapies, which make anticoagulation unsafe. Moreover, certain cancer therapeutics can increase the likelihood of bleeding. This is of particular concern with ibrutinib, which is known to increase the risk of bleeding via is effects on the glycogen VI collagen activation pathway as well as inhibition of platelet adhesion via von Willebrand's factor and glycoprotein 1B interactions.[28] In fact, warfarin is typically avoided in patients treated with ibrutinib owing to the increased rates of subdural hematomas. Although DOACs appear generally safe in these patients, a significant potential for drug-drug interactions exists. For example, the Factor Xa inhibitors interact with the cytochrome P450 system and the direct thrombin inhibitor, dabigatran is metabolized via p-glycoprotein. As such, their efficacy and safety can be significantly affected by various cancer therapeutics. Left atrial appendage occlusion devices may be an attractive option for

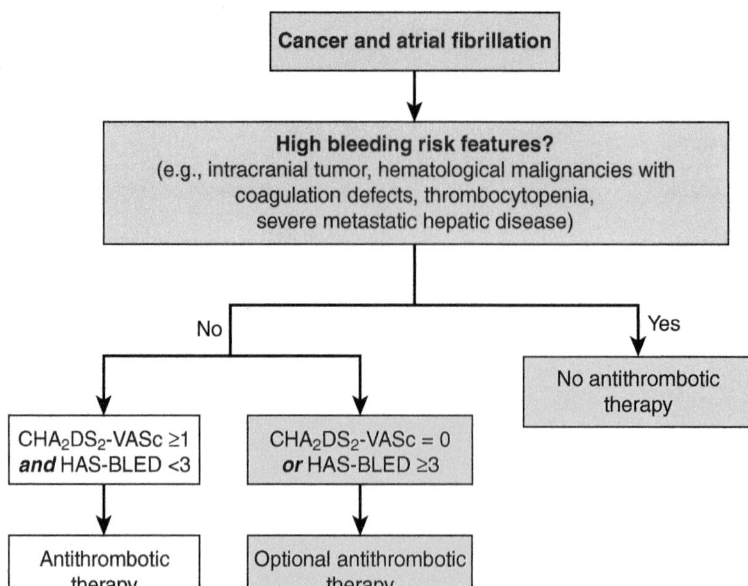

FIG. 19.2 A suggested anticoagulation approach for patients with cancer and with atrial fibrillation. (Modified from Farmakis D, Parissis J, Filippatos G. Insights into onco-cardiology: atrial fibrillation in cancer. *J Am Coll Cardiol.* 2014;63:945–953.)

those patients with cancer with chronic bleeding diatheses; however, these patients must be able to tolerate at least short-term anticoagulation and longer-term antiplatelet medications.[29] Last but not least, decisions on anticoagulation and stroke prevention strategies likely vary across the cancer continuum (Fig. 19.3).

Treatment of atrial fibrillation itself focuses on rate control versus rhythm control. It should be recognized that drug-drug interactions are also of significant concern in this setting, because nondihydropyridine calcium channel blockers also interact with the cytochrome P450 system and various antiarrhythmics can lead to significant QT prolongation, which can be augmented with numerous cancer drugs. An illustrating example is ibrutinib; verapamil and diltiazem are to be avoided in patients on this TKI because these calcium channel blockers are potent CYP3A4 inhibitors, and concomitant treatment can increase ibrutinib serum concentrations up to 900%. Likewise, amiodarone should be avoided because ibrutinib inhibits p-glycoprotein and may increase amiodarone serum concentrations. The preferred and first-line therapy should be a beta-blocker. Catheter ablation is an option; however, its safety and efficacy have not been specifically studied in patients with cancer. Given that the pathophysiology of cancer-associated AF may be different than in the general population, the benefits of ablation may not be as significant.[30]

QT PROLONGATION AND VENTRICULAR ARRHYTHMIAS

Ventricular arrhythmias occur less frequently than atrial arrhythmias; however, the potential for serous life-threatening complications is significant. Ventricular arrythmias, specifically torsades de pointes (TdP) can occur as a result of QT interval prolongation. Multiple cancer therapeutics are associated with QT prolongation; however, the actual arrhythmic risk remains quite low, especially if appropriate risk mitigation strategies, including electrolyte repletion and avoidance of other QT prolonging drugs, are employed. Ventricular arrhythmias can also occur in the absence of QT interval prolongation, either as a consequence of another CV toxicity such as ischemia, or via direct arrhythmogenesis to myocardial cells.

ANTHRACYCLINES

Although ventricular arrhythmias have been reported with anthracyclines, this occurs primarily in the setting of anthracycline-induced cardiomyopathy.

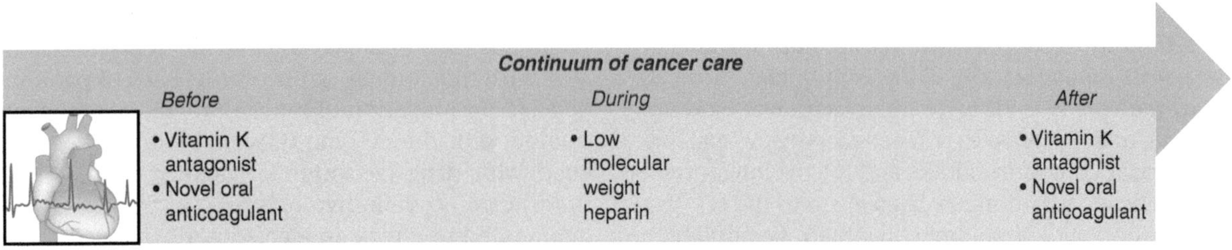

Continuum of cancer care		
Before	During	After
• Vitamin K antagonist • Novel oral anticoagulant	• Low molecular weight heparin	• Vitamin K antagonist • Novel oral anticoagulant

	VKA	LMWH	Novel oral anticoagulant
Reversibility	Vitamin K, FFP, prothrombin complex conc.	Protamine (but does not completely abolish the anti-Xa activ. of LMWH)	Idarucizumab (Praxbind) for dabigatran Andexanet alfa (Andexxa) if available or 4-factor prothrombin complex concentrate for all other
Drug-drug inter.	+++	+	+++
Reduced renal function	Preferred if ESRD w/HD	Caution if eGFR <30 mL/min, monitor F.Xa	Reduce rivaroxaban and endoxaban if eGFR 15–50 Reduce dabigatran
Reduced liver function	Not required	Not required	Not recommended with mod to sev. (rivaroxaban and endoxaban) severe (apixaban) liver dysfunction
Costs	Low	High	High
Comments	Inconvenience with recurrent INR checks	HIT Discomfort Challenging long-term	Lack of ample experience and publications in patients with cancer; Concerns for use in patients with GI (and GU) tract lesions

FIG. 19.3 Illustration of the preferred choices for specific anticoagulation therapies in patients with cancer and atrial fibrillation.

In a study by Mazur and colleagues,[6] 73.9% of patients with an anthracycline-induced cardiomyopathy experienced nonsustained ventricular tachycardia with 30.4% having either sustained ventricular tachycardia (VT) or ventricular fibrillation (VF). Similar results were reported by Fradley and colleagues[5] with an incidence of nonsustained VT, VT, or VF at 44.4%, which was similar to other nonischemic etiologies evaluated.[5] Anthracyclines have little direct effect on the ventricular conduction system and the risk of significant QT prolongation is rare.[31]

ARSENIC TRIOXIDE

Arsenic trioxide is used primarily in the treatment of acute promyelocytic leukemia. It has significant QT prolonging effects; in one study evaluating over 3000 electrocardiograms from 113 patients, 26% demonstrated a Fridercia-corrected QT interval of more than 500 msec. There were no reported episodes of TdP however.[32] Excellent risk mitigation strategies have minimized reported episodes of TdP. Despite the rare occurrence of ventricular arrhythmias with this therapeutic, the United States Food and Drug Administration has issued a Black Box warning for increased risk of sudden death.

FLUOROPYRIMIDINES

The majority of ventricular arrhythmias associated with 5-fluorouracil (5FU) and other fluoropyrimidines occur in the setting of myocardial ischemia from coronary vasospasm. Direct electrical toxicity is rare, with no evidence of significant QT prolonging effects. Whereas studies have suggested an increased burden of premature ventricular contractions (PVCs) within the first 24 hours of 5FU infusions, a subsequent meta-analysis failed to show a significantly increased risk of sustained ventricular arrhythmias.[33]

TYROSINE KINASE INHIBITORS

QT prolongation can be a significant issue with various TKIs, with multiple agents having standard or Black Box warnings for QT prolongation and sudden death. Despite this, documented adverse clinical events are quite rare. Unlike many pharmaceuticals that directly block potassium channels leading to delays in repolarization, TKIs likely affect intracellular pathways leading to increased late sodium current and decreased potassium current causing repolarization abnormalities and QT prolongation.

Significant attention has been given to the QT prolonging potential of nilotinib, sunitinib, vemurafenib, and vandetanib. Nilotinib is a BCR-ABL TKI used primarily in the treatment of chronic myeloid leukemia and sunitinib, a TKI used primarily in metastatic renal cell carcinoma. Vandetanib is used primarily in medullary thyroid cancer, whereas vandetanib is used to treat advanced melanoma. In phase 1 clinical trials of nilotinib, the mean QT prolongation was 5 to 15 msec. In the ENESTnd trial, no QT intervals greater than 500 msec nor episodes of TdP were reported.[34] The incidence of sunitinib-induced QT prolongation greater than 500 msec was 2.3%, with malignant arrhythmias occurring is less than 0.1% of treated patients.[7] Vandetanib carries a Black Box warning for QT prolongation and sudden cardiac death (SCD). In a meta-analysis of nine trials, the incidence of all grade QT prolongation was 16% to 18%, with a 3.7% to 12% incidence of high-grade prolongation.[35] Among patients treated with vemurafenib, 7% demonstrated a QT interval of more than 480 msec with 3% having a QT interval greater than 500 msec. A recent meta-analysis by Porta-Sanchez and colleagues[31] confirmed the QT prolonging potential of nilotinib, sunitinib, and vandetanib; however, it was not predictive of TdP or other life-threatening ventricular arrhythmias.

Ibrutinib is also associated with increased rates of ventricular arrhythmias, independent of QT prolongation. In fact, suggestion is that ibrutinib may lead to QT shortening. A study of the Federal Drug Administration Adverse Reporting System (FAERS) identified seven episodes of VT/VF and six cases of sudden cardiac death.[36] Guha and colleagues[37] reported the incidence of ibrutinib-associated ventricular arrhythmias at 678 per 100,000 person years, considerably higher than patients not taking the drug. The exact arrhythmogenic mechanism remains uncertain.

CYCLIN-DEPENDENT KINASE 4/6 INHIBITORS

Cyclin-dependent kinase 4/6 inhibitors disrupt cell cycle replication and are approved for the treatment of hormone-receptor-positive, HER2 negative advanced breast cancer. The QT prolonging potential is not class related as only ribociclib is associated with this finding. In one study, 3.3% of patients had QT prolongation of more than 480 msec when treated with the 600 mg dose. QT intervals shortened with drug cessation or dose reduction and there were no definitive episodes of SCD. It is recommended to check an electrocardiogram at baseline and again day 14 during the first cycle and the beginning of the second cycle. Therapy should be withheld if the QTcF is greater than 450 msec and stopped if the QTcF exceeds 480 msec.[38]

BRADYARRHYTHMIAS AND AUTONOMIC DYSFUNCTION

Bradyarrhythmias secondary to cancer therapeutics are relatively uncommon and rarely require intervention. Several agents are associated with heart rate slowing and/or heart block, including anaplastic lymphoma kinase (ALK) inhibitors, taxanes, and immune checkpoint inhibitors. Bradycardia is commonly observed with the ALK inhibitor crizotinib, a TKI used primarily to treat non–small-cell lung cancer, with an average decline in heart rate of 26.1 beats per minute.[39] In a retrospective study of 1053 patients, 42% of individuals experienced sinus bradycardia; however, only 9 patients required dose/treatment adjustment owing to associated symptoms.[40] Interestingly, the development of bradycardia was associated with enhanced antitumor response. Another ALK inhibitor, ceritinib, is also associated with bradycardia, but at lower rates, affecting approximately 3% of those treated with the drug.[41] A proposed mechanism for ALK inhibitor-induced bradycardia may be off-target effects leading to a decrease in the I_f (funny channel) currents in sinoatrial nodal cells.[40]

Bradycardia is also a frequently encountered with the taxanes, especially paclitaxel; however, it is rarely clinically significant. In one phase 2 study of patients with ovarian cancer receiving paclitaxel, 29% experienced asymptomatic bradycardia.[42] In another study of 140 patients, 1 person developed high degree atrioventricular (AV) block requiring pacemaker implantation.[43] Bradycardia from taxanes may be related to its off-target effects on the histamine receptor leading to conduction delay through the AV node and His/Purkinje system.[44]

Although myocarditis is the most common cardiotoxicity observed with immune checkpoint inhibitor

(ICI), arrhythmias including heart block can often be the initial manifestation of this process. In fact, in a large multicenter registry, an abnormal electrocardiogram and abnormal troponin were the most common findings associated with the development of major adverse cardiac events.[45] Complete heart block in the setting of ICI myocarditis should be managed aggressively with a low threshold for permanent pacemaker implantation along with anti-inflammatory treatment for the underlying disease process.[46]

Beyond bradycardia, autonomic dysfunction is another frequent complication of cancer therapeutics, particularly chest and neck radiation. For example, Hodgkin's lymphoma survivors who received thoracic radiation demonstrated increased resting heart rates and abnormal heart rate recovery and blood pressure response to exercise.[47] Patients who receive neck radiation are at risk for baroreceptor dysfunction, which can lead to multiple autonomic abnormalities. Chemotherapies can also be associated with autonomic abnormalities: studies have shown decreased heart rate variability after exposure to anthracyclines, even in the setting of normal left ventricle function.[48]

CARDIAC IMPLANTABLE ELECTRONIC DEVICES

Damage to cardiac implantable electronic devices (CIEDs), including pacemakers and defibrillators, from external beam ionizing radiation is quite rare. The overwhelming majority of patients with CIEDs can safely receive radiation. Nevertheless, certain precautions can be taken to ensure device and patient safety during radiation protocols. The amount of cardiac monitoring during radiation depends on the patient-specific factors, including pacemaker dependency and underlying medical conditions. Continuous electrocardiography should be considered in patients at high risk, such as those who are pacemaker dependent, along with device reprogramming to asynchronous mode or the application of a magnet.[49] For patients with implantable cardioverter defibrillators (ICDs), the use of a magnet or reprogramming to deactivate tachy-therapies is controversial because the risk of inappropriate shocks is exceedingly low.[50]

In patients with pacemakers who are receiving radiation with beam energy less than 10 MV, additional device evaluations during therapy are not indicated. If the radiation is greater than 10 MV, weekly device evaluation is recommended to ensure stable pacing and sensing parameters. Weekly device evaluation is also recommended in patients with ICDs receiving less than 10 MV of beam energy because ICDs are generally thought to be more sensitive to radiation damage. If the beam energy is greater than 10 MV, it is recommended that patients with ICDs undergo device evaluation after every fraction of radiation. For those at very high risk, a knowledgeable electrophysiologist should be readily available to assist with any clinical management issues.[50]

REFERENCES

1. O'Neal WT, Lakoski SG, Qureshi W, et al. Relation between cancer and atrial fibrillation (from the REasons for Geographic And Racial Differences in Stroke Study). *Am J Cardiol.* 2015;115(8):1090–1094. doi:10.1016/j.amjcard.2015.01.540.
2. Rahman F, Ko D, Benjamin EJ. Association of atrial fibrillation and cancer. *JAMA Cardiol.* 2016;1(4):384–386. doi:10.1001/jamacardio.2016.0582.
3. Amioka M, Sairaku A, Ochi T, et al. Prognostic significance of new-onset atrial fibrillation in patients with non-Hodgkin's lymphoma treated with anthracyclines. *Am J Cardiol.* 2016;118(9):1386–1389. doi:10.1016/j.amjcard.2016.07.049.
4. Kilickap S, Barista I, Akgul E, Aytemir K, Aksoy S, Tekuzman, G. Early and late arrhythmogenic effects of doxorubicin. *South Med J.* 2007;100(3):262–265. doi:10.1097/01.smj.0000257382.89910.fe.
5. Fradley MG, Viganego F, Kip K, et al. Rates and risk of arrhythmias in cancer survivors with chemotherapy-induced cardiomyopathy compared with patients with other cardiomyopathies. *Open Heart.* 2017;4(2):e000701. doi:10.1136/openhrt-2017-000701.
6. Mazur M, Wang F, Hodge DO, et al. Burden of cardiac arrhythmias in patients with anthracycline-related cardiomyopathy. *JACC Clin Electrophysiol.* 2017;3(2):139–150. doi:10.1016/j.jacep.2016.08.009.
7. Tamargo J, Caballero R, Delpon E. Cancer chemotherapy and cardiac arrhythmias: a review. *Drug Saf.* 2015;38(2):129–152. doi:10.1007/s40264-014-0258-4.
8. Feliz V, Saiyad S, Ramarao SM, et al. Melphalan-induced supraventricular tachycardia: incidence and risk factors. *Clin Cardiol.* 2011; 34(6):356–359. doi:10.1002/clc.20904.
9. Sureddi RK, Amani F, Hebbar P, et al. Atrial fibrillation following autologous stem cell transplantation in patients with multiple myeloma: incidence and risk factors. *Ther Adv Cardiovasc Dis.* 2012; 6(6):229–236. doi:10.1177/1753944712464102.
10. Tonorezos ES, Stillwell EE, Calloway JJ, et al. Arrhythmias in the setting of hematopoietic cell transplants. *Bone Marrow Transplant.* 2015;50(9):1212–1216. doi:10.1038/bmt.2015.127.
11. Petrini I, Lencioni M, Ricasoli M, et al. Phase II trial of sorafenib in combination with 5-fluorouracil infusion in advanced hepatocellular carcinoma. *Cancer Chemother Pharmacol.* 2012;69(3):773–780. doi:10.1007/s00280-011-1753-2.
12. Lipton JH, Chuah C, Guerci-Bresler A, et al. Ponatinib versus imatinib for newly diagnosed chronic myeloid leukaemia: an international, randomised, open-label, phase 3 trial. *Lancet Oncol.* 2016;17(5):612–621. doi:10.1016/S1470-2045(16)00080-2.
13. Kantarjian HM, Cortes JE, Kim DW, et al. Bosutinib safety and management of toxicity in leukemia patients with resistance or intolerance to imatinib and other tyrosine kinase inhibitors. *Blood.* 2014;123(9):1309–1318. doi:10.1182/blood-2013-07-513937.
14. Fradley MG, Gliksman M, Emole J, et al. Rates and risk of atrial arrhythmias in patients treated with ibrutinib compared with cytotoxic chemotherapy. *Am J Cardiol.* 2019;124(4):539–544. doi:10.1016/j.amjcard.2019.05.029.
15. Wiczer TE, Levine LB, Brumbaugh J, et al. Cumulative incidence, risk factors, and management of atrial fibrillation in patients receiving

ibrutinib. *Blood Adv.* 2017;1(20):1739–1748. doi:10.1182/bloodadvances.2017009720.

16. Shah N, Rochlani Y, Pothineni NV, Paydak, H. Burden of arrhythmias in patients with multiple myeloma. *Int J Cardiol.* 2016;203:305–306. doi:10.1016/j.ijcard.2015.10.083.
17. Atrash S, Tullos A, Panozzo S, et al. Cardiac complications in relapsed and refractory multiple myeloma patients treated with carfilzomib. *Blood Cancer J.* 2015;5:e272. doi:10.1038/bcj.2014.93.
18. Lee DH, Fradley MG. Cardiovascular complications of multiple myeloma treatment: evaluation, management, and prevention. *Curr Treat Options Cardiovasc Med.* 2018;20(3):19. doi:10.1007/s11936-018-0618-y.
19. Siegel JP, Puri RK. Interleukin-2 toxicity. *J Clin Oncol.* 1991;9(4):694–704. doi:10.1200/JCO.1991.9.4.694.
20. Heinzerling L, Ott PA, Hodi FS, et al. Cardiotoxicity associated with CTLA4 and PD1 blocking immunotherapy. *J Immunother Cancer.* 2016;4:50. doi:10.1186/s40425-016-0152-y.
21. Bonifant CL, Jackson HJ, Brentjens RJ, Curran KJ. Toxicity and management in CAR T-cell therapy. *Mol Ther Oncolytics.* 2016;3:16011. doi:10.1038/mto.2016.11.
22. January CT, Wann LS, Calkins H, et al. 2019 AHA/ACC/HRS focused update of the 2014 AHA/ACC/HRS guideline for the management of patients with atrial fibrillation: a report of the American College of Cardiology/American Heart Association task force on clinical practice guidelines and the Heart Rhythm Society in Collaboration with the Society of Thoracic Surgeons. *Circulation.* 2019;140(2):e125–e151. doi:10.1161/CIR.0000000000000665.
23. D'Souza M, Carlson N, Fosbol E, et al. CHA2DS2-VASc score and risk of thromboembolism and bleeding in patients with atrial fibrillation and recent cancer. *Eur J Prev Cardiol.* 2018;25(6):651–658. doi:10.1177/2047487318759858.
24. Hu WS, Lin CL. Impact of atrial fibrillation on the development of ischemic stroke among patients with cancer classified by CHA2DS2-VASc score-a nationwide cohort study. *Oncotarget.* 2018;9(7):7623–7630. doi:10.18632/oncotarget.24143.
25. Melloni C, Dunning A, Granger CB, et al. Efficacy and safety of apixaban versus warfarin in patients with atrial fibrillation and a history of cancer: insights from the ARISTOTLE trial. *Am J Med.* 2017;130(12):1440–1448.e1441. doi:10.1016/j.amjmed.2017.06.026.
26. Fanola CL, Ruff CT, Murphy SA, et al. Efficacy and safety of edoxaban in patients with active malignancy and atrial fibrillation: analysis of the ENGAGE AF - TIMI 48 trial. *J Am Heart Assoc.* 2018;7(16):e008987. doi:10.1161/JAHA.118.008987.
27. Shah S, Norby FL, Datta YH, et al. Comparative effectiveness of direct oral anticoagulants and warfarin in patients with cancer and atrial fibrillation. *Blood Adv.* 2018;2(3):200–209. doi:10.1182/bloodadvances.2017010694.
28. Levade M, David E, Garcia C, et al. Ibrutinib treatment affects collagen and von Willebrand factor-dependent platelet functions. *Blood.* 2014;124(26):3991–3995. doi:10.1182/blood-2014-06-583294.
29. Rhea IB, Lyon AR, Fradley MG. Antiscoagulation of cardiovascular conditions in the patient with cancer: review of old and new therapies. *Curr Oncol Rep.* 2019;21(5):45. doi:10.1007/s11912-019-0797-z.
30. Rhea I, Burgos PH, Fradley MG. Arrhythmogenic anticancer drugs in cardio-oncology. *Cardiol Clin.* 2019;37(4):459–468. doi:10.1016/j.ccl.2019.07.011.
31. Porta-Sanchez A, Gilbert C, Spears D, et al. Incidence, diagnosis, and management of QT prolongation induced by cancer therapies: a systematic review. *J Am Heart Assoc.* 2017;6(12):e007724. doi:10.1161/JAHA.117.007724.
32. Roboz GJ, Ritchie EK, Carlin RF, et al. Prevalence, management, and clinical consequences of QT interval prolongation during treatment with arsenic trioxide. *J Clin Oncol.* 2014;32(33):3723–3728. doi:10.1200/JCO.2013.51.2913.
33. Abdel-Rahman O. 5-Fluorouracil-related cardiotoxicity: findings from five randomized studies of 5-fluorouracil-based regimens in metastatic colorectal cancer. *Clin Colorectal Cancer.* 2019;18(1):58–63. doi:10.1016/j.clcc.2018.10.006.
34. Kim TD, le Coutre P, Schwarz M, et al. Clinical cardiac safety profile of nilotinib. *Haematologica.* 2012;97(6):883–889. doi:10.3324/haematol.2011.058776.
35. Zang J, Wu S, Tang L, et al. Incidence and risk of QTc interval prolongation among patients with cancer treated with vandetanib: a systematic review and meta-analysis. *PLoS One.* 2012;7(2):e30353. doi:10.1371/journal.pone.0030353.
36. Lampson BL, Yu L, Glynn RJ, et al. Ventricular arrhythmias and sudden death in patients taking ibrutinib. *Blood.* 2017;129(18):2581–2584. doi:10.1182/blood-2016-10-742437.
37. Guha A, Derbala MH, Zhao Q, et al. Ventricular arrhythmias following ibrutinib initiation for lymphoid malignancies. *J Am Coll Cardiol.* 2018;72(6):697–698. doi:10.1016/j.jacc.2018.06.002.
38. Spring LM, Zangardi ML, Moy B, Bardia A. Clinical management of potential toxicities and drug interactions related to cyclin-dependent kinase 4/6 inhibitors in breast cancer: practical considerations and recommendations. *Oncologist.* 2017;22(9):1039–1048. doi:10.1634/theoncologist.2017-0142.
39. Ou SH, Tong WP, Azada M, Siwak-Tapp C, Dy J, Stiber JA. Heart rate decrease during crizotinib treatment and potential correlation to clinical response. *Cancer.* 2013;119(11):1969–1975. doi:10.1002/cncr.28040.
40. Ou SH, Tang Y, Polli A, Wilner KD, Schnell, P. Factors associated with sinus bradycardia during crizotinib treatment: a retrospective analysis of two large-scale multinational trials (PROFILE 1005 and 1007). *Cancer Med.* 2016;5(4):617–622. doi:10.1002/cam4.622.
41. Khozin S, Blumenthal GM, Zhang L, et al. FDA approval: ceritinib for the treatment of metastatic anaplastic lymphoma kinase-positive non-small cell lung cancer. *Clin Cancer Res.* 2015;21(11):2436–2439. doi:10.1158/1078-0432.CCR-14-3157.
42. McGuire WP, Rowinsky EK, Rosenshein NB, et al. Taxol: a unique antineoplastic agent with significant activity in advanced ovarian epithelial neoplasms. *Ann Intern Med.* 1989;111(4):273–279. doi:10.7326/0003-4819-111-4-273.
43. Rowinsky EK, McGuire WP, Guarnieri T, Fisherman JS, Christian MC, Donehower RC. Cardiac disturbances during the administration of taxol. *J Clin Oncol.* 1991;9(9):1704–1712. doi:10.1200/JCO.1991.9.9.1704.
44. Arbuck SG, Strauss H, Rowinsky E, et al. A reassessment of cardiac toxicity associated with Taxol. *J Natl Cancer Inst Monogr.* 1993;(15):117–130.
45. Mahmood SS, Fradley MG, Cohen JV, et al. Myocarditis in patients treated with immune checkpoint inhibitors. *J Am Coll Cardiol.* 2018;71(16):1755–1764. doi:10.1016/j.jacc.2018.02.037.
46. Johnson DB, Balko JM, Compton ML, et al. Fulminant myocarditis with combination immune checkpoint blockade. *N Engl J Med.* 2016;375(18):1749–1755. doi:10.1056/NEJMoa1609214.
47. Groarke JD, Tanguturi VK, Hainer J, et al. Abnormal exercise response in long-term survivors of Hodgkin lymphoma treated with thoracic irradiation: evidence of cardiac autonomic dysfunction and impact on outcomes. *J Am Coll Cardiol.* 2015;65(6):573–583. doi:10.1016/j.jacc.2014.11.035.
48. Lakoski SG, Jones LW, Krone RJ, Stein PK, Scott JM. Autonomic dysfunction in early breast cancer: incidence, clinical importance, and underlying mechanisms. *Am Heart J.* 2015;170(2):231–241. doi:10.1016/j.ahj.2015.05.014.
49. Hurkmans CW, Knegjens JL, Oei BS, et al. Management of radiation oncology patients with a pacemaker or ICD: a new comprehensive practical guideline in The Netherlands. Dutch Society of Radiotherapy and Oncology (NVRO). *Radiat Oncol.* 2012;7:198. doi:10.1186/1748-717X-7-198.
50. Zecchin M, Severgnini M, Fiorentino A, et al. Management of patients with cardiac implantable electronic devices (CIED) undergoing radiotherapy: a consensus document from Associazione Italiana Aritmologia e Cardiostimolazione (AIAC), Associazione Italiana Radioterapia Oncologica (AIRO), Associazione Italiana Fisica Medica (AIFM). *Int J Cardiol.* 2018;255:175–183. doi:10.1016/j.ijcard.2017.12.061.

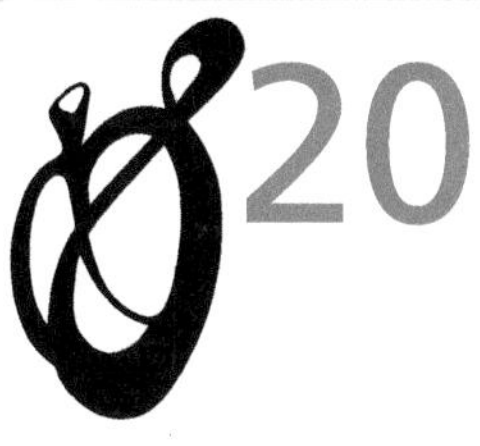

20 Hypertension and Renal Disease During Anti-Cancer Therapies

SANDRA M.S. HERRMANN, STEPHEN J.H. DOBBIN, JOERG HERRMANN, RHIAN M. TOUYZ, AND NINIAN N. LANG

Acute kidney injury in the cancer patient

Cancer (patient)-related causes

Prerenal
- Hypercalcemia
- Testing (e.g., IV contrast)
- Cardiomyopathy/heart failure (e.g., low output)

Intrarenal
- Lymphomatous infiltration
- Light chain (LC) cast nephropathy
- LC deposition disease (LCDD)
- Heavy chain DD
- Proximal LC tubulopathy
- Monoclonal gammopathy of renal significance (MGRS)
- Membranous nephropathy (e.g., solid tumors)
- Minimal change disease (e.g., hematologic malignancies)
- Prolonged hypotension

Postrenal
- Retroperitoneal fibrosis
- Tumor ureteral obstruction
- Nephrolithiasis
- Benign prostate hypertrophy
- Prostate, cervical cancer

Treatment-related causes

Prerenal
- Sepsis
- Volume depletion/ blood loss
- Veno-occlusive disease/hepatic sinusoidal obstructive syndrome
- Capillary leak syndrome (IL-2)

Intrarenal
- Tumor lysis syndrome
- Proximal tubular injury (e.g., Cisplatin)
- ATN (e.g., Ifosfamide, Imatinib)
- Crystal nephropathy (e.g., Methotrexate)
- AIN (e.g., VEGF-I, ICI)
- TMA (e.g., VEGF-I, Cisplatin, Gemcitabine)

Postrenal
- Bladder outlet obstruction, e.g., secondary to hemorrhagic cystitis with cyclophosphamide

CHAPTER OUTLINE

KEY POINTS

- Blood pressure measurement is part of the routine assessment during clinic or hospital-delivered cancer care, but should also be measured at home where possible, especially in patients receiving oral cancer therapy, such as vascular endothelial growth factor inhibitors (VEGFIs; weekly during the first cycle, then every 2 to 3 weeks).
- The treatment goal during VEGFI therapy should be less than 130/80 mm Hg, ideally, and not above 140/90 mm Hg in general, balancing risk and benefit of cardiovascular and oncologic treatment.
- Cancer therapies can usually be continued if blood pressure elevation is in the absence of clinically evident end-organ effects and can be managed with antihypertensive drugs.
- Non-dihydropyridine calcium channel antagonists (diltiazem, verapamil) should be avoided in patients on VEGF and Bruton's tyrosine kinase inhibitors because of drug-drug interactions.
- Angiotensin converting enzyme (ACE) inhibitors and angiotensin receptor blocker (ARBs) should be used carefully in patients with cancer at risk of or with evident volume depletion.
- Hypertension should prompt an evaluation of renal function in patients with cancer, including assessment for proteinuria, because it might be part of a broader syndrome.
- Worsening renal function, acute on chronic, or acute kidney injury (AKI) is not uncommon; categories include prerenal, intrarenal, and postrenal factors as seen in the general population, but with some unique nuances relating mainly to cancer therapies.
- The development of AKI should prompt a nephrology, ideally onco-nephrology, consultation as well as multidisciplinary discussions on cancer therapy.

HYPERTENSION RISK DURING ANTI-CANCER THERAPIES

VEGF Inhibitors

Most cancer therapeutics that have been associated with hypertension have an antiangiogenic, vascular effect in common. The classic examples of this are VEGFIs. Indeed, the introduction of VEGFIs highlighted the importance of blood pressure management in the context of cancer therapy.[1] VEGFI treatment causes an increase in blood pressure in almost all patients (up to 60% to 80% of patients in clinical trials).[2] In a carefully characterized registry cohort, 73% of patients with renal cell cancer receiving targeted therapy (mainly VEGFI), developed cardiovascular toxicity, 55% of which was accounted for by hypertension.[3] VEGFI-associated hypertension develops quickly, and may be difficult to treat, interferring with the delivery of optimal anti-cancer VEGFI therapy.[1,4–7] In addition to the acute effects of hypertension, as patients survive longer and receive VEGFIs for prolonged periods, the risk of chronic end-organ effects of hypertension, including myocardial ischaemia and infarction, heart failure, renal dysfunction, and stroke, are of increasing concern.[1]

Variability in the definitions used for clinical trial reporting, together with blood pressure thresholds that are greater than those in evidence-based hypertension guidelines, means that the incidence of VEGFI-associated hypertension may be underestimated.[1,7,8] Additionally, patients with complicated hypertension or a history of cardiovascular disease are usually excluded from clinical trials and accordingly the *real world* incidence of VEGFI-associated hypertension may be higher than reported.[1,7] There have, however, been efforts to improve standardization of the definition of VEGFI-associated hypertension, with recommendations that such a diagnosis requires that the blood pressure be greater than 140/90 mm Hg on two to three occasions at least one week apart for most patients. The threshold for diagnosis is lower (130/80 mm Hg) for patients with additional cardiovascular risk factors, such as diabetes mellitus or renal impairment.[1,9,10] These definitions are based in large part on earlier guidelines where blood pressure targets were set at 140/90 mm Hg. However, many major current guidelines have lowered the definition of hypertension to a cutoff of 130/80 mm Hg[11–14] and, accordingly, the definition of VEGFI-induced hypertension may also require modification. Based on the effect of VEGFI on the endothelium and the vasculature, these patients can be viewed as being at higher risk in general.

Within hours to days of starting treatment with VEGFIs, blood pressure rises in a dose-dependent manner.[1,2,15] This is potentiated when multiple anti-angiogenic agents are used in combination. In patients with renal cell cancer treated with sunitinib, blood pressure increased by an average of 14/11 mm Hg in the first week of treatment and by 22/17 mm Hg in the second week. This effect was persistent during sunitinib treatment, but reversed rapidly once VEGFI was withdrawn.[2] The rapid and early rise in blood pressure can provoke acute complications, for example, in patients not previously 'conditioned' to the effects of hypertension an acute rise in blood pressure can precipitate acute end-organ complications, such as stroke, myocardial ischaemia, heart failure, and acute kidney injury at a lower threshold than might be expected in patients with long-standing hypertension.[16] Posterior reversible leukoencephalopathy can occur, although this is rare (<1% of patients treated with VEGFI). Clinical signs and symptoms include headache, confusion, seizures, and visual impairment. Magnetic resonance T2-weighed imaging of the brain reveals edema, classically within the posterior fossa.[17] The underlying pathophysiology seems to be related to the combination of hypertension, impaired cerebral autoregulation and cerebrovascular permeability/endothelial dysfunction.[1] Importantly, with early recognition/diagnosis, prompt treatment of hypertension, and withdrawal of VEGFI therapy, the, prognosis is favorable.

The mechanisms responsible for VEGFI-associated hypertension remain incompletely defined, but alterations in vascular tone appear to be of fundamental importance. Proposed mechanisms include endothelial dysfunction, oxidative stress, upregulation of the endothelin-1 system, activation of the renin angiotensin aldosterone system, capillary rarefaction, and vascular remodelling as well as renal dysfunction with impaired sodium handling and increased salt sensitivity. There is a complex relationship between these various factors, and the relative contribution of each mechanism may vary at different stages in the progression of acute hypertensive effects through to sustained and chronically elevated blood pressures. Combination of VEGFI and other anti-cancer drugs may amplify hypertension and renal toxicity. For instance, in patients with hepatocellular carcinoma, treatment with combination VEGFI (bevacizumab) and programmed death 1 inhibitors (atezolizumab), was associated with a higher rate of hypertension and proteinuria than in patients treated with VEGFI (sorafenib) alone.[18]

Conflicting evidence exists regarding risk factors predisposing patients to VEGFI-induced hypertension. Conventional cardiovascular risk factors, including older age (>65 years), previous history of hypertension, smoking, elevated body mass index, and possibly hypercholesterolemia have been linked with an increased risk of VEGF-induced hypertension.[1,19] However, other studies have suggested that these factors and others, including a history of vascular disease, reduced renal function, and family history of hypertension or cardiovascular disease are not predictive.[6,20]

As hypertension associated with VEGFI agents occurs as a pharmacodynamic on-target effect,[21] it has been proposed that it may reflect effective inhibition of the VEGF signalling pathway and could be gauged as an indicator of the therapeutic response.[22] Indeed, supportive evidence indicates that the development of VEGFI-associated hypertension is associated with one to two years greater progression-free and overall survival.[21,22] In light of this association between the development of hypertension and improved anti-cancer responses, it has been suggested that VEGFI-induced hypertension could be used to define the optimal biologically active doses of VEGFI drugs. However, this suggestion should be considered cautiously and the development of hypertension should not be used as a measure to guide the maximum possible dose of VEGFI agents for individual patients.[21]

Non-VEGFIs

Although VEGFIs represent the class of anti-cancer drugs most associated with treatment-induced hypertension, it may also be encountered as a result of other anti-cancer agents, including platinum-based therapies, proteasome inhibitors, and mammalian target of rapamycin (mTOR) inhibitors and as a result of corticosteroid therapy, either alone or as adjuvant therapy.[23,24]

Platinum-Based Therapies

Hypertension is a well-recognized complication of cisplatin-based chemotherapy, noted in 14% to 53% of patients even many years after the completion of therapy.[24,25] It is believed that endothelial dysfunction is the main cause of cisplatin-induced hypertension.[26]

Platinum compounds also cause dose-dependent and frequently irreversible nephrotoxicity.[27] The pathophysiologic mechanisms responsible for this are thought to be similar to those seen in the development of hypertension, with endothelial dysfunction as a major factor. In support of this theory, microalbuminuria, a sensitive marker of endothelial dysfunction, is present in up to 22% of patients at least 10 years after cisplatin-based chemotherapy for metastatic testicular cancer.[24,26] Furthermore, patients with microalbuminuria following cisplatin-based chemotherapy have higher blood pressures than those who do not.[24]

Proteasome Inhibitors

Hypertension has been associated with each of the proteasome inhibitors currently in use (bortezomib, carfilzomib, and ixazomib), with the majority of cases being low-grade and reversible. Carfilzomib is the most potent anti-myeloma drug in this class and is also most commonly associated with hypertension.[28] In a head-to-head comparsion of bortezomib-based therapy *versus* carfilzomib-based therapy, grade 1 or 2 hypertension was seen in 6% of patients treated with bortezomib and in 16% of those in the carfilzomib treatment arm. Grade 3 hypertension was evident in 3% and 9% of patients treated with bortezomib and carfilzomib, respectively.[29] Proteasome inhibitor-associated hypertension may be a reflection of reduced nitric oxide bioavailability, with the blood pressure rise often being further exacerbated by the use of corticosteroids.

Mammalian Target of Rapamycin (mTOR) Inhibitors

Mammalian target of rapamycin inhibitors, such as everolimus, sirolimus, and temsirolimus have antitumor activity against a number of malignancies, particularly advanced renal cell carcinoma and breast cancer. Clinical evidence also derives from their widespread use following solid organ transplantation[30] hypertension in up to 30% of patients receiving everolimus and almost 40% of patients treated with sirolimus.[30] The incidence of hypertension as an adverse effect of mTOR inhibitors used in the treatment of malignancy is less well described, although it could be expected to be similarly high. These agents are also associated with the development of proteinuria and edema.[31]

Monitoring Blood Pressure During Cancer Treatment

Although blood pressure control is important for patients receiving any form of cancer therapy, the rapid and potentially substantial rise in response to VEGFI means that this group should be considered a particularly high-risk group for whom specific strategies apply (Table 20.1).

In addition to blood pressure monitoring at baseline prior to beginning VEGFI therapy, blood pressure should be monitored regularly throughout treatment. Monitoring is particularly relevant in the early stages of treatment when the risk of acute rises in blood pressure is greatest.[20,32] It is recommended that blood pressure be monitored on a weekly basis during the first cycle of treatment and at least every two to three weeks thereafter.[10]

Office blood pressures should be measured based on clinical guidelines,[11,12,14,33] where 3 measurements should be made at least 3 minutes apart and an average taken of the two last readings. Measurements should be made using an appropriately calibrated device with a correctly sized cuff and the patient sitting at rest for 5 minutes.[33,34] Home blood pressure monitoring may be appropriate for some patients. If introduced, it is important to provide patients with a blood pressure diary, instructions on accurate self-measurement, and criteria for

TABLE 20.1 **Monitoring and Treatment During and After VEGF Inhibitor Therapy**

All patients should undergo baseline assessment of blood pressure and renal function.	
Blood pressure should be monitored regularly during treatment:	• Weekly measurements in first cycle • 2–3 weekly throughout treatment • Home blood pressure monitoring where appropriate
VEGFI-induced hypertension diagnosed if blood pressure:	• >140/90 mm Hg • >130/80 mm Hg and high risk of cardiovascular disease • >140/90 mm Hg with an increase in diastolic blood pressure by >20 mm Hg associated with symptoms
If VEGFI-induced hypertension is diagnosed:	• Referral to cardiovascular-oncology specialist should be considered • ACE inhibitor/ARB or dihydropyridine calcium channel antagonist as first line treatment • Dihydropyridine calcium channel antagonist and ACEi/ARB used in combination if control not achieved • Addition of diuretics, beta blockers, and NO donors may have a role in controlling resistant hypertension • Dose reduction of VEGFI or temporary withdrawal should be considered in cases of severe or symptomatic hypertension
Management of complications of VEGFI-induced hypertension:	• Urgent referral to cardiovascular-oncology specialist • VEGFI therapy should be discontinued • Left ventricular dysfunction or heart failure is treated with ACEi and beta blockers • Myocardial ischemia and infarction should be managed with as short a period of antiplatelet therapy as is safely possible
If VEGFI-induced proteinuria is diagnosed:	• Referral to nephrologist should be considered • Asymptomatic proteinuria may not require any intervention • Strive for tight blood pressure control • ACEi/ARB treatment may be beneficial in the context of hypertension • Progressive renal dysfunction should prompt withdrawal of VEGFI treatment

Following completion of VEGFI treatment, blood pressure monitoring should continue, and anti-hypertensive treatment may require dose reduction or withdrawal over time.
ACEi, Angiotensin-converting enzyme inhibitor; *ARB,* angiotensin receptor blocker; *VEGFI,* vascular endothelial growth factor inhibitor.

blood pressure readings that should prompt them to seek attention from their oncologist or medical practitioner. Ideally, blood pressure should be measured by ambulatory blood pressure monitoring during the first week of commencing VEGFI treatment and during each cycle of therapy.

Blood Pressure Treatment Thresholds

In patients commencing anti-cancer treatment, it is important to maintain a robust approach to blood pressure control, both before and during treatment. Prior to commencing VEGFI therapy, anti-hypertensive treatment should be started in patients with blood pressure above the target levels outlined previously. Where possible, adequate blood pressure control, according to relevant hypertension guidelines, should be achieved before starting treatment. However, this may not always be clinically possible, especially if there is an urgency to commence anti-cancer treatment. Therefore, the decisions regarding timing of anti-cancer therapy and optimization of cardiovascular status and blood pressure control should be made on an individual basis with input from both oncologists and cardiovascular physicians.[10,35]

Although we recommend a target blood pressure less than 130/80 mm Hg prior to commencing VEGFI therapy during treatment, anti-hypertensive therapy should only be commenced to maintain blood pressure less than 140/90 mm Hg. This is in line with the European Society of Cardiology position paper, and National Cancer Institute Drug Steering Committee's recommendations.[10,36] This more lenient blood pressure target during therapy is suggested to reduce the need for delay or interruption of VEGFI therapy and to reduce the risk of iatrogenic hypotension.

In addition, a diagnosis of VEGI-related hypertension should be considered in patients who do not fulfil these blood pressure definitions, but who have a rise of above 20 mm Hg in blood pressure following the initiation of VEGFI therapy. The acute rise in pressure in these patients puts them among the patients at highest risk of hypertensive complications.[10,20] All current recommendations for diagnosis and treatment in this patient group are based on expert opinion and general consensus rather than robust clinical evidence.

In line with the published Common Terminology Criteria for Adverse Events (version 5.0), hypertension is graded 1 to 5 based on severity, with increased grade mandating more intensive blood pressure-lowering therapy, often with more than one drug, as well as increased frequency of blood pressure monitoring and consideration of hospitalization in severe cases.

Treatment of Hypertension During Anti-Cancer Therapy

Careful consideration of drug pharmacokinetics and pharmacodynamics is important when choosing an appropriate anti-hypertensive agent, as well as taking comorbid conditions and potential side-effects into account (Table 20.2). Notably, non-dihydropyridine calcium channel antagonists (e.g., verapamil and diltiazem) have the potential for cytochrome P450 (CYP 450) inhibition. They should be avoided in patients receiving VEGFI because they are metabolized *via* CYP 450 and high circulating concentrations of VEGFI can occur as a consequence.[22,36] Choice of anti-hypertensive agents generally follows national guidelines for first-line treatment of hypertension and currently no clinical evidence indicates superiority of one agent over another.[35–37] Angiotensin-converting enzyme inhibitors (ACEis), angiotensin receptor blockers (ARBs) or dihydropyridine calcium channel antagonists tend to be the drugs most frequently used to treat VEGFI-associated hypertension. The use of ACEi/ARBs is despite the lack of robust evidence for a major role of the renin-angiotensin-aldosterone system in the development of VEGFI-induced hypertension. The frequency of their use partly reflects their widespread use in the treatment of essential hypertension and not a specific action toward a clear pathophysiologic mechanism. However, the beneficial endothelial and anti-proteinuria effects provided by ACEi/ARBs suggest that there may be a role for these agents in patients with diabetic nephropathy, left ventricular systolic dysfunction, or VEGFI-induced proteinuria. ACEi/ARBs may not be appropriate in patients receiving concomitant chemotherapy regimens that are renally excreted, those with renovascular disease, or with a tendency toward hyperkalemia.

Dihydropyridine calcium channel antagonists (amlodipine and nifedipine) have great potency reducing arterial smooth muscle cell contractility in the blood vessels. Their efficacy for controlling hypertension induced by bevacizumab has been demonstrated in patients with metastatic non-small-cell lung, colorectal, and ovarian cancers.[38]

It is frequently necessary to use combination therapy with two or more anti-hypertensive agents to achieve target goals of blood pressure control in patients with VEGFI-induced hypertension.[37] The combination of ACEi (or ARB) and dihydropyridine calcium channel antagonist is accepted as the first choice combination for use.[35,36,39] Other anti-hypertensive agents, including diuretics and beta blockers, have also been shown to be effective.[40] Mineralocorticoid receptor antagonists, such as eplerenone and spironolactone, are increasingly used in patients with treatment-resistant hypertension,[41] and therefore may be useful in the management of VEGFI-induced hypertension in some patients.

Given the proposed underlying mechanisms for the development of VEGFI-associated hypertension, it is not surprising that NO donors are of proven efficacy in the treatment of VEGFI-associated hypertension,[42] but they have not found a place as first-line therapy for VEGFI-associated hypertension. Evidence for their clinical utility is related to case reports, but the anti-hypertensive effect appears to be maintained for at least six or seven months. Longer term data are lacking and the potential for tachyphylaxis is not fully defined. In light of the mechanistic role of endothelin-1 in the hypertensive response to VEGFI therapy, it has been suggested that endothelin receptor antagonism may be a therapeutic option for some patients.[43] Although potentially promising, these strategies are in the early stages of development and require further evaluation in clinical studies.

As highlighted in all major hypertension guidelines nonpharmacologic treatment should be a cornerstone of treating patients with cancer therapy-associated hypertension. Lifestyle modification, including smoking cessation, reduced alcohol intake, weight control, exercise, and healthy diet, should be combined with pharmacologic interventions. Patients should be screened for and treated as necessary for obstructive sleep apnea. Adequate pain control is also important. Agents, which may

TABLE 20.2 **Summary of the Recommended Anti-Hypertensive Agents and Their Use in the Treatment of Vascular Endothelial Growth Factor-Induced Hypertension: Their Indications and Advantages, and Any Cautions or Contraindications.**

DRUG CLASS	THERAPY STAGE	EXAMPLES	ADVANTAGES/ INDICATIONS	PATIENT-SPECIFIC CAUTIONS/ CONTRAINDICATIONS	GENERAL CAUTIONS/ CONTRAINDICATIONS
ACE inhibitors	1/2	• Captopril • Enalapril • Lisinopril • Perindopril • Ramipril • Trandolapril	• Younger patients (<55 years) • Proteinuria • Diabetic nephropathy • Left ventricular dysfunction • Rapid onset of action	• Renal impairment • Hyperkalemia • Coadministration/ titration with renal clearance–dependent agents (e.g., cisplatin and pemetrexed)	• Renovascular disease • Peripheral vascular disease
Angiotensin II receptor antagonists	1/2	• Candesartan • Irbesartan • Losartan • Valsartan	• ACE inhibitor-related cough • Younger patients (<55 years) • Proteinuria • Diabetic nephropathy • Left ventricular dysfunction • Rapid onset of action	• Coadministration/ titration with renal clearance–dependent agents (e.g., cisplatin and pemetrexed) • Renal impairment • Hyperkalemia	• Renovascular disease • Peripheral vascular disease
Dihydropyridine calcium channel antagonists	1/2	• Amlodipine • Lercanidipine	• Older patients (>55 years) • Isolated systolic hypertension	• Peripheral edema	• Slow onset of action
Thiazide or loop diuretics	3/4	• Bendroflumethiazide • Hydrochlorothiazide • Indapamide • Furosemide • Torsemide	• Older patients (>55 years) • Isolated systolic hypertension • Secondary stroke prevention	• Hypercalcemia • Hypokalemia • QT prolonging drugs	• Gout • Sulfa allergy • Renal impairment
β-blockers	3/4	• Atenolol • Bisoprolol • Carvedilol • Metoprolol	• Ischemic heart disease (esp., early years after myocardial infarction, angina) • Left ventricular dysfunction • Anxiety	• Asthenia; malaise; fatigue • QT interval prolonging drugs	• Bradycardia • Heart block • Asthma / chronic obstructive pulmonary disease • Decompensated heart failure
Mineralocorticoid receptor antagonists	3/4	• Eplerenone • Spironolactone	• Resistant hypertension • Left ventricular dysfunction	• Renal impairment • Hyperkalemia	• Gynecomastia (spironolactone)
Nitric oxide donors	3/4	• Isosorbide mononitrate	• Resistant hypertension • Ischemic heart disease	• Postural hypotension	• Tolerance with chronic use

ACE, Angiotensin-converting enzyme.

contribute to hypertension should be avoided. This includes nonsteroidal anti-inflammatory agents, corticosteroids, erythropoietin, and sympathomimetic agents.[35]

Interruption or Dose Reduction of VEGFI

VEGFI-induced hypertension is a reversible process and, in addition to interventions with anti-hypertensive drug therapy, VEGFI dose reduction or temporary withdrawal may be required or considered in order to control hypertension. These measures should be considered only in cases of severe or symptomatic hypertension. If VEGFI therapy is suspended, it is typically for at least four weeks, although bevacizumab and aflibercept have longer half-lives than the tyrosine kinase inhibitors types of VEGFI and require to be withdrawn for a longer period. This allows time for adequate blood pressure controll, with input from a hypertension specialist. After temporary cessation of VEGFI treatment, it is usually reintroduced at the same or a reduced dose.[35]

Notably, some VEGFI regimens (e.g., sunitinib) have *off periods*, where treatment is temporarily withheld. It is important to be attentive to the development of symptomatic rebound hypotension during these periods, and anti-hypertensive therapy may need to be down-titrated in these periods. A particular concern during these period is for the precipitation of "water-shed" cerebral ischemia. Furthermore, on completion of VEGFI therapy, antihypertensives may also require down-titration or withdrawal.

ACUTE KIDNEY INJURY

Kidney injury (KI) is a common complication in patients with cancer who are on active therapy, occurring in 17.5% of patients within one year and in 27% in 5 years.[44–48] The highest incidence rates have been reported in patients with kidney cancer and multiple myeloma (44% and 26%, respectively), but is also noted in more than 10% of patients with bladder cancer, liver cancer, and leukemia. The risk of KI is highest in the first 90 days following systemic therapy and some studies suggest that the it might be even more common in contemporary practice. For instance, in Ontario, Canada, the annual incidence of AKI in patients with cancer on systemic therapy increased from 18 to 52 per 1000 person-years from 2007 to 2014. Advanced cancer stage, chronic kidney disease (CKD), and diabetes were also identified as risk factors for AKI in patients with cancer. Other studies outlined that patients who are receiving treatment for high-risk myelodysplastic syndrome or acute leukemia, or who underwent hematopoietic cell transplantation or nephrectomy (for renal cell carcinoma) are at highest risk.

Most studies indicate that patients with cancer who develop AKI, particularly those who require renal replacement therapy (RRT), have a higher risk of mortality. Overall severity of illness, age, and functional status are contributing factors and the presence of cancer alone should not be considered an absolute exclusion criterion for RRT. RRT was required in 5.1% of patients within one year of AKI onset. AKI in patients with cancer on active therapy has also been linked to longer lengths of hospital stay and costs as well as lower remission rates. Furthermore, AKI can lead to cardiovascular complications, especially increased risk of future heart failure hospitalizations.

Acute kidney injury in patients with cancer can be caused by the same factors as found in the general population as well as some that are specific to the cancer population (Table 20.3). In many cases, AKI is multifactorial in these patients. Prerenal etiologies most commonly account for AKI in patients with cancer, often volume depletion as a consequence of chemotherapy-related nausea, vomiting, diarrhea, and/or diuretic use. Medications that affect renal autoregulation, such as ACEi and ARBs, can exacerbate the risk and severity of prerenal AKI. For the cardio-oncologist the risks of kidney dysfunction associated with these drugs needs to be considered, especially in patients with advanced malignancy and those at high risk of volume depletion during chemotherapy. A hepatorenal-like syndrome secondary to sinusoidal obstruction syndrome (veno-occlusive disease) can be seen in patients who have undergone myeloablative allogeneic hematopoietic cell transplantation.

Several specific intrinsic renal causes of AKI, in addition to the common ones of hypotension-related acute tubular necrosis (ATN), need to be considered in patients with cancer. Among the most unique etiologies is the infiltration/deposition of cancer cells or their products. Light chain cast nephropathy is a classic example, seen in patients with monoclonal gammopathy including multiple myeloma, Waldenström macroglobulinemia, lymphoma, and chronic lymphocytic leukemia (CLL). Lights chains produced in excess are filtrated in the glomeruli, but then cause injury to the medullary tubular cells and precipitate as casts within the tubule leading to obstruction.

Renal parenchymal invasion has been reported in patients with multiple myeloma (plasma cells) and is most commonly noted with rapidly growing hematologic malignancies, such as lymphoma or acute leukemia. In fact, in as many as 60% of patients with lymphoma lymphomatous invasion of the kidneys will be seen on autopsy. The majority of these are clinically silent because a considerable burden of compromise of the function of both kidneys would need to be present for renal failure to become evident by standard means of assessment. However, parenchymal infiltration can present with the syndrome of AKI, proteinuria, and/or hematuria, and bilaterally enlarged kidneys on renal imaging. A

TABLE 20.3 Pathomechanistic Approach to Nephrotoxicities in Patients With Cancer

TYPE OF INJURY	LOCATION	MECHANISM	CLINICAL CORRELATES
Prerenal		Volume depletion	Nausea, vomiting, diarrhea Decreased oral uptake (anorexia or mucositis)
		Decreased effective arterial blood volume	Shock, sepsis, heart failure, cirrhosis, effusion/ascites Capillary leak syndrome (increased IL-2 levels, engraftment syndrome 10 to 20 days after HSCT) Hepatic sinusoidal obstruction syndrome <3 weeks after HSCT
		Glomerular hemodynamics	Hypercalcemia Calcineurin inhibitors Abdominal compartment syndrome
Intrarenal	Glomerular	Paraneoplastic	TMA (gastric, breast, prostate, and lung cancer, lymphoma, HLH) Hepatic sinusoidal obstruction syndrome <3 weeks after HSCT MCD, FSGS: Hodgkin, lymphohistiocytosis (HLH)
		Drug-induced	TMA (VEGF inhibitors, TKIs, gemcitabine, mitomycin-C, cisplatin, IFN, mTOR inhibitors, radiation therapy, 6–12 months after) FSGS (IFN, pamidronate, TKIs, mTOR inhibitors) MCD (IFN) Immune complex GN (pegfilgrastim, filgrastim)
		Dysproteinemia	MIDD (MM > MGRS > CLL:LCDD > HCDD; k LC > l LC; nodular mesangial sclerosis + GBM and TBM Ig or LC deposits) MPGN (monoclonal capillary Ig deposits in MM, MGRS, CLL, WM) PGNMID (GN with endocapillary proliferation, usually IgG3-k) Cryoglobulinemia (type I in WM, CLL, MM; type II in B-cell lymphoma)
		Amyloidosis	AL amyloid (secondary to plasma cell dyscrasias, incl. MM; l LC > k LC, can also deposit in the tubule-interstitium, leading to increased serum creatinine without significant proteinuria) AA amyloid (secondary to deposition of serum amyloid A (e.g., with hepatocellular and renal cell carcinoma, Hodgkin and non-Hodgkin lymphoma, and hairy cell leukemia)
		Post-HSCT	MN > MCD TMA (>30 days after HSCT)
	Tubular	ATN	Shock, sepsis HLH Drug toxicity (cisplatin > carboplatin > oxaliplatin, ifosfamide, pemtrexed, imatinib, BRAF inhibitors, clofarabine, carfilzomib, mTOR inhibitors)
		Intratubular	TLS (more common in hematologic malignancies) Cast nephropathy (MM > WM and CLL, triggered by prerenal causes, hypercalcemia, NSAIDs, IV contrast; less likely with serum-free light chains <70 mg/dL) Drug-induced crystal deposition (methotrexate) Fanconi syndrome (complete/incomplete, LCDD, ifosfamide, cisplatin) Phosphaturia (imatinib) Magnesium wasting (platinum drugs, anti-EGFR antibodies) Nephrogenic diabetes insipidus (ifosfamide, cisplatin)
	Interstitial	Infiltration	MM, lymphoma, leukemia
		Drug-induced AIN	ICI and VEGF inhibitors, esp., TKIs
		Post-HSCT	BK virus-associated nephropathy Adenovirus-associated AIN
Postrenal		Ureteral obstruction	Tumor invasion Retroperitoneal fibrosis Ureteral stenosis induced by BK virus or adenovirus post HSCT
		Bladder outlet obstruction	Bladder cancer, prostate cancer Chronic cystitis Blood clots

AA, Amyloid A; *AIN,* acute interstitial nephritis; *AL,* amyloid light chain; *CLL,* chronic lymphocytic leukemia; *FSGS,* focal segmental glomerulosclerosis; *GBM,* glomerular basement membrane; *GN,* glomerulonephritis; *HCDD,* heavy chain deposit disease; *HLH,* hemophagocytic lymphohistiocytosis; *HSCT,* hematopoietic stem cell transplantation; *ICI,* immune checkpoint inhibitors; *IFN,* interferon; *Ig,* immunoglobulin; *IL,* interleukin; *IV,* intravenous; *LC,* light chain; *LCDD,* light chain deposition disease; *MCD,* minimal chain disease; *MGRS,* monoclonal gammopathy of renal significance; *MIDD,* monoclonal immunoglobulin deposition disease; *MM,* multiple myeloma; *MN,* membranous nephropathy; *MPGN,* membranoproliferative glomerulonephritis; *mTOR,* mammalian target of rapamycin; *NSAID,* nonsteroidal anti-inflammatory drug; *PGNMID,* proliferative glomerulonephritis with monoclonal immunoglobulin G deposits; *TBM,* tubular basement membrane; *TKI,* tyrosine kinase inhibitor; *TLS,* tumor lysis syndrome; *TMA,* thrombotic microangiopathy; *VEGF,* vascular endothelial growth factor; *WM,* Waldenström macroglobulinemia.

kidney biopsy can confirm the diagnosis, although this is not always required. It is to be emphasized that this syndrome should be recognized promptly, because it may respond well to therapy aimed at the underlying primary malignancy. Resolution of AKI with anti-cancer therapy would strongly support that lymphomatous infiltration of the kidney was the underlying cause. The mechanisms by which renal parenchymal infiltration causes AKI are unclear, but it may involve compression of the renal tubules and microvasculature, leading to tubular obstruction and ischemia. AKI caused by metastases of extrarenal solid tumors is very rare (if occurring, usually pulmonary, gastric, or breast carcinoma) and it usually reflects widespread loss of parenchyma.

Tumor lysis syndrome (TLS) is considered an oncologic emergency. It is caused by degradation (lysis) of a large volume of tumor cells with release of large amounts of intracellular contents into the systemic circulation, resulting in hyperkalemia, hyperuricemia, hyperphosphatemia, and hypocalcemia. AKI in this setting results from the formation of crystals composed of uric acid, calcium phosphate, and/or xanthine. These crystals can cause intratubular obstruction, inflammation, and a reduction in glomerular filtration rate. TLS is most commonly observed in patients with high-grade lymphomas (such as Burkitt lymphoma) or leukemias after initiation of chemotherapy, although it may develop spontaneously or with treatment of other cancers that have a high proliferative rate or large tumor burden.

NEPHROTOXICITY OF CANCER DRUGS

Drug-induced nephrotoxicity is an important cause of AKI in patients with cancer and can be seen with conventional chemotherapeutic agents as well as newer targeted and immunotherapies (Fig. 20.1).[44,49,50] The most important will be reviewed here, based on the

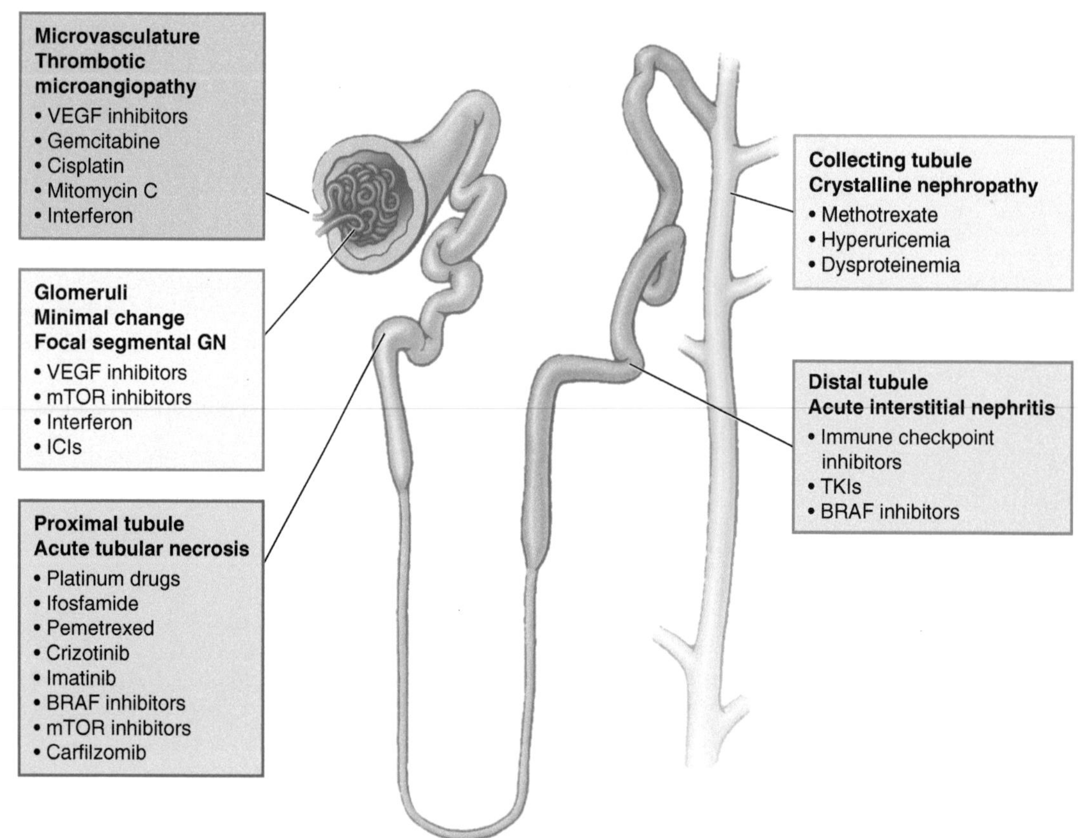

FIG. 20.1 Illustration of cancer therapy-induced nephrotoxicity by site of action/injury. *GN,* Glomerulonephritis; *ICI,* immune checkpoint inhibitors; *mTOR,* mammalian target of rapamycin; *TKI,* tyrosine kinase inhibitor; *VEGF,* vascular endothelial growth factor. (Used with permission of Mayo Foundation for Medical Education and Research. All rights reserved.)

main target of injury within the kidney: the renal microvasculature, glomeruli, tubules, and/or interstitium.

Renal Vasculature: Antineoplastic Drugs Associated With Thrombotic Microangiopathy Syndromes

Thrombotic microangiopathy (TMA) presents clinically as microangiopathic hemolytic anemia, thrombocytopenia, hypertension, and AKI with hematuria and proteinuria. Neurologic abnormalities and gastrointestinal symptoms can be seen as well. The pathologic characteristic is intrarenal or systemic microvascular thrombi, with endothelial swelling and microvascular obstruction. TMA may be associated with the primary cancer, especially gastric carcinoma, followed by breast and lung carcinomas, or, more likely, with therapeutic regimens, including drug therapies, radiation therapy, and hematopoietic cell transplantation. Among drug therapies, the classic examples are VEGF inhibitors, gemcitabine, and mitomycin C. It is less frequently seen with bleomycin, cisplatin, and 5-fluorouracil.

Bevacizumab

It is not surprising that AKI is associated with VEGF inhibitors, because VEGF is produced by renal visceral epithelial cells and binds to VEGF receptors located on glomerular endothelium, mesangium, and peritubular capillaries.[21] Local VEGF production maintains normal functioning of all of these cell types, including injury repair and cell turnover. Importantly, there is crosstalk between the glomerular endothelium and epithelium, maintaining the integrity of the filtration barrier. In rodent studies, a single dose of an anti-VEGF antibody was sufficient to cause a two- to three-fold increase in proteinuria.[23] Renal histopathology revealed glomerular endothelial cell swelling, vacuolization, and detachment, as well as disruption of epithelial cell slit diaphragms. Immunohistochemistry also showed downregulation of nephrin, which was partially restored with administration of recombinant VEGF. Reports on bevacizumab use in patients likewise confirm the onset of proteinuria (even to the degree of nephrotic syndrome) after three or more months of therapy. Half of these patients will have hypertension and AKI: in the original series, all had TMA on histology. This seems to be the predominant histopathologic feature, although a number of renal lesions, including focal segmental glomerulosclerosis (FSGS), mebranoproliferative glomerulonephritis (GN), glomerular endotheliosis, cryoglobulinemic GN, nonspecific immune complex GN, and acute interstitial nephritis have been described with angiogenesis inhibitor drugs. Importantly, proteinuria, hypertension, and AKI generally improve on withdrawal of bevacizumab.

Gemcitabine

Anaplastic lymphoma kinase from gemcitabine use, which is well documented, primarily relates to TMA. Hypertension, microangiopathic hemolytic anemia, and ischemic skin lesions may be present. Peripheral edema and heart failure can also be seen. Of interest, gemcitabine TMA can have a delayed onset (median time to diagnosis 8 months after initiation of therapy). Of further interest, new or worsening hypertension is not an uncommon feature and usually precedes the diagnosis of TMA in all cases. In some series, the severity of hypertension correlates with poorer outcome. The mechanism by which TMA induces hypertension is likely glomerular ischemia induced by microvascular capillary obstruction. Therapy is mainly supportive, including drug discontinuation, antihypertensive therapy, and dialysis, when needed. Most cases show partial or full recovery, approximately one-quarter will remain dialysis-dependent.

Glomerulus: Podocytopathy

Chronic interferon (IFN) therapy can lead to acute and chronic renal disease with nephrotic range proteinuria. Several pathologic forms have been described, including minimal change disease, FSGS, and collapsing FSGS. IFN therapy discontinuation inconsistently leads to recovery; steroids do not seem to be helpful. The mechanism of podocyte injury with IFN remains to be defined.

Tubules: Acute Tubular Injury

Cisplatin is a classic nephrotoxic drug that can injure multiple renal compartments in a dose-dependent manner, including blood vessels, glomeruli, and, most commonly, renal tubular cells. AKI secondary to cisplatin can present as a functional decline in glomerular filtration rate as TMA or, most commonly, as acute tubular necrosis. Tubulopathies without AKI present as isolated proximal tubulopathy (proteinuria and phosphate wasting) or Fanconi syndrome. Sodium wasting can lead to hypovolemia, orthostasis, and

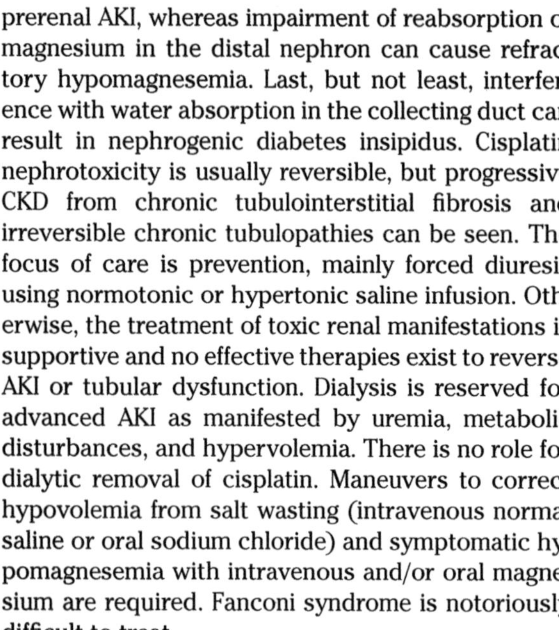

prerenal AKI, whereas impairment of reabsorption of magnesium in the distal nephron can cause refractory hypomagnesemia. Last, but not least, interference with water absorption in the collecting duct can result in nephrogenic diabetes insipidus. Cisplatin nephrotoxicity is usually reversible, but progressive CKD from chronic tubulointerstitial fibrosis and irreversible chronic tubulopathies can be seen. The focus of care is prevention, mainly forced diuresis using normotonic or hypertonic saline infusion. Otherwise, the treatment of toxic renal manifestations is supportive and no effective therapies exist to reverse AKI or tubular dysfunction. Dialysis is reserved for advanced AKI as manifested by uremia, metabolic disturbances, and hypervolemia. There is no role for dialytic removal of cisplatin. Maneuvers to correct hypovolemia from salt wasting (intravenous normal saline or oral sodium chloride) and symptomatic hypomagnesemia with intravenous and/or oral magnesium are required. Fanconi syndrome is notoriously difficult to treat.

Ifosfamide

Nephrotoxicity is a major side effect of ifosfamide, mediated primarily by injury to the renal tubular cells. AKI and tubulopathies akin to cisplatin can be seen. Prior cisplatin exposure is a risk factor, as is preexisting CKD and cumulative doses more than 90 mg/m^2. Preventive options other than dose reduction are limited and treatment is mainly supportive: electrolyte supplementation, renal function monitoring, and dialysis, as indicated. In addition to CKD and end-stage renal disease, long-term complications include a permanent proximal tubulopathy and isolated renal phosphaturia in up to 20%.

Pemetrexed

AKI has been noted with high-dose pemetrexed therapy (600 mg/m^2). Usually only minimal proteinuria is seen and most cases are reversible, but CKD can evolve, likely relating to the extent of primarily chronic tubulointerstitial fibrosis and tubular atrophy. In addition, acute tubular necrosis, acute interstitial nephritis, renal tubular acidosis, and nephrogenic diabetes insipidus can be seen.

Tubules: Magnesium Wasting

Cetuximab

Cetuximab is a chimeric monoclonal antibody against EGF receptor (EGFR), which interferes with EGFR-enabled reabsorption of magnesium in the distal convoluted tubule, leading to magnesium wasting. Nearly all patients have some decline in magnesium serum concentrations with cetuximab and more than one-half develop hypomagnesemia. Older age and baseline magnesium concentration are risk factors. Severe hypomagnesemia can lead to hypokalemia and hypocalcemia. Intravenous repletion of magnesium is the main intervention, along with calcium and potassium repletion, as required. Discontinuation of cetuximab leads to resolution of magnesium wasting over approximately 4 to 6 weeks.

Tubules: Crystal Nephropathy

Methotrexate

Nephrotoxicity can be a complication of high-dose methotrexate therapy (1 to 12 g/m^2).

Methotrexate-induced AKI primarily results from precipitation of methotrexate/7-hydroxy-methotrexate in the distal tubules causing acute tubular injury. Risk factors include intravascular volume depletion, reduced urine output, acidic urine, and reduced GFR at baseline ($<$60 mL/min). Prevention is focused on volume repletion before/during drug infusion, appropriate drug dosing, and alkalization of the urine (pH 7.1). Leucovorin is administered 24 to 36 hours after methotrexate therapy to reduce nonmalignant cell injury. When there is concern about an increased risk of methotrexate toxicity, glucarpidase may be used in order to cleave methotrexate to noncytotoxic metabolites. Although high-flux hemodialysis can be used to clear methotrexate from the circulation, it is associated with immediate postdialysis plasma rebound.

Postrenal Causes

Post-renal causes of AKI in patients with cancer are more common than in the general population and can be the consequence of intratubular, extrarenal, or urinary tract obstruction.

Intratubular obstruction may be caused by crystals (uric acid, xanthine, hypoxanthine, or calcium phosphate) or light chain casts. Crystallization of drugs, such as methotrexate, can also be responsible. Maintaining a high urine output with intravenous fluids is the best preventive measure, but it may require further careful consideration in patients with cancer with heart failure or left ventricular dysfunction.

Extrarenal obstruction can be caused by a wide range of malignancies, most commonly those arising in the gastrointestinal and genitourinary tracts, and especially cancer of the bladder, prostate, uterus, or cervix. Extrarenal obstruction usually indicates metastatic disease. Conversely, malignancy should be considered in any patient not known to have cancer who presents with bilateral urinary tract obstruction that is not associated with kidney stones. Renal imaging studies typically show dilatation of the collecting system in one or both kidneys (hydronephrosis) in this setting. Conversely, severe hydronephrosis may not be evident if ureteral obstruction is caused by retroperitoneal tumor or fibrosis (which may itself be secondary to malignancy).

Urinary tract obstruction can also be unrelated to the malignancy (e.g., benign prostatic hyperplasia) and urinary retention should be excluded in any patient with reduced urine output.

Renal Disease and Hematopoietic Stem Cell Transplantation (HSCT)

Renal failure is a common complication after HSCT. It has been reported in 50% to 75% of patients after myeloablative allogeneic HSCT; half of these require dialysis. In comparison, renal failure is seen in 40% of patients after non-myeloablative allogenic HSCT and in 25% of patients following autologous HSCT with a dialysis rate of 10% or less. In terms of timelines, renal failure is more insidious (over three months) with autologous HSCT compared with myoablative HSCT (within the first 3 weeks). This relates to the higher intensity conditioning regimens used for myeloablative HSCT, the occurrence of veno-occlusive disease (VOD), graft-versus-host disease and, importantly, the need for immunosuppression with calcineurin inhibitors.

The etiology of HSCT-related renal failure varies by time from transplantation. In the first days after HSCT, tumor lysis syndrome and myelotoxicity pose a risk without proper prophylaxis and cryopreservation. Other early risk factors over the first few weeks include a prerenal state owing to volume depletion (vomiting and diarrhea, as a result of conditioning regimens, and acute graft-versus-host disease), or calcineurin inhibitors. Acute tubular necrosis caused by nephrotoxic agents (amphotericin B, aminoglycosides, intravenous contrast, and calcineurin inhibitors), hemorrhagic or septic shock. Obstructive uropathy can develop in the setting of severe hemorrhagic cystitis (owing to cyclophosphamide).

The most common cause of severe renal failure after myeloablative HSCT, however, is VOD, a unique form of the hepatorenal syndrome commonly associated with regimens that include cyclophosphamide, busulfan, and/or total body irradiation. It generally emerges in the first 30 days after HSCT. In the first stage, sodium retention predominates with low urinary sodium concentration and severe water retention and hyponatremia. Weight gain, edema, and ascites are the clinical consequences. In the second stage, jaundice and right upper quadrant pain follow. In the third stage, renal failure is seen in approximately 50% and can be precipitated by renal insults, such as sepsis or nephrotoxins. Some degree of renal insufficiency, however, is present in almost all patients with VOD. Therapy is supportive and resolution usually occurs unless there is progressive hepatic and renal failure, which carry 100% mortality by day 100 after HSCT.

ACKNOWLEDGMENTS

Rhian M. Touyz is supported by a British Heart Foundation (BHF) Chair Award (CH/12/429762) and Stephen J.H. Dobbin is funded through the BHF Research Excellence Award (RE/13/5/30177).

REFERENCES

1. Small HY, Montezano AC, Rios FJ, Savoia C, Touyz RM. Hypertension due to antiangiogenic cancer therapy with vascular endothelial growth factor inhibitors: understanding and managing a new syndrome. *Can J Cardiol.* 2014;30(5):534–543. doi:10.1016/j.cjca.2014.02.011.
2. Azizi M, Chedid A, Oudard S. Home blood-pressure monitoring in patients receiving sunitinib. *N Engl J Med.* 2008;358(1):95–97. doi:10.1056/NEJMc072330.
3. Hall PS, Harshman LC, Srinivas S, Witteles RM. The frequency and severity of cardiovascular toxicity from targeted therapy in advanced renal cell carcinoma patients. *JACC Heart Fail.* 2013;1(1):72–78. doi:10.1016/j.jchf.2012.09.001.
4. Robinson ES, Khankin EV, Karumanchi SA, Humphreys BD. Hypertension induced by vascular endothelial growth factor signaling pathway inhibition: mechanisms and potential use as a biomarker. *Semin Nephrol.* 2010;30(6):591–601. doi:10.1016/j.semnephrol.2010.09.007.
5. Bair SM, Choueiri TK, Moslehi J. Cardiovascular complications associated with novel angiogenesis inhibitors: emerging evidence and evolving perspectives. *Trends Cardiovasc Med.* 2013;23(4):104–113. doi:10.1016/j.tcm.2012.09.008.
6. Robinson ES, Matulonis UA, Ivy P, et al. Rapid development of hypertension and proteinuria with cediranib, an oral vascular endothelial growth factor receptor inhibitor. *Clin J Am Soc Nephrol.* 2010;5(3):477–483. doi:10.2215/CJN.08111109.
7. Cameron AC, Touyz RM, Lang NN. Vascular complications of cancer chemotherapy. *Can J Cardiol.* 2016;32(7):852–862. doi:10.1016/j.cjca.2015.12.023.

8. Nazer B, Humphreys BD, Moslehi J. Effects of novel angiogenesis inhibitors for the treatment of cancer on the cardiovascular system: focus on hypertension. *Circulation*. 2011;124(15):1687–1691. doi:10.1161/CIRCULATIONAHA.110.992230.
9. Abi Aad S, Pierce M, Barmaimon G, Farhat FS, Benjo A, Mouhayar E. Hypertension induced by chemotherapeutic and immunosuppresive agents: a new challenge. *Crit Rev Oncol Hematol*. 2015; 93(1):28–35. doi:10.1016/j.critrevonc.2014.08.004.
10. Maitland ML, Bakris GL, Black HR, et al. Initial assessment, surveillance, and management of blood pressure in patients receiving vascular endothelial growth factor signaling pathway inhibitors. *J Natl Cancer Inst*. 2010;102(9):596–604. doi:10.1093/jnci/djq091.
11. Whelton PK, Carey RM, Aronow WS, et al. 2017 ACC/AHA/AAPA/ABC/ACPM/AGS/APhA/ASH/ASPC/NMA/PCNA Guideline for the prevention, detection, evaluation, and management of high blood pressure in adults: executive summary. *J Am Soc Hypertens*. 2018;71(6):1269–1324. doi:10.1016/j.jash.2018.06.010.
12. Leung AA, Daskalopoulou SS, Dasgupta K, et al. Hypertension: Canada's 2017 Guidelines for diagnosis, risk assessment, prevention, and treatment of hypertension in adults. *Can J Cardiol*. 2017;33(5):557–576. doi:10.1016/j.cjca.2017.03.005.
13. Williams B, :>Mancia G, Spiering W, et al. 2018 Practice guidelines for the management of arterial hypertension of the European Society of Hypertension (ESH) and the European Society of Cardiology (ESC). *Blood Press*. 2018;39(33):3021–3104. doi:10.1080/08037051.2018.1527177.
14. Bress AP, Colantonio LD, Cooper RS, et al. Potential cardiovascular disease events prevented with adoption of the 2017 American College of Cardiology/American Heart Association Blood Pressure Guideline. *Circulation*. 2019;139(1):24–36. doi:10.1161/CIRCULATIONAHA.118.035640.
15. Chu TF, Rupnick MA, Kerkela R, et al. Cardiotoxicity associated with tyrosine kinase inhibitor sunitinib. *Lancet*. 2007;370(9604): 2011–2019. doi:10.1016/S0140-6736(07)61865-0.
16. Guiga H, Decroux C, Michelet P, et al. Hospital and out-of-hospital mortality in 670 hypertensive emergencies and urgencies. *J Clin Hypertens*. 2017;19(11):1137–1142. doi:10.1111/jch.13083.
17. Hamid M, Ghani A, Micaily I, Sarwar U, Lashari B, Malik F. Posterior reversible encephalopathy syndrome (PRES) after bevacizumab therapy for metastatic colorectal cancer. *J Community Hosp Intern Med Perspect*. 2018;8(3):130–133. doi:10.1080/20009666.2018.1478563.
18. Finn RS, Qin S, Ikeda M, et al. Atezolizumab plus bevacizumab in unresectable hepatocellular carcinoma. *N Engl J Med*. 2020;382: 1894–1905. doi:10.1056/NEJMoa1915745.
19. Touyz RM, Herrmann SMS, Herrmann J. Vascular toxicities with VEGF inhibitor therapies—focus on hypertension and arterial thrombotic events. *J Am Soc Hypertens*. 2018;12(6):409–425. doi:10.1016/j.jash.2018.03.008.
20. Maitland ML, Kasza KE, Karrison T, et al. Ambulatory monitoring detects sorafenib-induced blood pressure elevations on the first day of treatment. *Clin Cancer Res*. 2009;15(19):6250–6257. doi:10.1158/1078-0432.CCR-09-0058.
21. Snider KL, Maitland ML. Cardiovascular toxicities: clues to optimal administration of vascular endothelial growth factor signaling pathway inhibitors. *Target Oncol*. 2009;4(2):67–76. doi:10.1007/s11523-009-0106-0.
22. Rini BI, Cohen DP, Lu DR, et al. Hypertension as a biomarker of efficacy in patients with metastatic renal cell carcinoma treated with sunitinib. *J Natl Cancer Inst*. 2011;103(9):763–773. doi:10.1093/jnci/djr128.
23. Małyszko J, Młyszko M, Kozlowski L, Kozlowska K, Małyszko J. Hypertension in malignancy—an underappreciated problem. *Oncotarget*. 2018;9:20855–20871. doi:10.18632/oncotarget.25024.
24. Sagstuen H, Aass N, Fosså SD, et al. Blood pressure and body mass index in long-term survivors of testicular cancer. *J Clin Oncol*. 2005;23(22):4980–4990. doi:10.1200/JCO.2005.06.882.
25. De Vos FYFL, Nuver J, Willemse PHB, et al. Long-term survivors of ovarian malignancies after cisplatin-based chemotherapy: cardiovascular risk factors and signs of vascular damage. *Eur J Cancer*. 2004;40(5):696–700. doi:10.1016/j.ejca.2003.11.026.
26. Nuver J, Smit AJ, Sleijfer DT, et al. Microalbuminuria, decreased fibrinolysis, and inflammation as early signs of atherosclerosis in long-term survivors of disseminated testicular cancer. *Eur J Cancer*. 2004;40(5):701–706. doi:10.1016/j.ejca.2003.12.012.
27. Fosså SD, Aass N, Winderen M, Börmer OP, Olsen DR. Long-term renal function after treatment for malignant germ-cell tumours. *Ann Oncol*. 2002;13(2):222–228. doi:10.1093/annonc/mdf048.
28. Siegel D, Martin T, Nooka A, et al. Integrated safety profile of single-agent carfilzomib: experience from 526 patients enrolled in 4 phase II clinical studies. *Haematologica*. 2013;98:1753–1761. doi:10.3324/haematol.2013.089334.
29. Dimopoulos MA, Moreau P, Palumbo A, et al. Carfilzomib and dexamethasone versus bortezomib and dexamethasone for patients with relapsed or refractory multiple myeloma (ENDEAVOR): and randomised, phase 3, open-label, multicentre study. *Lancet Oncol*. 2016;17(1):27–38. doi:10.1016/S1470-2045(15)00464-7.
30. Kaplan B, Qazi Y, Wellen JR. Strategies for the management of adverse events associated with mTOR inhibitors. *Transplant Rev*. 2014;28(3):126–133. doi:10.1016/j.trre.2014.03.002.
31. Pallet N, Legendre C. Adverse events associated with mTOR inhibitors. *Expert Opin Drug Saf*. 2012;12(2):177–186. doi:10.1517/14740338.2013.752814.
32. Kappers MHW, Van Esch JHM, Sleijfer S, Danser AJ, Van Den Meiracker AH. Cardiovascular and renal toxicity during angiogenesis inhibition: clinical and mechanistic aspects. *J Hypertens*. 2009;27(12):2297–2309. doi:10.1097/HJH.0b013e3283309b59.
33. Williams B, Mancia G, Spiering W, et al. 2018 ESC/ESH Guidelines for the management of arterial hypertension. The Task Force for the management of arterial hypertension of the European Society of Cardiology and the European Society of Hypertension. *J Hypertens*. 2018;36(10):1953–2041. doi:10.1097/HJH.0000000000001940.
34. James PA. Evidence-based guideline for the management of high blood pressure in adults. *JAMA*. 2014;311(5):507–520. doi:10.1001/jama.2013.284427.
35. Kalaitzidis RG, Elisaf MS. Uncontrolled hypertension and oncology: clinical tips. *Curr Vasc Pharmacol*. 2017;16(1):23–29. doi:10.2174/1570161115666170414121436.
36. Zamorano JL, Lancellotti P, Muñoz DR, et al. 2016 ESC position paper on cancer treatments and cardiovascular toxicity developed under the auspices of the ESC committee for practice guidelines: the task force for cancer treatments and cardiovascular toxicity of the european society of cardiology (ESC). *Russ J Cardiol*. 2017;143(3):105–139.
37. Copur MS, Obermiller A. An algorithm for the management of hypertension in the setting of vascular endothelial growth factor signaling inhibition. *Clin Colorectal Cancer*. 2011;10(3):151–156. doi:10.1016/j.clcc.2011.03.021.
38. Mir O, Coriat R, Ropert S, et al. Treatment of bevacizumab-induced hypertension by amlodipine. *Invest New Drugs*. 2012;30(2):702–707. doi:10.1007/s10637-010-9549-5.
39. NICE. Hypertension in adults: diagnosis and management. *Guidel - Summ Clin Guidel Prim Care*. 2017;59–65. https://www.nice.org.uk/guidance/cg127/resources/hypertension-in-adults-diagnosis-and-management-pdf-35109454941637.
40. Pasquier E, Street J, Pouchy C, et al. Β-blockers increase response to chemotherapy via direct antitumour and anti-angiogenic mechanisms in neuroblastoma. *Br J Cancer*. 2013;108(12):2485–2494. doi:10.1038/bjc.2013.205.
41. Calhoun DA, Jones D, Textor S, et al. Resistant hypertension: diagnosis, evaluation, and treatment: a scientific statement from the American Heart Association professional education committee of the council for high blood pressure research. *Hypertension*. 2008;117(25):e510–526. doi:10.1161/CIRCULATIONAHA.108.189141.
42. Kruzliak P, Kovacova G, Pechanova O. Therapeutic potential of nitric oxide donors in the prevention and treatment of angiogenesis-inhibitor-induced hypertension. *Angiogenesis*. 2013;16(2):289–295. doi:10.1007/s10456-012-9327-4.
43. Lankhorst S, Kappers MHW, Van Esch JHM, et al. Treatment of hypertension and renal injury induced by the angiogenesis inhibitor sunitinib preclinical study. *Hypertension*. 2014;64(6):1282–1289. doi:10.1161/HYPERTENSIONAHA.114.04187.
44. Rosner MH, Perazella MA. Acute kidney injury in patients with cancer. *N Engl J Med*. 2017;376(18):1770–1781. doi:10.1056/NEJMra1613984.
45. Perazella MA, Rosner MH. Acute kidney injury in patients with cancer. *Oncology* (Williston Park). 2018;32(7):351–359.

46. Rosner MH, Perazella MA. Acute kidney injury in the patient with cancer. *Kidney Res Clin Pract.* 2019;38(3):295–308. doi:10.23876/j.krcp.19.042.
47. Izzedine H, Perazella MA. Anticancer drug-induced acute kidney injury. *Kidney Int Rep.* 2017;2(4):504–514. doi:10.1016/j.ekir.2017.02.008.
48. Lam AQ, Humphreys BD. Onco-nephrology: AKI in the patient with cancer. *Clin J Am Soc Nephrol.* 2012;7(10):1692–1700. doi:10.2215/CJN.03140312.
49. Perazella MA, Shirali AC. Nephrotoxicity of cancer immunotherapies: past, present and future. *J Am Soc Nephrol.* 2018;29(8):2039–2052. doi:10.1681/ASN.2018050488.
50. Perazella MA. Onco-nephrology: renal toxicities of chemotherapeutic agents. *Clin J Am Soc Nephrol.* 2012;7(10):1713–1721. doi:10.2215/CJN.02780312.

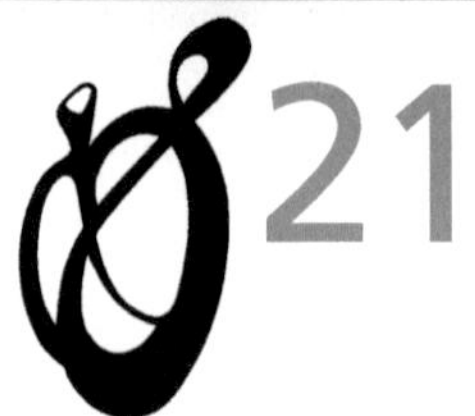

21 Pulmonary Disease During Cancer Therapy

YEVGENIYA MOGILEVSKAYA AND ALEXANDER GEYER

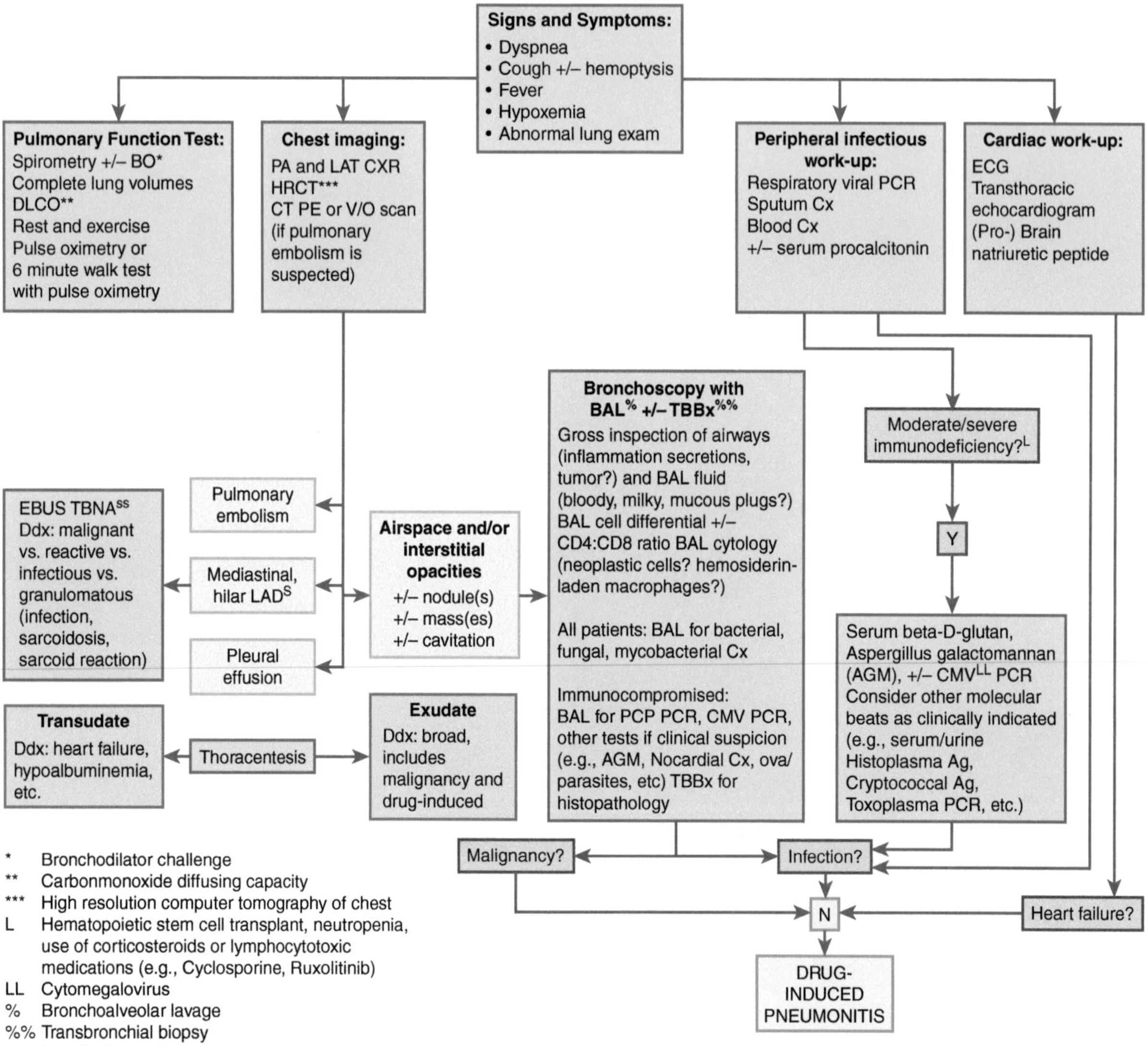

Signs and Symptoms:
- Dyspnea
- Cough +/– hemoptysis
- Fever
- Hypoxemia
- Abnormal lung exam

Pulmonary Function Test:
Spirometry +/– BO*
Complete lung volumes
DLCO**
Rest and exercise
Pulse oximetry or
6 minute walk test
with pulse oximetry

Chest imaging:
PA and LAT CXR
HRCT***
CT PE or V/O scan
(if pulmonary
embolism is
suspected)

Peripheral infectious work-up:
Respiratory viral PCR
Sputum Cx
Blood Cx
+/– serum procalcitonin

Cardiac work-up:
ECG
Transthoracic
echocardiogram
(Pro-) Brain
natriuretic peptide

Pulmonary embolism

Mediastinal, hilar LAD[S]

Pleural effusion

EBUS TBNA[ss]
Ddx: malignant
vs. reactive vs.
infectious vs.
granulomatous
(infection,
sarcoidosis,
sarcoid reaction)

Airspace and/or interstitial opacities
+/– nodule(s)
+/– mass(es)
+/– cavitation

Bronchoscopy with BAL[%] +/– TBBx[%%]
Gross inspection of airways (inflammation secretions, tumor?) and BAL fluid (bloody, milky, mucous plugs?) BAL cell differential +/– CD4:CD8 ratio BAL cytology (neoplastic cells? hemosiderin-laden macrophages?)

All patients: BAL for bacterial, fungal, mycobacterial Cx

Immunocompromised:
BAL for PCP PCR, CMV PCR, other tests if clinical suspicion (e.g., AGM, Nocardial Cx, ova/parasites, etc) TBBx for histopathology

Moderate/severe immunodeficiency?[L]

Y

Serum beta-D-glutan, Aspergillus galactomannan (AGM), +/– CMV[LL] PCR
Consider other molecular beats as clinically indicated (e.g., serum/urine Histoplasma Ag, Cryptococcal Ag, Toxoplasma PCR, etc.)

Transudate
Ddx: heart failure,
hypoalbuminemia,
etc.

Thoracentesis

Exudate
Ddx: broad,
includes
malignancy and
drug-induced

Malignancy?

Infection?

Heart failure?

N

DRUG-INDUCED PNEUMONITIS

* Bronchodilator challenge
** Carbonmonoxide diffusing capacity
*** High resolution computer tomography of chest
L Hematopoietic stem cell transplant, neutropenia, use of corticosteroids or lymphocytotoxic medications (e.g., Cyclosporine, Ruxolitinib)
LL Cytomegalovirus
% Bronchoalveolar lavage
%% Transbronchial biopsy
s Lymphadenopathy
ss Endoabronchial ultrasound with transbronchial needle aspirate

CHAPTER OUTLINE

KEY POINTS

- Pulmonary complications in patients with cancer may involve any intrathoracic structures
- Differential diagnosis of parenchymal infiltrates in patients with cancer includes infection, inflammation, neoplastic involvement, and other miscellaneous diagnoses (e.g., pulmonary edema).
- Clinical presentation of drug-induced pneumonitis ranges from asymptomatic infiltrates to hypoxemic respiratory failure
- Drug-induced pneumonitis is a diagnosis of exclusion; its work-up includes laboratory and imaging studies with bronchoscopy reserved for cases when infectious, neoplastic, and miscellaneous (e.g., heart failure) causes cannot otherwise be excluded
- Treatment of drug-induced pneumonitis involves temporary or permanent discontinuation of the presumed offending agent and initiation of corticosteroids if there are significant symptoms or pulmonary functional impairment (e.g., reduced vital or diffusing capacity)
- Lung injury is an important dose-limiting factor in chest radiation therapy
- Radiation pneumonitis generally occurs one to six months following completion of therapy and may be asymptomatic or present with dyspnea, hypoxemia or, rarely, respiratory failure
- Radiographic findings typically progress from ground glass opacities to patchy consolidation to fibrosis and volume loss, and usually develop within the field of radiation
- Treatment of radiation pneumonitis with steroids is indicated in the presence of symptoms, hypoxemia, or significant pulmonary function abnormalities
- Organizing pneumonia is a rare complication of radiation therapy described predominantly after breast radiation. Radiographic opacities occur outside the radiation field and may be migratory. This process usually responds to steroids, but a prolonged taper may be required

OVERVIEW OF PULMONARY COMPLICATIONS OF CANCER THERAPY AND THEIR EVALUATION

Pulmonary complications in patients who have cancer may involve any intrathoracic structures, including the airways, lung parenchyma, pulmonary vasculature, and pleura. They may be caused by a direct neoplastic involvement or result from the untoward effects of cancer therapy. Owing to the sheer breadth of the differential diagnosis, it is helpful to categorize pulmonary conditions afflicting these patients. For example, a quartet of *infection*, *inflammation*, *malignancy*, and *miscellaneous causes* provides a useful frame of reference.

Many patients present with symptoms such as dyspnea and cough (with or without hemoptysis), sometimes in conjunction with fever or hypoxemia. Physical examination may reveal tachypnea, crackles, or wheezes. Often, however, a respiratory disorder will come to light incidentally, as a result of routine body imaging revealing an abnormality, such as nodule(s), ground glass opacities, or consolidations. Whether demonstrating an incidental finding or obtained as part of a diagnostic evaluation, cross-sectional chest imaging plays a key role in developing a differential diagnosis. Pulmonary function testing can identify and stage the severity of an obstructive or restrictive ventilatory deficit as well as diffusion impairment and is particularly useful to monitor response to therapy. Cardiac evaluation with an electrocardiogram (ECG), transthoracic echocardiogram, and/or serum levels of (Pro-)brain natriuretic peptide is often required to identify or rule out a cardiac condition (e.g., congestive heart failure) as the cause of respiratory symptoms and imaging abnormalities. Noninvasive microbiologic investigation is an integral component of evaluation. Specific tests depend on the clinical suspicion and the level of immunodeficiency. They may include a respiratory viral polymerase chain reaction panel, sputum (induced if necessary), and blood culture for bacterial pathogens and serum procalcitonin, urinary streptococcal and legionella antigens, serum beta-D-glucan, aspergillus galactomannan, cytomegalovirus DNA, and others.

More invasive testing may become necessary if the above investigations do not result in a diagnosis. Thoracentesis is usually performed to elucidate the etiology of a pleural effusion that may be transudative (often from heart failure, renal failure, or fluid overload) or exudative (e.g., malignant, parapneumonic). Bronchoscopy with bronchoalveolar lavage and, when safe, transbronchial biopsies are useful primarily to identify pathogens or neoplastic lung disease. When malignancy, infection, and heart failure are excluded as the causes of abnormal chest imaging, drug (or radiation) induced lung injury is usually presumed. It is, in other words, a diagnosis of exclusion.

PULMONARY TOXICITY ASSOCIATED WITH ANTINEOPLASTIC AGENTS

Pneumonitis

Drug-induced pneumonitis is among the most common pulmonary complications of cancer therapeutics. A comprehensive and continuously updated list of drugs (including cancer drugs) reported to cause pneumonitis can be found at pneumotox.com. Pneumonitis may present with asymptomatic airspace opacities on computed tomography (CT) imaging or be associated with symptoms of cough, dyspnea, fevers, and hypoxemia. Life-threatening respiratory failure can occur. Severe drug-induced pneumonitis can lead to pulmonary fibrosis and permanent impairment of lung function.

Except for a few chemotherapeutic agents (e.g., bleomycin), the details of the pathophysiology of lung injury are unknown. Various mechanisms of pulmonary toxicity have been proposed, based on the mechanisms of action of different classes of therapeutic agents. These include a direct toxic effect on alveolar epithelial cells, the induction of an inflammatory immunologic response and endothelial cell injury, or activation causing capillary leak syndrome.[1] In the presence of clinical-radiographic characteristics consistent with drug-induced pneumonitis, the diagnosis rests on excluding other causes, particularly infection, neoplastic lung involvement, and cardiogenic pulmonary edema. Bronchoscopy with bronchoalveolar lavage and, if possible, transbronchial biopsy, plays an important role in the process of excluding infection and malignancy when such determination cannot be made on clinical, laboratory, and imaging findings alone. Histopathologic examination, when available, may demonstrate nonspecific interstitial pneumonitis, organizing pneumonia, hypersensitivity pneumonitis, various stages of diffuse alveolar damage, and, in the later stages, pulmonary fibrosis. No histopathologic findings are diagnostic and their interpretation must be guided by clinical correlation.

Treatment of drug-induced pneumonitis depends on its severity. In mild (e.g., subtle ground glass opacities, mild or no symptoms, and/or mildly abnormal pulmonary function tests) or asymptomatic cases, observation with or without discontinuation of the offending agent may be appropriate. More severe cases often require systemic corticosteroids and permanent discontinuation of the drug. Often patients are receiving multiple antineoplastic medications and it may be difficult to identify the culprit. Rechallenge with some or all the potential offenders rarely may be undertaken under careful observation with or without accompanying systemic steroids. Duration of treatment with steroids (usually oral prednisone) may last from several weeks to 3 to 12 months, depending on the severity of pneumonitis and its response to therapy. Occasionally, additional immunosuppressive therapies may be required, either to achieve an adequate response (e.g., infliximab in the case of immune checkpoint inhibitor-induced pneumonitis) or to maintain it (e.g., azithromycin or mycophenolate mofetil as a steroid-sparing agent in treatment of organizing pneumonia).

In addition to drug-induced pneumonitis, other diffuse parenchymal lung diseases associated with antineoplastic therapies include diffuse alveolar hemorrhage (see below) pulmonary alveolar proteinosis (busulfan, dasatinib, imatinib, leflunomide, sirolimus), pleuroparenchymal fibroelastosis (bleomycin, alkylating agents), differentiation syndrome (all-transretinoic acid, arsenic trioxide, enasidenib, ivosidenib, gilteritinib), and periengraftment respiratory distress syndrome (after hematopoietic stem cell transplant [HSCT]).

Pleural Effusion

Pleural effusions can occur because of drug-induced capillary leak (e.g., gemcitabine), congestive heart failure (e.g., anthracyclines), pulmonary venoocclusive disease (e.g., after HSCT) or as a result of direct drug toxicity (e.g., dasatinib). Dasatinib, especially at higher doses (>100 mg/day) is associated with pleural effusions.[2] The mechanisms of this form of toxicity are poorly understood, but pleural effusions are usually exudative with high lymphocyte count suggesting an inflammatory basis to fluid accumulation. When other causes of pleural disease are excluded, management may involve simple observation with or without interruption/discontinuation of dasatinib therapy, thoracentesis (repeated if necessary), and indwelling catheter placement. Diuretics and steroids can be used on a case-by-case basis, but are of limited value in our opinion.

Pulmonary Vascular Complications

Pulmonary vascular complications include venous thromboembolism (VTE), pulmonary hemorrhage, pulmonary arterial hypertension, and pulmonary venoocclusive disease.

Venous thromboembolism has been described in association with anastrozole, bevacizumab, cisplatin, dovitinib, everolimus, granulocyte-macrophage colony-stimulating factor, lapatinib, lenvatinib, lenalidomide, methotrexate, pembrolizumab, sirolimus, sunitinib, tamoxifen, and thalidomide (pneumotox.com). Patients with cancer are at increased risk of VTE and it may be difficult to distinguish the underlying predisposition from drug-induced effects. Recommendations for VTE treatment in such patients have been published.[3]

Diffuse alveolar hemorrhage has been described in association with bevacizumab, bortezomib, carfilzomib, crizotinib, cyclophosphamide, cytosine arabinoside, docetaxel, erlotinib, etoposide, everolimus, fludarabine, gefitinib, gemcitabine, gemtuzumab, imatinib, irinotecan, lenalidomide, methotrexate, mitomycin, nilotinib, osimertinib, pemetrexed, rituximab, sirolimus, post-HSCT, and sunitinib (pneumotox.com). Treatment involves discontinuation of the offending agent, supplemental oxygen, and correction of thrombocytopenia or coagulopathy, if present. The role of steroids, aminocaproic acid, tranexamic acid, and activated factor VII is not well defined.[4]

Pulmonary arterial hypertension has been associated with the BCR-Abl tyrosine kinase inhibitor I) dasatinib (and, less commonly, bosutinib, nilotinib, ponatinib). Other agents include alemtuzumab, bevacizumab, gemcitabine, leflunomide, mitomycin, ruxolitinib, and thalidomide (pneumotox.com). Recommendations for the management of tyrosine kinase inhibitor-related pulmonary hypertension were published by Weatherald and colleagues.[5]

Pulmonary venoocclusive disease (PVOD) has occurred in patients treated with bleomycin, cyclophosphamide, gemcitabine, melphalan, fludarabine, busulfan, and nitrosoureas, with or without radiation therapy to the chest (pneumotox.com). Diagnosis of PVOD requires a high index of suspicion because presentation may be subtle and easily confused with congestive heart failure (dyspnea, hypoxemia, pleural effusions, thickened interlobular septa on CT imaging). Echocardiogram will often reveal new pulmonary hypertension with no evidence of left ventricular dysfunction, but right heart catheterization may be needed to fully exclude it. Surgical lung biopsy is the gold standard for diagnosing PVOD, but often it is not performed because of the patient's ill health. Treatment is similar to those of patients with group 1 pulmonary arterial hypertension, but the risk of pulmonary edema in response to pulmonary arterial vasodilation is significant. The condition is often rapidly progressive and fatal despite therapy. Lung transplantation is not an option for patients with active cancer.

RADIATION-INDUCED LUNG INJURY

Radiation-induced lung injury (RILI) is an important dose-limiting factor in radiation directed to the thorax; it typically affects patients treated for lung cancer, breast cancer, or lymphoma, or those who receive total body irradiation for bone marrow transplant preparation.[6] The reported incidence of RILI is 5% to 25%, 5% to 10%, and 1% to 5% in patients undergoing chest radiation therapy for lung cancer, mediastinal lymphoma, and breast cancer, respectively.

Three pathophysiologic types can be distinguished. Classic radiation pneumonitis, which entails injury within the field of radiation owing to the direct cytotoxic action of ionizing radiation on lung cells, can progress to pulmonary fibrosis. Sporadic radiation pneumonitis mimics hypersensitivity pneumonitis and patients usually present with severe dyspnea and injury outside the field of radiation. Last, but not least, radiation-induced organizing pneumonia presents with infiltrates, often migratory and outside of the field of radiation, and it predominantly is seen with breast radiation (rarely with mediastinal or spine radiation). It usually responds well to steroid therapy which may, however, be prolonged owing to frequent relapses.[7]

Risk factors for radiation-induced lung injury can be divided into radiation-related, disease-related, and host-related as outlined (Table 21.1). The clinical presentation varies from asymptomatic to life-threatening respiratory failure. The main symptoms include dyspnea and dry, nonproductive cough, with low-grade fevers occurring less than 10% of the time; hemoptysis is rare. The physical examination may be normal or demonstrate adventitious lung sounds corresponding to a consolidation. The severity is graded according to factors established by the Radiation Therapy Oncology Group (Table 21.2).

TABLE 21.1 Risk Factors for Radiation-Induced Lung Injury

RADIATION RISK FACTORS	DISEASE RISK FACTORS	HOST RISK FACTORS
• % Total lung volume receiving ≥20 Gy (V20), ≥30%	• Refractory or relapsed disease (lymphoma)	• Age 50 years
• % Total lung volume receiving ≥5 Gy (V5), ≥65%	• Supraclavicular field (breast cancer)	• Autoimmune disease
• Mean total dose >20 Gy	• Bulky disease	• Interstitial lung disease
• Absolute volume lung spared >5 Gy (AVS5), <500 mL	• Chemotherapy	• Former or current smoker
• Target location: lower lobe	• Reirradiation	• COPD

COPD, Chronic obstructive pulmonary disease.

TABLE 21.2 Grades of Severity of Radiation-Induced Lung Injury According to the Radiation Therapy Oncology Group

GRADE	DEFINITION
I	Asymptomatic or mild symptoms (dry cough); slight radiographic appearances
II	Moderate symptomatic fibrosis or pneumonitis (severe cough); low-grade fever, patchy radiographic appearances
III	Severe symptomatic fibrosis or pneumonitis; dense radiographic changes
IV	Severe respiratory insufficiency/continuous oxygen/assisted ventilation

In general, radiation pneumonitis occurs one to six months following completion of radiation therapy. Serologic tests are nonspecific and may include an elevated white blood cell count, erythrocyte sedimentation rate, or C-reactive protein. Chest CT scan is the preferred imaging with the typical features being (1) ground glass opacities representing early radiation pneumonitis a few weeks after therapy completion, (2) patchy areas of consolidation in the later phases, and (3) linear scarring with consolidation and volume loss when fibrosis develops. These findings typically occur in the field of radiation. Although radiation pneumonitis is a clinical diagnosis, bronchoscopy and lung biopsy allow exclusion of other causes of lung injury, such as infection or disease progression. Pulmonary function tests typically show a restrictive patter with decreased lung volumes, compliance, forced vital capacity, and diffusing capacity.

The management varies by degree of severity. For very mild symptoms, clinical observation can be considered. For significantly symptomatic patients, a treatment course of prednisone 1 mg/kg/day for 2 to 4 weeks, followed by a slow taper over 6 to 12 weeks is recommendable. Patient frequently experience substantial symptomatic relief along with resolution of radiographic findings. However, relapse is possible following steroid taper and patients must be closely monitored. No established therapy exists to treat pulmonary fibrosis caused by radiation-induced lung injury, but clinical trials are ongoing using nintedanib, a multikinase inhibitor, and pirfenidone, an antifibrotic.

REFERENCES

1. Cortes JE, Jimenez CA, Mauro MJ, Geyer A, Pinilla-Ibarz J, Smith BD. Pleural effusion in dasatinib-treated patients with chronic myeloid leukemia in chronic phase: identification and management. *Clin Lymphoma Myeloma Leuk.* 2017;17(2):78–82.
2. Farge D, Frere C, Connors JM, et al. 2019 international clinical practice guidelines for the treatment and prophylaxis of venous thromboembolism in patients with cancer. *Lancet Oncol.* 2019;20(10):e566–e581.
3. Rathi NK, Tanner AR, Dinh A, et al. Low-, medium- and high-dose steroids with or without aminocaproic acid in adult hematopoietic SCT patients with diffuse alveolar hemorrhage. *Bone Marrow Transplant.* 2015;50(3):420–426.
4. Weatherald J, Chaumais MC, Montani D. Pulmonary arterial hypertension induced by tyrosine kinase inhibitors. *Curr Opin Pulm Med.* 2017;23(5):392–397.
5. Hanania AN, Mainwaring W, Ghebre YT, Hanania NA, Ludwig M. Radiation-induced lung injury: assessment and management. *Chest.* 2019;156(1):150–162.
6. Otani K, Seo Y, Ogawa K. Radiation-induced organizing pneumonia: a characteristic disease that requires symptom oriented management. *Int J Mol Sci.* 2017;18(2):281.
7. Stover DE, Gulati CM, Geyer AI, Kaner RJ. Pulmonary toxicity. In DeVita VT Jr, Lawrence TS, Rosenberg SA, eds. *DeVita, Hellman, and Rosenberg's Cancer: Principles and Practice of Oncology.* 10th ed. Philadelphia: Wolters Kluwer; 2015.

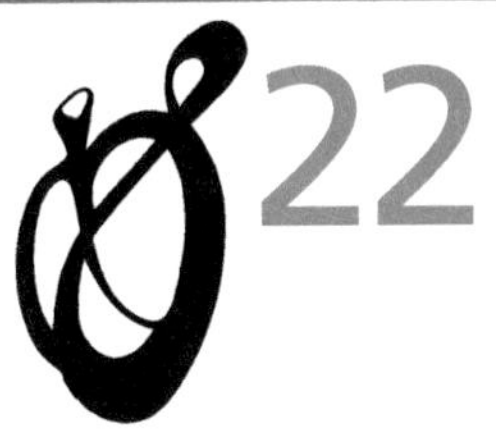

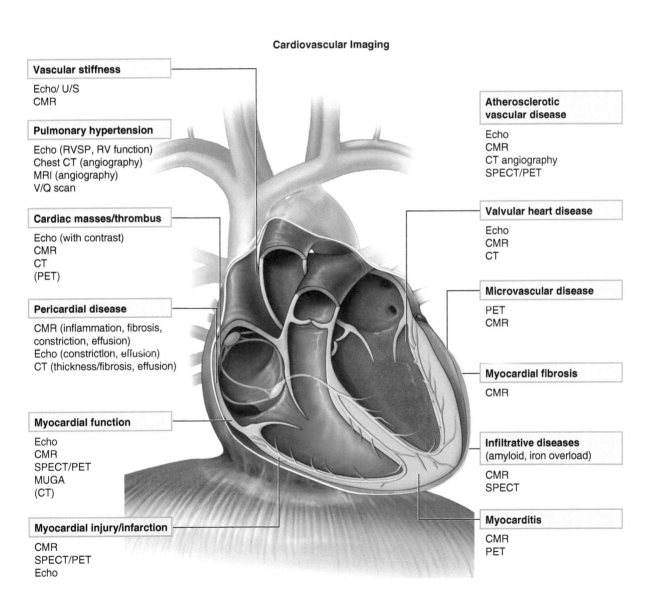

22 Cardiovascular Testing in Patient with Cancer

BÉNÉDICTE LEFEBVRE AND BONNIE KY

Cardiovascular Imaging

Vascular stiffness
Echo/ U/S
CMR

Pulmonary hypertension
Echo (RVSP, RV function)
Chest CT (angiography)
MRI (angiography)
V/Q scan

Cardiac masses/thrombus
Echo (with contrast)
CMR
CT
(PET)

Pericardial disease
CMR (inflammation, fibrosis, constriction, effusion)
Echo (constriction, effusion)
CT (thickness/fibrosis, effusion)

Myocardial function
Echo
CMR
SPECT/PET
MUGA
(CT)

Myocardial injury/infarction
CMR
SPECT/PET
Echo

Atherosclerotic vascular disease
Echo
CMR
CT angiography
SPECT/PET

Valvular heart disease
Echo
CMR
CT

Microvascular disease
PET
CMR

Myocardial fibrosis
CMR

Infiltrative diseases (amyloid, iron overload)
CMR
SPECT

Myocarditis
CMR
PET

CHAPTER OUTLINE

KEY POINTS

- New imaging modalities play a central role in identifying cardiovascular complications. Cardiotoxicity can manifest in a number of ways, depending on the agent, and can include disease states such as heart failure and cardiomyopathy, coronary artery disease, coronary vasospasm, myocarditis, pericardial constriction, and pulmonary hypertension. In light of the many potential cardiovascular diseases (CVD), a broad range of cardiovascular imaging modalities is needed to best serve the needs in the cancer population (Table 22.1).
- When choosing an imaging technique, a nonradiating cardiovascular imaging method is preferred if comparable in terms of accuracy, cost, and convenience (Table 22.2).
- Given its great accessibility and low cost, echocardiography is the recommended method for serial evaluation of left ventricular ejection fraction (LVEF), ideally with three-dimensional (3D) quantitation. The use of global longitudinal strain (GLS) is also strongly encouraged.
- One of the most studied deformation parameters, GLS holds utility in detecting preclinical changes during cancer therapy. It is predictive of subsequent declines in LVEF.[1–3] However, high image quality and consistent acquisition and analyses platforms are critical for comparisons over time. Moreover, ongoing research is aimed at determining the incremental utility of GLS over conventional parameters.
- Cardiac magnetic resonance (CMR), which is the gold standard for the evaluation of LVEF, allows also for the detailed assessment of cardiac morphology, including measures of myocardial injury, which may be particularly relevant to cancer therapy cardiotoxicity. Cost, access, and technical requirements limit its widespread use.
- The use of one modality for serial assessment of LVEF throughout cancer therapy evaluation is recommended to limit variability.

ECHOCARDIOGRAPHY

Given multiple advantages, including accessibility, relatively low cost, lack of ionizing radiation, and portability, echocardiography is an essential tool and the cornerstone for the assessment of cancer therapy complications. Although at times limited owing to poor acoustic windows, echocardiography is versatile and can provide comprehensive information on both cardiac structure and function. These include parameters related to left and right ventricular size, systolic function (left ventricular ejection fraction [LVEF] and right ventricular fractional area change), and measures of cardiac mechanics such as global longitudinal strain (GLS), diastolic function, valve disease, and pericardial disease. Echocardiography can also be used to gain insight into cardiac hemodynamics, as well as in the diagnosis of ischemia. In the following section, we focus primarily on the echocardiographic assessment of left ventricular systolic function and left ventricular cardiac mechanics and briefly discuss the role of echocardiography in diagnosing pericardial, valvular, and coronary artery disease as well as its use in hemodynamic assessment.

Evaluation of Cardiac Systolic Function and Mechanics

Prior to starting cancer therapy, baseline LVEF evaluation by echocardiography should be assessed with the best technique available. The American Society of Echocardiography (ASE) and the European Association of Cardiovascular Imaging (EACVI) recommend the modified biplane Simpson's method.[4] However, it is difficult to diagnose small, nearly subclinical changes in LV function by using two-dimensional (2D) measurements.[4] Previous studies comparing different transthoracic echocardiogram techniques demonstrated that 2D echocardiography LVEF quantitation by Simpson's method can only distinguish changes in LVEF on the order of approximately 10%.[5,6] Compared with 2D methods, which has a temporal variability (as defined by the standard error) of 0.049 (95% CI, 0.045–0.054), for serial evaluation of LVEF in patients with cancer over one year, noncontrast three-dimensional (3D) echocardiography has a variability of 0.028 (95% CI, 0.025–0.031).[6,7] 3D-derived left ventricular volumes are more precise, accurate, and reproducible and do not rely on geometric assumptions.[6,8] However, to obtain accurate 3D volumes, there is still a need for high-quality images and advanced training and time for image post-processing.

Echocardiography can be limited owing to poor acoustic windows, which may be worsened in patients with cancer following radiation or surgery (mastectomy). If the quality of the image is suboptimal as defined as two or more nonvisualized contiguous segments, microbubble contrast (Optison, Definity, or Lumason) should be used, as recommended by the ASE guidelines to help in improving endocardial border detection.[4] Echocardiographic contrast can also be used to improve the diagnostic yield of associated complications of cardiomyopathy and of cancer, such as intracardiac thrombus.

Limitations of LVEF assessment also include its inability to identify small changes in cardiac function or robustly identify patients at increased risk for the development of cancer therapeutics-related cardiac dysfunction (CTRCD). However, a growing body of literature supports the use of myocardial mechanics and deformation, and in particular, strain assessment to detect subclinical changes in cardiac function. Global longitudinal strain, one of the most studied deformation parameters, has been shown to be predictive of subsequent declines in LVEF.[1–3,9] GLS is typically derived from the apical two-, three-, and four-chamber images. In a prospective study of 81 women with breast cancer receiving trastuzumab, an 11% (95% CI, 8.3%–14.6%) reduction in GLS derived from the apical two- and four-chamber views predicted future cardiotoxicity with a sensitivity of 65% and a specificity of 94%.[3] Based largely on this study and others, the ASE and the EACVI recommended that a change of more than 15% in GLS during cancer therapy is significant and should be interpreted as abnormal.[7] Of note, the use of the same vendor and analysis software for the follow up of serial GLS are also of importance, and several factors that can influence strain values need to be recognized (Fig. 22.1). GLS is highly dependent on image quality. Furthermore, GLS is load dependent (like LVEF) and a function of chamber size and hypertrophy. There is an important need to demonstrate appropriate quality control prior to the use of strain. The SUCCOUR (Strain sUrveillance of Chemotherapy for improving Cardiovascular Outcomes) trial did not meet its primary endpoint at 1 year and the clinical management implications of GLS remain to be defined.[10]

Circumferential motion contributes substantially more to LVEF than longitudinal motion[11] and may also be highly relevant to cardio-oncology. In a prospective study of 135 patients with breast cancer receiving doxorubicin and/or trastuzumab, every 1% worsening in the circumferential strain, patient had an increased odds of developing CTRCD by 17% to 23% ($P < .001$).[12] In comparison, for every 1% worsening in the longitudinal strain, there was a 3% to 25% increased odds of developing CTRCD ($P = .037$).[12] The role of circumferential strain in the cardio-oncology population is an area of active investigation.

3D measurement of cardiac mechanics is also an interesting and promising area of study. In a study of 142 patients with breast cancer receiving anthracyclines, with or without trastuzumab, a decrease in 3D measures of LVEF, GLS, and global circumferential strain was more marked than changes in analogous 2D-derived parameters during anthracycline chemotherapy; it was associated with subsequent declines in LVEF.[13] 3D-derived LV strain is a new technique that incorporates data from all the layers of the myocardium. Its role in detecting subclinical cardiotoxicity is an area of active research. However, widespread feasibility of 3D echocardiography remains a limitation.[8]

Cardiac Structure and Hemodynamic Assessment

Echocardiography can also be used to diagnose pericardial disease, including effusions, which can be a consequence of metastatic disease, drug exposure, infection, or a consequence of radiation with subsequent pericardial constriction.[7] Echocardiography is also important in assessing valvular function. Indeed, radiation may result in abnormal valve morphology and cause valvular regurgitation

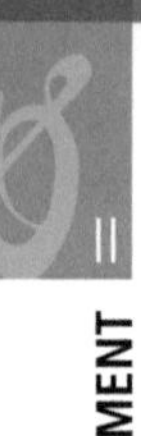

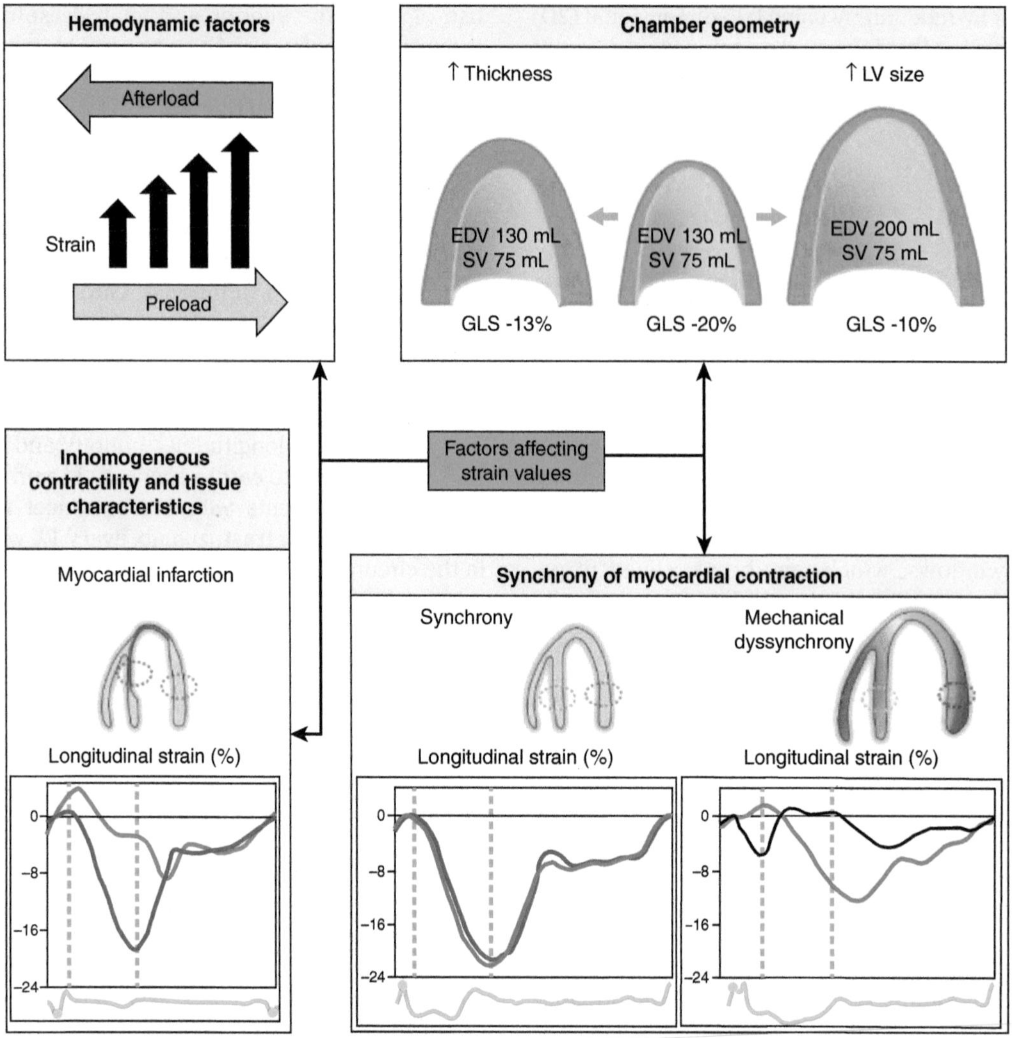

FIG. 22.1 Strain values are significantly influenced by loading conditions, chamber geometry, conduction delays, and tissue characteristics. The strain curves illustrate typical findings: *blue* indicates normal segments, *purple* indicates infarcted segment, *yellow* indicates early activated (septal) segment, reindicates late activated (lateral) segment. *Dashed green* lines indicate aortic valve opening and closure. *EDV,* End-diastolic volume; *GLS,* global longitudinal strain; *SV,* stroke volume. (Voigt J-U, Cvijic M. 2- and 3-Dimensional myocardial strain in cardiac health and disease. *JACC Cardiovasc Imaging.* 2019;12(9):1849–1863.)

or stenosis.[14] Patients with cancer are also at risk of developing valvular endocarditis, either secondary to bacteremia or marantic disease. Echocardiography plays a central role in assessing for vegetations. In cases of poor acoustic windows, transesophageal echocardiography is used to better assess valvular dysfunction, and identify valvular endocarditis, either of the infective or marantic subtype.

Assessment of right ventricular function and pulmonary pressures is also important, because some newer cancer therapies, including tyrosine kinase inhibitors and proteasome inhibitors, have been associated with the development of pulmonary hypertension.[15,16] Serial pulmonary arterial systolic pressure measurement is recommended whenever using medications such as dasatinib.[17]

Echocardiography can also be readily used to assess diastolic function. E/e′, the ratio between early mitral inflow velocity (E) and mitral annular early diastolic velocity (e′), can be used to estimate LV filling pressures and LV compliance. A recent systematic review and meta-analysis[18] reported that four diastolic function variables were associated with a long-term risk of cardiotoxicity in patients treated with doxorubicin. Changes in mitral E (odds ratio [OR], 3.4; 95% CI, 1.5–7.8; P = .003), mitral E/A, the ratio of early mitral inflow velocity (E) and late diastolic transmitral flow velocity (A), (OR, 4.3; 95% CI, 2.1–8.9; $P < .0001$), lateral E′ (OR, 3.7; 95% CI, 1.5–9.4; $P < .005$) and lateral S′, the peak tissue Doppler imaging systolic velocity, (OR, 2.7; 95% CI, 1.2–5.8; $P = .01$) were all significantly associated with a subsequent decrease in systolic function. It is of critical importance not only to understand the potential changes in diastolic function with cardiotoxic cancer therapy, but also to determine if changes in diastolic function are associated with an increased risk of heart failure with reduced or preserved ejection fraction, as they are in the general population.[19] This is an area of active research. Assessment of diastolic function should be performed when evaluating patients with cancer as per the ASE guidelines.[7]

Stress Echocardiography

Stress echocardiography with exercise or pharmacologic stress (e.g., dobutamine) is an excellent tool to diagnose ischemia. It can also be used to assess for contractile reserve and severity of valvular disease with low-flow, low-gradient severe aortic stenosis.[7,20] In a small study of 49 cases of breast cancer with patients undergoing high-dose chemotherapy, a decrease in contractile reserve, as defined by difference between peak and rest LVEF in absolute units by five or more units, was a predictor of a subsequent decline in LVEF.[21] The sensitivity and specificity of stress echocardiography is 88% and 83%, respectively for obstructive coronary artery disease.[22]

In conclusion, echocardiography is an affordable, accessible, and safe imaging technique to assess baseline and serial LVEF during cancer therapy. GLS should be used whenever possible to identify preclinical changes in ventricular function, especially in patients receiving cardiotoxic cancer therapy who are at increased risk for CTRCD. Echocardiography can also be used to gain important insight into pericardial disease, valvular disease, cardiac hemodynamics, and ischemia.

CARDIAC MAGNETIC RESONANCE (CMR) IMAGING

Cardiac Function Assessment

A study by Armstrong and colleagues[23] compared the use of 2D-derived measures of LVEF by echocardiography with CMR-derived measures in cancer survivors. This study demonstrated that 2D echocardiography overestimated LVEF by 5%. Also, transthoracic echocardiography had a sensitivity of 25% and a false–negative rate of 75% in detecting LVEF less than 50% when compared with CMR. 3D echocardiographic assessment of LVEF had better performance and similar to CMR ($P = .08$), with a sensitivity of 53% and a false–negative rate of 47%. Furthermore, 11% of the 114 patients were classified as having a LVEF less than 50% when using CMR instead of 2D echocardiography.[23,24] Based on these data, the authors recommended to consider a multimodality approach, including CMR, in a high-risk population when LVEF by 2D transthoracic echocardiography was quantified between 50% and 59%.

In general, CMR imaging is a precise technique that can be used to assess a broad range of early and late complications of cardiac cancer therapy, such as declines in left and right ventricular systolic ejection function (LVEF, RVEF), myocarditis, valve dysfunction or pericarditis. Although considered the gold standard modality to measure LVEF, given its lack of geometric assumptions (the endocardium in systole and diastole is contoured in multiple short axis slices from base to apex), the use of CMR is typically not considered as first-line given accessibility and cost issues. Complete evaluation with CMR is also time-consuming compared with other modalities. Patients who suffer from claustrophobia or have metallic devices may not be able to tolerate this procedure. However, CMR may now be performed in patients with pacemakers and defibrillators. Protocols, as reported in the 2017 Heart Rhythm Society (HRS) Expert consensus document,[25] have been developed to define the safe conduct of CMR with specific cardiovascular implantable electronic devices, but only at 1.5 Tesla so far (Class IIa indication). CMR must not be performed in patients with abandoned pacemaker or implantable cardioverter defibrillator leads, lead remnants, fractured leads, or surgically implanted epicardial leads. In those with breast cancer, tissue expanders that may be used in breast reconstruction contain a magnetic infusion port that may heat or migrate during MRI. Despite demonstration of feasibility and relative safety in a few small studies, there are case reports demonstrating harm and tissue expanders are still deemed unsafe and contraindicated as it pertains to MRI.[26–29]

However, if transthoracic echocardiogram images are suboptimal for adequate diagnosis, the use of CMR for LVEF and LV volumes is warranted. CMR measurements are highly accurate with superior intraobserver and interobserver reproducibility, and CMR offers high spatial and temporal resolution.[30] CMR can also identify small or subclinical LVEF changes and is used to elucidate reproducibly the impact of LV volumes on changes in LVEF, which is particularly relevant in the cancer population, where patients may be volume depleted or overloaded. However, the lack of studies identifying its use in robustly identifying measures of early and subclinical LV systolic dysfunction in the context of potential cardiotoxic cancer therapy currently makes CMR a limited modality,[7,24,31] although a number of studies are underway to accomplish this objective.

For example, CMR-derived measures of longitudinal and circumferential strain may be used to detect subclinical changes in LVEF, although this method is mostly used for research purposes. In a prospective study by Ong and colleagues[32] where 41 women with HER2+ breast cancer were treated with trastuzumab, in combination with anthracyclines in 56% of those, a substantial decrease in longitudinal and circumferential strain at 6 and 12 months was correlated with small changes in LVEF (Pearson's $r = -0.60$ for GLS and -0.75 for GCS; $P < .001$).[32] Jolly and colleagues[33] studied mid-wall circumferential strain obtained by CMR in the context of cardiotoxic chemotherapy in 72 adult subjects, which demonstrated a strong correlation between the decrease in circumferential strain and LVEF ($r = -0.61$; $P < .0001$). Another study[34] evaluated 46 long-term survivors of childhood cancer up to 27 years after their cancer therapy in which they were treated with a cumulative anthracycline dose 200 mg/m^2 or more. All had normal systolic function, both on transthoracic echocardiogram and on CMR. However, significant abnormalities were seen in circumferential, longitudinal, and regional peak circumferential strains in multiple segments compared with normal subjects (circumferential strain $-14.9\% \pm 1.4\%$ vs. $-19.5\% \pm 2.1\%$; $P < .001$) and (longitudinal strain ($-13.5\% \pm 1.9\%$ vs. $17.3\% \pm 1.4\%$; $P < .001$) in cancer survivors and controls, respectively).[34]

Cardiac Structure Assessment

With high spatial and temporal resolution, CMR is useful in the detection of pericardial diseases such as constriction, metastases, or tumor invasion to the parietal or visceral pericardium. Importantly, CMR is also used to characterize the myocardium in cases of infiltrative or inflammatory processes, such as amyloidosis, iron-overload cardiomyopathy, or myocarditis. Primary amyloidosis that may be associated with multiple myeloma can present with concentric left ventricle hypertrophy, restrictive ventricular filling pattern, subendocardial, focal or patchy late gadolinium enhancement (LGE), elevated native T1 relaxation time, higher extracellular volume and a typical black blood pool pattern.[24,35,36] Iron-overload cardiomyopathy that can be primary from hemochromatosis or secondary from repetitive blood transfusions is characterized by short T2-star (T2*).[37,38]

Myocarditis is another important complication of cancer therapy that can be potentially life threatening. Agents, such as cyclophosphamide, cytarabine, immune checkpoint inhibitors, tyrosine kinase inhibitors, and even anthracyclines, have been implicated in myocarditis.[7,39–41] As the signs and symptoms can be quite variable, ranging from fatigue, chest discomfort, subtle electrocardiographic changes, arrhythmias, and abnormal cardiac biomarkers, to changes in cardiac function with nonspecific regional wall motion abnormalities, cardiogenic shock and even cardiac arrest, it is important to have robust strategies to diagnose myocarditis. CMR allows for detailed tissue characterization and can detect changes, including fibrosis and edema. The Lake Louise Consensus Criteria[42] published in 2009, have been established as part of the diagnostic criteria for myocarditis. When at least two of the three criteria are present, a systematic review showed a diagnosis accuracy of 78% for sensitivity and 88% of specificity, with an area-under-the-curve of 83%.[43] The Updated Lake Louise Criteria[44] suggest the presence of one T1-based and one T2-based criteria can be used to diagnosis acute or active inflammation with increased specificity.[44,45]

CMR has also been used to define the structural changes that occur with anthracycline use. The use of contrast with gadolinium allows for the characterization of the myocardium, including fibrosis. An abnormal increase in T1 and extracellular volume (ECV), both potentially indicative of diffuse fibrosis, was observed in a cross-sectional analyses of a small cohort of 54 cancer survivors, at 3 years after anthracycline use, independent of other cardiovascular comorbid conditions.[46] Another small study of 42 patients previously treated with anthracyclines (median 84 months prior) demonstrated increased

ECV compared with age- and gender-matched controls (0.36 ± 0.03 vs. 0.28 ± 0.02; $P < .001$).[47] Early changes in contrast-enhanced T1-weighted signal intensities have also been observed within 3 months after anthracycline-based chemotherapy, potentially indicative of subclinical injury.[48] A recent basic translational study conducted in pigs receiving intracoronary doxorubicin showed that the first sign of reversible cardiotoxicity in this animal cohort was an increased in T2 signal, demonstrating cellular edema. This change occurred early during treatment (6 weeks) at a reversible stage and without any change in other markers, including T1, ECV, or left ventricular motion defects.[49]

Late gadolinium enhancement is another important prognostic factor used in the diagnosis and management of cardiomyopathy; it has been validated against endomyocardial biopsy for the diagnosis of myocardial fibrosis or scar.[50] However, a cross-sectional study of 91 patients with anthracycline-induced cardiomyopathy who underwent CMR found that only 6% of the subjects had LGE positivity despite a mean LVEF of 36 ± 8%.[51]

CMR may be used to identify and quantify valvular disease. In this context, CMR is Class I indication by the American College of Cardiology/American Heart Association 2014 Valvular heart disease guideline.[20] It can assess valve thickening secondary to radiation and be used to calculate precisely flow regurgitation in valvular insufficiency. CMR can also be useful to diagnose complications of cardiomyopathy, such as a LV thrombus, if it is not well-visualized with contrast-enhanced transthoracic echocardiogram imaging. Additionally, CMR can help in the identification of catheter thrombus or endocarditis and can aid in the workup of cardiac masses.

Stress Cardiac Magnetic Resonance

High-resolution myocardial perfusion CMR (stress-induced with adenosine infusion) has been shown to diagnose flow-limiting epicardial coronary artery lesions and has high correlation with fractional flow reserve (FFR). Thus, stress CMR offers a noninvasive modality to ascertain significant coronary artery disease.[52] Many studies have also validated this method in the emergency room setting of patients at intermediate risk with acute coronary syndrome.[53–55]

In summary, CMR offers numerous new techniques and image sequences for the diagnosis of the different cancer therapy complications. CMR allows for the detailed assessment of various cardiac structures and remains the gold standard for the evaluation of LVEF. However, its cost, accessibility, technical requirements, and study duration limit its use.

NUCLEAR IMAGING

Multigated Acquisition Scan (MUGA)

Multigated acquisition scan, also called equilibrium radionuclide angiogram, technetium-labeled red blood cells, or blood pool scan, was the conventional method of choice of determining LVEF in the late 1970s and has been widely used, standardized, and studied. Although it has largely fallen out of favor given the use of radiation and lack of incremental information beyond LVEF,[7,56,57] it is still a very sensitive and reproducible modality for LVEF assessment. However, the evaluation of LVEF by MUGA exposes a patient to 5 to 10 mSV per evaluation.[7,58] This can increase up to 15 mSV when combined with myocardial perfusion imaging.[59]

A study by Bellenger and colleagues[30] compared the mean LVEF derived by MUGA and echocardiography and showed that the values calculated by radionuclide ventriculography were inferior to 2D echocardiogram and CMR (24 ± 9%, 31% ± 10%, and 30% ± 11%, respectively). These results reinforced the point that LVEF values vary across imaging modalities and, thus, are not interchangeable during the assessment of cardiotoxicity. Another study by Huang and colleagues[57] studied 75 patients with cancer who had assessment of LVEF within 30 days with both MUGA and CMR methods. Although the mean MUGA LVEF was only slightly lower than the mean CMR LVEF (48.5% vs. 50.0%), MUGA misclassified 26 patients (35%) as having an LVEF of less than 50%.

The latest guidelines from the Society of Nuclear Medicine[60] report normal resting MUGA LVEF ranges between 50% and 80%. Based on these reference values, the ASE and EACVI (7) have noted prior indications for the use of MUGA in the context of anthracycline-based chemotherapy, as outlined in Table 22.1. However, as alluded to the use of MUGA has fallen out of favor given increased radiation exposure.

TABLE 22.1 Overview of Cardiac Imaging Recommendations

CANCER THERAPY	MONITORING RECOMMENDATION	REFERENCE
Anthracyclines	**Echo**	
	Recommended for those with symptoms of heart failure	ASCO [1]
	Recommended for surveillance of those undergoing treatment; frequency based on clinical discretion	ASCO [1]
	Recommended to perform in asymptomatic patients 6–12 months after completion of therapy in those felt to be at a higher risk for CTRCD	ASCO [1]
	LVEF measurement at baseline and during treatment (frequency not defined) (2D/3D) and GLS with treatment or risk factor modification at LVEF ≥60%, 50%–59%, 40%–49%, and <40%	Liu et al. [2]
	LVEF at baseline and at end of treatment. Regular LVEF monitoring if cumulative dose exceeds 240 mg/m^2. Recommendation based on use of 2D echocardiogram and GLS	SEOM [3] ESC [4]
	Measurement of LVEF at baseline, every 3 months during chemotherapy, at the end of treatment (within 1 month), every 3 months during the first year after chemotherapy, every 6 months during the following 4 years, and yearly afterward	Cardinale et al. [5]
	CMR	
	Recommended instead of echo only if echo unavailable or not technically feasible	ASCO [1]
	Recommendation is to perform in asymptomatic patients 6–12 months after completion of therapy in those felts to be at a higher risk for CTRCD and not a good candidate for echocardiogram	ASCO [1]
	Utility of CMR over LVEF monitoring in terms of myocardial fibrosis and inflammation quantification	Jordan et al. [6]
	Multigated acquisition scan (MUGA)	
	Recommended instead of echo only if echo unavailable or not technically feasible and CMR unavailable	ASCO [1]
	Recommended to perform in asymptomatic patients 6–12 months after completion of therapy in those felt to be at a higher risk for CTRCD and not a good candidate for echocardiogram and CMR unavailable	ASCO [1]
	LVEF >50% at baseline 1. Measurement at 250–300 mg/m^2 2. Measurement at 450 mg/m^2 3. Measurement before each dose above 450 mg/m^2 4. Discontinue therapy if LVEF decreases by ≥10% from baseline and <50%	ASNC [7]
	LVEF <50% at baseline 1. Do not treat if LVEF is <30% 2. Serial measurement before each dose 3. Discontinue therapy is LVEF decreases by ≥10% from baseline or LVEF ≤30%	ASNC [7]
Trastuzumab	**Echo**	
	Recommended for surveillance of patients with metastatic breast cancer receiving trastuzumab	ASCO [1]
	Recommended: 1. Baseline evaluation of LVEF 2. Repeat measurement of LVEF every 3 months while on treatment 3. Repeat echo at 4 week intervals if therapy is withheld for significant LVEF decline. The caveat to this recommendation is that ASCO does not endorse holding treatment unless deemed clinically necessary by oncologist (E, evidence quality: insufficient) 4. Every 6 months for the immediate 2-year period after completing the regimen	SEOM [3] ASCO [1] Manufacturer [8,9]
	Transthoracic echocardiograms that includes comprehensive 2D, 3D, and strain imaging in patients with LVEF 40%–49% and no HF signs or symptoms 1. Baseline 2. After starting HER2 targeted therapy every 6 weeks for 2 assessments 3. Every 3 months during the study 4. Asymptomatic absolute decline in LVEF of ≥10% points from baseline or to ≤35%, HER2 targeted therapy held with a confirmatory echocardiogram at 2–4 weeks 5. Repeat echo at the end of treatment and 6 months after end of treatment	SAFE, HEaRt study [10,11]
Immune checkpoint inhibitors	1. Echo recommended with signs/symptoms of myocarditis, pericarditis, arrhythmias, impaired ventricular function with heart failure, and vasculitis 2. Additional testing guided by cardiology may include stress testing, cardiac MRI, and cardiac catheterization	ASCO [12]

TABLE 22.1 Overview of Cardiac Imaging Recommendations—cont'd

CANCER THERAPY	MONITORING RECOMMENDATION	REFERENCE
Tyrosine kinase inhibitors	**Echo**	
	1. Recommended baseline echo with follow up at 1 months and every 3 months while on therapy with VEGF or VEGF receptor inhibitors (the authors recognize lack of sufficient data)	ASE/EACVI [13]
	2. Recommended stress echo in risk stratifying patients with intermediate or high pretest probability of CAD who are to undergo tyrosine kinase inhibitor therapy, particularly sorafenib and sunitinib	
Radiation therapy	**Echo**	
	Baseline and repeated echo after radiation therapy involving the heart are recommended for the diagnosis and follow up of valvular heart disease 1. Annual echocardiogram if symptomatic valvular disease 2. Screening echocardiogram 10 years after radiation therapy and every 5 years thereafter in asymptomatic patients	ASE/EACVI [14]
	Cardiac MRI	
	Recommended in those with suboptimal echocardiography or discrepant results	ESC [4]
	Coronary CT angiography/calcium artery calcium score	
	Reasonable to perform ≥5 years after radiotherapy, and further workup (e.g., coronary angiography, functional testing) is indicated for risk stratification if there is concern for severe ischemic heart disease	SCAI [15]
	SPECT	ASE [14]
	1. Reasonable to screen for CAD with a functional noninvasive stress test 5–10 years after radiation exposure in asymptomatic individuals deemed a high risk for radiation-induced heart disease 2. Repeat stress testing can be planned every 5 years if the first examination does not show inducible ischemia	
Prior exposure (not currently on therapy)	**Echo**	
	Recommended for those with symptoms of heart failure	ASCO [1]
	CMR	
	Recommended instead of echo only if echo unavailable or not technically feasible	ASCO [1]
Potentially cardiotoxic therapy	**Echo**	
	LVEF measurement at baseline and during$ treatment (2D/3D) and GLS with treatment or risk factor modification at LVEF ≥60%, 50%–59%, 40%–49%, and <40%	Liu et al. [2]

ASCO, American Society of Clinical Oncology; *ASE*, American Society of Echocardiography; *ASNC*, American Society of Nuclear Cardiology; *CAD*, coronary artery disease; *CMR*, cardiac magnetic resonance imaging; *CTRCD*, cancer therapeutics-related cardiac dysfunction; *EACVI*, European Association of Cardiovascular Imaging; *ESC*, European Society of Cardiology; *GLS*, global longitudinal strain; *LVEF*, left ventricular ejection fraction; *SCAI*, Society for Cardiovascular Angiography and Interventions; *MRI*, magnetic resonance imaging; *SEOM*, Spanish Society of Medical Oncology; *SPECT*, single-photon emission computed tomography; *VEGF*, vascular endothelial growth factor.

REFERENCES

[1] Armenian SH, Lacchetti C, Barac A, et al. Prevention and monitoring of cardiac dysfunction in survivors of adult cancers: American Society of Clinical Oncology Clinical Practice Guideline. *J Clin Oncol.* 2017;35(8):893–911.

[2] Liu J, Banchs J, Mousavi N, et al. Contemporary role of echocardiography for clinical decision making in patients during and after cancer therapy. *JACC Cardiovasc Imaging.* 2018;11(8):1122–1131.

[3] Virizuela JA, García AM, de Las Peñas R, et al. SEOM clinical guidelines on cardiovascular toxicity (2018). *Clin Transl Oncol Off Publ Fed Span Oncol Soc Natl Cancer Inst Mex.* 2019;21(1):94–105.

[4] Zamorano JL, Lancellotti P, Rodriguez Muñoz D, et al. 2016 ESC position paper on cancer treatments and cardiovascular toxicity developed under the auspices of the ESC Committee for practice guidelines: the task force for cancer treatments and cardiovascular toxicity of the European Society of Cardiology (ESC). *Eur Heart J.* 2016;37(36):2768–2801.

[5] Cardinale D, Colombo A, Bacchiani G, et al. Early detection of anthracycline cardiotoxicity and improvement with heart failure therapy. *Circulation.* 2015;131(22):1981–1988.

[6] Jordan JH, Todd RM, Vasu S, Hundley WG, et al. Cardiovascular magnetic resonance in the oncology patient. *JACC Cardiovasc Imaging.* 2018;11(8):1150–1172.

[7] Russell RR, Alexander J, Jain D, et al. The role and clinical effectiveness of multimodality imaging in the management of cardiac complications of cancer and cancer therapy. *J Nucl Cardiol.* 2016;23(4):856–884.

[8] Herceptin Hylecta. Genentech-Manufacturer Information. https://www.gene.com/download/pdf/herceptin_hylecta_prescribing.pdf. Accessed September 19, 2021.

[9] Perjeta. Genentech-Manufacturer Information. https://www.gene.com/download/pdf/perjeta_prescribing.pdf. Accessed September 19, 2021.

[10] Lynce F, Barac A, Tan MT, et al. SAFE-HEaRt: rationale and design of a pilot study investigating cardiac safety of HER2 targeted therapy in patients with HER2-positive breast cancer and reduced left ventricular function. *Oncologist.* 2017;22(5):518–525.

[11] Lynce F, Barac A, Geng X, et al. Prospective evaluation of the cardiac safety of HER2-targeted therapies in patients with HER2-positive breast cancer and compromised heart function: the SAFE-HEaRt study. *Breast Cancer Res Treat.* 2019;175(3):595–603.

[12] Brahmer JR, Lacchetti C, Schneider BJ, et al. Management of immune-related adverse events in patients treated with immune checkpoint inhibitor therapy: American Society of Clinical Oncology clinical practice guideline. *J Clin Oncol.* 2018;36(17):1714–1768.

[13] Plana JC, Galderisi M, Barac A, et al. Expert consensus for multimodality imaging evaluation of adult patients during and after cancer therapy: a report from the American Society of Echocardiography and the European Association of Cardiovascular Imaging. *Eur Heart J Cardiovasc Imaging.* 2014;15(10):1063–1693.

[14] Lancellotti P, Nkomo VT, Badano LP, et al. Expert consensus for multi-modality imaging evaluation of cardiovascular complications of radiotherapy in adults: a report from the European Association of Cardiovascular Imaging and the American Society of Echocardiography. *Eur Heart J Cardiovasc Imaging.* 2013;14(8):721–740.

[15] Iliescu C, Grines CL, Herrmann J, et al. SCAI expert consensus statement: evaluation, management, and special considerations of cardio-oncology patients in the cardiac catheterization laboratory (Endorsed by the Cardiological Society of India, and Sociedad Latino Americana de Cardiologıa Intervencionista). *Catheter Cardiovasc Interv.* 2016;87(5):895–899.

(From Biersmith MA, Tong MS, Guha A, et al. Multimodality cardiac imaging in the era of emerging cancer therapies. *J Am Heart Assoc.* 2020;9(2):e013755. https://doi.org/10.1161/JAHA.119.013755. Used with the permission of John Wiley & Sons.])

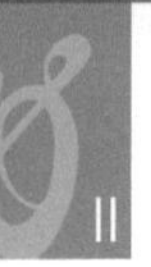

Nuclear Single-Photon Emission Computed Tomography (SPECT)

Nuclear stress testing imaging can also be useful in patients with suspected coronary artery disease and in identifying ischemic territories. Stress myocardial perfusion imaging with single-photon emission computed tomography with the radioisotopes Tc-99m sestamibi, Tc-99m tetrofosmin, and, less commonly, thallium-201 (T1-201) can detect regional wall motion abnormalities and/or flow-limiting coronary artery perfusion deficits.[22] It can be performed with exercise or pharmacologically induced stress with a vasodilator (adenosine, dipyridamole, or regadenoson) or an inotrope (dobutamine). In noncancer populations, false–negative rates of up to 15% have been reported largely secondary to the presence of balanced ischemia with multivessel coronary artery disease.[22]

Positive Emission Tomography

With higher spatial and temporal resolution than MUGA and SPECT, positron emission tomography (PET) is the gold standard to assess myocardial metabolism and myocardial perfusion. Myocardial perfusion imaging with PET can quantify myocardial blood flow and coronary flow reserve.[22] Rubidium-82 (^{82}RB PET) is superior in patients with a high body mass index ($\geq$30 kg/m^2) owing to its greater penetration and accuracy in quantifying myocardial blood flood with very low radiation exposure.[61] Studies have shown that myocardial blood flow can be a surrogate for myocardial dysfunction, both at the macro- and microcirculation and it predicts future adverse cardiac events.[62,63] Fluorine-18-fluorodeoxyglucose (^{18}F-FDG)-PET is another technique used in the diagnosis of tumors, but it can also characterize vascular disease.[64] By being a glucose analog, ^{18}F-FDG-PET uptake is related to intense metabolic activities, such as inflammation. However, the myocardium also has a high metabolic rate and this modality cannot adequately assess for coronary atherosclerosis or vasculitis, but it is used primarily for larger vessel disease, such as that of the aorta.[64] Another radiotracer, F-sodium fluoride (^{18}F-NaF), has also been studied as a technique to identify microcalcifications in the vasculature. Unfortunately, only a small percentage of plaques demonstrate increased uptake of this radiotracer and this technique is limited in its sensitivity to detect small plaques.[65,66] Thus, more data and prospective studies are needed for a better understanding of their potential role in the routine care of patients with cancer. Furthermore, some studies have shown the feasibility of conducting FDG-PET in order to assess myocardial inflammation such as myocarditis. In head-to-head comparison with CMR in 65 patients, FDG-PET showed a sensitivity of 74% and a specificity of 97%, with a diagnostic accuracy of 87%.[67] A dietary preparation of low carbohydrates for at least 24 hours is essential to improve the diagnosis.

CARDIAC COMPUTER TOMOGRAPHY (CT)

Cardiac computer tomography is used in the evaluation of coronary artery disease, either with angiography to assess the degree of stenosis or coronary artery calcium to assess for plaque burden. It can also characterize pericardial disease, given its excellent spatial resolution, and assess LVEF. However, owing to radiation, it is not recommended for the routine evaluation of LVEF.

Technically, CT angiography is limited by radiation exposure (up to 24 mSV) and the need for lower, regular heart rates to provide adequate image quality.[22,68] This modality tends to overestimate calcific lesions and underestimate soft plaques owing to partial volume averaging and calcium blooming artifacts. However, coronary artery calcium score with the Agatston score has a low radiation dose of about 1 mSV and may be used in patients as a means of risk stratification.[22] In the general population, a number of studies have linked the presence of coronary artery calcium with an increased risk of cardiovascular events. One study showed that a positive calcium score was associated with a five-fold increased risk in fatal and nonfatal coronary artery disease events and a three-fold increased risk in any cardiovascular disease events. A score of more than 100 was associated with early death.[69] Another study of almost 10,000 patients showed that a coronary artery calcium score of 0 in low-to-intermediate risk individuals is a potent predictor of survival over a 15-year period.[70] A high calcium score is also useful to ascertain the diagnosis of low-gradient severe aortic stenosis where a score of 2000 Agatston Units (AU) or greater in men and 1200 AU or greater in women suggestive of severe aortic stenosis.[71–73] Finally, fractional flow reserve CT (FFR-CT) identifies hemodynamically

TABLE 22.2 Strengths and Limitations of Different Imaging Modalities for Diagnosis and Monitoring of Cardiotoxicity

IMAGING MODALITY	VOLUME/ FUNCTION ASSESSMENT	TISSUE/MASS CHARACTERIZATION	MYOCARDITIS/ INFLAMMATION	VALVE DISEASE	PERICARDIAL DISEASE	CORONARY DISEASE/ ISCHEMIA	RADIATION EXPOSURE	REPRODUCIBILITY/ ACCURACY	COST	AVAILABILITY
2D echo	+	+	0	+++	++	0	None	+	+	+++
3D echo	++	++	0	+++	+	0	None	++	+	++
Stress echo	++	0	0	++	+	+++	None	++	++	++
CMR	+++[a]	+++[b]	+++	++	+++	+++	None	+++	+++	++
PET	++	++	+++	0	++	+++	+++	+++	+++	+
Nuclear[b]	++	+	+	0	++	++	+++	++	+	++
CTCA	+	+	0	+	++	+++[c]	+/++	+++	++	++

[a]Established gold standard.
[b]Includes SPECT, MUGA.
[c]CTCA is the only noninvasive test that provides anatomic information with regard to presence of coronary disease. All other modalities rely on functional assessment.
+++, Excellent diagnostic accuracy or features/ high cost; ++, intermediate diagnostic accuracy or features/intermediate cost; +, reasonable diagnostic accuracy or features/low cost; 0, unable to diagnose; *2D echo,* 2-dimensional echocardiography; *3D echo,* 3-dimensional echocardiography; *CMR,* cardiac magnetic resonance; *CTCA,* computed tomography coronary angiogram; *PET,* positron emission tomography; *Stress echo,* stress echocardiography.
From Seraphim A, Westwood M, Bhuva AN, et al. Advanced imaging modalities to monitor for cardiotoxicity. *Curr Treat Options Oncol.* 2019;20(9):73.

significant coronary lesions in a noninvasive manner.[74] Although a very promising method of identifying culprit lesions, it is however costly and not accessible to all centers. Its specific role in the cancer population remains to be determined.

CONCLUSION

With the rapid development of new cancer treatments, there is a growing burden of cardiovascular disease, secondary to both the "off-target" effects of therapies, but also secondary to the increase in cancer survival rates. This has resulted in a greater need for the diagnosis and treatment of common comorbid conditions in this population, and in particular, cardiovascular disease.

In terms of diagnostic modalities, echocardiography is a portable, low-cost, widely accessible modality and is the method of choice and most widely used technique for serial evaluation of LVEF (Table 22.2). The use of deformation indices, such as global longitudinal strain, allows for the earlier detection of subclinical changes in cardiac function; however, factors that impact strain values need to be considered. GLS, as with LVEF, is still load dependent and highly dependent on image quality (Fig. 22.1). Ongoing clinical studies are aimed at determining if there is incremental clinical utility to the use of GLS. CMR, despite being the gold standard for LVEF evaluation, has limited use owing to high cost and unequal access. It is however an excellent modality for tissue characterization and allows also for the detailed assessment of cardiac morphology. Nuclear imaging is useful for the diagnosis and risk stratification of coronary artery disease. With repeated LVEF assessment required throughout the course of cancer therapy (before, during, and after), these techniques are not recommended owing to radiation exposure. CT is an excellent tool to diagnose coronary artery disease with FFR-CT and predict cardiovascular outcomes with coronary artery calcium score. Finally, given the variability across modalities, the use of one method for serial assessment of LVEF throughout cancer therapy evaluation is strongly recommended. A summary of the recommendations for cardiac imaging in patients undergoing cancer therapy is provided in Table 22.1.

REFERENCES

1. Sawaya H, Sebag IA, Plana JC, et al. Assessment of echocardiography and biomarkers for the extended prediction of cardiotoxicity in patients treated with anthracyclines, taxanes, and trastuzumab. *Circ Cardiovasc Imaging*. 2012;5(5):596–603.
2. Sawaya H, Sebag IA, Plana JC, et al. Early detection and prediction of cardiotoxicity in chemotherapy-treated patients. *Am J Cardiol*. 2011;107(9):1375–1380.
3. Negishi K, Negishi T, Hare JL, Haluska BA, Plana JC, Marwick TH. Independent and incremental value of deformation indices for prediction of trastuzumab-induced cardiotoxicity. *J Am Soc Echocardiogr*. 2013;26(5):493–498.
4. Lang RM, Badano LP, Mor-Avi V, et al. Recommendations for cardiac chamber quantification by echocardiography in adults: an update from the American Society of Echocardiography and the European Association of Cardiovascular Imaging. *J Am Soc Echocardiogr*. 2015;28(1):1–39.e14.
5. Otterstad JE, Froeland G, St. John Sutton M, Holme I. Accuracy and reproducibility of biplane two-dimensional echocardiographic measurements of left ventricular dimensions and function. *Eur Heart J*. 1997;18(3):507–513.
6. Thavendiranathan P, Grant AD, Negishi T, Plana JC, Popović ZB, Marwick TH. Reproducibility of echocardiographic techniques for sequential assessment of left ventricular ejection fraction and volumes. *J Am Coll Cardiol*. 2013;61(1):77–84.
7. Plana JC, Galderisi M, Barac A, et al. Expert consensus for multimodality imaging evaluation of adult patients during and after cancer therapy: a report from the American Society of Echocardiography and the European Association of Cardiovascular Imaging. *J Am Soc Echocardiogr*. 2014;27(9):911–939.
8. Santoro C, Arpino G, Esposito R, et al. 2D and 3D strain for detection of subclinical anthracycline cardiotoxicity in breast patients with cancer: a balance with feasibility. *Eur Heart J Cardiovasc Imaging*. 2017;18(8):930–936.
9. Stoodley PW, Richards DAB, Hui R, et al. Two-dimensional myocardial strain imaging detects changes in left ventricular systolic function immediately after anthracycline chemotherapy. *Eur J Echocardiogr*. 2011;12(12):945–952.
10. Negishi T, Thavendiranathan P, Negishi K, et al. Rationale and design of the strain surveillance of chemotherapy for improving cardiovascular outcomes. *JACC Cardiovasc Imaging*. 2018;11(8):1098–1105.
11. Stokke TM, Hasselberg NE, Smedsrud MK, et al. Geometry as a confounder when assessing ventricular systolic function: comparison between ejection fraction and strain. *J Am Coll Cardiol*. 2017;70(8):942–954.
12. Narayan HK, French B, Khan AM, et al. Noninvasive measures of ventricular-arterial coupling and circumferential strain predict cancer therapeutics–related cardiac dysfunction. *JACC Cardiovasc Imaging*. 2016;9(10):1131–1141.
13. Zhang KW, Finkelman BS, Gulati G, et al. Abnormalities in 3-dimensional left ventricular mechanics with anthracycline chemotherapy are associated with systolic and diastolic dysfunction. *JACC Cardiovasc Imaging*. 2018;11(8):1059–1068.
14. Lancellotti P, Nkomo VT, Badano LP, et al. Expert consensus for multi-modality imaging evaluation of cardiovascular complications of radiotherapy in adults: a report from the European Association of Cardiovascular Imaging and the American Society of Echocardiography. *J Am Soc Echocardiogr*. 2013;26(9):1013–1032.
15. Montani D, Bergot E, Günther S, et al. Pulmonary arterial hypertension in patients treated by dasatinib. *Circulation*. 2012;125(17):2128–2137.

16. Grandin EW, Ky B, Cornell RF, Carver J, Lenihan DJ. Patterns of cardiac toxicity associated with irreversible proteasome inhibition in the treatment of multiple myeloma. *J Card Fail.* 2015; 21(2):138–144.
17. Zamorano JL, Lancellotti P, Rodriguez Muñoz D, et al. 2016 ESC position paper on cancer treatments and cardiovascular toxicity developed under the auspices of the ESC Committee for practice guidelines: the task force for cancer treatments and cardiovascular toxicity of the European Society of Cardiology (ESC). *Eur Heart J.* 2016;37(36):2768–2801.
18. Nagiub M, Nixon JV, Kontos MC. Ability of nonstrain diastolic parameters to predict doxorubicin-induced cardiomyopathy: a systematic review with meta-analysis. *Cardiol Rev.* 2018;26(1):29–34.
19. Kane GC, Karon BL, Mahoney DW, et al. Progression of left ventricular diastolic dysfunction and risk of heart failure. *JAMA.* 2011;306(8)856–863. doi:10.1001/jama.2011.1201
20. Nishimura RA, Otto CM, Bonow RO, et al. 2014 AHA/ACC guideline for the management of patients with valvular heart disease: a report of the American College of Cardiology/American Heart Association task force on practice guidelines. *J Thorac Cardiovasc Surg.* 2014;148(1):e1–e132.
21. Civelli M, Cardinale D, Martinoni A, et al. Early reduction in left ventricular contractile reserve detected by dobutamine stress echo predicts high-dose chemotherapy-induced cardiac toxicity. *Int J Cardiol.* 2006;111(1):120–126.
22. Mangla A, Oliveros E, Williams KA, Kalra DK. Cardiac imaging in the diagnosis of coronary artery disease. *Curr Probl Cardiol.* 2017;42(10):316–366.
23. Armstrong GT, Plana JC, Zhang N, et al. Screening adult survivors of childhood cancer for cardiomyopathy: comparison of echocardiography and cardiac magnetic resonance imaging. *J Clin Oncol.* 2012;30(23):2876–2884.
24. Jordan JH, Todd RM, Vasu S, Hundley WG. Cardiovascular magnetic resonance in the oncology patient. *JACC Cardiovasc Imaging.* 2018;11(8):1150–1172.
25. Indik JH, Gimbel JR, Abe H, et al. 2017 HRS expert consensus statement on magnetic resonance imaging and radiation exposure in patients with cardiovascular implantable electronic devices. *Heart Rhythm.* 2017;14(7):e97–e153.
26. Nava MB, Bertoldi S, Forti M, et al. Effects of the magnetic resonance field on breast tissue expanders. *Aesthetic Plast Surg.* 2012;36(4):901–907.
27. Marano AA, Henderson PW, Prince MR, Dashnaw SM, Rohde CH. Effect of MRI on breast tissue expanders and recommendations for safe use. *J Plast Reconstr Aesthet Surg.* 2017;70(12):1702–1707.
28. Thimmappa ND, Prince MR, Colen KL, et al. Breast tissue expanders with magnetic ports: clinical experience at 1.5 T. *Plast Reconstr Surg.* 2016;138(6):1171–1178.
29. Dibbs R, Culo B, Tandon R, St Hilaire H, Shellock FG, Lau FH. Reconsidering the "MR Unsafe" breast tissue expander with magnetic infusion port: a case report and literature review. *Arch Plast Surg.* 2019;46(4):375–380.
30. Bellenger NG, Burgess MI, Ray SG, et al. Comparison of left ventricular ejection fraction and volumes in heart failure by echocardiography, radionuclide ventriculography and cardiovascular magnetic resonance; are they interchangeable? *European heart J.* 2000;21(16):1387–1396.
31. Wassmuth R, Lentzsch S, Erdbruegger U, et al. Subclinical cardiotoxic effects of anthracyclines as assessed by magnetic resonance imaging-a pilot study. *Am Heart J.* 2001;141(6):1007–1013.
32. Ong G, Brezden-Masley C, Dhir V, et al. Myocardial strain imaging by cardiac magnetic resonance for detection of subclinical myocardial dysfunction in breast patients with cancer receiving trastuzumab and chemotherapy. *Int J Cardiol.* 2018;261:228–233.
33. Jolly MP, Jordan JH, Meléndez GC, McNeal GR, D'Agostino RB, Hundley WG. Automated assessments of circumferential strain from cine CMR correlate with LVEF declines in patients with cancer early after receipt of cardio-toxic chemotherapy. *J Cardiovasc Magn Reson.* 2017;19(1):59.
34. Toro-Salazar OH, Gillan E, O'Loughlin MT, et al. Occult cardiotoxicity in childhood cancer survivors exposed to anthracycline therapy. *Circ Cardiovasc Imaging.* 2013;6(6):873–880.
35. Tuzovic M, Yang EH, Baas AS, et al. Cardiac amyloidosis: diagnosis and treatment strategies. *Curr Oncol Rep.* 2017;19(7):46.
36. Zhao L, Fang Q. Recent advances in the noninvasive strategies of cardiac amyloidosis. *Heart Fail Rev.* 2016;21(6):703–721.
37. Anderson LJ, Holden S, Davis B, et al. Cardiovascular T2-star (T2*) magnetic resonance for the early diagnosis of myocardial iron overload. *Eur Heart J.* 2001;22(23):2171–2179.
38. Pennell DJ. T2* magnetic resonance and myocardial iron in thalassemia. *Ann N Y Acad Sci.* 2005;1054:373–378.
39. Mahmood SS, Fradley MG, Cohen JV, et al. Myocarditis in patients treated with immune checkpoint inhibitors. *J Am Coll Cardiol.* 2018;71(16):1755–1764.
40. Neilan TG, Rothenberg ML, Amiri-Kordestani L, et al. Myocarditis associated with immune checkpoint inhibitors: an expert consensus on data gaps and a call to action. *Oncologist.* 2018;23(8):874–878.
41. Schmidinger M, Zielinski CC, Vogl UM, et al. Cardiac toxicity of sunitinib and sorafenib in patients with metastatic renal cell carcinoma. *J Clin Oncol.* 2008;26(32):5204–5212.
42. Friedrich MG, Sechtem U, Schulz-Menger J, et al. Cardiovascular magnetic resonance in myocarditis: a JACC white paper. *J Am Coll Cardiol.* 2009;53(17):1475-1487.
43. Kotanidis CP, Bazmpani MA, Haidich AB, Karvounis C, Antoniades C, Karamitsos TD. Diagnostic accuracy of cardiovascular magnetic resonance in acute myocarditis. *JACC Cardiovasc Imaging.* 2018;11(11):1583–1590.
44. Ferreira VM, Schulz-Menger J, Holmvang G, et al. Cardiovascular magnetic resonance in nonischemic myocardial inflammation. *J Am Coll Cardiol.* 2018;72(24):3158–3176.
45. Friedrich MG. Cardiovascular magnetic resonance for myocardial inflammation: Lake Louise versus mapping? *Circ Cardiovasc Imaging.* 2018;11(7):e008010.
46. Jordan JH, Vasu S, Morgan TM, et al. Anthracycline-associated T1 mapping characteristics are elevated independent of the presence of cardiovascular comorbidities in cancer survivors. *Circ Cardiovasc Imaging.* 2016;9(8):e004325. doi:10.1161/CIRCIMAGING.115.004325.
47. Neilan TG, Coelho-Filho OR, Shah RV, et al. Myocardial extracellular volume by cardiac magnetic resonance imaging in patients treated with anthracycline-based chemotherapy. *Am J Cardiol.* 2013;111(5):717–722.
48. Jordan JH, D'Agostino RB, Hamilton CA, et al. Longitudinal assessment of concurrent changes in left ventricular ejection fraction and left ventricular myocardial tissue characteristics after administration of cardiotoxic chemotherapies using T1-weighted and T2-weighted cardiovascular magnetic resonance. *Circ Cardiovasc Imaging.* 2014;7(6):872–879.
49. Galán-Arriola C, Lobo M, Vílchez-Tschischke JP, et al. Serial magnetic resonance imaging to identify early stages of anthracycline-induced cardiotoxicity. *J Am Coll Cardiol.* 2019;73(7): 779–791.
50. Lurz P, Eitel I, Adam J, et al. Diagnostic performance of CMR imaging compared with EMB in patients with suspected myocarditis. *JACC Cardiovasc Imaging.* 2012;5(5):513–524.
51. Neilan TG, Coelho-Filho OR, Pena-Herrera D, et al. Left ventricular mass in patients with a cardiomyopathy after treatment with anthracyclines. *Am J Cardiol.* 2012;110(11):1679–1686.
52. Lockie T, Ishida M, Perera D, et al. High-resolution magnetic resonance myocardial perfusion imaging at 3.0-tesla to detect hemodynamically significant coronary stenoses as determined by fractional flow reserve. *J Am Coll Cardiol.* 2011;57(1):70–75.
53. Miller CD, Case LD, Little WC, et al. Stress CMR reduces revascularization, hospital readmission, and recurrent cardiac testing in intermediate-risk patients with acute chest pain. *JACC Cardiovasc Imaging.* 2013;6(7):785–794.
54. Cury RC, Shash K, Nagurney JT, et al. Cardiac magnetic resonance with T2-weighted imaging improves detection of patients with acute coronary syndrome in the emergency department. *Circulation.* 2008;118(8):837–844.
55. Ingkanisorn WP, Kwong RY, Bohme NS, et al. Prognosis of negative adenosine stress magnetic resonance in patients presenting to an emergency department with chest pain. *J Am Coll Cardiol.* 2006; 47(7):1427–1432.
56. Plana JC, Thavendiranathan P, Bucciarelli-Ducci C, Lancellotti P. Multimodality imaging in the assessment of cardiovascular toxicity in the patient with cancer. *JACC Cardiovasc Imaging.* 2018;11(8):1173–1186.
57. Huang H, Nijjar PS, Misialek JR, et al. Accuracy of left ventricular ejection fraction by contemporary multiple gated acquisition

scanning in patients with cancer: comparison with cardiovascular magnetic resonance. *J Cardiovasc Magn Reson.* 2017;19(1):34.
58. Ong DS, Scherrer-Crosbie M, Coelho-Filho O, Francis SA, Neilan TG. Imaging methods for detection of chemotherapy-associated cardiotoxicity and dysfunction. *Expert Rev Cardiovasc Ther.* 2014;12(4):487–497.
59. Chen J, Einstein AJ, Fazel R, et al. Cumulative exposure to ionizing radiation from diagnostic and therapeutic cardiac imaging procedures. *J Am Coll Cardiol.* 2010;56(9):702–711.
60. Scheiner J, Sinusas A, Wittry MD, et al. Society of Nuclear Medicine Procedure Guideline for Gated Equilibrium Radionuclide Ventriculography. 2002. http://snmmi.files.cms-plus.com/docs/Gated Equilibrium Radionuclide Ventriculography 3.0.pdf.
61. Chatal J-F, Rouzet F, Haddad F, Bourdeau C, Mathieu C, Le Guludec D. Story of rubidium-82 and advantages for myocardial perfusion PET imaging. *Front Med (Lausanne).* 2015;2:65.
62. Ziadi MC, deKemp RA, Williams KA, et al. Impaired myocardial flow reserve on rubidium-82 positron emission tomography imaging predicts adverse outcomes in patients assessed for myocardial ischemia. *J Am Coll Cardiol.* 2011;58(7):740–748.
63. Farhad H, Dunet V, Bachelard K, Allenbach G, Kaufmann PA, Prior JO. Added prognostic value of myocardial blood flow quantitation in rubidium-82 positron emission tomography imaging. *Eur Heart J Cardiovasc Imaging.* 2013;14(12):1203–1210.
64. Moghbel M, Al-Zaghal A, Werner TJ, Constantinescu CM, Høilund-Carlsen PF, Alavi A. The role of PET in evaluating atherosclerosis: a critical review. *Semin Nucl Med.* 2018;48(6):488–497.
65. Joshi NV, Vesey AT, Williams MC, et al. 18F-fluoride positron emission tomography for identification of ruptured and high-risk coronary atherosclerotic plaques: a prospective clinical trial. *Lancet.* 2014;383(9918):705–713.
66. Dweck MR, Chow MWL, Joshi NV, et al. Coronary arterial 18F-sodium fluoride uptake. *J Am Coll Cardiol.* 2012;59(17):1539–1548.
67. Nensa F, Kloth J, Tezgah E, et al. Feasibility of FDG-PET in myocarditis: comparison to CMR using integrated PET/MRI. *J Nucl Cardiol.* 2018;25(3):785–794.
68. Anderson JL, Adams CD, Antman EM, et al. 2011 ACCF/AHA focused update incorporated into the ACC/AHA 2007 guidelines for the management of patients with unstable angina/non-ST-elevation myocardial infarction: a report of the American College of Cardiology Foundation/American Heart Association task force on practice guidelines. *Circulation.* 2011;123(18):e426–e579.
69. Carr JJ, Jacobs DR, Terry JG, et al. Association of coronary artery calcium in adults aged 32 to 46 years with incident coronary heart disease and death. *JAMA Cardiol.* 2017;2(4):391–399.
70. Valenti V, Ó Hartaigh B, Heo R, et al. A 15-year warranty period for asymptomatic individuals without coronary artery calcium. *JACC Cardiovasc Imaging.* 2015;8(8):900–909.
71. Aggarwal SR, Clavel MA, Messika-Zeitoun D, et al. Sex differences in aortic valve calcification measured by multidetector computed tomography in aortic stenosis. *Circ Cardiovasc Imaging.* 2013;6(1):40–47.
72. Clavel M-A, Messika-Zeitoun D, Pibarot P, et al. The complex nature of discordant severe calcified aortic valve disease grading: new insights from combined Doppler echocardiographic and computed tomographic study. *J Am Coll Cardiol.* 2013;62(24):2329–2338.
73. Clavel M-A, Burwash IG, Pibarot P. Cardiac imaging for assessing low-gradient severe aortic stenosis. *JACC Cardiovasc Imaging.* 2017;10(2):185–202.
74. Pijls NHJ, de Bruyne B, Peels K, et al. Measurement of fractional flow reserve to assess the functional severity of coronary-artery stenoses. *N Engl J Med.* 1996;334(26):1703–1708.

PART III

Cardiovascular Disease Management After Cancer Treatment

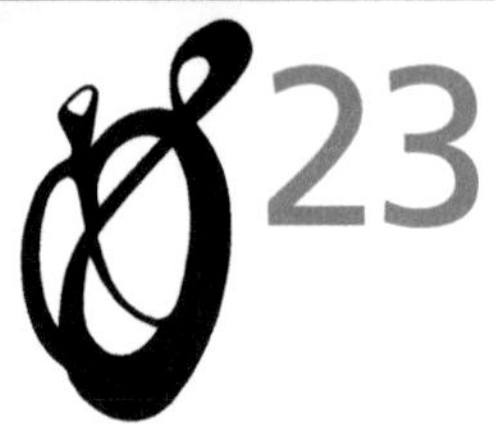

23 Key Points of Cardio-Oncology Evaluation After Cancer Therapy

JOERG HERRMANN

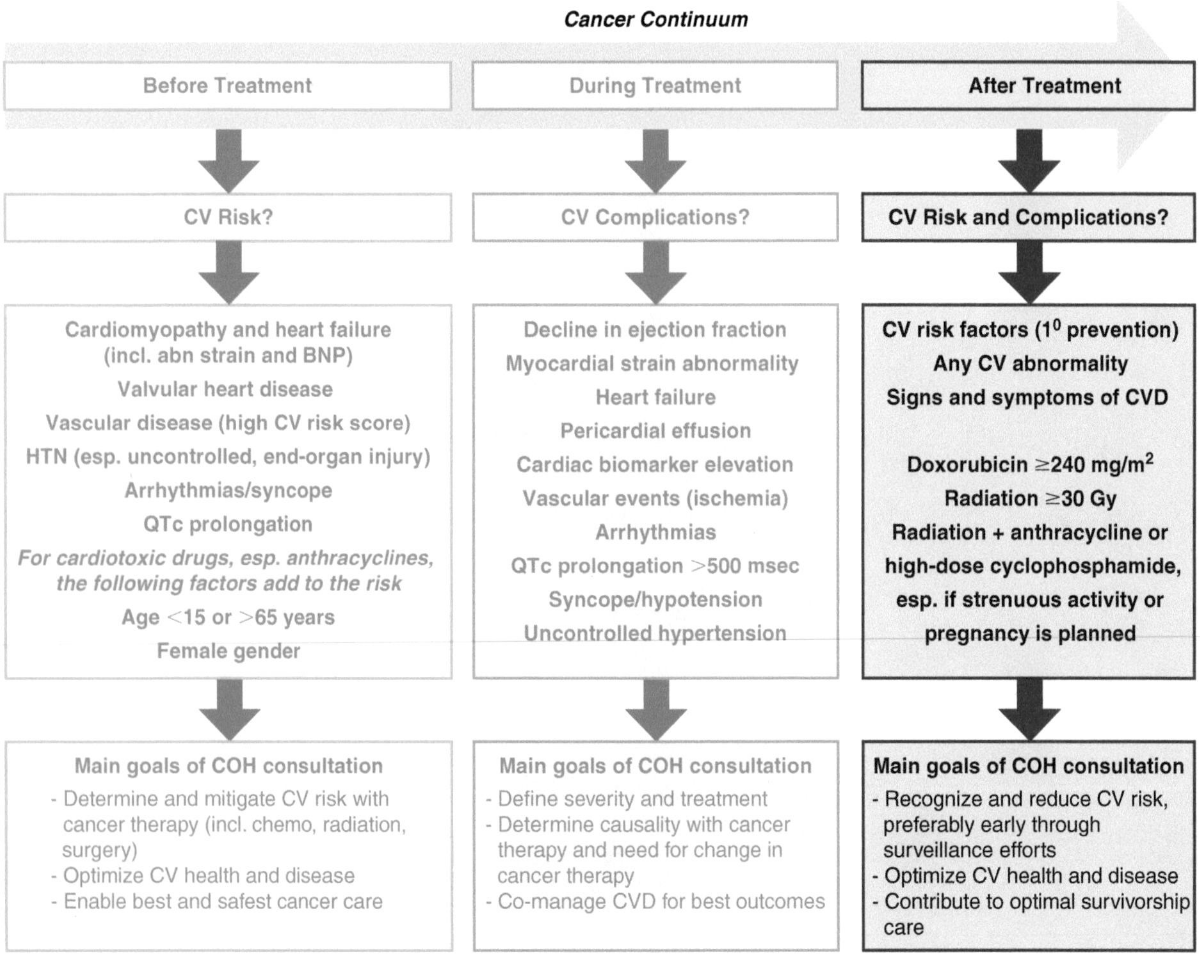

Cancer Continuum

Before Treatment	During Treatment	**After Treatment**
CV Risk?	CV Complications?	**CV Risk and Complications?**
Cardiomyopathy and heart failure (incl. abn strain and BNP) Valvular heart disease Vascular disease (high CV risk score) HTN (esp. uncontrolled, end-organ injury) Arrhythmias/syncope QTc prolongation *For cardiotoxic drugs, esp. anthracyclines, the following factors add to the risk* Age <15 or >65 years Female gender	Decline in ejection fraction Myocardial strain abnormality Heart failure Pericardial effusion Cardiac biomarker elevation Vascular events (ischemia) Arrhythmias QTc prolongation >500 msec Syncope/hypotension Uncontrolled hypertension	**CV risk factors (1^0 prevention)** **Any CV abnormality** **Signs and symptoms of CVD** **Doxorubicin ≥240 mg/m^2** **Radiation ≥30 Gy** **Radiation + anthracycline or high-dose cyclophosphamide, esp. if strenuous activity or pregnancy is planned**
Main goals of COH consultation - Determine and mitigate CV risk with cancer therapy (incl. chemo, radiation, surgery) - Optimize CV health and disease - Enable best and safest cancer care	Main goals of COH consultation - Define severity and treatment - Determine causality with cancer therapy and need for change in cancer therapy - Co-manage CVD for best outcomes	**Main goals of COH consultation** - Recognize and reduce CV risk, preferably early through surveillance efforts - Optimize CV health and disease - Contribute to optimal survivorship care

KEY POINTS

- The main objective of the posttherapy evaluation of patients with cancer is to identify cardiovascular (CV) risk and complications of cancer therapy.
- Patients may present with the chronic phase of complications encountered during cancer therapy (e.g., constrictive pericarditis following acute pericarditis).
- Patients may also present with the asymptomatic or symptomatic phase of late-onset complications of cancer therapy (e.g., cardiomyopathy and heart failure after anthracycline therapy or myocardial, pericardial, valvular, or vascular disease after radiation therapy).
- Surveillance efforts differ by type of cancer therapy exposure and their expected CV toxicity profile (e.g., cardiac function imaging for therapies with cardiotoxicity risk, vascular testing for therapies with vascular toxicity risk). Central to all preventive efforts is the optimization of CV health and CV risk factors and cardio-oncology rehabilitation programs are emerging.
- Integration of CV disease aspects into a cancer survivorship plan is recommendable.

Survivorship, namely the period after completion of cancer therapy, has not received as much attention as it deserves. Decades ago, this was, indeed, not much of a consideration, but in view of the ever-improving survival statistics, this is radically changing. In fact, a review of cancer versus cardiovascular (CV) mortality trends of 28 malignancies from the 1970s into the current era showed that cancer-related mortality continues to dominate outcomes in only one-third of malignancies. In the other two-thirds, cancer-related mortality has declined so much that it reaches or is surpassed by cardiovascular-related mortality. Management of CV disease in patients with cancer is therefore becoming more and more important.

Central to the best possible long-term outcomes is to optimize CV health and CV risk factor control, a topic that is emphasized in the first chapter in this section. This is followed by an overview of the long-term CV complications of chemotherapy and radiation therapy. The specific disease entities that can be encountered in cancer survivors are subsequently covered, and this section concludes with a chapter on cardiac rehabilitation, thereby going full circle to healthy lifestyle coaching and recommendable multidimensional and multidisciplinary efforts for the best possible long-term outcomes.

Much more remains to be done in the area of survivorship, in particular high-quality studies that inform on the best and most cost-effective modes of surveillance and prevention of the various disease entities that can reduce the quality and duration of life for cancer survivors. As most of the efforts in clinical cancer care have been directed to the active treatment period with cardio-oncology not being an exception in this regard, each cardio-oncology program will have to make an active effort addressing the question how to integrate cancer survivorship efforts into clinical practice. It will be of utmost importance to the patients.

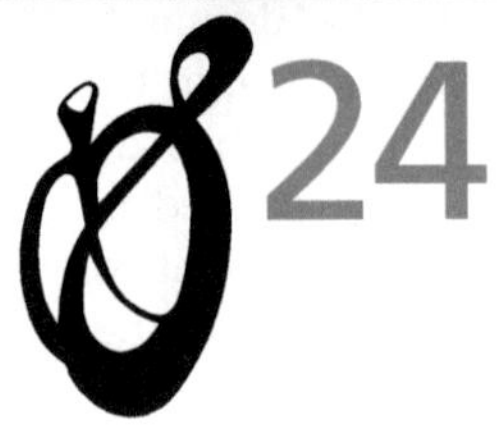

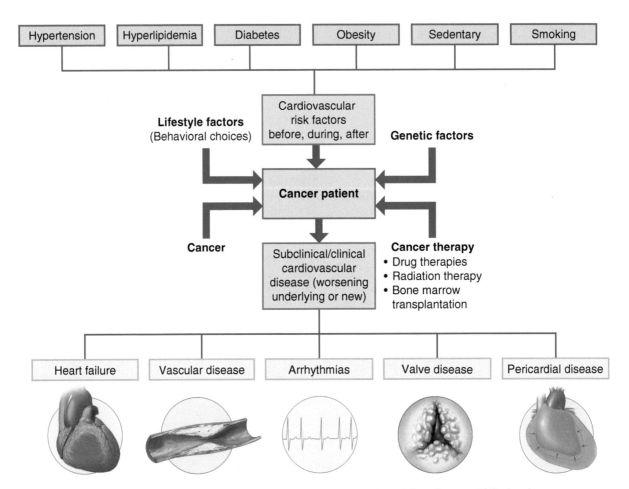

24 Cancer Survivorship and Comorbidity Disease Risk After Cancer Treatment

SUPARNA C. CLASEN, LAVANYA KONDAPALLI, AND JOSEPH R. CARVER

Hypertension
Hyperlipidemia
Diabetes
Obesity
Sedentary
Smoking

Cardiovascular risk factors before, during, after

Lifestyle factors (Behavioral choices)

Genetic factors

Cancer patient

Cancer

Cancer therapy
- Drug therapies
- Radiation therapy
- Bone marrow transplantation

Subclinical/clinical cardiovascular disease (worsening underlying or new)

Heart failure
Vascular disease
Arrhythmias
Valve disease
Pericardial disease

Simple, semi-complex, and complex surveillance based on risk and co-morbidity burden

CHAPTER OUTLINE

KEY POINTS

- Cancer survivors are a growing population
- Age at time of cancer treatment, health behaviors, comorbid conditions, genetics, and cancer treatment all weigh into the cardiovascular risk assessment of cancer survivors
- Anthracycline chemotherapy, mediastinal radiation, cranial radiation, Bcr-Abl tyrosine kinase inhibitor therapy, testicular cancer treatment, androgen deprivation therapy for prostate cancer, and pregnancy are among the areas of heightened cardiovascular concern in the treatment of survivors; there is no "safe" dose of potentially cardiotoxic cancer treatment
- Aggressive cardiovascular risk factor modification is the central tenet of cardiac survivorship care
- Cardiovascular risk calculators and guidelines exist, but mainly for childhood cancer survivors, and dedicated prospective surveillance and intervention studies in adult cancer survivors are needed

POPULATIONS AT RISK

Progress in cancer diagnosis and therapy has led to growing numbers of cancer survivors, with over 15 million survivors currently in the United States, soon to reach and exceed 20 million. Cancer survivors are a heterogeneous group of patients who may have had preexisting cardiac conditions or risk factors and who may have received a wide spectrum of treatments (e.g., chemotherapies with various drug and dosing combinations, radiation therapy, and bone marrow transplantation) that influence the risk of late cardiotoxicity. Cancer "survivorship" is likewise a heterogeneous term that refers to the patient once cancer treatment has commenced. There are emerging categories of cancer survivorship, namely extended survivorship and permanent survivorship. Extended survivorship begins at the end of the initial cancer treatment and includes months to early years after treatment, with a focus on monitoring and treating immediate effects of cancer treatment. Permanent survivorship begins several years after treatment and can vary, depending on cancer type, with a focus on the long-term effects of cancer treatment. This heterogeneity, coupled with the potentially long asymptomatic latency period from treatment completion to symptomatic recognition, has made developing universally accepted guidelines for surveillance and prevention a challenge.

Childhood Patients with Cancer

In 2013, there were an estimated 420,000 survivors of childhood cancer in the United States, with the number expected to increase to 500,000 by 2020. More than 80% of children treated for cancer are now surviving more than 5 years posttreatment and multiple medical conditions can develop as long-term and late effects of cancer treatment.[1] Importantly, childhood cancer survivors not only have more extensive morbidities, they also have an increased and premature mortality.[2] In regards to cardiovascular (CV) disease, childhood patients with cancer have a 15 times higher risk of heart failure (HF), a 10 times higher risk of coronary artery disease (CAD), and a 9 times higher risk of stroke than their siblings, for instance.[3] Notably, exposure to 250 mg/m^2 or more of doxorubicin or its equivalence increases the relative hazard of heart failure, pericardial disease, and valvular abnormalities by a factor of two to five compared with non-exposure.[4,5] Cardiac radiation treatment (RT) exposure of 15 Gy has been shown to increase the relative hazard of heart failure, myocardial infarction, pericardial disease, and valvular abnormalities by two- to six-fold compared with no RT exposure.[4,6]

Notably, these data stem from the premodern radiation therapy era. For currently treated patients, these data may be an overstatement of cardiovascular (CV) risk, but for the large population of survivors of pediatric cancer who continue to age into adulthood, these risk numbers represent their potential for late cardiac disease. The risk of HF after anthracyclines and RT has been said to be dose-dependent.[5] However, no "safe" dose of anthracycline or RT exists to preclude the development of late CV effects and that risk is lifelong.[7]

This risk is further modified by the presence and control of cardiovascular risk factors. As shown from data from the Childhood Cancer Survivor Study,[6] the risk of any cardiac event increased with an increasing number of cardiovascular risk factors. Hypertension, in particular, significantly increases the risk for coronary artery disease (RR, 6.1), heart failure (RR, 19.4), valvular disease (RR, 13.6), and arrhythmia (RR, 6.0; all P values <.01). The combined effect of chest-directed radiotherapy plus hypertension resulted in potentiation of risk for each of the major cardiac events beyond expected values (Fig. 24.1). Hypertension was independently associated with the risk of cardiac death (RR, 5.6; 95% CI, 3.2 to 9.7).[6]

Adolescents and Young Adults With Cancer

Cancer survivorship and disease risk in the adolescent and young adult (AYA) subgroup has its own unique challenges for treatment and long-term health and is often overlooked.[8] The AYA group is defined as those diagnosed with cancer between 15 and 39 years of age with a heterogeneous diagnosis of cancer ranging from leukemia, lymphoma, germ cell tumors, sarcomas, breast, and thyroid cancer. Treatment of patients in this subgroup requires an understanding of the interplay between risk

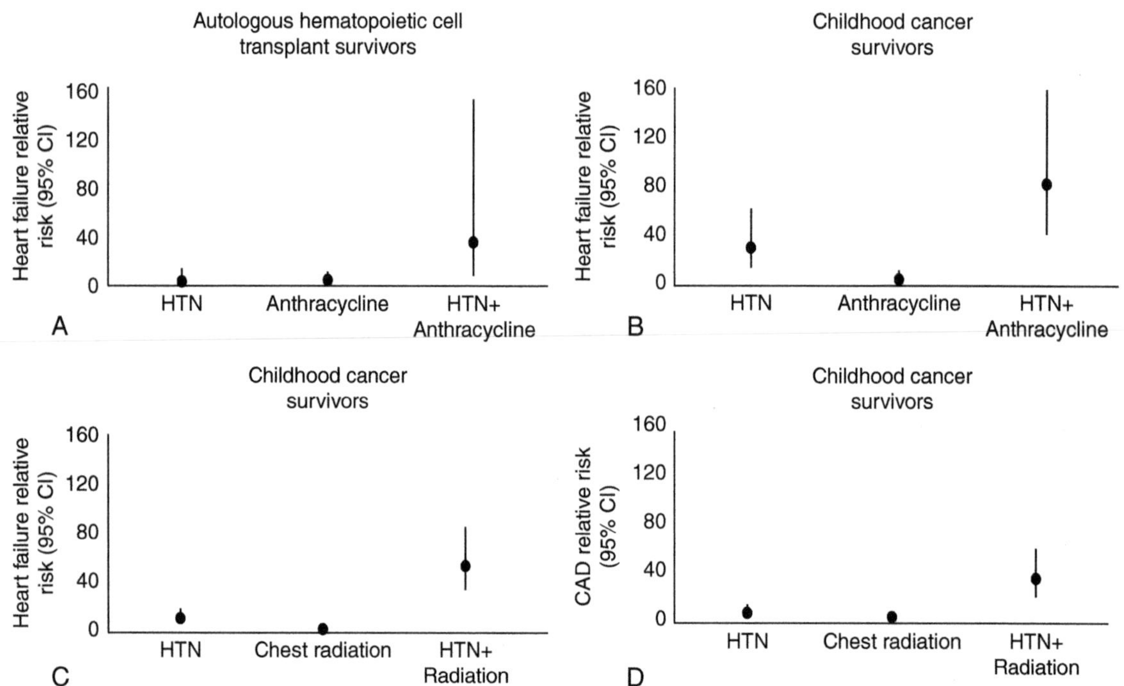

FIG. 24.1 Potentiation of cardiovascular risk by the combination of hypertension (*HTN*) and anthracycline therapy in survivors of hematopoietic cell transplantation. The same is seen after radiation therapy in childhood cancer survivors; cardiovascular risk factors potentiate the risk of heart failure and coronary artery disease (*CAD*). (**A**, Adapted from Armenian SH, Sun C-L, Shannon T, et al. Incidence and predictors of congestive heart failure after autologous hematopoietic cell transplantation. *Blood*. 2011;118(23):6023–6029.) And in childhood cancer survivors (**B–D**, Adapted from Armstrong GT, Oeffinger KC, Chen Y, et al. Modifiable risk factors and major cardiac events among adult survivors of childhood cancer. *J Clin Oncol*. 2013;31(29):3673–3680.)

behaviors (smoking, binge drinking, obesity, lack of physical activity), socioeconomic vulnerabilities,[9] and chronic conditions (cardiovascular disease [CVD], hypertension, diabetes mellitus, and treatment-related disability). In one retrospective cohort study using the Kaiser Permanente Southern California database, 5673 AYA patients diagnosed with cancer from 1998 to 2009 were compared with 57,617 controls.[8] Chao and colleagues[8] found that AYA cancer survivors had a more than two-fold increased risk of developing CVD (adjusted incidence rate ratio, 2.37; 95% CI, 1.93 to 2.93) when compared with patients without cancer. The highest risk of developing CVD was seen in survivors of leukemia and breast cancer (adjusted incidence rate ratio, 4.23; 95% CI, 1.73 to 10.31; and 3.63; 95% CI, 2.41 to 5.47, respectively).[8] Cancer survivors who developed CVD had an 11-fold higher mortality rate than survivors without CVD. Hypertension was the most common and most potent CVD risk factor.[8]

Another population-based study from the California Cancer Registry and state hospital discharge data of 79,176 AYA patients diagnosed with 14 first primary cancers in the period 1996–2012 demonstrated an approximate 2.8% incidence of developing CVD.[9] Survivors of central nervous system cancer (7.3%), acute lymphoid leukemia (6.9%), acute myeloid leukemia (6.8%), and non-Hodgkin lymphoma (4.1%) had the highest 10-year CVD incidence. Interestingly, in multivariable models, African-Americans (hazard ratio [HR], 1.55; 95% CI, 1.33 to 1.81; vs. non-Hispanic caucasians), those with public/no health insurance (HR, 1.78; 95% CI, 1.61 to 1.96; vs. private), and those who resided in lower socioeconomic status neighborhoods had a higher CVD risk. These sociodemographic differences in CVD incidence were apparent across most cancer sites. The mortality rate was ≥ eight-fold among AYAs who developed CVD. These studies highlight the nuances between both risk/sociodemographic and inherent cardiovascular effects.

Adult Patients With Cancer

Anthracycline-induced cardiac dysfunction and heart failure is now a well-recognized long-term effect of cancer therapy. Anthracycline chemotherapy (e.g., doxorubicin, epirubicin, daunorubicin, mitoxantrone) is the cornerstone of the treatment of lymphoma, sarcoma, and breast cancer. Reported incidence rates of anthracycline cardiotoxicity have varied widely owing to differences in patient populations, differences in therapy and dose exposures, as well as follow-up strategies and times. For example, in those with breast cancer, one group found that cardiotoxicity occurred mainly within the first year after anthracycline-containing therapy at a rate of approximately 9% and was associated with anthracycline dose and left ventricular ejection fraction (LVEF) at the end of treatment.[10,11] On the contrary, a cohort study of 142 lymphoma cases, in which the patients received doxorubicin-based chemotherapy (median cumulative dose of 300 mg/m^2) at least 5 years prior (median 8 years), noted that only one patient developed heart failure with an EF less than 30%,[12] but decreased fractional shortening (<25%) was seen in 28% of the patients. One important issue has been the lack of a uniform definition of cardiotoxicity. In a recent consensus statement, cancer therapy-related cardiac dysfunction is defined as a decrease in LVEF by more than 10 percentage points from baseline to a value of less than 53%. Imaging and monitoring of cardiac dysfunction are discussed elsewhere in this book. However, we emphasize that that anthracycline-induced cardiac dysfunction can occur at any time and low-dose anthracycline does not eliminate the risk of cardiac dysfunction.

Cardiac late effects are increased in patients exposed to anthracycline and chest radiation. The use of therapeutic radiation also can lead to the spectrum of radiation-induced heart (RIHD) disease, including CAD, HF, valvular heart disease, pericardial disease, conduction abnormalities, autonomic dysfunction, and sudden cardiac death (see Chapter 26). Risk factors for RIHD in addition to concomitant adjuvant anthracycline-based chemotherapy include doses more than 30 Gy, fractionated dose more than 2 Gy/day, a large volume of irradiated heart, younger age at exposure, and longer time after exposure.[13] Patient-specific factors include age more than 65 years and the presence of comorbid conditions (i.e., diabetes, hypertension, and preexisting cardiac disease). Notably, existing data on incidence rates date to the premodern era of radiation therapy and may overestimate the risk of cardiotoxicity compared with patients being treated today.[14] However, there does not seem to be a "safe" dose threshold and even patients treated with chest radiation today require optimal cardiovascular care.[15,16]

As outlined by the Early Breast Cancer Trialists' Collaborative Group, rates of major coronary events

TABLE 24.1 Outline of the Three Cardinal Cancer Survivorship Populations

SURVIVOR POPULATION	AGE AT CANCER DIAGNOSIS (YEARS)	SPECIAL CONSIDERATIONS
Childhood	<15	Increased morbidities and premature mortality compared with siblings
AYA	15–39	Developmental stages, psychosocial forces, high-risk behaviors may impact health
Adult	>39	Existing comorbidities may influence risk of cardiotoxicity from cancer therapy

AYA, Adolescents and young adults.

increased linearly with the mean dose to the heart by 7.4% per Gray (95% CI, 2.9–14.5; $P < .001$), and event rates were higher, even in those with just one additional cardiovascular risk factor. The increase in risk was apparent within the first 5 years after RT and continued into the third decade after treatment completion.[16] Patients with Hodgkin lymphoma experience an even higher long-term cumulative risk of RIHD, and the third patient group with high long-term survival rates and notable impact of radiation treatment are patients with testicular cancer.[17] Mediastinal irradiation in these patients was found to be associated with a 3.7-fold (95% CI, 2.2- to 6.2-fold) increased myocardial infarction (MI) risk compared with surgery alone, whereas infradiaphragmatic irradiation was not associated with an increased MI risk. Cisplatin-based chemotherapy, particularly the BEP (bleomycin, etoposide, and platinum) regimen, in these patients also needs to be taken into consideration, with a 5.7-fold higher risk (95% CI, 1.9- to 17.1-fold) for coronary artery disease compared with surgery only and a 3.1-fold higher risk (95% CI, 1.2- to 7.7-fold) for MI compared with age-matched control.[18] Survivorship recommendations by age group are outlined in Table 24.1.

MANAGEMENT OF CARDIOVASCULAR (CV) RISK FACTORS

A number of cardiovascular diseases can be seen in the various cancer survivorship populations. Children Oncology Group guidelines emphasize the significance of CV risk factor control and this holds true for all cancer survivors. CV risk factors not only increase the risk of vascular disease, but also cardiomyopathy/heart failure. The operational model is that of multiple hits affecting the cardiovascular system. This reduces the cardiovascular reserves and fosters progression from at risk to asymptomatic and eventually clinically evident disease states, best known as Stages A–D of heart failure. One of the key goals when seeing cancer survivors in follow up should be to prevent any possible progression of CV disease and optimal CV risk factor control is integral in this regard. Furthermore, given commonalities, control of risk factors is expected to reduce the risk of recurrent malignancy as well. Thus, the CV risk factor status should be assessed each year in a cancer survivor, especially in those exposed to cancer therapies with long-term cardiovascular toxicity potential (Table 24.2). Importantly, the impact of multiple risk factors is at least additive.[6] Indeed, childhood cancer survivors who were exposed to anthracyclines and then developed hypertension were at a risk of developing cardiomyopathy and HF beyond what can be seen with either risk factor alone and can be expected based on a simple addtive effect.

Although our focus is cardiovascular comorbidity disease risk, cancer survivors are at risk for other noncardiovascular comorbid conditions as well; for example, pneumonitis or pulmonary fibrosis from bleomycin (see Chapter 21). The Children's Oncology Group provides guidelines by body system and cancer treatment with recommendations for long-term follow up of childhood and AYA

TABLE 24.2 Recommendations for Cardiovascular Risk Factor Surveillance

	ANNUALLY	EVERY 2–3 YEARS	EVERY 5 YEARS
Physical examination, assessment, and management of cardiovascular risk	X		
Discussion of potential cardiovascular late effects	X		
Lipid profile and HbA1c		X	
Left ventricular function assessment (e.g., echocardiogram or cardiac magnetic resonance imaging)			X[a]

[a]After initial left ventricular function assessment within 1 year of completion of cancer treatment.

survivors (http://survivorshipguidelines.org/). As previously mentioned, AYA survivors are a particularly vulnerable group because they are at a point of transition in their lives (e.g., graduation, first job, marriage, moving from a pediatrician to an internist), may not have health insurance, or may not have access to high-quality survivorship care.[19] AYA cancer survivors compared with noncancer patients self-reported higher rates of smoking, obesity, disability, poor mental and physical health, and lack of medical care because of cost. Fertility challenges are common for men and women who have undergone cancer treatment. Anxiety, depression, and posttraumatic stress are all well-studied late and long-term effects of cancer treatment. Cognitive dysfunction, also referred to as "chemo brain," cancer-related fatigue, and pain syndromes are common among cancer survivors. A retrospective, population-wide cohort study matching cancer survivors with controls found the rate of opioid prescribing was 1.22 times higher among survivors (adjusted relative rate, 1.22; 95% CI, 1.11 to 1.34) and that a higher opioid prescribing rate was still seen in survivors 10 or more years from their cancer diagnosis.[20]

Lifestyle

There are well-accepted guidelines to intervene and treat obesity, smoking, and a sedentary lifestyle in survivors. These should be the initial focus for every survivor and reinforced at every visit. Particular aspects of the importance of exercise are captured in the chapters on exercise and rehabilitation (see Chapters 13 and 34). Patients with cancer, including survivors, should be informed about the risks of and cautioned against a sedentary lifestyle.

Hypertension

Hypertension may be the most important modifiable risk factor for late cardiotoxicity in cancer survivors. Data from childhood cohort studies show that there is an age-specific cumulative prevalence of hypertension in survivors that increases sharply with age. Survivors of childhood cancer in the St. Jude Lifetime Cohort Studies had rates of hypertension greater than 70% by the age of 50, which was 2.6 times higher than expected.[21]

Cancer treatment can also lead to hypertension as a late effect. Long-term follow-up studies from Norway in men with testicular cancer treated from 1980 to 1994 show that those exposed to platinum-containing chemotherapies had higher age-adjusted systolic blood pressure (SBP) and diastolic blood pressure (DBP) and had increased odds for hypertension at follow up compared with those with testicular cancer treated with surgery alone.[18,22]

Vascular endothelial growth factor inhibitors and small molecule tyrosine kinase inhibitors have been associated with the *de novo* development of hypertension and/or acceleration of existing hypertension. Although an acute effect, the persistence of these abnormities is not uncommon and requires monitoring, vigilance, and treatment modification into survivorship.

Regardless of the primary cancer treated, achieving control of blood pressure to guideline targets is critical. Given the importance of the association between hypertension and cardiovascular mortality, we recommend guideline-driven screening and management (see Chapter 32).

Hyperlipidemia

Anticancer therapies can result in lipid abnormalities during and after cancer treatment. The extent and duration of dyslipidemia are related to the type of anticancer therapy. For example, in testicular cancer, acute lipid profile changes secondary to cisplatin-containing chemotherapy[23] as well as long-term changes[18] have been seen. In a 20-year follow-up study of men with testicular cancer, approximately 8% of survivors experienced atherosclerotic disease and there was an approximately two-fold increased risk with exposure to chemotherapy and radiation when compared with surgical treatment (RT: HR, 2.3; 95% CI, 1.04 to 5.3; chemotherapy: HR, 2.6; 95% CI, 1.1 to 5.9; RT/chemotherapy: HR, 4.8; 95% CI, 1.6 to 14.4). Treatment with BEP alone had a 5.7-fold higher risk (95% CI, 1.9- to 17.1-fold) for coronary artery disease compared with surgery only and a 3.1-fold higher risk (95% CI, 1.2- to 7.7-fold) for myocardial infarction compared with the general population.[18]

In adults with breast cancer on aromatase inhibitors, a meta-analysis of seven randomized control studies demonstrated that longer duration of aromatase inhibitor use was associated with increased odds of developing cardiovascular disease (OR, 1.26; 95% CI, 1.10 to 1.43; $P < .001$; number

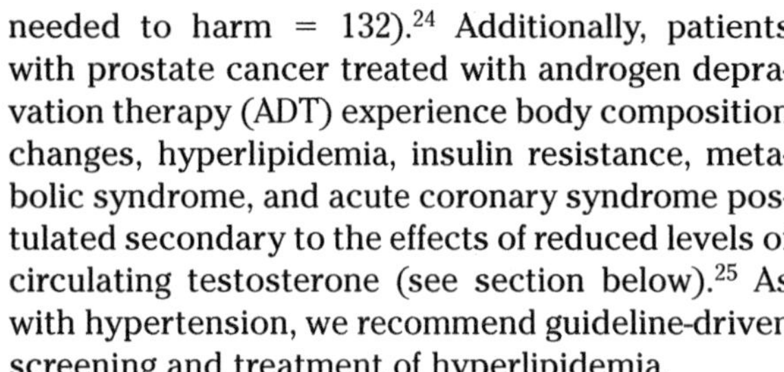

needed to harm = 132).[24] Additionally, patients with prostate cancer treated with androgen depravation therapy (ADT) experience body composition changes, hyperlipidemia, insulin resistance, metabolic syndrome, and acute coronary syndrome postulated secondary to the effects of reduced levels of circulating testosterone (see section below).[25] As with hypertension, we recommend guideline-driven screening and treatment of hyperlipidemia.

Metabolic Syndrome

The metabolic syndrome is defined by a constellation of cardiovascular risk factors, such as central obesity, insulin resistance, hyperglycemia, hypertension, high plasma triglyceride levels, and low plasma high-density lipoprotein (HDL) cholesterol levels, which predispose to type-2-diabetes and atherosclerotic disease. The diagnosis of metabolic syndrome has been associated with increased future cardiovascular risk. Due to their increased risk of future CV disease and events, the metabolic syndrome has gained attention in the cancer survivorship population.[26] This was first described in a study of 50 male survivors of childhood cancer, who, compared with 50 age- and sex-matched controls, had an increased rate of obesity relative weight, >120%; (OR, 4.5; 95% CI, 1.3 to 15.8; $P = .01$) fasting hyperinsulinemia (> 111 pmol/L; OR, 3.0; 95% CI, 1.0 to 8.6; $P = .04$), and reduced HDL cholesterol (< 1.07 mmol/L; OR, 7.9; 95% CI, 2.2 to 29.6; $P < .001$). A combination of obesity, hyperinsulinemia, and low HDL cholesterol was seen in 16% of cancer survivors but in none of the controls ($P = .01$).[27,28] In a larger meta-analysis of cross-sectional studies on metabolic syndrome in cancer survivors by Jung and colleagues,[29] it was found that, compared with healthy controls, cancer survivors were at an increased risk of metabolic syndrome with an OR of 1.84 (95% CI, 1.14 to 2.97; I^2, 80.5%). There were variations in the prevalence of metabolic syndrome components, depending on the type of malignancy and cancer-therapy exposure. In particular, survivors of hematologic malignancies, such as acute lymphocytic leukemia (ALL) and leukemia, especially following allogeneic bone marrow transplant, had an increased prevalence of metabolic syndrome: 39% of those given a combination of chemotherapy and cranial or whole-body irradiation (or both) and up to 8% of those given chemotherapy alone.[26,30]

Additional Cardiovascular Risk Factor Aspects in Cancer Survivors

The mechanism behind the metabolic syndrome in cancer survivors is not yet fully known, but is likely related to a complex interplay of genetic factors, environmental factors, and cancer-treatment exposure. There have been several postulated mechanisms of hormonal disturbances based on studies from childhood cancer survivors: disturbance of the hypothalamus-pituitary-axis (HPA) and growth hormone deficiency (GH), thyroid hormone disturbances, and sex-hormone disturbances. Additionally, in the adult population, men undergoing ADT have adverse cardio-metabolic changes related to body composition changes, hyperlipidemia, insulin resistance, and metabolic syndrome, and are at an increased risk of coronary events.[25,31,32]

Disturbance of the Hypothalamus-Pituitary Axis

The hypothalamus and pituitary are particularly sensitive to radiation therapy and the severity and frequency of hormonal insufficiency and deficiencies correlate with total radiation dose. The growth hormone axis has been shown to be the most vulnerable and perturbations to this axis can occur in isolation without other endocrine disturbances at radiation therapy doses even less than 30 Gy.[33] Talvensaari and colleagues[28] were the first to demonstrate that survivors of childhood cancer had lower growth-hormone levels. GH deficiency is the most common endocrine dysfunction in survivors treated with cranial radiotherapy and is associated with obesity.[26,34] Childhood survivors of ALL and brain cancer have a two- to three-fold higher likelihood of developing obesity (BMI ≥ 30 mg/kg) after brain radiation therapy compared with the normal population. A retrospective cohort analysis of the Childhood Cancer Survivor Study comparing 1765 adult survivors of childhood ALL with 2565 adult siblings of childhood cancer survivors demonstrated that age- and race-adjusted OR for obesity in survivors treated with cranial radiation doses 20 Gy or greater compared with siblings was 2.59 for females (95% CI, 1.88 to 3.55; $P < .001$) and 1.86 for males (95% CI, 1.33 to 2.57; $P < .001$). The OR for obesity was greatest among females diagnosed at 0 to 4 years of age and treated with radiation doses 20 Gy or greater (OR, 3.81; 95% CI, 2.34 to 5.99; $P < .001$). An increased risk of obesity was not seen with chemotherapy alone or with cranial radiation doses of 10 to 19 Gy.[34] Additional small studies have shown associations of growth-hormone deficiency in cancer survivors,[30] but remain limited in number of studies, variability in follow-up duration, and detailed comparisons with healthy counterparts. At higher radiation doses (30 to 50 Gy), there can be deficiencies in the gonadotropin, adrenocorticotropin, and thyrotropin axes, and doses higher than 60 Gy can cause pan hypopituitarism.[26,33] Moreover, the effects of cranial radiotherapy have been associated with other metabolic disturbances, including dyslipidemia and insulin resistance in young-adult survivors of ALL, although the underlying mechanism remains to be fully elucidated.[35] These data suggest that survivors treated with cranial or cranial-spinal radiation are at elevated risk for metabolic syndrome and, as a result, possibly early atherosclerosis.

Androgen Deprivation Therapy and Issues in Survivorship

Patients with prostate cancer treated with androgen deprivation therapy in the form of gonadotropin-releasing hormone agonists have an increased risk of metabolic syndrome, diabetes mellitus, and cardiovascular disease.[25,31] Currently, six months of ADT and RT are the standard treatment for unfavorable-risk prostate cancer. Hypogonadism resulting from ADT is associated with decreased muscle mass and strength, increased fat mass,[36] sexual dysfunction, vasomotor symptoms, decreased quality of life, anemia, and bone loss.[32] Data on ADT therapy associated with increased risk for cardiovascular-associated mortality have been mixed, with multiple early studies showing an increased risk of incident nonfatal MI,[37] stroke, and other cardiovascular events. However, a meta-analysis by Nguyen and colleagues[38] did not show an increased risk of cardiovascular deaths.

In 2010 the American Heart Association (AHA) and American Cancer Society (ACS) issued an advisory on ADT use.[39] In men with prostate cancer, concurrent comorbidity is often present, independent of the actual exposure to ADT, which may result in adverse cardiovascular outcomes. To address these discrepancies, there are several ongoing and recently completed randomized control studies to assess the effect of ADT in patients with prostate cancer. From a practical management standpoint, vigilant monitoring and aggressive management of hypertension and hyperlipidemia, as well as lifestyle modifications achieving an ideal weight, smoking cessation, and exercise should be part of the regular evaluation and management of men on ADT.

SPECIAL ISSUES IN CANCER SURVIVORSHIP

Pregnancy

Pregnancy in young women who are childhood survivors of cancers has unique challenges.[40,41] The offspring of women who received chemotherapy and pelvic irradiation are at risk for preterm delivery, increased risk of miscarriage, and low birthweight.

The maternal cardiovascular risks of pregnancy are directly related to the physiology of pregnancy. Pregnancy increases the workload on the heart: blood volume, heart rate, and cardiac output increase, coupled with a decrease in systemic vascular resistance. Cardiac output begins to increase as early as 5 weeks of gestation and peaks at 28 weeks. With these changes and the added CV hemodynamic stress, survivors who have received anthracyclines and/or chest RT are at risk of progression from the at risk (Stage A) to the symptomatic (Stage C) and advanced/end-stage (Stage D) stages of heart failure.

Labor and delivery add additional hemodynamic stress, mainly owing to dynamic fluid shifts. With each uterine contraction during labor, an additional 300 to 500 mL of blood enters the general circulation. Competing hemodynamic stress emerges from anesthesia as epidural block leads to peripheral vasodilatation with changes in blood pressure. Postdelivery, residual uterine blood volume increases the already expanded overall blood volume. Thus, management centers on fluid and blood volume.

The first step to address regarding pregnancy in cancer survivors is preconception counseling about potential risks and expectations. Although no official guidelines exist, we recommend maternal echocardiography, either prior to contemplated pregnancy or early in the first trimester (baseline) and repeated after 28 weeks when blood volume reaches its prelabor and delivery maximum. From the standpoint of biomarkers, we only measure troponin or NT-proBNP with symptoms that might suggest LV dysfunction; no evidence indicates that these biomarkers elevate in uncomplicated pregnancies.

Second Malignancies Requiring Potentially Cardiotoxic Treatment

Cancer survivors are at an increased risk of developing secondary cancers that may require additional potentially cardiotoxic chemotherapy. For example, a patient treated for Hodgkin lymphoma with anthracycline and mediastinal radiation in childhood can develop left-sided breast cancer, which may best be treated with anthracyclines and left breast radiation. Although there is a myriad of issues with second malignancies, from a cardiac standpoint concern is that the tumor burden and effects may lead to "stage progression" from Stage A heart failure. Cumulative anthracycline dose and radiation dose to the heart are also of concern. Decisions must be individualized and, whereas they are beyond the scope of this discussion, referral to a cardio-oncology specialist is recommended.

PREDICTORS OF LATE EFFECTS

Because every patient with cancer exposed to cardiotoxic treatment does not develop late cardiovascular toxicities, the future understanding and management of cardiovascular diseases in cancer survivors has to expand beyond our current management guidelines. We need a better understanding of the genetics for individuals and need predictive modeling tools for all survivors.

Genetic Predictors of Late Effects

There are emerging data for the pharmacogenomic prediction of anthracycline-induced cardiotoxicity. Genetic variants in the anthracycline metabolism pathway have been implicated to increase cardiovascular toxicity. Multiple genetic variants in *SLC28A3*, *RARG*, *UGT1A6*, and other genes have been associated with anthracycline-induced cardiotoxicity.[42] These and other predictors of genetic predisposition to cardiomyopathy remain intriguing research avenues and more work is needed to translate risk from genetic polymorphisms to clinical practice.

Predictive Modeling Tools

To date, robust evidence-based clinical paradigms for cardiotoxicity prediction have been sparse. Recently, data from large cohort studies have been used to develop predictive models for determining heart failure and cardiovascular toxicity risk in childhood cancer survivors.[43–45] For instance, the Childhood Cancer Survivor Study (CCSS) used readily available demographic and cancer treatment characteristics from the Childhood Cancer Survivor Study (CCSS) to predict individual risk of heart failure, ischemic heart disease, and stroke among 5-year survivors of childhood cancer. In particular, these risk scores are based on a standard prediction model that includes sex, chemotherapy, and radiotherapy (cranial, neck, and chest) exposures. The CCSS prediction model has distinct low-, moderate-, and high-risk groups for development of heart failure, ischemic heart disease, and stroke by 50 years of age (accessible at https://ccss.stjude.org/tools-and-documents/calculators-and-other-tools/ccss-cardiovascular-risk-calculator.html). These CCSS models have been validated in European cohorts and have been an important first step in the ability to predict adverse outcomes.

SURVEILLANCE RECOMMENDATIONS: WHAT TESTS AND HOW OFTEN?

Long-term CV surveillance after cancer treatment has been based on expert consensus (Table 24.3).

For clinical care, several themes consistently emerge for both pediatric and adult survivors who have received potentially cardiotoxic therapy:

1. The risk is lifelong and increases over time.
2. Higher risk populations can be identified based on treatment dosing (Chapter 27, Table 27.1).[46]
3. The risk is generally proportional to the cumulative anthracycline and/or RT dose, but can occur at any dose of either.
4. The combination of anthracycline and mediastinal RT increases risk as does treatment at a young age.
5. There should be documentation of LV systolic function within a year of treatment completion.
6. It is reasonable, in asymptomatic survivors, to image patients every 5 years with the same imaging technique originally used.

TABLE 24.3 **Cardiotoxicity Surveillance Guidelines**

Childhood and AYA Cancer Survivors
Children's Oncology Group Survivorship Guidelines survivorshipguidelines.org
Recommendations for cardiomyopathy surveillance for survivors of childhood cancer: a report from the International Late Effects of Childhood Cancer Guideline Harmonization Group[46]
Adult Cancer Survivor Guidelines
Survivorship, Version 2.2018, National Comprehensive Cancer Network Clinical Practice Guidelines in Oncology
Prevention and Monitoring of Cardiac Dysfunction in Survivors of Adult Cancers: American Society of Clinical Oncology Clinical Practice Guideline[47]
Expert consensus for multimodality imaging evaluation of adult patients during and after cancer therapy: a report from the American Society of Echocardiography and the European Association of Cardiovascular Imaging[48]
European Society of Cardiology Position Paper on cancer treatments and cardiovascular toxicity[49]
European Society of Medical Oncology Consensus Paper on Management of Cardiac Disease in Patients with Cancer Throughout Oncological Treatment[50]

AYA, Adolescents and young adults.

7. At each visit, a detailed CV history and clinical examination should be focused on subtle changes in functional status and/or physical examination.
8. At each interaction, traditional cardiac risk factors should be identified and aggressively managed with an emphasis on healthy lifestyle (e.g., refrains from smoking, emphasis on a healthy diet and regular exercise).
9. Collaborations between primary care, oncology, and cardio-oncology are critical to survivorship care.
10. At every opportunity, provide information/reinforcement counseling regarding the potential late CV effects of cancer treatment.
11. Treatment completion care plans are important to the navigation of long-term survivorship care.[42–46,48]

The risk for CAD after RT is real. No universally accepted recommendations exist for screening beyond clinical assessment. Regular exercise testing, with or without imaging (echocardiogram/nuclear imaging), and/or noninvasive coronary imaging (coronary computed tomography angiography) are techniques available. At this time, we do not recommend routine screening in the absence of even a subtle change in exercise performance. However, we have a low threshold for stress testing/imaging for any exercise-associated symptoms or chest pain.

As per the ACC/AHA Heart Failure guidelines, these patients are considered to be at a high risk for the development of heart failure (Stage A) and therefore screening with an LVEF assessment is appropriate on a 5-year basis. Because other illnesses may unmask reduced cardiac reserve in patients with prior anthracycline or RT exposure, there is a low threshold for additional screening of LV function and more aggressive screening should be done for any change in symptoms, clinical examination, or functional status.[6,48]

Although every survivor who received potentially cardiotoxic treatment is considered Stage A, factors may define a "high-risk" survivor who may need more frequent/aggressive surveillance. One risk stratification tool from the American Society of Clinical Oncology's Clinical Practice Guidelines emphasizes the need for a thorough clinical screening for heart failure within one year after completing anthracycline therapy for "high-risk" survivors. Once again, we emphasize that lifelong follow up is needed for the delayed consequences of radiation and chemotherapy.

REFERENCES

1. Robison LL, Hudson MM. Survivors of childhood and adolescent cancer: life-long risks and responsibilities. *Nat Rev Cancer.* 2014;14(1):61–70.
2. Bhakta N, Liu Q, Ness KK, et al. The cumulative burden of surviving childhood cancer: an initial report from the St Jude Lifetime Cohort Study (SJLIFE). *Lancet.* 2017;390(10112):2569–2582.
3. Oeffinger KC, Mertens AC, Sklar CA, et al. Chronic health conditions in adult survivors of childhood cancer. *N Engl J Med.* 2006;355(15):1572–1582.
4. Mulrooney DA, Yeazel MW, Kawashima T, et al. Cardiac outcomes in a cohort of adult survivors of childhood and adolescent cancer: retrospective analysis of the Childhood Cancer Survivor Study cohort. *BMJ.* 2009;339:b4606.
5. van der Pal HJ, van Dalen EC, van Delden E, et al. High risk of symptomatic cardiac events in childhood cancer survivors. *J Clin Oncol.* 2012;30(13):1429–1437.
6. Armstrong GT, Oeffinger KC, Chen Y, et al. Modifiable risk factors and major cardiac events among adult survivors of childhood cancer. *J Clin Oncol.* 2013;31(29):3673–3680.
7. Hudson MM, Ness KK, Gurney JG, et al. Clinical ascertainment of health outcomes among adults treated for childhood cancer. *JAMA.* 2013;309(22):2371–2381.
8. Chao C, Xu L, Bhatia S, et al. Cardiovascular disease risk profiles in survivors of adolescent and young adult (AYA) cancer: the Kaiser Permanente AYA Cancer Survivors Study. *J Clin Oncol.* 2016;34(14): 1626–1633.
9. Keegan THM, Kushi LH, Li Q, et al. Cardiovascular disease incidence in adolescent and young adult cancer survivors: a retrospective cohort study. *J Cancer Surviv.* 2018;12(3):388–397.
10. Cardinale D, Colombo A, Lamantia G, et al. Anthracycline-induced cardiomyopathy: clinical relevance and response to pharmacologic therapy. *J Am Coll Cardiol.* 2010;55(3):213–220.
11. Cardinale D, Colombo A, Bacchiani G, et al. Early detection of anthracycline cardiotoxicity and improvement with heart failure therapy. *Circulation.* 2015;131(22):1981–1988.
12. Hequet O, Le QH, Moullet I, et al. Subclinical late cardiomyopathy after doxorubicin therapy for lymphoma in adults. *J Clin Oncol.* 2004;22(10):1864–1871.
13. Adams MJ, Lipshultz SE, Schwartz C, Fajardo LF, Coen V, Constine L. Radiation-associated cardiovascular disease: manifestations and management. *Semin Radiat Oncol.* 2003;13(3):346–356.
14. Aleman BM, Moser EC, Nuver J, et al. Cardiovascular disease after cancer therapy. *Eur J Cancer Suppl.* 2014;12(1):18–28.
15. Darby SC, Ewertz M, McGale P, et al. Risk of ischemic heart disease in women after radiotherapy for breast cancer. *N Engl J Med.* 2013;368(11):987–998.
16. Darby S, McGale P, Correa C, et al. Effect of radiotherapy after breast-conserving surgery on 10-year recurrence and 15-year breast cancer death: meta-analysis of individual patient data for 10,801 women in 17 randomised trials. *Lancet.* 2011;378(9804):1707–1716.
17. van den Belt-Dusebout AW, Nuver J, de Wit R, et al. Long-term risk of cardiovascular disease in 5-year survivors of testicular cancer. *J Clin Oncol.* 2006;24(3):467–475.
18. Haugnes HS, Wethal T, Aass N, et al. Cardiovascular risk factors and morbidity in long-term survivors of testicular cancer: a 20-year follow-up study. *J Clin Oncol.* 2010;28(30):4649–4657.
19. Overholser L, Kilbourn K, Liu A. Survivorship issues in adolescent and young adult oncology. *Med Clin North Am.* 2017;101(6):1075–1084.
20. Sutradhar R, Lokku A, Barbera L. Cancer survivorship and opioid prescribing rates: a population-based matched cohort study among individuals with and without a history of cancer. *Cancer.* 2017;123(21):4286–4293.
21. Gibson TM, Li Z, Green DM, et al. Blood pressure status in adult survivors of childhood cancer: a report from the St. Jude Lifetime Cohort Study. *Cancer Epidemiol Biomarkers Prev.* 2017;26(12):1705–1713.
22. Sagstuen H, Aass N, Fosså SD, et al. Blood pressure and body mass index in long-term survivors of testicular cancer. *J Clin Oncol.* 2005;23(22):4980–4990.
23. Raghavan D, Cox K, Childs A, Grygiel J, Sullivan D. Hypercholesterolemia after chemotherapy for testis cancer. *J Clin Oncol.* 1992;10(9):1386–1389.
24. Amir E, Seruga B, Niraula S, Carlsson L, Ocaña A. Toxicity of adjuvant endocrine therapy in postmenopausal breast patients with cancer: a systematic review and meta-analysis. *J Natl Cancer Inst.* 2011;103(17):1299–1309.
25. Kintzel PE, Chase SL, Schultz LM, O'Rourke TJ. Increased risk of metabolic syndrome, diabetes mellitus, and cardiovascular disease in men receiving androgen deprivation therapy for prostate cancer. *Pharmacotherapy.* 2008;28(12):1511–1522.
26. de Haas EC, Oosting SF, Lefrandt JD, Wolffenbuttel BH, Sleijfer DT, Gietema JA. The metabolic syndrome in cancer survivors. *Lancet Oncol.* 2010;11(2):193–203.
27. Talvensaari KK, Knip M, Lanning P, Lanning M. Clinical characteristics and factors affecting growth in long-term survivors of cancer. *Med Pediatr Oncol.* 1996;26(3):166–172.
28. Talvensaari KK, Lanning M, Tapanainen P, Knip M. Long-term survivors of childhood cancer have an increased risk of manifesting the metabolic syndrome. *J Clin Endocrinol Metab.* 1996;81(8):3051–3055.
29. Jung HS, Myung SK, Kim BS, Seo HG. Metabolic syndrome in adult cancer survivors: a meta-analysis. *Diabetes Res Clin Pract.* 2012;95(2):275–282.
30. Gurney JG, Ness KK, Sibley SD, et al. Metabolic syndrome and growth hormone deficiency in adult survivors of childhood acute lymphoblastic leukemia. *Cancer.* 2006;107(6):1303–1312.
31. Shastri BR, Yaturu S. Metabolic complications and increased cardiovascular risks as a result of androgen deprivation therapy in men with prostate cancer. *Prostate Cancer.* 2011;2011:391576.
32. Collins L, Basaria S. Adverse effects of androgen deprivation therapy in men with prostate cancer: a focus on metabolic and cardiovascular complications. *Asian J Androl.* 2012;14(2):222–225.
33. Darzy KH, Shalet SM. Hypopituitarism following radiotherapy. *Pituitary.* 2009;12(1):40–50.
34. Oeffinger KC, Mertens AC, Sklar CA, et al. Obesity in adult survivors of childhood acute lymphoblastic leukemia: a report from the Childhood Cancer Survivor Study. *J Clin Oncol.* 2003;21(7):1359–1365.
35. Janiszewski PM, Oeffinger KC, Church TS, et al. Abdominal obesity, liver fat, and muscle composition in survivors of childhood acute lymphoblastic leukemia. *J Clin Endocrinol Metab.* 2007; 92(10):3816–3821.
36. Smith MR, Finkelstein JS, McGovern FJ, et al. Changes in body composition during androgen deprivation therapy for prostate cancer. *J Clin Endocrinol Metab.* 2002;87(2):599–603.
37. D'Amico AV, Denham JW, Crook J, et al. Influence of androgen suppression therapy for prostate cancer on the frequency and timing of fatal myocardial infarctions. *J Clin Oncol.* 2007;25(17):2420–2425.
38. Nguyen PL, Je Y, Schutz FA, et al. Association of androgen deprivation therapy with cardiovascular death in patients with prostate cancer: a meta-analysis of randomized trials. *JAMA.* 2011; 306(21):2359–2366.
39. Levine GN, D'Amico AV, Berger P, et al. Androgen-deprivation therapy in prostate cancer and cardiovascular risk: a science advisory from the American Heart Association, American Cancer Society, and American Urological Association: endorsed by the American Society for Radiation Oncology. *Circulation.* 2010; 121(6):833–840.
40. Blatt J. Pregnancy outcome in long-term survivors of childhood cancer. *Med Pediatr Oncol.* 1999;33(1):29–33.
41. Green DM, Whitton JA, Stovall M, et al. Pregnancy outcome of female survivors of childhood cancer: a report from the Childhood Cancer Survivor Study. *Am J Obstet Gynecol.* 2002;187(4):1070–1080.
42. Aminkeng F, Ross CJ, Rassekh SR, et al. Recommendations for genetic testing to reduce the incidence of anthracycline-induced cardiotoxicity. *Br J Clin Pharmacol.* 2016;82(3):683–695.
43. Rahman A. Prediction model for heart failure in childhood cancer survivors. *Lancet Oncol.* 2014;15(12):e537.
44. Chow EJ, Chen Y, Kremer LC, et al. Individual prediction of heart failure among childhood cancer survivors. *J Clin Oncol.* 2015; 33(5):394–402.

45. Chow EJ, Chen Y, Hudson MM, et al. Prediction of ischemic heart disease and stroke in survivors of childhood cancer. *J Clin Oncol.* 2018;36(1):44–52.
46. Armenian SH, Hudson MM, Mulder RL, et al. Recommendations for Cardiomyopathy Surveillance for Survivors of Childhood Cancer: a report from the International Late Effects of Childhood Cancer Guideline Harmonization Group. *Lancet Oncol.* 2015;16(3): e123–e136.
47. Armenian SH, Lacchetti C, Barac A, et al. Prevention and monitoring of cardiac dysfunction in survivors of adult cancers: American Society of Clinical Oncology clinical practice guideline. *J Clin Oncol.* 2017;35(8):893–911.
48. Plana JC, Galderisi M, Barac A, et al. Expert consensus for multimodality imaging evaluation of adult patients during and after cancer therapy: a report from the American Society of Echocardiography and the European Association of Cardiovascular Imaging. *Eur Heart J Cardiovasc Imaging.* 2014;15(10):1063–1093.
49. Zamorano JL, Lancellotti P, Rodriguez Muñoz D, et al. 2016 ESC position paper on cancer treatments and cardiovascular toxicity developed under the auspices of the ESC Committee for practice guidelines: the task force for cancer treatments and cardiovascular toxicity of the European Society of Cardiology (ESC). *Eur Heart J.* 2016;37(36):2768–2801.
50. Curigliano C, Lenihan D, Fradley M, et al. Management of cardiac disease in patients with cancer throughout oncological treatment: ESMO consensus recommendations. *Ann Oncol.* 2020;31(2): 171–190.

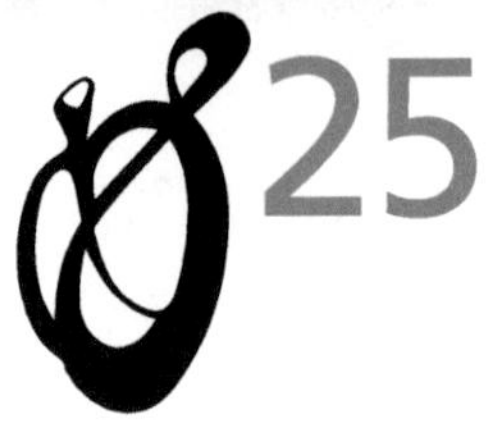

25 Long-Term Complications of Chemotherapy

JENNIFER E. LIU, KATHERINE LEE CHUY, ANTHONY YU, AND RICHARD STEINGART

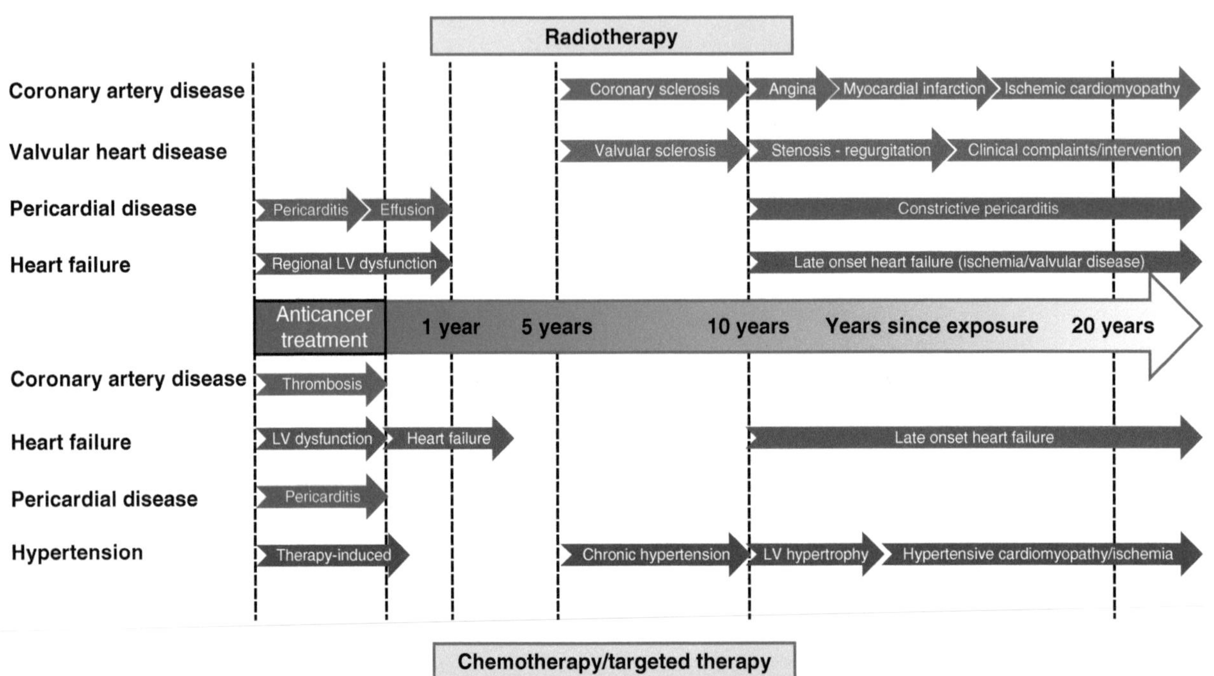

CHAPTER OUTLINE

KEY POINTS

- Despite improvement in cancer survival, many cancer survivors have shortened life spans owing to the late effects of cardiovascular disease (CVD) from their cancer and its treatment
- Cancer therapeutics can lead to a wide spectrum of acute and long-term cardiovascular complications owing to on-target and off-target effects
- Anthracyclines are the best studied anticancer therapy associated with cardiotoxicity with established risk of cardiomyopathy and heart failure that can manifest 10 to 20 years after treatment
- Traditional cardiovascular (CV) risk factors are more prevalent in many cancer survivors than in the general population and are strongly associated with adverse cardiovascular outcomes
- Although intervention trials are lacking, CV risk factors are clearly rationale targets for primary and secondary efforts

Advances in cancer treatment have resulted in significant improvement in patient survival, transforming once-fatal cancers into chronic diseases. As a result, there are currently more than 15 million cancer survivors in the United States and this number is expected to grow as early cancer screening improves, treatments advance, and the population ages. Despite this improvement in cancer survival, many cancer survivors have shortened life spans owing to the late effects of cardiovascular disease from their cancer and its treatment. Understanding how to improve the prevention, recognition, and treatment of long-term cardiovascular complications of cancer and its therapies has become an important priority. Although many cancer therapies can have long-term cardiovascular consequences, this chapter focuses on widely employed agents that have been shown to have adverse effects on the cardiovascular system. It is important to acknowledge that many newer therapies have significantly improved cancer survival where the long-term cardiovascular effects are not yet known.

ANTHRACYCLINES

Anthracyclines are widely used chemotherapeutic agents in pediatric and adult hematologic and solid malignancies. It is estimated that over half of childhood cancer survivors have received prior anthracycline treatment. Chronic progressive cardiomyopathy is the most common presentation of anthracycline-induced cardiotoxicity. Acute cardiotoxicity is seen in less than 1% of pediatric patients, which manifests as transient and reversible left ventricular (LV) dysfunction within the first week of treatment, although persistent changes may be seen with higher cumulative doses.[4] Early nonspecific electrocardiogram changes, conduction abnormalities, and arrhythmias can occur in 10% to 30% of patients; they are often transient.[1,2]

Anthracycline cardiomyopathy is typically a dilated cardiomyopathy with thinned LV walls and abnormal systolic and diastolic indices, which in childhood survivors, can progress over the longer term to a restrictive cardiomyopathy.[3,4] New, more sensitive assessments using echocardiographic global longitudinal strain or cardiac magnetic resonance imaging identify a greater proportion of childhood and adult cancer survivors with cardiac dysfunction.[4,5] It is therefore unclear whether the traditional classification into early- and late-onset anthracycline cardiotoxicity as distinct entities is justified. Rather, there may be a continuous process of maladaptive LV remodeling that ranges from subtle and asymptomatic LV dysfunction to dilated and/or restrictive cardiomyopathy to severe systolic LV dysfunction and advanced heart failure (Fig. 25.1).[1,6]

Decades of follow up on childhood cancer survivors show that as many as 60% develop cardiac dysfunction on echocardiography by 6 years,[3] and almost 10% develop clinical heart failure by 20 to 30 years,[7] with risk persisting over 30 years after treatment.[8] The only consistent risk factor for development of anthracycline-induced cardiomyopathy is the cumulative anthracycline dose. Among childhood cancer survivors exposed to cumulative anthracycline doses (<400 mg/m^2), the incidence of cardiomyopathy was 11% and increased to 100% for cumulative doses (>800 mg/m^2) at a median of 7 years, with severity increasing with time.[9] Compared with cancer survivors without anthracycline exposure, among survivors exposed to more than 300 mg/m^2, the risk was 27 times greater at a mean follow-up period of 9 years.[10] Interestingly, an estimated three-fold increased risk has been demonstrated even with low cumulative dose exposure just above 100 mg/m^2, suggesting that there is no safe anthracycline dose.[5,10] Although less common, pericardial disease is another chronic complication of

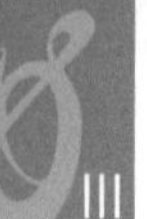

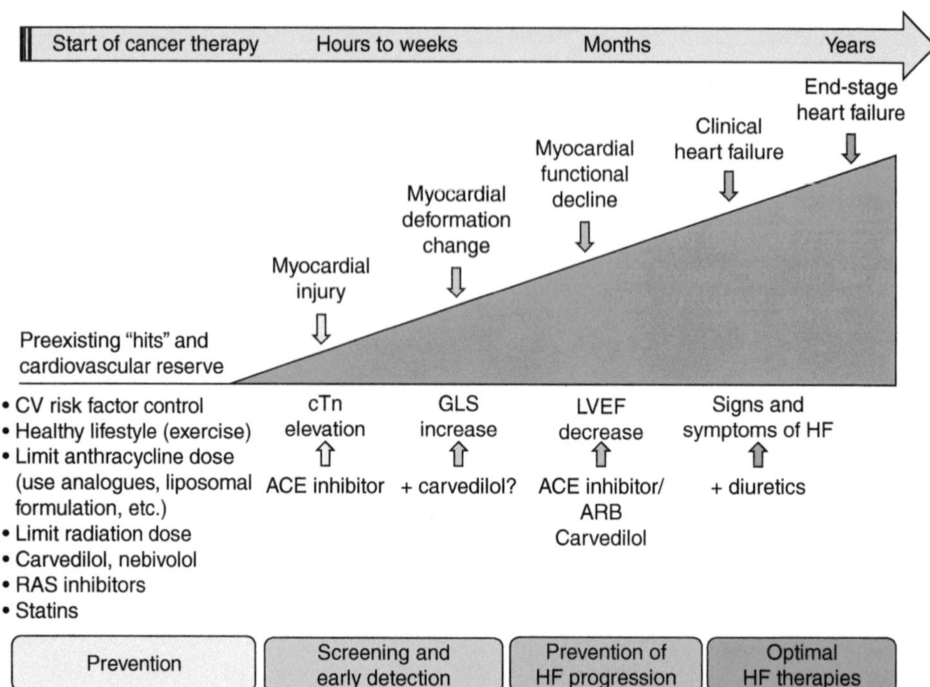

FIG. 25.1 Schematic representation of cardiotoxicity progression over time and directed prevention, screening, detection, and treatment. *ACEI*, Angiotensin-converting enzyme inhibitors; *ARB*, angiotensin receptor blockers; *cTN*, cardiac troponin; *CV*, cardiovascular; *GLS*, global longitudinal strain; *HF*, heart failure; *LVEF*, left ventricular ejection fraction; *RAS*, renin-angiotensin system. (Modified from Cardinale D, Biasillo G, Cipolla CM. Curing cancer, saving the heart: a challenge that cardiooncology should not miss. *Curr Cardiol Rep*. 2016;18(6):51. https://doi.org/10.1007/s11886-016-0731-z.)

high-dose anthracycline treatment.[7] In addition, a decline in exercise capacity that can be independent of measured indices of systolic function (e.g., ejection fraction [EF]) and impaired exercise hemodynamics has been shown in long-term follow up of childhood cancer survivors.[5] Similar trends are seen among adult cancer survivors. Cardiotoxicity, defined as a reduction in LV EF from baseline of more than 10% to less than 50%, occurs at a median time of 3.5 months after treatment, with most cases presenting within the first year.[6] Rates of symptomatic heart failure on treatment increased with cumulative anthracycline dose, to almost 50% at 700 mg/m^2.[11] About 20% of lymphoma survivors at cumulative doses above 250 mg/m^2 had evidence of cardiac dysfunction at 9 years, 7 times higher compared with the noncancer population.[4] Compared with lymphoma survivors who received low cumulative doses (<150 mg/m^2), those who received 250 mg/m^2 or more had almost a 10-fold risk of developing symptomatic heart failure at 5 years.[12]

Additional risk factors for anthracycline-induced cardiomyopathy include length of follow up, age at treatment (especially <5 and >65 years of age), female gender, genetic polymorphism in anthracycline metabolism, concomitant cardiotoxic agents, chest radiation, and preexisting cardiovascular conditions[10–13]-especially hypertension, which has been demonstrated in both childhood and adult cancer survivors to intensify the risk by 7-to 12-fold (see Chapter 24, Figure 24.1).[12,14] At least in some patient groups, when detected and treated early, anthracycline-related cardiac dysfunction can be mitigated, if not completely reversed.[6] Specific recommendations for long-term screening in adult cancer survivors are not defined. Key consensus statements are provided in Chapters 7 and 27.

TARGETED HER2 THERAPY

Human epidermal growth factor 2 (HER2, also known as erbB2) is a cell-surface tyrosine kinase receptor that has been implicated in the development of many human cancer types, most notably breast cancer. Amplification or overexpression of HER2 is found in approximately 15% to 20% of primary invasive breast cancers and is associated with an aggressive cancer phenotype and poor clinical outcomes. Trastuzumab, a humanized monoclonal antibody against the extracellular domain of HER2, improves outcomes for patients with early-stage[15,16] and metastatic HER2-positive breast cancer.[17] Many other targeted anti-HER2 therapies have since been developed, including pertuzumab, ado-trastuzuamab emtansine (TDM-1), lapatinib, and neratinib. Growing evidence indicates that therapies targeting HER2 may be effective in treating other nonbreast malignancies, such as gastric or gastroesophageal junction cancer, ovarian cancer, and lung cancer.[18,19]

In a pivotal trial of concurrent anthracycline- and trastuzumab-based therapy for metastatic breast cancer, symptomatic and asymptomatic cardiac dysfunction was observed in 27% of patients and severe heart failure (New York Heart Association class III or IV) was observed in 16% of patients.[17] With administration of trastuzumab sequentially after completion of anthracyclines and implementation of routine cardiac monitoring during trastuzumab treatment, the incidence of early cardiac dysfunction and severe heart failure has decreased to 7.1% to 18.6% and 0.4% to 4.1%, respectively.[15,16,20,21] The risk of cardiotoxicity is further decreased when anti-HER2 therapy is administered without anthracyclines. In a study of adjuvant paclitaxel and trastuzumab for patients with node-negative HER2-positive breast cancer, 3.2% developed asymptomatic cardiac dysfunction and 0.5% developed symptomatic heart failure.[22]

In contrast to anthracycline-associated cardiotoxicity, partial improvement of LV function is often observed with interruption or discontinuation of anti-HER2 therapy. Nonetheless, a reduction in LVEF compared with baseline can persist after completion of trastuzumab therapy, and patients may be at risk for late clinical cardiac events.[16,23] Indeed, several registry-based analyses have outlined a persistent and cumulatively increasing risk of heart failure in patients treated with trastuzumab, whereas clinical trials have indicated that the cardiac risk is confined to the active treatment period (e.g., HERA trial).[24] At present, it is not clearly defined if trastuzumab exposure is associated with late (posttherapy) development of heart failure or other clinically relevant long-term sequelae, such as decreased cardiorespiratory fitness as women age, whether such presentations are confined to those with reversible or irreversible declines in cardiac function during trastuzumab therapy, or if such sequelae could start even years after therapy.

VEGF SIGNALING PATHWAY INHIBITORS

Angiogenesis inhibitors are effective as anticancer therapies by depriving tumors of vascular supply. They are used to treat a wide variety of solid tumors, including colorectal cancer, renal cell cancer, non–small-cell lung cancer, thyroid cancer, and hepatocellular carcinoma. Vascular endothelial growth factor (VEGF) is the most heavily studied and targeted angiogenesis factor for cancer treatment. Current strategies to inhibit the VEGF signaling pathway include monoclonal antibodies (e.g., bevacizumab, ramucirumab) or small molecular tyrosine kinase inhibitors (TKIs) (e.g., sunitinib, sorafenib, pazopanib).[25] Hypertension is a class effect of VEGF signaling pathway inhibitors (VSPIs), and results from both on-target and off-target effects. Some of the proposed mechanisms of VSPI-induced hypertension include decreased nitric oxide signaling, increased endothelin-1 secondary to endothelial dysfunction, and microcapillary rarefaction (reduction in the capillary bed density).[26] VSPI-induced hypertension typically develops within 1 week of initiation of therapy, and generally resolves within 1 to 2 weeks of discontinuation of VSPI treatment. Management of VSPI-induced hypertension (HTN) with antihypertensive medications is important to prevent short- and long-term cardiovascular effects, such as renal impairment, left ventricular systolic dysfunction, arrhythmia, and thrombosis/hemorrhage.

OTHER TYROSINE KINASE INHIBITORS

Tyrosine kinase inhibitors targeting BCR-ABL1 have significantly improved patient survival in patients with chronic myelogenous leukemia. Differences in the off-target kinase inhibition profiles of newer generation BCR-ABL TKIs, such as dasatinib, nilotinib, bosutinib, and ponatinib, are hypothesized to account for the distinct toxicity profiles of each agent. For example, treatment with dasatinib has been associated with severe drug-induced pulmonary arterial hypertension in a French PH Registry; the majority of patients do not achieve a complete clinical or hemodynamic recovery despite discontinuation of therapy.[27] In contrast, nilotinib and ponatinib have been associated with an increased risk of coronary, cerebrovascular, and peripheral arterial vascular events which, in turn, will adversely affect longer term cardiovascular outcomes.[28,29] Patients receiving BCR-ABL TKIs should undergo a careful cardiovascular (CV) risk assessment and aggressive control of modifiable risk factors. It may be reasonable to consider prophylactic aspirin and/or statin therapy among patients with high CV risk profiles or those requiring treatment with high-risk TKIs, such as nilotinib or ponatib.

PLATINUM- BASED CHEMOTHERAPY

The platinum-based drugs cisplatin, carboplatin, and oxaliplatin belong to a larger class of alkylating agents used to treat numerous cancers, including bladder, ovarian, lung, head and neck, and testicular cancer. Cisplatin-based chemotherapy is standard systemic treatment for germ cell tumors (GCTs), with 5-year survival rates exceeding 90%. Cisplatin is associated with acute and late cardiovascular side effects, including HTN, myocardial ischemia and infarction, thromboembolism, and cerebrovascular disease.[30] Although the endothelial toxic effects appear central, the exact molecular mechanism has not been well defined. Markers of inflammation and endothelial dysfunction have been noted in patients with testicular cancer during cisplatin chemotherapy including fibrinogen, Von Willebrand factor, C-reactive protein, and tissue-type plasminogen activator.[31] Microalbuminuria, a marker of systemic vascular dysfunction prognostic of cardiovascular outcome, has been shown to persist late after cisplatin treatment in 22% of testicular cancer survivors. Thromboembolic events have been reported in 9% of patients with GCT during cisplatin chemotherapy. Long-term survivors of GCT treated with cisplatin have a significantly increased risk of late-onset cardiovascular disease (CVD) compared with an age-matched population. The reported incidence of coronary artery disease in survivors of testicular cancer ranges from 5.6% to 6.7% with relative risks of 1.4 to as high as 7.1.[32] Increased CVD mortality has also been reported in GCT survivors with a 1.6-fold increased risk at a median follow up of 10 years. A recent study reported a significant 5.3-fold increase in CVD mortality during the first year after cisplatin chemotherapy, which dramatically decreased after one year as compared with surgery alone, underscoring the importance of attention to acute toxic effects of cisplatin chemotherapy.[33] CV risk factors, including HTN, hypercholesterolemia, insulin resistance, and metabolic syndrome, have also been shown to be more prevalent in testicular cancer survivors compared with age-matched controls.[30] The multiple hit hypothesis has been proposed to explain the pathophysiology of CVD in GCT survivors where multiple factors interact synergistically to increase the CVD risk. These include chemotherapy-induced vascular injury, changes in metabolic homeostasis, and prolonged retention of serum platinum.[34]

ANTIESTROGEN THERAPY

Endocrine therapy with tamoxifen or third-generation aromatase inhibitors (AIs) is used in women with hormone-receptor positive-breast cancer[35] as adjuvant therapy in early disease or as first-line therapy in advanced disease. Tamoxifen is a selective estrogen-receptor modulator with both agonist and antagonist actions, whereas AIs interfere with endogenous estrogen production in adipose tissue.[35,36] AIs have shown superior disease benefit over tamoxifen, although a few studies have shown higher CV risk with AIs over tamoxifen.[37–39] Although the absolute incidence of ischemic heart disease (IHD; <5%) and CV death (1%) among patients on AIs remains low,[37,40] an analysis of randomized, controlled trials estimates a 19% increased risk for CV disease and a 30% increased risk of IHD.[40] A closer look reveals nonsignificant higher trends for IHD with AIs versus tamoxifen in some of the included studies[37,38] and significantly decreased risk between tamoxifen and placebo or no treatment.[41–43] Therefore, the findings may be driven by benefit with tamoxifen rather than harm with AIs, attributed in part to favorable lipid profile changes with tamoxifen.[35,40] Incident HTN has been shown to be higher with AIs across studies—up to 13%[37]—and, in addition, evidence of significant vascular dysfunction has been demonstrated.[44] On the other hand, tamoxifen is associated with greater risks of pulmonary emboli and cerebrovascular events.[37,41]

ANDROGEN DEPRIVATION THERAPY

Androgen deprivation therapy (ADT) remains the mainstay of management of hormone-sensitive advanced prostate cancer; it involves lowering serum testosterone to induce hypogonadism, either through bilateral orchiectomy or pharmacologic agents: gonadotropin-releasing hormone (GnRH) agonists with or without androgen receptor blockers, GnRH antagonists, and the newer antiandrogens abiraterone and enzalutamide, with GnRH agonists being the most commonly used agents.[42]

ADT is associated with decreased insulin sensitivity, worse glucose control in patients with diabetes mellitus, and up to a 60% increased risk of developing diabetes mellitus.[43] Studies have shown that approximately 70% of patients with prostate cancer on ADT develop sarcopenic obesity, a disproportionate decrease in lean body mass and an increase in primarily subcutaneous fat mass.[42,43] Given these changes, up to 75% of patients develop a distinct form of metabolic syndrome, with accumulation of subcutaneous instead of abdominal fat, an increase in high-density lipoprotein, but without significant increase in blood pressure.[43,45,46] A range of CV events associated with ADT, including IHD, ventricular arrhythmia or sudden cardiac death, cerebrovascular events, peripheral artery disease, and venous thromboembolism has been shown in observational studies, with up to 11% and 16% greater risk of myocardial infarction and sudden cardiac death, respectively.[47] Comparison of the GnRH antagonist degarelix versus GnRH agonists suggests that degarelix has a better CV safety profile.[48]

The CV and metabolic effects associated with both AIs and ADT have not been shown to cause a concomitant increase in CV mortality[39,49,50] and the question remains as to how much the cardiometabolic effects translate into clinical events in this population. However, as postmenopausal women and patients with prostate cancer are already at high CV risk, the CV risks of treatment must be balanced against expected therapeutic benefits.

CONCLUSIONS

The evidence that cancer survivors are at significant risk for long-term complications of CVD is beyond dispute. Over past decades, curative regimens have become less cardio toxic.[2] But traditional CV risk factors are highly prevalent in cancer survivors and are strongly associated with adverse cardiovascular outcomes.[14] Prospective trials of risk factor intervention are lacking in these patients. Despite that, CV risk factors are clearly rationale targets for primary and secondary prevention efforts. After a brief "rest period" after completion of cancer care, we recommend that the oncology survivorship group reeducate the patient and their significant others about the potential challenges that cardiovascular disease can present to their health going forward. Basics of diet, smoking, alcohol, exercise, and blood pressure and lipid control should be emphasized. Referral to the cardiovascular clinic is offered for further patient education or for more advanced testing as the clinical presentation warrants.

REFERENCES

1. Lipshultz SE, Alvarez JA, Scully RE. Anthracycline associated cardiotoxicity in survivors of childhood cancer. *Heart*. 2008;94(4):525–533.
2. Buza V, Rajagopalan B, Curtis AB. Cancer treatment-induced arrhythmias: focus on chemotherapy and targeted therapies. *Circ Arrhythm Electrophysiol*. 2017;10(8):e005443.
3. Lipshultz SE, Lipsitz SR, Sallan SE, et al. Chronic progressive cardiac dysfunction years after doxorubicin therapy for childhood acute lymphoblastic leukemia. *J Clin Oncol*. 2005;23(12):2629–2636.
4. Armenian SH, Mertens L, Slorach C, et al. Prevalence of anthracycline-related cardiac dysfunction in long-term survivors of adult-onset lymphoma. *Cancer*. 2018;124(4):850–857.
5. Armstrong GT, Joshi VM, Ness KK, et al. Comprehensive Echocardiographic detection of treatment-related cardiac dysfunction in adult survivors of childhood cancer: results From the St. Jude Lifetime Cohort Study. *J Am Coll Cardiol*. 2015;65(23):2511–2522.
6. Cardinale D, Colombo A, Bacchiani G, et al. Early detection of anthracycline cardiotoxicity and improvement with heart failure therapy. *Circulation*. 2015;131(22):1981–1988.
7. Mulrooney DA, Yeazel MW, Kawashima T, et al. Cardiac outcomes in a cohort of adult survivors of childhood and adolescent cancer: retrospective analysis of the Childhood Cancer Survivor Study cohort. *BMJ*. 2009;339:b4606.
8. Armstrong GT, Kawashima T, Leisenring W, et al. Aging and risk of severe, disabling, life-threatening, and fatal events in the childhood cancer survivor study. *J Clin Oncol*. 2014;32(12):1218–1227.
9. Steinherz LJ, Steinherz PG, Tan CTC, Heller G, Murphy L. Cardiac Toxicity 4 to 20 years after completing anthracycline therapy. *N Engl J Med*. 1991;266(12):1672–1677.
10. Blanco JG, Sun CL, Landier W, et al. Anthracycline-related cardiomyopathy after childhood cancer: role of polymorphisms in carbonyl reductase genes—a report from the Children's Oncology Group. *J Clin Oncol*. 2012;30(13):1415–1421.
11. Swain SM, Whaley FS, Ewer MS. Congestive heart failure in patients treated with Doxorubicin: a retrospective analysis of three trials. *Cancer*. 2003;97(11):2869–2879.
12. Armenian SH, Sun CL, Shannon T, et al. Incidence and predictors of congestive heart failure after autologous hematopoietic cell transplantation. *Blood*. 2011;118(23):6023–6029.
13. Armenian SH, Ding Y, Mills G, et al. Genetic susceptibility to anthracycline-related congestive heart failure in survivors of haematopoietic cell transplantation. *Br J Haematol*. 2013;163(2):205–213.
14. Armstrong GT, Oeffinger KC, Chen Y, et al. Modifiable risk factors and major cardiac events among adult survivors of childhood cancer. *J Clin Oncol*. 2013;31(29):3673–3680.

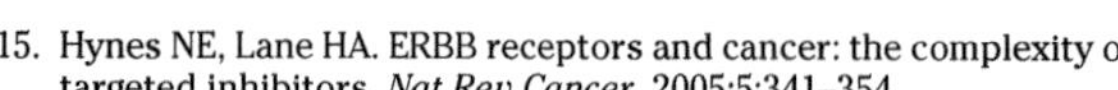

15. Hynes NE, Lane HA. ERBB receptors and cancer: the complexity of targeted inhibitors. *Nat Rev Cancer.* 2005;5:341–354.
16. Slamon DJ, Clark GM, Wong SG, Levin WJ, Ullrich A, McGuire WL. Human breast cancer: correlation of relapse and survival with amplification of the HER-2/neu oncogene. *Science.* 1987;235:177–182.
17. Romond EH, Perez EA, Bryant J, et al. Trastuzumab plus adjuvant chemotherapy for operable HER2-positive breast cancer. *N Engl J Med.* 2005;353:1673–1684.
18. Bang YJ, Van Cutsem E, Feyereislova A, et al. Trastuzumab in combination with chemotherapy versus chemotherapy alone for treatment of HER2-positive advanced gastric or gastro-oesophageal junction cancer (ToGA): a phase 3, open-label, randomised controlled trial. *Lancet.* 2010;376:687–697.
19. Peters S, Zimmermann S. Targeted therapy in NSCLC driven by HER2 insertions. *Transl Lung Cancer Res.* 2014;3:84–88.
20. Piccart-Gebhart MJ, Procter M, Leyland-Jones B, et al. Trastuzumab after adjuvant chemotherapy in HER2-positive breast cancer. *N Engl J Med.* 2005;353:1659–1672.
21. Tan-Chiu E, Yothers G, Romond E, et al. Assessment of cardiac dysfunction in a randomized trial comparing doxorubicin and cyclophosphamide followed by paclitaxel, with or without trastuzumab as adjuvant therapy in node-positive, human epidermal growth factor receptor 2-overexpressing breast cancer: NSABP B-31. *J Clin Oncol.* 2005;23:7811–7819.
22. Tolaney SM, Barry WT, Dang CT, et al. Adjuvant paclitaxel and trastuzumab for node-negative, HER2-positive breast cancer. *N Engl J Med.* 2015;372:134–141.
23. Romond EH, Jeong JH, Rastogi P, et al. Seven-year follow-up assessment of cardiac function in NSABP B-31, a randomized trial comparing doxorubicin and cyclophosphamide followed by paclitaxel (ACP) with ACP plus trastuzumab as adjuvant therapy for patients with node-positive, human epidermal growth factor receptor 2-positive breast cancer. *J Clin Oncol.* 2012;30:3792–3799.
24. de Azambuja E, Procter MJ, van Veldhuisen DJ, et al. Trastuzumab-associated cardiac events at 8 years of median follow-up in the Herceptin adjuvant trial (BIG 1-01). *J Clin Oncol.* 2014;32:2159–2165.
25. Li W, Croce K, Steensma DP, McDermott DF, Ben-Yehuda O, Moslehi J. Vascular and metabolic implications of novel targeted cancer therapies: focus on Kinase inhibitors. *J Am Coll Cardiol.* 2015;66:1160–1178.
26. Maitland ML, Bakris GL, Black HR, et al. Initial assessment, surveillance, and management of blood pressure in patients receiving vascular endothelial growth factor signaling pathway inhibitors. *J Natl Cancer Inst Monogr.* 2010;102(9):596–604.
27. Montani D, Bergot E, Gunther S, et al. Pulmonary arterial hypertension in patients treated by dasatinib. *Circulation.* 2012;125:2128–2137.
28. Giles FJ, Mauro MJ, Hong F, et al. Rates of peripheral arterial occlusive disease in patients with chronic myeloid leukemia in the chronic phase treated with imatinib, nilotinib, or non-tyrosine kinase therapy: a retrospective cohort analysis. *Leukemia.* 2013;27:1310–1315.
29. Cortes JE, Kim DW, Pinilla-Ibarz J, et al. A phase 2 trial of ponatinib in Philadelphia chromosome-positive leukemias. *N Engl J Med.* 2013;369:1783–1796.
30. Hanna N, Einhorn LH. Testicular cancer: a reflection on 50 years of discovery. *J Clin Oncol.* 2014;32(28):3085–3092.
31. Meinardi MT, Gietema JA, van der Graaf WT, et al. Cardiovascular morbidity in long-term survivors of metastatic testicular cancer. *J Clin Oncol.* 2000;18(8):1725–1732.
32. Nuver J, Smit AJ, van der Meer J, et al. Acute chemotherapy-induced cardiovascular changes in patients with testicular cancer. *J Clin Oncol.* 2005;23(36):9130–9137.
33. Feldman DR, Schaffer WL, Steingart RM. Late cardiovascular toxicity following chemotherapy for germ cell tumors. *J Natl Compr Canc Netw.* 2012;10(4):537–544.
34. Fung C, Fossa SD, Milano MT, Sahasrabudhe DM, Peterson DR, Travis LB. Cardiovascular disease mortality after chemotherapy or surgery for testicular nonseminoma: a population-based study. *J Clin Oncol.* 2015;33(28):3105–3115.
35. Esteva FJ, Hortobagyi GN. Comparative assessment of lipid effects of endocrine therapy for breast cancer: implications for cardiovascular disease prevention in postmenopausal women. *Breast.* 2006;15:301–312.
36. Foglietta J, Inno A, de Iuliis F, et al. Cardiotoxicity of aromatase inhibitors in breast patients with cancer. *Clin Breast Cancer.* 2016;17(1):11–17.
37. Arimidex T, Alone or in Combination Trialists' Group. Comprehensive side-effect profile of anastrozole and tamoxifen as adjuvant treatment for early-stage breast cancer: long-term safety analysis of the ATAC trial. *Lancet Oncol.* 2006;7(8):633–643.
38. Bliss JM, Kilburn LS, Coleman RE, et al. Disease-related outcomes with long-term follow-up: an updated analysis of the intergroup exemestane study. *J Clin Oncol.* 2012;30(7):709–717.
39. van de Velde CJH, Rea D, Seynaeve C, et al. Adjuvant tamoxifen and exemestane in early breast cancer (TEAM): a randomised phase 3 trial. *Lancet.* 2011;377(9762):321–331.
40. Khosrow-Khavar F, Filion KB, Al-Qurashi S, et al. Cardiotoxicity of aromatase inhibitors and tamoxifen in postmenopausal women with breast cancer: a systematic review and meta-analysis of randomized controlled trials. *Ann Oncol.* 2017;28(3):487–496.
41. Davies C, Pan J, Godwin J, et al. Long-term effects of continuing adjuvant tamoxifen to 10 years versus stopping at 5 years after diagnosis of oestrogen receptor-positive breast cancer: ATLAS, a randomised trial. *Lancet.* 2013;381:805–816.
42. Gupta D, Lee Chuy K, Yang JC, Bates M, Lombardo M, Steingart RM. Cardiovascular and metabolic effects of androgen-deprivation therapy for prostate cancer. *J Oncol Pract.* 2018;14(10):580–588.
43. Tzortzis V, Samarinas M, Zachos I, Oeconomou A, Pisters L, Bargiota A. Adverse effects of androgen deprivation therapy in patients with prostate cancer: focus on metabolic complications. *Hormones.* 2017;16(2):115–123.
44. Blaes A, Beckwith H, Florea N, et al. Vascular function in breast cancer survivors on aromatase inhibitors: a pilot study. *Breast Cancer Res Treat.* 2017;166(2):541–547.
45. Gupta D, Salmane C, Slovin S, Steingart RM. Cardiovascular complications of androgen deprivation therapy for prostate cancer. *Curr Treat Options Cardiovasc Med.* 2017;19(8):61.
46. Levine GN, D'Amico AV, Berger P, et al. Androgen-deprivation therapy in prostate cancer and cardiovascular risk: a science advisory from the American Heart Association, American Cancer Society, and American Urological Association: endorsed by the American Society for Radiation Oncology. *Circulation.* 2010;121(6):833–840.
47. Zareba P, Duivenvoorden W, Leong DP, Pinthus JH. Androgen deprivation therapy and cardiovascular disease: what is the linking mechanism? *Ther Adv Urol.* 2016;8(2):118–129.
48. Sciarra A, Fasulo A, Ciardi A, et al. A meta-analysis and systematic review of randomized controlled trials with degarelix versus gonadotropin-releasing hormone agonists for advanced prostate cancer. *Medicine (Baltimore).* 2016;95(27):e3845.
49. Nguyen PL, Je Y, Schutz FAB, et al. Association of androgen deprivation therapy with cardiovascular death in patients with prostate cancer. *JAMA.* 2011;306(21):2359–2366.
50. Amir E, Seruga B, Niraula S, Carlsson L, Ocana A. Toxicity of adjuvant endocrine therapy in postmenopausal breast patients with cancer: a systematic review and meta-analysis. *J Natl Cancer Inst.* 2011;103(17):1299–1309.

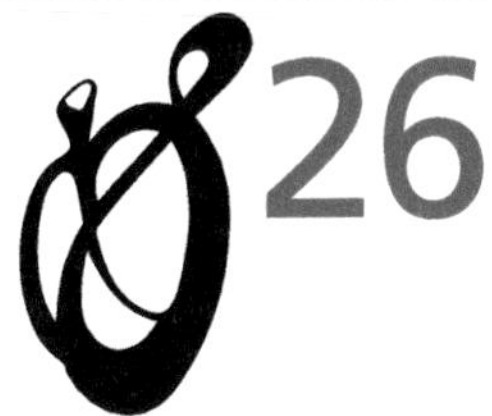

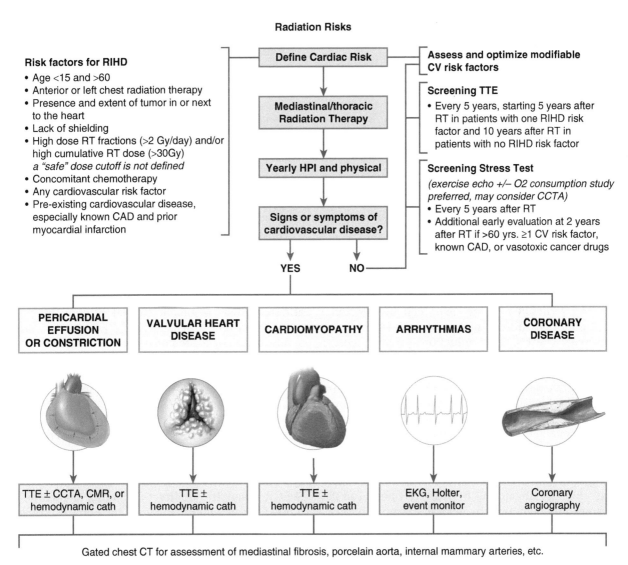

26 Long-Term Consequences of Radiation Therapy

WILLIAM FINCH, MIRELA TUZOVIC, AND ERIC H. YANG

Radiation Risks

Define Cardiac Risk

Risk factors for RIHD
- Age <15 and >60
- Anterior or left chest radiation therapy
- Presence and extent of tumor in or next to the heart
- Lack of shielding
- High dose RT fractions (>2 Gy/day) and/or high cumulative RT dose (>30Gy)
  a "safe" dose cutoff is not defined
- Concomitant chemotherapy
- Any cardiovascular risk factor
- Pre-existing cardiovascular disease, especially known CAD and prior myocardial infarction

Assess and optimize modifiable CV risk factors

Mediastinal/thoracic Radiation Therapy

Screening TTE
- Every 5 years, starting 5 years after RT in patients with one RIHD risk factor and 10 years after RT in patients with no RIHD risk factor

Yearly HPI and physical

Screening Stress Test
(exercise echo +/– O2 consumption study preferred, may consider CCTA)
- Every 5 years after RT
- Additional early evaluation at 2 years after RT if >60 yrs. ≥1 CV risk factor, known CAD, or vasotoxic cancer drugs

Signs or symptoms of cardiovascular disease?

YES / **NO** (NO → screening TTE and screening stress test)

YES →

PERICARDIAL EFFUSION OR CONSTRICTION	**VALVULAR HEART DISEASE**	**CARDIOMYOPATHY**	**ARRHYTHMIAS**	**CORONARY DISEASE**
TTE ± CCTA, CMR, or hemodynamic cath	TTE ± hemodynamic cath	TTE ± hemodynamic cath	EKG, Holter, event monitor	Coronary angiography

Gated chest CT for assessment of mediastinal fibrosis, porcelain aorta, internal mammary arteries, etc.

For interventional planning (catheter-based and/or surgical Heart Team approach)

CAD, Coronary artery disease; *CCTA*, coronary computed tomography; *CMR*, cardiac magnetic resonance imaging; *CV*, cardiovascular; *EKG*, electrocardiogram; *Gy*, gray; *HPI*, history of present illness; *RIHD*, radiation-induced heart disease; *RT*, radiation therapy; *TTE*, transthoracic echocardiography.

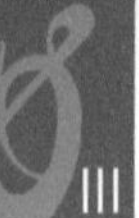

CHAPTER OUTLINE

KEY POINTS

- Patients with cancer who are exposed to radiation therapy are at increased risk for numerous cardiac complications, including cardiomyopathy, valve disease, pericardial disease, arrhythmias, conduction abnormalities, autonomic dysfunction, and coronary artery disease that usually occur years, if not decades, following therapy.
- Patients with prior mediastinal or thoracic radiation should be screened for signs or symptoms of cardiac disease and modifiable cardiovascular risk factors on an at least annual basis.
- Even in patients with a history of radiation therapy but no signs and symptoms of cardiovascular disease serial screening with a transthoracic echocardiogram and functional/anatomic assessment is recommended; the timing is based on patient- and treatment-specific risk factors.
- If radiation-induced heart disease is diagnosed, treatment is typically the same as that provided for the general population; however, treatment outcomes (i.e., pharmacologic, percutaneous, surgical) may be worse in patients who have had radiation therapy owing to common involvement of multiple heart structures and thus the presence of multiple heart disease processes at once as well as multiple other complications and comorbid conditions acquired during cancer treatment.

Radiation therapy (RT) as a component of cancer treatment is a significant cause of cardiac complications during survivorship. It is most commonly reported after external beam RT (EBRT) for breast cancer or Hodgkin lymphoma (HL) but may also be seen with RT for gastric, esophageal, or lung cancer. All structures of the heart can be affected, including pericardium, myocardium, heart valves, coronary arteries, and conduction system. Accordingly, the spectrum of radiation-induced heart disease (RIHD) is quite broad and includes acute and constrictive pericarditis, (typically restrictive) cardiomyopathy, valvular heart disease (VHD), coronary artery and microvascular disease, heart block, and autonomic dysfunction. A number of these disease processes can ultimately present in heart failure (HF) as the final common pathway (Fig. 26.1). The individual disease elements of RIHD and their treatment will be reviewed herein first, followed by an outline of general screening efforts and preventive recommendations.

CORONARY ARTERY DISEASE

Coronary atherosclerosis in RIHD typically matches radiation dose exposure in location and severity. With RT for HL, ostial disease of both the right and left coronary arteries are the most classic lesions, whereas after RT for left-sided breast cancer the mid (and distal) left anterior descending coronary artery (LAD) is most commonly involved.[1,2] The clinical presentation of radiation-induced coronary atherosclerosis is similar to that of conventional coronary artery disease (CAD), presenting with stable angina or acute coronary syndrome.[3] For diagnosis, single photon emission computerized tomography myocardial perfusion imaging (SPECT MPI) has indicated perfusion defects in as many as 70% of patients 5 years after RT for breast cancer.[4] However, limited data exist regarding the sensitivity or specificity of SPECT MPI in this specific population and cited data are reflective of other radiation techniques. Positron emission tomography (PET) MPI may be a reasonable alternative to SPECT, given the ability to quantify myocardial blood flow. In comparison with nuclear MPI, stress echocardiography has lower sensitivity but higher specificity the diagnosis of radiation-induced CAD (Table 26.1).[5]

Coronary artery calcium scoring, and coronary computed tomography angiography (CCTA) are gaining increasing interest and may play a larger role for the diagnosis of CAD after RT in the future.

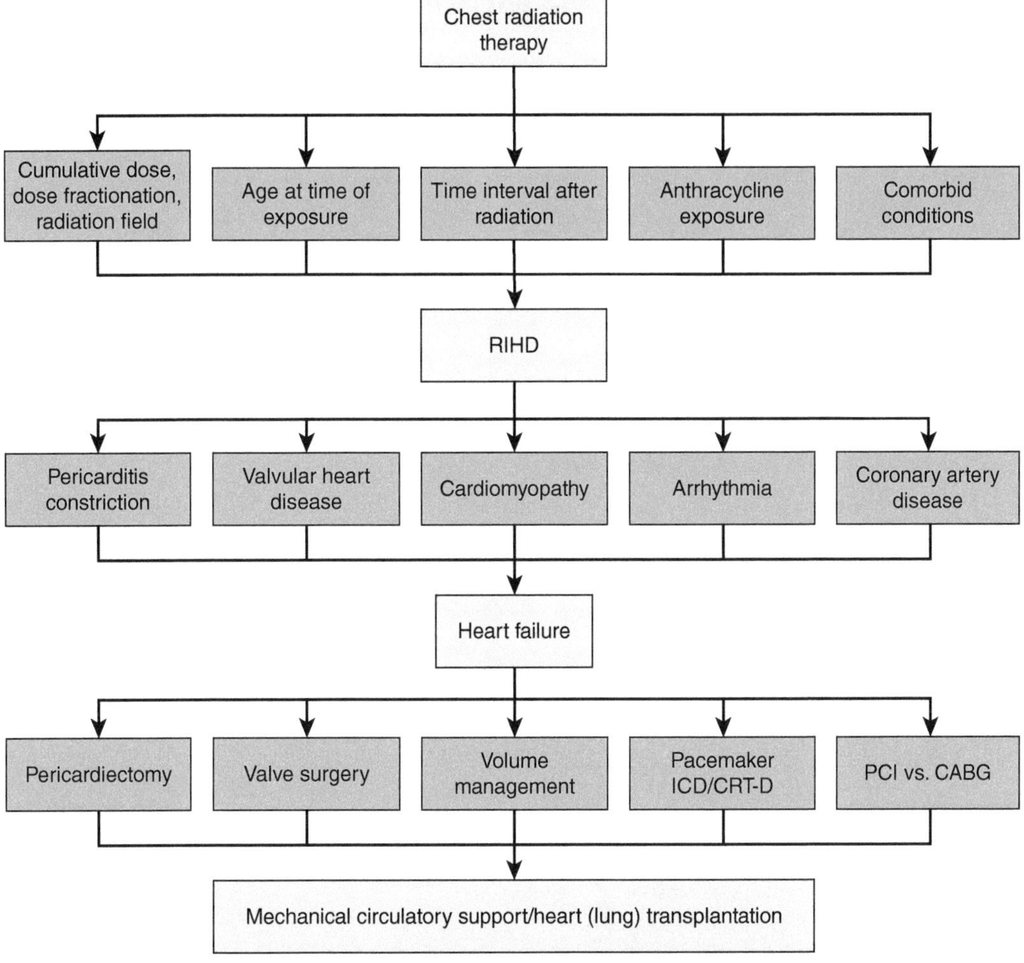

FIG. 26.1 The spectrum of radiation-induced heart disease (*RIHD*), which can culminate in the "common final pathway" of heart failure (HF) presentation. Treatment modalities are directed toward the disease aspects. *CABG,* Coronary artery bypass grafting; *CRT-D,* cardiac resynchronization therapy defibrillator; *ICD,* implantable cardioverter defibrillator; *PCI,* percutaneous coronary intervention. (From Finch W, Lee MS, Yang EH. Radiation-induced heart disease: long-term manifestations, diagnosis, and management. In: Herrmann J, ed. *Clinical Cardiooncology.* 1st ed. Elsevier; 2016.)

In a small cohort study, coronary artery calcium score following mediastinal RT for HL was higher in those with than in those without obstructive CAD (median score of 439 vs. 68), and a score of 0 had a negative predictive value for symptomatic CAD of 100%.[6] Using CTA, another study found a 24% prevalence of CAD in 119 patients who had undergone mediastinal RT as children.[7] Both calcified and noncalcified plaques were seen, primarily in the proximal coronary arteries (57% included the proximal LAD) and mostly non-obstructive. Coronary CTA has thus been attributed a higher sensitivity and negative predictive value for CAD than stress testing. As in general practice, however, catheter-based coronary angiography remains the gold standard for the detection of CAD.

Management of CAD in cases of radiation therapy is not specifically addressed in United States guidelines on management of acute coronary syndrome and stable ischemic heart disease, however, the same principles apply. Revascularization using either percutaneous coronary intervention or coronary artery bypass graft surgery may be necessary when critical stenoses are present; the need for concomitant valve or pericardial surgery may influence the decision.[8] A noteworthy concern is limited usability of the internal mammary arteries after chest radiation; however, a study of 125 patients

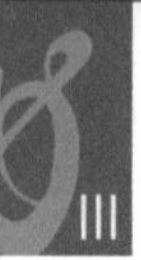

TABLE 26.1 Differential applicability of Imaging Techniques for the Detection and Follow Up of Radiation-Induced Heart Disease

	ECHOCARDIOGRAPHY	CARDIAC CMR	CARDIAC CT	STRESS ECHOCARDIOGRAPHY	ERNA/SPECT PERFUSION
Pericardial Disease					
Effusion—screening and positive diagnosis	++++	++	+	−	−
Effusion—follow up	++++	+	−	−	−
Constriction—screening and positive diagnosis	++++	++++	++	−	−
Myocardial Disease					
LV systolic dysfunction	++++ (1st line, contrast echocardiography if poor acoustic window)	++++	+	++++ (contractile reserve assessment)	++++/++++ (if analysis of function and perfusion needed)
LV diastolic dysfunction	++++	+	−	+	++/+
LV dysfunction—follow up	++++ (1st line, contrast echocardiography if poor acoustic window)	+	−	++ (contractile reserve assessment)	++/++
Myocardial fibrosis	−	++++	+	−	−
Valve Disease					
Positive diagnosis and severity assessment	++++	++	++	++	−
Follow up	++++	+	−	++	−
Coronary Artery Disease					
Positive diagnosis	+ (if resting wall-motion abnormalities)	++++ (stress CMR[b])	++++ (CT angio[a])	++++ (exercise or dobutamine[b])	+/++++
Follow up	+	+	++	++++ (1st line)	+/++

[a]For anatomic evaluation, an excellent negative predictive value.
[b]For functional evaluation.
Angio, Angiography; *CMR,* cardiac magnetic resonance; *CT,* computed tomography; *ERNA,* equilibrium radionuclide angiocardiography; *SPECT,* single-photon emission CT; *LV,* left ventricular.
++++: highly valuable; ++: valuable; +: of interest; −: of limited interest.

who had undergone mediastinal irradiation did not identify vessel fibrosis or significant histologic damage.[9,10] Still, there might be merit in evaluating the internal mammary arteries by conventional or CT angiography before cardiac surgery.

VALVULAR HEART DISEASE

Cardiac valvular abnormalities are common following mediastinal RT (Fig. 26.2 and 28.3), with significant valve disease (defined as mild or greater aortic regurgitation; or moderate or greater mitral or tricuspid regurgitation; or aortic stenosis) in 29% of asymptomatic patients starting 2 years after RT, compared with 4% of age- and gender-matched controls.[11] This rate increases significantly over time to 42% at 14 years and over 60% after 20 years postirradiation in high exposure cohorts, such as patients with lymphoma. Moderate or greater valvular disease is most commonly observed of the aortic and mitral valves, and regurgitation occurs more often than stenosis of these valves. The risk of radiation-induced valvular disease is greatest when the radiation dose exceeds 25 Gy.[12,13]

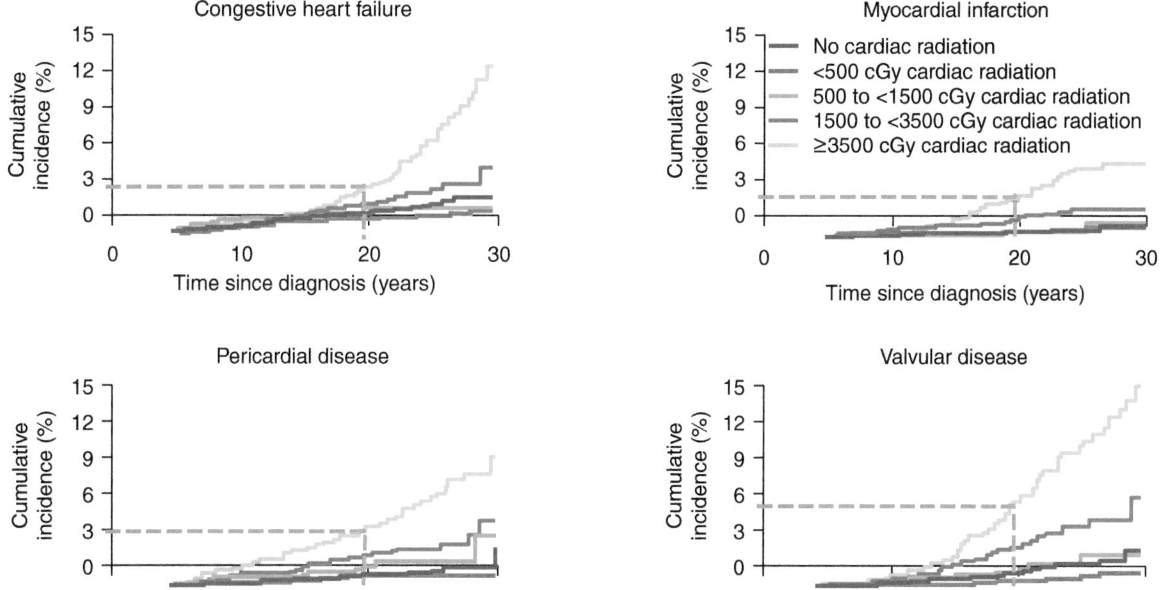

FIG. 26.2 Cumulative incidence of the various aspects of radiation-induced heart disease in childhood cancer survivors. Notice the dose dependency and timeline of 15 years from diagnosis for clinical appearance. (From Mulrooney DA, Yeazel MW, Mertens AC, et al. Cardiac outcomes in a cohort of adult survivors of childhood and adolescent cancer: retrospective analysis of the Childhood Cancer Survivor Study cohort. *BMJ.* 2009;339:b4606, with permission.)

When valve disease is symptomatic or other indications for replacement are present, surgical management is indicated, according to standard valve guidelines (see Chapter 28).[14,15] Patients with RIHD undergoing valve surgery have a relatively high rate of morbidity and mortality after valve surgery (30-day mortality of 12%).[14,15] Because mediastinal RT can result in comorbidities that can result in prohibitively high surgical risk (e.g., frozen mediastinum or porcelain aorta), percutaneous valve therapies may be preferable in many cases.[13] Of note, the Society of Thoracic Surgeons (STS) risk score as a standard tool for surgical risk assessment in patients with aortic stenosis underestimates the risk of surgical aortic valve replacement (SAVR) in this population. Transcatheter aortic valve replacements have been used successfully in patients with severe aortic stenosis whose radiation-induced mediastinal and pulmonary fibrosis precluded surgery. In several nonrandomized analyses, patients who underwent transcatheter aortic valve replacement had a higher survival rate after valve replacement compared with patients who underwent surgical aortic valve replacement.[16] More recently, percutaneous edge-to-edge mitral valve repair, with technologies such as MitraClip (Abbott Medical, Abbott Park, IL), has been used for radiation-induced mitral regurgitatio.[17] One potential concern after MitraClip for RT-induced mitral regurgitation is that if there is ongoing reactive damage to the mitral apparatus, delayed mitral stenosis may occur; however, at 6 months postprocedure there was nearly a 90% rate of improved New York Heart Association (NYHA) functional class.[17]

CARDIOMYOPATHY

Direct damage to the myocardium from radiotherapy may result in cardiomyopathy even in the absence of significant epicardial CAD or VHD. Prior thoracic radiation exposure increases the risk of HF substantially (hazard ratio [HR], 2.7 to 7.4 for HL and HR, 1.5 to 2.4 for breast cancer).[18] Radiation-induced cardiomyopathy (RICM) more commonly presents as HF with preserved ejection fraction.[18] For patients with breast cancer receiving radiotherapy, the odds ratio of developing HF per log of mean cardiac radiation dose is 16.9 (3.9 to 73.7) for HF with preserved ejection fraction (EF), and 3.17 (0.8 to 13.0) for HF with reduced EF.[19] Studies measuring diastolic function in long-term survivors of HL who received RT have, however, shown inconsistent results and many have found none or only mild changes in diastolic parameters.[18]

Patients who develop RICM present similar to those with HF from any other causes. The effects of radiation are synergistic with anthracycline chemotherapy, resulting in doubling of the risk of heart failure compared with RT alone.[20–22] Myocardial fibrosis, which is a hallmark of RICM, can be seen in a patchy or diffuse distribution on cardiac magnetic resonance (see Table 26.1).[23] Echocardiography, including strain imaging using speckle tracking, can be helpful in identifying radiation-induced myocardial dysfunction.[24] Global longitudinal strain may become abnormal before the ejection fraction declines, which is typically reduced compared with controls, but still in the normal range. Fibrosis within the myocardium and endocardium may additionally result in diastolic dysfunction.[25] When HF with reduced ejection fraction is present, therapy for cardiomyopathy does not differ from that of nonradiation-induced cardiomyopathies. In patients with advanced RICM, orthotopic heart transplantation is a last resort; however, it should be noted that mediastinal fibrosis may increase the operative risk significantly.[26] Last but not least, all patients presenting with HF after chest RT should be evaluated for all possible radiation toxicities, including CAD, VHD, and pericardial disease, which can present as or at least contribute to HF in these patients.

PERICARDIAL DISEASE

In the early era of mantle radiation for HL high radiation doses resulted not infrequently in acute pericarditis (up to 60% incidence in early studies) often with pericardial effusions and risk of cardiac tamponade.[27] Pericardiocentesis or surgical approaches may be required in the latter case, and nonsteroidal antiinflammatory drugs take center stage in the management of the acute inflammation and pericardial irritation. Long-term complications may include pericardial fibrosis resulting in constrictive pericarditis (CP), which may be delayed to more than 20 years after RT.[28–30] CP caused by mediastinal RT has similar symptoms and physical examination findings; diagnostic evaluation and management is likewise similar to CP owing to other causes.[29] The most notable distinction from other etiologies is that RT-induced CP has been associated with a significantly higher long-term mortality.[31] This is exemplified in patients undergoing pericardiectomy: 5-year mortality is 2.5 times higher in patients who have RT versus those who have not (90% vs. 36%).[31,32] When CP is present along with valvular disease, perioperative mortality is increased to as high as 40% at 30 days.[14,15] Thus, if symptomatic CP is present in patients with cancer after RT, candidacy for pericardiectomy needs to be carefully considered, and not too early and not too late, owing to considerable perioperative mortality.

PERIPHERAL ARTERY DISEASE

Thoracic radiation or RT for head and neck cancers may include the carotid or subclavian arteries in the radiation field.[33] In patients with RT for HL, 7% of patients were found to have carotid or subclavian atherosclerosis causing at least 40% stenosis after 20 years. Additionally, 4% developed transient ischemic attack or stroke only 5.6 years (median) after RT. The median radiation dose to the low-cervical region in patients who developed carotid or subclavian stenosis was 44 Gy. In patients with head and neck cancers even higher doses may be encountered (approaching 56 Gy in one study).[34] In these patients, carotid stenosis rates are as high as 79% at a median of 9.2 years after RT, compared with a reference of 21%. The (relative) risk of stroke after neck RT for either HL or head and neck cancer is five to six times higher than that seen in siblings or the general population.[35] The risk of stroke is increased regardless of whether the head and neck cancer type is associated with smoking.[35] In this population, carotid or subclavian artery stenting, carotid endarterectomy, and subclavian artery bypass grafting are all potential therapies.[33] In patients with RT exposure for breast cancer treatment, there is an increase in arterial stiffness (measured by the augmentation index and carotid-radial pulse-wave velocity) in the arm ipsilateral to the radiation site compared with the contralateral arm, suggesting direct and localized vascular damage as a result of RT.[36]

ARRHYTHMIAS AND AUTONOMIC DYSFUNCTION

Fibrosis of the conduction system, including the bundle branches, His bundle, and the atrioventricular node, may occur after thoracic RT.[11] Other factors associated with conduction disease in these patients include right coronary artery disease and calcification of the aortomitral curtain.[37–39] When complete heart block occurs, syncope is the most common clinical presentation in symptomatic patients and it may require pacemaker implantation. Patients after chest radiation may also be at higher risk of atrial fibrillation.

Autonomic dysfunction with a reduction in parasympathetic tone and an increase in sympathetic tone may be observed after mediastinal RT,[40] translating into higher resting heart rates and heart rate variability and reduced baroreflex sensitivity. For instance, patients who had received RT (median dose of 38 Gy at a median follow-up time of 19 years) for HL are noted to have a higher resting heart rate than HL patients without RT and a higher rate of abnormal heart rate recovery (31.9% vs. 9.3%) at one minute of recovery after Bruce protocol stress testing. Abnormal heart rate response in this study was noted to be associated with a higher risk of all-cause mortality (HR, 4.60; 95% CI, 1.62 to 13.02). Additionally, RT for nasopharyngeal carcinoma has been associated with reduced heart rate response to deep breathing or the Valsalva manuever.[41] The authors hypothesize this may be related to fibrosis of the carotid artery walls with resultant stiffening of baroreceptors. Although fibrotic changes are less likely to revert, aerobic exercise may reduce autonomic imbalance by various mechanisms, last but not least by reconditioning.[42]

PREVENTION AND SCREENING FOR RIHD

Although dose reduction efforts including radiation protection blocks, advanced planning techniques, and involved field radiation have had a significant impact on reducing the risk, RIHD remains a concern and warrants screening efforts. Even more, practices nowadays will still have to care for patients exposed to high-dose chest RT in the past.

Patients who have had RT should be seen annually as part of a survivorship plan regardless of the presence of symptoms (Table 26.2). Biomarkers and cardiac enzymes have limited use at this time, primarily owing to a lack of data as to how they should be applied.[43] Screening efforts for RIHD thus remain primarily imaging-based. The American Society of Echocardiography and European Association of Cardiovascular Imaging (ASE/EACVI), the Society for Cardiac Angiography and Intervention (SCAI), and the International Cardio-Oncology Society (IC-OS) have released screening guidelines for RIHD (Central Illustration).[44,5] The guiding principles are to screen for asymptomatic coronary artery and VHD, CP, and cardiomyopathy in patients who are at high risk for RIHD, especially those who have received at least 30 Gy of radiation (plus or minus additional risk factors). Recommendations include echocardiography and stress test starting 5 to 10 years after RT, then every 2 to 5 years, depending on risk (see Table 26.2).

The ASE/EACVI guidelines do not specify the choice of noninvasive stress tests, whereas SCAI recommends exercise echocardiogram as the preferred test.[44,5] When stress echocardiography is used, consideration should be given to a concomitant oxygen consumption study because it tests the cardiopulmonary axis, given the potential involvement of the lung fields and related changes after chest radiation. Another alternative mentioned by the SCAI guidelines is coronary CTA for screening, assessing the overall burden of CAD. This aspect is given further attention in the IC-OS guidelines, which recommend the use of CAC and CCTA for (earlier) visualization of evolving CAD in patients after RT.[5] If the screening tests identify evidence of cardiovascular disease, then additional diagnostic imaging should be pursued, including diagnostic catheterization, coronary angiography, cardiac magnetic resonance (CMR), or computed tomography, as appropriate.[44] CMR may be an important diagnostic tool for the detection of RIHD. In one study where CMR was performed in HL survivors at a median time of 24 years following RT, 70% of patients had significant abnormalities. These abnormalities included valvular dysfunction, reduction in left ventricular EF, late myocardial enhancement, and perfusion deficits[45] Contrast-enhanced MRI is excellent for the diagnosis of acute pericarditis by demonstrating pericardial enhancement.

Deformation imaging with strain is a sensitive way to detect myocardial dysfunction; it is widely used in the assessment of oncology patients,

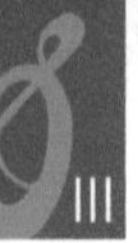

TABLE 26.2 Screening Recommendation for Asymptomatic Patients With Cardiac Radiation Exposure (for the SCAI algorithm, please see Central Illustration)

Screening for CAD

European Society of Medical Oncology consensus statement
- evaluation for CAD/ ischemia, even if asymptomatic, starting at 5 years post-treatment and then at least every 3-5 years thereafter

EACVI/ASE consensus statement
- Functional noninvasive stress test
- Screening recommended in high-risk patients*
- Starting 5 to 10 years after radiation exposure
- Reassess every 5 years
- Annual cardiovascular history and examination

International Cardio-Oncology Society consensus statement
- Comprehensive cardiovascular history and physical exam annually
- Review available CT imaging for atherosclerotic calcifications as available
- Screening for CAD with coronary artery calcium, coronary CT angiography, or functional stress testing in patients without documented atherosclerosis on prior evaluations
- Starting 5 years after radiation exposure
- Repeat screening at 5 year intervals, depending on the patient's overall cardiovascular risk

Screening for noncoronary atherosclerotic disease

EACVI/ASE consensus statement
- carotid artery ultrasonography in patients with neurologic signs or symptoms

International Cardio-Oncology Society consensus statement

After head and/or neck radiation
- Auscultation for carotid bruits during their routine physical examination
- Screening for signs and symptoms of dysautonomia on follow-up physical examinations (including orthostatic vital signs)
- Review of available CT scans for carotid calcifications to aid in identification of asymptomatic atherosclerosis
- Carotid ultrasound to screen for development of asymptomatic atherosclerotic plaque
- Initial evaluation as early as 1 y post-radiation in higher risk patients (determined by radiation dose and CV risk)
- Follow-up every 3 to 5 y can be useful to guide preventive therapy

After abdominal or pelvic radiation
- Review of available CT scans for aortic and iliofemoral calcifications to identify atherosclerosis can be useful
- Evaluation for radiation nephropathy and/or renal artery stenosis in patients with worsening renal function and/or systemic hypertension can be useful

Screening for valvular disease

European Society of Medical Oncology consensus statement
- evaluation for valvular disease, even if asymptomatic, starting at 5 years post-treatment and then at least every 3-5 years thereafter

EACVI/ASE consensus statement
- Echocardiogram
- Starting 5 years after radiation in high-risk patients*
- Starting 10 years after radiation in all others
- Reassess every 5 years
- Annual cardiovascular history and examination

International Cardio-Oncology Society consensus statement
- Comprehensive cardiovascular history and physical exam annually
- Screening recommended for patients who received RT with the heart in the radiation field
- Starting at 5 years post RT
- Reassess every 3-5 years

Screening for cardiac dysfunction/cardiomyopathy

American Society of Clinical Oncology Clinical Practice Guideline
- Echocardiogram
- Screening recommended for high-dose radiotherapy (≥ 30 Gy) where the heart is in the treatment field or lower-dose anthracycline (eg, doxorubicin < 250 mg/m^2, epirubicin < 600mg/m^2) in combination with lower-dose RT (< 30 Gy) where the heart is in the treatment field
- Starting during and/or 6 to 12 months after completion of cancer-directed therapy
- Regular evaluation of cardiovascular risk factors including smoking, hypertension, diabetes, dyslipidemia, and obesity

TABLE 26.2 **Screening Recommendation for Asymptomatic Patients With Cardiac Radiation Exposure (for the SCAI algorithm, please see Central Illustration)—cont'd**

International Late Effects of Childhood Cancer Guideline Harmonization Group
- Screening recommended for individuals treated with ≥ 35 Gy of chest radiation or anthracycline ≥ 100mg/m2 + ≥ 15 Gy of radiation, and screening may be reasonable for moderate doses (15 Gy to 35 Gy)
- Echocardiogram, cardiac MRI, radionuclide angiography
- Starting no later than 2 years after completion of cardiotoxic therapy for high-risk survivors
- Repeat at 5 years after diagnosis
- Reassess every 5 years (can consider more frequent surveillance for high-risk individuals)
- Screening for modifiable cardiovascular risk factors

International Cardio-Oncology Society consensus statement
- Echocardiogram (or cardiac MRI) screening recommended for patients at risk of cardiomyopathy
- Starting as early as 6-12 months after radiation therapy in high-risk patients**
- In all patients in whom the heart is in the radiation field, an echocardiogram within 5 years post RT is recommended
- Reassessment every 5 years by echocardiogram and NT-proBNP levels can be useful

Table 5. Screening recommendation for asymptomatic patients with cardiac radiation exposure. *High-risk patients were defined as having had anterior or left chest irradiation as well as one of the following risk factors: dose greater than 30 Gy, dose fraction greater than 2 Gy, age less than 50 years, lack of shielding, concomitant anthracyclines, cardiovascular risk factors, or known cardiac disease.
**Patients at high-risk for radiation-associated cardiac disease defined as those with: 1) mediastinal radiotherapy ≥30 Gy with the heart in the treatment field; 2) lower dose radiotherapy (<30 Gy) with anthracycline exposure; 3) patients aged <50 years and longer time since RT; 4) high dose of radiation fractions (>2 Gy/d); 5) presence and extent of tumor in or next to the heart; 6) presence of CV risk factors; and 7) pre-existing CV disease
CT, Computed tomography; *EACVI/ASE*, European Association of Cardiovascular Imaging/American Society of Echocardiography.
van Leeuwen-Segarceanu EM, Bos W-JW, Dorresteijn LD, et al. Screening Hodgkin lymphoma survivors for radiotherapy induced cardiovascular disease. *Cancer Treat Rev.* 2011:37(5):391–403.

particularly those undergoing treatment with anthracyclines.[46] Evidence indicates that strain is abnormal in patients with cancer who have had radiation exposure. One study measured strain values in those patients with breast cancer receiving either right- or left-sided chest radiotherapy prior to, immediately after, and 2 months following therapy. Regional strain changes were noted immediately and at the 2 month follow up in patients with left-sided breast cancer; however, this was not seen in patients with right-sided breast cancer.[47]

The right ventricle (RV) is also affected as a result of RT in patients with cancer; however, few studies have evaluated the extent and mechanism of these changes. It is likely that the same mechanisms of myocardial fibrosis, endothelial dysfunction, and oxidative stress known to contribute to left ventricular dysfunction, valve disease, pericardial diseases, and CAD also affect RV function and structure. RV wall thickness appears reduced in patients who have received chemotherapy alone or a combination of chemotherapy and low- or high-dose RT. The effect of RT on RV systolic function remains unclear, with some studies showing a decrease whereas others show no significant change.[48]

PREVENTIVE DRUG THERAPIES

Evidence regarding the prevention of cardiotoxicity owing to radiation exposure is limited and no agents are approved for the prevention or treatment of RIHD. The role of preventive medications, including (high-dose) statins, antiplatelet agents, angiotensin-converting enzyme inhibitors (ACEi) and angiotensin-receptor blockers (ARB), is unclear. Indeed, renin-angiotensin aldosterone system inhibitors (both ACEi and ARBs) and HMG-CoA reductase inhibitors (statins) have been shown to prevent both cardiac fibrosis and damage to other organs after radiation in experimental studies though not universally.[49,50] Importantly, there is paucity of data in humans, but a study evaluating the effects of statin therapy on arterial endothelial function in acute lymphoblastic leukemia or non-Hodgkin lymphoma survivors is on-going. Certainly, cardiovascular risk factors amplify the burden of radiation in terms of risk of ischemic heart disease and acute coronary events (Fig. 26.3) as well as HF and even VHD (see Chapter 24, Fig. 24.1). Pristine control of controllable risk factors is therefore paramount, including the use of ACEi/ARBs and statins, when indicated, and in keeping with their positive effect on vascular health and atherosclerosis.

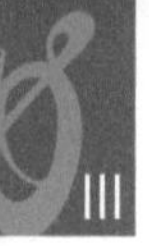

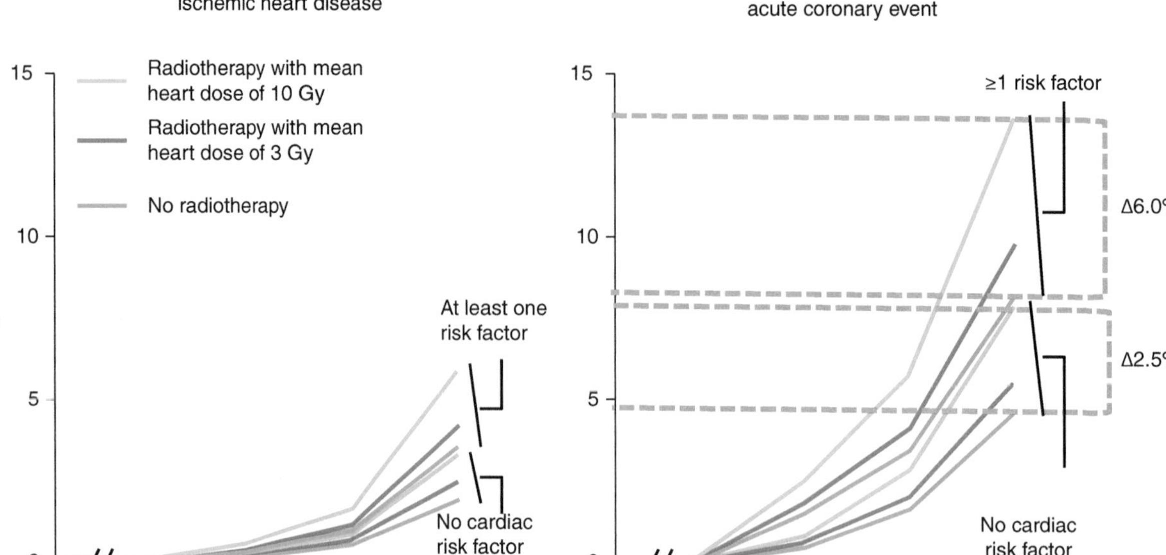

FIG. 26.3 Cumulative risk of death from ischemic heart disease (*left*) and of at least one acute coronary event (*right*) in patients after chest radiation for breast cancer. (From Darby SC, Ewertz M, McGale P, et al. Risk of ischemic heart disease in women after radiotherapy for breast cancer. *N Engl J Med.* 2013;368:977).

FUTURE AVENUES

Although there is a continued focus in the literature on the cardiovascular manifestations of RT, existing studies do not provide much insight into preventative strategies that reduce the development of RIHD. Whereas there are mixed data on the effects of traditional medications for the management of conventional cardiovascular risk factors and diseases, there is a paucity of randomized, controlled clinical trial data in patients who have had radiation. In addition, the precise timing of these therapies in patients having had chest RT, as well as accompanying surveillance strategies for cardiovascular toxicity, remain unknown. Multidisciplinary collaborations between cardiology and oncology are essential to establish registries and clinical trials to assess long-term outcomes and the impact of surveillance and proposed pharmacologic intervention and strategies. Whereas the landscape of cancer treatment continues to evolve, including RT techniques, many questions and challenges remain for the field of cardio-oncology to investigate in order to provide evidence-based care for the detection and treatment of radiation treatment-induced manifestations of cardiovascular disease.

REFERENCES

1. Nilsson G, Holmberg L, Garmo H, et al. Distribution of coronary artery stenosis after radiation for breast cancer. *J Clin Oncol.* 2012;30:380–386.
2. Cheng YJ, Nie XY, Ji CC, et al. Long-trm cardiovascular risk after radiotherapy in women with breast cancer. *J Am Heart Assoc.* 2017;6(5):e005633.
3. Santoro F, Ferraretti A, Centola A, et al. Early clinical presentation of diffuse, severe, multi-district atherosclerosis after radiation therapy for Hodgkin lymphoma. *Int J Cardiol.* 2013;165:373–374. doi:10.1016/j.ijcard.2012.08.027.
4. Marks LB, Yu X, Prosnitz RG, et al. The incidence and functional consequences of RT-associated cardiac perfusion defects. *Int J Radiat Oncol Biol Phys.* 2005;63:214–223.
5. Mitchell JD, Cehic DA, Morgia M, Bergrom C, Toohey J, Guerrero PA, Ferencik M, Kikuchi R, Carver JR, Zaha VG, Alvarez-Cardona JA, Szmit S, Daniele AJ, Lopez-Mattei J, Zhang L, Herrmann J, Nohria A, Lenihan DJ, Dent SF. Cardiovascular Manifestations From Therapeutic Radiation: A Multidisciplinary Expert Consensus Statement From the International Cardio-Oncology Society. JACC CardioOncol. 2021 Sep 21;3(3):360–380. doi: 10.1016/j.jaccao.2021.06.003. PMID: 34604797; PMCID: PMC8463721.
6. Andersen R, Wethal T, Gunther A, et al. Relation of coronary artery calcium score to premature coronary artery disease in survivors >15 years of Hodgkin's lymphoma. *Am J Cardiol.* 2010; 105:149–152.
7. Kupeli S, Hazirolan T, Varan A, et al. Evaluation of coronary artery disease by computed tomography angiography in patients treated for childhood Hodgkin's lymphoma. *J Clin Oncol.* 2010;28:1025–1030.
8. Handler CE, Livesey S, Lawton PA. Coronary ostial stenosis after radiotherapy: angioplasty or coronary artery surgery? *Br Heart J.* 1989;61:208–211.
9. Gansera B, Schmidtler F, Angelis I, et al. Quality of internal thoracic artery grafts after mediastinal irradiation. *Ann Thorac Surg.* 2007;84:1479–1484.

10. Khan MH, Ettinger SM. Post mediastinal radiation coronary artery disease and its effects on arterial conduits. *Catheter Cardiovasc Interv*. 2001;52:242–248.
11. Heidenreich PA, Hancock SL, Lee BK, et al. Asymptomatic cardiac disease following mediastinal irradiation. *J Am Coll Cardiol*. 2003;42:743–749.
12. Cella L, Liuzzi R, Conson M, et al. Dosimetric predictors of asymptomatic heart valvular dysfunction following mediastinal irradiation for Hodgkin's lymphoma. *Radiother Oncol*. 2011;101:316–321.
13. Janelle GM, Mnookin SC, Thomas JJ, et al. Surgical approach for a patient with aortic stenosis and a frozen mediastinum. *J Cardiothorac Vasc Anesth*. 2003;17:770–772.
14. Handa N, McGregor CG, Danielson GK, et al. Valvular heart operation in patients with previous mediastinal radiation therapy. *Ann Thorac Surg*. 2001;71:1880–1884.
15. Crestanello JA, McGregor CG, Danielson GK, et al. Mitral and tricuspid valve repair in patients with previous mediastinal radiation therapy. *Ann Thorac Surg*. 2004;78:826–831.
16. Zhang D, Guo W, Al-Hijji MA, et al. Outcomes of patients with severe symptomatic aortic valve stenosis after chest radiation: transcatheter versus surgical aortic valve replacement. *J Am Heart Assoc*. 2019;8:e012110.
17. Scarfo I, Denti P, Citro R, Buzzatti N, Alfieri O, La Canna G. MitraClip for radiotherapy-related mitral valve regurgitation. *Hellenic J Cardiol*. 2019;60:232–238.
18. Nolan MT, Russell DJ, Marwick TH. Long-term risk of heart failure and myocardial dysfunction after thoracic radiotherapy: a systematic review. *Can J Cardiol*. 2016;32(7):908–920.
19. Saiki H, Petersen IA, Scott CG, et al. Risk of heart failure with preserved ejection fraction in older women after contemporary radiotherapy for breast cancer. *Circulation*. 2017;135(15):1388–1396.
20. Billingham ME, Bristow MR, Glatstein E, et al. Adriamycin cardiotoxicity: endomyocardial biopsy evidence of enhancement by irradiation. *Am J Surg Pathol*. 1977;1:17–23.
21. Aleman BM, van den Belt-Dusebout AW, De Bruin ML, et al. Late cardiotoxicity after treatment for Hodgkin lymphoma. *Blood*. 2007;109:1878–1886.
22. Shapiro CL, Hardenbergh PH, Gelman R, et al. Cardiac effects of adjuvant doxorubicin and radiation therapy in breast patients with cancer. *J Clin Oncol*. 1998;16:3493–3501.
23. Umezawa R, Ota H, Takanami K, et al. MRI findings of radiation-induced myocardial damage in patients with oesophageal cancer. *Clin Radiol*. 2014;69:1273–1279.
24. Tsai HR, Gjesdal O, Wethal T, et al. Left ventricular function assessed by two-dimensional speckle tracking echocardiography in long-term survivors of Hodgkin's lymphoma treated by mediastinal radiotherapy with or without anthracycline therapy. *Am J Cardiol*. 2011;107:472–477.
25. Heidenreich PA, Hancock SL, Vagelos RH, et al. Diastolic dysfunction after mediastinal irradiation. *Am Heart J*. 2005;150.977–982.
26. Uriel N, Vainrib A, Jorde UP, et al. Mediastinal radiation and adverse outcomes after heart transplantation. *J Heart Lung Transplant*. 2010;29:378–381.
27. Cohn KE, Stewart JR, Fajardo LF, et al. Heart disease following radiation. *Medicine*. 1967;46:281–298.
28. Ling LH, Oh JK, Schaff HV, et al. Constrictive pericarditis in the modern era: evolving clinical spectrum and impact on outcome after pericardiectomy. *Circulation*. 1999;100:1380–1386.
29. Greenwood RD, Rosenthal A, Cassady R, et al. Constrictive pericarditis in childhood due to mediastinal irradiation. *Circulation*. 1974;50:1033–1039.
30. Applefeld MM, Cole JF, Pollock SH, et al. The late appearance of chronic pericardial disease in patients treated by radiotherapy for Hodgkin's disease. *Ann Intern Med*. 1981;94:338–341.
31. George TJ, Arnaoutakis GJ, Beaty CA, et al. Contemporary etiologies, risk factors, and outcomes after pericardiectomy. *Ann Thorac Surg*. 2012;94:445–451.
32. Bertog SC, Thambidorai SK, Parakh K, et al. Constrictive pericarditis: etiology and cause-specific survival after pericardiectomy. *J Am Coll Cardiol*. 2004;43(8):1448.
33. Hull MC, Morris CG, Pepine CJ, et al. Valvular dysfunction and carotid, subclavian, and coronary artery disease in survivors of Hodgkin lymphoma treated with radiation therapy. *JAMA*. 2003;290:2831–2837.
34. Lam WW, Leung S, So NM, et al. Incidence of carotid stenosis in nasopharyngeal carcinoma patients after radiotherapy. *Cancer*. 2001;92:2357–2363.
35. Dorresteijn LD, Kappelle AC, Boogrd W, et al. Increased risk of ischemic stroke after radiotherapy on the neck in patients younger than 60 years. *J Clin Oncol*. 2001;20:282–288.
36. Vallerio P, Sarno L, Stucchi M, et al. Long-term effects of radiotherapy on arterial stiffness in breast cancer women. *Am J Cardiol*. 2016;118(5):771–776.
37. de Waard DE, Verhorst PM, Visser CA. Exercise-induced syncope as late consequence of radiotherapy. *Int J Cardiol*. 1996;57:289–291.
38. Orzan F, Brusca A, Gaita F, et al. Associated cardiac lesions in patients with radiation-induced complete heart block. *Int J Cardiol*. 1993;39:151–156.
39. Santoro F, Ieva R, Lupo P, et al. Late calcification of the mitral-aortic junction causing transient complete atrio-ventricular block after mediastinal radiation of Hodgkin lymphoma: multimodal visualization. *Int J Cardiol*. 2012;155:e49–e50.
40. Groarke JD, Tanguturi VK, Hainer J, et al. Abnormal exercise response in long-term survivors of Hodgkin lymphoma treated with thoracic irradiation. *J Am Coll Cardiol*. 2015;65:573–583.
41. Huang CC, Huang TL, Hsu HC, et al. Long-term effects of neck irradiation on cardiovascular autonomic function: a study in nasopharyngeal carcinoma patients after radiotherapy. *Muscle Nerve*. 2013;47:344–350.
42. Scott JM, Jones LW, Hornsby WE, et al. Cancer therapy-induced autonomic dysfunction in early breast cancer: implications for aerobic exercise training. *Int J Cardiol*. 2014;171(2):e50–e51.
43. Nellessen U, Zingel M, Hecker H, et al. Effects of radiation therapy on myocardial cell integrity and pump function: which role for cardiac biomarkers? *Chemotherapy*. 2010;56:147–152.
44. Iliescu CA, Grines CL, Herrmann J, et al. SCAI Expert consensus statement: evaluation, management, and special considerations of cardio-oncology patients in the cardiac catheterization laboratory (endorsed by the Cardiological Society of India, and Sociedad Latino Americana de Cardiologıa Intervencionista). *Catheter Cardiovasc Interv*. 2016;87:E202–E223.
45. Machann W, Beer M, Breunig M, et al. Cardiac magnetic resonance imaging findings in 20-year survivors of mediastinal radiotherapy for Hodgkin's disease. *Int J Radiat Oncol Biol Phys*. 2011;79(4):1117–1123.
46. Plana JC, Galderisi M, Barac A, et al. Expert consensus for multimodality imaging evaluation of adult patients during and after cancer therapy: a report from the American Society of Echocardiography and the European Association of Cardiovascular Imaging. *J Am Soc Echocardiogr*. 2014;27(9):911–939.
47. Erven K, Jurcut R, Weltens C, et al. Acute radiation effects on cardiac function detected by strain rate imaging in breast patients with cancer. *Int J Radiat Oncol Biol Phys*. 2011;79(5):1444–1451.
48. Tadic M, Cuspidi C, Hering D, et al. Radiotherapy-induced right ventricular remodeling: The missing piece of the puzzle. *Arch Cardiovasc Dis*. 2017;110(2):116–123.
49. van der Veen SJ, Ghobadi G, de Boer RA, et al. ACE inhibition attenuates radiation-induced cardiopulmonary damage. *Radiother Oncol*. 2015;114:96–103.
50. Zhang K, He X, Zhou Y, et al. Atorvastatin ameliorates radiation-induced cardiac fibrosis in rats. *Radiat Res*. 2015;184(6):611–620.

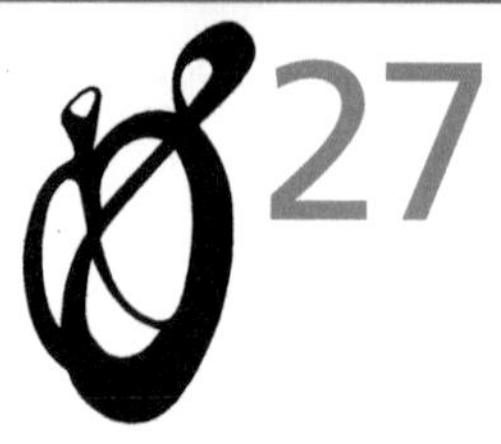

27 Prevention and Management of Cardiomyopathy and Heart Failure in Cancer Survivors

JOSE A. ALVAREZ-CARDONA AND DANIEL J. LENIHAN

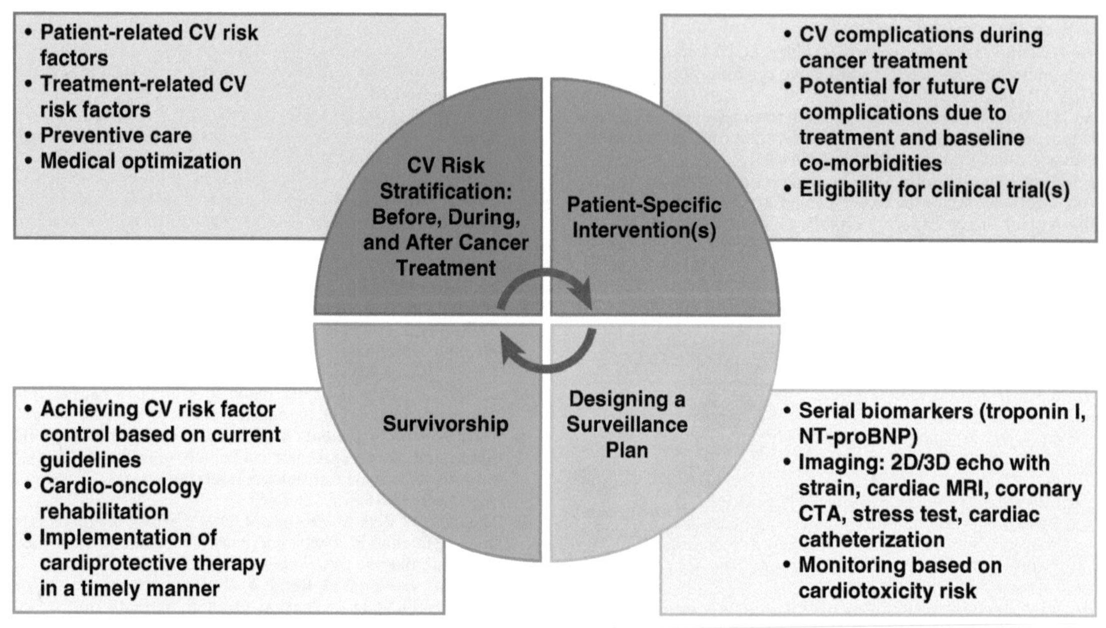
• Patient-related CV risk factors
• Treatment-related CV risk factors
• Preventive care
• Medical optimization
CV Risk Stratification: Before, During, and After Cancer Treatment
Patient-Specific Intervention(s)
• CV complications during cancer treatment
• Potential for future CV complications due to treatment and baseline co-morbidities
• Eligibility for clinical trial(s)
Survivorship
Designing a Surveillance Plan
• Achieving CV risk factor control based on current guidelines
• Cardio-oncology rehabilitation
• Implementation of cardiprotective therapy in a timely manner
• Serial biomarkers (troponin I, NT-proBNP)
• Imaging: 2D/3D echo with strain, cardiac MRI, coronary CTA, stress test, cardiac catheterization
• Monitoring based on cardiotoxicity risk

CHAPTER OUTLINE

KEY POINTS

- Cancer survivors should be followed for cardiomyopathy (CM) or heart failure (HF) as a continuation of care, with CV risks ascertained before treatment, and any cardiac disease emerging during and after cancer therapy
- The most effective surveillance tools and the frequency of testing are not well defined
- The frequency of surveillance is yet to be determined in adult cancer survivors; for childhood cancer survivors there are at least proposed guidelines
- How to respond appropriately to abnormal findings has not been rigorously defined in any clinical trials to date
- The overall goal is to enhance optimal long-term outcomes with a comprehensive, multidisciplinary approach that may be best organized by a survivorship clinic

The essential key to prevent heart disease in cancer survivors is identifying those at increased risk of developing cardiac dysfunction (heart failure with reduced ejection fraction [HFrEF] or heart failure with preserved ejection fraction [HFpEF]) in a timely manner (according to American Society of Clinical Oncology) high/low cardiotoxicity risk determination see Chapter 7). The anticipation of an increased cardiovascular (CV) risk should be based on the individual's exposure to potentially cardiotoxic cancer therapy (including chest radiation) and the additional presence of CV risk factors that may have been present prior to or developed during or after cancer treatment. Efforts should be directed at identifying the etiology, mechanism, and severity of a patient's symptoms, recognizing that heart failure (HF) is a heterogeneous and complex syndrome. Early detection of left ventricular (LV) dysfunction utilizing a combination of imaging (e.g., echocardiography, cardiac magnetic resonance imaging, and computed tomography) as well as the timely use of cardiac biomarkers (e.g., N-terminal pro-brain natriuretic peptide [NT-proBNP], troponin I) allows the prompt initiation of cardioprotective therapy, which translates into significant recovery of cardiac function or prevention of HF.[1]

Once cardiac dysfunction is detected, the next step is classifying the patient as having either HFrEF (LV ejection fraction [EF] ≤40%), HFpEF (LVEF ≥50%) or borderline HFpEF (LVEF 41% to 49%), recognizing that some patients may be asymptomatic and the only evidence of LV dysfunction is an abnormal cardiac function test or elevated natriuretic peptide level.[2] Symptomatic patients with HF should be treated according to the American College of Cardiology and American Heart Association guidelines (Figs. 27.1 and 27.2).[4] Several surveillance

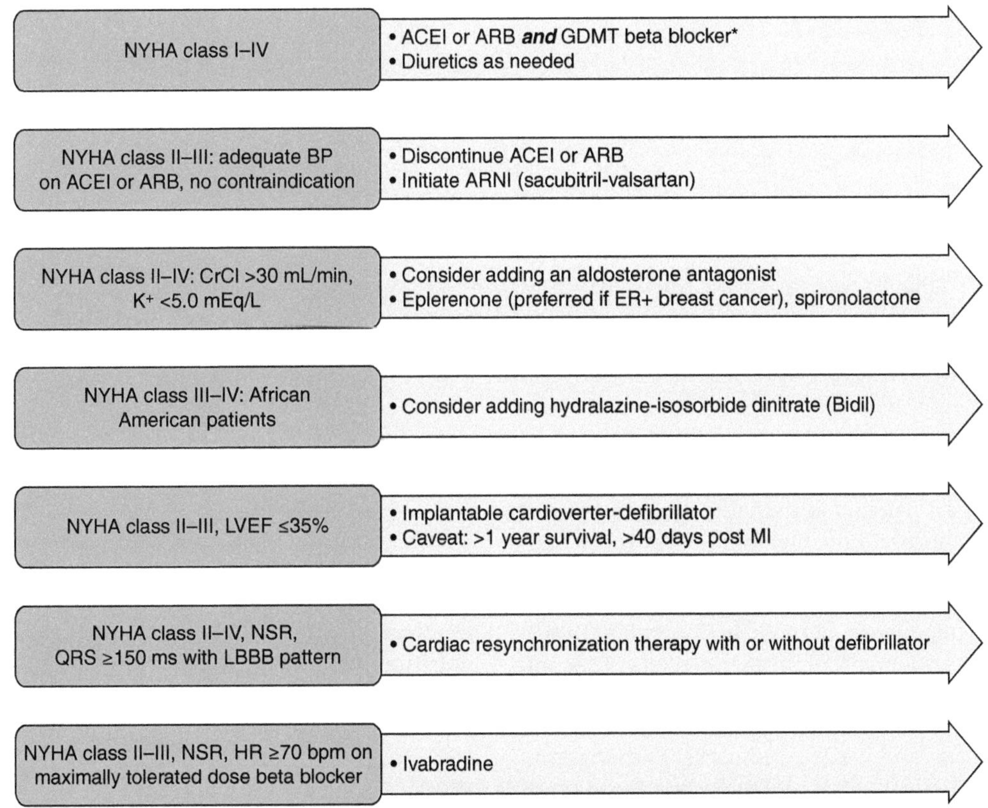

FIG. 27.1 Treatment of HFrEF (ACC/AHA stage B/C) in patients with current or prior HF symptoms.[3,4] *ACC*, American College of Cardiology; *AHA*, American Heart Association; *ER+*, estrogen receptor positive; *HF*, heart failure; *HFrEF*, heart failure with reduced ejection fraction.

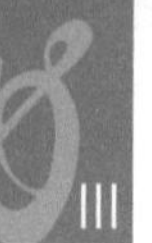

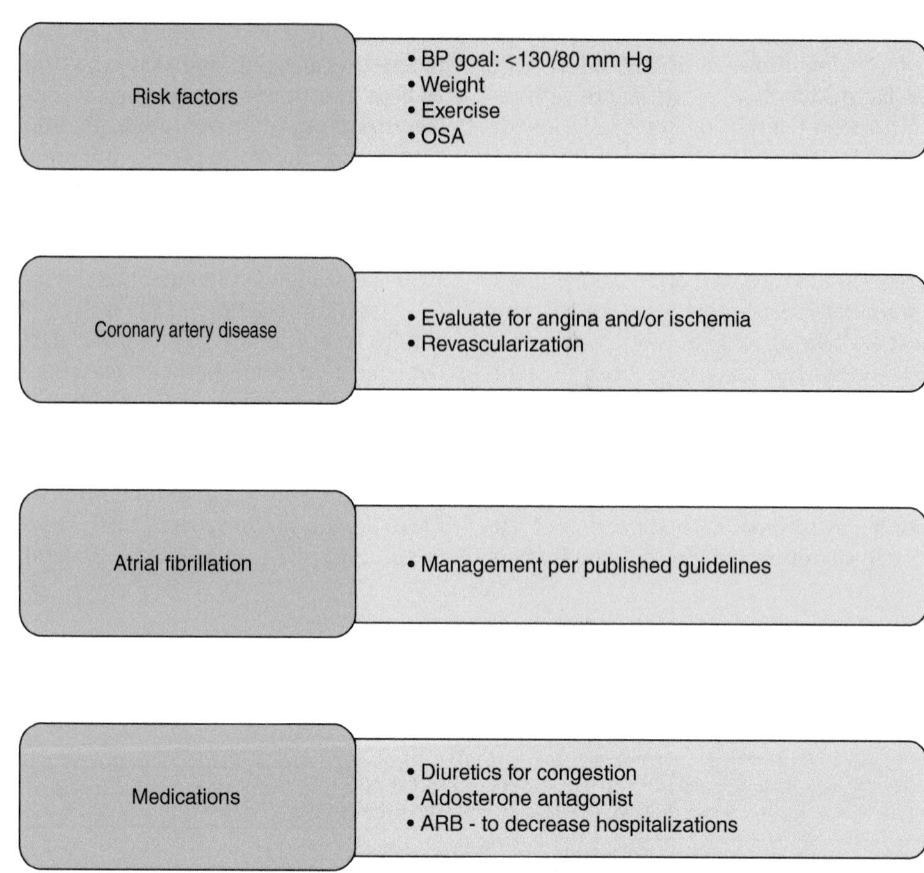

FIG. 27.2 Treatment of HFpEF Stage C.[4] *HFpEF,* Heart failure with preserved ejection fraction.

recommendations for childhood cancer survivors were released over time and harmonized by an international expert panel in 2015 (Table 27.1).[5–7] The full set of recommendations, including postcancer care for adult cancer survivors by the American Society of Clinical Oncology and the European Society of Medical Oncology were outlined in Chapter 7 (Tables 7.2 and 7.3). A summary of these three sets of recommendations for cardiac surveillance in cancer survivors is provided in Table 27.2. These emphasize the role of imaging and cardiac biomarkers when monitoring such patients. It is ultimately the decision of the treating physician to determine the frequency of and the exact tools to be utilized for proper surveillance in cancer survivorship based on any comorbid conditions of the patient and intensity of prior cancer treatments.

ADVANCED HF THERAPY IN CANCER SURVIVORS

Decisions about pursuing advanced HF therapies in cancer survivors is complex and should consider the type of malignancy, risk of recurrence, type of treatment received, current functional capacity, and nutritional status, among other factors. Early identification of patients progressing to stage D HF is based on different factors: need for intravenous inotropes, New York Heart Association class IIIB or IV symptoms, persistently elevated natriuretic peptide levels, evidence of end-organ dysfunction, left ventricular ejection fraction (LVEF) 35% or greater, recurrent defibrillator shocks, more than one HF hospitalization in the past year, edema despite escalating doses of diuretics, hypotension, tachycardia, and

TABLE 27.1 **2015 International Late Effects of Childhood Cancer Guideline Harmonization Group Recommendations for Cardiomyopathy Surveillance for Survivors of Childhood Cancer**[15]

General Recommendations

- Survivors treated with anthracyclines or chest radiation or both and their health care providers should be aware of the risk of cardiomyopathy.

Who Needs Cardiomyopathy Surveillance?

Anthracycline Exposure

- Cardiomyopathy surveillance is recommended for survivors treated with high dose (≥250 mg/m^2) anthracyclines.
- Cardiomyopathy surveillance is reasonable for survivors treated with moderate dose (≥100 to <250 mg/m^2) anthracyclines.
- Cardiomyopathy surveillance may be reasonable for survivors treated with low dose (<100 mg/m^2) anthracyclines.

Radiation Exposure

- Cardiomyopathy surveillance is recommended for survivors treated with high dose (≥35 Gy) chest radiation.
- Cardiomyopathy surveillance may be reasonable for survivors treated with moderate dose (≥15 to <35 Gy) chest radiation.
- No recommendation can be formulated for cardiomyopathy surveillance for survivors treated with low dose (<15 Gy) chest radiation with conventional fractionation.

Anthracycline and Radiation Exposure

- Cardiomyopathy surveillance is recommended for survivors treated with moderate to high dose anthracyclines (≥100 mg/m^2) and moderate to high dose chest radiation (≥15 Gy).

What Surveillance Modality Should be Used?

- Echocardiography is recommended as the primary cardiomyopathy surveillance modality for assessment of left ventricular systolic function in survivors treated with anthracyclines or chest radiation.
- Radionuclide angiography or cardiac magnetic resonance imaging may be reasonable for cardiomyopathy surveillance in at-risk survivors for whom echocardiography is not technically feasible or optimal.
- Assessment of cardiac blood biomarkers (e.g., natriuretic peptides) in conjunction with imaging studies may be reasonable in instances where symptomatic cardiomyopathy is strongly suspected or in individuals who have borderline cardiac function during primary surveillance.
- Assessment of cardiac blood biomarkers is not recommended as the only strategy for cardiomyopathy surveillance in at-risk survivors.

At What Frequency Should Surveillance be Performed for High- Risk Survivors?

- Cardiomyopathy surveillance is recommended for high-risk survivors to begin no later than 2 years after completion of cardiotoxic therapy, repeated at 5 years after diagnosis and continued every 5 years thereafter.
- More frequent cardiomyopathy surveillance is reasonable for high-risk survivors.
- Lifelong cardiomyopathy surveillance may be reasonable for high-risk survivors.

At What Frequency Should Surveillance be Performed for Moderate- or Low-Risk Survivors?

- Cardiomyopathy surveillance is reasonable for moderate- and low-risk survivors to begin no later than 2 years after completion of cardiotoxic therapy, repeated at 5 years after diagnosis and continue every 5 years thereafter.
- More frequent cardiomyopathy surveillance may be reasonable for moderate- and low-risk survivors.
- Lifelong cardiomyopathy surveillance may be reasonable for moderate- and low-risk survivors.

At What Frequency Should Surveillance be Performed for Survivors who are Pregnant or Planning to Become Pregnant?

- Cardiomyopathy surveillance is reasonable before pregnancy or in the first trimester for all female survivors treated with anthracyclines or chest radiation.
- No recommendations can be formulated for the frequency of ongoing surveillance in pregnant survivors who have normal left ventricular systolic function immediately before or during the first trimester of pregnancy.

What Should be Done when Abnormalities are Identified?

- Cardiology consultation is recommended for survivors with asymptomatic cardiomyopathy following treatment with anthracyclines or chest radiation.

What Advice Should be Given Regarding Physical Activity and Other Modifiable Cardiovascular Risk Factors?

- Regular exercise, as recommended by the American Heart Association and European Society of Cardiology (ESC), offers potential benefits to survivors treated with anthracyclines or chest radiation.
- Regular exercise is recommended for survivors treated with anthracyclines or chest radiation who have normal left ventricular systolic function.
- Cardiology consultation is recommended for survivors with asymptomatic cardiomyopathy to define limits and precautions for exercise.

Continued

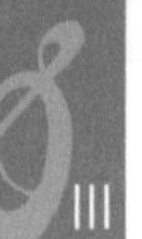

TABLE 27.1 2015 International Late Effects of Childhood Cancer Guideline Harmonization Group Recommendations for Cardiomyopathy Surveillance for Survivors of Childhood Cancer[15]—cont'd

- Cardiology consultation may be reasonable for high-risk survivors who plan to participate in high-intensity exercise to define limits and precautions for physical activity.
- Screening for modifiable cardiovascular risk factors (hypertension, diabetes, dyslipidemia, and obesity) is recommended for all survivors treated with anthracyclines or chest radiation so that necessary interventions can be initiated to help avert the risk of symptomatic cardiomyopathy.

Recommendation Grading

- Strong recommendation, with a low degree of uncertainty (high-quality evidence)
- Moderate level recommendation (moderate quality evidence)
- Moderate level recommendation (weak quality evidence)
- Recommendation against a particular intervention, with harms outweighing benefits

TABLE 27.2 Summary of the Suggested Surveillance and Treatment Strategies in Adult Cancer Survivors[a]

History and Physical Examination

- At least annually and preferably by a cardiologist or health care provider with cardio-oncology expertise (in particular, careful attention to signs and symptoms of heart failure [HF])
- Address any preexisting or new cardiovascular risk factors
- Emphasize the importance of a heart-healthy lifestyle including diet and exercise

Individuals With Clinical Signs or Symptoms Concerning for Left Ventricular (LV) Dysfunction or HF

- 2D or 3D echocardiogram with strain imaging and contrast as needed
- Cardiac MRI (with gadolinium contrast) if echocardiogram is not available or technically limited
- Serum cardiac biomarkers: troponin I or T, brain natriuretic peptide (BNP), NT-proBNP
- Referral to a cardio-oncologist based on abnormal findings
- Asymptomatic LV dysfunction or HF due to cancer therapy: medical treatment with angiotensin-converting enzyme inhibitor or angiotensin receptor blocker) and/or beta blocker, and regular cardiovascular evaluation (e.g., annually, if asymptomatic) should be continued indefinitely, regardless of improvement in cardiac function or symptoms; any decision to withdraw guideline-based medical therapy should only be done after a period of stability, no active cardiac risk factors, and no further active cancer therapy

Asymptomatic Patients at Increased Risk for LV Dysfunction

- 2D or 3D echocardiogram with strain imaging and contrast between 6 and 12 months, 2 years, and possibly periodically thereafter after completion of cardiotoxic treatment (either high cumulative anthracycline dose (doxorubicin equivalent ≥250 mg/m^2 or low cumulative anthracycline dose or trastuzumab and at least 1, certainly if 2 or more additional risk factors including hypertension, dyslipidemia, diabetes mellitus, obesity, smoking, family history of cardiomyopathy, age >60–65 years, low-normal LVEF (50%–54%) or structural heart disease, e.g., moderate or severe valvular heart disease at baseline, history of other cardiovascular comorbidities (i.e., atrial fibrillation or coronary artery disease)
- Cardiac MRI (with gadolinium contrast) if echocardiogram is not available or technically limited
- Consider periodic assessment of serum cardiac biomarkers (troponin I or T, NT-proBNP or BNP) at the time of cardiac function assessments
- Consider the combination of an imaging diagnostic test and serum cardiac biomarkers (troponin I or T, NT-proBNP or BNP) if risk of cardiac dysfunction or HF is considered high
- For patients with a history of mediastinal or chest radiation, evaluation for coronary artery disease and myocardial ischemia as well as valvular heart disease is recommended, even if asymptomatic, starting at 5 years posttreatment and then at least every 3–5 years thereafter
- Referral to a cardio-oncologist if asymptomatic LV dysfunction or abnormal biomarkers are detected
- Treatment for LV dysfunction or HF as above

[a]Based on the recommendations of ASCO, ESMO, and the National Comprehensive Cancer Network (NCCN; "https://www.nccn.org/guidelines/guidelines-detail?category=3&id=1466" https://www.nccn.org/guidelines/guidelines-detail?category=3&id=1466).

ASCO, American Society of Clinical Oncology; *ESMO*, European Society of Medical Oncology; *LVEF*, left ventricular ejection fraction; *MRI*, magnetic resonance imaging; *NT-proBNP*, N-terminal pro-brain natriuretic peptide.

progressive intolerance of optimal guideline-directed medical therapy.[3] These are all indicators that a patient should be evaluated for advanced HF therapies.

Durable mechanical circulatory support and heart transplantation are viable options for cancer survivors. Some of the challenges encountered in patients with chemotherapy-induced cardiomyopathies include the need for more right ventricular assist device support (19% vs. 11% vs. 6%; $P = .006$) compared with patients with nonischemic and ischemic cardiomyopathy (CM), and a higher risk of bleeding. Nonetheless, they still have a similar survival compared with patients without a history of chemotherapy.[8] In a retrospective study by Oliveira and colleagues patients who had had a heart transplant with history of chemotherapy-induced CM had a short- and long-term survival comparable to that of patients with a nonischemic CM. Survival at 1, 3, and 5 years was 86%, 79%, and 71%, respectively. Although these patients had a higher incidence of posttransplant infection and malignancies, survival was not affected.[9] Another retrospective analysis also showed a favorable 10-year postheart transplant survival in patients who had doxorubicin-related cardiomyopathy.[10] Cancer survivors with HF benefit from the same therapies as patients without cancer.

CARDIO-ONCOLOGY REHABILITATION

Cardiac rehabilitation provides a structured wellness program that focuses on prescriptive exercise, medical evaluation, nutritional counseling, cardiac risk factor modification, and behavioral interventions.[11] Meta-analyses have demonstrated that cardiac rehabilitation reduces hospital admissions while improving survival and health-related quality of life in patients with coronary artery disease.[12] The effects of cancer treatment extend beyond the heart and affect other systems, including the musculoskeletal system. It is recognized that patients with cancer experience a decline in cardiorespiratory fitness affecting their quality of life and overall survival.[13–15] For example, women with breast cancer have been shown to have significant impairment in cardiopulmonary function with an average peak oxygen consumption (VO_2 peak) 27% less than that of age-matched sedentary but otherwise healthy women without a history of breast cancer.[13] Engaging in vigorous exercise has been shown to improve mortality in adult survivors of childhood cancer, supporting its role in the care of cancer survivors.[16] A cardio-oncology rehabilitation algorithm was recently published by the American Heart Association and should serve as a platform for clinicians.[17]

REFERENCES

1. Cardinale D, Colombo A, Bacchiani G, et al. Early detection of anthracycline cardiotoxicity and improvement with heart failure therapy. *Circulation.* 2015;131:1981–1988.
2. Yancy CW, Jessup M, Bozkurt B, et al. 2013 ACCF/AHA guideline for the management of heart failure: executive summary: a report of the American College of Cardiology Foundation/American Heart Association Task Force on practice guidelines. *Circulation.* 2013;128:1810–1852.
3. Yancy CW, Januzzi Jr JL, Allen LA, et al. 2017 ACC expert consensus decision pathway for optimization of heart failure treatment: answers to 10 pivotal issues about heart failure with reduced ejection fraction: a report of the American College of Cardiology Task Force on expert consensus decision pathways. *J Am Coll Cardiol.* 2018;71:201–230.
4. Yancy CW, Jessup M, Bozkurt B, et al. 2017 ACC/AHA/HFSA focused update of the 2013 ACCF/AHA guideline for the management of heart failure: a report of the American College of Cardiology/American Heart Association Task Force on Clinical Practice Guidelines and the Heart Failure Society of America. *Circulation.* 2017;136:e137–e161.
5. Armenian SH, Hudson MM, Mulder RL, et al. Recommendations for cardiomyopathy surveillance for survivors of childhood cancer: a report from the International Late Effects of Childhood Cancer Guideline Harmonization Group. *Lancet Oncol.* 2015;16:e123–e136.
6. Armenian SH, Lacchetti C, Barac A, et al. Prevention and monitoring of cardiac dysfunction in survivors of adult cancers: American Society of Clinical Oncology clinical practice guideline. *J Clin Oncol.* 2017;35:893–911.
7. Curigliano C, Lenihan D, Fradley M, et al. Management of cardiac disease in patients with cancer throughout oncological treatment: ESMO consensus recommendations. *Ann Oncol.* 2020;31:171–190.
8. Oliveira GH, Dupont M, Naftel D, et al. Increased need for right ventricular support in patients with chemotherapy-induced cardiomyopathy undergoing mechanical circulatory support: outcomes from the INTERMACS Registry (Interagency Registry for Mechanically Assisted Circulatory Support). *J Am Coll Cardiol.* 2014;63:240–248.
9. Oliveira GH, Hardaway BW, Kucheryavaya AY, Stehlik J, Edwards LB, Taylor DO. Characteristics and survival of patients with chemotherapy-induced cardiomyopathy undergoing heart transplantation. *J Heart Lung Transplant.* 2012;31:805–810.
10. Lenneman AJ, Wang L, Wigger M, et al. Heart transplant survival outcomes for adriamycin-dilated cardiomyopathy. *Am J Cardiol.* 2013;111:609–912.
11. Franklin BA, Brinks J. Cardiac rehabilitation: underrecognized/underutilized. *Curr Treat Options Cardiovasc Med.* 2015;17:62.
12. Anderson L, Oldridge N, Thompson DR, et al. Exercise-cased cardiac rehabilitation for coronary heart disease: Cochrane systematic review and meta-analysis. *J Am Coll Cardiol.* 2016;67:1–12.
13. Jones LW, Courneya KS, Mackey JR, et al. Cardiopulmonary function and age-related decline across the breast cancer survivorship continuum. *J Clin Oncol.* 2012;30:2530–2537.
14. Peel AB, Barlow CE, Leonard D, DeFina LF, Jones LW, Lakoski SG. Cardiorespiratory fitness in survivors of cervical, endometrial, and ovarian cancers: The Cooper Center Longitudinal Study. *Gynecol Oncol.* 2015;138:394–397.
15. Peel AB, Thomas SM, Dittus K, Jones LW, Lakoski SG. Cardiorespiratory fitness in breast patients with cancer: a call for normative values. *J Am Heart Assoc.* 2014;3:e000432.
16. Scott JM, Li N, Liu Q, et al. Association of exercise with mortality in adult survivors of childhood cancer. *JAMA Oncol.* 2018;4:1352–1358.
17. Gilchrist SC, Barac A, Ades PA, et al. Cardio-oncology rehabilitation to manage cardiovascular outcomes in patients with cancer and survivors: a scientific statement from the American Heart Association. *Circulation.* 2019;139:e997–e1012.

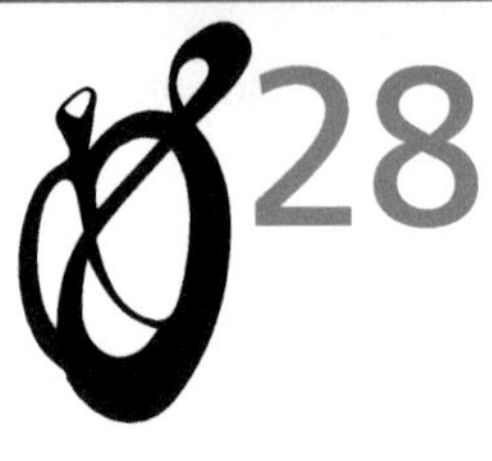

28 Structural Heart Disease Prevention and Management in Cancer Survivors

VUYISILE T. NKOMO, DIMITRI J. MAAMARI, AND JAE K. OH

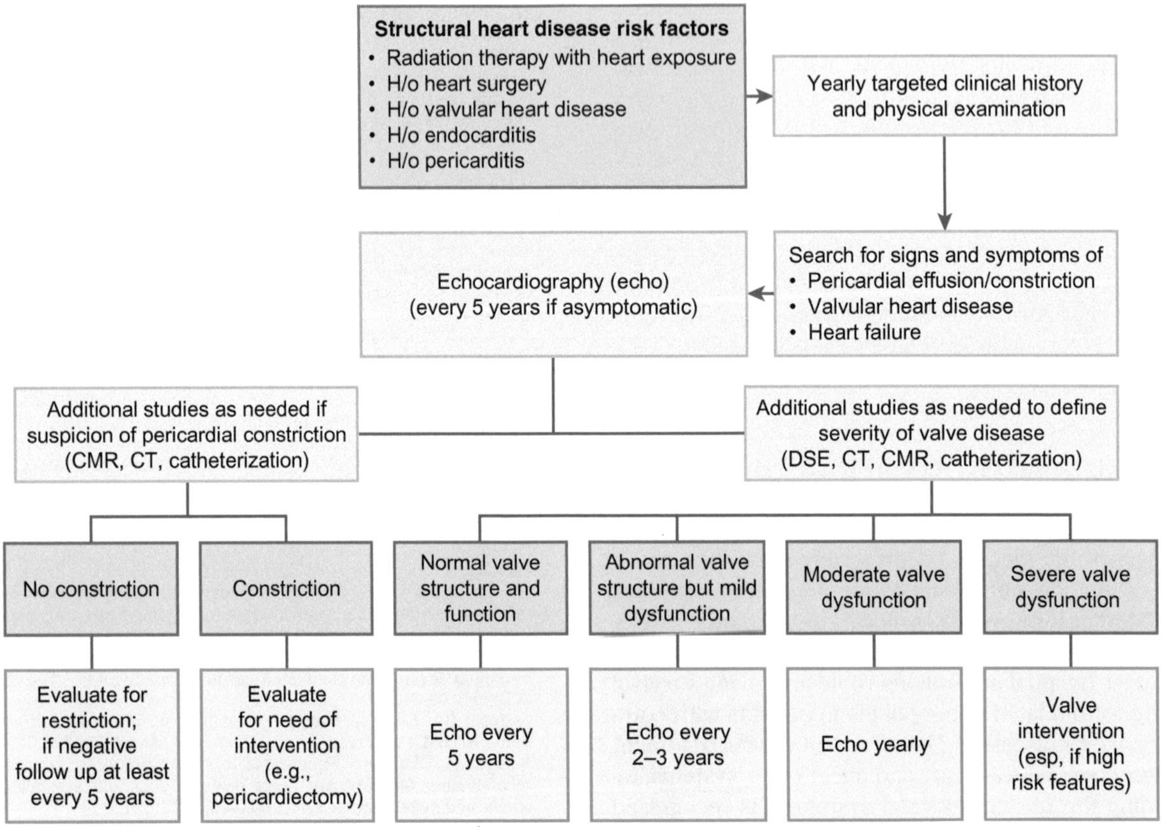

Structural heart disease risk factors
- Radiation therapy with heart exposure
- H/o heart surgery
- H/o valvular heart disease
- H/o endocarditis
- H/o pericarditis

→ Yearly targeted clinical history and physical examination

→ Search for signs and symptoms of
- Pericardial effusion/constriction
- Valvular heart disease
- Heart failure

→ Echocardiography (echo) (every 5 years if asymptomatic)

→ Additional studies as needed if suspicion of pericardial constriction (CMR, CT, catheterization)
- No constriction → Evaluate for restriction; if negative follow up at least every 5 years
- Constriction → Evaluate for need of intervention (e.g., pericardiectomy)

→ Additional studies as needed to define severity of valve disease (DSE, CT, CMR, catheterization)
- Normal valve structure and function → Echo every 5 years
- Abnormal valve structure but mild dysfunction → Echo every 2–3 years
- Moderate valve dysfunction → Echo yearly
- Severe valve dysfunction → Valve intervention (esp, if high risk features)

CHAPTER OUTLINE

KEY POINTS

- Structural heart disease in cancer survivors can appear early, but typically appears late (often >10 years) after cancer treatment, especially in its symptomatic form
- Chest radiation therapy increases the risk of structural heart disease in cancer survivors, including pericardial and valvular heart disease
- Prognosis and management depend on the severity of structural heart disease, stage of malignancy, and burden of comorbidity
- The benefits of intervention (e.g., aortic valve replacement in case of severe aortic stenosis) extends to patients with cancer
- Commonly used calculators such as the Society of Thoracic Surgeons Predicted Risk of Mortality (PROM) score may underestimate the surgery-related risk in patients with cancer, especially after radiation therapy
- A heart team evaluation is paramount in the treatment of cancer survivors with structural heart disease and decision making should be shared with the patient

PERICARDIAL DISEASE

The spectrum of pericardial disease in patients with cancer is covered in Chapter 16.

Most of the presentations occur around the time of cancer diagnosis or treatment. However, patients who experienced an episode of acute pericarditis during the initial cancer treatment are at risk of developing chronic recurrent/relapsing pericarditis.[1] One important aspect, especially in cancer survivors, is to define and treat the underlying cause beyond cancer and cancer therapies, including infections, uremia, or collagen vascular disease. Radiation therapy involving the heart is an important etiology and, in fact, pericarditis is not uncommon in these patients, as illustrated in childhood cancer survivors (Fig. 28.1).[2] Although outcomes for pericardiectomy have improved, patients with radiation-induced constrictive pericarditis continue to do most poorly.[3] Proper recognition and management is therefore important.

Constrictive pericarditis usually can be diagnosed by echocardiography and/or cardiac catheterization (Fig. 28.2).[4] An important differentiation is restrictive cardiomyopathy and it is important to define to the best of one's ability whether pericardiectomy will improve signs and symptoms, especially in view of a surgical mortality risk in the order of 6% to 12%. Patients with only a mild to moderate increase in central venous pressure and little or no edema can be followed clinically. Volume management is a key element in all patients with constriction, avoiding both hyper- as well as hypovolemia. On the other hand, patients with advanced stages of constrictive pericarditis, especially low cardiac output syndrome and cachexia, may no longer be candidates for surgery because the surgical risk is extremely high and the benefit, if any, is small.

VALVE DISEASE

Similar to pericardial disease, valvular heart disease is an important long-term consequence in patients who have undergone radiation therapy to the chest (see also Chapter 26). In fact, it is one of the most frequent cardiovascular diseases in survivors of Hodgkin lymphoma (Fig. 28.3).[5] Some studies suggest that not only radiation exposure, but also anthracycline exposure increases the risk of valvular heart disease in these and in other patients.[6,7]

Classic radiation-induced heart disease includes fibrosis and calcification of the aortic and mitral valves and surrounding structures, with sparing of the mitral leaflet tips and commissures. The reported incidence of clinically significant valve disease following radiation exposure is 1% at 10 years; 5% at 15 years; and 6% at 20 years.[7] The incidence increases significantly after more than 20 years following irradiation; mild aortic regurgitation (AR) up to 45%, moderate AR up to 10%, aortic stenosis up to 16%, and mild mitral regurgitation up to 48%.[8]

Risk factors for development of valve disease after cancer treatment include younger age at time of initial cancer, cardiovascular risk factors, high-dose radiation, anterior or left chest radiation without shielding, and adjuvant chemotherapy.[8] The dominant lesions in radiation-induced valvular heart disease are calcific stenosis of the aortic and mitral valves that is usually associated with some degree of valvular regurgitation. Tricuspid valve regurgitation is a less-common complication, but it can occur as a direct result of radiation-related damage or from right ventricular pacemaker-lead impingement often placed for radiation-related brady-arrhythmias.

Guidelines recommend aortic valve replacement when the degree of aortic valve stenosis is severe

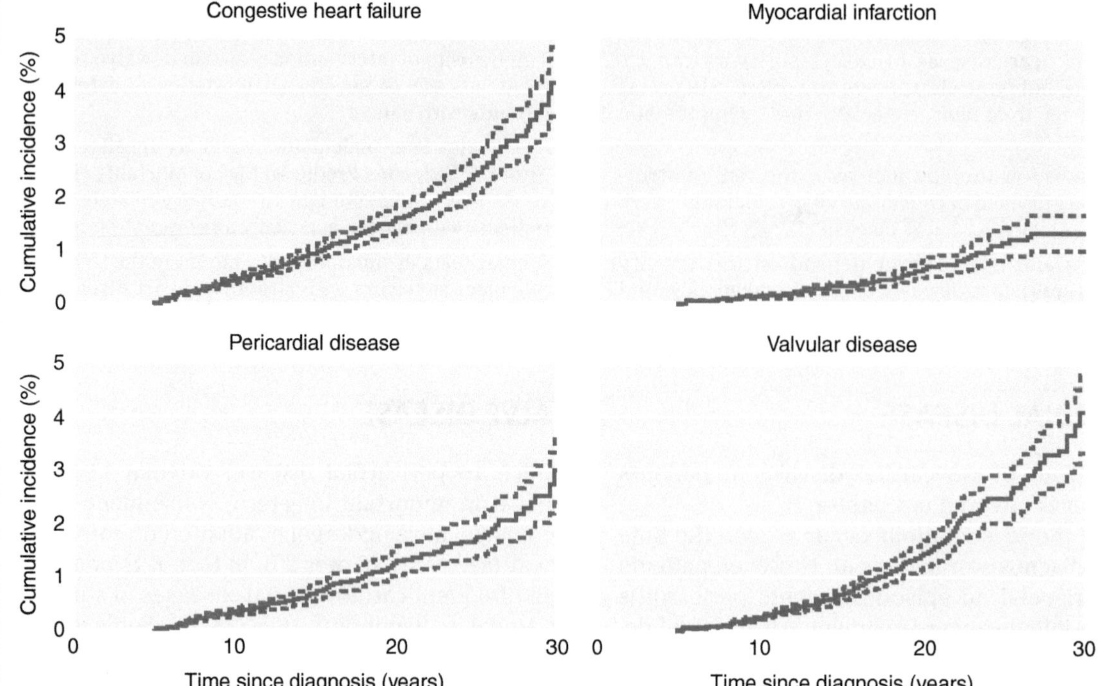

FIG. 28.1 Cumulative incidence and 95% confidence interval of cardiac disorders as displayed among childhood cancer survivors. (From Mulrooney DA, Yeazel MW, Kawashima T, et al. Cardiac outcomes in a cohort of adult survivors of childhood and adolescent cancer: retrospective analysis of the Childhood Cancer Survivor Study cohort. *BMJ.* 2009;339:b4606.)

and the patient is symptomatic or has reduced left ventricular systolic dysfunction with left ventricular ejection fraction less than 50%. Transcatheter aortic valve replacement is emerging as a dominant form of aortic valve replacement, but some patients still require surgical aortic valve replacement when there are technical limitations to transcatheter aortic valve replacement, such as inappropriately small or large aortic valve annulus size, presence of concomitant severe coronary artery disease not amenable to percutaneous intervention, or an indication for surgery beyond aortic valve replacement. Also, heavy calcification of the left ventricular outflow tract is a risk for perivalvular regurgitation after transcatheter aortic valve replacement.[9–11] Transcatheter aortic valve replacement is a particularly appealing alternative in patients with previous radiation to the chest because of often associated radiation-induced calcification of the thoracic aorta.

Mitral annulus and leaflet calcification, with sparing of the leaflet tips, is a classic feature of radiation-induced mitral valve stenosis. Leaflet calcification associated with reduction in mitral valve opening area of 1.5 cm^2 or less is considered severe mitral stenosis.[12,13] Severe mitral annulus calcification may or may not be associated with severe mitral inflow obstruction, and multimodality imaging is recommended for detailed evaluation of the extent and distribution of mitral annulus calcification, as well as hemodynamic severity of mitral inflow obstruction. Invasive hemodynamic cardiac catheterization is recommended in symptomatic patients when the predominant lesion is mitral annulus calcification because symptoms may be related more to concomitant diastolic dysfunction or left atrial stiffness, where mitral valve replacement will be of no benefit and may be harmful.[13] Severe mitral annulus calcification complicates mitral valve surgery because the mitral valve is not repairable and there is high risk of suboptimal results or complications with mitral valve replacement. Percutaneous mitral valve replacement is an emerging form of treatment for severe mitral annulus calcification,[14] but symptoms must first be confirmed to be related to severe mitral annulus calcification obstruction before embarking on this

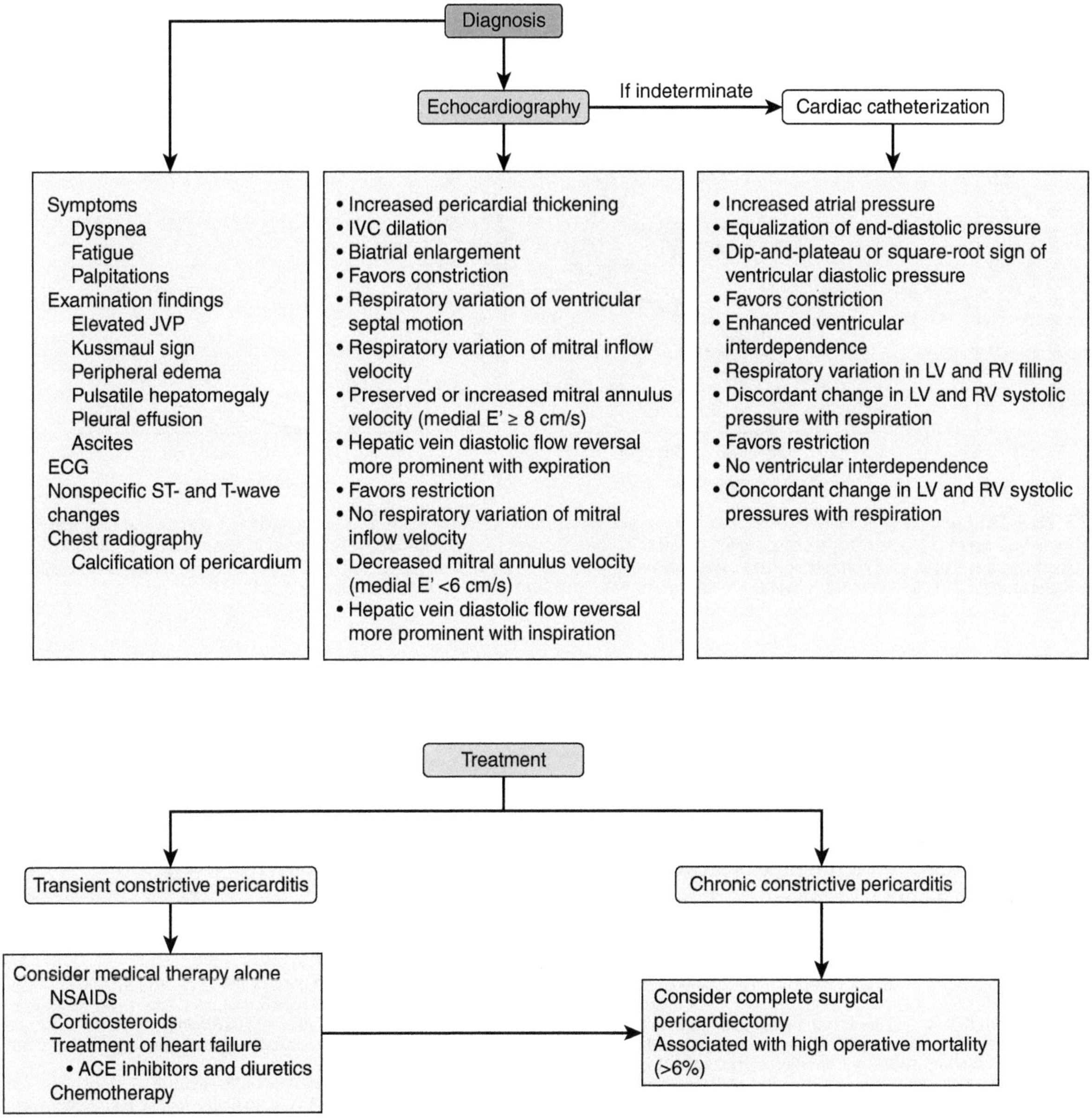

Diagnosis
Echocardiography
If indeterminate
Cardiac catheterization
Symptoms
Dyspnea
Fatigue
Palpitations
Examination findings
Elevated JVP
Kussmaul sign
Peripheral edema
Pulsatile hepatomegaly
Pleural effusion
Ascites
ECG
Nonspecific ST- and T-wave changes
Chest radiography
Calcification of pericardium
• Increased pericardial thickening
• IVC dilation
• Biatrial enlargement
• Favors constriction
• Respiratory variation of ventricular septal motion
• Respiratory variation of mitral inflow velocity
• Preserved or increased mitral annulus velocity (medial E' ≥ 8 cm/s)
• Hepatic vein diastolic flow reversal more prominent with expiration
• Favors restriction
• No respiratory variation of mitral inflow velocity
• Decreased mitral annulus velocity (medial E' <6 cm/s)
• Hepatic vein diastolic flow reversal more prominent with inspiration
• Increased atrial pressure
• Equalization of end-diastolic pressure
• Dip-and-plateau or square-root sign of ventricular diastolic pressure
• Favors constriction
• Enhanced ventricular interdependence
• Respiratory variation in LV and RV filling
• Discordant change in LV and RV systolic pressure with respiration
• Favors restriction
• No ventricular interdependence
• Concordant change in LV and RV systolic pressures with respiration
Treatment
Transient constrictive pericarditis
Chronic constrictive pericarditis
Consider medical therapy alone
NSAIDs
Corticosteroids
Treatment of heart failure
• ACE inhibitors and diuretics
Chemotherapy
Consider complete surgical pericardiectomy
Associated with high operative mortality (>6%)

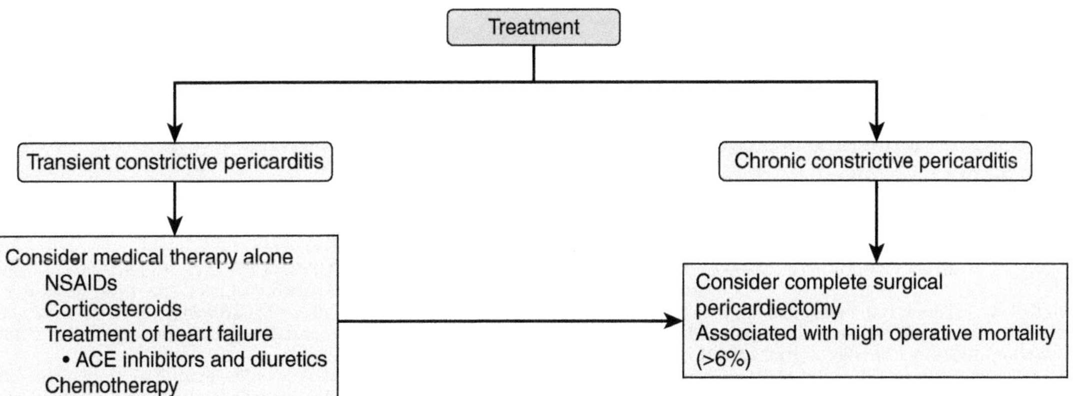

FIG. 28.2 Overview of the diagnosis and management of constrictive pericarditis. *ACE,* Angiotensin-converting enzyme; ECG, electrocardiography; IVC, inferior vena cava; JVP, jugular venous pressure; LV, left ventricle; NSAID, nonsteroidal anti-inflammatory drug; RV, right ventricle. (From Khandaker MH, Espinosa RE, Nishimura RA, et al. Pericardial disease: diagnosis and management. *Mayo Clin Proc.* 2010;85(6):572–593. doi:10.4065/mcp.2010.0046. PMID: 20511488; PMCID: PMC2878263.)

procedure; hemodynamic cardiac catheterization plays a key role in this regard.[6] Heart team evaluation is mandatory and preprocedural planning prior to percutaneous mitral valve replacement includes multimodality imaging to determine percutaneous valve size as well as risk of left ventricular outflow tract obstruction.[15] Three-dimensional prototyping is also useful in preprocedural planning.[16] An alternative to percutaneous implantation of mitral valve includes direct transatrial surgical implantation of a transcatheter heart valve which allows for surgical modification of the procedure,

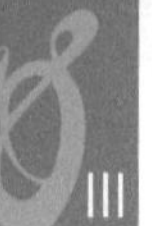

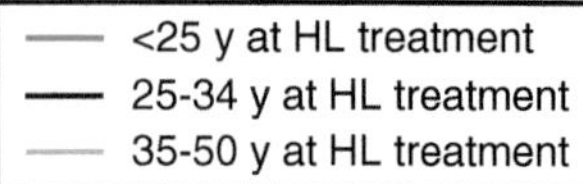

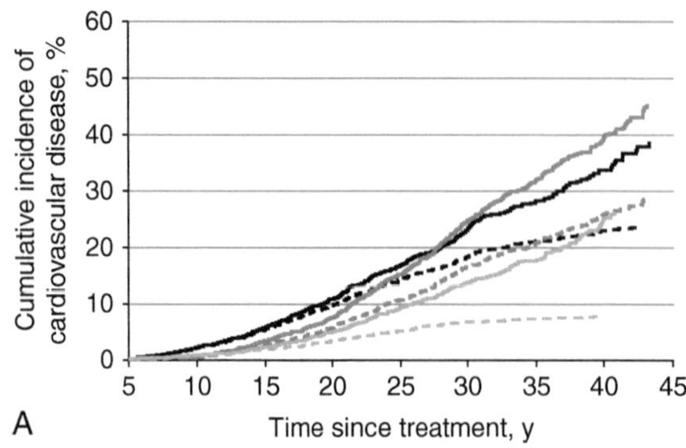

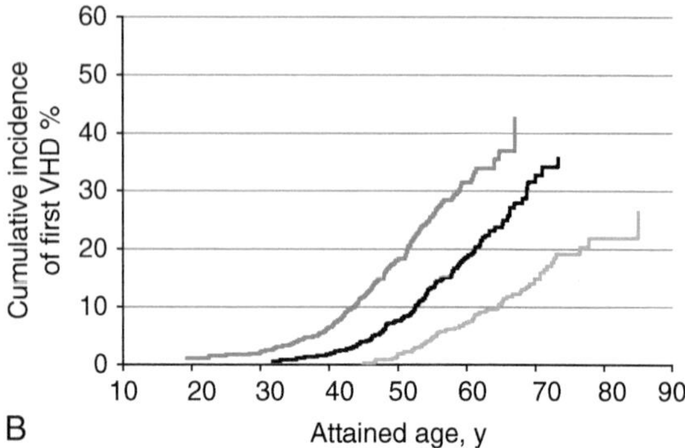

FIG. 28.3 (A) Cumulative incidences of all and first cardiovascular disease (with death from any cause as a competing risk). **(B)** Cumulative incidence of valvular heart disease (*VHD*) by attained age for different groups of age at Hodgkin lymphoma (*HL*) diagnosis (with death from any cause as a competing risk). (From van Nimwegen FA, Schaapveld M, Janus CPM, et al. Cardiovascular disease after Hodgkin lymphoma treatment: 40-year disease risk. *JAMA Intern Med.* 2015;175(6):1007–1017. doi:10.1001/jamainternmed.2015.1180.)

such as debulking of mitral annulus calcification or resection of the anterior mitral valve leaflet to prevent dynamic left ventricular outflow tract obstruction or pericardial patch closure of a perivalvular leak.[17,18]

Mitral valve bypass with a left atrial to left ventricular conduit is a potential alternative in properly selected patients.[19–22] At the time of valve surgery, a consideration should be given to a prophylactic pericardiectomy.

REFERENCES

1. Imazio M, Colopi M, De Ferrari GM. Pericardial diseases in patients with cancer: contemporary prevalence, management and outcomes. *Heart.* 2020;106(8):569–574. doi:10.1136/heartjnl-2019-315852.
2. Mulrooney DA, Yeazel MW, Kawashima T, et al. Cardiac outcomes in a cohort of adult survivors of childhood and adolescent cancer: retrospective analysis of the Childhood Cancer Survivor Study cohort. *BMJ.* 2009;339:b4606. doi:10.1136/bmj.b4606.
3. Murashita T, Schaff HV, Daly RC, et al. Experience with pericardiectomy for constrictive pericarditis over eight decades. *Ann Thorac Surg.* 2017;104(3):742–750. doi:10.1016/j.athoracsur.2017.05.063.
4. Khandaker MH, Espinosa RE, Nishimura RA, et al. Pericardial disease: diagnosis and management. *Mayo Clin Proc.* 2010;85(6):572–593. doi:10.4065/mcp.2010.0046.
5. van Nimwegen FA, Schaapveld M, Janus CP, et al. Cardiovascular disease after Hodgkin lymphoma treatment: 40-year disease risk. *JAMA Intern Med.* 2015;175(6):1007–1017. doi:10.1001/jamainternmed.2015.1180.
6. Murbraech K, Wethal T, Smeland KB, et al. Valvular dysfunction in lymphoma survivors treated with autologous stem cell transplantation: national cross-sectional study. *JACC Cardiovasc Imaging.* 2016;9(3):230–239. doi:10.1016/j.jcmg.2015.06.028.
7. Cohn KE, Stewart JR, Fajardo LF, et al. Heart disease following radiation. *Medicine (Baltimore).* 1967;46(3):281–298.
8. Lancellotti P, Nkomo VT, Badano LP, et al. Expert consensus for multi-modality imaging evaluation of cardiovascular complications of radiotherapy in adults: a report from the European Association of Cardiovascular Imaging and the American Society of Echocardiography. *J Am Soc Echocardiogr.* 2013;26(9):1013–1032.
9. Maeno Y, Abramowitz Y, Yoon SH, et al. Relation between left ventricular outflow tract calcium and mortality following transcatheter aortic valve implantation. *Am J Cardiol.* 2017;120(11):2017–2024.
10. Hansson NC, Leipsic J, Pugliese F, et al. Aortic valve and left ventricular outflow tract calcium volume and distribution in transcatheter aortic valve replacement: influence on the risk of significant paravalvular regurgitation. *J Cardiovasc Comput Tomogr.* 2018; 12(4):290–297.
11. Choi JW, Al'Aref SJ, Baskaran L, Leipsic JA. Left ventricular outflow tract calcium and TAVR—the tip of the iceberg? *J Cardiovasc Comput Tomogr*, 2020;14:42–43.
12. Nishimura RA, Otto CM, Bonow RO, et al. 2014 AHA/ACC guideline for the management of patients with valvular heart disease: a report of the American College of Cardiology/American Heart Association task force on practice guidelines. *J Am Coll Cardiol.* 2014;63(22):e57–e185.
13. Nishimura RA, Otto CM, Bonow RO, et al. 2017 AHA/ACC focused update of the 2014 AHA/ACC guideline for the management of patients with valvular heart disease: a report of the American College of Cardiology/American Heart Association task force on clinical practice guidelines. *J Am Coll Cardiol.* 2017;70(2):252–289.
14. Reddy YNV, Murgo JP, Nishimura RA. Complexity of defining severe "stenosis" from mitral annular calcification. *Circulation.* 2019; 140(7):523–525.
15. Guerrero M, Eleid M, Foley T, Said S, Rihal C. Transseptal transcatheter mitral valve replacement in severe mitral annular calcification (transseptal valve-in-MAC). *Ann Cardiothorac Surg.* 2018;7(6): 830–833.
16. Eleid MF, Foley TA, Said SM, Pislaru SV, Rihal CS. Severe mitral annular calcification: multimodality imaging for therapeutic strategies and interventions. *JACC Cardiovasc Imaging.* 2016;9(11):1318–1337.
17. El Sabbagh A, Eleid MF, Matsumoto JM, et al. Three-dimensional prototyping for procedural simulation of transcatheter mitral valve replacement in patients with mitral annular calcification. *Catheter Cardiovasc Interv.* 2018;92(7):E537–E549.

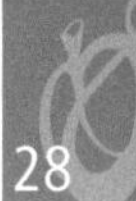

18. El Sabbagh A, Eleid MF, Foley TA, et al. Direct transatrial implantation of balloon-expandable valve for mitral stenosis with severe annular calcifications: early experience and lessons learned. *Eur J Cardiothorac Surg*. 2018;53(1):162–169.
19. Stone GW, Lindenfeld J, Abraham WT, et al. Transcatheter mitral-valve repair in patients with heart failure. *N Engl J Med*. 2018;379(24): 2307–2318.
20. Said SM. Mitral valve bypass: another extra-anatomic solution for another tiger territory? *J Thorac Cardiovasc Surg*. 2019;157(4):e147–e148.
21. Said SM, Schaff HV. An alternate approach to valve replacement in patients with mitral stenosis and severely calcified annulus. *J Thorac Cardiovasc Surg*. 2014;147(6):e76–e78.
22. López-Rodríguez FJ, Arnáiz-García ME, Barreiro-Pérez M, González-Santos JM. Left atrial to left ventricular valved conduit for a calcified mitral annulus and ascending aorta. *J Thorac Cardiovasc Surg*. 2019;157(4):e143–e145.

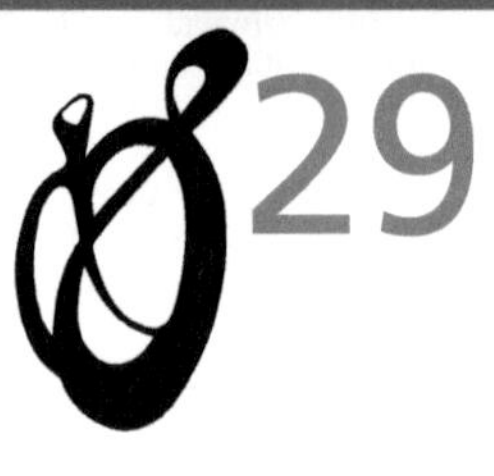

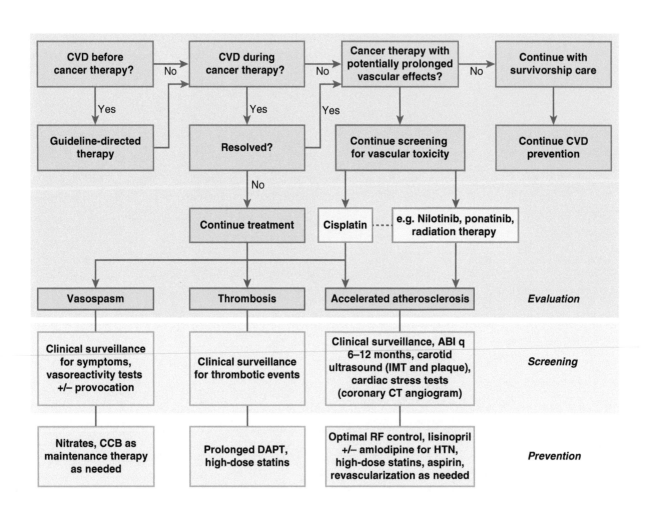

29 Vascular Disease Prevention and Management After Cancer Therapy

JOERG HERRMANN

CVD before cancer therapy?
No
Yes
Guideline-directed therapy
CVD during cancer therapy?
No
Yes
Resolved?
Yes
No
Continue treatment
Cancer therapy with potentially prolonged vascular effects?
No
Continue with survivorship care
Continue CVD prevention
Continue screening for vascular toxicity
Cisplatin
e.g. Nilotinib, ponatinib, radiation therapy

Evaluation
Vasospasm
Thrombosis
Accelerated atherosclerosis

Screening
Clinical surveillance for symptoms, vasoreactivity tests +/– provocation
Clinical surveillance for thrombotic events
Clinical surveillance, ABI q 6–12 months, carotid ultrasound (IMT and plaque), cardiac stress tests (coronary CT angiogram)

Prevention
Nitrates, CCB as maintenance therapy as needed
Prolonged DAPT, high-dose statins
Optimal RF control, lisinopril +/– amlodipine for HTN, high-dose statins, aspirin, revascularization as needed

CHAPTER OUTLINE

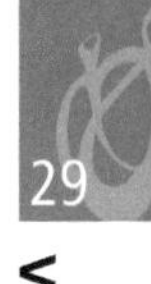

KEY POINTS

- Vascular disease after completion of cancer therapy can be due to (1) the continuum of preexisting vascular disease and/or (2) as a new development owing to cancer therapy exposure.
- The first category requires optimal, guideline-directed therapies in the overall context of the patient's care, conditions, and goals.
- The second category needs definition of the contributing role of the cancer therapy, thereby allowing for appropriate management.
- Cancer therapies, such as cisplatin, BCR-ABL inhibitors, and radiation, can have a direct long-lasting effect on the vasculature.
- Vascular changes can also be an indirect consequence of cancer and its therapy (e.g., via reduction in physical activity, weight increase, hypothyroidism, kidney disease).
- Promoting vascular health and preventing vascular disease is a key mandate.
- For patients requiring treatment, this is to be disease- and guideline-directed.

Historically vascular disease after cancer therapy had not been a topic of relevance given the generally very poor survival prognosis of many malignancies. This has changed over the past two decades. An illustrating example is chronic myeloid leukemia (CML), the prognosis of which has changed completely.[1] The advent of inhibitors that target the molecular arrangement underlying this disease has provided a "cure."[2] Indeed, as long as patients are responding to therapy they enjoy a life expectancy similar to their peers and, in fact, they are more likely to die of non-CML diseases, one of these being vascular disease.[3] In addition to this specific example, it has also been recognized that in general cardiovascular disease (CVD), including myocardial infarction and stroke, has a significant impact on the overall outcome of patients with cancer (**Fig. 29.1**).[4]

GENERAL CONSIDERATIONS

Vascular disease after completion of cancer therapy can be caused by (1) the continuum of vascular disease that was present even before the cancer treatment, and/or (2) the new development of vascular disease during or after completion of cancer therapy. This distinction helps with the direction of therapy. Whereas the first scenario requires follow up and treatment in keeping with published guidelines, the second scenario must take into account the uniqueness of the cancer therapy the patient has received. For instance, vascular toxicity risk with cancer therapeutics such as 5-FU is expected to be limited to the time of exposure.[9] On the contrary, cisplatin and BCR-ABL inhibitors, such as nilotinib and ponatinib, as well as radiation therapy can have long-lasting effects even beyond the active treatment period.[9,10] These nuances have implications for the association of vascular presentations with the cancer therapy and the duration of preventive efforts. For example, it would be unlikely that a patient develops chest pain one year after colon cancer treatment because of 5-FU exposure. Rather, it is more likely that the patient is experiencing progression of underlying coronary artery disease (CAD) that is now becoming clinically apparent. In this setting, contrary to the acute 5-FU therapy scenario, vasodilator therapy would not be the first line of management. As in the other two chapters of vascular diseases in patients with cancer, there is merit to focus on the three main modes of presentation as follow up, screening, prevention, and treatment differ. Cultivating an understanding of the most likely clinical course in any given patient and focusing on the underlying mechanism (i.e., a pathophysiology directed approach) is likely the most efficient and effective way. At the same time, there needs to be an openness of mind for differential diagnoses, the impact of additional factors, and the comorbidities of the patient that can contribute to the presentations.

FOLLOW-UP SCREENING

The three principal presentations of arterial vascular disease to pay particular attention to during follow up are the same as outlined in the related Chapters 8 and 17: vasospasm, thrombosis, and accelerated atherosclerosis.

Typical vasospasm is not common, but some patients with cancer can remain sensitive for Raynaud's for a long time and others can experience chest pain owing to altered vasoreactivity, for many years. Beyond the larger-sized arteries alterations of the

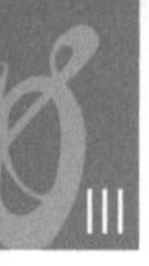

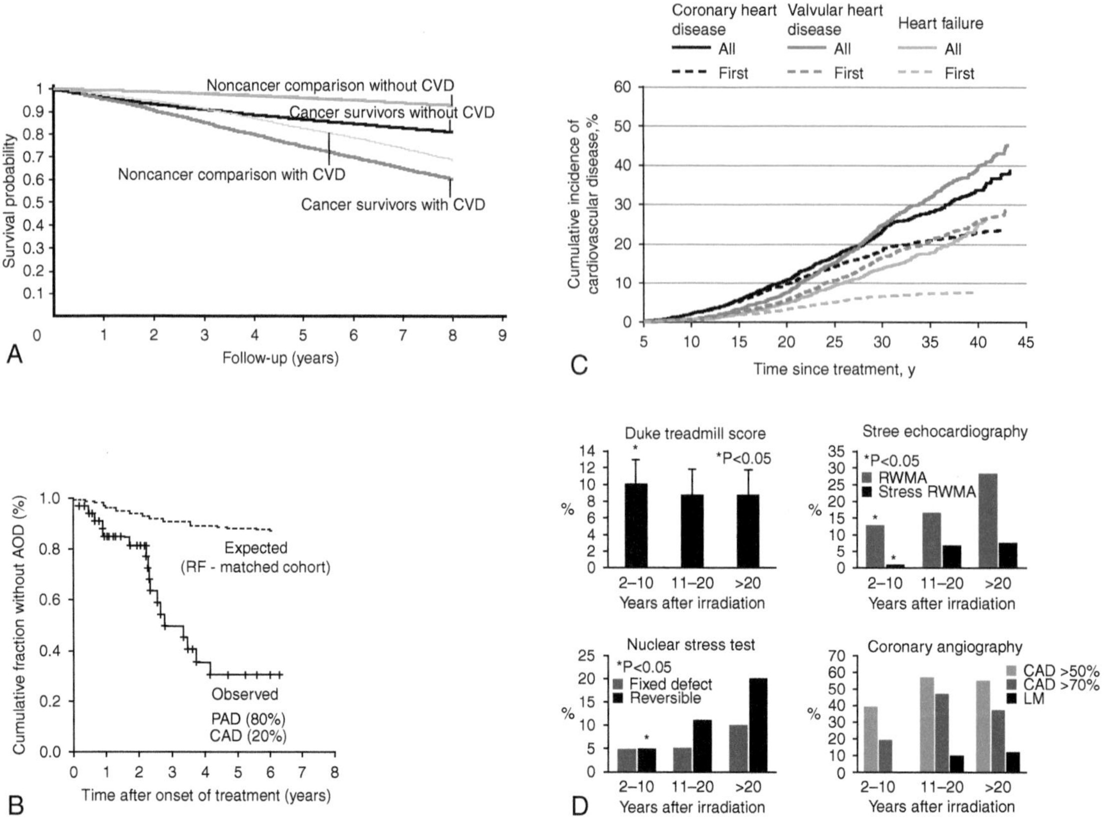

FIG. 29.1 A. Survival of patients without cancer and cancer survivors with and without concomitant cardiovascular disease (CVD).[4] **B.** Cumulative incidence of arterial occlusive disease in patients with chronic myeloid leukemia on nilotinib (observed) versus risk factor-matched controls. Peripheral arterial disease is four times more commonly seen than coronary artery disease.[5] **C.** Cumulative incidence of CVD after chest radiation in patients with Hodgkin lymphoma.[6] **D.** Burden of coronary artery disease in patients with Hodgkin lymphoma after mediastinal radiation.[7]

microcirculation can play an important role. Proactive screening is usually not done as the incidence rates are not very high and there is no longer the critical aspect of continuation and completion of cancer therapy. Enabling oncologic and hematologic therapy, minimizing therapy interruptions and therapy cessations is an important goal before and during cancer therapy. This is no longer relevant after therapy and the trigger for evaluations are signs and symptoms whose differential diagnoses include abnormal peripheral or central vasoreactivity. Raynaud's is usually very easy to define.[11,12] Coronary vasospasm should be suspected in patients presenting with chest pain, provoked by mental stress, cold exposure, and other factors, not necessarily with exercise and occurring at unusual times such as early morning hours.[13] ST segment elevation can be seen and it responds to vasodilator therapy as does the chest pain. In case of microvascular angina the chest pain is even more atypical, not only in terms of provoking factors but also in terms of duration (possibly for hours at a time) and associated symptoms (commonly dyspnea).[14]

The risk of *arterial thrombosis* as a consequence of cancer therapy usually does not persist.[15] Although not confined mechanistically to thrombosis alone, the risk of myocardial infarction and stroke in patients with cancer is highest in the first year and subsides gradually over the course of the second year after diagnosis.[15] This may be due to the reduction in tumor burden and the procoagulant state. Furthermore, the effects of most cancer therapies that could increase the thrombotic risk are wearing off, with the exception of cisplatin. Circulating levels of cisplatin can remain detectable for decades after completion of cancer therapy.[16] Radiation therapy is the other modality with a long-term effect on the vasculature, which at times can lead to thrombosis as a consequence of accelerated atherosclerosis.[17] As with abnormal vasoreactivity, proactive screening for thrombosis is usually not done. The evaluation is driven by signs and symptoms that include thrombosis as the underlying cause. The precise diagnosis is then made by vascular imaging, in most cases angiography. An intraluminal filling defect is the classic angiographic sign. This may not be present in case of spontaneous resolution or embolization of the thrombus. A careful assessment of the distal vasculature is very important in this setting and in general. Truncation of side branches and the distal segments is diagnostic as is slow flow, which is indicative of microcirculatory impairment.

Accelerated atherosclerosis is the leading entity in terms of vascular risk after completion of cancer therapy. The risk is particularly high in patients who received BCR-ABL inhibitors or radiation therapy (see **Fig. 29.1**).[8] These patients may benefit from preemptive screening using ankle-brachial index (ABI), carotid ultrasound, and noninvasive coronary imaging and stress tests (**Fig. 29.2**). For patients who received radiation therapy, which testing modality to use depends on the location of radiation therapy. Consensus guidelines recommend a cardiac stress test every 5 years in patients with defined high-risk features (Chapter 26). As cardiovascular risk factors add to the risk, regular screening for these is recommended.[8]

TREATMENT

With improving survival outcomes more and more patients with cancer approach their peers without

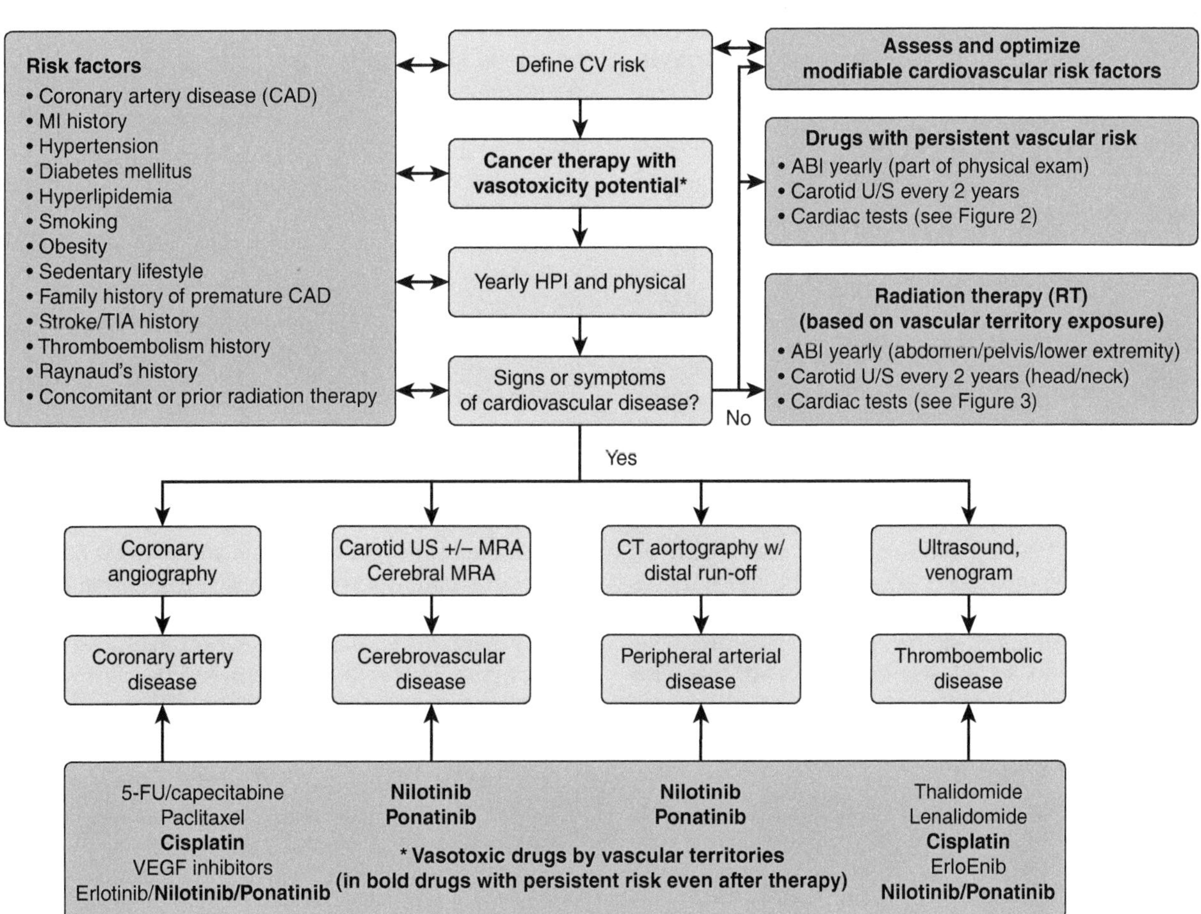

FIG. 29.2 Society of Cardiovascular Angiography and Intervention screening algorithm for vascular disease in at-risk patients with cancer.[8]

cancer in terms of management needs. The unique impact of cancer and its treatment is diminishing over time and management becomes more reactive than proactive. Accordingly, general societal treatment recommendations apply, but with some considerations (https://www.nature.com/articles/s41569-020-0347-2#Sec24).[18]

For patients with *vasospasm or altered vasoreactivity (paradoxic vasoconstriction)* vasodilators such as nitrates and calcium channel blockers (CCBs) are mainstay therapy. CCBs are more effective in cases of microcirculatory involvement (microvascular angina).[14] They are also usually first-line therapy for patients with Raynaud's, especially slow-release/long-acting dihydropyridine CCB, such as nifedipine XL.[19] Importantly, beta-blockers should be used very carefully with caution in these patients. If any need to be used, carvedilol as a combined alpha-/beta-blocker is the preferred choice. The treatment of microvascular angina and altered epicardial vasoreactivity can be challenging as well. Symptoms can be resistant and certain downstream consequences, such as arrhythmias, need to be resolved. Multiple drugs may need to be used sequentially or in combination to accomplish these goals. In these cases a thorough reevaluation is useful, including an assessment of all signs and symptoms with which the patient initially presented as well as vasoreactivity studies. For instance, patients with ventricular tachycardia episodes in the setting of documented epicardial vasospasm need to be reevaluated for the resolution of arrhythmias (and vasospasm) on therapy. Otherwise they require implantable cardioverter-defibrillator (ICD) placement, and one may opt to do so in any patient who has presented with a related cardiac arrest. Although theoretically a treatable course, the dynamics can become unpredictable and patients may lose response to therapy (i.e., recurrent chest pain on nitrate-CCB combination therapy). In these cases reevaluation is useful to determine if there is now a greater contribution of the microvasculature. This usually requires an invasive evaluation approach for differentiation.[14] Alteration of pain reception can be a contributing factor that should be addressed in a multidisciplinary approach (pain clinic, antidepressant use, spinal cord stimulator evaluation).[20]

In case of an *arterial thrombotic event* patients are to be treated per guidelines with options including anticoagulation, fibrinolysis, antiplatelet therapy, and revascularization.[21,22] It is important to define the underlying cause. Although the thrombotic risk declines after successful cancer treatment, thromboembolism remains of differential diagnostic concern. Deep venous thrombosis in the setting of a patent foramen ovale (PFO), marantic endocarditis, atrial fibrillation, or a left ventricular thrombus can lead to thromboembolic acute coronary, cerebrovascular, or peripheral vascular syndromes and require anticoagulation therapy. Documented plaque ruptures with subsequent *in situ* thrombosis are treated with antiplatelet and revascularization strategies. Thrombectomy is recommended mainly for certain patient populations with stroke and also for those with acute limb ischemia, although thrombolytic therapy remains the first strategy to consider in these patients.[23–25] On the contrary, thrombectomy is no longer universally recommended for coronary lesions in view of higher stroke rates and no decisive coronary/myocardial ischemic benefit.[26] Surgery is to be considered if the location and/or extent of disease are unfavorable for a percutaneous approach.[27] Erosions are not revascularized in the absence of significant plaque burden compromising luminal dimensions. However, dual antiplatelet therapy should be recommended. Based on current American College of Cardiology/American Heart Association (ACC/AHA) guidelines, dual antiplatelet therapy (DAPT) should be continued for one year in patients with acute coronary syndrome (ACS), thereafter guided by risk calculators.[28]

Patients, who present with *accelerated atherosclerosis (progressive arterial occlusive disease),* treatment is in keeping with societal guidelines. Optimal medical therapy is a key element, including the most optimal control of lipid levels, blood pressure, and glucose. High-intensity statin therapy is advisable and angiotensin-converting enzyme inhibitor and amlodipine for blood pressure control in these patients.[29] Metformin used to be and may very well still be the lowest cost, first-line antidiabetic drug of choice for patients with CVD, given improved outcome data.[30] However, two other classes of drugs have emerged (sodium-glucose cotransporter 2 inhibitor and glucagon-like peptide-1 receptor agonists) that were found to reduce CV events, but mainly cardiac rather than vascular events (i.e., not necessarily a reduction in myocardial infarction, stroke, and revascularization rates).[30] The importance of exercise cannot be over-emphasized. It is a key element in the management of peripheral arterial disease and may outperform stenting in patients with limited coronary artery disease.[31] Its beneficial effect extends to the entire arterial tree, as does optimal medial drug therapy, fostering stabilization of atherosclerotic plaques and the reduction of further growth of stenoses. Revascularization, however, may become necessary in those patients whose symptoms cannot be adequately controlled with medications and in those who show clear signs of detrimental consequences of non-revascularized (stable) lesions, such as cardiac function decline with exercise. In the setting of symptomatically uncontrolled or prognostically relevant myocardial ischemia, revascularization is to be entertained and the decision for a percutaneous or surgical approach should be in line with current guidelines.[27,32,33]

PREVENTION

In the cancer survivor population, the emphasis of prevention is on optimal CV risk factor control and optimal health metrics. These efforts would reduce the risk of all three outlined vascular disease presentations. Importantly, patients without cancer but with CVD have a worse prognosis than cancer survivors without CVD, and patients affected by both, cancer and CVD, do the worst.[4] Intriguingly, adherence to optimal diet, exercise, and body weight targets decreases the risk of both CVD and cancer.[34] Even more, there is a graded (dose) response between the number of AHA health metrics met and the incidence (risk) of CVD and cancer, especially colon, breast, and lung cancer.[35] Thus, preventive lifestyle efforts have multiple benefits in cancer survivors, decreasing not only their risk for CVD but also (recurrent) malignancies.[36]

Specific disease-oriented preventive efforts in cancer survivors with *vasospasm* are directed to the avoidance or at least reduction of symptomatic episodes and thus are part of the overall treatment plan. Identification and avoidance of triggers is an important element. Continuation of vasodilator and supplemental therapy (ranolazine, sildenafil, anti-alpha-agonist adrenergic, and pain modulation) even once symptom control is accomplished is important.[20] Medications should be titrated off only very slowly. The effect might be monitored with vasoreactivity studies, assuming they reliably indicate changes before the development of symptoms.

For patients with *thrombosis* preventive efforts are mainly secondary prevention efforts and are directed toward improving endothelial health and reducing the risk of thrombus formation. For the long-term (1 year past event) use of DAPT, the presumed antiischemic benefit must be weighed against the bleeding risk. Calculators for both are available, developed though in non-patients with cancer. The use of the DAPT score and the long-term dynamics of (stent) thrombotic risk after percutaneous coronary intervention were recently defined in patients with patients with cancer.[37–40] The use of these calculators may need to be validated in those with cancer and the long-term dynamics of thrombotic risk in these patients remain to be defined.

For patients with or at high risk of *accelerated atherosclerosis/progressive arterial occlusive disease* (e.g., secondary to treatment with radiation therapy, BCR-ABL inhibitors, and possibly cisplatin) optimal primary and secondary prevention efforts should be implemented. These include high-dose statins even in the absence of hyperlipidemia and angiotensin-converting enzyme inhibitors or amlodipine if hypertensive (with an ideal blood pressure goal of <130/80 mmHg, and a definite blood pressure goal of <140/90 mmHg for all). Patients should adhere to physical exercise recommendation and 150 minutes of moderate intensity exercise, such as brisk walking for 30 minutes 5 times a week, suffices. The body weight should be normal and the diet rich in fruits and vegetables. Smoking is absolutely prohibited. ABIs, carotid intima-media thickness (IMT), and stress tests may be used to follow serially the patients and to detect disease before signs and symptoms develop. The cost of these tests needs to be taken into consideration, but a reasonable schedule might be ABIs every 6 to 12 months, carotid IMT every 2 years, and cardiac stress test every 5 years.[8]

REFERENCES

1. Thompson PA, Kantarjian HM, Cortes JE. Diagnosis and treatment of chronic myeloid leukemia in 2015. *Mayo Clin Proc.* 2015;90(10):1440–1454.
2. Quintas-Cardama A, Kantarjian H, Cortes J. Imatinib and beyond—exploring the full potential of targeted therapy for CML. *Nat Rev Clin Oncol.* 2009;6(9):535–543.
3. Druker BJ, Guilhot F, O'Brien SG, et al. Five-year follow-up of patients receiving imatinib for chronic myeloid leukemia. *N Engl J Med.* 2006;355(23):2408–2417.
4. Armenian SH, Xu L, Ky B, et al. Cardiovascular disease among survivors of adult-onset cancer: a community-based retrospective cohort study. *J Clin Oncol.* 2016;34(10):1122–1130.
5. Hadzijusufovic E, Albrecht-Schgoer K, Huber K, et al. Nilotinib-induced vasculopathy: identification of vascular endothelial cells as a primary target site. *Leukemia.* 2017;31(11):2388–2397.
6. van Nimwegen FA, Schaapveld M, Janus CP, et al. Cardiovascular disease after Hodgkin lymphoma treatment: 40-year disease risk. *JAMA Intern Med.* 2015;175(6):1007–1017.
7. Heidenreich PA, Schnittger I, Strauss HW, et al. Screening for coronary artery disease after mediastinal irradiation for Hodgkin's disease. *J Clin Oncol.* 2007;25(1):43–49.

8. Iliescu CA, Grines CL, Herrmann J, et al. SCAI expert consensus statement: evaluation, management, and special considerations of cardio-oncology patients in the cardiac catheterization laboratory (endorsed by the Cardiological Society of India, and Sociedad Latino Americana de Cardiologıa Intervencionista). *Catheter Cardiovasc Interv.* 2016;87(5):E202–E223.
9. Herrmann J. Tyrosine kinase inhibitors and vascular toxicity: impetus for a classification system? *Curr Oncol Rep.* 2016;18(6):33.
10. Valent P, Hadzijusufovic E, Schernthaner GH, Wolf D, Rea D, le Coutre P. Vascular safety issues in CML patients treated with BCR/ABL1 kinase inhibitors. *Blood.* 2015;125(6):901–906.
11. Wigley FM. Clinical practice. Raynaud's phenomenon. *N Engl J Med.* 2002;347(13):1001–1008.
12. Wigley FM, Flavahan NA. Raynaud's phenomenon. *N Engl J Med.* 2016;375(6):556–565.
13. Lanza GA, Careri G, Crea F. Mechanisms of coronary artery spasm. *Circulation.* 2011;124(16):1774–1782.
14. Herrmann J, Kaski JC, Lerman A. Coronary microvascular dysfunction in the clinical setting: from mystery to reality. *Eur Heart J.* 2012;33(22):2771–2782b.
15. Navi BB, Reiner AS, Kamel H, et al. Risk of arterial thromboembolism in patients with cancer. *J Am Coll Cardiol.* 2017;70(8):926–938.
16. Gietema JA, Meinardi MT, Messerschmidt J, et al. Circulating plasma platinum more than 10 years after cisplatin treatment for testicular cancer. *Lancet.* 2000;355(9209):1075–1076.
17. Darby SC, Ewertz M, McGale P, et al. Risk of ischemic heart disease in women after radiotherapy for breast cancer. *N Engl J Med.* 2013;368(11):987–998.
18. Herrmann J. Vascular toxic effects of cancer therapies. *Nat Rev Cardiol.* 2020;17:503–522. doi:10.1038/s41569-020-0347-2.
19. Goundry B, Bell L, Langtree M, Moorthy A. Diagnosis and management of Raynaud's phenomenon. *BMJ.* 2012;344:e289.
20. Crea F, Camici PG, Bairey Merz CN. Coronary microvascular dysfunction: an update. *Eur Heart J.* 2014;35(17):1101–1111.
21. O'Gara PT, Kushner FG, Ascheim DD, et al. 2013 ACCF/AHA guideline for the management of ST-elevation myocardial infarction: a report of the American College of Cardiology Foundation/American Heart Association Task Force on Practice Guidelines. *J Am Coll Cardiol.* 2013;61(4):e78–e140.
22. Amsterdam EA, Wenger NK, Brindis RG, et al. 2014 AHA/ACC Guideline for the Management of Patients with Non-ST-Elevation Acute Coronary Syndromes: a report of the American College of Cardiology/American Heart Association Task Force on practice guidelines. *J Am Coll Cardiol.* 2014;64(24):e139–e228.
23. Powers WJ, Derdeyn CP, Biller J, et al. 2015 American Heart Association/American Stroke Association focused update of the 2013 guidelines for the early management of patients with acute ischemic stroke regarding endovascular treatment: a guideline for healthcare professionals from the American Heart Association/American Stroke Association. *Stroke.* 2015;46(10):3020–3035.
24. Powers WJ, Rabinstein AA, Ackerson T, et al. 2018 Guidelines for the early management of patients with acute ischemic stroke: a guideline for healthcare professionals from the American Heart Association/American Stroke Association. *Stroke.* 2018;49(3):e46–e110.
25. Gerhard-Herman MD, Gornik HL, Barrett C, et al. 2016 AHA/ACC guideline on the management of patients with lower extremity peripheral artery disease: a report of the American College of Cardiology/American Heart Association Task Force on Clinical Practice Guidelines. *J Am Coll Cardiol.* 2017;69(11):e71–e126.
26. Levine GN, Bates ER, Blankenship JC, et al. 2015 ACC/AHA/SCAI focused update on primary percutaneous coronary intervention for patients with st-elevation myocardial infarction: an update of the 2011 ACCF/AHA/SCAI guideline for percutaneous coronary intervention and the 2013 ACCF/AHA guideline for the management of st-elevation myocardial infarction: a report of the American College of Cardiology/American Heart Association Task Force on Clinical Practice Guidelines and the Society for Cardiovascular Angiography and Interventions. *Circulation.* 2016;133(11):1135–1147.
27. Neumann FJ, Sousa-Uva M, Ahlsson A, et al. 2018 ESC/EACTS Guidelines on myocardial revascularization. *EuroIntervention.* 2019;14(14):1435–1534.
28. Levine GN, Bates ER, Bittl JA, et al. 2016 ACC/AHA guideline focused update on duration of dual antiplatelet therapy in patients with coronary artery disease: a report of the American College of Cardiology/American Heart Association Task Force on Clinical Practice Guidelines: an update of the 2011 ACCF/AHA/SCAI guideline for percutaneous coronary intervention, 2011 ACCF/AHA Guideline for Coronary Artery Bypass Graft Surgery, 2012 ACC/AHA/ACP/AATS/PCNA/SCAI/STS guideline for the diagnosis and management of patients with stable ischemic heart disease, 2013 ACCF/AHA guideline for the management of st-elevation myocardial infarction, 2014 AHA/ACC guideline for the management of patients with non-st-elevation acute coronary syndromes, and 2014 ACC/AHA guideline on perioperative cardiovascular evaluation and management of patients undergoing noncardiac surgery. *Circulation.* 2016;134(10):e123–e155.
29. Touyz RM, Herrmann SMS, Herrmann J. Vascular toxicities with VEGF inhibitor therapies. Focus on hypertension and arterial thrombotic events. *J Am Soc Hypertens.* 2018;12(6):409–425.
30. Sattar N, Petrie MC, Zinman B, Januzzi Jr JL. Novel diabetes drugs and the cardiovascular specialist. *J Am Coll Cardiol.* 2017;69(21):2646–2656.
31. Hambrecht R, Walther C, Möbius-Winkler S, et al. Percutaneous coronary angioplasty compared with exercise training in patients with stable coronary artery disease: a randomized trial. *Circulation.* 2004;109(11):1371–1378.
32. Levine GN, Bates ER, Blankenship JC, et al. 2011 ACCF/AHA/SCAI guideline for percutaneous coronary intervention: a report of the American College of Cardiology Foundation/American Heart Association Task Force on Practice Guidelines and the Society for Cardiovascular Angiography and Interventions. *Catheter Cardiovasc Interv.* 2013;82(4):E266–E355.
33. Hillis LD, Smith PK, Anderson JL, et al. 2011 ACCF/AHA guideline for coronary artery bypass graft surgery: executive summary: a report of the American College of Cardiology Foundation/American Heart Association Task Force on Practice Guidelines. *Circulation.* 2011;124(23):2610–2642.
34. Ford ES, Bergmann MM, Kröger J, et al. Healthy living is the best revenge: findings from the European Prospective Investigation Into Cancer and Nutrition-Potsdam study. *Arch Intern Med.* 2009;169(15):1355–1362.
35. Rasmussen-Torvik LJ, Shay CM, Abramson JG, et al. Ideal cardiovascular health is inversely associated with incident cancer: the Atherosclerosis Risk In Communities study. *Circulation.* 2013;127(12):1270–1275.
36. Squires RW, Shultz AM, Herrmann J. Exercise training and cardiovascular health in patients with cancer. *Curr Oncol Rep.* 2018;20(3):27.
37. Yeh RW, Secemsky EA, Kereiakes DJ, et al. Development and validation of a prediction rule for benefit and harm of dual antiplatelet therapy beyond 1 year after percutaneous coronary intervention. *JAMA.* 2016;315(16):1735–1749.
38. Costa F, van Klaveren D, James S, et al. Derivation and validation of the predicting bleeding complications in patients undergoing stent implantation and subsequent dual antiplatelet therapy (PRECISE-DAPT) score: a pooled analysis of individual-patient datasets from clinical trials. *Lancet.* 2017;389(10073):1025–1034.
39. Tantry US, Navarese EP, Myat A, Gurbel PA. Selection of P2Y12 inhibitor in percutaneous coronary intervention and/or acute coronary syndrome. *Prog Cardiovasc Dis.* 2018;60(4–5):460–470.
40. Guo W, Fan X, Lewis BR, et al. Patients with cancer have a higher risk of thrombotic and ischemic events after percutaneous coronary intervention. *JACC Cardiovasc Interv.* 2021;14(10):1094–1105.

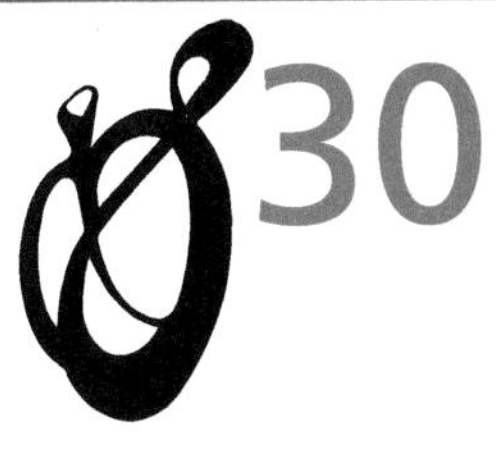

30 Prevention of VTE After Initial Presentation and Cancer Treatment

ROBERT D. MCBANE II

Patients with cancer with VTE

Risk of recurrent VTE
- 20% within the initial 6 months of AC, annual rate as high as 30%

Risk factors
- Cancer type (lung, pancreas, brain, ovarian, MDS, advanced type)
- Premature discontinuation of anticoagulation?

Management
- Increase in LMWH dose (by 20–25%) in patients treated with LMWH
- Switch from VKA to LMWH in patients treated with VKA; and
- Inferior vena cava filter insertion with continued anticoagulant therapy, unless contraindicated

Cancer survivor

Long-term risk of VTE
- In childhood patients with cancer:
- 4+/–0.5 % at 30 years, 2-fold higher than siblings

Risk factors

Female
Low or high BMI
Cisplatin exposure
Recurrent or secondary cancer

Management
- Lifelong DOACs

CHAPTER OUTLINE

KEY POINTS

- In patients with cancer with venous thromboembolism (VTE), the risk of VTE recurrence is increased six-fold with an annual rate as high as 30% in the absence of anticoagulation and as high as 20% even within the initial 6 months on anticoagulation therapy.
- The majority of VTEs occur within the first months of cancer diagnosis.
- Several additional risk score tools have been developed that expand the timeframe of prediction from 2.5 (Khorana score) to 6 months, but await external validation and assessment of suitability for long-term prediction in survivorship.
- The rate of VTE recurrence differs significantly by cancer type, stage of disease, and stage progression over time; specific risk factors include brain, lung, pancreatic, or ovarian cancer; myeloproliferative or myelodysplastic disorders; stage IV cancer; cancer stage progression; or leg paresis.
- If outlined risk factors are present, it is likely best to continue anticoagulation (premature discontinuation of anticoagulation should be avoided).
- The original and modified Ottawa prediction scores were developed to risk stratify for recurrent VTE; among the variables included in the score, female gender and lung cancer increase the risk, whereas breast cancer and stage I (/II) decrease the risk.
- The risk for VTE remains increased in cancer survivors, especially in childhood cancer survivors who face a 25-fold higher risk than their siblings without disease.

INTRODUCTION

Cancer accounts for up to 20% of venous thromboembolic events occurring in the community, increasing the risk of venous thromboembolism (VTE) by a factor of 4 (without chemotherapy) to 7 (with chemotherapy).[1–5] The likelihood of developing VTE is highest during the first 3 months after the cancer diagnosis and the majority of thrombotic events occur within the first year.[5] For patients with cancer-associated VTE, approximately half have metastatic disease at the time of VTE diagnosis.[5] With nearly 2 million Americans given a new cancer diagnosis each year and an estimated nearly 20 million cancer survivors in the United States alone, there is a large burden of potential cancer-related VTE to manage.[1]

This topic gains further significance based on the fact that thromboembolic events, including VTE, are a leading cause of death among cancer outpatients; patients with cancer with VTE have a 3-fold and 8-fold higher risk of death than patients with cancer but no VTE and patients with VTE but no cancer, respectively.[6–8] Those surviving face a high risk of VTE recurrence, as high as 30% annually in the absence of anticoagulation therapy and as high as 20% after 6 months on therapy. This chapter focuses on this risk of recurrent VTE in patients with active cancer and the risk of VTE in cancer survivors. Management of acute VTE is covered in **Chapter 18**.

PATIENT AND TUMOR-SPECIFIC RISK OF VTE

A number of variables have been implicated in the pathogenesis of thrombosis in patients with cancer and, most importantly, these pertain to the initial diagnosis (cancer type, site, and stage, i.e., biological aggressiveness) and treatment period: cancer-specific prothrombotic activity, cancer-directed systemic therapy and surgery (but not radiation therapy), hospitalization with associated immobility, and central venous catheters used for chemotherapy delivery.[5,9–12] The procoagulant potential, however, can persist beyond the acute period. For instance, childhood cancer survivors remain at increased risk for VTE for life[13]; in fact, VTE was the most common cardiovascular disease in German childhood cancer survivors.[14]

Tools capable of identifying individuals at highest risk are, in general, useful clinically to direct preventive strategies, such as the Khorana score (Chapter 9).[15] Several attempts have been made to improve upon the Khorana score by adding biomarker and genetic information (Table 30.1).[16–19] The Vienna Cancer and Thrombosis Study (CATS) Score system added two thrombosis biomarkers, fibrin D-dimer and soluble p-selectin, to the Khorana variables.[16] The advantage of this tool is added precision for the identification of patients with cancer at very high risk of thrombosis. Using this tool, the cumulative probability of VTE after 6 months was 35% for

TABLE 30.1 Risk Prediction Tools/Scores for VTE in Patients with Cancer

TOOL	VARIABLES	POINTS	C-STATISTIC	VTE RATES BY RISK	TIMEFRAME	EXTERNAL VALIDATION
Khorana[15]	**Cancer-specific risk** • Very high (gastric, pancreatic) • High (lung, lymphoma, gynecology, genitourinary) **Laboratory, prechemotherapy** • Platelet count (> 350,000,mm^2) • Leukocyte count (> 11,000/mm^2) • Hemoglobin (< 10 m/dL) or erythropoietin use **BMI** ≥ 35 kg/m^2 **Risk summary** High 3; Intermediate 1–2; Low 0	 2 1 1 1 1 1	0.7	**Low** (0) 0.3% to 0.8% **Intermediate** (1–2) 1.8% to 2.0% **High** (≥ 3) 6.7% to 7.1%	2.5 mos	Yes
Vienna CATS[16]	• Khorana score • Fibrin D-dimer (≥ 1.44 μg/mL) • Soluble p-selectin (≥ 53.1 ng/mL)	1—6 1 1	0.58	Scores 0 = 1.0% 1 = 4.4% 2 = 3.5% 3 = 10.3% 4 = 20.3% ≥ 5 = 35%	6 mos	No
PROTECHT[17]	• Khorana score (BMI excluded) • Platinum chemotherapy • Gemcitabine therapy	1—5 1 1	0.59	**Low** (≤ 2) 7.4% **High** (≥ 3) 34%	4 mos	No
CONKO[18]	• Khorana score (BMI excluded) • World Health Organization performance	1—5 1	0.53			No
COMPASS CAT[19]	• Anthracycline or hormonal Rx • Time since cancer diagnosis ≤ 6 mos • Central venous line • Advanced cancer stage • Cardiovascular risk factors (2 factors: PAD, stroke, CAD, hypertension, dyslipidemia, DM, obesity) • Recent hospitalization • Personal history of VTE • Platelet count (≥ 350,000/mm^2)	6 4 3 2 5 5 1 1	0.85	**Low/Intermediate** (≤ 6) 1.7% **High** (≥7) 13.3%	6 mos	No

VTE, venous thromboembolism; DVT, deep venous thrombosis; PE, pulmonary embolism; LMWH, low molecular weight heparin.

patients with the highest risk (scores ≥ 5) with a positive predictive value of 42.9%. For the patients at very low risk (score = 0), the 6-month cumulative VTE rate was 1.0% with a negative predictive value of 99.0%. This tool has not yet been externally validated. The PROTECHT score (PROphylaxis of Thrombo Embolism during CHemoTherapy) adds more granularity to chemotherapy agents employed.[16] Platinum-based chemotherapy or gemcitabine therapy each gain points using this tool. The body mass index (BMI) criteria was removed from scoring. The CONKO tool adds World Health Organization performance score metrics to the Khorana variables.[17] The COMPASS–CAT risk assessment tool variables include anthracycline or antihormonal therapy, time since cancer diagnosis, central venous catheter, cancer stage, cardiovascular risk factors, recent hospitalization, personal history of VTE, and platelet counts.[19] The rates of VTE at 6 months were 1.7% for patients at low to intermediate risk and 13.3% for those at high risk. Taken together, each risk assessment tool has advantages and limitations; ideally, these tools would identify those individuals at highest risk of developing VTE for whom DVT prophylaxis would be useful in the ambulatory setting as well as those at very low risk for whom anticoagulant prophylaxis would add more harm than benefit.

Translating these efforts to (long-term) cancer survivors and risk prediction of recurrent VTE have not been as advanced, but a cohort study from

Olmsted County, Minnesota and the Ottawa prediction scores of recurrent VTE provide some guidance (Figs. 30.1 and 30.2).[20,21] As shown in the Olmsted County study, the risk of recurrent VTE remains rather steady over the course of a decade (see Fig. 30.1). Overall recurrent VTE is seen not only among patients with cancer types at the top of the pyramid of thrombotic risk potential, namely brain

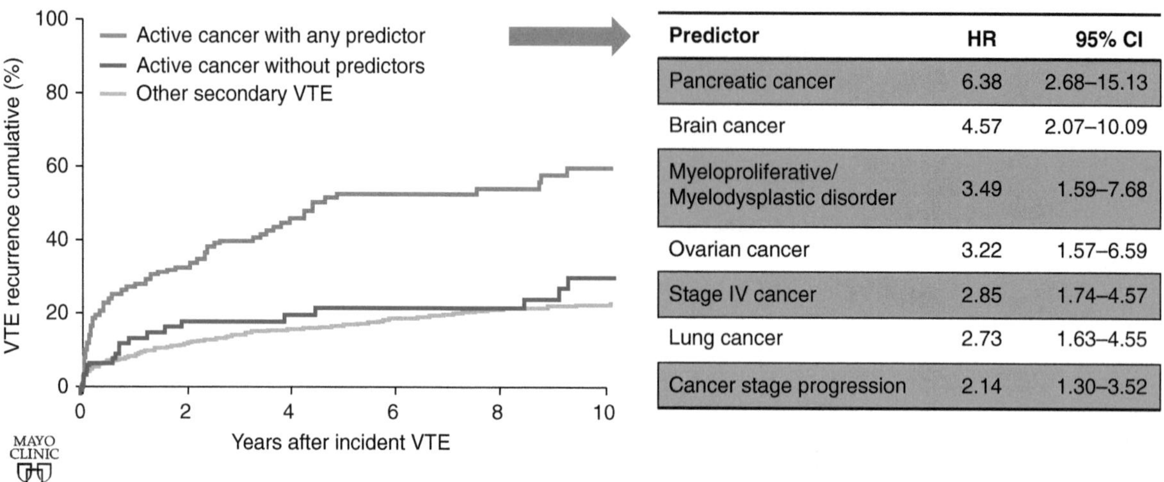

Predictor	HR	95% CI
Pancreatic cancer	6.38	2.68–15.13
Brain cancer	4.57	2.07–10.09
Myeloproliferative/ Myelodysplastic disorder	3.49	1.59–7.68
Ovarian cancer	3.22	1.57–6.59
Stage IV cancer	2.85	1.74–4.57
Lung cancer	2.73	1.63–4.55
Cancer stage progression	2.14	1.30–3.52

FIG. 30.1 Risk of VTE in patients with cancer after cancer and/or venous thromboembolism (VTE); cumulative event curve and risk factors for recurrent VTE are shown in a patient cohort from Olmsted Country.

Ottawa risk prediction score

Variable	Points
Female	1
Lung cancer	1
Breast cancer	-1
TNM* stage I	-2
Previous VTE	1
Recurrent VTE risk category	
Low (≤0)	-3 to 0
High (≥1)	1 to 3

Modififed ottawa risk prediction score

Variable	Points
Female	1
Lung cancer	1
Breast cancer	-1
Cancer stage I+II	-1
Previous VTE	1
Recurrent VTE risk category	
Low (≤–1)	-3 to 0
Intermediate	0
High (≥1)	1 to 3

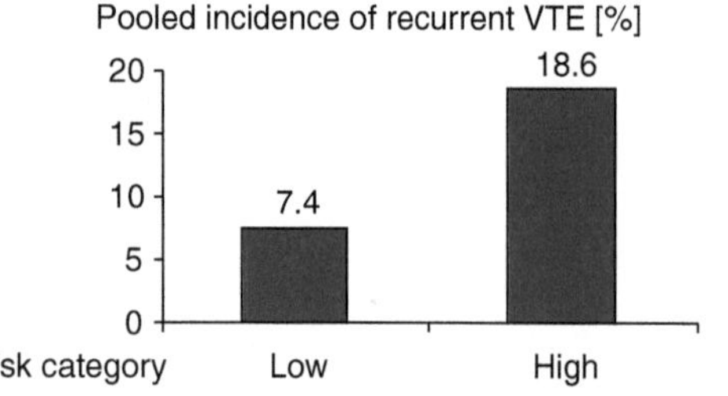

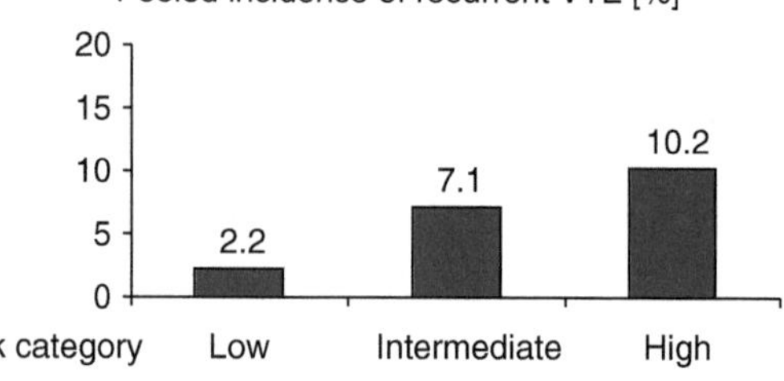

FIG. 30.2 Outline of the original and modified Ottawa prediction score for recurrent venous thromboembolism (VTE) and the associated recurrent VTE rate by risk category based on a meta-analysis of validation studies.

and pancreas cancer, but also lung and ovarian cancer as well as myeloproliferative and myelodysplastic disorders.[12] As with incident VTE, recurrent VTE risk is lower with stage I disease and highest with progressive and stage IV disease. Additional factors for recurrent VTE to consider include hormonal therapy in both sexes, although women in general seem to face a higher risk of recurrent VTE. Furthermore, age, residual thrombosis, surgical procedures, immobility, hospital and nursing home stay, and infections appear to add incremental risk.[9] Extremes of body weight, both high and low BMI, have been shown to confer an increased risk of VTE in patients with cancer as well.[9,20,22] Finally, centrally placed venous catheters also increase the risk of VTE for their dwell-time.[9]

The only validated tools available for risk prediction of recurrent VTE are the original and the modified Ottawa predictions scores (see Fig. 30.2)[21]. As outlined in a recent meta-analysis of the available data from the original and validation studies, the original Ottawa score is best suited to identify patients at high risk of recurrent VTE (49.3% of the population) with 70% sensitivity and 50% specificity.[22] The modified Ottawa prediction score, on the other hand, seems to be the one most valuable in identifying patients at low risk of VTE recurrence (19% of the external validation set) with a sensitivity of 90% and a specificity of 50%. An important aspect is the fact that these numbers were obtained from patients on anticoagulation therapy. Thus, these data may help in guiding decisions on anticoagulation therapy after 6 months. This being said, 12% of patients overall and nearly 1 in 5 in the high-risk group still had recurrent VTE while on anticoagulation, underscoring the general predisposition of patients with cancer even while their malignancies are being treated.

In cancer survivors, data on long-term VTE risk have very recently been reported by the German CVSS and the St. Jude childhood cancer survivor studies (Fig. 30.3).[13,14] These showed a persistently elevated risk of VTE in childhood cancer survivors, averaging approximately two-fold higher than in siblings and the general population over three to four4 decades. Risk factors for VTE in cancer survivors included female sex, cisplatin therapy, L-asparaginase, high or low BMI,

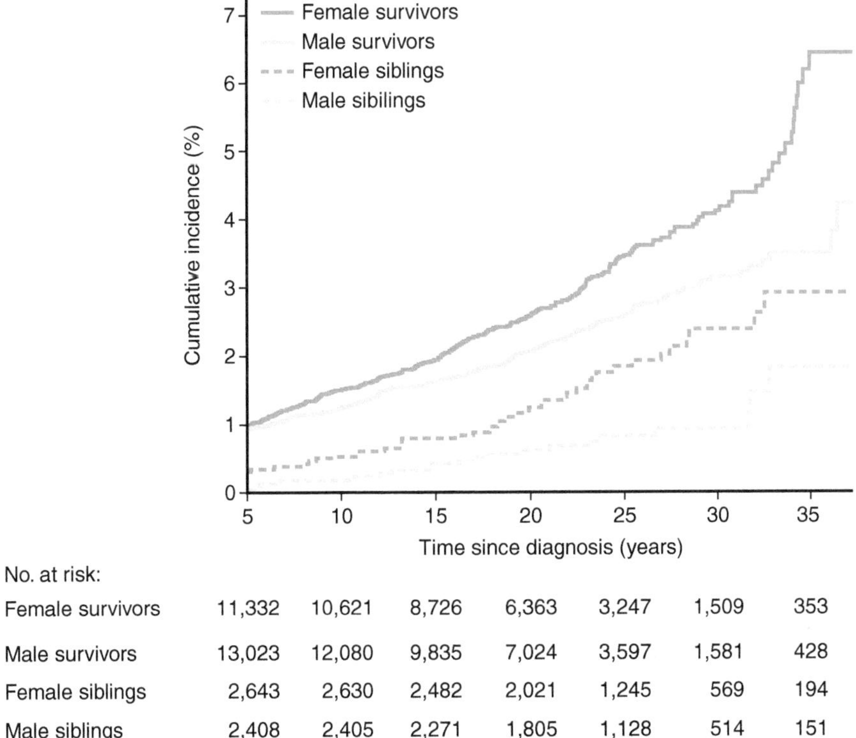

No. at risk:

Female survivors	11,332	10,621	8,726	6,363	3,247	1,509	353
Male survivors	13,023	12,080	9,835	7,024	3,597	1,581	428
Female siblings	2,643	2,630	2,482	2,021	1,245	569	194
Male siblings	2,408	2,405	2,271	1,805	1,128	514	151

FIG. 30.3 Cumulative incidence of male and female childhood cancer survivors overall (left) and combined with stratified subgroup analysis (right). (Reproduced with permission from Madenci AL, Weil BR, Liu Q, et al. Long-term risk of venous thromboembolism in survivors of childhood cancer: a report from the Childhood Cancer Survivor Study_*J Clin Oncol*. 2018;36:3144–3151.)

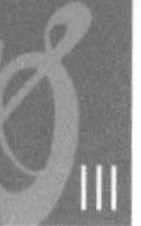

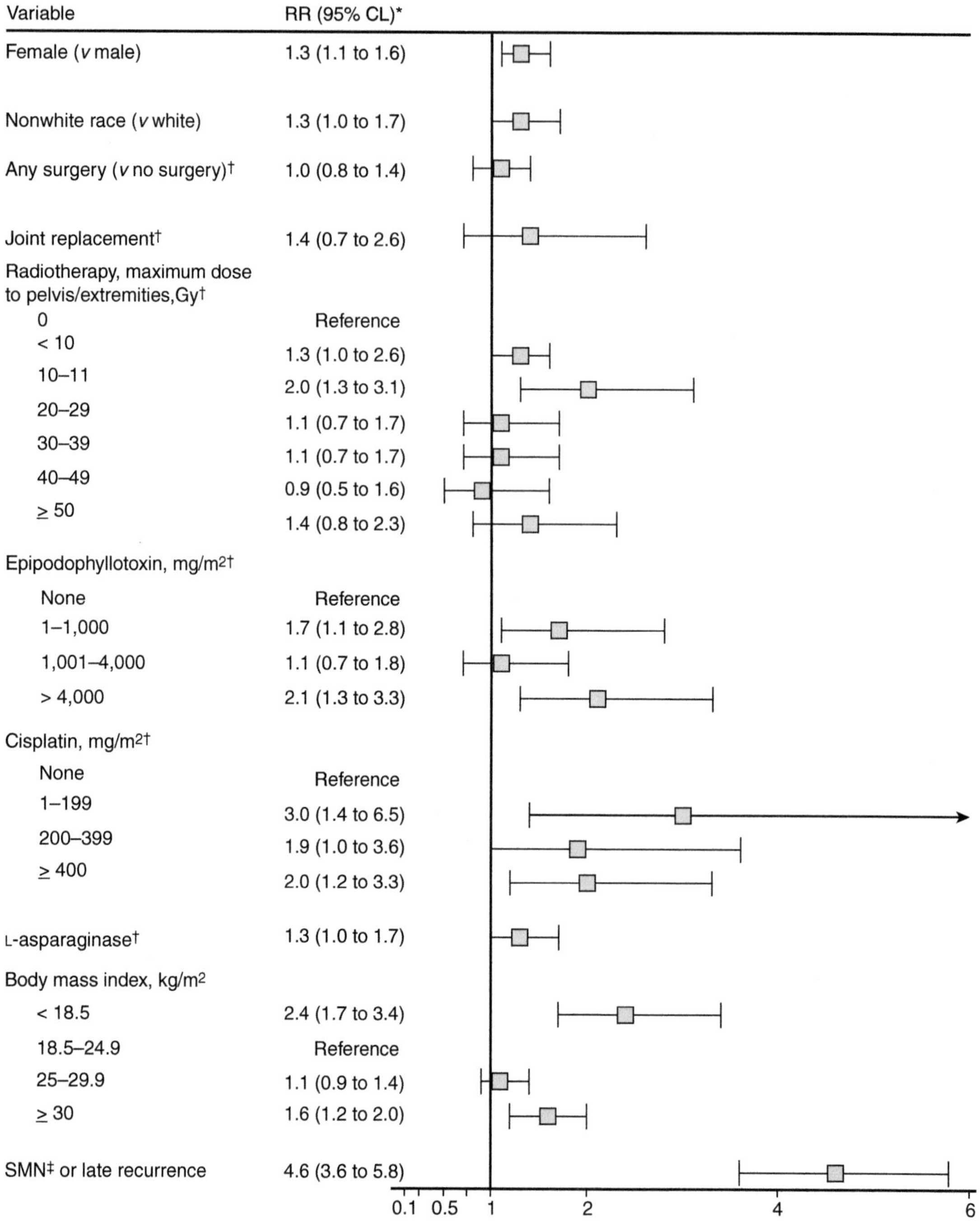

Variable	RR (95% CL)*
Female (*v* male)	1.3 (1.1 to 1.6)
Nonwhite race (*v* white)	1.3 (1.0 to 1.7)
Any surgery (*v* no surgery)†	1.0 (0.8 to 1.4)
Joint replacement†	1.4 (0.7 to 2.6)
Radiotherapy, maximum dose to pelvis/extremities,Gy†	
0	Reference
< 10	1.3 (1.0 to 2.6)
10–11	2.0 (1.3 to 3.1)
20–29	1.1 (0.7 to 1.7)
30–39	1.1 (0.7 to 1.7)
40–49	0.9 (0.5 to 1.6)
≥ 50	1.4 (0.8 to 2.3)
Epipodophyllotoxin, mg/m2†	
None	Reference
1–1,000	1.7 (1.1 to 2.8)
1,001–4,000	1.1 (0.7 to 1.8)
> 4,000	2.1 (1.3 to 3.3)
Cisplatin, mg/m2†	
None	Reference
1–199	3.0 (1.4 to 6.5)
200–399	1.9 (1.0 to 3.6)
≥ 400	2.0 (1.2 to 3.3)
L-asparaginase†	1.3 (1.0 to 1.7)
Body mass index, kg/m2	
< 18.5	2.4 (1.7 to 3.4)
18.5–24.9	Reference
25–29.9	1.1 (0.9 to 1.4)
≥ 30	1.6 (1.2 to 2.0)
SMN‡ or late recurrence	4.6 (3.6 to 5.8)

0.1 0.5 1 2 4 6

FIG. 30.3,cont'd

late cancer recurrence or secondary malignancy, and limb-sparing therapies in patients with osteosarcoma. VTE was associated with a two-fold increased risk of late mortality.

PREVENTION OF RECURRENT VTE AND VTE IN CANCER SURVIVOR

In cancer survivors, as with outpatient ambulatory patients with cancer, the use of primary prophylaxis is not recommended, with the exception of those at high risk, based on the Khorana score (values ≥ 2) or those with myeloma receiving immunomodulatory therapy.[23–25] This is even in view of several important trials that have highlighted the reduction in VTE risk, albeit in patients with active cancer (Table 30.2)[26–30]. The increased risk of bleeding and overall cost-effectiveness needs to be considered, and the risk-benefit in cancer survivors versus those with active cancer is not clear.

TABLE 30.2 **VTE Prevention Trials in Patients with Cancer**

TRIAL	SIZE	DESIGN	DRUG	PRIMARY OUTCOME	FOLLOW UP DURATION	PRIMARY OUTCOMES
PROTECHT[26]	1150	Randomized (2:1), double blind, placebo controlled	Nadroparin 3800 IU daily vs. placebo	Symptomatic DVT, PE, or fatal PE composite	Up to 4 months	• Nadroparin resulted in lower thromboembolic rates (2% vs. 3.9%). • Similar major bleeding (0.7% vs 0%). • Similar mortality at 1 year (43.3% vs. 40.7%)
SAVE-ONCO[27]	3212	Randomized, double blind, placebo controlled	Semuloparin 20 mg daily vs. Placebo	Symptomatic DVT, PE, or fatal PE composite.	3.5 months	• Semuloparin resulted in lower VTE rates (1.2% vs. 3.4%). • Similar major bleeding (1.2% vs. 1.1%) • Similar mortality (43.4% vs. 44.5%)
FRAGMATIC[28]	2202	Randomized, open label	Dalteparin 5000 IU daily mg daily vs. No LMWH	Overall survival Time to event endpoint	23.1 month median follow up	• The trial did not reach its intended number of events for the primary analysis. • Similar mortality rates (90% vs. 93%) • Similar metastasis-free survival at 1 year (16.2% vs. 14.9%) • Dalteparin resulted in lower VTE rates (5.5% vs. 9.7%). • Similar major bleeding (0.1% vs. 0.5%)
AVERT[29]	574	Randomized, double blind, placebo controlled	Apixaban 2.5 mg twice daily vs. placebo	Confirmed proximal DVT or PE	6 months	• Apixaban resulted in lower VTE rates (4.2% vs. 10.2%). • Major bleeding was greater in apixaban (3.5% vs. 1.8%). • Similar mortality (12.2% vs. 9.8%)
CASSINI[30]	1080	Randomized, double blind, placebo controlled	Rivaroxaban 10 mg daily vs. placebo	Composite proximal DVT, PE, or death	6 months	• 49 patients (4.5%) were not randomized owing to baseline DVT at screening. • The primary composite endpoint was similar (6.0% vs. 8.8%) at 180 days. • The primary composite endpoint was lower in patients on rivaroxaban during the intervention period (2.6% vs. 6.4%). • Major bleeding rates were similar (1% vs. 2%). • Similar mortality (20% vs. 23.8%)

DVT, deep venous thrombosis; *PE*, pulmonary embolism; *LMWH*, low molecular weight heparin.

It is important to emphasize guideline recommendations that anticoagulant therapy should continue in patients with VTE as long as their cancer is deemed active. Avoidance of premature cessation of anticoagulant therapy may be regarded as the single most important advice. Decision-making for continued therapy after 6 months of anticoagulation can be challenging. Although cancer is associated with a high risk of recurrent VTE, the rate of recurrence differs significantly by cancer type, stage of disease, and stage progression over time. For the following patient characteristics, it is likely best to continue anticoagulation: patients with brain, lung, pancreatic, or ovarian cancer; myeloproliferative or myelodysplastic disorders; stage IV cancer; cancer stage progression; or leg paresis. Anticoagulation options could include continued low molecular weight (LMW) heparin (dalteparin or enoxaparin), apixaban (or other oral novel direct factor inhibitors), or warfarin. For patients without these characteristics, decision-making is less clear. Balancing the risk of recurrent thrombosis, the risk of major bleeding and patient-specific preferences are most appropriate. Contributing factor should be eliminated when feasible. For instance, centrally placed venous catheters should be removed when no longer needed. The benefits of antihormonal therapy should be balanced with the risks. Inactivity should be avoided and targeting a normal BMI should be a priority. Patients with cancer who discontinue anticoagulation should receive proper VTE prophylaxis during periods of vulnerability, including major surgery and major trauma or prolonged immobilization. There are no data on serial screening for subclinical thrombosis. Data on screening for residual thrombosis from the DACUS study indicate that patients without residual thrombus have a low recurrent VTE rate (< 3%) (see treatment chapter).[31] For those with residual thrombus after 6 months, which was the majority (70%) of patients, recurrent VTE was 20% plus or minus 2% regardless of continuation or discontinuation of anticoagulation, which reiterates the needs to define best therapy for these patients.

SUMMARY

Venous thromboembolism is a common and important complication of cancer. Patients with cancer are at high risk of recurrent VTE, and this risk persists over years. Risk factors have been identified with two leading models: the Ottawa prediction score and the Olmsted County model. Any risk factor identified in the Olmsted model increases the risk of recurrent VTE by a factor of 3, whereas a positive Ottawa score signifies an increased risk of 19%. How to manage screen-positive patients is unknown at this point given the lack of clinical trials in this area. Certainly, anticoagulation should not be discontinued prematurely in patients with cancer with VTE, and decision-making after 6 months of anticoagulation should be done carefully with shared decision-making. Reduction of any modifiable risk factor is an important step (i.e., minimizing the time of antihormonal therapy, central catheter placement, and immobility). For cancer therapies that have been associated with a thrombotic risk (see **Chapter 8,** Tables 8.1 and 8.2), the duration of effect is not expected to be long-lasting with the exception of cisplatin, circulating levels of which can remain elevated for decades.

REFERENCES

1. Cancer Statistics. National Cancer Institute. Updated: April 27, 2018.
2. Heit JA, Silverstein MD, Mohr DN, Petterson TM, O'Fallon WM, Melton LJ 3rd. Risk factors for deep vein thrombosis and pulmonary embolism: a population-based case-control study. *Arch Intern Med.* 2000;160:809–815.
3. Heit JA, O'Fallon WM, Petterson TM, et.al. 3rd. Relative impact of risk factors for deep vein thrombosis and pulmonary embolism: a population-based study. *Arch Intern Med.* 2002;162:1245-1248.
4. Braekkan SK, Borch KH, Mathiesen EB, Njølstad I, Wilsgaard T, Hansen JB. Body height and risk of venous thromboembolism: the Tromsø Study. *Am J Epidemiol.* 2010;171:1109-1115.
5. Blom JW, Doggen CJ, Osanto S, Rosendaal FR. Malignancies, prothrombotic mutations, and the risk of venous thrombosis. *JAMA.* 2005;293:715–722.
6. Sørensen HT, Mellemkjaer L, Olsen JH, Baron JA. Prognosis of cancers associated with venous thromboembolism. *N Engl J Med.* 2000;343:1846–1850.
7. Khorana AA, Francis CW, Culakova E, Kuderer NM, Lyman GH. Thromboembolism is a leading cause of death in patients with cancer receiving outpatient chemotherapy. *J Thromb Haemost.* 2007;5:632–634.
8. Chew, HK, Wun T, Harvey D, Zhou H, White RH. Incidence of venous thromboembolism and its effect on survival among patients with common cancers. *Arch Intern Med.* 2006;166:458–464.
9. Ashrani AA, Gullerud RE, Petterson TM, Marks RS, Bailey KR, Heit JA. Risk factors for incident venous thromboembolism in active patients with cancer: a population based case-control study. *Thromb Res.* 2016;139:29–37.
10. Blom JW, Vanderschoot JP, Oostindi®r MJ, Osanto S, van der Meer FJ, Rosendaal FR. Incidence of venous thrombosis in a large cohort of 66,329 patients with cancer: results of a record linkage study. *J Thromb Haemost.* 2006;4:529–535.
11. Cronin-Fenton DP, Søndergaard F, Pedersen LA, et al. Hospitalisation for venous thromboembolism in patients with cancer and the general population: a population-based cohort study in Denmark, 1997–2006. *Br J Cancer.* 20108;103:947–953.
12. Petterson TM, Marks RS, Ashrani AA, Bailey KR, Heit JA.– Risk of site-specific cancer in incident venous thromboembolism: a population-based study. *Thromb Res.* 2015;135:472–478.

13. Madenci AL, Weil BR, Liu Q, et al. Weldon. Long-term risk of venous thromboembolism in survivors of childhood cancer: a report from the Childhood Cancer Survivor Study._*J Clin Oncol.* 2018;36:3144–3151
14, Faber J, Wingerter A, Neu MA, et al. Burden of cardiovascular risk factors and cardiovascular disease in childhood cancer survivors: data from the German CVSS-study. *Eur Heart J.* 2018;39:1555–1562.
15. Ay C, Dunkler D, Marosi C, et al. Prediction of venous thromboembolism in patients with cancer. *Blood.* 2010;116:5377–5382.
16. Verso M, Agnelli G, Barni S, Gasparini G, LaBianca R. A modified Khorana risk assessment score for venous thromboembolism in patients with cancer receiving chemotherapy: the Protecht score. *Intern Emerg Med.* 2012;7:291–292.
17. Pelzer U, Sinn M, Stieler J, Riess H. Primary pharmacological prevention of thromboembolic events in ambulatory patients with advanced pancreatic cancer treated with chemotherapy? *Dtsch Med Wochenschr.* 2013;138:2084–2088.
18. Gerotziafas GT, Taher A, Abdel-Razeq H, et al. A predictive score for thrombosis associated with breast, colorectal, lung, or ovarian cancer: the prospective COMPASS-cancer-associated thrombosis study. *Oncologist.* 2017;22:1222–1231.
19. Louzada ML, Carrier M, Lazo-Langner A, et al. Development of a clinical prediction rule for risk stratification of recurrent venous thromboembolism in patients with cancer-associated venous thromboembolism. *Circulation.* 2012;126:448–454.
20. Chee CE, Ashrani AA, Marks RS, et al. Predictors of venous thromboembolism recurrence and bleeding among active patients with cancer: a population-based cohort study. *Blood.* 2014;123:3972–3978.
21. Khorana AA, Francis CW, Culakova E, Kuderer NM, Lyman GH. Frequency, risk factors, and trends for venous thromboembolism among hospitalized patients with cancer. *Cancer.* 2007;110:2339–2346.
22. Khorana AA, Kuderer NM, Culakova E, Lyman GH, Francis C-W. Development and validation of a predictive model for chemotherapy-associated thrombosis. *Blood.* 2008;111:4902–4907.
23. Delluc A, Miranda S, den Exter P, et al. Accuracy of the Ottawa score in risk stratification of recurrent venous thromboembolism in patients with cancer-associated venous thromboembolism. A systematic review and meta-analysis. *Haematologica.* 2019 Jul 4. pii: haematol.2019.222828. doi: 10.3324/haematol.2019.222828. [Epub ahead of print].
24. Napolitano M, Saccullo G, Malato A, et al. Optimal duration of low molecular weight heparin for the treatment of cancer-related deep vein thrombosis: the Cancer-DACUS Study. *J Clin Oncol.* 2014;32:3607–3612.
25. Ay C, Dunkler D, Marosi C, et al. Prediction of venous thromboembolism in patients with cancer. *Blood.* 2010;116:5377–5382.
26. Verso M, Agnelli G, Barni S, Gasparini G, LaBianca R. A modified Khorana risk assessment score for venous thromboembolism in patients with cancer receiving chemotherapy: the Protecht score. *Intern Emerg Med.* 2012;7:291–292.
27. Pelzer U, Sinn M, Stieler J, Riess H. Primary pharmacological prevention of thromboembolic events in ambulatory patients with advanced pancreatic cancer treated with chemotherapy? *Dtsch Med Wochenschr.* 2013;138:2084–2088.
28. Gerotziafas GT, Taher A, Abdel-Razeq H, et al. A predictive score for thrombosis associated with breast, colorectal, lung, or ovarian cancer: the prospective COMPASS-cancer-associated thrombosis study. *Oncologist.* 2017;22:1222–1231.

31 Arrhythmia Prevention and Management in Cancer Survivors

MICHAEL FRADLEY

Patient with cancer

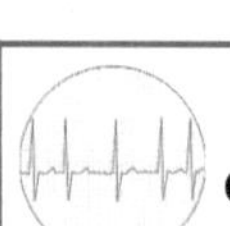

Atrial Fibrillation and Other Atrial Arrhythmias
• Esp. with chest radiation, cardiomyopathy, or hypertension
• Often underrecognized (screening?)
• Rate versus rhythm control?
• Anticoagulation decisions?
• Management per society guidelines

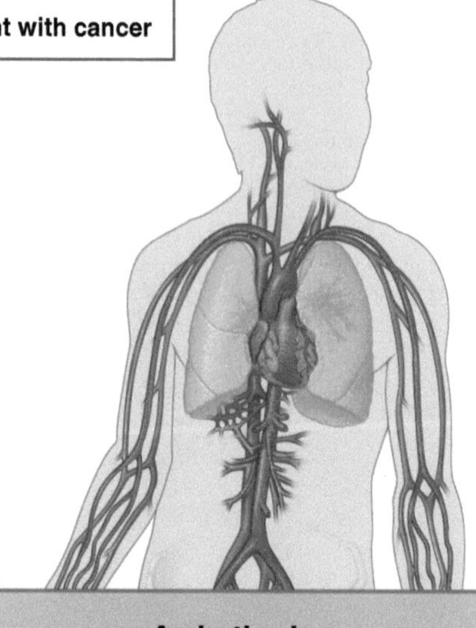

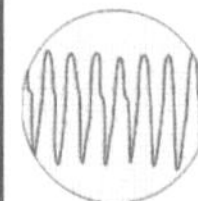

QT Prolongation and Ventricular Arrhythmias
• Esp. with therapy-induced cardiomyopathy, coronary artery disease, renal disease
• Need for additional studies?
• Anti-arrhythmic +/– device therapy?
• Management per society guidelines
Arrhythmias after cancer therapy

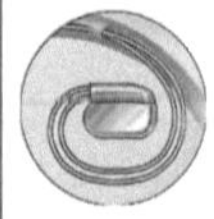

Cardiac Implantable Devices (pacemaker, ICD)
• Adjustment to programming based on therapy (radiation) and clinical presentation
• ICD, CRT-D, pacemaker indication?
• Device infection?
• Management per society guidelines

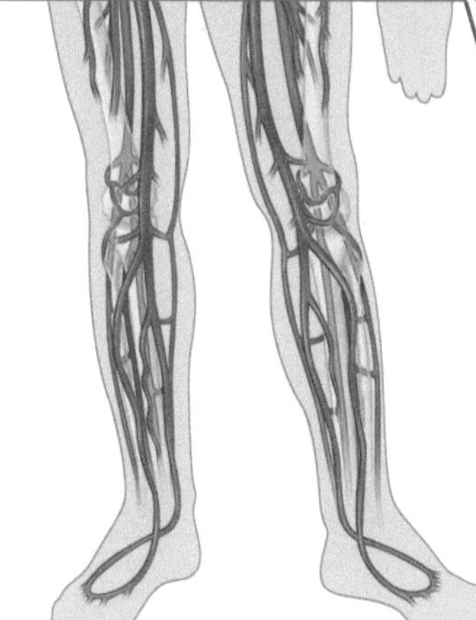

Bradyarrhythmias and Autonomic Dysfunction
• Esp. after chest or neck radiation, drug-induced neurotoxicity
• Need for additional studies?
• Need for medical or device therapy?
• Any modifiable cause or factor?
• Management per society guidelines

CHAPTER OUTLINE

KEY POINTS

- Cancer survivors are at risk of developing arrhythmias, often not diagnosed until clinically evident, and at times with life-threatening consequences.
- The long-term risk of recurrent arrhythmias once in remission and after cessation of cancer therapies is unknown.
- Arrhythmias occur with similar frequency in patients with chemotherapy-induced cardiomyopathy and other forms of left ventricular dysfunction.
- Cardiac resynchronization demonstrates benefit in patients with chemotherapy-induced cardiomyopathy.
- Autonomic dysfunction is frequently encountered in cancer survivors treated with chemotherapy and/or radiation.

It is well established from multiple epidemiologic studies that cardiovascular (CV) disease is more common in cancer survivors than in the general population. Although attention is frequently given to ischemic heart disease and heart failure, arrhythmias are also significantly increased in the survivorship population, with an incidence of 1.3% by age 45 based on data from the Childhood Cancer Survivors Study.[1] Unfortunately, risk factors for the development of arrhythmias in cancer survivors are not well established, which makes the development of screening and prevention strategies more challenging.

ATRIAL AND VENTRICULAR ARRHYTHMIAS IN CANCER SURVIVORS

Atrial arrhythmias, particularly atrial fibrillation (AF), are well described cardiotoxicities of many different cancer therapeutics including cytotoxic and targeted therapeutics (Table 31.1). However, little is known about the long-term risk of recurrent arrhythmias once the offending agent has been stopped. Thus far it is unclear if the development of arrhythmias while taking a cancer therapeutic increases the likelihood of future recurrent episodes. In patients on ibrutinib, for instance, the risk seems to reside with those who either have a history of AF or are otherwise at risk of AF.[2] Thus, at least these patients have the substrate for AF, which then emerges with triggers related to the malignancy and/or therapy.

TABLE 31.1 Cancer Treatments Frequently Associated With Atrial Arrhythmias

DRUG	CLASS	FREQUENCY
Doxorubicin	Anthracycline	10.3%
Melphalan	Alkylating	13%
Gemcitabine	Antimetabolite	8%
Carfilzomib	Proteasome inhibitor	3.8%
Interleukin-2	Immunotherapy	13%
Sorafenib	Tyrosine kinase inhibitor	5%
Ibrutinib	Bruton's tyrosine kinase inhibitor	14%

Such suggestive but nonconfirmed persistent risk estimates lead to significant management dilemmas, especially as it relates to anticoagulation. It is not clear if patients with an elevated stroke risk as determined by their CHA_2DS_2-VASc score (≥2 in men, and ≥3 in women, see Fig. 19.1), should receive long-term anticoagulation if the arrhythmia only occurred while taking their cancer therapeutic. Given these uncertainties, the ARCHER trial (Clinicaltrials.gov – NCT04118530) was designed to evaluate the long-term risk of recurrent atrial fibrillation in stem cell transplant survivors with elevated stroke risk who developed new-onset AF after conditioning chemotherapy. Patients who meet the inclusion criteria will have a subcutaneous implantable loop recorder inserted to monitor for recurrent arrhythmias. The data from this trial will help to inform our decisions on the long-term management of these patients.

If atrial or ventricular tachyarrhythmias are observed in cancer survivors, the evaluation and treatment of these patients should follow the same guidelines and recommendations as those for the general population. In the setting of AF, patients with an elevated CHA_2DS_2-VASc score should be started on anticoagulation to minimize the risk of thromboembolism, if deemed to be at a low bleeding risk (Fig. 19.2). Just like for other cardiovascular diseases, management of AF anticoagulation in cancer survivors increasingly matches those without cancer further out from malignancy and therapy. Rate versus rhythm control strategies should be considered based on the presence of additional symptoms or CV abnormalities. An evaluation for cardiomyopathy and/or ischemic heart disease should be initiated if arrhythmias (especially ventricular arrhythmias) are observed in patients with long-term CV risk who have received treatments (i.e., anthracyclines, chest radiation).[3,4]

Several studies have evaluated the arrhythmic burden in patients with chemotherapy-induced cardiomyopathy. Historically, this type of nonischemic cardiomyopathy was thought to portend a worse prognosis when compared with other etiologies.[5] Arrhythmias were thought to be one potential reason for this observation. More recently however, a large retrospective study from the Mayo Clinic suggested similar outcomes between cancer survivors with an anthracycline-mediated cardiomyopathy, and other types of left ventricular dysfunction. Specifically, no significant difference was found in overall survival, freedom from heart transplantation, or freedom from implantable cardioverter defibrillator (ICD) therapies in the different groups. Moreover, intracardiac device evaluation revealed nonsustained ventricular tachycardia to be the most common arrhythmia in patients with anthracycline-mediated cardiomyopathy (73.9%), followed by AF (56.6%) and sustained ventricular tachycardia (VT) or ventricular fibrillation (30.4%). These values did not significantly differ between the different groups.[6] A related study by Fradley and colleagues[7] reported similar results. When comparing patients with chemotherapy-induced cardiomyopathy with patients with other forms of nonischemic cardiomyopathy no significant difference was seen in atrial or ventricular arrhythmias. Patients with an ischemic cardiomyopathy demonstrated higher rates and risk of both nonsustained ventricular tachycardia and the combined outcome of sustained VT or ventricular fibrillation however.[7] It remains essential to monitor for and treat arrhythmias routinely if they are observed in these patients.

AUTONOMIC DYSFUNCTION AND BRADYARRHYTHMIA

Electrocardiographic abnormalities, especially resting sinus tachycardia, and autonomic dysfunction are increasingly recognized cardiovascular complications of cancer survivors (see Fig. 31.1). Impaired autonomic function is associated with increased rates of both short- and long-term CV disease and mortality (see Fig. 31.2). Patients with symptomatic tachycardia can be treated with atrioventricular (AV) nodal blocking agents, whereas hypotension can be managed with hydration and salt consumption, as well as pharmacologically with midodrine, fludrocortisone, and droxidopa. Nevertheless, controlled studies assessing the utility of these interventions in cancer survivors are lacking. Chemotherapies, especially anthracyclines, have been associated with the development of autonomic dysfunction. In a study of 47 patients with breast cancer with normal left ventricular (LV) function, resting heart rate was significantly elevated in patients three years after anthracycline chemotherapy compared with age-matched controls.[8] In another study, 50% of patients with breast cancer treated with anthracyclines and trastuzumab developed sinus tachycardia (heart rate >110 bpm) compared with 0% of the control patients.[9] The exact time course for the development of autonomic dysfunction after exposure to anthracyclines is not clear.

Radiation is also associated with the development of abnormalities of the autonomic nervous system. Evidence suggests dose-related damage, with increased prevalence of abnormal heart rate recovery at higher radiation doses. Among patients with Hodgkin lymphoma, those who had received thoracic radiation were found to have a significant increase in resting heart rate and heart rate recovery compared with matched control patients. In addition, patients who had received radiation therapy had reduced exercise tolerance and increased all-cause mortality.[10] In a related study, childhood Hodgkin lymphoma survivors were more likely to have an elevated resting heart rate and blunted blood pressure and heart rate

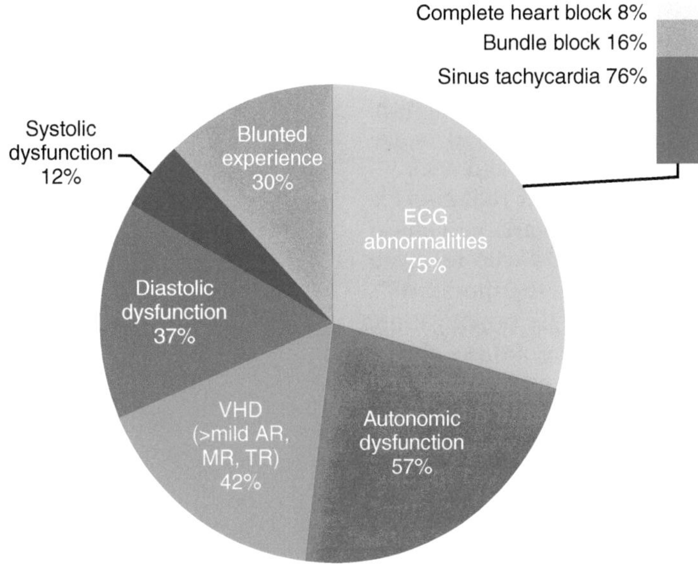

FIG. 31.1 Cardiovascular abnormalities in 48 long-term (median 16.5 years) survivors of Hodgkin lymphoma.[11]

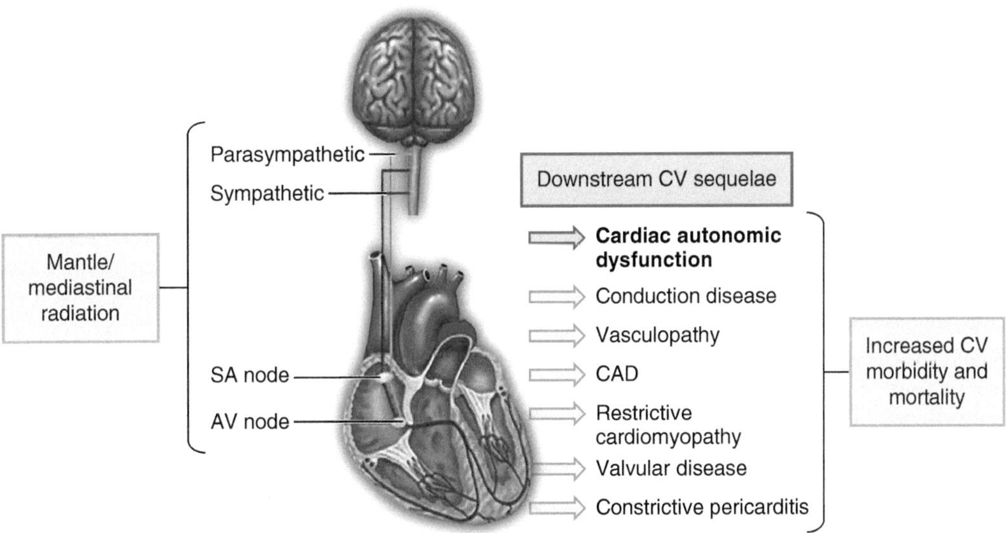

Outcome	Elevated resting heart rate*	Abnormal heart rate recovery**
Exercise duration	−1.1 ± 0.3 (P = .001)	−1.0 ± 0.4 (P = .006)
Mortality, HR (95% CI)	0.99 (0.40–2.45)	5.50 (1.97–15.36)

*relative to patients without elevated resting heart rate; **with normal heart rate recovery

FIG. 31.2 Cardiovascular consequences of radiation therapy (RT) in survivors of Hodgkin lymphoma. Increased prevalence of elevated resting heart rate and abnormal heart rate recovery is noted, relative to controls, and these abnormalities contribute to decreased exercise tolerance, and abnormal heart rate recovery is associated with increased mortality among patients who have had RT. *AV,* Atrioventricular; *SA,* sinoatrial. (From Groarke JD, Tanguturi VK, Hainer J, et al. Abnormal exercise response in long-term survivors of Hodgkin lymphoma treated with thoracic irradiation: evidence of cardiac autonomic dysfunction and impact on outcomes. *J Am Coll Cardiol*. 2015;65(6):573–583.)

response to exercise.[11] Additionally, autonomic dysfunction can occur in patients receiving head and neck radiation owing to baroreceptor damage. For example, heart rate response to deep breathing or Valsalva maneuver was diminished in patients receiving radiation to the head and neck.[12]

Electrocardiographic changes after radiation exposure have been reported, with variable clinical relevance. In a study of 25 patients who received more than 45 grays of radiation to the thorax, 48% developed T-wave abnormalities, QTc prolongation, and poor R-wave progression. Most of these abnormalities resolved on subsequent evaluations and none of the patients required intervention for these findings.[13] Bundle branch blocks as well as complete heart block have also been reported in long-term survivors of Hodgkin lymphoma after chest radiation therapy, though these are far less common than sinus tachycardia (Fig. 31.1).

CARDIAC IMPLANTABLE ELECTRONIC DEVICES IN CANCER SURVIVORS

Implantable cardiac devices should be considered in cancer survivors based on the same standard indications for the general population. Although the overall benefit of device-based therapy in patients with nonischemic cardiomyopathy has been called into question based on data from recent large studies,[14] ICD implantation remains a class I indication in patients who develop a chemotherapy-induced cardiomyopathy with an ejection fraction of 35% despite optimal medical therapy.[15] Moreover, in the setting of a prolonged QRS duration, the addition of cardiac resynchronization therapy (CRT) can be beneficial to certain patients (Table 31.2).[15] Nevertheless, patients with chemotherapy-induced cardiomyopathy have been significantly underrepresented in the majority of ICD and CRT trials. As such, the definite benefits of CRT to this unique population have been established only recently.

Several recent studies have evaluated the role of CRT in the setting of chemotherapy-induced cardiomyopathy. A retrospective study of four patients demonstrated improvement in left ventricular ejection fraction (LVEF) and parameters of reverse remodeling, along with a reduction in heart failure symptoms.[16] A follow-up study of 18 patients with anthracycline-induced cardiomyopathy implanted with a CRT device demonstrated significant improvements in ejection fraction, left ventricular end-diastolic and end-systolic diameters, and New York Heart Association (NYHA) functional class.[17] These studies served as the foundation for the MADIT-CHIC study, a prospective multicenter trial evaluating the benefit of CRT in chemotherapy-induced cardiomyopathy. Thirty patients were enrolled from 12 centers with established cardio-oncology programs. Patients with low LVEF (≤35%) owing to chemotherapy, NYHA class II-IV heart failure symptoms, and wide QRS, were implanted with a CRT. Subjects were followed for 6 months to assess for changes in LVEF and overall improvement in clinical symptoms. Patients with CRT experienced a statistically significant improvement in mean LVEF of 10.6% (95% confidence interval [CI], 8.0, 13.3) at 6 months along with 37 mL mean reduction in LV end-systolic volume, and 32 mL reduction in LV end-diastolic volume. Additionally, 41% of patients improved their NYHA functional status at 6 months,

TABLE 31.2 Indications for Cardiac Resynchronization Defibrillator Implantation

Class I
• LVEF ≤35% • LBBB with QRS ≥150 ms • NYHA Class II-IV
Class IIa
• LVEF ≤35% • LBBB with QRS 120–149 ms • NYHA Class II-IV
• LVEF ≤35% • Non-LBBB with QRS ≥150 ms • NYHA Class III-IV
• LVEF ≤35% • Anticipated RV pacing >40%
Class IIb
• LVEF <30% owing to ischemic cardiomyopathy • LBBB with QRS ≥150 ms • NYHA Class I
• LVEF <35% • Non-LBBB with QRS 120–149 ms • NYHA Class III-IV
• LVEF <35% • Non-LBBB with QRS ≥150 ms • NYHA Class II

LBBB, Left bundle branch block; *LVEF*, left ventricular ejection fraction; *NYHA*, New York Heart Association; *RV*, right ventricular.
Adapted from Tracy CM, Epstein AE, Darbar D, et al. 2012 ACCF/AHA/HRS focused update of the 2008 Guidelines for Device-Based Therapy of Cardiac Rhythm Abnormalities: a report of the American College of Cardiology Foundation/American Heart Association Task Force on Practice Guidelines and the Heart Rhythm Society. [corrected]. *Circulation*. 2012;126(14):1784–1800. doi:10.1161/CIR.0b013e3182618569.

with no deaths and only one heart failure event.[18] Based on these data, CRT should be strongly considered in patients with chemotherapy-induced cardiomyopathy who meet traditional criteria for implantation. In this context, it is pertinent that the American College of Cardiology Foundation/American Heart Association {AHA} guidelines recommended neither ICD nor CRT if the expected life expectancy is less than 1 year, whereas the European Society of Cardiology [ESC] guidelines set a limitation by life expectancy for ICD therapy but not for CRT and CRT-P is favored in patients with advanced heart failure and major comorbid conditions, including severe renal failure, frailty, and cachexia (Herrmann, 2020, see supplemental content).[19]

REFERENCES

1. Armstrong GT, Oeffinger KC, Chen Y, et al. Modifiable risk factors and major cardiac events among adult survivors of childhood cancer. *J Clin Oncol.* 2013;31(29):3673–3680. doi:10.1200/JCO.2013.49.3205.
2. Wiczer TE, Levine LB, Brumbaugh J, et al. Cumulative incidence, risk factors, and management of atrial fibrillation in patients receiving ibrutinib. *Blood Adv.* 2017;1(20):1739–1748. doi:10.1182/bloodadvances.2017009720.
3. January CT, Wann LS, Alpert JS, et al. 2014 AHA/ACC/HRS guideline for the management of patients with atrial fibrillation: a report of the American College of Cardiology/American Heart Association Task Force on practice guidelines and the Heart Rhythm Society. *Circulation.* 2014;130(23):e199–e267. doi:10.1161/CIR.0000000000000041.
4. January CT, Wann LS, Calkins H, et al. 2019 AHA/ACC/HRS focused update of the 2014 AHA/ACC/HRS guideline for the management of patients with atrial fibrillation: a report of the American College of Cardiology/American Heart Association Task Force on Clinical Practice Guidelines and the Heart Rhythm Society in collaboration with the Society of Thoracic Surgeons. *Circulation.* 2019;140(2):e125–e151. doi:10.1161/CIR.0000000000000665.
5. Felker GM, Thompson RE, Hare JM, et al. Underlying causes and long-term survival in patients with initially unexplained cardiomyopathy. *N Engl J Med.* 2000;342(15):1077–1084. doi:10.1056/NEJM200004133421502.
6. Mazur M, Wang F, Hodge DO, et al. Burden of cardiac arrhythmias in patients with anthracycline-related cardiomyopathy. *JACC Clin Electrophysiol.* 2017;3(2):139–150. doi:10.1016/j.jacep.2016.08.009.
7. Fradley MG, Viganego F, Kip K, et al. Rates and risk of arrhythmias in cancer survivors with chemotherapy-induced cardiomyopathy compared with patients with other cardiomyopathies. *Open Heart.* 2017;4(2):e000701. doi:10.1136/openhrt-2017–000701.
8. Jones LW, Haykowsky M, Pituskin EN, et al. Cardiovascular reserve and risk profile of postmenopausal women after chemoendocrine therapy for hormone receptor—positive operable breast cancer. *Oncologist.* 2007;12(10):1156–1164. doi:10.1634/theoncologist.12-10-1156.
9. Jones LW, Haykowsky M, Peddle CJ, et al. Cardiovascular risk profile of patients with HER2/neu-positive breast cancer treated with anthracycline-taxane-containing adjuvant chemotherapy and/or trastuzumab. *Cancer Epidemiol Biomarkers Prev.* 2007;16(5):1026–1031. doi:10.1158/1055-9965.EPI-06-0870.
10. Groarke JD, Tanguturi VK, Hainer J, et al. Abnormal exercise response in long-term survivors of Hodgkin lymphoma treated with thoracic irradiation: evidence of cardiac autonomic dysfunction and impact on outcomes. *J Am Coll Cardiol.* 2015;65(6):573–583. doi:10.1016/j.jacc.2014.11.035.
11. Adams MJ, Lipsitz SR, Colan SD, et al. Cardiovascular status in long-term survivors of Hodgkin's disease treated with chest radiotherapy. *J Clin Oncol.* 2004;22(15):3139–3148. doi:10.1200/JCO.2004.09.109.
12. Huang CC, Huang TL, Hsu HC, et al. Long-term effects of neck irradiation on cardiovascular autonomic function: a study in nasopharyngeal carcinoma patients after radiotherapy. *Muscle Nerve.* 2013;47(3):344–350. doi:10.1002/mus.23530.
13. Gomez DR, Yusuf SW, Munsell MF, et al. Prospective exploratory analysis of cardiac biomarkers and electrocardiogram abnormalities in patients receiving thoracic radiation therapy with high-dose heart exposure. *J Thorac Oncol.* 2014;9(10):1554–1560. doi:10.1097/JTO.0000000000000306.
14. Kober L, Thune JJ, Nielsen JC, et al. Defibrillator implantation in patients with nonischemic systolic heart failure. *N Engl J Med.* 2016;375(13):1221–1230. doi:10.1056/NEJMoa1608029.
15. Tracy CM, Epstein AE, Darbar D, et al. 2012 ACCF/AHA/HRS focused update of the 2008 guidelines for device-based therapy of cardiac rhythm abnormalities: a report of the American College of Cardiology Foundation/American Heart Association Task Force on Practice Guidelines and the Heart Rhythm Society [corrected]. *Circulation.* 2012;126(14):1784–1800. doi:10.1161/CIR.0b013e3182618569.
16. Ajijola OA, Nandigam KV, Chabner BA, et al. Usefulness of cardiac resynchronization therapy in the management of doxorubicin-induced cardiomyopathy. *Am J Cardiol.* 2008;101(9):1371–1372. doi:10.1016/j.amjcard.2007.12.037.
17. Rickard J, Kumbhani DJ, Baranowski B, et al. Usefulness of cardiac resynchronization therapy in patients with adriamycin-induced cardiomyopathy. *Am J Cardiol.* 2010;105(4):522–526. doi:10.1016/j.amjcard.2009.10.024.
18. Singh JP, Solomon SD, Fradley MG, et al. Association of cardiac resynchronization therapy with change in left ventricular ejection fraction in patients with chemotherapy-induced cardiomyopathy. *JAMA.* 2019;322(18):1799–1805. doi:10.1001/jama.2019.16658.
19. Herrmann J. Adverse cardiac effects of cancer therapies: cardiotoxicity and arrhythmia. *Nat Rev Cardiol.* 2020;17:474–502. doi:10.1038/s41569-020-0348-1.

32 Hypertension and Renal Failure Prevention and Management After Cancer Therapy

NINIAN N. LANG, STEPHEN J.H. DOBBIN, SANDRA M.S. HERRMANN, JOERG HERRMANN, AND RHIAN M. TOUYZ

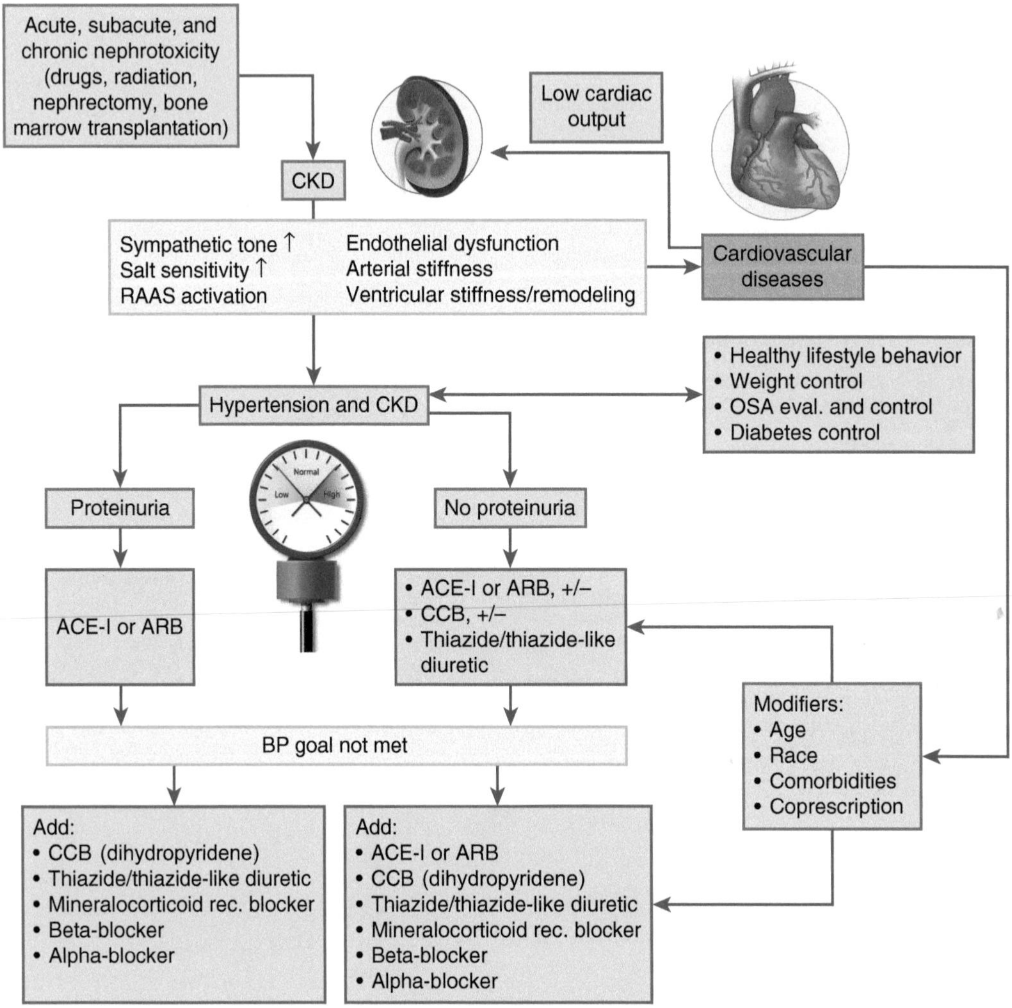

Acute, subacute, and chronic nephrotoxicity (drugs, radiation, nephrectomy, bone marrow transplantation)

Low cardiac output

CKD

Sympathetic tone ↑
Salt sensitivity ↑
RAAS activation
Endothelial dysfunction
Arterial stiffness
Ventricular stiffness/remodeling

Cardiovascular diseases

Hypertension and CKD

- Healthy lifestyle behavior
- Weight control
- OSA eval. and control
- Diabetes control

Normal
Low
High

Proteinuria

No proteinuria

ACE-I or ARB

- ACE-I or ARB, +/–
- CCB, +/–
- Thiazide/thiazide-like diuretic

Modifiers:
- Age
- Race
- Comorbidities
- Coprescription

BP goal not met

Add:
- CCB (dihydropyridene)
- Thiazide/thiazide-like diuretic
- Mineralocorticoid rec. blocker
- Beta-blocker
- Alpha-blocker

Add:
- ACE-I or ARB
- CCB (dihydropyridene)
- Thiazide/thiazide-like diuretic
- Mineralocorticoid rec. blocker
- Beta-blocker
- Alpha-blocker

CHAPTER OUTLINE

KEY POINTS

- Hypertension is an important cardiovascular risk factor in cancer survivors and it potentiates the risk of heart failure in patients previously exposed to cardiotoxic chemotherapy or mediastinal radiation
- Regular routine blood pressure surveillance is an important measure in cancer survivorship with blood pressure goals that match the 2017 American College of Cardiology/American Heart Association (ACC/AHA) guidelines (<130/80 mm Hg)
- First-line therapies for hypertension include inhibitors of the renin angiotensin aldosterone system and dihydropyridine calcium channel blockers (amlodipine, nifedipine), alone or in combination
- In patients with left ventricular systolic dysfunction, heart failure, or prior myocardial infarction preference should be for renin angiotensin aldosterone system inhibitors as well as beta-blockers, especially carvedilol or bisoprolol
- Chronic kidney disease (CKD) can be the consequence of acute kidney injury during cancer therapy, and the longer-term effects of cancer therapies (especially cisplatin, ifosfamide, kidney radiation, nephrectomy, and hematopoietic stem cell transplantation [HSCT]), as well as hypertension and diabetes
- CKD commonly occurs after HSCT (myeloablative > non-myeloablative allogeneic > autologous); CKD, which is also more common after allogenic HSCT, is attributable to subacute thrombotic microangiopathy related to calcineurin inhibitors, higher intensity nephrotoxic chemotherapy, graft-versus-host disease, and/or total body radiation
- Long-term surveillance of renal function should be an integral component of the care of cancer survivors; prevention of renal dysfunction is a priority, also in view of its implications for cardiovascular diseases in cancer survivors

HYPERTENSION

As outlined in Chapters 11 and 20, cessation/withdrawal of cancer therapy can lead to complete resolution of blood pressure derangements in patients with hypertension induced or aggravated by cancer therapies. However, blood pressure elevation can persist. Among the chemotherapeutics associated with a long-term risk of hypertension are the platinum drugs, ifosfamide, and calcineurin inhibitors after stem cell transplantation. A reduction in the capillary bed paired with chronic induction of inflammation and oxidative stress might explain why cisplatin can lead to blood pressure elevation in the long term. The patient group best studied in this regard is survivors of testicular cancer. Compared with healthy controls, testicular cancer survivors are at a 40% higher risk of developing hypertension, even when adjusting for age.[1] This risk is highest in those who received cisplatin therapy, especially at dosages greater than 850 mg/m^2 (OR, 2.4; 95% CI, 1.4 to 4.0).[1] Moreover, cancer survivors can develop essential hypertension and/or cardiometabolic disease, especially with aging. Patients with obesity and wide neck circumference should be evaluated for obstructive sleep apnea, an important risk factor for hypertension.[2,3] Thus, hypertension in a cancer survivor should prompt a comprehensive assessment of potential underlying causes, which includes renal and other secondary etiologies.

The impact of hypertension on cardiovascular and overall outcomes in childhood cancer survivors is significant, with an increased risk of cardiovascular events and cardiovascular diseases. In patients exposed to radiation therapy or anthracyclines, who become hypertensive, the increased risk for heart failure is amplified.[4] Radiation exposure to the chest and anthracycline use should be considered as additional risk factors for cardiovascular events in the population of adult cancer survivors. Recognition, evaluation, and optimal treatment of hypertension in cancer survivors is thus extremely important.

In patients previously exposed to abdominal radiotherapy, renal radiation injury may aggravate hypertension control and severity. In patients with head and neck cancer or malignancy in the upper chest, radiation therapy and surgery can lead to injury of the carotid baroreceptors. This can cause blood pressure variability, including hypertension and orthostatic hypotension as well as tachycardia.

Management of Hypertension in Cancer Survivors

Despite the increasing clinical need for robust guidelines for long-term monitoring and management of cardiovascular risk factors and disease in cancer survivors, particularly as cancer treatments continue to improve clinical outcomes, these remain sparse. Clinical guidelines currently focus on cardiovascular screening prior to or during treatment or on monitoring of cardiac function.[5,6] The most comprehensive recommendations for long-term monitoring of cardiovascular disease and risk factors have been aimed at long-term survivors of hematologic malignancies who have undergone bone marrow transplantation.[7,8] These recommend regular screening for cardiovascular risk factors following the completion of anticancer treatment, including obesity, hypertension, and diabetes. However, recommendations for the wider cancer survivor population are lacking.

In patients who develop hypertension following the completion of anticancer therapies, the increased risks of cardiovascular events and end-organ damage favor stricter blood pressure control, and we recommend a target blood pressure of less than 130/80 mm Hg. In addition to antihypertensive medications, lifestyle modifications, such as dietary measures and physical activity, are important to reduce cardiovascular risk. First-line treatment regimens should follow conventional hypertension management guidelines.[2,3] These recommend angiotensin-converting enzyme inhibitors/angiotensin II receptor blockers (ACEi/ARBs) and dihydropyridine calcium channel blockers (CCB) in the first instance, either alone or in combination, although thiazide diuretics may also be used. ACEi/ARB should be preferred in patients with left-ventricular systolic dysfunction, heart failure, or prior myocardial infarction. Beta-blockers are generally recommended as second-line therapies, but of particular use in patients with left-ventricular dysfunction or coronary artery disease, both of which may be prevalent in cancer survivors. Other secondary medications include loop diuretics, mineralocorticoid receptor antagonists, and alpha-blockers, which may be beneficial in patients with resistant hypertension.

RENAL DISEASE

Survivors of cancer may develop chronic kidney disease (CKD) for many reasons, both related and unrelated to the malignancy and its treatment (Table 32.1), as well as previous episodes of acute kidney injury (AKI). In childhood cancer survivors after a median follow up of 18 years, nephrectomy, abdominal irradiation, high-dose cisplatin, and high-dose ifosfamide were found to be independent risk factors for impaired renal function, whereas cyclophosphamide or methotrexate were not.[9] In adults, ifosfamide and cisplatin are likewise associated with a permanent decline in renal function.[10] These changes occur early during therapy, often after the first cycle. Thereafter no further decline in renal function is usually seen with cisplatin, whereas a slow, gradual drop in renal function can be seen with ifosfamide, even more than 2 years out from therapy.

In addition to a reduction in glomerular filtration rate (commonly evident as an increase in serum creatinine or cystatin C), proteinuria and nephrotic syndrome are important to recognize and indicative of glomerular disease. A renal biopsy can aid in the diagnostic work-up and guide therapy. Patients with renal cell carcinoma are at long-term risk of reduced renal function because a large percentage have underlying CKD and a reduced renal functional reserve. Even among those with a normal renal function before radial nephrectomy, one-third will develop AKI postoperatively, which increases the risk for CKD more than four-fold. With partial nephrectomy, the risk of AKI is 20%. Obstructive nephropathy needs to be considered as a postrenal cause for CKD in cancer survivors.

CHRONIC KIDNEY DISEASE AFTER HEMATOPOIETIC STEM CELL THERAPY

CKD, which is an important long-term complication of hematopoietic stem cell therapy (HSCT), is found in 15% to 20% of survivors after allogeneic HSCT—mainly related to low-grade renal thrombotic microangiopathy.[11] Although more fulminant courses can be seen, the typical presentation is that of slowly

TABLE 32.1 Potential Late Effects of Nephrotoxicity of Cancer Therapies and Recommendations Provided in the Children's Oncology Group Long-Term Follow-Up Guidelines

THERAPEUTIC EXPOSURE	POTENTIAL LATE EFFECT	RISK FACTORS	HIGHEST RISK FACTORS	HEALTH COUNSELING/FURTHER CONSIDERATIONS
Ifosfamide	Renal toxicity Glomerular toxicity (decreased GFR) Tubular toxicity (renal tubular acidosis, hypophosphatemia, hypokalemia, hypomagnesemia, Fanconi syndrome, rickets)	Host factors • Younger age at treatment • Single kidney Treatment factors • Higher cumulative dose • Combined with other nephrotoxins: • Cisplatin • Carboplatin • Aminoglycosides • Amphotericin • Immunosuppressants • Methotrexate • Radiation impacting the kidney Medical conditions: • Tumor infiltration of the kidney • Preexisting renal impairment • Nephrectomy	Host factors • Age <5 years at time of treatment Treatment factors • Ifosfamide dose ≥60 mg/m² • Renal radiation dose ≥15 Gy	Electrolyte supplements for patients with persistent electrolyte wasting. Nephrology consultation for patients with hypertension, proteinuria or progressive renal insufficiency Category = 1
Carboplatin Cisplatin	Renal toxicity Glomerular injury Tubular injury Renal insufficiency	Host factors • Single kidney Treatment factors • Combined with other nephrotoxins: • Ifosfamide • Aminoglycosides • Amphotericin • Immunosuppressants • Methotrexate • Radiation impacting the kidney Medical conditions: • Diabetes mellitus • Hypertension • Nephrectomy	Treatment factors • Cisplatin dose ≥200 mg/m² • Renal radiation dose ≥15 Gy	In patients with salt-wasting tubular dysfunction, educate that low magnesium levels potentiate coronary atherosclerosis. Electrolyte supplements for patients with persistent electrolyte wasting. Nephrology consultation for patients with hypertension, proteinuria or renal insufficiency.
Methotrexate	Renal toxicity Acute toxicities predominate	Host factors • Single kidney Treatment factors • Combined with other nephrotoxins: • Cisplatin/carboplatin • Ifosfamide • Aminoglycosides • Amphotericin • Immunosuppressants • Radiation impacting the kidney	Treatment factors • Treatment before 1970	Nephrology consultation for patients with hypertension, proteinuria, or renal insufficiency. Category = 2A

Continued

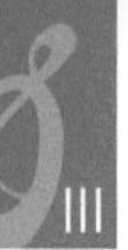

TABLE 32.1 Potential Late Effects of Nephrotoxicity of Cancer Therapies and Recommendations Provided in the Children's Oncology Group Long-Term Follow-Up Guidelines—cont'd

THERAPEUTIC EXPOSURE	POTENTIAL LATE EFFECT	RISK FACTORS	HIGHEST RISK FACTORS	HEALTH COUNSELING/FURTHER CONSIDERATIONS

Radiation whole abdomen
All upper abdominal fields
TBI
	Renal toxicity
	Renal insufficiency
	Hypertension
		Host factors
		• Bilateral Wilms tumor
		• Single kidney
		Treatment factors
		• Radiomimetic chemotherapy
		• Radiation dose ≥10 Gy
		• TBI combined with radiation to the kidney
		• Combined with other nephrotoxins:
		  • Cisplatin
		  • Carboplatin
		  • Ifosfamide
		  • Aminoglycosides
		  • Amphotericin
		  • Immunosuppressants
		Medical conditions:
		• Diabetes mellitus
		• Hypertension
		• Nephrectomy
			Treatment factors
			• Radiation dose ≥15 Gy
			• TBI ≥6 Gy in single fraction
			• TBI ≥12 Gy fractionated
				Nephrology consultation for patients with hypertension, proteinuria or renal insufficiency.
				Category = 1

Nephrectomy	Renal toxicity
	Renal insufficiency
	Hypertension
	Proteinuria
	Hydrocele (males only)
		Treatment factors
		• Combined with other nephrotoxins:
		  • Cisplatin
		  • Carboplatin
		  • Ifosfamide
		  • Aminoglycosides
		  • Amphotericin
		  • Immunosuppressants
		  • Methotrexate
		  • Radiation impacting the kidney
				Discuss contact sports, bicycle safety (e.g., avoiding handlebar injuries) and proper use of seatbelts (i.e., wearing lap belts around hips). Counsel to use NSAIDs with caution.
				Nephrology consultation for patients with hypertension, proteinuria or renal insufficiency.
				Category = 1

GFR, Glomerular filtration rate; *NSAIDs*, nonsteroidal antiinflammatory drugs; *TBI*, total body irradiation.
From Jones DP, Spunt SL, Green D, Springate JE; Children's Oncology Group. Renal late effects in patients treated for cancer in childhood: a report from the Children's Oncology Group. *Pediatr Blood Cancer*. 2008;51(6):724–731. doi:10.1002/pbc.21695.

rising serum creatinine values, hypertension, and anemia out of proportion to the level of kidney disease. Peripheral smear may reveal schistocytosis, low serum haptoglobin, and platelet counts with elevated lactate dehydrogenase. Urine analysis can show proteinuria and hematuria of variable degree, whereas renal imaging is usually unremarkable. Renal biopsy usually is not required to guide management and only performed if other forms of glomerular disease are expected, for example, membranous nephropathy with nephrotic syndrome-type presentations. Thrombotic microangiopathy (TMA) after HSCT is thought to be provoked by endothelial injury at the time of conditioning, especially radiation therapy, and then modulated by graft-versus-host disease, infections, and medications. The time course for renal failure typical of radiation-induced kidney damage is often many months after HSCT because kidney cells have a much slower turnover than mucosal cells and thus manifest radiation damage much later. Renal shielding with total body radiation serves an important role in prevention. Most patients who develop CKD after abdominal radiation received doses above 20 Gy. The role of ACEi/ARBs is yet to be defined.

CALCINEURIN INHIBITOR TOXICITY

Long-term use of calcineurin inhibitors (cyclosporine and tacrolimus) very likely contributes to CKD, as well after solid organ transplantation and autoimmune disease.[11] Akin to the well-described interaction after kidney transplantation, calcineurin inhibitors are thought to exacerbate TMA in patients after HSCT.

Their role after allogenic HSCT is to reduce acute and chronic graft-versus-host disease. Therapy is usually limited to one year or less, which reduces the CKD risk and the dose of calcineurin inhibitor dose should be minimized as much as possible.

MANAGEMENT OF HSCT-RELATED CKD

Hypertension control is important for any patient with CKD, and especially after HSCT in view of their (potential) comorbidity burden. Angiotensin-converting enzyme or angiotensin receptor blockade may be preferred and should be used if proteinuria is present. These receptors retard progression of radiation nephropathy in animal models. This recommendation holds even if with a risk of hyperkalemia, which should be followed and counteracted by a low-potassium diet, diuretics, and possibly low-dose sodium polystyrene. Plasma exchange may be used for TMA after HSCT, but the evidence base is not strong. Patients who have had HSCT and are on dialysis may have a worse prognosis than other patients on dialysis. Renal transplantation is to be considered on an individual basis. Those who receive a renal allograft from the same donor as their original HSCT will need minimal or no immunosuppression as a result of immunologic tolerance of the allograft.[11]

ACKNOWLEDGMENTS

Rhian M. Touyz is supported by a British Heart Foundation (BHF) chair award (CH/12/429762) and Stephen J.H. Dobbin is funded through the BHF Research Excellence Award (RE/13/5/30177).

REFERENCES

1. Sagstuen H, Aass N, Fosså SD, et al. Blood pressure and body mass index in long-term survivors of testicular cancer. *J Clin Oncol.* 2005;23(22):4980–4990. doi:10.1200/JCO.2005.06.882.
2. Whelton PK, Carey RM, Aronow WS, et al. 2017 ACC/AHA/AAPA/ABC/ACPM/AGS/APhA/ASH/ASPC/NMA/PCNA guideline for the prevention, detection, evaluation, and management of high blood pressure in adults: a report of the American College of Cardiology/American Heart Association task force on clincial practice guidelines. *J Am Coll Cardiol.* 2018;71(19):e127–e248. doi:10.1016/j.jash.2018.06.010.
3. Williams B, Mancia G, Spiering W, et al. 2018 Practice guidelines for the management of arterial hypertension of the European Society of Hypertension and the European Society of Cardiology: ESC/ESH task force for the management of arterial hypertension. *J Hypertens.* 2018;36(12):2284–2309. doi:10.1097/HJH.0000000000001961.
4. Khanna A, Pequeno P, Gupta S, et al. Increased risk of all cardiovascular disease subtypes among childhood cancer survivors: population-based matched cohort study. *Circulation.* 2019;140(12):1041–1043. doi:10.1161/CIRCULATIONAHA.119.041403.
5. Curigliano G, Lenihan D, Fradley M, et al. Management of cardiac disease in patients with cancer throughout oncological treatment: ESMO consensus recommendations. *Ann Oncol.* 2020;31(2):171–190. doi:10.1016/j.annonc.2019.10.023.
6. Armenian SH, Lacchetti C, Barac A, et al. Prevention and monitoring of cardiac dysfunction in survivors of adult cancers: American Society of Clinical Oncology clinical practice guideline. *J Clin Oncol.* 2017;35(8):893–911. doi:10.1200/JCO.2016.70.5400.
7. Defilipp Z, Duarte RF, Snowden JA, et al. Metabolic syndrome and cardiovascular disease following hematopoietic cell transplantation: screening and preventive practice recommendations from CIBMTR and EBMT. *Bone Marrow Transplant.* 2017;52(2):173–182. doi:10.1038/bmt.2016.203.
8. Armenian SH, Chemaitilly W, Chen M, et al. National Institutes of Health Hematopoietic Cell Transplantation Late Effects Initiative: the cardiovascular disease and associated risk factors working group report. *Biol Blood Marrow Transplant.* 2017;23(2):201–210. doi:10.1016/j.bbmt.2016.08.019.
9. Jones DP, Spunt SL, Green D, Springate JE; Children's Oncology Group. Renal late effects in patients treated for cancer in childhood: a report from the Children's Oncology Group. *Pediatr Blood Cancer.* 2008;51(6):724–731. doi:10.1002/pbc.21695.
10. Dekkers IA, Blijdorp K, Cransberg K, et al. Long-term nephrotoxicity in adult survivors of childhood cancer. *Clin J Am Soc Nephrol.* 2013;8(6):922–929. doi:10.2215/CJN.09980912.
11. Humphreys BD, Soiffer RJ, Magee CC. Renal failure associated with cancer and its treatment: an update. *J Am Soc Nephrol.* 2005;16(1):151–161. doi:10.1681/ASN.2004100843.

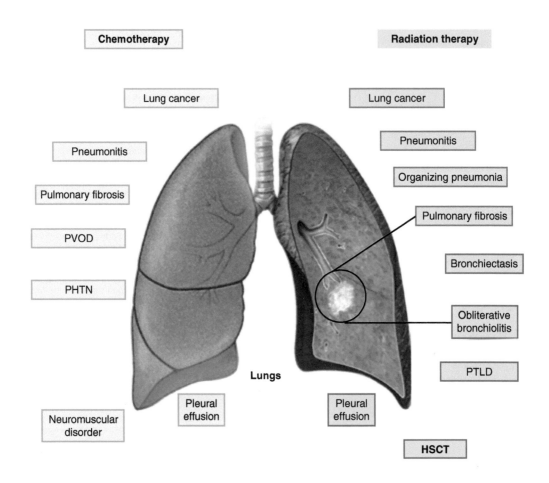

33 Monitoring for and Management of Delayed Complications After Cancer Therapy

YEVGENIYA MOGILEVSKAYA AND ALEXANDER GEYER

Chemotherapy

Lung cancer

Pneumonitis

Pulmonary fibrosis

PVOD

PHTN

Neuromuscular disorder

Pleural effusion

Lungs

Radiation therapy

Lung cancer

Pneumonitis

Organizing pneumonia

Pulmonary fibrosis

Bronchiectasis

Obliterative bronchiolitis

PTLD

Pleural effusion

HSCT

CHAPTER OUTLINE

KEY POINTS

- Several different delayed pulmonary complications can occur after chemotherapy, radiation therapy, and stem cell transplantation.
- Pulmonary fibrosis is the most common delayed parenchymal process and needs to be distinguished from organizing pneumonia, which may develop months after therapy and, unlike fibrosis, is usually reversible with steroids.
- Obliterative bronchiolitis is a rare but serious complication that develops several months to years after hematopoietic stem cell transplantation in patients with chronic graft versus host disease; initially it may be asymptomatic, recognizable only on screening spirometry and with a variable response to immunosuppressive treatment.
- Bronchiectasis may develop as a result of fibrosis or recurrent infection and, when symptomatic, requires a combination of respiratory hygiene (e.g., inhaled bronchodilators and mucolytics, mechanical mucus clearance maneuvers) and antimicrobials for management.
- Pulmonary arterial hypertension is associated with certain pharmacologic cancer agents, particularly with dasatinib and, less commonly, with other tyrosine kinase inhibitors (bosutinib, nilotinib, ponatinib) and cancer therapeutics such as alemtuzumab, bevacizumab, gemcitabine, leflunomide, mitomicin, ruxolitinib, and thalidomide.
- Pulmonary venoocclusive disease is a rare complication of cytotoxic and myeloablative therapies and can easily be missed owing to its subtle presentation suggestive of mild congestive heart failure.
- Pleural effusions are common in patients with cancer with the differential diagnosis including complications of cancer therapy (e.g., dasatinib), malignant pleural effusion, volume overload, and congestive heart failure.
- Secondary intrathoracic malignancies, including lung cancer and posttransplant lymphoproliferative neoplasm, may arise several months to years after cancer therapy.

INTRODUCTION

The lungs are a common site of neoplastic involvement—both primary and metastatic. Moreover, given the large surface area of the alveolar–capillary interface, lungs are a common site for idiosyncratic drug toxicities that often are difficult to distinguish from infections, postsurgical inflammatory or radiation therapy (RT) associated processes, and neoplastic involvement itself.[1] Pulmonary complications of cancer treatment may occur during (early) or after (delayed) therapy. Delayed complications include diseases of lung parenchyma (pneumonitis, pulmonary fibrosis), airways (obliterative bronchiolitis, bronchiectasis), vasculature (pulmonary hypertension, pulmonary venoocclusive disease), pleural (serositis, effusion), neuromuscular system (weakness, diaphragm paralysis), and secondary malignancy (Central Illustration).

PARENCHYMAL DISEASE

Parenchymal lung disease has been reported with a variety of chemotherapeutic and biologic agents (e.g., bleomycin, mitomycin-C, carmustine, busulfan, and cyclophosphamide.[2] Bleomycin lung toxicity is one of the most common and best characterized. Bleomycin-induced pneumonitis (BIP) may occur during therapy or after 6 months or more.[3] Common symptoms include dyspnea, cough, and fever. Imaging usually demonstrates interstitial infiltrates and/or opacities. Patients with BIP tend to respond to corticosteroids starting at 0.5 to 1.0 mg/kg/day of prednisone or equivalent for a month followed by a taper over 3 to 6 months. BIP can progress to pulmonary fibrosis and is associated with an increased mortality among testicular cancer survivors.[4] Other chemotherapies associated with the late complication of pulmonary fibrosis include busulfan, carmustine, and lomustine. Corticosteroid treatment has little benefit in pulmonary fibrosis, except potentially during an acute exacerbation.

RT-induced pneumonitis typically occurs several months after completion of therapy for lung, breast, and esophageal cancers as well as bone metastases, Hodgkin and non-Hodgkin lymphoma, or total body irradiation for leukemia. Symptoms are similar to those of drug-induced pneumonitis. With the exception of breast radiation-induced organizing pneumonia, airspace opacities occur within the field of radiation.[1] Steroids may be helpful in expediting resolution of symptoms. Radiation-induced pulmonary fibrosis develops between 6 and 24 months after therapy. Some patients may be asymptomatic, whereas others may present with progressive dyspnea and cough. Pulmonary function tests demonstrate a restrictive deficit and diffusion impairment. Steroids are of little benefit in RT-induced fibrosis.

AIRWAY DISEASE

Bronchiolitis obliterans has been reported between 3 months and 3 years following a hematopoietic stem cell transplantation (HSCT) and is a manifestation of chronic graft versus host disease.[5] Patients present with subacute dyspnea with or without a cough. Because symptom onset may be insidious, leading to a delay in diagnosis, routine monitoring with spirometry at 6 months, and 1 and 2 years posttransplant is recommended. The gold standard for diagnosis is surgical biopsy demonstrating chronic inflammation, fibrosis, and obliteration of small airways; however, pulmonary function testing (obstructive ventilatory deficit) and chest computed tomography (mosaic attenuation of lung parenchyma accentuated on expiration) with the exclusion of other etiologies in the appropriate clinical context may be used to make the diagnosis. Treatment involves immunosuppression, inhaled bronchodilators, and montelukast. Lung transplant has been used in refractory cases.

Bronchiectasis is a permanent dilatation of airways. It may develop in the setting of cancertherapy-associated pulmonary fibrosis, as a result of recurrent pulmonary infections, or as a late sequelae of bronchiolitis obliterans.[2] Symptoms include dyspnea and a productive cough. Periods of stability may be punctuated by acute exacerbations, with fevers and increased mucus purulence and/or volume. Pulmonary function testing may demonstrate an obstructive pattern. Chest computed tomography imaging may demonstrate dilated bronchi, mucus impaction, and mosaic attenuation from air trapping. Pulmonary hygiene with the help of mucus clearance devices, inhaled bronchodilators, and antibiotics are the mainstay of therapy.

VASCULAR DISEASE

Pulmonary vascular disease secondary to chemotherapy or RT includes pulmonary arterial hypertension and pulmonary venoocclusive disease (PVOD). Patients may present with exertional dyspnea and hypoxemia. Pulmonary hypertension can be seen after exposure to alkylating agents such as cyclophosphamide and tyrosine kinase inhibitors such as dasatinib.[6]

Several chemotherapeutic agents, such as bleomycin, carmustine, and mitomycin, have been associated with PVOD. PVOD has also been reported after HSCT. This diagnosis requires a high index of suspicion. Echocardiogram can suggest the possibility of pulmonary hypertension, but right-side heart catheterization is often necessary to confirm it and distinguish between pulmonary arterial and pulmonary venous hypertension. Surgical lung biopsy is the gold standard for diagnosing PVOD. Management remains unclear and is based on anecdotal evidence of benefit of glucocorticoids. Pulmonary vasodilators have to be used with extreme caution in PVOD owing to the risk of inducing pulmonary edema.

PLEURAL DISEASE

Pleural effusions may be noticed secondary to chemotherapy and RT and may occur at any time from 2 months to up to 5 years with certain medications, such as the BCR-Abl tyrosine kinase inhibitor dasatinib.[7] The mechanism is not entirely understood, but it may involve a serositis-like reaction. Exclusion of heart failure, infection, and malignancy is necessary before the effusion can be attributed to the side effects of cancer therapy. Treatment may entail temporarily or permanently discontinuing the offending agent or reducing the dose (dasatinib). Sometimes administration of glucocorticoids and/or diuretics may be of value. In case of recurrence, an indwelling pleural catheter or pleurodesis may be attempted.[7]

Pleural effusions are common after HSCT, with an estimated incidence of 10% at 1 year and 12% at 5 years posttransplant and they are associated with graft versus host disease and impaired survival,[8,9] More than 50% of these effusions are exudative. A minority of patients have accompanying pericardial effusions. Immunosuppressive therapy usually leads to resolution.

NEUROMUSCULAR DISEASE

Chemotherapy has been shown to result in sensory and motor neuropathy. Doxorubicin has been well documented to cause skeletal muscle weakness, which may occur during treatment or several months after treatment.[10] The mechanism is thought to be secondary to oxidative stress resulting in muscular weakness and fatigue.

Treatment with checkpoint inhibitors, such as ipilimumab and nivolumab, may result in neurotoxicity, including a Guillain-Barre syndrome-like reaction and may cause respiratory muscle weakness. These adverse reactions may be noted at any point in the course of treatment, but have typically been noted up to 4 months following treatment.[10] Symptoms may include supine dyspnea and hypoxemia. Diagnosis may be made with pulmonary function testing demonstrating a restrictive defect or a decrease in forced vital capacity in supine position as well as decreased negative inspiratory flow. There is a decrease in maximal inspiratory and expiratory pressure. Diaphragmatic ultrasound may reveal decreased diaphragmatic excursion. Nerve conduction studies and autoimmune antibody testing can corroborate the diagnosis. Treatment includes discontinuation of the offending drug. Corticosteroids in high doses may be administered. In cases of severe respiratory failure plasmapheresis or administration of immunoglobulins may be required.

SECONDARY INTRATHORACIC MALIGNANCY

Cancer survivors are at an increased risk of secondary tumors as a result of treatment with chemotherapy or RT. Lung cancer accounts for a notable proportion of these secondary neoplasms.[11] History of use of alkylating agents and chest RT as well as cigarette smoking are the main risk factors.[12]

Posttransplant lymphoproliferative disorders (PTLD) are lymphoid and/or plasmacytic proliferations that occur in the setting of allogeneic HSCT as a result of immunosuppression with or without concurrent reactivation of Epstein-Barr virus. Over 80% of PTLD develop in the first year posttransplant, with more than half presenting with extranodal masses, including tumors of the lung.[13]

LONG-TERM MONITORING AND PREVENTION OF COMPLICATIONS

Although specific guidelines exist to monitor for cancer recurrence (e.g., computed tomographic chest every 6 months for 2 years and then annually for lung cancer,[14] limited literature is available to guide clinicians in monitoring for delayed pulmonary toxicity of cancer therapies.

For childhood cancer survivors at risk for pulmonary fibrosis owing to treatment with bleomycin, busulfan, carmustine, or lomustine (especially in conjunction with chest RT or total body irradiation), the Children's Oncology Group recommends yearly pulmonary examination and, if pulmonary dysfunction is detected, yearly PFT (http://www.survivorshipguidelines.org, last accessed March 3, 2020).

For childhood cancer survivors with a history of chest RT, guidelines from the Children's Oncology Group recommend yearly pulmonary examinations and discussion of imaging surveillance with computed tomography of the chest (http://www.survivorshipguidelines.org, last accessed March 3, 2020). Smoking cessation counseling and, when appropriate, assistance with pharmacotherapy should be provided to all smoking cancer survivors.

The United States Advisory Committee on Immunization Practices (ACIP) recommends annual influenza vaccination of all individuals 6 months of age and older. For cancer survivors younger than 65 years of age, an *inactivated* influenza vaccine is recommended. Individuals over 65 years of age should receive the high-dose trivalent inactivated influenza vaccine. *Live attenuated* vaccine should *not* be used in persons with chronic medication conditions and immunocompromized individuals (https://www.cdc.gov/vaccines/hcp/acip-recs/vacc-specific/flu.html, last accessed March 3, 2020).

Two types of pneumococcal vaccine are approved in the United States: a pneumococcal polysaccharide vaccine (Pneumovax 23) and a pneumococcal protein-conjugate vaccine (Prevnar 13). No specific recommendations are available for cancer survivors and, therefore, we recommend adhering to the general guidelines available from the ACIP (https://www.cdc.gov/vaccines/hcp/acip-recs/vacc-specific/pneumo.html, last accessed March 3, 2020). For healthy adults 65 and older, Pneumovax 23 alone is recommended. Adults younger than 65 with medical condition (e.g., chronic heart, lung, or liver disease; diabetes; smoking; alcohol use disorder) should also receive Pneumovax 23. For adults older than 19 years of age with severe immunocompromising conditions (e.g., asplenia, use of immunosuppressive medication, HIV, cerebrospinal leak, cochlear implants, or a history of invasive pneumococcal disease) both Prevnar 13 and Pneumovax 23 are recommended and should be administered in that sequence and at least 8 weeks apart.

Additional recommendations may evolve as viral pandemics emerge. This is illustrated in COVID-19. The National Comprehensive Cancer Network among other provide guidance on vaccinations, which are indicated including and especially in immunocompromised individuals. Delays may apply for patients who underwent hematopoetic stem cell transplantation or CAR T-cell therapy (https://www.nccn.org/docs/default-source/covid-19/2021_covid-19_vaccination_guidance_v4-0.pdf?sfvrsn=b483da2b_70, last accessed 10/14/2021)

REFERENCES

1. Abid SH, Malhotra V, Perry MC. Radiation-induced and chemotherapy-induced pulmonary injury. *Curr Opin Oncol.* 2001;13(4):242–248. doi:10.1097/00001622-200107000-00006.
2. Mertens AC, Yasui Y, Liu Y, et al. Pulmonary complications in survivors of childhood and adolescent *cancer.* A report from the Childhood Cancer Survivor Study. *Cancer.* 2002;95(11):2431–2441. doi:10.1002/cncr.10978.
3. White DA, Stover DE. Severe bleomycin-induced pneumonitis. Clinical features and response to corticosteroids. *Chest.* 1984;86(5):723–728. doi:10.1378/chest.86.5.723.
4. Fossa SD, Gilbert E, Dores GM, et al. Noncancer causes of death in survivors of testicular cancer. *J Natl Cancer Inst.* 2007;99(7):533–544. doi:10.1093/jnci/djk111.
5. Bergeron A, Chevret S, de Latour RP, et al. Noninfectious lung complications after allogeneic haematopoietic stem cell transplantation. *Eur Respir J.* 2018;51(5):1–13. doi:10.1183/1399–3003.02617–2017.
6. Ranchoux B, Günther S, Quarck R, et al. Chemotherapy-induced pulmonary hypertension: role of alkylating agents. *Am J Pathol.* 2015;185(2):356–371. doi: 10.1016/j.ajpath.2014.10.021.
7. Chen E, Itkin M. Thoracic duct embolization for chylous leaks. *Semin Intervent Radiol.* 2011;28(1):63–74. doi:10.1055/s-0031-1273941.
8. Armstrong GT, Liu Q, Yasui Y, et al. Late mortality among 5-year survivors of childhood cancer: a summary from the Childhood Cancer Survivor Study. *J Clin Oncol.* 2009;27(14):2328–2338. doi:10.1200/JCO.2008.21.1425.
9. Ugai T, Hamamoto K, Kimura S, et al. A retrospective analysis of computed tomography findings in patients with pulmonary complications after allogeneic hematopoietic stem cell transplantation. *Eur J Radiol.* 2015;84(12):2663–2670. doi:10.1016/j.ejrad.2015.08.020.
10. Spain L, Walls G, Julve M, et al. Neurotoxicity from immune-checkpoint inhibition in the treatment of melanoma: a single centre experience and review of the literature. *Ann Oncol.* 2017;28(2):377–385. doi:10.1093/annonc/mdw558.
11. Bright CJ, Reulen RC, Winter DL, et al. Risk of subsequent primary neoplasms in survivors of adolescent and young adult cancer (Teenage and Young Adult Cancer Survivor Study): a population-based, cohort study. *Lancet Oncol.* 2019;20(4):531–545. doi:10.1016/S1470-2045(18)30903-3.
12. Turcotte LM, Liu Q, Yasui Y, et al. Chemotherapy and risk of subsequent malignant neoplasms in the Childhood Cancer Survivor Study Cohort. *J Clin Oncol.* 2019;37(34):3310–3319. doi:10.1200/JCO.19.00129.
13. Nalesnik MA, Jaffe R, Starzl TE, et al. The pathology of posttransplant lymphoproliferative disorders occurring in the setting of cyclosporine A-prednisone immunosuppression. *Am J Pat–hol.* 1988;133(1):173–192.
14. Schneider BJ, Ismaila N, Aerts J, et al. Lung cancer surveillance after definitive curative-intent therapy: ASCO Guideline. *J Clin Oncol.* 2010;38(7):753–766. doi:10.1200/JCO.19.02748.

34 Cardio-Oncology Rehabilitation for Patients with Cancer and Survivors

RAY W. SQUIRES

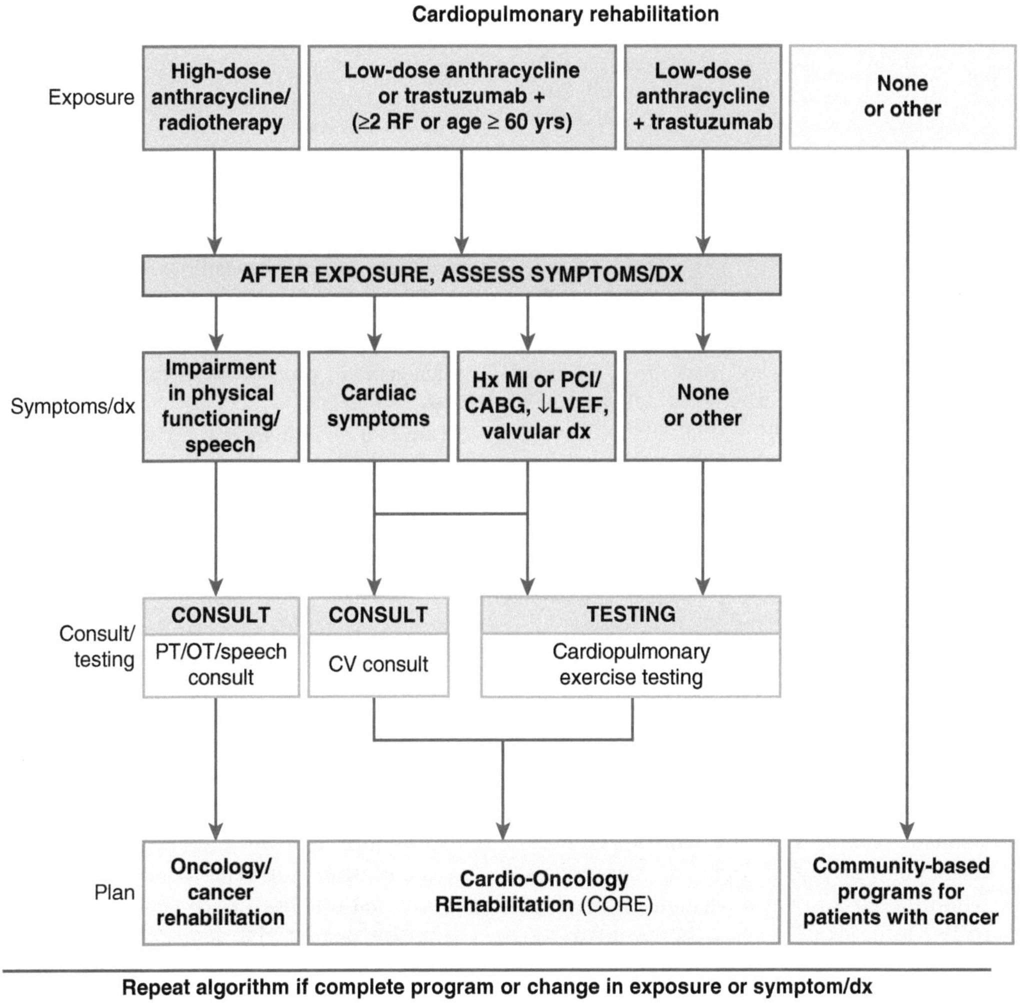

Cardiopulmonary rehabilitation

Exposure
High-dose anthracycline/ radiotherapy
Low-dose anthracycline or trastuzumab + (≥2 RF or age ≥ 60 yrs)
Low-dose anthracycline + trastuzumab
None or other
AFTER EXPOSURE, ASSESS SYMPTOMS/DX
Symptoms/dx
Impairment in physical functioning/ speech
Cardiac symptoms
Hx MI or PCI/ CABG, ↓LVEF, valvular dx
None or other
Consult/ testing
CONSULT
PT/OT/speech consult
CONSULT
CV consult
TESTING
Cardiopulmonary exercise testing
Plan
Oncology/ cancer rehabilitation
Cardio-Oncology REhabilitation (CORE)
Community-based programs for patients with cancer
Repeat algorithm if complete program or change in exposure or symptom/dx

(From Gilchrist SC, Barac A, Ades PA et al. Cardio-oncology rehabilitation to manage cardiovascular outcomes in patients with cancer and survivors: a scientific statement from the American Heart Association. *Circulation.* 2019;139(21):139 e997–e1012.)

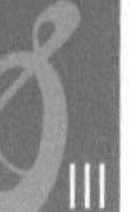

CHAPTER OUTLINE

KEY POINTS

- Patients with cancer experience an increased risk of developing cardiovascular diseases owing, in part, to the direct effects of cancer treatments (cardiotoxicity), a high prevalence of standard cardiovascular risk factors, and deconditioning associated with a decrease in cardiorespiratory fitness.
- Cardiorespiratory fitness, which is inversely related to cardiovascular risk, is approximately 30% lower in patients with cancer than in healthy persons.
- In breast cancer survivors, a strong, graded relationship between the amount of habitual physical activity and the incidence of coronary artery disease and heart failure has been established. Patients in the top tertile of physical activity experience an approximately 35% reduction in cardiovascular endpoints.
- Exercise training guidelines have been published for patients with cancer but are achieved by less than one third of patients. Exercise training in patients with cancer results in reduction in symptoms and improvement in quality of life and cardiorespiratory fitness.
- A 2019 American Heart Association scientific statement, endorsed by the American Cancer Society, recommends partnering with existing multidimensional, interdisciplinary cardiac rehabilitation programs to provide cardio-oncology rehabilitation (CORE).
- CORE will include standard cardiac rehabilitation components and interventions, as follows, with cancer-specific features: patient assessment; nutrition counseling; management of weight, blood pressure, blood lipids, and diabetes; tobacco cessation; psychosocial management; physical activity counseling; and exercise training.
- CORE is a novel concept in the care of patients with cancer. Widespread implementation will require development of a robust evidence base and a strategy for reimbursement.

INTERRELATIONSHIP OF CANCER AND CARDIOVASCULAR DISEASES

There are approximately 17 million survivors of cancer in the United States.[1] Many of these patients are at increased risk of noncancer maladies, primarily cardiovascular diseases, such as coronary artery disease and chronic heart failure. Persons who survive at least 5 years beyond a cancer diagnosis experience a 1.3- to 3.6-fold increase in cardiovascular mortality and a 1.7- to 18.5-fold risk of developing cardiovascular diseases.[2,3] With current treatments, improvements in cancer-specific mortality have resulted in cardiovascular diseases becoming more problematic for cancer survivors. Some of the heightened cardiovascular risk is owing to age-related pathology, direct effects of cancer treatments (cardiotoxicity), and indirect effects of cancer treatment, such as deconditioning and an increase in body fat stores.[4]

Cancer and cardiovascular disease are interrelated and share common risk factors, such as cigarette smoking, a diet rich in animal fat, dyslipidemia, obesity, chronic inflammation, sedentary lifestyle, and diabetes mellitus.[5,6] Preexisting cardiovascular disease is present in approximately 20% to 30% of patients with cancer.[5] Compared with healthy controls, those with cancer report reduced health-related quality of life with persistent fatigue as a common feature. Cancer-related fatigue is general in nature, not relieved by rest or sleep, and may persist for months to years after remission.[7]

Cardiovascular risk factors that are present before a cancer diagnosis are strong predictors of chemotherapy and radiation-related cardiovascular diseases.[8–10] In addition, cancer survivors are more likely than healthy controls to have hypertension and diabetes.[11] For 2-year survivors of adult-onset cancer, survivors with at least two cardiovascular risk factors had a higher risk of cardiovascular diseases (incidence rate ratio 1.8 to 2.6) compared with healthy controls. There was a 3.8-fold increased risk of all-cause mortality in cancer survivors who developed cardiovascular diseases compared with survivors without cardiovascular diseases.[11]

EXERCISE CAPACITY (CARDIORESPIRATORY FITNESS) IS REDUCED IN PATIENTS WITH CANCER AND IMPROVES WITH EXERCISE TRAINING

Exercise capacity of patients with cancer is, on average, approximately 70% of that of healthy individuals.[12] Multiple factors are responsible for reduced exercise tolerance and fatigue, such as deconditioning resulting from inactivity, cancer-related impaired skeletal muscle energy metabolism, anorexia, anemia, dehydration, skeletal muscle fiber atrophy, systemic inflammation, and cardiac dysfunction, many of which result from the multisystem detrimental effects of cancer or its treatments (surgery, chemotherapy, radiation therapy, hormonal therapy).[13]

The single best measure of cardiovascular function, health, and reserve is peak oxygen uptake (VO_2peak), also called cardiorespiratory fitness, measured from expiratory gas exchange during graded exercise to maximal effort (cardiopulmonary exercise testing).[14] Cardiorespiratory fitness is inversely related to cardiovascular risk. The survival benefit for each increase of 3.5 mL/kg/min in VO_2peak (1 metabolic equivalent of task [MET]) is 10% to 25%.[15] Exercise training after treatment for cancer generally results in improvement in exercise capacity with a reduction of dyspnea, deconditioning, and fatigue.[14] In studies that measured VO_2peak, the treatment effect was in the order of an increase of 3 to 5 mL/kg/min in peak VO_2. In addition, exercise training during breast cancer treatment results in an improvement in VO_2peak of 2 to 3 mL/kg/min.[14]

EXERCISE TRAINING IMPROVES PROGNOSIS FOR PATIENTS WITH CANCER AND EXERCISE GUIDELINES HAVE BEEN PUBLISHED BUT ARE NOT WIDELY FOLLOWED

The prognostic value of exercise training for clinical cardiovascular events in patients with cancer has recently been investigated. An analysis of two large prospective cohort studies in patients with breast cancer confirmed a strong, graded relationship between exercise training dose and the incidence of coronary artery disease and heart failure. Patients in the top tertile of physical activity (>24.5 MET-h per week) experienced a 30% to 37% reduction in cardiovascular endpoints.[16]

Exercise training guidelines have been formulated and published for patients with cancer and survivors but are achieved by less than one third of patients.[17] It is estimated that only 10% of patients are physically active during, and only 20% to 30% are active after, cancer treatment.[17]

CARDIO-ONCOLOGY REHABILITATION: PARTNERING WITH EXISTING CARDIAC REHABILITATION PROGRAMS TO IMPROVE SYMPTOMS, CARDIORESPIRATORY FITNESS, AND CARDIOVASCULAR HEALTH IN PATIENTS WITH CANCER

A system is needed that augments the usual clinical care of patients with cancer and provides guidance for exercise training and control of cardiovascular risk factors. Fortunately, such a system currently exists in the form of outpatient cardiac rehabilitation (CR) programs in North America.

Cardiac rehabilitation is defined as "the provision of comprehensive long-term services involving medical evaluation, prescriptive exercise, cardiac risk factor modification, and education, counseling, and behavior intervention."[18] The objectives of CR are to increase cardiorespiratory fitness, reduce angina symptoms, facilitate cardiovascular risk reduction, improve psychosocial well-being, reduce recurrent hospitalizations, and decrease morbidity and mortality from cardiovascular diseases.[19] Referral to CR is a class I American Heart Association/American College of Cardiology Foundation guideline recommendation for patients with acute coronary syndroms[20] and is a clinical performance measure.[21] Reimbursement for CR is available for patients with acute coronary syndromes, as well as for percutaneous coronary intervention, coronary artery bypass graft surgery, stable angina pectoris, lower extremity symptomatic peripheral artery disease, heart failure with reduced left ventricular ejection fraction, heart valve surgery, and heart transplantation.[22] Reimbursement for CR currently requires that CR services be provided in a medical facility (center-based program). Figure 34.1 provides an overview of the elements and outcomes of CR in patients with cancer and replace with the new reference for Fig. 34.1. It can be appreciated that CR is multidimensional and requires an interdisciplinary team approach that may include physicians, advanced practice providers, exercise physiologists, nurses, dietitians, physical therapists, psychologists, social workers, nicotine dependence counselors, and others, as needed.[23]

A 2019 American Heart Association scientific statement, endorsed by the American Cancer Society, provides a rationale for the use of CR to provide supervised exercise training and ancillary services to patients with cancer and survivors (Table 34.1).[24] The paper introduces the concept of cardio-oncology rehabilitation (CORE), which is the process of identifying those patients with cancer at high risk for cardiovascular pathology and the use of CR facilities and staff to address the unique clinical courses of patients with cancer. The scientific statement endorses the American Society of Clinical Oncology clinical practice guideline criteria for identifying patients at heightened cardiovascular risk[25]:

1. Treatment with high-dose anthracycline (e.g., doxorubicin ≥250 mg/m^2, epirubicin ≥600 mg/m^2), or high-dose radiotherapy ≥30 Gy when the heart is in the treatment field or lower-dose anthracycline in combination with lower-dose radiotherapy;
2. Treatment with lower-dose anthracycline or trastuzumab alone plus the presence of two or more cardiovascular risk factors (smoking, hypertension, diabetes mellitus, obesity, dyslipidemia), older age (>60 years) at cancer treatment, or compromised cardiac function (history of myocardial infarction, borderline or low left ventricular ejection fraction, moderate valvular disease); or
3. Treatment with lower-dose anthracycline followed by trastuzumab.

These criteria serve as a starting point for referral to CORE. The expertise of the cardiologist and oncologist is critically important in terms of evaluating the patient's underlying risk for treatment-related cardiovascular disease.[25] Pediatric patients should also be considered for CORE on the basis of prior high-risk exeposures.[26] The Central Illustration provides an algorithm for referral to CORE and oncology/cancer rehabilitation. The CORE algorithm is based on the patient's underlying risk of cardiac dysfunction, cardiac symptoms, or cardiovascular disease history,

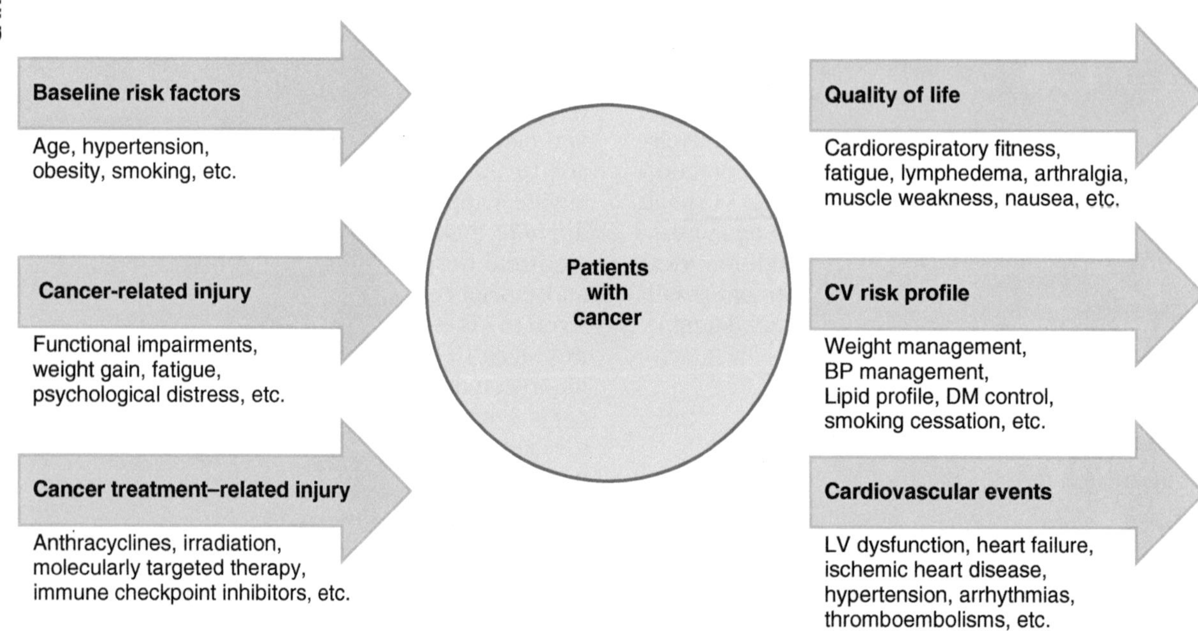

FIG. 34.1 Potential benefits of cardiac rehabilitation for patients with cancer. *BP,* Blood pressure; *CV,* cardiovascular; *DM,* diabetes mellitus; *LV,* left ventricular. (Modified from Sase K, Kida K, Furukawa Y. Cardio-oncology rehabilitation-challenges and opportunities to improve cardiovascular outcomes in patients with cancer and survivors. *J Cardiol.* Dec 2020;67(6):559–567.)

TABLE 34.1 **Studies of Exercise on Clinical and CVD Outcomes in Patients With Cancer in the Adjuvant and Postadjuvant Setting**

SETTING	CLINICAL OUTCOMES	CARDIOVASCULAR OUTCOMES
Adjuvant		
Breast	↓ CVD events ↓ CAD mortality	↑ ↔ ↓ CRF ↓ LVEF
Prostate		↑ CRF
Colorectal		↑ CRF
Mixed (meta-analysis)		↑ CRF
Postadjuvant		
Breast	↓ CVD events ↓ All-cause mortality	↔ ↑ CRF ↑ Vascular function
Prostate		↑ CRF ↑ Vascular function ↔ Lipid profile ↔ Blood pressure
ASCC	↓ CVD events ↓ All-cause mortality	
Testicular		↑ CRF ↑ Vascular function ↑ Framingham Risk Score
Colorectal	↓ All-cause mortality	↑ ↔ CRF
Leukemia		↑ CRF
Lymphoma		↑ CRF
Mixed (meta-analysis)		↑ CRF

Downward-pointing arrow (↓) indicates a decrease; upward-pointing arrow (↑) indicates an increase; and sideways-pointing arrow (↔) indicates no change. *ASCC,* Adult survivors of childhood cancer; *CAD,* coronary artery disease; *CRF,* cardiorespiratory fitness; *CVD,* cardiovascular disease; *LVEF,* left ventricle ejection fraction.

Reprinted with permission from Gilchrist SC, Barac A, Ades PA, et al. Cardio-oncology rehabilitation to manage cardiovascular outcomes in patients with cancer and survivors: a scientific statement from the American Heart Association. *Circulation*. 2019;139:e997–e1012 © 2019 American Heart Association, Inc.

and not by a specific point in the cancer continuum.[24] Thus, patients may enter CORE at the time of active treatment, in the survivorship setting, or at any time after a cancer diagnosis in patients with existing cardiovascular diseases or in those patients who develop cardiac symptoms. Referrals to CORE should arise from the treating provider (oncologist, internist, cardiologist).[24] For patients with treatment-related frailty; musculoskeletal, neurologic, or cognitive issues; and bone loss, referral to a physical medicine & rehabilitation specialist for cancer rehabilitation before starting CORE is recommended.

The CR model is eminently applicable to cancer care for several reasons: supervised exercise training with the goal of improving cardiorespiratory fitness and cardiovascular outcomes; measurement and modification/control of cardiovascular risk factors; individualized care for each patient in terms of exercise and medical therapy; and surveillance to communicate with providers regarding changes in patient status, such as symptoms and vital signs.[24]

Cardiac rehabilitation staff providing CORE will require additional knowledge to administer patient-specific exercise training based on each patient's health status, treatments received, and specific risks associated with cancer type.[24] Table 34.2 lists metrics to assess exercise training safety. The American College of Sports Medicine has developed a credentialing process for exercise physiologists who work with patients who have cancer: the Certified Cancer

Exercise Trainer.[13] Table 34.3 provides the traditional components of CR with cancer-specific considerations for CORE. Physicians and advanced practice providers should partner with an oncologist to provide critical components of the medical evaluation.

To date, six studies have investigated the feasibility and utility of the CR model for patients with cancer and survivors.[24] Investigators demonstrated that the CR model can improve cardiorespiratory fitness, skeletal muscular strength, and quality of life in cancer survivors.

Information for the development of an individualized exercise program for patients with cancer enrolled in CORE is provided in Chapter 13 and by Squires and colleagues.[13] Specific recommendations are given for the role of graded exercise testing for safety screening and guidance in exercise prescription, as well as for the following prescriptive exercise factors:

- Frequency of exercise sessions: 2 to 5 sessions/week.
- Intensity of effort: moderate to vigorous.
- Duration of training: 20 to 60 minutes per session.

TABLE 34.2 Safety Considerations for Exercise Training in CORE

NORMAL TESTING
CPET Resting BP ≤ 160/90 mm Hg[a] Normal BP response to exercise No inducible ischemia No atrial or ventricular arrhythmias Maintain normal O_2 saturations No symptoms[b]
6-min walk test Resting blood pressure ≤160/90 mm Hg[a] Maintain normal O_2 saturations
Laboratory studies Absence of severe anemia (<8.0 g/dL) Absolute neutrophil count > 500 mm Platelet count >50,000/μL
No Baseline Symptoms
Acute nausea during exercise Vomiting within 24 h Disorientation Blurred vision
Ongoing Cancer Complications
Acute infection Acute metabolic disease[c] New-onset lymphedema Mental or physical impairment to exercise Initial wound healing after surgery Bone or brain metastasis[d]
Displays Exercise Knowledge
Understands functions of aerobic and resistance equipment Demonstrates correct form on equipment Understands perceived exertion and heart rate goals; performs exercise accordingly

[a]If elevated, recheck after 5 minutes. If still elevated, then reschedule CPET after patient is seen by provider to adjust BP medications.
[b]Symptoms, such as dyspnea, chest pain, or dizziness, or other cardiac symptoms during exercise deemed abnormal by supervising physician.
[c]Examples include abnormal thyroid function, uncontrolled diabetes mellitus, and electrolyte abnormalities.
[d]For patients with bone or brain metastases, a plan in CORE needs to include a consultation with oncology rehabilitation to establish a patient-specific safe exercise plan.
BP, Blood pressure; *CORE,* cardio-oncology rehabilitation; *CPET,* cardiopulmonary exercise testing.

TABLE 34.3 **Components of Cardiac Rehabilitation (CR) With Cancer-Specific CORE Features**

CR	CORE
Patient assessment	Review cancer therapies and potential side effects Assess health conditions impairing exercise Assess for lymphedema, ostomy, and infection risks Review for metastatic disease, presence/stage, and readiness for exercise vs. cancer rehabilitation if bony metastasis Review complete blood cell count Screen for depression, fatigue, and quality of life Perform cardiopulmonary assessment
Nutrition counseling	Cancer-specific nutritional recommendations (e.g., National Comprehensive Cancer Network) Involve dietitians who specialize in cancer
Weight management	Assess weight management issues—weight loss, loss of lean muscle mass, and gain in fat mass—that are cancer specific Tailor aerobic and resistance training accordingly
BP management	Review chemotherapeutic agents and molecularly targeted drugs causing hypertension, such as VEGF signaling pathway inhibitors Appropriately screen and reassess for those on active therapy
Lipid/lipoprotein management	Primary CVD prevention setting: ACC and AHA cholesterol guidelines for lipid management, which recommend statin therapy for CVD risk score ≥7.5% over a 10-year period Recognize setting when CVD risk score not valid
Diabetes mellitus management	Recognize chemotherapeutic agents that worsen glucose control
Tobacco cessation	Provide referral to smoking cessation program within cancer center
Psychosocial management	Develop referral network of social work and mental health professionals who support the care and treatment of patients with cancer
PA counseling	Emphasize the health risks of prolonged periods of sitting: goal is an increase in habitual lifestyle PA and a decrease in sedentary time
Exercise training	Aerobic and resistance exercise training prescription based on ACSM guidelines specific to patients with cancer Supervised exercise training in the CORE setting Incorporation of behavioral change strategies demonstrated effective for patients with cancer and survivors

ACC, American College of Cardiology; *ACSM,* American College of Sports Medicine; *AHA,* American Heart Association; *BP,* blood pressure; *CORE,* cardio-oncology rehabilitation; *CR,* cardiac rehabilitation; *CVD,* cardiovascular disease; *PA,* physical activity; and *VEGF,* vascular endothelial growth factor.
Reprinted with permission from Gilchrist SC, Barac A, Ades PA, et al. Cardio-oncology rehabilitation to manage cardiovascular outcomes in patients with cancer and survivors: a scientific statement from the American Heart Association. *Circulation.* 2019;139:e997–e1012.

- Types of exercise modalities: aerobic-walk, cycle, treadmill, etc.
- Progression of the dose of exercise: gradual increase to 150+ minutes/week of moderate intensity or 75+ minutes/week of vigorous intensity aerobic activity.
- Resistance exercise: 2 to 3 sessions/week; weight machines or free weights, elastic bands, etc., at a moderate level of effort.

CORE is a very new concept in the care of patients with cancer and, as such, presents considerable obstacles to be overcome for widespread implementation to occur. Unlike traditional CR performed in a medical facility, with third-party reimbursement for multiple cardiovascular diagnoses discussed previously, no reimbursement strategy is available to provide access for patients with cancer without a covered cardiovascular diagnosis to comprehensive CORE within the CR model.[24] In addition, existing CR program staff will require additional training in cancer-specific issues and the development of partnerships with oncologists and cardio-oncology trained cardiologists wherever possible. There are geographic variations in the distribution of CR programs in the United States and access to a program at a reasonable distance from home may pose a barrier to entry. New models for the delivery of CR services are being evaluated. In particular, CR-based components similar to those provided by center-based programs in locations more convenient and accessible to patients (in the patient's home or a local exercise facility with periodic contact with CR staff) appear attractive, but reimbursement is not currently available for CR services provided outside of a medical facility for patients with either cardiovascular diseases or cancer.[23,24]

Current knowledge gaps for CORE will require research in the following areas[24]:

1. Development of an evidence base for CORE with communication of the benefits to patients and families, clinicians, health systems, payers, and employers;
2. Demonstrate which patients are likely to benefit, including improved economic outcomes;
3. Identify the most effective and efficient models for delivery of CORE;
4. Test the impact of CORE on cardiac-specific outcomes in patients with cancer;
5. Create automatic or opt-out referral systems and stratify participation by cancer type, stage, and cardiovascular risk level to ensure participation by all who can benefit; and
6. Define and test the effects of embedding a small set of metrics in quality reporting.

SUMMARY

Patients with cancer are at increased risk for the development of coronary artery disease and heart failure owing to the effects of cancer treatments and the presence of cardiovascular risk factors. Exercise capacity is below normal and fatigue is a common and persistent problem for many patients. Exercise training reduces symptoms, improves quality of life, and reduces cardiovascular events. Despite publication of exercise training guidelines for patients with cancer, most patients are not physically active. The concept of cardio-oncology rehabilitation has recently been introduced. CORE proposes the use of existing cardiac rehabilitation programs to identify appropriate patients and to provide supervised exercise training and cardiovascular risk factor control. For widespread implementation of CORE to occur, the development of a robust evidence base and a reimbursement strategy is needed. In the future, efforts might advance to move from rehabilitation to prehabilitation and panhabilitation, as patients with cancer progress through the continuum of cancer care.

REFERENCES

1. https://cancercontrol.cancer.gov/ocs/statistics/statistics.html
2. Hooning MJ, Botma A, Aleman BM, et al. Long term risk of cardiovascular disease in 10-year survivors of breast cancer. *J Natl Cancer Inst.* 2007;99:365–375.
3. Chow EJ, Mueller BA, Baker KS, et al. Cardiovascular hospitalizations and mortality among recipients of hematopoietic stem cell transplantation. *Ann Intern Med.* 2011;155:21–32.
4. Baker KS, Ness KK, Steinberger J, et al. Diabetes, hypertension, and cardiovascular events in survivors of hematopoietic stem cell transplantation: a report from the Bone Marrow Transplantations Survivor Study. *Blood.* 2007;109:1765–1772.
5. Al-Kindi SG, Oliviera GH. Prevalence of preexisting cardiovascular disease in patients with different types of cancer: the unmet need for onco-cardiology. *Mayo Clin Proc.* 2016;91:81–83.
6. Koene RJ, Prizment AE, Blaes A, Konety SH. Shared risk factors in cardiovascular disease and cancer. *Circulation.* 2016;133: 1104–1114.
7. Hoffman M, Ryan JL, Figueroa-Mosley CD, et al. Cancer-related fatigue: the scale of the problem. *Oncologist.* 2007;12 (suppl 1):4–10.
8. Doyle JJ, Neugut AI, Jacobson JS, et al. Chemotherapy and cardiotoxicity in older breast patients with cancer: a population-based study. *J Clin Oncol.* 2005;23:8597–8605.
9. Perez EA, Suman VJ, Davidson NE, et al. Cardiac safety analysis of doxorubicin and cyclophosphamide followed by paclitazel with or without trastuzumab in the North Central Cancer Treatment Group N9831 adjuvant breast cancer trial. *J Clin Oncol.* 2008;26:1231–1238.
10. Darby SC, Ewertz M, McGale P, et al. Risk of ischemic heart disease in women after radiotherapy for breast cancer. *N Engl J Med.* 2013; 368:987–998.
11. Armenian SH, Xu L, Ky B, et al. Cardiovascular disease among survivors of adult-onset cancer: a community-based retrospective cohort study. *J Clin Oncol.* 2016;34:1122–1130.
12. Kenjale AA, Hornsby WE, Crowgey T, et al. Pre-exercise participation cardiovascular screening in a heterogenous cohort of adult patients with cancer. *Oncologist.* 2014;19:999–1005.
13. Squires RW, Shultz AM, Hermann J. Exercise training and cardiovascular health in patients with cancer. *Curr Oncol Rep.* 2018;20: 27–47.
14. Squires RW. Physical activity and exercise in cardiovascular prevention and rehabilitation. In: Yusuf S, Camm AJ, Fallen EL, Gersh B, eds. *Evidence Based Cardiology.* 3rd ed. Oxford: Wiley-Blackwell; 2010: pp. 190–200.
15. Ross R, Blair SN, Arena R, et al. Importance of assessing cardiorespiratory fitness in clinical practice: a case for fitness as a vital sign: a scientific statement from the American Heart Association. *Circulation.* 2016;134:e653–e699.
16. Jones LW, Habel LA, Weltzien E, et al. Exercise and risk of cardiovascular events in women with nonmetastatic breast cancer. *J Clin Oncol.* 2016;34:2743–2749.
17. Rock CL, Doyle C, Demark-Wahnefried W, et al. Nutrition and physical activity guidelines for cancer survivors. *CA Cancer J Clin.* 2012;62:243–274.
18. Wenger NK, Froelicher ES, Smith LK, et al. Cardiac rehabilitation as secondary prevention. Agency for Health Care Policy and Research and National Heart, Lung, and Blood Institute. *Clin Pract Guide Quick Ref Guide Clin.* 1995;52:1–23.
19. Franklin BA, Brinks J. Cardiac rehabilitation: underrecognized/ underutilized. *Curr Treat Options Cardio Med.* 2015;17:62.
20. Smith SC Jr, Benjamin EJ, Bonow RO, et al. AHA/ACCF secondary prevention and risk reduction therapy for patients with coronary and other atherosclerotic vascular disease: 2011 update: a guideline from the American Heart Association and American College of

Cardiology Foundation [published correction appears in Circulation 2015; 131:e408]. *Circulation.* 2011;124:2458–2473.

21. Thomas RJ, King M, Lui K, et al. AACVPR/ACCF/AHA 2010 update: performance measures on cardiac rehabilitation for referral to cardiac rehabilitation/secondary prevention services: a report of the American Association of Cardiovascular and Pulmonary Rehabilitation and the American College of Cardiology Foundation/American Heart Association Task Force on performance measures (Writing Committee to Develop Clinical Performance Measures for Cardiac Rehabilitation). *Circulation.* 2010;122:1342–1350.
22. Squires RW, Leth SE, Swere K, Thomas RJ. Standardizing outpatient cardiac rehabilitation practices in a large multistate medical system: a practice convergence project. *J Cardiopulm Rehabil.* 2019;3:124–128.
23. Thomas RJ, Beatty AL, Beckie TM, et al. AACVPR/AHA/ACC Scientific Statement: Home-based cardiac rehabilitation: a scientific statement from the American Association of Cardiovascular and Pulmonary Rehabilitation, the American Heart Association, and the American College of Cardiology. *Circulation.* 2019;140: e69–e89.
24. Gilchrist SC, Barac A, Ades PA, et al. Cardio-oncology rehabilitation to manage cardiovascular outcomes in patients with cancer and survivors: a scientific statement from the American Heart Association. *Circulation.* 2019;139:e997–e1012.
25. Armenian SH, Lacchetti C, Barac A, et al. Prevention and monitoring of cardiac dysfunction in survivors of adult cancers: American Society of Clinical Oncology clinical practice guideline. *J Clin Oncol.* 2017;35:893–911.
26. Berkman AM, Lakoski SG. Treatment, behavioral, and psychosocial components of cardiovascular disease risk among survivors of childhood and young adult cancer. *J Am Heart Assoc.* 2015;4: e001891.

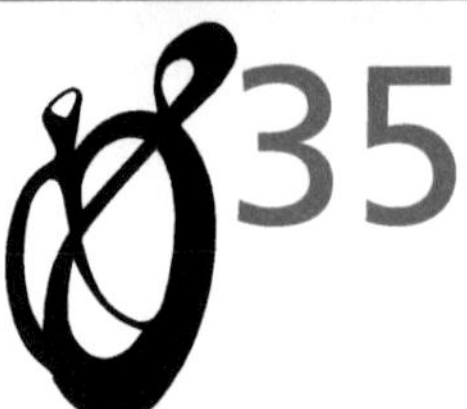

35 Breast Cancer

KATHRYN J. RUDDY AND PAUL V. VISCUSE

	Stage I	Stage II	Stage III	Stage IV
Stages	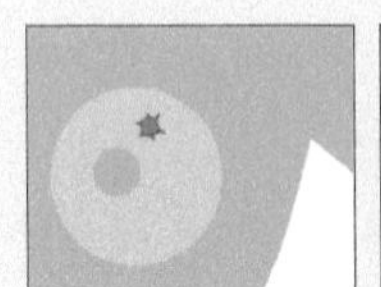	 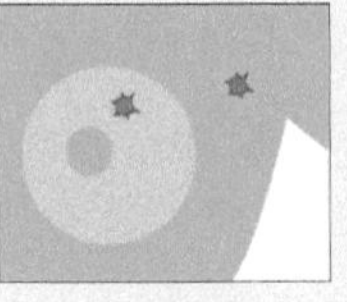	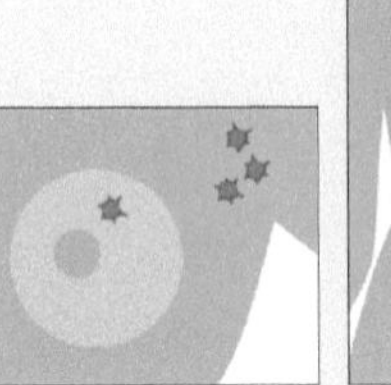	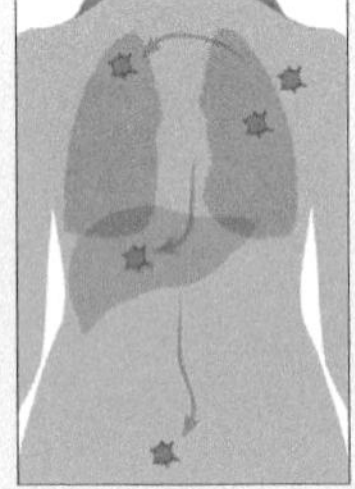
	Tumor in breast and/or regional lymph nodes but not in the rest of the body (standardly treated with curative intent)			Spread outside the breast and regional lymph nodes
Treatment	**Surgery** +/– radiation (usually recommended after lumpectomy, and sometimes offered after mastectomy if tumor is large and/or node-positive; fields depend on size/lymph node status) +/– neoadjuvant/adjuvan chemo (often 2–3 drugs concurrently; more likely recommended if tumor is HER2+, ER–, of high grade) +/– neoadjuvant/adjuvan endocrine tx (standard if tumor is ER+) +/– neoadjuvant/adjuvan trastuzumab (nearly always if HER2+)			Usually no surgery or radiation unless needed for palliation Systemic therapy is mainstay • Chemotherapy (often single agents in sequence) • Endocrine therapy (if ER+) • HER2-directed therapy (if HER2+) • Other targeted therapies (e.g., PARP inhibitors)
Prognosis	5-year survival 99%–100%	5-year survival 90%–99%	5-year survival 66%–98%	5-year survival 20%–25%

Potential CV toxicities

Radiation: coronary, valvular heart disease, pericarditis, cardiomyopathy, heart failure, arrhythmias

Chemotherapies:
- **Anthracyclines:** heart failure, asymptomatic cardiac function decline
- **Taxane:** arrhythmias (sinus bradycardia, conduction blocks), ischemia
- **Capecitabine:** acute coronary syndrome, variant angina, arrhythmias
- **Platinum:** angina, arterial and venous thrombotic events, hypertension

Endocrine therapies:
- Ovarian function suppression and surgical menopause may accelerate CV aging
- Tamoxifen seems to be associated with less hyperlipidemia and CAD than aromatase inhibitor

Trastuzumab: heart failure, asymptomatic cardiac function decline

PARP inhibitor: hyperlipidemia, hypertension, palpitations

CDK4/6 inhibitor: interstitial lung disease, pneumonitis; ribociclib: QTc prolongation

mTOR inhibitor: hypertension, arterial and venous thrombotic events, arrhythmias; interstitial lung disease, pneumonitis

CHAPTER OUTLINE

KEY POINTS

- Most common female cancer
- Median age at diagnosis is 62 years[1]
- Risk factors for breast cancer include increased age, early age at menarche, late age at first birth, late age at menopause, family history, *BRCA1/BRCA2* genes, alcohol use, hormone replacement therapy, and atypical hyperplasia on biopsy[2]
- Early stage disease has 5-year overall survival of approximately 90%; stage IV metastatic disease has 5-year overall survival of approximately 30%[3]
- Treatment varies based on stage, expression of human epidural growth factor 2 (HER2), expression of estrogen receptors or progesterone receptors (ER/PR), and presence of deleterious *BRCA* genes
- Radiation and systemic agents used in the treatment of breast cancer are associated with increased risk for various cardiovascular diseases

INCIDENCE

Approximately 200,000 new cases of breast cancer are discovered each year, which accounts for 15% of all new cancer cases (99% of which are in women, making this the most common female cancer). The incidence of localized disease is 62%, regional disease 31%, and 6% distant metastasis.[3] More than 3 million survivors of breast cancer are living in the United States.[1]

RISK FACTORS

Increased age is the largest risk factor; one-quarter of breast cancers occur in premenopausal women. Earlier age at menarche, later age at first birth, and later age at menopause place women at higher risk. Genetic risks for breast cancer include deleterious *BRCA* mutations and women are also at increased risk if they have a mother or sister with breast cancer. Other risk factors include hormone replacement therapy, alcohol use, breast density on mammography, and a history of a benign breast biopsy, especially if atypical hyperplasia. Use of contraceptive pills may also increase risk.[2]

PROGNOSIS

Approximately 41,000 deaths in 2018 were from breast cancer, representing 7% of all cancer deaths. Disease confined to the breast and/or regional lymph nodes has an estimated 5-year survival of approximately 90%. Metastasis outside the breast and regional lymph nodes has an estimated 5-year survival of approximately 30%.[3]

TREATMENT OVERVIEW

The treatment of breast cancer varies based on the stage at presentation and if the tumor overexpresses HER2neu receptor (HER2), estrogen receptor (ER), and/or progesterone receptor (PR). Patients with stage I–III disease (confined to the breast and/or regional lymph nodes) are typically treated with either breast-conserving surgery or mastectomy, with axillary lymph node sampling (often by sentinel node biopsy). Breast-conserving surgery generally requires subsequent radiation, whereas postmastectomy radiation is considered if tumor size more than 5 cm, surgical margins less than 1 mm, and/or regional nodal involvement. Chemotherapy is sometimes utilized in the neoadjuvant setting (before surgery) with or without adjuvant therapy (after surgery). For HER2-negative tumors, chemotherapy often includes combination therapy with cyclophosphamide plus either anthracycline or taxane (or both). For HER2-positive tumors, HER2-targeted agent(s) (e.g., trastuzumab, pertuzumab) are added to one of the following regimens: (1) anthracycline/cyclophosphamide followed or preceded by a taxane; (2) carboplatin with a taxane; or (3) taxane monotherapy (for small, node-negative tumors). Neoadjuvant chemotherapy is often offered if surgical staging information is not needed to inform the chemotherapy decision. Adjuvant chemotherapy can be offered if there is a poor response to neoadjuvant chemotherapy or if neoadjuvant chemotherapy was not given but is deemed to be potentially useful. Endocrine therapy is used, typically in the adjuvant setting, if the tumor is ER/PR positive. The treatment regimen is 5 to 10 years of an estrogen receptor antagonist (tamoxifen) or an aromatase inhibitor (e.g., letrozole, anastrozole, exemestane). Aromatase inhibitors are only effective in women without ovarian hormonal production. Premenopausal women at higher risk of recurrence may be offered bilateral salpingo-oophorectomy or ovarian function suppression with a gonadotropin-releasing hormone agonist (e.g., leuprolide, triptorelin, or goserelin) to allow treatment with aromatase inhibitor (which is slightly more effective than tamoxifen at reducing the risk of recurrence) or to improve the efficacy of tamoxifen.[4]

Patients with stage IV metastatic disease are generally treated with systemic therapy as opposed to surgery and radiation. For ER-positive and HER2-negative tumors without visceral crisis, multiple sequential lines of endocrine therapy are usually used to control disease as long as possible before chemotherapy is needed. Cyclin-dependent kinase (CDK) 4/6 inhibitors and mammalian target of rapamycin (mTOR) inhibitors are two classes of targeted therapies that are sometimes combined with endocrine therapies to increase time to progression on a given line of treatment. In patients with a deleterious *BRCA* mutation, olaparib, a polyadenosine 5-diphosphoribose polymerase (PARP) inhibitor, has been shown to be an effective targeted monotherapy by inducing synthetic lethality through the formation of double-stranded DNA breaks that cannot be accurately repaired due to *BRCA1/BRCA2* deficiency. For ER-negative, chemotherapy is used to control disease, and most patients are treated with multiple drugs sequentially over time, switching from one to another whenever disease progresses or intolerable side effects develop. Chemotherapy options include, but are not limited to, anthracyclines, taxanes, capecitabine, vinca alkaloids, platinums, and cyclophosphamide. Single agents are often administered (rather than combining multiple drugs) to minimize toxicities. HER2-targeted therapy (e.g., trastuzumab, pertuzumab, lapatinib) should be combined with endocrine therapy or chemotherapy in patients with HER2-positive disease.[4]

CARDIOVASCULAR RISK

Left breast and chest wall radiation therapy has been associated with a number of effects on the cardiovascular system. Coronary artery disease, the most common form of cardiac injury, involves complicated lesions typically involving the left anterior descending artery; it is typically noted years after radiation treatment. Pericarditis has been noted on acute presentation within weeks of radiation. Valvular disease had been seen many years after radiation with older regimens and most commonly has involved mixed stenosis and regurgitation of the aortic valve. However, this has become very rare with the standard doses presently administered for breast cancer. Heart failure with preserved ejection fraction can occur secondary to diastolic dysfunction from radiation-induced restrictive cardiomyopathy and may progress to systolic heart failure. Conduction system abnormalities may include a variety of arrhythmias and conduction blocks, but they are rarely clinically significant.[5–7]

Various chemotherapeutic agents commonly used in the treatment of breast cancer have been associated with various cardiovascular outcomes. Use of anthracycline chemotherapy (e.g., doxorubicin, daunorubicin, epirubicin, idarubicin) can lead to congestive heart failure or asymptomatic decline in left-ventricular ejection fraction. This can occur within the first year of treatment, but has also been described 10 to 20 years after treatment.[8] Taxanes (paclitaxel, docetaxel) have been associated with arrhythmias, such as sinus bradycardia and various conduction blocks, but these are rare and usually clinically insignificant (resolving with completion of therapy).[9] Capecitabine (fluoropyrimidines) use may result in acute coronary syndromes, variant angina, or asymptomatic electrocardiogram changes. Angiography is usually unrevealing, but vasospasm can be noted with variable nitroglycerin response.[9,10] Platinum-based therapy (i.e., cisplatin, carboplatin) has been associated with angina, acute myocardial infarction, hypertension, cardiomyopathy, and congestive heart failure.[9]

Increased cholesterol levels, hypertension, and palpitations have been noted with PARP inhibitor therapy.[11,12] Endocrine therapy with tamoxifen may be protective against hyperlipidemia and hypertension, whereas early menopause owing to salpingo-oophorectomy or use of medical ovarian function suppression may increase the risk of cardiovascular disease.[13] Congestive heart failure and asymptomatic left-ventricular ejection fraction decline may result from HER2-targeted therapy with trastuzumab.[14,15]

REFERENCES

1. Noone AM, Howlader N, Krapcho M, et al., eds. *SEER Cancer Statistics Review, 1975–2015*. Bethesda, MD: National Cancer Institute; 2018. Available at: https://seer.cancer.gov/csr/1975_2015/.
2. Clemons M, Goss P. Estrogen and the risk of breast cancer. *N Engl J Med*. 2001;344(4):276–285.
3. Siegel R, Miller K, Jemal A. Cancer statistics, 2019. *CA Cancer J Clin*. 2019;69:7–34.
4. National Comprehensive Cancer Network. *Breast Cancer* (Version 1.2018). Available at: https://www.nccn.org/professionals/physician_gls/pdf/breast.pdf. Accessed November 13, 2018.
5. Darby S, Ewertz M, McGale P, et al. Risk of ischemic heart disease in women after radiotherapy for breast cancer. *N Engl J Med*. 2013;368(11):987–998.
6. Darby S, Cutter D, Boerma M, et al. Radiation-related heart disease: current knowledge and future prospects. *Int J Radiat Oncol Biol Phys*. 2010;76(3):656–665.
7. Cuomo J, Sharma G, Conger P, Weintraub N. Novel concepts in radiation-induced cardiovascular disease. *World J Cardiol*. 2016;8(9):504.
8. McGowan J, Chung R, Maulik A, Piotrowska I, Walker J, Yellon D. Anthracycline chemotherapy and cardiotoxicity. *Cardiovasc Drugs Ther*. 2017;31(1):63–75.
9. Rosa G, Gigli L, Tagliasacchi M, et al. Update on cardiotoxicity of anti-cancer treatments. *Eur J Clin Invest*. 2016;46(3):264–284.
10. Layoun M, Wickramasinghe C, Peralta M, Yang E. Fluoropyrimidine-induced cardiotoxicity: manifestations, mechanisms, and management. *Curr Oncol Rep*. 2016;18(6):35
11. Swisher E, Lin K, Oza A, et al. Rucaparib in relapsed, platinum-sensitive high-grade ovarian carcinoma (ARIEL2 Part 1): an international, multicentre, open-label, phase 2 trial. *Lancet Oncol*. 2017;18(1):75–87.
12. Mirza M, Monk B, Herrstedt J, et al. Niraparib maintenance therapy in platinum-sensitive, recurrent ovarian cancer. *N Engl J Med*. 2016;375(22):2154–2164.
13. Khosrow-Khavar F, Filion K, Al-Qurashi S, et al. Cardiotoxicity of aromatase inhibitors and tamoxifen in post-menopausal women with breast cancer: a systematic review and meta-analysis of randomized controlled trials. *Ann Oncol*. 28(3);2016:487–496.
14. Suter T, Cook-Bruns N, Barton C. Cardiotoxicity associated with trastuzumab (Herceptin) therapy in the treatment of metastatic breast cancer. *The Breast*. 2004;13(3):173–183.
15. Tocchetti C, Ragone G, Coppola C, et al. Detection, monitoring, and management of trastuzumab-induced left ventricular dysfunction: an actual challenge. *Eur J Heart Fail*. 2012;14(2):130–137.

36 Gynecologic Malignancies

MEGHAN SHEA, SARA BOUBERHAN, AND STEPHEN A. CANNISTRA

Endometrial cancer

Stages	**Stage I** Tumor confined to uterus	**Stage II** Tumor invades cervix	**Stage III** Tumor invades serosa or adnexa or regional LN	**Stage IV** Invades adjacent organs or distant metastases
Treatment	• Often surgery alone	• Surgery • External beam pelvic radiation • Vaginal brachytherapy	• Surgery • Radiation to pelvis and involved LNs with cisplatin, then 4 cycles caroplatin/ paclitaxel	• Palliative chemotherapy: Cisplatin/paclitaxel • Pembrolizumab if MSI high
Prognosis	5-year survival 95%	5-year survival 95%	5-year survival 70%	5-year survival 20%
Potential CV toxicities		Local radiation side effects	**Liposomal doxorubicin:** cardiomyopathy and heart failure **Cisplatin:** arterial and venous thrombotic events, arrhythmias, electrolyte wasting, potential for volume overload, hypertension **Paclitaxel:** bradycardia, ischemia, hypotension, flushing **Immune checkpoint inhibitors:** myocarditis, cardiomypathy, pericarditis, arrhythmias, vasculitis, ischemic events	

FIGO Staging System for Endometrial (Uterine) Cancer and Treatment by Stage. FIGO, International Federation of Gynecology and Obstetrics; LN, lymph node; MSI, microsatellite instability; CV, cardiovascular; VO, volume overload.

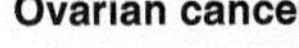

Ovarian cancer

Stages	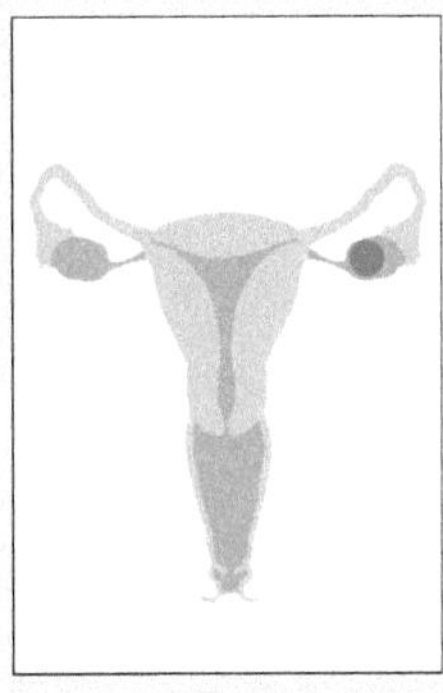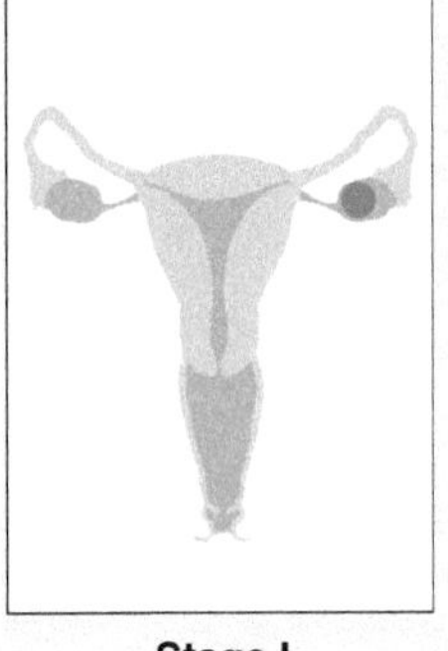 **Stage I** Tumor confined to ovary	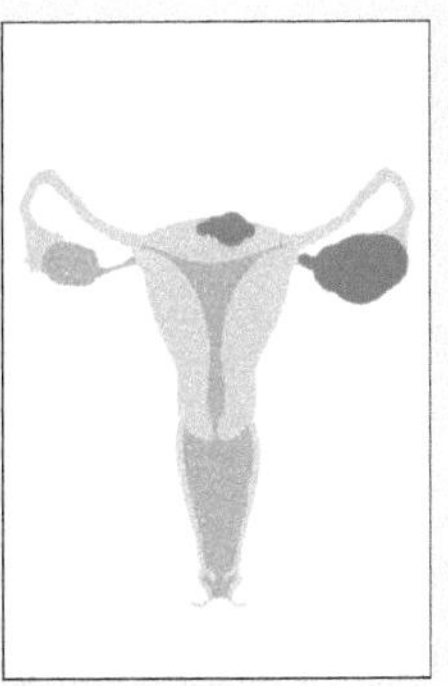 **Stage II** Tumor spreads within the pelvis	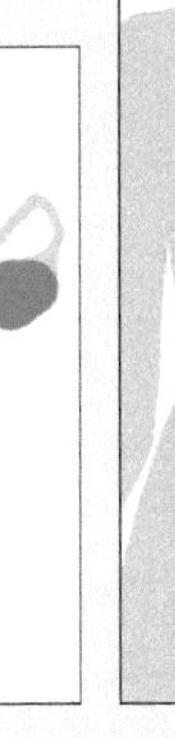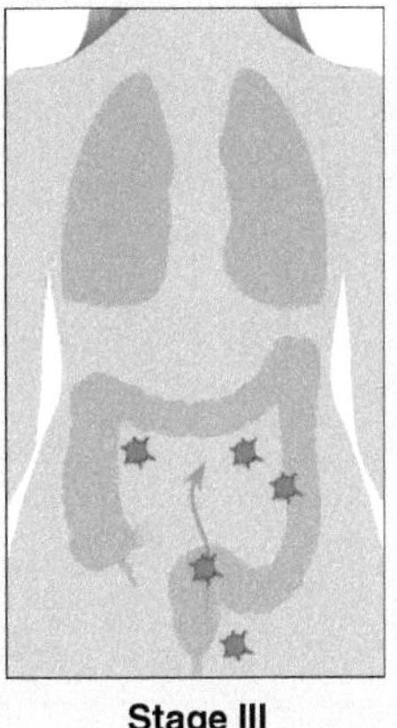 **Stage III** Tumor involves LN or extrapelvic peritoneum	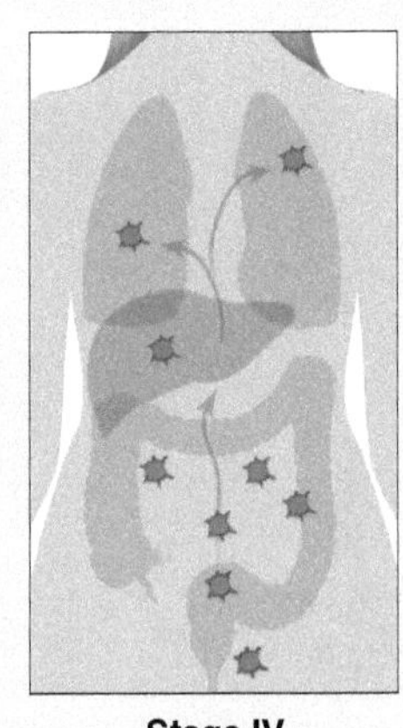 **Stage IV** Distant metastases
Treatment	• Surgery ± carboplatin and paclitaxel	• Surgery • Carboplatin/ paclitaxel	• Surgery • Carboplatin/ paclitaxel ± bevacizumab	• Surgery • Carboplatin/ paclitaxel ± bevacizumab
Prognosis	5-year survival 95%	5-year survival 80%	5-year survival 10%–30%	5-year survival <10%
Potential CV toxicities	**Carboplatin:** arterial and venous thrombotic events, arrhythmias, electrolyte wasting, potential for volume overload, hypertension **Paclitaxel:** bradycardia, ischemia, hypotension, flushing (less common than with cisplatin) **Bevacizumab:** hypertension, arterial and venous thrombotic events, bleeding, cardiomyopathy **Niraparib:** hypertension, arrhythmia, palpiations			

Continued

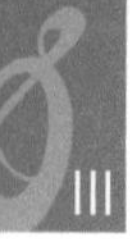

Cervical cancer

Stages	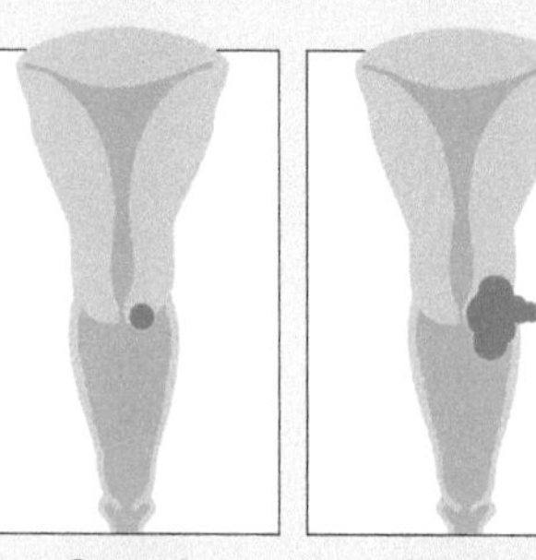 **Stage I** Tumor confined to cervix	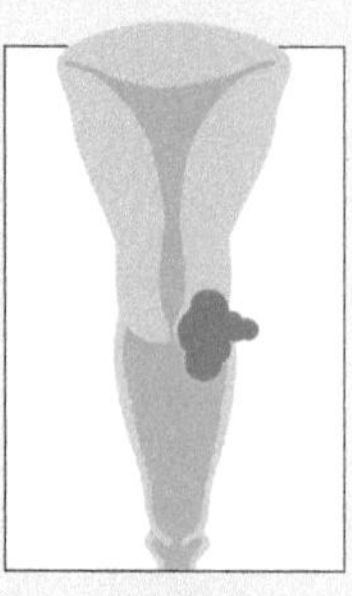 **Stage II** Tumor invades beyond cervix	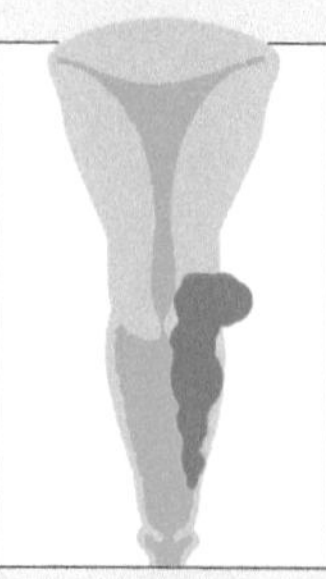 **Stage III** Tumor invades pelvic sidewall or regional LN	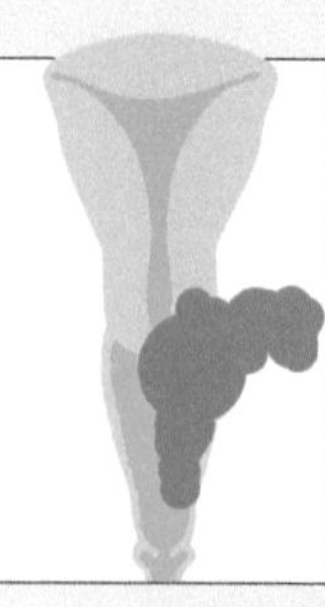 **Stage IV** Invades adjacent organs or distant metastases
Treatment	Surgery	Concurrent radiation and cisplatin chemotherapy	Concurrent radiation and cisplatin chemotherapy	Palliative chemotherapy (cisplatin/paclitaxel/ bevacizumab)
Prognosis	5-year survival 95%	5-year survival 85%	5-year survival 50%–60%	5-year survival 15%–20%
Potential CV toxicities	**Cisplatin:** arterial and venous thrombotic events, arrhythmias, electrolyte wasting, potential for volume overload, hypertension **Paclitaxel:** bradycardia, ischemia, hypotension, flushing **Bevacizumab:** hypertension, arterial and venous thrombotic events, bleeding, cardiomyopathy			

CHAPTER OUTLINE

ENDOMETRIAL CANCER

KEY POINTS ABOUT ENDOMETRIAL CANCER

- Most common gynecologic malignancy
- Median age at diagnosis is 62 years.
- Risk factors for typical endometrioid histology include obesity, younger age at menarche, family history, and exogenous estrogen exposure.
- Most patients (67%) present with early-stage disease.
- Treatment strategy and prognosis vary based on stage at presentation.
- Treatment is typically well tolerated from a cardiovascular standpoint.

Incidence

Approximately 63,230 new cases of cancer of the uterus (commonly of the endometrium, excluding cancers of the cervix) were reported in 2018.[1] Endometrial cancer incidence is rising, and mortality rates have not decreased.[2] It is most common in postmenopausal women, and the incidence increases with age, reaching 1 in 75 women by the eighth decade.[1]

Risk Factors

The incidence of endometrial cancer increases with age and is uncommon in women under age 40. In general, factors that increase exposure of estrogen, including obesity, younger age at menarche, late menopause, and nulliparity will increase the risk of developing endometrial cancer.[2,3] Additional risk factors include prior tamoxifen use (usually in the adjuvant setting for breast cancer), hypertension, diabetes mellitus, and Lynch syndrome (also known as hereditary nonpolyposis colorectal cancer).[3]

Prognosis

Patients with localized uterine cancer have a 94.9% 5-year survival. For those with regional spread to lymph nodes at the time of diagnosis, 5-year survival is estimated to be 68.6%. Unfortunately, the survival drops off dramatically for those with metastatic disease to 16.3% at 5 years.

Treatment Overview

The treatment for endometrial cancer varies based on the stage at presentation.[4] The endometrioid histology is the most common type of endometrial cancer, and its treatment is discussed below. Of note, rarer histologic subtypes of endometrial cancer can require alternative treatment strategies. Patients with stage IA disease (invasion to <50% of the myometrium) without other risk factors are often treated with surgery alone, and most patients will be cured without additional treatment.[5] Patients with more locally advanced disease that has not extended outside of the uterus (i.e., stages IB-II) are often treated with adjuvant radiation following surgery to decrease their risk of recurrent disease.[6] Patients with stage III disease often receive postoperative adjuvant radiation and chemotherapy, such as external beam radiation therapy with concurrent cisplatin as a radiation sensitizer, followed by carboplatin and paclitaxel.[7]

Patients presenting with metastatic disease are often treated with chemotherapy, typically carboplatin and paclitaxel, based on its efficacy and tolerability.[8] Carboplatin alternatively can be combined with liposomal doxorubicin.[9] Topotecan[10] and the antiangiogenic drug bevacizumab, which is a humanized monoclonal antibody against vascular endothelial growth factor (VEGF),[11] also have activity as single agents. Recent studies support the use of immune checkpoint inhibitors in tumors with high microsatellite instability (MSI-H), including endometrial cancers.[12,13] In this regard, the US Food and Drug Administration (FDA) has granted accelerated approval to the immune checkpoint inhibitor pembrolizumab for treatment of MSI high tumors of any histologic type that has progressed after standard therapy.

Cardiovascular Risk

Systemic treatments for endometrial cancer are typically well tolerated from a cardiovascular perspective. The drug-specific toxicities for the most commonly used antineoplastic agents (carboplatin, paclitaxel, liposomal doxorubicin, and pembrolizumab) are discussed below.

OVARIAN CANCER

KEY POINTS ABOUT OVARIAN CANCER

- Rare cancer with high mortality
- Median age at diagnosis is 63 years.

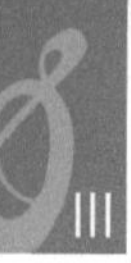

- Strongest risk factor is family history of ovarian or breast cancer.[14]
- Majority of patient have advanced disease at diagnosis (stage III or IV).
- Given the high risk of recurrence, patients often are treated with multiple lines of chemotherapy.
- Bevacizumab carries significant cardiovascular risks—hypertension, arterial or venous thromboembolism (Table 36.1).

Incidence

Ovarian cancer most often presents at an advanced stage with widespread disease within the peritoneum and/or distant metastases. High-grade serous carcinoma is the most common histology. The staging is determined surgically. In the United States in 2018, there were approximately 22,240 new cases of ovarian cancer diagnosed and 14,070 ovarian cancer deaths.[1] After endometrial cancer, it is the second most common gynecologic malignancy, but also the most lethal, owing to the fact that it presents at an advanced stage in the majority of patients. The median age at diagnosis is 63 years; it is most often diagnosed in women between 55 and 64 years.[1]

Risk Factors

The strongest clinical risk factor is a family history of ovarian or breast cancer, which may be a surrogate for germline mutation in high-risk genes such as *BRCA1* or *BRCA2*. In particular, women with a genetic predisposition, such as known carriers of *BRCA1/2* mutation or mutations in mismatch repair genes (Lynch syndrome) have the highest risk of developing this disease.[14] The US Preventive Services Task Forces currently recommends against routine screening for ovarian cancer,[15] although the role of screening continues to be evaluated, especially in women with a genetic predisposition. In that regard, for women with a known germline mutation that predisposes to a high risk of developing ovarian cancer (e.g., mutation in either *BRCA1* or *BRCA2*), a prophylactic bilateral oophorectomy is recommended once childbearing is complete.[16–18] Other risk factors include increasing age, polycystic ovarian syndrome,[19] infertility,[20] and endometriosis[21] (specifically for clear cell, endometrioid and low grade histology).

Prognosis

5-Year survival prognosis is 92.3% for patients with stage I ovarian cancer and 74% for those with stage II disease. In comparison, patients presenting with advanced disease fair much worse with 29.2% 5-year survival rate.

Treatment Overview

Given the recurrence rate of ovarian cancer, patients often receive multiple lines of chemotherapy. As seen in the central illustration, patients undergo upfront cytoreductive surgery followed by adjuvant chemotherapy with a platinum-based doublet. Standard treatment is carboplatin and paclitaxel, with the possible addition of bevacizumab in patients with advanced disease (stages III or IV). For patients with a *BRCA* germline mutation with advanced disease, olaparib maintenance is now approved following adjuvant chemotherapy.[22,23] For patients with advanced disease at presentation, relapse is a

TABLE 36.1 Systemic Cancer Treatments in Gynecologic Malignancies With Potential CV Side Effects

SYSTEMIC CANCER TREATMENTS	POTENTIAL CV SIDE EFFECTS
Bevacizumab	Hypertensive crisis (including posterior reversible leukoencephalopathy and CNS hemorrhage), cardiomyopathy, arterial embolism (CVA, MI), VTE. HTN occurs in up to 20% of patients receiving bevacizumab and is generally easy to manage with diuretics and ACE inhibitors, such as lisinopril
Paclitaxel	Rare sinus bradycardia (usually asymptomatic) Ventricular ectopy, conduction blocks, bradyarrythmias (rare)
Liposomal doxorubicin	EF decline, heart failure (rare compared with standard, nonliposomal doxorubicin)
Cisplatin/carboplatin	Volume overload, electrolyte disturbance, arrhythmias, arterial and venous thromboembolic events
Pembrolizumab	Myocarditis (rare), rarely pneumonitis that may be confused with a cardiac etiology for dyspnea
Niraparib	HTN, tachycardia, pneumonitis (rare)

ACE, Angiotensin-converting enzyme; *CNS*, central nervous system; *CV*, cardiovascular; *CVA*, cerebral vascular accident; *EF*, ejection fraction; *HTN*, hypertension; *MI*, myocardial infarction; *VTE*, venous thromboembolism.

common occurrence despite aggressive first-line chemotherapy. In this setting, the choice of second-line therapy at the time of relapse depends on the platinum-free interval. Patients who are platinum sensitive (platinum-free interval >6 months) proceed with combination platinum-based chemotherapy in an attempt to palliate symptoms and prolong survival, although cure is rarely achieved after disease recurrence. For patients with a platinum-free interval greater than 12 months a secondary cytoreduction approach is often considered,[24,25] followed by combination platinum-based chemotherapy. The regimens include carboplatin/paclitaxel/bevacizumab,[26] carboplatin/gemcitabine/bevacizumab,[27] or carboplatin/liposomal doxorubicin[28] followed by maintenance with a poly (ADP-ribose) polymerase (PARP) inhibitor, such as niraparib, olaparib, or rucaparib, or maintenance bevacizumab. If the patient is platinum resistant (platinum-free interval <6 months) then paclitaxel, liposomal doxorubicin or topotecan in combination with bevacizumab[29] is a reasonable approach. Third-line therapy often involves single agent therapy based on prior chemotherapy exposure, response, and treatment-related toxicities. Drugs in this setting include paclitaxel, liposomal doxorubicin, topotecan, bevacizumab, gemcitabine, pembrolizumab (for MSI-H tumors), or poly (ADP-ribose) polymerase inhibitors (for patients with *BRCA* mutation).[16]

Cardiovascular Risk

Systemic treatments for ovarian cancer are typically well tolerated from a cardiovascular perspective, although bevacizumab can cause significant cardiovascular risks in some patients (see Table 36.1).

CERVICAL CANCER

KEY POINTS ABOUT CERVICAL CANCER

- Incidence has decreased in developed countries, but continues to be high in resource-poor settings where screening is under-utilized.
- Median age at diagnosis is 50 years.
- Infection with high-risk human papillomavirus (HPV) strains is the most common cause
- 45% of patients diagnosed with invasive cervical carcinoma present with early-stage disease.
- Treatment strategy and prognosis vary based on stage at presentation.
- Treatment is typically well tolerated from a cardiovascular standpoint.

Incidence

Approximately 13,240 new cases of cervical cancer were diagnosed in the United States in 2018. The incidence of cervical cancer has decreased in the last three decades, whereas mortality rates during this time have not significantly declined.[1] Treatment options for cervical cancer remain limited and appropriate screening remains critical.

Risk Factors

High-risk HPV strains (16 and 18) are the most common cause of cervical cancer, and risk factors for the development of cervical cancer overlap with those for infection with high-risk HPV. In particular, higher number of sexual partners, younger age at first intercourse, higher parity, younger age at first pregnancy, and longer duration of oral contraceptive use have been identified as cervical cancer risk factors.[30] Smoking has also been associated with the development of squamous cell cervical carcinoma.[30]

Prognosis

The 5-year survival prognosis of localized stage cervical cancer is 91.7%. However, 5-year survival rates decrease with increasing extent of disease; 56% for those presenting with regionally advanced disease and 17.2% for those presenting with metastatic disease.

Treatment Overview

The treatment of cervical cancer varies by stage. Patients with stage IA disease are often treated with a simple hysterectomy. On the contrary, patients with stage IB-IIA disease who are candidates for surgical resection will be treated with a radical hysterectomy, which is a more aggressive surgical procedure involving removal of the uterus, parametria, top part of the vagina, and a radical node dissection.[31] Patients with early-stage disease with high-risk features require adjuvant therapy following surgery.[32,33] Patients who present with locally advanced disease (e.g., stages IIB and beyond), which by definition cannot be surgically resected with clean margins, are treated with concurrent cisplatin with radiation delivered with curative intent.[34,35] Patients with metastatic disease are often treated with palliative combination chemotherapy with cisplatin, paclitaxel, and bevacizumab.[36] Recently, the FDA granted approval to the immune checkpoint inhibitor pembrolizumab for treatment of cervical tumors that express programmed death ligand-1 (PD-L1; combined positive score ≥1) and progressed after chemotherapy.[37]

Cardiovascular Risk

Systemic treatments for cervical cancer are typically well tolerated from a cardiovascular perspective, although bevacizumab may carry a significant cardiovascular risk for some patients (see Table 36.1).

CARDIOVASCULAR SIDE EFFECTS OF SYSTEMIC CANCER TREATMENTS IN GYNECOLOGIC MALIGNANCIES

Cancer Treatments With Potential Cardiovascular Side Effects

Bevacizumab

Of the commonly used antineoplastic agents in gynecologic malignancies, bevacizumab carries the most significant cardiovascular risks, including hypertensive crisis, and arterial and venous thromboembolism. Hypertension is a class effect of vascular endothelial growth factor inhibitors. Prior to receiving VEGF inhibitors, all patients need to have controlled blood pressure. Many require adjustment and/or addition of antihypertensives while on therapy. The Investigational Drug Steering Committee of the National Cancer Institute (NCI) developed consensus recommendations for assessment, monitoring, and administration of angiogenesis inhibitors.[38] A significant increase in both diastolic and systolic blood pressure can arise in the first few weeks of therapy; thus, it is recommended to actively monitor and manage blood pressure with a goal less than 130/80 mm Hg for most patients and even lower goals for those with preexisting cardiovascular risk factors.[38] Bevacizumab increases the risk of thrombosis, both arterial and venous, with potentially fatal consequences in some patients, although the drug is generally well tolerated by most. Early diagnosis and discontinuation of the medication if a severe side effect occurs is key.[39,40] Bevacizumab rarely leads to heart failure. When cardiomyopathy occurs, patients should be evaluated for uncontrolled hypertension and ischemic heart disease.[41] Despite the risk of cardiomyopathy, no evidence supports routine monitoring with echocardiograms.[40]

Paclitaxel

Paclitaxel is typically well tolerated from a cardiovascular standpoint, but it has been known to cause multiple transient cardiac effects, including ventricular ectopy, sinus bradycardia, conduction blocks, and cardiac ischemia.[42] The most common cardiac effect is bradycardia, which typically remains without hemodynamic consequences and symptoms. Notably, no evidence exists of either cumulative cardiac toxicity over time or augmentation of anthracycline-associated cardiac toxicity. Cardiac monitoring is typically not performed during administration, but might be considered for patients with unstable cardiac status who nonetheless require paclitaxel for tumor control.

Liposomal Doxorubicin

Liposomal doxorubicin is typically well tolerated from a cardiovascular standpoint and demonstrates a different profile of toxicity than conventional doxorubicin. In patients receiving cumulative doses of 500 mg/m^2 or more of liposomal doxorubicin, the median drop in ejection fraction reported was 2%; 12% had a decline in ejection fraction of 10% or more.[43] Unlike the dose-dependence of conventional anthracycline toxicity, no correlation has been reported between the dose of liposomal doxorubicin administration and a change in LVEF.[43] Symptoms of congestive heart failure have been reported in <1% of patients receiving liposomal doxorubicin.[44] Nevertheless, monitoring for signs and symptoms of cardiomyopathy is often performed.

Cisplatin

Cisplatin can lead to hypertension and arterial and venous thrombotic events though relatively infrequently. Hypomagnesemia and hypokalemia are frequent side effects of cisplatin treatment[45] owing to renal tubular wasting, and patients on treatment should have their electrolytes monitored routinely. Owing to nephrotoxicity, cisplatin requires administration of pre- and posthydration, which can induce volume overload in patients with congestive heart failure.

Pembrolizumab

Pembrolizumab is an immune checkpoint inhibitor that enhances the immune response against tumors such as endometrial and ovarian cancers with MSI-high status and cervical cancers with evidence of PD-L1 expression as previously mentioned. The drug is typically well tolerated from a cardiovascular standpoint, and no cardiovascular adverse events were reported in a phase II study of pembrolizumab in MSI-H tumors.[12] However, autoimmune myocarditis, cardiomyopathy, heart failure, cardiac fibrosis, and cardiac arrest have all been reported following administration of immune checkpoint inhibitors.[46] Although rare, patients experiencing new cardiomyopathy or heart failure symptoms following the administration of immune checkpoint inhibitors like pembrolizumab should have their cardiac function evaluated.

Niraparib

Although generally well tolerated from a cardiovascular standpoint, niraparib has been associated with hypertension (19%) and palpitations (10%).[47] Blood pressure should be monitored routinely in patients receiving treatment.[22]

Cancer Treatments Without Known Potential Cardiovascular Side Effects

In comparison to niraparib, no cardiac adverse events (including hypertension and palpitations) were reported with patients on olaparib (package insert)[48] or rucaparib (package insert).[49] However, because these agents are relatively new, more prolonged follow up will be required to assess fully their toxicity profiles. Additionally, topotecan has not been found to have cardiovascular complications.[50]

REFERENCES

1. Benedet JL, et al. FIGO staging classifications and clinical practice guidelines in the management of gynecologic cancers. FIGO Committee on Gynecologic Oncology. *Int J Gynaecol Obstet.* 2000;70(2): 209–262.
2. Setiawan VW, et al. Type I and II endometrial cancers: have they different risk factors? *J Clin Oncol.* 2013;31(20):2607–2618.
3. Siegel RL, Miller KD, Jemal A. Cancer statistics, 2018. *CA Cancer J Clin.* 2018;68(1):7–30.
4. Smith RA, et al. American Cancer Society guidelines for the early detection of cancer: update of early detection guidelines for prostate, colorectal, and endometrial cancers. Also: update 2001—testing for early lung cancer detection. *CA Cancer J Clin.* 2001;51(1):38–75, quiz 77–80.
5. Creutzberg CL, et al. Surgery and postoperative radiotherapy versus surgery alone for patients with stage-1 endometrial carcinoma: multicentre randomised trial. PORTEC Study Group (Post Operative Radiation Therapy in Endometrial Carcinoma). *Lancet.* 2000;355(9213):1404–1411.
6. Keys HM, et al. A phase III trial of surgery with or without adjunctive external pelvic radiation therapy in intermediate risk endometrial adenocarcinoma: a Gynecologic Oncology Group study. *Gynecol Oncol.* 2004;92(3):744–751.
7. DeBoer SM, et al. Adjuvant chemoradiotherapy versus radiotherapy alone for women with high-risk endometrial cancer (PORTEC-3): final results of an international, open-label, multicentre, randomised, phase 3 trial. *Lancet Oncol.* 2018;19(3):295–309.
8. Hoskins PJ, et al. Paclitaxel and carboplatin, alone or with irradiation, in advanced or recurrent endometrial cancer: a phase II study. *J Clin Oncol.* 2001;19(20):4048–4053.
9. Pignata S, et al. A multicentre phase II study of carboplatin plus pegylated liposomal doxorubicin as first-line chemotherapy for patients with advanced or recurrent endometrial carcinoma: the END-1 study of the MITO (Multicentre Italian Trials in Ovarian Cancer and Gynecologic Malignancies) group. *Br J Cancer.* 2007; 96(11):1639–1643.
10. Wadler S, et al. Topotecan is an active agent in the first-line treatment of metastatic or recurrent endometrial carcinoma: Eastern Cooperative Oncology Group Study E3E93. *J Clin Oncol.* 2003;21(11): 2110–2114.
11. Aghajanian C, et al. Phase II trial of bevacizumab in recurrent or persistent endometrial cancer: a Gynecologic Oncology Group study. *J Clin Oncol.* 2011;29(16):2259–2265.
12. Le DT, et al. PD-1 blockade in tumors with mismatch-repair deficiency. *N Engl J Med.* 2015;372(26):2509–2520.
13. Le DT, et al. Mismatch repair deficiency predicts response of solid tumors to PD-1 blockade. *Science.* 2017;357(6349):409–413.
14. Jones MR, et al. Genetic epidemiology of ovarian cancer and prospects for polygenic risk prediction. *Gynecol Oncol.* 2017;147(3): 705–713.
15. Grossman DC, et al. Screening for ovarian cancer: US Preventive Services Task Force Recommendation Statement. *JAMA.* 2018;319(6): 588–594.
16. NCCN Guidelines. *Genetic/Familial High-risk Assessment: Breast and Ovarian.* NCCN Clinical Practice Guidelines in Oncology. Version 2.2019.
17. Kauff ND, et al. Risk-reducing salpingo-oophorectomy in women with a BRCA1 or BRCA2 mutation. *N Engl J Med.* 2002;346(21):1609–1615.
18. Walker JL, et al. Society of Gynecologic Oncology recommendations for the prevention of ovarian cancer. *Cancer.* 2015;121(13): 2108–2120.
19. Chittenden BG, et al. Polycystic ovary syndrome and the risk of gynaecological cancer: a systematic review. *Reprod Biomed Online.* 2009;19(3):398–405.
20. Ness RB, et al. Infertility, fertility drugs, and ovarian cancer: a pooled analysis of case-control studies. *Am J Epidemiol.* 2002;155(3): 217–224.
21. Pearce CL, et al. Association between endometriosis and risk of histological subtypes of ovarian cancer: a pooled analysis of case-control studies. *Lancet Oncol.* 2012;13(4):385–394.
22. Moore KN, Mirza MR, Matulonis UA. The poly (ADP ribose) polymerase inhibitor niraparib: management of toxicities. *Gynecol Oncol.* 2018;149(1):214–220.
23. Moore K, et al. Maintenance olaparib in patients with newly diagnosed advanced ovarian cancer. *N Engl J Med.* 2018;379(26): 2495–2505.
24. Al Rawahi T, et al. Surgical cytoreduction for recurrent epithelial ovarian cancer. *Cochrane Database Syst Rev.* 2013;(2):CD008765.
25. Lorusso D, et al. The role of secondary surgery in recurrent ovarian cancer. *Int J Surg Oncol.* 2012;2015:613980.
26. Coleman RL, et al. Bevacizumab and paclitaxel-carboplatin chemotherapy and secondary cytoreduction in recurrent, platinum-sensitive ovarian cancer (NRG Oncology/Gynecologic Oncology Group study GOG-0213): a multicentre, open-label, randomised, phase 3 trial. *Lancet Oncol.* 2017;18(6):779–791.

27. Aghajanian C, et al. OCEANS: a randomized, double-blind, placebo-controlled phase III trial of chemotherapy with or without bevacizumab in patients with platinum-sensitive recurrent epithelial ovarian, primary peritoneal, or fallopian tube cancer. *J Clin Oncol.* 2012;30(17):2039–2045.
28. Pujade-Lauraine E, et al. Pegylated liposomal doxorubicin and carboplatin compared with paclitaxel and carboplatin for patients with platinum-sensitive ovarian cancer in late relapse. *J Clin Oncol.* 2010;28(20):3323–3329.
29. Pujade-Lauraine E, et al. Bevacizumab combined with chemotherapy for platinum-resistant recurrent ovarian cancer: the AURELIA open-label randomized phase III trial. *J Clin Oncol.* 2014;32(13): 1302–1308.
30. Berrington DE González A, Green J; International Collaboration of Epidemiological Studies of Cervical Cancer. Comparison of risk factors for invasive squamous cell carcinoma and adenocarcinoma of the cervix: collaborative reanalysis of individual data on 8,097 women with squamous cell carcinoma and 1,374 women with adenocarcinoma from 12 epidemiological studies. *Int J Cancer.* 2007;120(4):885–891.
31. Somashekhar SP, Ashwin KR. Management of early stage cervical cancer. *Rev Recent Clin Trials.* 2015;10(4):302–308.
32. Peters WA, et al. Concurrent chemotherapy and pelvic radiation therapy compared with pelvic radiation therapy alone as adjuvant therapy after radical surgery in high-risk early-stage cancer of the cervix. *J Clin Oncol.* 2000;18(8):1606–1613.
33. Sedlis A, et al. A randomized trial of pelvic radiation therapy versus no further therapy in selected patients with stage IB carcinoma of the cervix after radical hysterectomy and pelvic lymphadenectomy: a Gynecologic Oncology Group Study. *Gynecol Oncol.* 1999;73(2):177–183.
34. Rose PG, et al. Concurrent cisplatin-based radiotherapy and chemotherapy for locally advanced cervical cancer. *N Engl J Med.* 1999;340(15):1144–1153.
35. Eifel PJ, et al. Pelvic irradiation with concurrent chemotherapy versus pelvic and para-aortic irradiation for high-risk cervical cancer: an update of radiation therapy oncology group trial (RTOG) 90-01. *J Clin Oncol.* 2004;22(5):872–880.
36. Tewari KS, et al. Improved survival with bevacizumab in advanced cervical cancer. *N Engl J Med.* 2014;370(8):734–743.
37. Frenel JS, et al. Safety and efficacy of pembrolizumab in advanced, programmed death ligand 1-positive cervical cancer: results from the Phase Ib KEYNOTE-028 Trial. *J Clin Oncol.* 2017;35(36):4035–4041.
38. Maitland ML, et al. Initial assessment, surveillance, and management of blood pressure in patients receiving vascular endothelial growth factor signaling pathway inhibitors. *J Natl Cancer Inst.* 2010; 102(9):596–604.
39. Hamnvik OP, et al. Clinical risk factors for the development of hypertension in patients treated with inhibitors of the VEGF signaling pathway. *Cancer.* 2015;121(2):311–319.
40. Tebbutt NC, et al. Risk of arterial thromboembolic events in patients with advanced colorectal cancer receiving bevacizumab. *Ann Oncol.* 2011;22(8):1834–1838.
41. Choueiri TK, et al. Congestive heart failure risk in patients with breast cancer treated with bevacizumab. *J Clin Oncol.* 2011;29(6): 632–638.
42. Rowinsky EK, et al. Cardiac disturbances during the administration of taxol. *J Clin Oncol.* 1991;9(9):1704–1712.
43. Safra T, et al. Pegylated liposomal doxorubicin (doxil): reduced clinical cardiotoxicity in patients reaching or exceeding cumulative doses of 500 mg/m^2. *Ann Oncol.* 2000;11(8):1029–1033.
44. O'Brien ME, et al. Reduced cardiotoxicity and comparable efficacy in a phase III trial of pegylated liposomal doxorubicin HCl (CAELYX/Doxil) versus conventional doxorubicin for first-line treatment of metastatic breast cancer. *Ann Oncol.* 2004;15(3):440–449.
45. Lam M, Adelstein DJ. Hypomagnesemia and renal magnesium wasting in patients treated with cisplatin. *Am J Kidney Dis.* 1986; 8(3):164–169.
46. Heinzerling L, et al. Cardiotoxicity associated with CTLA4 and PD1 blocking immunotherapy. *J Immunother Cancer.* 2016;4:50.
47. Mirza MR, et al. Niraparib maintenance therapy in platinum-sensitive, recurrent ovarian cancer. *N Engl J Med.* 2016;375(22): 2154–2164.
48. Pujade-Lauraine E, Ledermann JA, Selle F, et al. Olaparib tablets as maintenance therapy in patients with platinum-sensitive, relapsed ovarian cancer and a BRCA1/2 mutation (SOLO2/ENGOT-Ov21): a double-blind, randomised, placebo-controlled, phase 3 trial. *Lancet Oncol.* 18(9); 2017: 1274–1284.
49. Coleman RL, et al. Rucaparib maintenance treatment for recurrent ovarian carcinoma after response to platinum therapy (ARIEL3): a randomised, double-blind, placebo-controlled, phase 3 trial. *Lancet.* 2017;390:1949–1961.
50. Yeh ET, Bickford CL. Cardiovascular complications of cancer therapy: incidence, pathogenesis, diagnosis, and management. *J Am Coll Cardiol.* 2009;53(24):2231–2247.

37 Prostate and Testicular Cancer

PEDRO C. BARATA AND OLIVER SARTOR

Stages	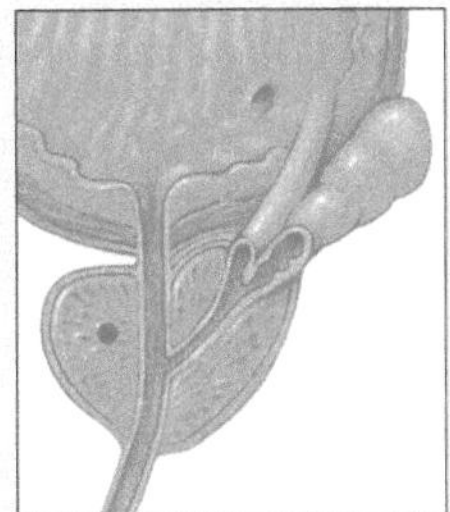 **Stage I** Small and only in the prostate (PSA < 10, Gleason < 7)	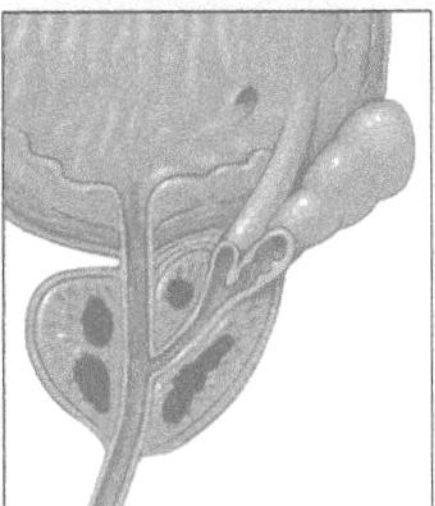 **Stage II** May be in both lobes, but still only prostate (any PSA, any Gleason)	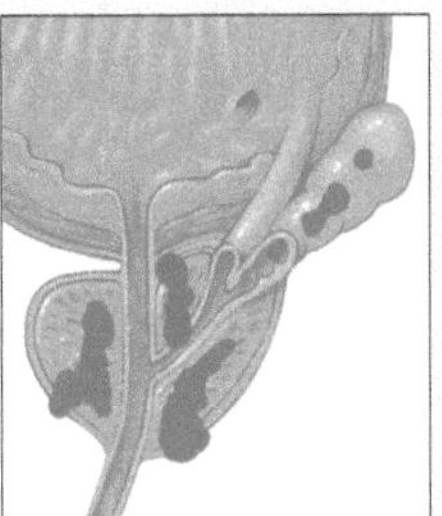 **Stage III** Spread to close by LNs or seminal vesicles (any PSA, any Gleason)	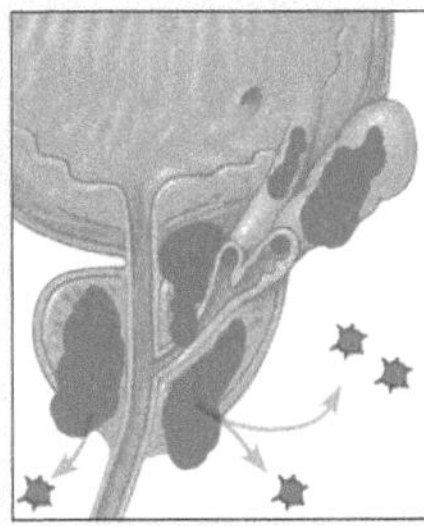 **Stage IV** Spread to other organs (any PSA, any Gleason)
Treatment	Active surveillance Surgery Radiotherapy	Surgery Radiotherapy + androgen deprivation therapy (ADT)	Surgery Radiotherapy + ADT (GnRH antagonist +/– antiandrogen)	ADT +/– novel hormonal agents Taxane-based chemotherapy Radium-223 Sipuleucel-T +/– local therapies
Prognosis	5-year survival 99%	5-year survival 99%	5-year survival 99%	5-year survival 29%

Potential CV toxicities

GnRH agonists (leuprolide, goserelin, triptorelin, buserelin, histrelin): ischemia, arrhythmias, thrombosis, edema, hypertension, QTc prolongation
GnRH antagonists (degarelix): hypertension, QTc prolongation
Anti-androgens (abiraterone, apalutamide, enzalutamid): hypertension, edema, arrhythmias, chest pain, heart failure, QTc prolongation
Sipuleucel-T: hypertension, arterial and venous thrombotic events
Docetaxel: hypotension, edema
Cabazitaxel: edema, arrhythmias, hypotension
Paclitaxel: bradycardia, ischemia
Mitoxantrone: edema, arrhythmias, ischemia, hypertension, heart failure
Platinum drugs: arterial and venous thrombotic events, arrhythmias

Stages	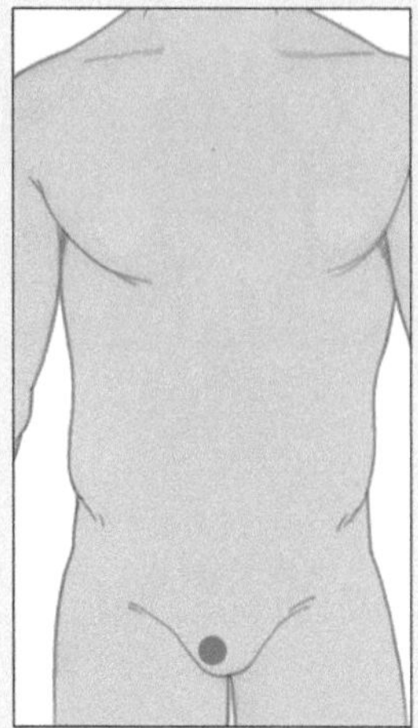 **Stage I** Cancer is found only in the testicle T1–4, no LN Serum tumor marker normal	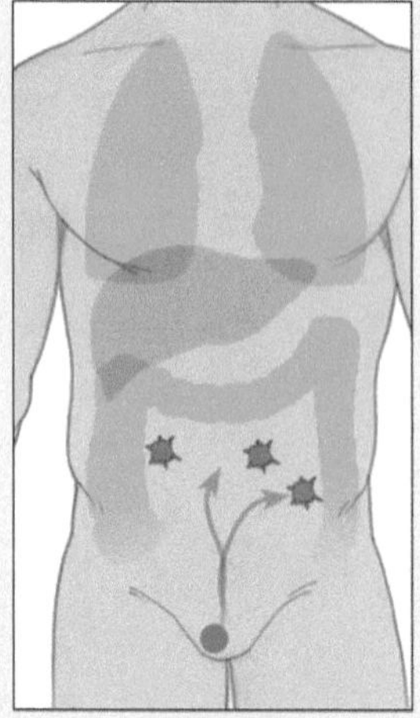 **Stage II** Cancer has spread to one or more LN in the abdomen LDH < 1.5 x normal hCG (seminoma, non-seminoma) <5000 AFP (non-seminoma) <1000	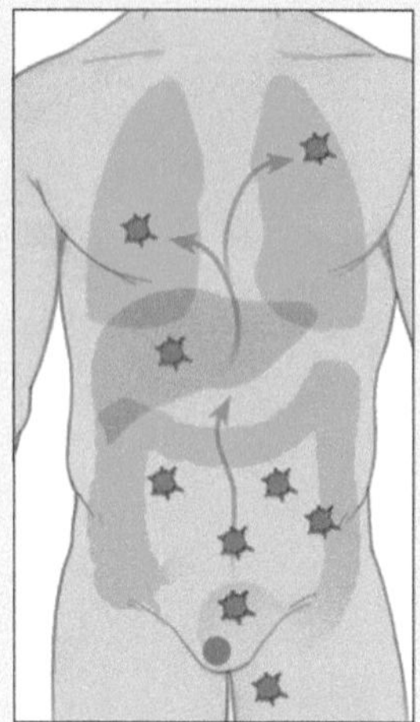 **Stage III** Cancer has spread beyond the lymph nodes in the abdomen
Treatment	Surgery (orchiectomy) Chemotherapy Radiotherapy (infra-diaphragmatic 20–30 Gy)	Surgery (orchiectomy) Chemotherapy Radiotherapy (infra-diaphragmatic 30–40 Gy)	Surgery (orchiectomy) Chemotherapy Radiotherapy (regional)
Prognosis	5-year survival 99%	5-year survival >95%	5-year survival 73%

Potential CV toxicities

Chemotherapy regimens:
BEP: bleomycin, etoposide, cisplatin; **EP:** etoposide, cisplatin; **VIP:** ifosfamide, etoposide, cisplatin
Bleomycin: ischemia events, Raynaud's, interstitial pneumonitis, pulmonary fibrosis
Etoposide: hypotension with rapid infusion
Cisplatin: arterial and venous thrombotic events, arrhythmias
Ifosfamide: arrhythmias, ECG (ST-T wave changes), cardiomyopathy
Radiation therapy: peripheral vascular disease

CHAPTER OUTLINE

KEY POINTS ABOUT TESTICULAR CANCER

- Worldwide, testicular cancer is a relatively rare cancer, accounting for 1% to 2% of all cancers (>52,000 new cases and almost 10,000 deaths worldwide every year); however, it is the most common cancer among men 15 to 40 years of age.
- Major risk factors for testicular cancer include congenital anomaly (cryptorchidism), as well as prior unilateral testicular cancer, HIV infection, and family history of testicular cancer.
- With treatment, 5-year survival rates exceed 95% for all stages. Stage I is often managed with surgery alone, whereas more advanced stages often include a combination of surgery (orchiectomy) and systemic cisplatin-based chemotherapy. Retroperitoneal lymphadenectomy and/or radiation therapy may also be offered to patients with nodal involvement.
- Treatment-related cardiovascular toxicities are associated in particular with the use cisplatin-based chemotherapy and radiation therapy.

Cardiovascular (CV) disease and cancer have consistently been the top two contributors to the burden of chronic disease and the leading causes of death in the United States.[1] Cancer treatments including chemotherapy, androgen-deprivation therapy and radiotherapy are associated with an increased risk of CV events. The incidence of cardiotoxicity varies by the type and duration of treatment received, and preexisting CV risk factors at baseline.[2]

This chapter provides a short overview of prostate and testicular cancer, their treatment and treatment-related CV toxicities.

TESTICULAR CANCER

Incidence

Testicular cancer is the most common cancer among men 15 to 40 years of age in the United States and Europe, and incidence has increased over the past several decades.[3]

Risk Factors

The etiology of germ-cell testicular cancer remains largely unknown. Several epidemiology studies support the association determined *in utero*, such as congenital anomaly (cryptorchidism), as well as prior unilateral testicular cancer, HIV infection, and a family history of testicular cancer.[4]

Diagnosis and Staging

Testicular tumors usually present as a nodule or painless swelling of one testicle, which may be noted incidentally by the patient or his sexual partner. In some cases, a man with prior atrophic testis will note a unilateral enlargement and may complain of a dull ache or heavy sensation in the lower abdomen or perianal or scrotal area.

Testicular cancer is staged using clinical and radiographic information that has treatment and prognosis implications. Staging is based on the primary tumor (T), lymph nodes (N), and distant metastases (M) (TNM) staging system developed by the American Joint Committee on Cancer and the Union for International Cancer Control, which applies to both seminomas and non-seminomatous germ cell tumors.

Treatment

Depending on the tumor stage, surgery alone (orchiectomy) or surgery followed by radiation therapy or systemic chemotherapy may be appropriate. Of note, most testicular cancers are germ cell tumors (seminoma and non-seminoma), which are among the most curable solid cancers, with 5-year survival rates exceeding 95% for all stages.[5] This is mainly because of the significant treatment advances, in particular, the inclusion of cisplatin in the chemotherapy regimens that can cure up to 80% of patients with disseminated germ cell tumors.[6]

Cisplatin or cis-diamminedichloroplatinum (II), is a well-known potent alkylating agent that acts by damaging the cell DNA. It is used in combination with (1) etoposide, (2) bleomycin and etoposide or (3) vinblastine and ifosfamide across all stages.[7]

Cardiovascular Risk

Cisplatin-based chemotherapy is associated with clinically important toxicities, including vascular toxicity, autonomic CV dysfunction, hypertension and hypotension, pericarditis, and arrhythmia.[8–10] Acute CV toxicity is hypothesized to be the consequence of direct damage to the vascular endothelium, and an increase in circulating von Willebrand factor levels or microalbuminuria may serve as signs of endothelial injury in this setting.[11,12] Vascular toxicity is also one of the most significant late consequences of cisplatin-based chemotherapy in the treatment of men with germ cell tumors. The 25-year risk of CV disease (CVD) is approximately 16%, and the risk of developing a major cardiac event is increased seven-fold.[12–14] These dynamics are supported further by a high burden of CV risk factors, including hypertension and hyperlipidemia, and the metabolic syndrome.[15,16] Of note, testicular cancer survivors have a two times higher age-adjusted risk of metabolic syndrome[17,18] Overall, CV mortality is increased in patients with testicular cancer treated with chemotherapy (HR 1.36, 95% CI, 1.07 to 1.78).[19] The risk for cardiac events is increased further in patients treated both with radiotherapy and cisplatin-based chemotherapy (relative risk: RR 2.4, 95% CI, 1.04 to 5.45). Herein, only a minority of patients received mediastinal radiotherapy and no increased risk was observed with other chemotherapy agents, such as bleomycin.[15] An increased risk of CVD after radiation has been best characterized in patients with breast cancer or non-Hodgkin lymphoma, but it has also been observed in those with testicular cancer who received both subdiaphragmatic and mediastinal radiation therapy.[16,20]

The current knowledge about long-term toxicities in patients with testicular cancer is based on treatments administered several decades ago. The optimization of therapies, including the use of modern radiation techniques, reductions in mediastinal irradiation, lowering cumulative doses of chemotherapy, and preferential use of active surveillance for those with low-risk disease will potentially reduce the risk of cardiac toxicity in this patient population. Following successful treatment, these patients will naturally need long-term follow up with a special focus on modifiable CVD risk factors. As outlined, these include hypertension, dyslipidemia, and diabetes, as well as counseling on diet, smoking cessation, and exercise.

KEY POINTS ABOUT PROSTATE CANCER

- Prostate cancer is the most common cancer in men, responsible for more than 31,600 deaths in 2019, in the United States.
- Major risk factors for prostate cancer include older age, positive family history of cancer, race/ethnicity, tall height, and lack of exercise/sedentary lifestyle.
- With treatment, 5-year survival rates are almost 100% for men with localized prostate cancer, whereas for those men diagnosed with locally advanced or metastatic disease, the 5-year survival rate is around 30%.
- Early stages are managed with surgery or radiation therapy alone or in combination with androgen-deprivation therapy; stage IV (advanced disease) is managed with systemic treatment that includes androgen-deprivation therapy in combination with novel hormonal agents, chemotherapy, and/or other therapies.
- Treatment-related cardiovascular toxicities are mainly associated with the inhibition of the androgen-signalling pathway.
- GnRH antagonists may be associated with fewer cardiovascular events compared with GnRH agonists.

PROSTATE CANCER

Incidence

Prostate cancer is the most common cancer in men, responsible for more than 31,600 deaths in 2019, in the United States.[21] Despite the decline in the incidence of localized disease, the number of patients diagnosed with metastatic prostate cancer has increased by almost 3% per year since 2012.[22]

Risk Factors

Established risk factors for prostate cancer include older age, positive family history of cancer, race/ethnicity, tall height, and lack of exercise/sedentary lifestyle.[23]

Diagnosis and Staging

With the introduction of prostate-specific antigen (PSA) and transrectal ultrasound (TRUS), the diagnosis of prostate cancer has moved from a condition that presented with locally advanced or metastatic disease to one that is found upon screening. As a consequence, with proper treatment, 5-year survival rates are almost 100% for men with localized or regional prostate cancer, whereas for those men diagnosed with locally advanced or metastatic disease, the 5-year survival rate is around 30%.[24]

A definitive diagnosis is based on biopsies from throughout the prostate, obtained with the use of either-TRUS or newer imaging techniques, such as magnetic resonance TRUS fusion imaging.

When the cancer is limited to the prostate, it is considered localized and potentially curable. However, disease may spread to bones or elsewhere outside the prostate, and a number of different therapies may be used alone or in combination to improve the clinical outcomes of patients.

Imaging for staging includes conventional techniques, such as MRI or computed tomography and bone scans, but newer and more sensitive imaging techniques, such as prostate-specific membrane antigen or fluciclovine-positron emission tomography scans, are emerging.

Treatment

Adenocarcinoma of prostate is a hormonally driven disease, and tumor growth is primarily dependent on androgens. After the Scottish surgeon John Hunter had reported the association between prostate growth and testicular function for the first time in the late 18th century, and Louis Mercier had performed the first orchiectomy for the treatment of enlarged prostate a few decades later (1857), androgen-deprivation therapy (ADT) intended to lower testosterone levels below 50 ng/dL became the cornerstone of medical treatment for metastatic disease after the studies from Charles Huggins and Clarence Hodges, in 1941. ADT is also the mainstay of treatment of localized disease, and approximately 40% of all prostate patients with cancer receive ADT within 6 months of diagnosis.[25] Surgery and radiation therapy are curative approaches to localized prostate cancer. ADT is also included in the treatment of localized disease in combination with radiation therapy.

The two central elements of ADT are GhRH agonists and antagonists. Novel andogren axis inhibitors have shown efficacy even in advanced stages.[26–28] This includes androgen synthesis inhibitors (abiraterone, enzalutamide, apalutamide, and darolutamide) have been developed and are now approved for the treatment of castration resistant non-metastatic and metastatic prostate cancer in association with ADT.

Chemotherapy with taxanes, which bind to and inhibit microtubule polymerization, thereby interrupting cell division (such as docetaxel and cabazitaxel), play an important role in the advanced setting.[29] Both agents have been shown to prolong clinical outcomes of men with metastatic castrate-sensitive (mCSPC) and metastatic castration-resistant prostate cancer and are often used in clinical practice.

Since the approval of docetaxel by the US Food and Drug Administration (FDA) in 2005, the management of patients with advanced prostate cancer has profoundly changed with the clinical development of these and other agents, including radionuclide-based therapies and a dendritic cell-based vaccine.[28,30–34] However, advanced prostate cancer is rarely curative, and ultimately most patients will die from progressive disease.

When radiation therapy is considered, it usually targets the prostate gland with(out) regional lymph nodes for curative purposes and spine and/or ribs for distant metastases.

Cardiovascular Risk

Cardiovascular disease is a major cause of non-cancer–related mortality in men with prostate cancer.[35] Large observational data have suggested that men treated with ADT are at an increased risk of cardiovascular events, including myocardial infarction and stroke.[36] Possible explanations for this increased risk may include metabolic changes, such as hyperglycemia and dyslipidemia, which are induced by ADT and are well-established risk factors for atherosclerosis.

To date, these observations have not been confirmed by prospective, randomized studies but were

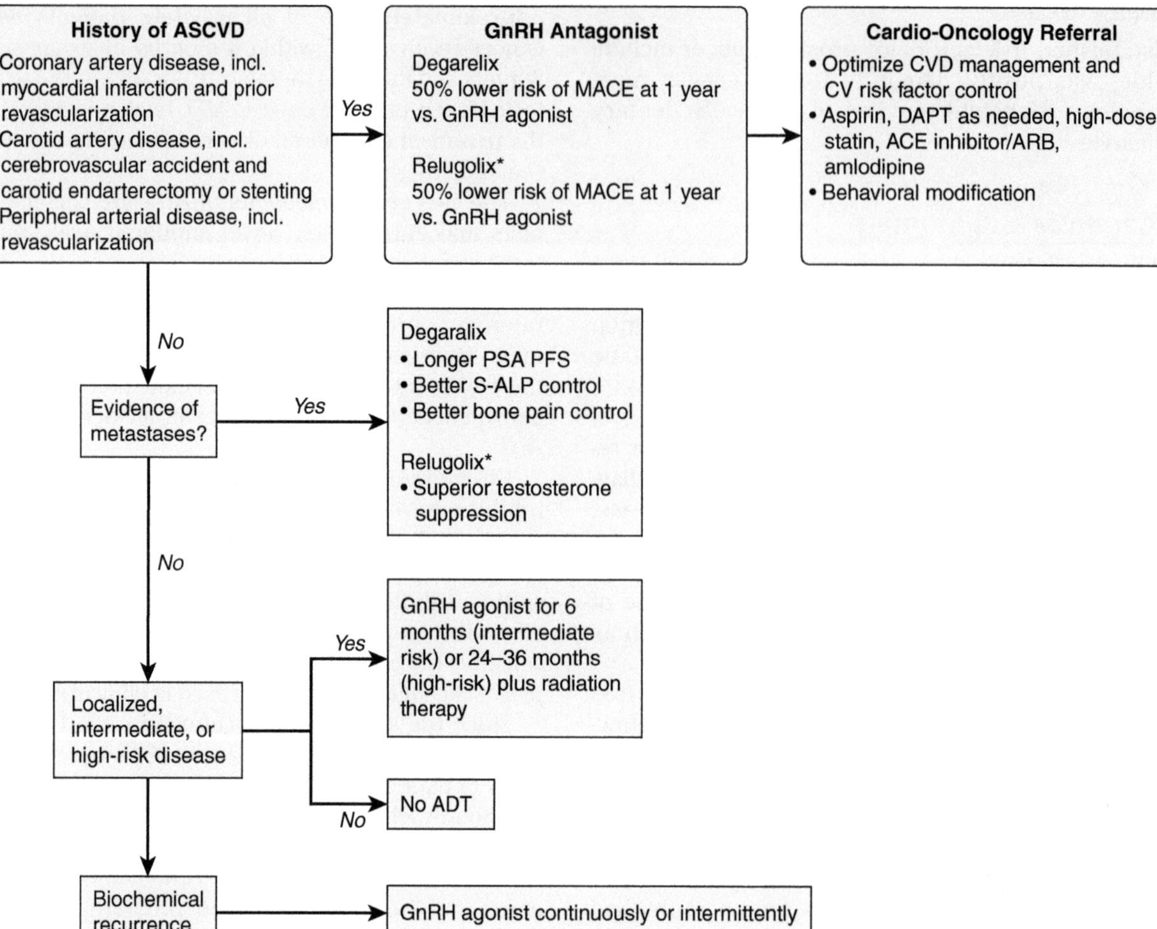

FIG 37.1 Cardiovascular (cardio-oncology) considerations in prostate patients with cancer. *ADT,* Androgen-deprivation therapy; *ASCVD,* atherosclerotic cardiovascular disease; *CV,* cardiovascular; *CVD,* cardiovascular disease; *GnRH,* gonadotropin-releasing hormone; *MACE,* major adverse cardiovascular events; *PSA,* prostate-specific antigen.

the basis for a joint statement by Cardiology and Oncology societies aiming to raise awareness to the association between ADT and cardiovascular disease and to promote management of cardiovascular issues as part of the overall management of ADT-receiving prostate patients with cancer.[36] A potential management approach is outlined in Figure 37.1.

The risk of CV events seems to be related to the presence or absence of preexisting CVD. Prior history of myocardial infarct or ischemic congestive heart failure was shown to be associated with an increased risk of all-cause mortality with neoadjuvant ADT prior to radiation therapy (HR 1.96, 95% CI, 1.04 to 3.71).[37] In a different study in the metastatic setting, men with two or more prior CV events experienced the greatest risk of additional CV events after starting ADT (HR 1.91, 95% CI, 1.66 to 2.20).[38] Of note, approximately one third of patients with metastatic prostate cancer have a history of CVD at the time of ADT. Thus, being cognizant of pre-ADT CVD and CV risk factors (as well as their implications for therapy) is an important part of prostate cancer management.

Although continuous ADT remains the gold standard, results from two phase III studies support intermittent ADT as a valid option based on better quality of life (QoL) and also a fewer number of CV events.[39–41] Duration of ADT seems to play a major role, but studies evaluating the incidence of CVD in patients treated with long-term ADT (18 to 36 months) for high-risk disease have not been conducted.

For metastatic disease, whereas most patients still receive an gonadotropin-releasing hormone (GnRH) agonist as the ADT of choice, newer GnRH antagonists may be associated with fewer cardiovascular events, but prospective validation of these findings is pending (NCT02663908). The HERO trial compared the outcomes of the oral GnRH antagonist relugolix versus the standard GnRH agonist leuprolide in patients with advanced prostate cancer.[42] Although relugolix was associated with a superior sustained suppression of testosterone at 48 weeks, the incidence of major adverse cardiovascular events (MACE) including myocardial infarction, central nervous system hemorrhage, and cerebrovascular conditions was numerically lower (3.6% and 2.8% for patients with and without MACE, respectively) than for patients treated with leuprolide (17.8% and 4.2% for patients with and without MACE, respectively). Based on these findings, the FDA approved relugolix (December 2020) for adults with advanced prostate cancer.

Similarly, the addition of an antiandrogen (e.g., bicalutamide) to ADT remains a valid option for selected patients, but it is associated with an absolute increase in CV event risk of 2% to 3% compared with ADT alone.

Novel androgen receptor inhibitors, such as abiraterone acetate and enzalutamide, may also increase the risk for CVD and atrial fibrillation.[43] Commonly, patients remain on abiraterone acetate/prednisone or enzalutamide for more than 12 months while on continuous ADT. Other novel hormonal agents are being successfully tested in this setting and are likely to be associated with similar CV risks.

Taxanes may potentiate the risk of left ventricular dysfunction when associated with other chemotherapy agents. Used as single agent therapy, they are rarely associated with CV events; heart failure occurs in less than 1%. Other chemotherapy drugs, such as anthracyclines, and/or targeted therapies, known to increase CV risk are not currently included in the treatment landscape of prostate cancer.

When radiation therapy is considered, it usually targets the prostate gland with(out) regional lymph nodes for curative purposes and spine and/or ribs for distant metastases. In the latter, radiosurgery is usually the preferred form of radiation delivered with minimal affectation of regional organs and not associated with a particular higher CV risk.

SURVIVORSHIP

With the development of more effective anticancer therapies, the number of survivors of cancer is rapidly growing.[44]

CVD is the leading cause of death in many survivors of cancer, and CV factors are more prevalent compared with age-matched controls.[1,45] Recognizing this increased risk and modifying risk factors remain the most effective strategies for prevention in this patient population (airway, breathing, circulation, disability, exposure [ABCD] approach approach). The atherosclerotic cardiovascular disease (ASCVD) risk calculator created by the American College of Cardiology and American Heart Association is the most widely used tool for risk discussions, and it is available online.

When patients complete curative treatment, some transition back to the traditional primary care team, whereas others continue to follow up with their oncologist. This transition is potentially challenging for logistical reasons, as shown by the high number of patients lost in this transition. Thus, survivorship recommendations for patients with multiple cancers, including prostate and testicular neoplasms, have been published with a focus on CVD prevention.[2,46]

Although cancer-specific guidelines do expand on the cancer-specific treatment effects on CVD, most of the CVD risk derives from the traditional CV risk factors. Consequently, the greatest reduction in risk is likely to be achieved with the primary prevention guidelines developed for the general population.

CONCLUSIONS

CVD is a frequent toxicity in patients diagnosed with genitourinary tumors, particularly associated with the use cisplatin-based regimens and radiation in testicular cancers and the inhibition of the androgen signalling pathway in prostate cancer.

The coordination between medical oncology and cardiology in identifying the patients who are at risk, and close monitoring of these patients during active treatment and enrollment in survivorship programs, are successful ways to prevent CVD and improve outcomes in cancer survivors.

REFERENCES

1. Weaver KE, Foraker RE, Alfano CM, et al. Cardiovascular risk factors among long-term survivors of breast, prostate, colorectal, and gynecologic cancers: a gap in survivorship care? *J Cancer Surviv*. 2013;7:253–261.
2. Chang HM, Moudgil R, Scarabelli T, et al. Cardiovascular complications of cancer therapy. Best practices in diagnosis, prevention, and management: Part 1. *J Am Coll Cardiol*. 2017;70:2536–2551.
3. Park JS, Kim J, Elghiaty A, et al. Recent global trends in testicular cancer incidence and mortality. *Medicine*. 2018;97:e12390–e12390.
4. McGlynn KA, Trabert B. Adolescent and adult risk factors for testicular cancer. *Nat Rev Urol*. 2012;9:339–349.
5. Nigam M, Aschebrook-Kilfoy B, Shikanov S, et al. Increasing incidence of testicular cancer in the United States and Europe between 1992 and 2009. *World J Urol*. 2015;33:623–631.
6. Williams SD, Birch R, Einhorn LH, et al. Treatment of disseminated germ-cell tumors with cisplatin, bleomycin, and either vinblastine or etoposide. *N Engl J Med*. 1987;316:1435–1440.
7. Motzer RJ, Agarwal N, Beard C, et al. Testicular cancer. *J Natl Compr Canc Netw*. 2009;7:672–693.
8. Patane S. Cardiotoxicity: cisplatin and long-term cancer survivors. *Int J Cardiol*. 2014;175:201–202.
9. Moore RA, Adel N, Riedel E, et al. High incidence of thromboembolic events in patients treated with cisplatin-based chemotherapy: a large retrospective analysis. *J Clin Oncol*. 2011;29:3466–3473.
10. Guglin M, Aljayeh M, Saiyad S, et al. Introducing a new entity: chemotherapy-induced arrhythmia. *Europace*. 2009;11:1579–1586.
11. Dieckmann KP, Struss WJ, Budde U. Evidence for acute vascular toxicity of cisplatin-based chemotherapy in patients with germ cell tumour. *Anticancer Res*. 2011;31:4501–4505.
12. Meinardi MT, Gietema JA, van der Graaf WT, et al. Cardiovascular morbidity in long-term survivors of metastatic testicular cancer. *J Clin Oncol*. 2000;18:1725–1732.
13. Carver JR, Szalda D, Ky B. Asymptomatic cardiac toxicity in long-term cancer survivors: defining the population and recommendations for surveillance. *Semin Oncol*. 2013;40:229–238.
14. van den Belt-Dusebout AW, Nuver J, de Wit R, et al. Long-term risk of cardiovascular disease in 5-year survivors of testicular cancer. *J Clin Oncol*. 2006;24:467–475.
15. Huddart RA, Norman A, Shahidi M, et al. Cardiovascular disease as a long-term complication of treatment for testicular cancer. *J Clin Oncol*. 2003;21:1513–1523.
16. Haugnes HS, Wethal T, Aass N, et al. Cardiovascular risk factors and morbidity in long-term survivors of testicular cancer: a 20-year follow-up study. *J Clin Oncol*. 2010;28:4649–4657.
17. Willemse PM, Burggraaf J, Hamdy NA, et al. Prevalence of the metabolic syndrome and cardiovascular disease risk in chemotherapy-treated testicular germ cell tumour survivors. *Br J Cancer*. 2013;109:60–67.
18. Zaid MA, Gathirua-Mwangi WG, Fung C, et al. Clinical and genetic risk factors for adverse metabolic outcomes in North American testicular cancer survivors. *J Natl Compr Canc Netw*. 2018;16:257–265.
19. Fung C, Fossa SD, Milano MT, et al. Cardiovascular disease mortality after chemotherapy or surgery for testicular nonseminoma: a population-based study. *J Clin Oncol*. 2015;33:3105–3115.
20. Terbuch A, Posch F, Annerer LM, et al. Long-term cardiovascular complications in stage I seminoma patients. *Clin Transl Oncol*. 2017;19:1400–1408.
21. Siegel RL, Miller KD, Jemal A. Cancer statistics, 2019. *CA Cancer J Clin*. 2019;69:7–34.
22. Kelly SP, Anderson WF, Rosenberg PS, et al. Past, current, and future incidence rates and burden of metastatic prostate cancer in the United States. *Eur Urol Focus*. 2018;4:121–127.
23. Gann PH. Risk factors for prostate cancer. *Rev Urol*. 2002;4(suppl 5): S3–S10.
24. Pascale M, Azinwi CN, Marongiu B, et al. The outcome of prostate patients with cancer treated with curative intent strongly depends on survival after metastatic progression. *BMC Cancer*. 2017;17:651–651.
25. Shahinian VB, Kuo YF, Gilbert SM. Reimbursement policy and androgen-deprivation therapy for prostate cancer. *N Engl J Med*. 2010;363:1822–1832.
26. James ND, de Bono JS, Spears MR, et al. Abiraterone for prostate cancer not previously treated with hormone therapy. *N Engl J Med*. 2017;377:338–351.
27. Fizazi K, Tran N, Fein L, et al. Abiraterone plus prednisone in metastatic, castration-sensitive prostate cancer. *N Engl J Med*. 2017; 377:352–360.
28. Beer TM, Armstrong AJ, Rathkopf DE, et al. Enzalutamide in metastatic prostate cancer before chemotherapy. *N Engl J Med*. 2014; 371:424–433.
29. Field JJ, Kanakkanthara A, Miller JH. Microtubule-targeting agents are clinically successful due to both mitotic and interphase impairment of microtubule function. *Bioorg Med Chem*. 2014;22: 5050–5059.
30. Kantoff PW, Hgano CS, Shore ND, et al. Sipuleucel-T immunotherapy for castration-resistant prostate cancer. *N Engl J Med*. 2010;363:411–422.
31. Parker C, Nilsson S, Heinrich D, et al. Alpha emitter radium-223 and survival in metastatic prostate cancer. *N Engl J Med*. 2013;369:213–223.
32. de Bono JS, Oudard S, Ozguroglu M, et al. Prednisone plus cabazitaxel or mitoxantrone for metastatic castration-resistant prostate cancer progressing after docetaxel treatment: a randomised open-label trial. *Lancet*. 2010;376:1147–1154.
33. Tannock IF, de Wit R, Berry WR, et al. Docetaxel plus prednisone or mitoxantrone plus prednisone for advanced prostate cancer. *N Engl J Med*. 2004;351:1502–1512.
34. Petrylak DP, Tangen CM, Hussain MHA, et al. Docetaxel and estramustine compared with mitoxantrone and prednisone for advanced refractory prostate cancer. *N Engl J Med*. 2004;351:1513–1520.
35. Lu-Yao GL, Albertsen PC, Moore DF, et al. Survival following primary androgen deprivation therapy among men with localized prostate cancer. *JAMA*. 2008;300:173–181.
36. Levine GN, D'Amico AV, Berger P, et al. Androgen-deprivation therapy in prostate cancer and cardiovascular risk: a science advisory from the American Heart Association, American Cancer Society, and American Urological Association: endorsed by the American Society for Radiation Oncology. *CA Cancer J Clin*. 2010;60:194–201.
37. Nanda A, Chen MH, Braccioforte MH, et al. Hormonal therapy use for prostate cancer and mortality in men with coronary artery disease-induced congestive heart failure or myocardial infarction. *JAMA*. 2009;302:866–873.
38. O'Farrell S, Garmo H, Holmberg L, et al. Risk and timing of cardiovascular disease after androgen-deprivation therapy in men with prostate cancer. *J Clin Oncol*. 2015;33:1243–1251.
39. Jin C, Fan Y, Meng Y, et al. A meta-analysis of cardiovascular events in intermittent androgen-deprivation therapy versus continuous androgen-deprivation therapy for prostate patients with cancer. *Prostate Cancer Prostatic Dis*. 2016;19:333–339.
40. Tsai H-T, Pfeiffer RM, Philips GK, et al. Risks of serious toxicities from intermittent versus continuous androgen deprivation therapy for advanced prostate cancer: a population based study. *J Urol*. 2017;197:1251–1257.
41. Hershman DL, Unger JM, Wright JD, et al. Adverse health events following intermittent and continuous androgen deprivation in patients with metastatic prostate cancer. *JAMA Oncol*. 2016;2:453–461.
42. Shore ND, Saad F, Cookson MS, et al. Oral relugolix for androgen-deprivation therapy in advanced prostate cancer. *N Engl J Med*. 2020;382:2187–2196.
43. Iacovelli R, Ciccarese C, Bria E, et al. The cardiovascular toxicity of abiraterone and enzalutamide in prostate cancer. *Clin Genitourin Cancer*. 2018;16:e645–e653.
44. Miller KD, Siegel RL, Lin CC, et al. Cancer treatment and survivorship statistics, 2016. *CA Cancer J Clin*. 2016;66:271–289.
45. Patnaik JL, Byers T, DiGuiseppi C, et al. Cardiovascular disease competes with breast cancer as the leading cause of death for older females diagnosed with breast cancer: a retrospective cohort study. *Breast Cancer Res*. 2011;13:R64.
46. Chang HM, Okwuosa TM, Scarabelli T, et al. Cardiovascular complications of cancer therapy. Best practices in diagnosis, prevention, and management: Part 2. *J Am Coll Cardiol*. 2017;70:2552–2565.

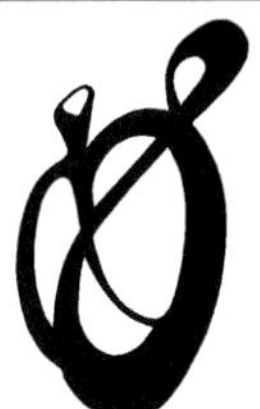

38 Renal and Urinary Bladder Cancer

ZHUOER XIE AND BRIAN A. COSTELLO

Stages	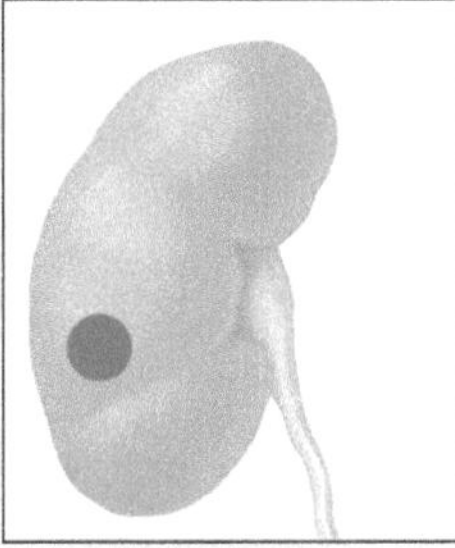 **Stage I** Tumor is 7 cm or less, is localized in kidney only	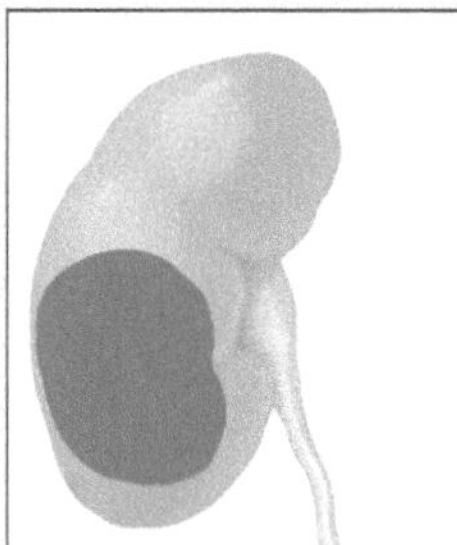 **Stage II** Tumor is larger than 7 cm and is found in kidney only	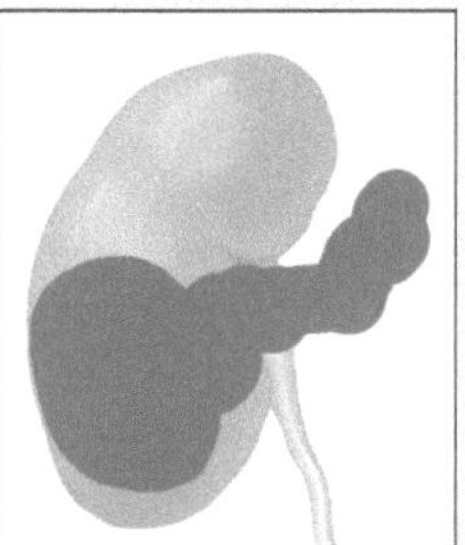 **Stage III** Tumor extends into major veins or perinephric tissues, but not into the ipsilateral adrenal gland and not beyond Gerota's fascia with negative LN or positive reginal LNs	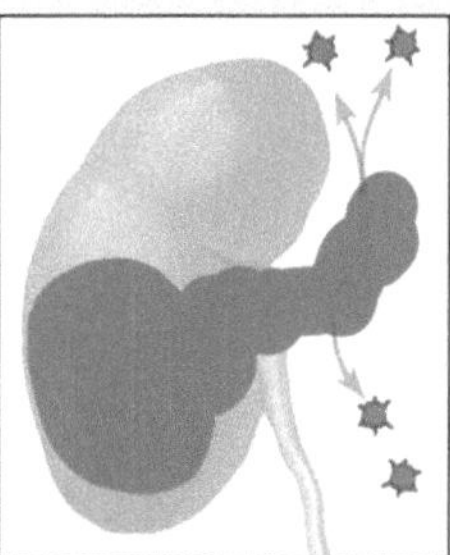 **Stage IV** Tumor invades beyond Gerota's fascia (including contiguous extension into the ipsilateral adrenal gland) with negative LN or any distant metastasis
Treatment	Radical nephrectomy Simple nephrectomy Partial nephrectomy	Radical nephrectomy Partial nephrectomy	Radical nephrectomy Partial nephrectomy	**Targeted or immunotherapy:** **Favorable risk disease:** • Pembrolizumab + axitinib • Sunitinib • Pazopanib **Intermediate/poor risk disease:** • Ipilimumab + nivolumab • Pembrolizumab + axitinib • Cabozantinib
Prognosis	5-year survival 92.6%	5-year survival 70%	5-year survival 70%	5-year survival 13%
Potential CV toxicities				**VEGF inhibitors:** hypertension, arterial and venous thromboembolic events, bleeding **Immune checkpoint inhibitors:** myocarditis, arrhythmias, cardiomyopathy, vasculitis, pericarditis, pericardial effusion

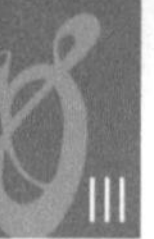

Stages	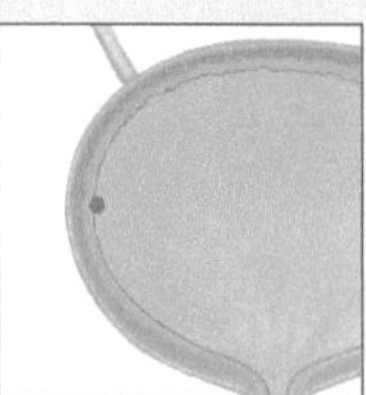 **Stage 0** Abnormal cells are found in the tissue lining the inside of the bladder	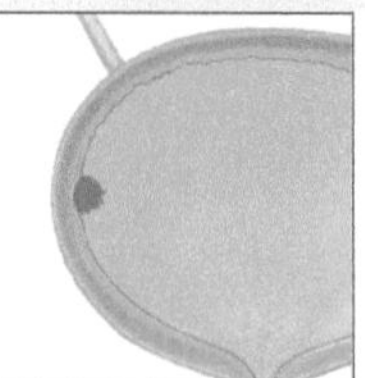 **Stage I** Cancer invades lamina propria (superficial connective tissue)	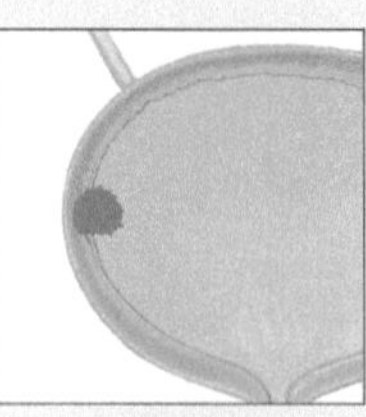 **Stage II** Cancer invades muscularis propria	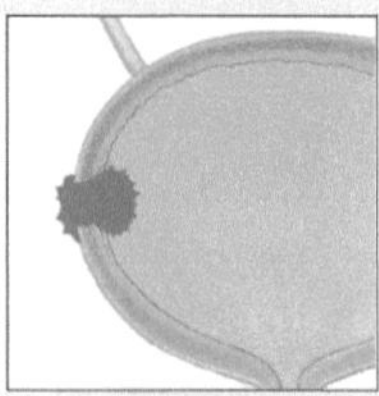 **Stage III** Tumor invades perivesical soft tissue or extravesical tumor invades directly into prostatic stroma, seminal vesicles, uterus, vagina with negative lymph node; or positive regional lymph node disease	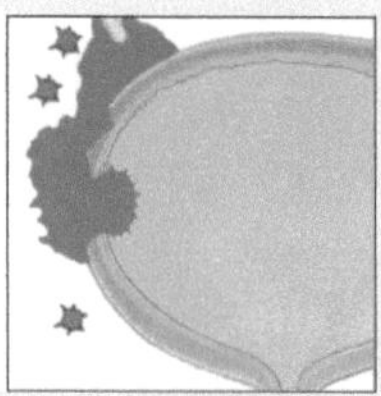 **Stage IV** Extravesical tumor invades pelvic wall or abdominal wall or any distant metastasis
Treatment	Observation Transurethral resection alone Transurethral resection followed by intravesical BCG or chemotherapy ± maintenance therapy Immunotherapy with BCG unresponsive high risk disease		Chemotherapy followed by radical or partial cystectomy Radical cystectomy External radiation therapy ± concurrent chemotherapy	LN negative patients: similar to stage II LN positive patients: initial treatment with chemotherapy or immunotherapy	Chemotherapy or immunotherapy
Prognosis	5-year survival 96%	5-year survival 70%	5-year survival 36.5%	5-year survival 36.5%	5-year survival 5.5%

Potential CV toxicities

Chemotherapy regimens:
MVAC: Methotrexate, Vinblastine, Doxorubicin, Cisplatin
GC: Gemcitabine, Cisplatin
CMV: Cisplatin, Methotrexate, Vinblastine
PGC: Paclitaxel, Gemcitabine, Cisplatin
Methotrexate: arterial and venous thrombotic events, hypotension, pericardial effusion, pericarditis
Vinblastine: ischemic events (all arterial territories), hypertension, Raynaud's phenomenon
Doxorubicin: cardiomyopathy
Cisplatin: hypertension, arterial and venous thrombotic events, arrhythmias
Gemcitabine: edema, ischemia events
Paclitaxel: bradycardia, ischemic events, edema, flushing
Immune checkpoint inhibitors: myocarditis, arrhythmias, cardiomyopathy, vasculitis, pericarditis, pericardial effusion

CHAPTER OUTLINE

KEY POINTS ABOUT BLADDER CANCER

- Smoking is the leading cause of bladder cancer in the United States.
- The median age at diagnosis is 73 years.
- Non-muscle invasive disease is treated with cystoscopic resection and intravesical therapy.
- Muscle invasive disease is treated with neoadjuvant cisplatin-based combination chemotherapy followed by cystectomy. If bladder preservation is desired or if the patient is not a surgical candidate, trimodality therapy with transurethral resection of bladder tumor (TURBT) followed by concurrent chemoradiation is recommended.
- For metastatic disease, cisplatin-based chemotherapy is the first-line therapy. Immunotherapy is indicated as the treatment of choice for some patients and has become standard second-line therapy in general.
- Cardiovascular side effects of systemic treatment have been reported, especially immunotherapy-associated cardiotoxicity.

BLADDER CANCER

Incidence

Bladder cancer is the most common malignancy involving the urinary system and the sixth most common malignancy in the United States. Approximately 81,400 cases of bladder cancer are diagnosed each year, typically.[1] In older individuals, with a median age at diagnosis of 73 years. Urothelial carcinoma is the most common histologic type in the United States and Western Europe.

Risk Factors

The most common risk factors for bladder cancer are cigarette smoking and various occupational exposures, such as dye, arsenic, and aromatic amines, most notably in the rubber/leather industries.[2] Schistosoma hematobium causes 50% of cases in developing countries. Other risk factors include male sex, white race, personal or family history of bladder cancer, prior chemotherapy with cyclophosphamide, pelvic radiation, chronic infection or irritation of the urinary tract, and certain medical conditions including obesity, diabetes, and human papillomavirus.[3,4]

Prognosis

For bladder cancer, 51% of patients present with *in situ* disease with a 95.8% 5-year survival, 34.1% with localized disease with a 5-year survival of 69.5%, and 7% with regional lymph node involvement with a 5-year survival of 36.3%. Five percent present with distant metastatic disease and the 5-year survival is 4.6%.

Treatment Overview

Nonmuscle invasion bladder cancer is generally managed with transuretheral resection of bladder tumor (TURBT) and intravesical bacillus Calmette-Guérin (BCG) or intravesical chemotherapy to reduce recurrence or delay progression of bladder cancer to a higher grade or stage.[5] The US Food and

Drug Administration (FDA) has also approved pembrolizumab for the treatment of patients with "BCG-unresponsive, high-risk, nonmuscle invasive bladder cancer with carcinoma *in situ* with or without papillary tumors who are ineligible for or have elected not to undergo cystectomy."[6]

For muscle invasive bladder cancer, neoadjuvant cisplatin-based chemotherapy followed by radical cystectomy with urinary diversion is considered the standard of care. A bladder-preserving approach is an alternative to cystectomy for patients who are medically unfit for surgery and those seeking an alternative to radical cystectomy. Maximal TURBT with concurrent chemoradiotherapy is recommended for this population.[7]

Role of Checkpoint Inhibitors

The FDA has approved the PD-L1 inhibitors atezolizumab, durvalumab, and avelumab as well as the PD-1 inhibitors nivolumab and pembrolizumab for patients with urothelial carcinoma. Pembrolizumab, atezolizumab, nivolumab, durvalumab, and avelumab are approved for the treatment of locally advanced or metastatic urothelial cell carcinoma that has progressed during or after platinum-based chemotherapy or that has progressed within 12 months of neoadjuvant or adjuvant platinum-containing chemotherapy, regardless of PD-L1 expression levels. Additionally, atezolizumab and pembrolizumab are approved as a first-line treatment option for patients with locally advanced or metastatic urothelial cell carcinoma who are not eligible for cisplatin-containing chemotherapy and whose tumors express PD-L1, or in patients who are not eligible for any platinum-containing chemotherapy regardless of PD-L1 expression.[8] As above, the most recent indication for pembrolizumab is refractory nonmuscle invasive bladder cancer.

Cardiovascular Risk

Cardiovascular Side Effects of Systemic Cancer Treatment in Bladder Cancer

Cisplatin

Cisplatin is typically well tolerated from a cardiovascular standpoint. Cardiotoxicity induced by cisplatin is rare (<1%), but has been reported.[9–11] Oxidative stress is an important mechanism of cardiotoxicity.[11] The manifestations include arrhythmias, myocarditis, cardiomyopathy, and congestive heart failure.[9,12] Elevated cardiac blood biomarkers during treatment require further clinical evaluation. Identifying early signs of cardiac damage could optimize the management of cardiotoxicity. Arterial and venous thrombotic events are other concerns with cisplatin therapy. Hypertension has also been noted in patients on platinum-based therapy.

Gemcitabine

Gemcitabine is generally not viewed as a cardiotoxic agent. Only a few case reports exist in literature about gemcitabine-induced cardiomyopathy.[13–15] Gemcitabine-associated peripheral edema is seen in 20% of patients, cardiac arrhythmia in 0.2% to 1.4%, reduction in left ventricular ejection fraction in 0.2%, and exudative pericarditis in 0.2%. Like cisplatin, gemcitabine can be toxic to the endothelium.

The development of peripheral edema is a nonspecific but multifactorial process that involves a combination of hydrostatic and oncotic forces, and/or vascular permeability changes. Other etiologies must be ruled out before attributing peripheral edema to gemcitabine.[16]

Discontinuation of gemcitabine therapy is appropriate if cardiotoxicity develops.

Checkpoint Inhibitors

Cancer immunotherapy with checkpoint inhibitors has revolutionized the management of a variety of malignancies, but can also produce immune-related adverse events. Based on the review of pharmaceutical safety databases, cardiovascular adverse events occur in less than 0.1% of patients receiving checkpoint inhibitors. The prevalence is higher (0.27%) when used in combination therapy.[17] The cardiotoxicity related to checkpoint inhibitors includes myocardial fibrosis, cardiomyopathy, heart failure, conduction abnormalities, vasculitis, myocarditis, pericarditis, arrhythmia, myocardial infarction, and cardiac arrest.[17–19]

It has been found that PD-1 and PD-L1 are expressed in human cardiomyocytes. Robust T-cell infiltration, activation, and clonal expansion have been observed in cardiomyocytes in patients receiving checkpoint inhibitors.[17] This is thought to play a role in cardiotoxicity related to checkpoint inhibitors.

The onset of cardiovascular side effects can be as soon as 2 weeks and as long as 32 weeks with a median onset of 10 weeks after medication initiation.[20] Signs and symptoms may include fatigue, chest pain, palpitation, peripheral edema, dyspnea, and pleural effusion.

Any grade of cardiac toxicity warrants workup and intervention. Initial workup includes an electrocardiogram, troponin, brain natriuretic peptide (BNP) and chest X-ray. Further diagnostic workup may include a stress test, cardiac catheterization, and cardiac magnetic resonance image. Checkpoint inhibitors should be held immediately and may need to be permanently discontinued. Management of cardiac symptoms should be based on American College of Cardiology/American Heart Association (ACC/AHA) guidelines. If the cardiotoxicity is felt to be caused by to immunotherapy, high-dose corticosteroids, such as methylprednisolone 1 g daily, may be necessary. The addition of mycophenolate, infliximab, or antithymocyte globulin may be considered if there is no immediate response to high-dose corticosteroids.[21]

RENAL CELL CARCINOMA

KEY POINTS ABOUT RENAL CELL CARCINOMA

- The median age at diagnosis is 64 years.
- Cigarette smoking, hypertension, and obesity are the most common risk factors for renal cell carcinoma.
- Localized disease is treated with partial or radical nephrectomy.
- Stage IV metastatic renal cell carcinoma is treated with systemic therapy.
- Cardiovascular side effects of systemic treatment have been reported.

Incidence

Kidney and renal pelvis cancers are the eighth most common malignancy in the United States.[22] Approximately 85% of kidney tumors are renal cell carcinoma (RCC), and approximately 70% of these have clear cell histology. A number of other RCC histologies are collectively termed "non-clear cell" RCC, including papillary and chromophobe, among others. Approximately 73,750 cases of RCC will be newly diagnosed in 2020 in the United States.[1] The median age at diagnosis is 64 years.[23] RCC is approximately 50% more common in men than in women.[24]

Risk Factors

The most common risk factors for RCC include cigarette smoking, hypertension, and obesity. Other risk factors include acquired cystic disease of the kidney, analgesic use, von Hippel-Lindau disease, previous chemotherapy, chronic hepatitis C infection, sickle cell disease, kidney stones, and occupational exposure to products such as cadmium, asbestos, and petroleum by-products.[25]

Prognosis

The overall 5-year survival rate of clear-cell RCC is 74.8%. Of patients, 65% present with localized disease and have a 5-year survival of 92.5%; 17% present with regional disease and 5-year survival is 69.6%; 16% present with metastatic disease and 5-year survival is 12%.

Prognostic models have been developed for risk stratification and systemic treatment guidance. The two most commonly used prognostic models are the International Metastatic Renal Cell Carcinoma Database Consortium model that was developed in the targeted therapy era[26] and an earlier model, the Memorial Sloan Kettering Score.[27] Both models stratify patients with metastatic RCC into favorable, intermediate, and poor risk groups.

Treatment Overview

Localized Disease: Stage I, II, or III Renal Cell Carcinoma

For patients with a resectable stage I, II, or III RCC, radical nephrectomy or partial nephrectomy are options. Partial nephrectomy is an alternative for some smaller, usually more peripheral tumors. A recent study showed improved survival with partial nephrectomy for patients with early stage kidney cancer.[28] The surgical approach for patients with stage II or III disease remains radical nephrectomy.[29] For elderly patients and those with multiple comorbid conditions, ablative techniques are an alternative.

Following complete resection of a localized RCC, no uniform consensus exists for using adjuvant therapy. Although there is an FDA approval for sunitinib in high-risk, resected RCC, many experts refrain from using adjuvant therapy outside of a clinical trial as a number of prior clinical trials in this setting have not shown benefit. No role was seen for radiation to the primary tumor.

Stage IV Disease Renal Cell Carcinoma

A unique feature of metastatic RCC is that consideration is given to removing the primary tumor, a so-called cytoreductive nephrectomy, for therapeutic purpose. Cytoreductive nephrectomy can be considered prior to systemic treatment or after it for selected patients, such as those with good performance status, potentially surgically resectable primary tumor mass, and no symptomatic metastatic disease.[30] More recently, data have showed that upfront sunitinib is not inferior to surgery plus sunitinib. So, patient selection and timing of any surgical intervention is very important.

For patients with favorable risk disease, sunitinib, pazopanib, or combination therapy with pembrolizumab and axitinib are first-line treatment options. For patients with intermediate or poor risk disease, combination therapy with ipilimumab plus nivolumab, pembrolizumab plus axitinib, or single agent cabozantinib are reasonable options.[31]

The FDA also approved the combination of avelumab plus axitinib for the frontline treatment of patients with advanced RCC in favorable, intermediate, and poor risk group.[32]

Bevacizumab is a recombinant humanized monoclonal antibody that binds and neutralizes circulating vascular endothelial growth factor (VEGF)-A. The combination of bevacizumab and interferon is available for the treatment of patients with metastatic RCC, but is rarely used either in combination or as single agents any longer.

Subsequent Therapy for Metastatic Renal Cell Carcinoma

Options for second-line therapies and beyond include VEGF receptor targeted therapy (cabozantinib, axitinib, sunitinib, or pazopanib), mammalian target of rapamycin (mTOR) inhibitors (everolimus, temsirolimus) and immunotherapy (single-agent nivolumab) in addition to selected drug combinations, such as interferon plus bevacizumab, and lenvatinib plus everolimus.

Cardiovascular Risk

Some patients with kidney cancer are more likely to die from cardiovascular disease than from cancer itself. Radical nephrectomy is associated with an increased risk of cardiovascular morbidity and mortality. Therefore, partial nephrectomy is preferred for early stage kidney cancer because it can achieve preserved renal function, reduce the frequency of cardiovascular events, and decrease overall mortality.[33–36]

Cardiovascular Side Effects of Systemic Cancer Treatment in Kidney Cancer

Tyrosine Kinase Inhibitors

Small molecule tyrosine kinase inhibitors (TKIs) have demonstrated antitumor activity. They not only target the VEGF receptor (VEGFR), but also inhibit platelet-derived growth factor receptor (PDGFR), fibroblast growth factor receptor (FGFR), epidermal growth factor receptor (EGFR), rearranged during transfection (RET), and c-KIT receptor.

Sunitinib

Sunitinib is an oral multitargeted TKI. The exact mechanism for sunitinib-associated cardiotoxicity remains unclear. However, VEGF signaling plays an important role in maintaining cardiac function and homeostasis.[37]

Sunitinib therapy has been associated with several cardiovascular toxicities including increased serum creatine kinase (49%), hypertension (15% to 39%), peripheral edema (≤24%), decreased left ventricular ejection fraction (11% to 16%), chest pain (13%), venous thromboembolism (4%), and cardiac failure (3%). Life-threatening adverse effects include hypertensive crisis and hemorrhage.[38] Studies show cardiovascular dysfunction is (mostly) reversible with careful cardiovascular and oncologic management.[37] Patients receiving therapy should be monitored closely for hypertension and reduced ejection fraction.[39]

Pazopanib

Pazopanib is another oral multitargeted TKI. It has similar efficacy as sunitinib. As with other VEGFR inhibitors, pazopanib is also associated with cardiovascular toxicity. Hypertension is the most common side effect (40% to 42%). Other cardiovascular side effects include conduction disturbances (bradycardia 2% to 19%, QT prolongation <2%, *torsades de pointes* <1%), peripheral edema (14%), systemic heart failure (11% to 13%), thrombotic events (5%), ischemic cardiac events (≤2%), and myocardial infarction (≤2%). Standard cardiovascular surveillance is needed to minimize potentially avoidable cardiovascular risk while undergoing treatment with pazopanib.[40]

Axitinib

Axitinib is a selective second-generation TKI targeting VEGFR, PDGFR, and c-KIT. Axitinib is well tolerated from a cardiotoxicity standpoint. Hypertension (17%) is a common treatment-related side effect; and uncontrolled hypertension can lead to serious cardiovascular events.[41,42]

Lenvatinib

Levantinib is a TKI targeting VEGFR, PDGFR, c-KIT, and RET. The most common side effects are hypertension (45% to 73%) and peripheral edema (14% to 21%).

Cabozantinib

Cabozantinib is a potent multi-targeted TKI against mesenchymal-epithelial transition factor and VEGFR. The mechanism of cabozantinib associated cardiovascular adverse effects is similar to other VEGFR inhibitors. Cabozantinib-associated cardiotoxicity includes hypertension (30% to 61%), hypotension (7%), thrombotic events (1% to 7%), and vascular disease (1%).

Bevacizumab

Bevacizumab, a monoclonal humanized antibody against VEGF, slows down the metastatic tissue growth via inhibiting microvascular growth. The cardiotoxicity associated with bevacizumab includes high-grade hypertension (4% to 35%), peripheral edema (15%), venous and arterial thromboembolism (5% to 11%), decreased left ventricular ejection fraction (10%), and cardiac ischemia.[43]

Bevacizumab-related hypertension can develop at any time during the treatment and there is a dose relationship. Hypertensive crisis or hypertensive encephalopathy can occur with a higher dose of bevacizumab. Patients who develop hypertension need to be treated with antihypertensive medication with the goal of blood pressure less than 140/90 mm Hg, preferably less than 130/80 mm Hg. A combination of antihypertensive drugs may be required with close monitoring the blood pressure. In case of resistant severe hypertension, bevacizumab may need to be discontinued.[43]

The risk factors for congestive heart failure include uncontrolled high blood pressure and previous exposure to cardiotoxic drugs, such as anthracyclines, which are commonly used in breast cancer or hematology malignancies.[44]

Everolimus

Everolimus is an oral mTOR inhibitor which binds to FK binding protein-12 and forms a complex that in turn binds and inhibits mTOR kinase. It also reduces angiogenesis by inhibiting VEGF and hypoxia-inducible factor expression. The most common cardiovascular toxicity associated with everolimus is hypertension (17% to 30%, with hypertensive crisis of 1%). Other cardiovascular toxicities include peripheral edema, hyperlipidemia, angina, atrial fibrillation, cardiac failure, deep vein thrombosis, and thrombotic events.[45]

Temsirolimus

Temsirolimus is another targeted inhibitor of mTOR that is administered intravenously. The cardiac toxicities associated with temsirolimus include edema (35%), chest pain (16%), hypertension (7%), venous thrombosis (2%), pericardial effusion (1%), and thrombophlebitis (1%), as well as hyperlipidemia.[46]

Ipilimumab

Ipilimumab is a cytotoxic T-lymphocyte antigen-4 blocking antibody. Cardiotoxic events related to ipilimumab have been reported in single cases with various presentations, including myocardial fibrosis, left ventricular dysfunction, myocarditis, heart failure, heart block, and cardiomyopathy.[47–49]

Checkpoint Inhibitors

Ipilimumab plus nivolumab, pembrolizumab plus axitinib, avelumab plus axitinib, and single-agent nivolumab are all approved for the treatment of metastatic RCC. Cardiotoxicity has been reported in patients with RCC treated with immune checkpoint inhibitors.

Checkpoint inhibitors occasionally are associated with cardiovascular adverse events. The prevalence is higher (0.27%) when used in combination therapy.[17] The manifestations of cardiotoxicity include myocardial fibrosis, cardiomyopathy, heart failure, conduction abnormalities, vasculitis, myocarditis, pericarditis, arrhythmia, myocardial infarction, and cardiac arrest.[17–19] It has been found that PD-1 and PD-L1 are expressed in human cardiomyocytes. Robust T-cell infiltration, activation, and clonal expansion were observed in cardiomyocytes in patients receiving checkpoint inhibitors.[17] This is thought to play a role in cardiotoxicity related to checkpoint inhibitors.

The onset of cardiovascular adverse events ranges from 2 to 32 weeks, with a median onset

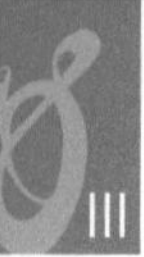

of 10 weeks after medication initiation.[20] Signs and symptoms may include fatigue, chest pain, palpitation, peripheral edema, dyspnea, and pleural effusion. Initial workup includes troponin, BNP, and chest X-ray. Further diagnostic workup may include a stress test, cardiac catheterization, and cardiac MRI. Checkpoint inhibitors should be held immediately. Management of cardiac symptoms should be based on ACC/AHA guidelines. High-dose corticosteroids may be necessary for immunotherapy related cardiotoxicity. Additional immunosuppressive agents, such as mycophenolate, may need to be considered if there is no immediate response to high-dose corticosteroids.[21]

Interferon

Cardiotoxicity related to interferon has been reported in case series. The most common presentations include cardiac arrhythmias, dilated cardiomyopathy, and ischemic heart disease. Cardiotoxicity may be reversible after discontinuing interferon.[50]

REFERENCES

1. Siegel RL, Miller KD, Jemal A. Cancer statistics, 2020. *CA Cancer J Clin.* 2020;70:7–30. doi:10.3322/caac.21590.
2. Freedman ND, Silverman DT, Hollenbeck AR, Schatzkin A, Abnet CC. Association between smoking and risk of bladder cancer among men and women. *JAMA.* 2011;306:737–745.
3. Xu Y, Huo R, Chen X, Yu X. Diabetes mellitus and the risk of bladder cancer: a PRISMA-compliant meta-analysis of cohort studies. *Medicine (Baltimore).* 2017;96:e8588.
4. DeGeorge KC, Holt HR, Hodges SC. Bladder cancer: diagnosis and treatment. *Am Fam Physician.* 2017;96:507–514.
5. Sylvester RJ, Van Der Meijden APM, Alfred Witjes J, Kurth K. Bacillus Calmette-Guerin versus chemotherapy for the intravesical treatment of patients with carcinoma in situ of the bladder: a meta-analysis of the published results of randomized clinical trials. *J Urol.* 2005;174:86–91.
6. Balar AV, Kulkarni GS, Uchio EM, et al. Keynote 057: Phase II trial of pembrolizumab (pembro) for patients (pts) with high-risk (HR) nonmuscle invasive bladder cancer (NMIBC) unresponsive to bacillus calmette-guérin (BCG). *J Clin Oncol.* 2020;37:350–350.
7. Vale CL. Neoadjuvant chemotherapy in invasive bladder cancer: update of a systematic review and meta-analysis of individual patient data. *Eur Urol.* 2005;48:202–206.
8. Kamat AM, Bellmunt J, Galsky MD, et al. Society for Immunotherapy of Cancer consensus statement on immunotherapy for the treatment of bladder carcinoma. *J Immunother Cancer.* 2017;5:68.
9. Hu Y, Sun B, Zhao B, et al. Cisplatin-induced cardiotoxicity with midrange ejection fraction: a case report and review of the literature. *Medicine (Baltimore).* 2018;97:e13807.
10. De Bree E, Van Ruth S, Schotborgh CE, Baas P, Zoetmulder FAN. Limited cardiotoxicity after extensive thoracic surgery and intraoperative hyperthermic intrathoracic chemotherapy with doxorubicin and cisplatin. *Ann Surg Oncol.* 2007;14:3019–3026.
11. Demkow U, Stelmaszczyk-Emmel A. Cardiotoxicity of cisplatin-based chemotherapy in advanced non–small cell lung patients with cancer. *Respir Physiol Neurobiol.* 2013;187:64–67.
12. Hanchate LP, Sharma SR, Madyalkar S. Cisplatin induced acute myocardial infarction and dyslipidemia. *J Clin Diagn Res.* 2017;11: OD05–OD07.
13. Khan MF, Gottesman S, Boyella R, Juneman E. Gemcitabine-induced cardiomyopathy: a case report and review of the literature. *J Med Case Rep.* 2014;220.
14. Mohebali D, Matos J, Chang JD. Gemcitabine induced cardiomyopathy: a case of multiple hit cardiotoxicity. *ESC Heart Fail.* 2017; 4:71–74.
15. Alam S, Illo C, Ma YT, Punia P. Gemcitabine-induced cardiotoxicity in patients receiving adjuvant chemotherapy for pancreatic cancer: a case Series. *Case Rep Oncol.* 2018;11:221–227.
16. Azzoli CG, Miller VA, Ng KK, et al. Gemcitabine-induced peripheral edema. *Am J Clin Oncol.* 2003;26:247–251.
17. Johnson DB, Balko JM, Compton ML, et al. Fulminant myocarditis with combination immune checkpoint blockade. *N Engl J Med.* 2016;375:1749–1755.
18. Varricchi G, Galdiero MR, Marone G, et al. Cardiotoxicity of immune checkpoint inhibitors. *ESMO Open.* 2017;2:e000247.
19. Champiat S, Lambotte O, Barreau E, et al. Management of immune checkpoint blockade dysimmune toxicities: a collaborative position paper. *Ann Oncol.* 2016;27:559–574.
20. Jain V, Bahia J, Mohebtash M, Barac A. Cardiovascular complications associated with novel cancer immunotherapies. *Curr Treat Options Cardiovasc Med.* 2017;19:36.
21. Brahmer JR, Lacchetti C, Schneider B, et al. Management of immune-related adverse events in patients treated with immune checkpoint inhibitor therapy: American Society of Clinical Oncology clinical practice guideline. *J Clin Oncol.* 2018;36:1714–1768.
22. Siegel RL, Miller KD, Jemal A. Cancer statistics, 2019 (US statistics). *CA Cancer J Clin.* 2019;69:7–34.
23. Kidney and Renal Pelvis Cancer. Cancer Stat Facts. https://seer.cancer.gov/statfacts/html/kidrp.html.
24. Siegel R, Jemal A. Cancer facts & figures. *Health Policy (New York).* 2010;1:1–68.
25. Cumberbatch MG, Rota M, Catto JWF, La Vecchia C. The role of tobacco smoke in bladder and kidney carcinogenesis: a comparison of exposures and meta-analysis of incidence and mortality risks. *Eur Urol.* 2016;70:458–466.
26. Heng DYC, Xie W, Regan MM, et al. Prognostic factors for overall survival in patients with metastatic renal cell carcinoma treated with vascular endothelial growth factor-targeted agents: results from a large, multicenter study. *J Clin Oncol.* 2009;27:5794–5799.
27. Motzer RJ, Bacik J, Murphy BA, Russo P, Mazumdar M. Interferon-alfa as a comparative treatment for clinical trials of new therapies against advanced renal cell carcinoma. *J Clin Oncol.* 2002;20: 289–296.
28. Tan HJ, Norton EC, Ye Z, et al. Long-term survival following partial vs radical nephrectomy among older patients with early-stage kidney cancer. *JAMA.* 2012;307:1629–1635.
29. Luo JH, Zhou FJ, Xie D, et al. Analysis of long-term survival in patients with localized renal cell carcinoma: laparoscopic versus open radical nephrectomy. *World J Urol.* 2010;28:289–293.
30. Culp SH, Tannir NM, Abel EJ, et al. Can we better select patients with metastatic renal cell carcinoma for cytoreductive nephrectomy? *Cancer.* 2010;116:3378–3388.
31. DiGiulio S. Kidney cancer. *NCCN Clin Pract Guidel Oncol.* 2012;5: 13–14.
32. Motzer RJ, Penkow K, Haanen J, et al. Avelumab plus axitinib versus sunitinib for advanced renal-cell carcinoma. *N Engl J Med.* 2019;380:1103–1115.
33. Thompson RH, Boorjian SA, Lohse CM, et al. Radical nephrectomy for pT1a renal masses may be associated with decreased overall survival compared with partial nephrectomy. *J Urol.* 2008;179: 468–471, discussion 472–473.
34. Weight CJ, Larson BT, Gao T, et al. Elective partial nephrectomy in patients with clinical T1b renal tumors is associated with improved overall survival. *Urology.* 2010;76:631–637.
35. Huang WC, Elkin EB, Levey AS, Jang TL, Russo P. Partial nephrectomy versus radical nephrectomy in patients with small renal tumors: is there a difference in mortality and cardiovascular outcomes? *J Urol.* 2009;181:55–62.
36. Kim SP, Thompson RH, Boorjian SA, et al. Comparative effectiveness for survival and renal function of partial and radical nephrectomy for localized renal tumors: a systematic review and meta-analysis. *J Urol.* 2012;188:51–57.

37. Narayan V, Keefe S, Haas N, et al. Prospective evaluation of sunitinib-induced cardiotoxicity in patients with metastatic renal cell carcinoma. *Clin Cancer Res.* 2017;23:3601–3609.
38. Schmidinger M, Zielinski CC, Vogl UM, et al. Cardiac toxicity of sunitinib and sorafenib in patients with metastatic renal cell carcinoma. *J Clin Oncol.* 2008;26:5204–5212.
39. Chu TF, Rupnick MA, Kerkela R, et al. Cardiotoxicity associated with tyrosine kinase inhibitor sunitinib. *Lancet.* 2007;370:2011–2019.
40. Pinkhas D, Ho T, Smith S. Assessment of pazopanib-related hypertension, cardiac dysfunction and identification of clinical risk factors for their development. *Cardio-Oncology.* 2017;3:5.
41. Gunnarsson O, Pfanzelter NR, Cohen RB, Keefe SM. Evaluating the safety and efficacy of axitinib in the treatment of advanced renal cell carcinoma. *Cancer Management and Research.* 2015;7:65–73.
42. Rini BI, de La Motte Rouge T, Harzstark AL, et al. Five-year survival in patients with cytokine-refractory metastatic renal cell carcinoma treated with axitinib. *Clin Genitourin Cancer.* 2013;11:107–114.
43. Economopoulou P, Kotsakis A, Kapiris I, Kentepozidis N. Cancer therapy and cardiovascular risk: focus on bevacizumab. *Cancer Manag Res.* 2015;7:133–143.
44. Miller KD, Chap LI, Holmes FA, et al. Randomized phase III trial of capecitabine compared with bevacizumab plus capecitabine in patients with previously treated metastatic breast cancer. *J Clin Oncol.* 2005;23:792–799.
45. Hedhli N, Russell KS. Cardiotoxicity of molecularly targeted agents. *Curr Cardiol Rev.* 2012;7:221–233.
46. Bellmunt J, Szczylik C, Feingold J, Berkenblit A, Strahs A. Temsirolimus safety profile and management of toxic effects in patients with advanced renal cell carcinoma and poor prognostic features. *Ann Oncol.* 2008;19:1387–1392.
47. Voskens CJ, Goldinger SM, Loquai C, et al. The price of tumor control: an analysis of rare side effects of anti-CTLA-4 therapy in metastatic melanoma from the ipilimumab network. *PLoS One.* 2013;8:e53745.
48. Heinzerling L, Ott PA, Hodi FS, et al. Cardiotoxicity associated with CTLA4 and PD1 blocking immunotherapy. *J Immunother Cancer.* 2016;4:50.
49. Roth ME, Muluneh B, Jensen BC, Madamanchi C, Lee CB. Left ventricular dysfunction after treatment with ipilimumab for metastatic melanoma. *Am J Ther.* 2016;23:e1925–e1928.
50. Sonnenblick M, Rosin A. Cardiotoxicity of interferon: a review of 44 cases. *Chest.* 1991;99:557–561. doi:10.1378/chest.99.3.557.

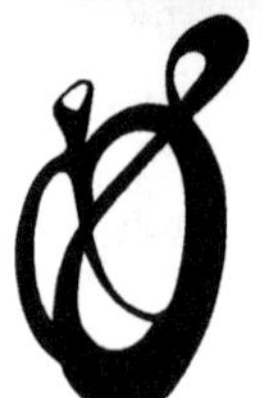

39 Lung Cancer

PRIYANKA MAKKAR AND ALEXANDER GEYER

	Non–small cell lung cancer (NSCLC)				Small cell lung cancer	
Stages				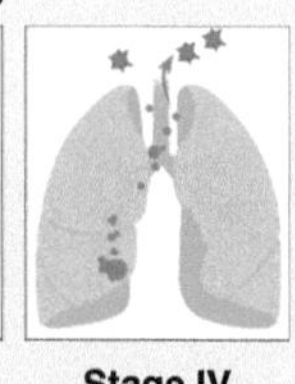	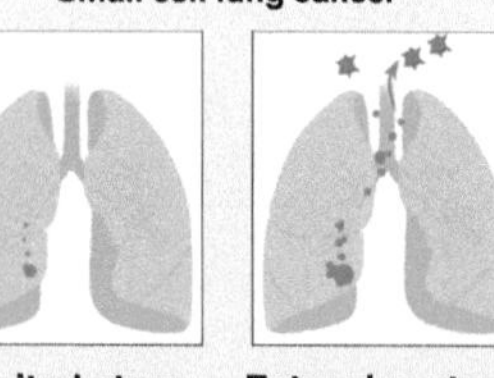	
	Stage I IA ≤3 cm IB >3 but <5 cm or involves main bronchus but ≤2 cm of trachea, or visceral pleura, or atelectasis or obstructive pneumonitis beyond hilar region	**Stage II** >5 to ≤7 cm or local pulmonary and bronchial lymph nodes (LNs)	**Stage III** Any size, any local or regional spread, but not to the other lung or distant spread	**Stage IV** Spread to the other lung, distant LNs and other organs, pleural or pericardial effusion	**Limited stage** Tumor confined to the ipsilateral hemi-thorax and regional nodes; able to be included in a single tolerable radiotherapy port	**Extensive stage** Tumor beyond the boundaries of limited disease including distant metastases, malignant pericardial, or pleural effusions, and contralateral supraclavicular and contralateral hilar involvement
Treatment	Surgery For stage IB: + adjuvant chemotherapy for high risk patients *: cisplatin + pemetrexed if nonsquamous, or gemcitabine, vinorelbine, or docetaxel if squamous	Surgery + adjuvant chemotherapy (as for high risk stage IB)* For stage IIB ± radiation or surgery + concurrent chemoradiation	Chemotherapy ± radiation For stage IIIA surgery*	Chemotherapy + targeted molecular therapy* ± immune checkpoint inhibitor (if PD-L1 +)	Surgery No LN involvement: surgery + adjuvant chemotherapy* ± radiation therapy LN involvement: chemotherapy* + radiation therapy *platinum-based, typ. cisplatin + etoposide	Surgery Platinum-based chemotherapy Brain metastasis, SVC syndrome, cord compression: radiation therapy to symptomatic sites
			*If EGFR mutant: osimertinib, gefitinib, erlotinib If ALK translocation: + crizotinib			
Prognosis	5-year survival 68%–92%	5-year survival 53%–60%	5-year survival 13%–36%	5-year survival 0%–10%	5-year survival 10%–13%	5-year survival 1%–3%

Potential CV toxicities

NSCLC:

- **Cisplatin:** hypertension, arterial and venous thrombosis, arrhythmias
- **Gemcitabine:** edema, vascular events/ischemia
- **Vinorelbine:** chest pain/ischemia
- **Doxetaxel:** hypotension, arrhythmias
- **Osimertinib:** QTc prolongation, cardiomyopathy
- **Gefitinib:** usually none
- **Erlotinib:** chest pain, arterial and venous thrombosis, edema, arrhythmias
- **Crizotinib:** edema, bradycardia, QTc prolongation, pulmonary embolism
- **Imnmune checkpoint inhibitors:** myocarditis
- **Radiation:** radiation-induced heart disease, autonomic dysfunction

Small cell lung cancer:

- **Cisplatin:** see NSCLC
- **Etoposide:** hypotension with rapid infusion

Limited stage:

- Irinorectan may be used instead of cisplatin (edema, hypotension, thromboembolism)
- Paclitaxel may be used instead of cisplatin (bradycardia, ischemia, edema, hypotension)

Extensive stage:

- ICI (atezolizumab, durvalumab, or pembrolizumab) in addition to platinum-etoposide: see NSCLC
- **Radiation:** see NSCLC

CHAPTER OUTLINE

KEY POINTS

- Lung cancer is the most common cancer worldwide (12.3% of newly diagnosed cancers in 2018) with non–small cell lung cancer (NSCLC) and small cell lung cancer (SCLC) accounting for 85% of the cases.
- Cigarette smoking is the primary risk factor for the development of lung cancer. Other risk factors include older age, family history of lung cancer, exposure to environmental agents, such as radon and asbestos, prior radiation therapy, and a history of pulmonary fibrosis.
- The 5-year survival for patients with NSCLC stage I-A1 disease is 92%, whereas it is 10% for patients with stage IV-A disease. Surgical removal of the tumor offers the best long-term survival and is an option up to stage IIIA.
- For patients with SCLC, the 5-year survival rate for those with limited stage disease is 10% to 13% and for those with extensive disease is 1% to 2%. Addition of radiation therapy and prophylactic intracranial radiation has also been shown to prolong survival in patient with limited stage SCLC. Chemotherapy is an integral part for all patients as a disseminated disease.
- Tyrosine kinase inhibitor-based targeted therapy for specific driver gene mutations, such as EGFR, ALK, ROS-1, BRAFV600E results in better survival as compared with standard chemotherapy, but is associated with cardiotoxicity. Similarly, immune checkpoint inhibitors, used in the absence of driver mutation and presence of tumor PDL-1 expression, can lead to cardiomyopathy and myocarditis with high fatality risk.

EPIDEMIOLOGY

Lung cancer is the most common cancer worldwide with 2.1 million new cases diagnosed and 1.7 million deaths in 2018.[1] Being tightly linked to cigarette smoking, the incidence and mortality of lung cancer follow the smoking trends across the world. In the industrialized countries, smoking rates peaked first in men, followed by women and so did the incidence of lung cancer. After the institution of comprehensive tobacco control programs, both smoking rates and the incidence of lung cancer have been declining there. For example, in the United States, the incidence of lung cancer peaked in the 1980s, followed by a decline, with a similar pattern in women following 20 years later. Lung cancer deaths in the United States have been declining at an average of 2.9% annually in men and half that in women. A similar pattern is expected to play out in the developing nations, although increasing air pollution and other region-specific factors (e.g., the use of indoor biofuel) will likely affect the incidence and prognosis of lung cancer in these countries.[2]

RISK FACTORS AND SCREENING

Besides smoking, even secondhand smoking, as the most common and important risk factor, various other lifestyle and environmental factors have been identified as risk factors for the development of lung cancer, including radon, radiation, asbestos, pulmonary fibrosis, and HIV.[3,4] Prior to the year 2011, screening for lung cancer was not recommended, given that no mortality benefit had ever been demonstrated. However, after the National Lung Screening Trial, which compared computed tomography (CT) of chest with chest X-ray in heavy smokers showed a 20% mortality benefit, the United States Preventive Task Force recommended screening for lung cancer with low dose (CT) in patients 55 to 77 years of age with at least a 30-pack year smoking history who were active smokers or had quit within the last 15 years.[5,6]

DIAGNOSIS AND STAGING

Small cell (SCLC) and non–small cell lung cancer (NSCLC) are the two distinct categories of lung cancer with NSCLC accounting for 85% of the cases. Initial evaluation of lung cancer includes clinical, laboratory, and radiographic studies followed by biopsy.[7] Clinical manifestation of lung cancer include cough, hemoptysis, chest pain, dyspnea, weight loss, and clubbing. Cough, the most common symptom, is mainly seen in squamous cell and small cell lung cancer because of central airway involvement.[8–10] Pulmonary function testing can be useful in patients presenting with dyspnea caused by lung cancer. In addition to uncovering underlying chronic obstructive pulmonary disease, it can show flattening of the inspiratory and/or expiratory loop from tumor in the trachea or from vocal cord paralysis.[11] Additional intrathoracic effects of lung cancer include pleural involvement, superior vena cava syndrome, and Pancoast syndrome. Other presenting symptoms may include paraneoplastic syndromes, which are distant effects not directly related to the tumor, invasion, obstruction, or metastases. Common paraneoplastic syndromes associated with lung cancer include hypercalcemia, syndrome of inappropriate antidiuretic hormone secretion (most commonly seen in SCLC), and a varied range of neurologic manifestations that include, but are not limited to, Lambert-Eaton myasthenic syndrome, cerebellar ataxia, limbic encephalitis, and autonomic neuropathy.[12–14] Other paraneoplastic syndromes include hypertrophic osteoarthropathy, dermatomyositis, polymyositis, and Cushing's syndrome (seen most commonly with SCLC and carcinoid tumors).[15]

The clinical staging of lung cancer starts with imaging studies, usually with contrast-enhanced CT of the chest, with extension to include liver and adrenal glands. Imaging studies to identify the highest clinical stage help guide where biopsy needs to be performed.[7,16] No large randomized trials have clearly shown survival benefits or reduction of futile thoracotomy with the use of whole-body positron emission tomography (PET) scans, thus a CT-guided approach to determine the initial clinical stage is recommended. Both CT and PET imaging are limited in their ability to appropriately stage NSCLC (sensitivity and specificity of CT scan is 55% and 81% and that of PET scan is 80% and 88%, respectively).[16,17] Routine imaging for distant metastases is not indicated, unlike SCLC, where MRI of the brain is indicated in all patients. Tissue biopsy is needed for definitive diagnosis of lung cancer. Site selection is important and would ideally result in the highest clinical stage if positive, as well as providing adequate tissue for immunohistochemical and genetic studies. Bronchoscopy with endobronchial ultrasound-transbronchial needle aspiration (EBUS-TBNA) has emerged as the most commonly used technique given its high accuracy in central tumors and most mediastinal lymph nodes.[18] EBUS for diagnosis of lung cancer has a sensitivity of 91.17%, a specificity of 100.0%, and a negative predictive value of 92.9%.[19] Other diagnostic modalities include image guided transthoracic needle biopsy, advanced bronchoscopic techniques (e.g., electromagnetic navigational bronchoscopy), mediastinoscopy and video-assisted thoracoscopic surgery (VATS). Complete staging is important for prognostication and treatment selection options. The 8th edition TNM staging system is currently in use for NSCLC.[20] SCLC is commonly divided into limited stage (LS) and extensive stage (ES). LS is defined as disease that is limited to ipsilateral hemithorax and regional lymph nodes; ES extends beyond.

TREATMENT

Treatment depends on tumor histology, extent of disease, and patient characteristics. The major histologic subtypes of NSCLC include squamous cell carcinoma, large cell carcinoma, and most commonly adenocarcinoma. In patients with stage I or stage II disease, complete surgical resection is the preferred approach if the patient is a surgical candidate. VATS is associated with decreased operative morbidity and a faster recovery compared with the traditional open thoracotomy.[21] In patients who have high risk stage IB disease and patients with stage II disease, adjuvant chemotherapy is indicated. Radiation therapy for patients with stage I and stage II disease is indicated only in patients with positive surgical margins. For patients with stage I or stage II disease who are not surgical candidates, definitive radiation therapy is an option, and stereotactic body radiation therapy is preferred for patients with tumor size less than 5 cm.[22] Stage III NSCLC is very heterogenous in its presentation and prognosis and thus an algorithmic management approach is not appropriate. A combination of two local therapies (surgery and radiation) followed by systemic chemotherapy is generally used after a multidisciplinary discussion.[23] Patients with stage I, II, and III disease are generally treated with curative intent. For those with stage IV disease, the goal of treatment is to prolong life and maintain quality of life and this is done so with systemic therapy. Before the initiation of therapy, the key factor to take into consideration is the presence or absence of driver mutation and programmed cell death ligand 1 (PDL-1) expression. In patients with PDL-1 expression of 50% or higher, pembrolizumab is preferred as monotherapy.[24] For those with PDL-1 expression less than 50%, chemotherapy along with pembrolizumab is being used.[25] When driver mutations, such as epidermal growth factor receptor (EGFR), anaplastic lymphoma kinase (ALK) fusion oncogene, KRAS, and so forth are present, specific inhibitors should be incorporated into the therapeutic regimen.[26] Prognosis depends on the stage of disease, with a 5-year survival rate ranging from 92% for stage I to 0 to 10% for stage IV NSCLC.

Small cell carcinoma is a poorly differentiated neuroendocrine tumor, often disseminated. In patients with LS disease without mediastinal lymph node involvement surgical resection is still the initial treatment of choice. If pathologic lymph node (pLN) involvement is discovered, adjuvant chemoradiation is recommended; if no pLN is found, adjuvant chemotherapy alone is recommended. Chemoradiotherapy is the treatment of choice in patients with mediastinal lymph node involvement. Prophylactic cranial radiation is given to all patients with LS SCLC.[27] Initial management of ES SCLC depends on the presence of brain metastasis. In the absence of brain metastasis, PDL-1 inhibitor along with a platinum-based drug and etoposide followed by whole brain radiotherapy is the initial treatment of choice. In contrast, in the presence of symptomatic brain metastasis, whole brain radiotherapy followed by PDL-1 inhibitor along with a platinum-based drug and etoposide is the treatment of choice.[28] With contemporary chemoradiotherapy and prophylactic cranial irradiation, median survival is around 17 months and the 5-year survival rate is about 20%.

CARDIOVASCULAR AND PULMONARY TOXICITY

Cardiovascular diseases are the most common cancer therapy side effects with concern that they may lead to early morbidity and mortality in cancer survivors. Radiation therapy can have acute and more profound long-term effects (Chapters 4 and 26).[29] Cisplatin-based chemotherapy is associated with vascular toxicity (see Chapters 8, 17, and 29).

Tyrosine kinase inhibitors are used in patients with NSCLC with targetable driver mutations. These include osimertinib, erlotinib, gefitinib, and afatinib for patients with EGFR mutations. A decline in cardiac function (incidence <10%) and QTc prolongation (<10%) are substantial concerns with osimertinib, whereas erlotinib shows more of a vascular toxicity profile with chest pain as the most common presentation (<20%) and especially in combination with gemcitabine, arterial and venous thrombotic events, as well as arrhythmias and syncopal events and edema. Crizotinib, ceritinib, and alectinib are used in patients with ALK gene rearrangements; all of them are known for their risk of bradycardia (4% to 14%), as well as the risk for QTc prolongation, especially crizotinib and ceritinib (4% to 12%), syncope (1% to 3%), and pulmonary embolism (1% to 10%). Entrectinib and crizotinib have been used when ROS proto-oncogene-1 (ROS1) rearrangements are confirmed; the greatest CV risks for entrectinib include hypotension (18%) as well as cardiac failure (3%), QTc prolongation (3%), syncope (4%), and pulmonary embolism (4%). Capmatinib, which is approved by the US Food and Drug Administration for adult patients with a mesenchymal-epithelial transition factor (MET) exon-14-skipping mutation, is notorious for causing peripheral edema (52%). Crizotinib, capmatinib, and cabozantinib have also been used as a MET inhibitors. Cabozantinib, in distinction to others, causes hypertension in up to 60% of patients and is confronted with all other risks of VEGF inhibitors. Selpercatinib is an approved rearranged during transfection (RET) inhibitor with the risk of hypertension (35%) and QTc prolongation. For patients with BRAF (V600E) mutations, combination therapy with BRAF and MEK inhibitors is the preferred treatment strategy; dabrafenib plus trametinib was a cardiotoxicity risk (decline in ejection fraction) in 3% and up to 11%, respectively, even by more than 20% points in 5% of patients on trametinib. Hypertension and QTc prolongation are additional concerns. Entrectinib (see above) and larotrectinib are used in patients with neurotrophic tyrosine receptor kinase (NTRK) fusion; in distinction to the former, the latter is associated with hypertension (11%).

Immune checkpoint inhibitor, even monotherapy, has been linked to cardiomyopathy and myocarditis in particular (Chapter 54).[30]

The lung is also a frequent target of toxicity related to radiotherapy, standard chemotherapy, and immunotherapy. Radiation therapy-induced pneumonitis is a dose-limiting toxicity. The risk of developing radiation pneumonitis depends on various patient-related factors, concurrent administration of chemotherapy, and treatment-related factors, including dosimetry. Treatment includes supportive management of cough and dyspnea, and the use of steroids with slow taper over 3 to 6 months.[31] The patterns of lung toxicity secondary to chemotherapy include parenchymal lung diseases, pleural disease, pulmonary vascular disease, pulmonary fibrosis, and airway disease. The temporal relationship with chemotherapy administration and exclusion of other etiologies are required for the diagnosis of chemotherapy-induced pulmonary disease.[32] The incidence of immunotherapy-related pneumonitis ranges from 2.7% to 5.0%. The incidence does not vary between individual immunotherapies; however, the risk increases with the combination of immunotherapeutic agents. The severity of injury varies from mild to severe. In mild cases, the patient is treated with temporary cessation of the drug with or without the addition of steroids and patients can be re-challenged once symptoms resolve with multidisciplinary discussion between the pulmonologist and oncologist. However, in more severe cases, steroids are always required, and patients are not re-challenged with the drug.[33]

REFERENCES

1. Siegel RL, Miller KD, Jemal A. Cancer statistics, 2019. *CA Cancer J Clin.* 2019;69(1):7–34.
2. Barta JA, Powell CA, Wisnivesky JP. Global epidemiology of lung cancer. *Ann Glob Health.* 2019;85(1):8.
3. de Groot PM, Wu CC, Carter BW, Munden RF. The epidemiology of lung cancer. *Transl Lung Cancer Res.* 2018;7(3):220–233.
4. Hubbard R, Venn A, Lewis S, Britton J. Lung cancer and cryptogenic fibrosing alveolitis. A population-based cohort study. *Am J Respir Crit Care Med.* 2000;161(1):5–8.
5. Aberle DR, Adams AM, Berg CD, et al. Reduced lung-cancer mortality with low-dose computed tomographic screening. *N Engl J Med.* 2011;365(5):395–409.
6. Humphrey LL, Deffebach M, Pappas M, et al. Screening for lung cancer with low-dose computed tomography: a systematic review to update the US Preventive Services Task Force recommendation. *Ann Intern Med.* 2013;159(6):411–420.
7. Rivera MP, Mehta AC, Wahidi MM. Establishing the diagnosis of lung cancer: diagnosis and management of lung cancer, 3rd ed: American College of Chest Physicians evidence-based clinical practice guidelines. *Chest.* 2013;143(suppl 5):e142S–e165S.
8. Chute CG, Greenberg ER, Baron J, Korson R, Baker J, Yates J. Presenting conditions of 1539 population-based lung patients with cancer by cell type and stage in New Hampshire and Vermont. *Cancer.* 1985;56(8):2107–2111.
9. Hyde L, Hyde CI. Clinical manifestations of lung cancer. *Chest.* 1974;65(3):299–306.
10. Kocher F, Hilbe W, Seeber A, et al. Longitudinal analysis of 2293 NSCLC patients: a comprehensive study from the TYROL registry. *Lung Cancer.* 2015;87(2):193–200.
11. O'Donnell DE, Lam M, Webb KA. Spirometric correlates of improvement in exercise performance after anticholinergic therapy in chronic obstructive pulmonary disease. *Am J Respir Crit Care Med.* 1999;160(2):542–549.
12. Hiraki A, Ueoka H, Takata I, et al. Hypercalcemia-leukocytosis syndrome associated with lung cancer. *Lung Cancer.* 2004;43(3):301–307.
13. List AF, Hainsworth JD, Davis BW, et al. The syndrome of inappropriate secretion of antidiuretic hormone (SIADH) in small-cell lung cancer. *J Clin Oncol.* 1986;4(8):1191–1198.
14. Honnorat J, Antoine JC. Paraneoplastic neurological syndromes. *Orphanet J Rare Dis.* 2007;2:22.
15. Ilias I, Torpy DJ, Pacak K, et al. Cushing's syndrome due to ectopic corticotropin secretion: twenty years' experience at the National Institutes of Health. *J Clin Endocrinol Metab.* 2005;90(8):4955–4962.
16. Silvestri GA, Gonzalez AV, Jantz MA, et al. Methods for staging non-small cell lung cancer: diagnosis and management of lung cancer, 3rd ed: American College of Chest Physicians evidence-based clinical practice guidelines. *Chest.* 2013;143(suppl. 5):e211S–e250S.
17. Pak K, Park S, Cheon GJ, et al. Update on nodal staging in non-small cell lung cancer with integrated positron emission tomography/computed tomography: a meta-analysis. *Ann Nucl Med.* 2015;29(5):409–419.
18. Navani N, Nankivell M, Lawrence DR, et al. Lung cancer diagnosis and staging with endobronchial ultrasound-guided transbronchial needle aspiration compared with conventional approaches: an open-label, pragmatic, randomised controlled trial. *Lancet Respir Med.* 2015;3(4):282–289.
19. Fernandez-Bussy S, Labarca G, Canals S, et al. Diagnostic yield of endobronchial ultrasound-guided transbronchial needle aspiration for mediastinal staging in lung cancer. *J Bras Pneumol.* 2015;41(3):219–224.
20. Goldstraw P, Chansky K, Crowley J, et al. The IASLC lung cancer staging project: proposals for revision of the TNM stage groupings in the forthcoming (eighth) edition of the TNM classification for lung cancer. *J Thorac Oncol.* 2016;11(1):39–51.
21. Mentzer SJ, DeCamp MM, Harpole DH Jr, Sugarbaker DJ. Thoracoscopy and video-assisted thoracic surgery in the treatment of lung cancer. *Chest.* 1995;107(suppl 6):298s–301s.
22. Woody NM, Stephans KL, Marwaha G, Djemil T, Videtic GM. Stereotactic body radiation therapy for non-small cell lung cancer tumors greater than 5 cm: safety and efficacy. *Int J Radiat Oncol Biol Phys.* 2015;92(2):325–331.
23. Huber RM, De Ruysscher D, Hoffmann H, Reu S, Tufman A. Interdisciplinary multimodality management of stage III nonsmall cell lung cancer. *Eur Respir Rev.* 2019;28(152):190024.
24. Reck M, Rodríguez-Abreu D, Robinson AG, et al. Pembrolizumab versus chemotherapy for PD-L1-positive non-small-cell lung cancer. *N Engl J Med.* 2016;375(19):1823–1833.
25. Yu H, Boyle TA, Zhou C, Rimm DL, Hirsch FR. PD-L1 expression in lung cancer. *J Thorac Oncol.* 2016;11(7):964–975.
26. Zhu QG, Zhang SM, Ding XX, He B, Zhang HQ. Driver genes in non-small cell lung cancer: characteristics, detection methods, and targeted therapies. *Oncotarget.* 2017;8(34):57680–57692.
27. Gaspar LE, Gay EG, Crawford J, et al. Limited-stage small-cell lung cancer (stages I-III): observations from the National Cancer Data Base. *Clin Lung Cancer.* 2005;6(6):355–360.
28. Agra Y, Pelayo M, Sacristan M, et al. Chemotherapy versus best supportive care for extensive small cell lung cancer. *Cochrane Database Syst Rev.* 2003(4):CD001990.
29. Jaworski C, Mariani JA, Wheeler G, Kaye DM. Cardiac complications of thoracic irradiation. *J Am Coll Cardiol.* 2013;61(23):2319–2328.
30. Herrmann J, Lerman A, Sandhu NP, et al. Evaluation and management of patients with heart disease and cancer: cardio-oncology. *Mayo Clin Proc.* 2014;89(9):1287–1306.
31. Jain V, Berman AT. Radiation pneumonitis: old problem, new tricks. *Cancers.* 2018;10(7):222.
32. Yoh K, Kenmotsu H, Yamaguchi Y, et al. Severe interstitial lung disease associated with amrubicin treatment. *J Thorac Oncol.* 2010;5(9):1435–1438.
33. Topalian SL, Hodi FS, Brahmer JR, et al. Safety, activity, and immune correlates of anti-PD-1 antibody in cancer. *N Engl J Med.* 2012;366(26):2443–2454.

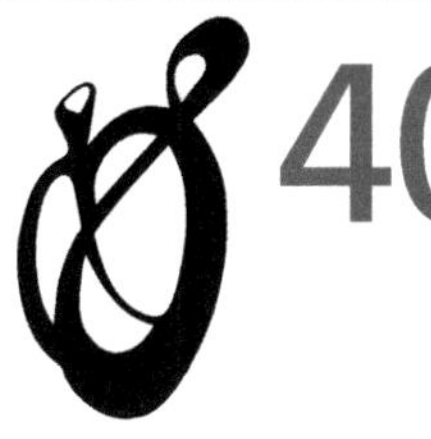

40 Colorectal Cancer

JASVINDER KAUR, JASKANWAL DEEP SINGH SARA, AND AXEL GROTHEY

Stages	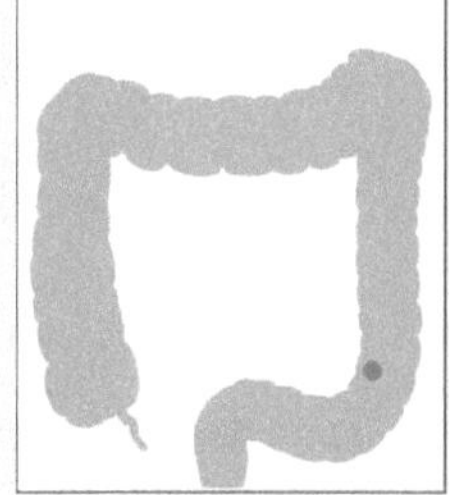 **Stage I** Contained within wall of colon/ rectum T1: Tumor invades submucosa T2: Tumor invades muscularis propria	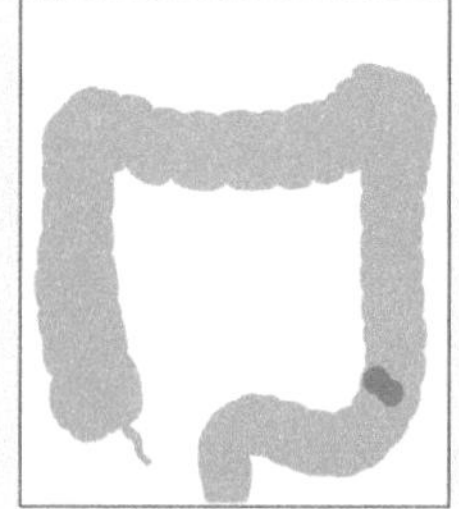 **Stage II** Penetration through wall of colon/rectum, no lymph node metastases	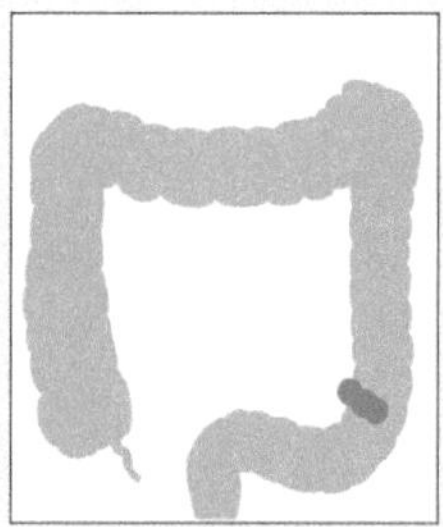 **Stage III** Lymph node involvement, no distant metastasis	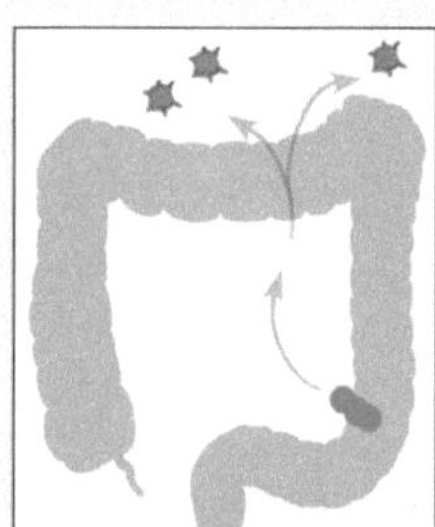 **Stage IV** Metastasis to distant organs and/ or peritoneum
Treatment	Surgery	Surgery ± adjuvant chemotherapy for high risk stage II cancers (fluoropyrimidine single agent, sometimes fluoropyrimidine + oxaliplatin)	Surgery with chemotherapy (commonly fluoropyrimidine + oxaliplatin, sometimes fluoropyrimidine single agent)	Chemotherapy with or without biologic agents Surgery (metastasectomy and primary tumor resection) in some patients with limited metastatic disease (resected stage IV)
Prognosis	5-year survival >90%	5-year survival 80%–90%	5-year survival 60%–80% (very variable depending on sub-stage)	5-year survival Resected stage IV 50%–60% Otherwise 10%–15%
Potential CV toxicities		**Fluorouracil (5-FU):** vasospasm, chest pain, arrhythmia, cardiac failure **Oxaliplatin:** edema, chest pain, thromboembolism **Irinotecan:** edema, hypotension, thromboembolism **VEGF inhibitors:** hypertension, arterial and venous thrombotic events, bleeding **EGFR antibodies:** cetuximab (US box warning for cardiopulmonary arrest), thrombotic events **BRAF inhibitors:** QTc prolongation, hypertension, edema, atrial fibrillation, vasculitis **MEK inhibitors:** edema, hypertension, cardiomyopathy, thromboembolism **Immune checkpoint inhibitors:** myocarditis, cardiomyopathy		

CHAPTER OUTLINE

KEY POINTS: ABOUT COLORECTAL CANCER

- Colorectal cancer is the second leading cause of cancer death in the United States.
- Decreasing incidence in those over 50 years of age, but rising incidence in younger adults.
- Median age of diagnosis is 71 years.
- 5% to 10% of patients have well-defined genetic predisposition (e.g., Lynch syndrome)
- Postoperative adjuvant therapy routinely recommended for patients with stage III, and some patients with stage II disease.
- In patients with localized rectal cancer, neoadjuvant (preoperative) radiation plus chemotherapy is standard of care.
- Some patients with limited metastatic spread can undergo surgery of metastases with curative intent.
- Medical therapy includes chemotherapeutic agents, targeted biologics, and immunotherapy, depending on molecular profile.
- Cardiovascular toxicities in colorectal patients with cancer are seen in particular with fluoropyrimidines, bevacizumab, immune checkpoint inhibitors.

INCIDENCE AND RISK FACTORS

In the United States, nearly 150,000 cases of colorectal cancer are being diagnosed in 2020, with slightly more than one-third of patients dying from this disease, making it the second leading cause of cancer death.[1] It is the fourth most common cancer-related cause of death worldwide.

Regardless of other risk factors, nearly 70% of patients are over 65 years of age. This is pertinent in the context of discussing the management of this cancer with chemotherapy or targeted agents. Age and the physiologic changes associated with it, as well as other medical conditions, which become more common with increasing age undoubtably have an impact on the treatment, in particular with drugs, which have cardiovascular side effects. In recent years, however, an increased incidence and mortality of colorectal cancer has been observed in younger patients, potentially associated with changes in lifestyle factors (e.g., diet, obesity).[1] In contrast, the mortality of older patients has gradually decreased, conceivably as a result of screening programs.

Several hereditary syndromes, comorbid conditions, and lifestyle conditions have been identified that increase the risk of colorectal cancer (Table 40.1).[2]

PRESENTATION

Clinical symptoms upon presentations vary, based on the location of the primary tumor (right- or left-sided colon cancer, rectum) and the presence of metastatic disease. A common symptom is blood per rectum (not infrequently initially misdiagnosed as related to hemorrhoids), change in bowel habits with

TABLE 40.1 Factors That Increase the Risk of Colon Cancer

Hereditary Polyposis Syndromes
• Familial adenomatosis polyposis coli (FAP) • Peutz-Jeghers syndrome • Juvenile polyposis
Hereditary Nonpolyposis Syndromes
• Hereditary nonpolyposis colorectal cancer (HNPCC: Lynch syndrome)
Others
• Inflammatory bowel disease • Prior colon cancer • Prior polyps • First-degree relative diagnosed when younger than age 50 • Western diet • Alcohol • Sedentary lifestyle • Obesity • Diabetes

emergence of constipation, or, especially for more distal tumors, alternating constipation and diarrhea, pain either in the area of the primary tumor or metastases (like right-upper quadrant abdominal pain in the context of liver metastases), and ascites. Increasingly cancers are identified via active screening programs with several testing modalities available (three stool-based and four direct visualization tests).[3]

INITIAL WORKUP

Standard history, examination, and laboratory tests, including full blood count and liver and renal function; also, preoperative evaluation of the serum marker carcinoembryonic antigen (CEA). The CEA level can have a prognostic value in the preoperative setting (>5 ng/dL suggests a worse prognosis). An increased preoperative value not normalized after 1 month following surgical resection may indicate persistent disease.[4] Sequential CEA levels are predominantly useful for posttreatment follow up. If the diagnostic endoscopy has been incomplete owing to obstruction at the site of the primary tumor, it will have to be completed after the cancer has been resected not to miss a secondary primary cancer or adenomatous polyps.

IMAGING STAGING

Computed tomography (CT) of the chest, abdomen, and pelvis is performed as a minimum. Magnetic resonance imaging (MRI) is mandatory for local staging of rectal cancers. An MRI can also be useful as imaging modality for liver metastases considered for surgical resection. In a similar way, a positron emission tomography/CT scan can identify extrahepatic metastases (e.g., peritoneal disease or retroperitoneal lymph nodes), which would change the plan of metastasectomy of liver and limited lung metastases.

PROGNOSIS

The prognosis and choice of therapy depends heavily on the anatomic staging, which is expressed in the TNM staging classification. Specific TNM categories are summarized in American Joint Committee on Cancer stages I–IV with subgroups.[5] Of note, for an adequate assessment of the lymph node status, at least 12 should be retrieved and examined.

TREATMENT OVERVIEW

Management depends on initial radiologic and, if appropriate, surgical staging and pathology. The 5-year survival for localized cancers (stage I/II) is 80% to more than 90%; with spread to regional nodes 5-year survival is 60% to 80%; and with distant spread, it falls to 10% to 15%, unless surgical resection of metastases can be performed.[1,6]

EARLY STAGE DISEASE (STAGES I–III)

For patients with stage II and III colon cancers, surgical resection is routinely the first step in the management of the disease. Subsequently, adjuvant chemotherapy can be considered based on stage and risk factors. No adjuvant therapy is recommended for stage I and low-risk stage II cancers.

For stage III cancers, a survival benefit associated with adjuvant 5-fluorouracil (5-FU)-based therapy was initially established in 1990.[7] At that time a 12 months' duration of 5-FU plus levamisole became standard of care in the adjuvant setting. Subsequently, 6 months of a combination of 5-FU plus leucovorin (LV or folinic acid as biomodulator of 5-FU activity) were found to be at least equally effective.[8] In 2004, a combination of infusional plus bolus 5-FU plus oxaliplatin (FOLFOX) showed superiority over 5-FU/LV in stage III colon cancer so that FOLFOX was widely adopted as adjuvant therapy, at least for patients under the age of 70.[9,10] The combination of capecitabine, an oral 5-FU prodrug plus oxaliplatin (CAPOX) emerged as an alternative standard adjuvant therapy in stage III cancers.[11] In the context of potential cardiotoxicity associated with 5-FU and derivates it is important to note that infusional 5-FU and daily oral capecitabine both carry the risk of coronary vasospasms independent of cardiac comorbidities. 5-FU delivered as bolus injection without protracted administration has a much lower risk of vasospasms.[12] A combination of bolus 5-FU/LV plus oxaliplatin (FLOX) has also been established as appropriate adjuvant therapy in stage III colon cancers, but with a more severe noncardiac toxicity profile (esp., diarrhea) compared with FOLFOX.[13] For patients who develop coronary vasospasms on adjuvant therapy with FOLFOX or CAPOX might be considered for FLOX if their cancer-related risk of recurrence outweighs the potential cardiac risk of being re-exposed to 5-FU, even in bolus form.[12]

More recently, a large international collaboration investigated if 3 months of oxaliplatin-containing treatment was noninferior to 6 months in 12,834 patients with stage III colon cancer.[14] Unexpectedly, noninferiority was confirmed for the vast majority of patients treated with CAPOX, but if FOLFOX was chosen as adjuvant therapy, most patients required a 6 months duration of therapy. These data have affected guideline recommendations in various countries. Especially for low-risk stage III cancers, 3 months of adjuvant CAPOX can now be considered standard adjuvant therapy.

PRINCIPLE OF RESECTION OF DISTANT METASTASES

If the disease is inoperable and nonresectable, either owing to staging as advanced disease or patient factors, then systemic treatment aimed at symptom control/prevention and prolongation of life is considered. In certain situations, advanced disease at limited sites, such as liver or lung, can be potentially operable/curable after systemic chemotherapy with the intention of downstaging to allow for surgery.[6] This would be referred to as "conversion therapy" in contrast to "neoadjuvant treatment" in which systemic therapy is administered in patients with resectable metastases. In a neoadjuvant setting the systemic therapy is mainly meant to obtain information on tumor biology (i.e., response to therapy) and to treat micrometastatic disease as early as possible.

MOLECULAR TESTING

All patients with colorectal cancer should have *RAS* and *RAF* mutation testing carried out, either from the tissue from their surgical resection or from tissue from a suitable biopsy (e.g., of a liver metastasis). The *KRAS* or *NRAS* oncogene is mutated in approximately 50% of colorectal cancers, and *RAS* mutations in exon 2, 3, and 4 are negative predictors of response to antiepidermal growth factor receptor antibodies.[15,16]

Testing for microsatellite instability (MSI) via polymerase chain reaction, next generation sequencing (NGS), or mismatch repair deficiency (MMR-D) via immunohistochemistry (IHC) is recommended for all colorectal cancers independent of stage and age. Patients with MMR-D/MSI-H cancers should be evaluated for the presence of the hereditary Lynch syndrome.[17] In addition, in stage II disease, these cancers have excellent prognosis and do not require adjuvant therapy.[18] In stage IV disease, MMR-D/MSI-H cancers are known to respond to immunotherapy with PD-1 antibodies or a combination of a PD-1 antibody plus a CTLA-4 antibody.[19,20]

PALLIATIVE THERAPY

The main goal of palliative medical therapy for patients with stage IV disease is to extend their life and maintain their quality of life as long as possible. Various anticancer agents have shown efficacy in metastatic colorectal cancer, as single agents, or more commonly, in combination. One of the guiding principles for treatment algorithms is that patients benefit from being exposed to all active agents over time.[21] The choice of first-line treatment is guided by patient characteristics (e.g., age, performance status, comorbidities, socioeconomic factors) and anatomic tumor parameters (e.g., extent of tumor burden, location of metastases, location of the primary tumor), and increasingly molecular parameters, such as *RAS* and *BRAF* mutation status, MSI/MMR status, and HER-2 expression. The choice of first-line therapy is important because it sets in motion a treatment algorithm which will eventually move on to second- and third-line therapies which changing of treatment regimens from line to line.

Table 40.2 details first-line treatment options based on molecular parameters, location of the primary tumor (sidedness), and preferred indication.[22]

Table 40.3 lists the currently used agents in the management of colorectal cancer with their mode of administration, indication, and key side-effects, with emphasis on their cardiotoxic potential.

RECTAL CANCER

The management of early stage rectal cancer is guided by the principle to minimize the risk of local recurrence. The anatomic difference between colon

TABLE 40.2 Medical Treatment Options in the First-Line Management of Metastatic Colorectal Cancer

REGIMEN	SIDEDNESS RESTRICTION	MOLECULAR RESTRICTION	PREFERRED INDICATION
Cape + BEV	None	None	Elderly patients, low-volume disease
FOLFOX/CAPOX/FOLFIRI + BEV	None	None	
FOLFOXIRI + BEV	None	None	Aggressive cancers (e.g., *BRAF* mutated, right-sided)
FOLFOX/FOLFIRI + EGFR mAb	Left-sided[a]	*RAS/BRAF* wt (HER-2 neg?)	Standard of care for left-sided *RAS/ BRAF* wt cancers
FOLFOXIRI + EGFR mAb	Left-sided[a]	*RAS/BRAF* wt (HER-2 neg?)	Left-sided cancers with high tumor load
PD-1 mAb or anti-PD-1 plus anti-CTLA-4 combination	None	MMR-D/MSI-H	Patients with MMR-D/MSI-H cancers not considered for chemotherapy
EGFR mAb plus BRAFi (encorafenib)	None	*BRAF* V600E mutation	Data in first-line pending

[a]Left-sided cancers: distal to the splenic colon flexure.
BEV, Bevacizumab; *BRAF,* b-raf or v-raf murine sarcoma viral oncogene homolog B1; *BRAFi,* BRAF inhibitor; *Cape,* capecitabine; *CTLA-4,* cytotoxic T lymphocyte-associated antigen-4; *EGFR,* epidermal growth factor receptor; *HER-2,* human EGFR-2; *mAb,* monoclonal antibody; *MMR-D,* mismatch repair deficiency; *MSI-H,* microsatellite instability-high; *PD-1,* programmed cell death protein 1; *wt,* wild-type.
For names of chemotherapy regimens see Chapter 54.

TABLE 40.3 Agents Used in the Management of Colorectal Cancer

AGENT CLASS	AGENT	ADMINISTRATION	COMMON USE	TREATMENT SETTING	MAIN SIDE EFFECTS
Cytotoxic Agents					
Fluoropyrimidine	5-FU (bolus)	IV over 2 min	Part of combination therapies with oxaliplatin (FOLFOX) and irinotecan (FOLFIRI)	Adjuvant and palliative	Mucositis, neutropenia. Less diarrhea and **coronary vasospasms** than infusional 5-FU
	5-FU (infusional)	IV in a protracted way over days	Part of combination therapies with oxaliplatin (FOLFOX), irinotecan (FOLFIRI), or both (FOLFOXIRI); parallel to radiation	Adjuvant and palliative	Diarrhea, **coronary vasospasms** (more common than with bolus 5-FU)
	Capecitabine	Oral (5-FU prodrug)	Single agent or in combination with oxaliplatin (less commonly in combination with irinotecan); parallel to radiation	Adjuvant and palliative	Diarrhea, hand-foot-syndrome, **coronary vasospasms** (more common than with bolus 5-FU)
	Trifluridine/ tipiracil (TAS-102)	Oral (combination of active agent—trifluridine—and inhibitor of degradation—tipiracil)	Single agent in third- or fourth-line setting, sometimes in combination with bevacizumab	Palliative	Neutropenia
Other cytotoxic agents	Irinotecan	IV	Part of combination therapies with 5-FU (FOLFIRI) and oxaliplatin (FOLFOX-IRI), single agent activity	Palliative	Neutropenia, diarrhea, fatigue, cholinergic syndrome
	Oxaliplatin	IV	Part of combination therapies with 5-FU (FOLFOX) or capecitabine (CAPOX) and irinotecan (FOLFOXIRI)	Adjuvant and palliative	Sensory neuropathy, diarrhea, neutropenia (mainly in combination with bolus 5-FU), thrombocytopenia

Continued

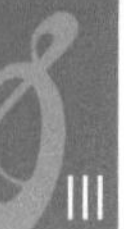

TABLE 40.3 **Agents Used in the Management of Colorectal Cancer—cont'd**

AGENT CLASS	AGENT	ADMINISTRATION	COMMON USE	TREATMENT SETTING	MAIN SIDE EFFECTS
Biologic Agents					
Large molecule VEGF inhibitors	Bevacizumab	IV	Added to cytotoxic regimes (e.g., FOLFOX/CAPOX, FOLFIRI, FOLFOXIRI) or single agent fluoropyrimidine	Palliative	**Hypertension** (best treated with Ca-antagonists and ACE inhibitors), proteinuria, rare bowel perforation
	Ramucirumab	IV	Added to cytotoxic regimes (e.g., FOLFIRI)	Palliative	**Hypertension** (best treated with Ca-antagonists and ACE inhibitors), proteinuria, rare bowel perforation
	Ziv-Aflibercept	IV	Added to cytotoxic regimes (e.g., FOLFIRI)	Palliative	**Hypertension** (best treated with Ca-antagonists and ACE inhibitors), proteinuria, diarrhea, rare bowel perforation
EGFR antibodies	Cetuximab	IV	Added to cytotoxic regimen, single agent activity; restricted to *RAS*-wild-type cancers	Palliative	Skin rash, diarrhea, hypomagnesemia, allergic reaction
	Panitumumab	IV	Added to cytotoxic regimen, single agent activity; restricted to *RAS*-wild-type cancers	Palliative	Skin rash, diarrhea, hypomagnesemia
HER-2 inhibitors	Trastuzumab[a]	IV	Later-line therapy for HER-2 overexpressing cancers in combination with either pertuzumab or lapatinib	Palliative	Diarrhea, nausea, **cardiomyopathy**
	Pertuzumab[a]	IV	Later-line therapy for HER-2 overexpressing cancers in combination with trastuzumab	Palliative	Diarrhea, nausea, **cardiomyopathy**
	Lapatiniba	Oral	Later-line therapy for HER-2 overexpressing cancers in combination with trastuzumab	Palliative	Skin rash, diarrhea, nausea, **cardiomyopathy**
Small Molecule Kinase Inhibitors					
Multikinase inhibitor (incl. VEGF-R)	Regorafenib	Oral	Single agent in third- or fourth-line setting	Palliative	Hand-foot single reaction, fatigue, hypertension (as anti-VEGF effect), diarrhea
BRAF inhibitor	Vemurafenib[a]	Oral	In combination with EGFR antibody in BRAF V600E mutated cancers	Palliative	Diarrhea, photosensitivity, skin rash
BRAF inhibitor	Encorafenib	Oral	In combination with EGFR antibody in *BRAF* V600E mutated cancers	Palliative	Diarrhea, skin rash
MEK inhibitor	Binimetinib[a]	Oral	In combination with EGFR antibody and BRAF inhibitor in *BRAF* V600E mutated cancers	Palliative	Diarrhea, skin rash, retinopathy, **cardiomyopathy**

TABLE 40.3 **Agents Used in the Management of Colorectal Cancer—cont'd**

AGENT CLASS	AGENT	ADMINISTRATION	COMMON USE	TREATMENT SETTING	MAIN SIDE EFFECTS
Immunotherapy					
Anti-PD-1 antibody	Pembrolizumab	IV	Single agent in MSI-H/MMR-D cancers	Palliative	Immune-related adverse events including rare **myocarditis**
	Nivolumab	IV	Single agent or combination with ipilimumab in MSI-H/MMR-D cancers	Palliative	Immune-related adverse events including. rare **myocarditis**
Anti-CTLA-4 antibody	Ipilimumab	IV	Combination with nivolumab in MSI-H/MMR-D cancers	Palliative	Immune-related adverse events, commonly diarrhea, rare **myocarditis**

[a]Not FDA approved (as of April 2020), but listed in some treatment guidelines (NCCN).
5-FU, 5-Fluorouracil; *BRAF*, b-raf or v-raf murine sarcoma viral oncogene homolog B1; *CTLA-4*, cytotoxic T lymphocyte-associated antigen-4; *EGFR*, epidermal growth factor receptor; *HER-2*, human EGFR-2; *MEK*, mitogen-activated protein kinase; *MMR-D*, mismatch repair deficiency; *MSI-H*, microsatellite instability-high; *PD-1*, programmed cell death protein 1; *VEGF(-R)*, vascular endothelial growth factor (receptor).
For names of chemotherapy regimens see Chapter 54.

and rectal cancer relates to the fact that the rectum is embedded in pelvic tissue so that surgical approaches are different from those in colon cancer. MRI has been established as the best way to stage rectal cancer regarding tumor extension and lymph node involvement, which is critical for treatment planning. Surgical standard of care is a total mesorectal excision, either in form of a sphincter-preserving, low-anterior resection for cancers located in the mid-upper rectum or abdominoperineal resection with placement of a permanent colostomy for low-lying rectal cancers.[23] To reduce the risk of local recurrence, radiation therapy is commonly applied to the pelvis in conjunction with a fluoropyrimidine-based chemotherapy as radiation sensitizer to a total dose of 50.4 Gy in 28 fractions. A pivotal randomized trial demonstrated that preoperative, neoadjuvant radiochemotherapy was more efficient in reducing local tumor recurrence than a postoperative, adjuvant approach.[24] In addition, neoadjuvant therapy was associated with a lower rate of acute and chronic complications and thus is considered standard of care now. For patients with stage II and III cancers, adjuvant, postoperative chemotherapy is commonly administered with either a fluoropyrimidine alone or in combination with oxaliplatin to lower the risk of systemic recurrence. The guiding consideration regarding the choice and duration of adjuvant chemotherapy mirrors the situation in colon cancer. Recently, three new strategies have made inroads into rectal cancer management. Instead of long-term chemoradiation, a short-course radiation-alone therapy of 5×5 Gy can be applied, which has shown similar efficacy in terms of local tumor control.[25] Secondly, the concept of total neoadjuvant therapy has been increasingly embraced in major centers, which implies that all planned medical and radiation therapy, including the previously postoperatively administered adjuvant chemotherapy, is now part of the preoperative treatment plan.[26,27] This approach has been shown to generate complete pathologic responses in about 30% of patients so that in patients with an excellent response and no evidence of residual cancer after neoadjuvant therapy, nonoperative strategies with close follow up and monitoring are now considered.[28] This concept is obviously of particular value for patients who would otherwise require abdominoperineal resection as surgery.

The medical management of metastatic rectal cancer follows the same guidelines as that for metastatic colon cancer.

CARDIOVASCULAR RISKS

Systemic therapies used in colon and rectal cancer are generally well tolerated from a cardiovascular perspective. Table 40.3 highlights the potential cardiovascular risks of some of the agents used. Because fluoropyrimidines form the backbone for various chemotherapy regimens and are used as radiation sensitizers in the management of rectal cancer, coronary vasospasm, which can occur with protracted either intravenous or oral delivery of 5-fluorouracil are some of the more frequently encountered cardiac complications. In addition, vascular endothelial growth factor (VEGF) inhibitors, such as bevacizumab, are known to induce hypertension, which is commonly responsive to standard antihypertensive medications.[29] Immune checkpoint inhibitors, which are used in MSI-H/MMR-D colorectal cancers, can induce myocarditis as a severe, but fortunately rare complication.[30]

REFERENCES

1. Siegel RL, Miller KD, Goding Sauer A, et al. Colorectal cancer statistics, 2020. *CA Cancer J Clin.* 2020;70:145–164.
2. Ballester V, Cruz-Correa M. How and when to consider genetic testing for colon cancer? *Gastroenterology.* 2018;155(4):955–959.
3. Force USPST, Bibbins-Domingo K, Grossman DC, et al. Screening for colorectal cancer: US Preventive Services Task Force recommendation statement. *JAMA.* 2016;315(23):2564–2575.
4. Saito G, Sadahiro S, Kamata H, et al. Monitoring of serum carcinoembryonic antigen levels after curative resection of colon cancer: cutoff values determined according to preoperative levels enhance the diagnostic accuracy for recurrence. *Oncology (Williston Park).* 2017;92(5):276–282.
5. Jessup J, Goldberg R, Asare E, et al. Colon and rectum. In: Amin MB, Edge SB, Greene FL, et al., eds. *AJCC Cancer Staging Manual.* 8th ed. Chicago IL: American Joint Committee on Cancer, Springer; 2017.
6. Nordlinger B, Sorbye H, Glimelius B, et al. EORTC liver metastases intergroup randomized phase III study 40983: long-term survival results. *ASCO Meet Abstr.* 2012;30(Suppl 15):3508.
7. Moertel CG, Fleming TR, Macdonald JS, et al. Levamisole and fluorouracil for adjuvant therapy of resected colon carcinoma. *N Engl J Med.* 1990;322(6):352–358.
8. Haller DG, Catalano PJ, Macdonald JS, et al. Phase III study of fluorouracil, leucovorin, and levamisole in high-risk stage II and III colon cancer: final report of intergroup 0089. *J Clin Oncol.* 2005; 23(34):8671–8678.
9. Andre T, Boni C, Mounedji-Boudiaf L, et al. Oxaliplatin, fluorouracil, and leucovorin as adjuvant treatment for colon cancer. *N Engl J Med.* 2004;350(23):2343–2351.
10. Andre T, Boni C, Navarro M, et al. Improved overall survival with oxaliplatin, fluorouracil, and leucovorin as adjuvant treatment in stage II or III colon cancer in the MOSAIC trial. *J Clin Oncol.* 2009;27(19):3109–3116.
11. Haller DG, Tabernero J, Maroun J, et al. Capecitabine plus oxaliplatin compared with fluorouracil and folinic acid as adjuvant therapy for stage III colon cancer. *J Clin Oncol.* 2011;29(11):1465–1471.
12. Chakrabarti S, Sara J, Lobo R, et al. Bolus 5-flurouracil (5-FU) in combination with oxaliplatin is safe and well tolerated in patients who experienced coronary vasospasm with infusional 5-FU or capecitabine. *Clin Colorectal Cancer.* 2019;18(1):52–57.
13. Kuebler JP, Wieand HS, O'Connell MJ, et al. Oxaliplatin combined with weekly bolus fluorouracil and leucovorin as surgical adjuvant chemotherapy for stage II and III colon cancer: results from NSABP C-07. *J Clin Oncol.* 2007;25(16):2198–21204.
14. Grothey A, Sobrero AF, Shields AF, et al. Duration of adjuvant chemotherapy for stage III colon cancer. *N Engl J Med.* 2018;378(13): 1177–1188.
15. Douillard JY, Oliner KS, Siena S, et al. Panitumumab-FOLFOX treatment and RAS mutations in colorectal cancer. *N Engl J Med.* 2013;369(11):1023–1034.
16. Amado RG, Wolf M, Peeters M, et al. Wild-type KRAS is required for panitumumab efficacy in patients with metastatic colorectal cancer. *J Clin Oncol.* 2008;26(10):1626–1634.
17. Lindor NM, Burgart LJ, Leontovich O, et al. Immunohistochemistry versus microsatellite instability testing in phenotyping colorectal tumors. *J Clin Oncol.* 2002;20(4):1043–1048.
18. Ribic CM, Sargent DJ, Moore MJ, et al. Tumor microsatellite-instability status as a predictor of benefit from fluorouracil-based adjuvant chemotherapy for colon cancer. *N Engl J Med.* 2003;349(3):247–257.
19. Le DT, Uram JN, Wang H, et al. PD-1 blockade in tumors with mismatch-repair deficiency. *N Engl J Med.* 2015;372(26):2509–2520.
20. Overman MJ, Lonardi S, Wong KYM, et al. Durable clinical benefit with nivolumab plus ipilimumab in DNA mismatch repair-deficient microsatellite instability-high metastatic colorectal cancer. *J Clin Oncol.* 2018;36(8):773–779.
21. Grothey A, Sargent D, Goldberg RM, Schmoll HJ. Survival of patients with advanced colorectal cancer improves with the availability of fluorouracil-leucovorin, irinotecan, and oxaliplatin in the course of treatment. *J Clin Oncol.* 2004;22(7):1209–1214.
22. Tejpar S, Stintzing S, Ciardiello F, et al. Prognostic and predictive relevance of primary tumor location in patients with RAS wild type metastatic colorectal cancer: retrospective analyses of the CRYSTAL and FIRE-3 trials. *JAMA Oncol.* 2017;3(2):194–201.
23. Quirke P, Steele R, Monson J, et al. Effect of the plane of surgery achieved on local recurrence in patients with operable rectal cancer: a prospective study using data from the MRC CR07 and NCIC-CTG CO16 randomised clinical trial. *Lancet.* 2009;373(9666):821–828.
24. Sauer R, Becker H, Hohenberger W, et al. Preoperative versus postoperative chemoradiotherapy for rectal cancer. *N Engl J Med.* 2004;351(17):1731–1740.
25. Kapiteijn E, Marijnen CA, Nagtegaal ID, et al. Preoperative radiotherapy combined with total mesorectal excision for resectable rectal cancer. *N Engl J Med.* 2001;345(9):638–646.
26. Fokas E, Allgauer M, Polat B, et al. Randomized phase II trial of chemoradiotherapy plus induction or consolidation chemotherapy as total neoadjuvant therapy for locally advanced rectal cancer: CAO/ARO/AIO-12. *J Clin Oncol.* 2019;37(34):3212–3222.
27. Cisel B, Pietrzak L, Michalski W, et al. Long-course preoperative chemoradiation versus 5 × 5 Gy and consolidation chemotherapy for clinical T4 and fixed clinical T3 rectal cancer: long-term results of the randomized Polish II study. *Ann Oncol.* 2019;30(8): 1298–1303.
28. Dossa F, Chesney TR, Acuna SA, Baxter NN. A watch-and-wait approach for locally advanced rectal cancer after a clinical complete response following neoadjuvant chemoradiation: a systematic review and meta-analysis. *Lancet Gastroenterol Hepatol.* 2017;2(7): 501–513.
29. Kozloff MF, Berlin J, Flynn PJ, et al. Clinical outcomes in elderly patients with metastatic colorectal cancer receiving bevacizumab and chemotherapy: results from the BRiTE observational cohort study. *Oncology (Williston Park).* 2010;78(5–6): 329–39.
30. Wang Y, Zhou S, Yang F, et al. Treatment-related adverse events of PD-1 and PD-L1 inhibitors in clinical trials: a systematic review and meta-analysis. *JAMA Oncol.* 2019;5(7):1008–1019.

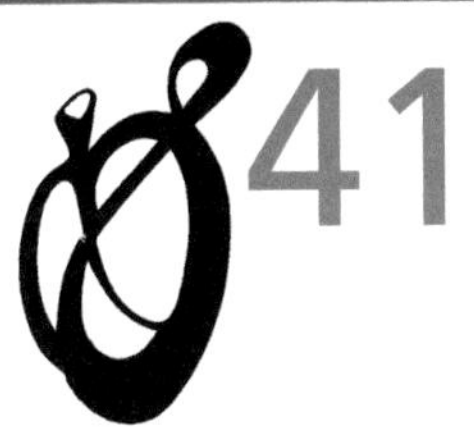

41 Esophageal and Gastric Cancer

THORVARDUR R. HALFDANARSON, MOHAMED BASSAM SONBOL, JASON S. STARR, AND CHRISTOPHER L. HALLEMEIER

Esophageal Cancer Stages	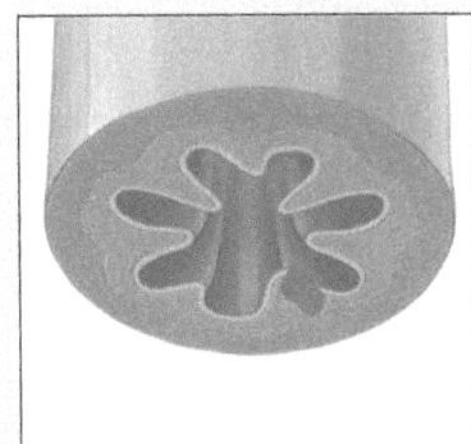	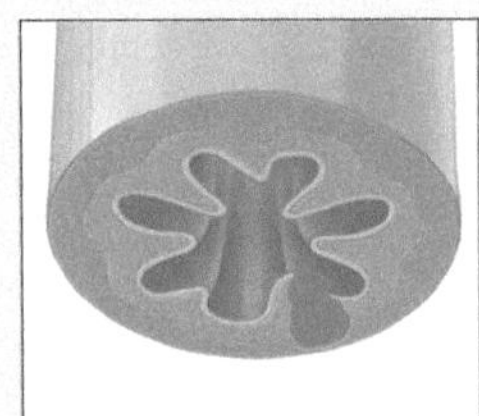	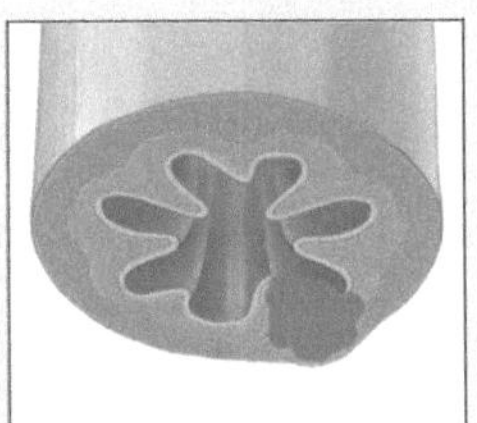	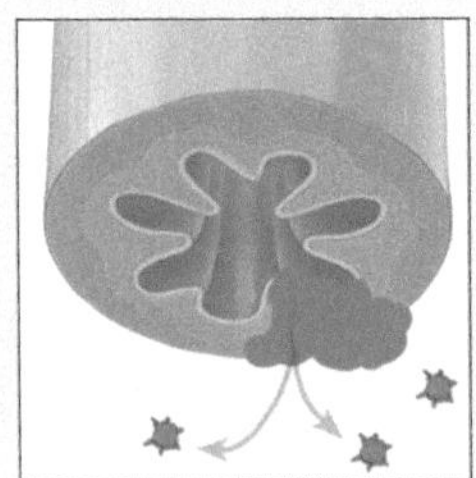
	Stage I Tumor extension no more than to the muscularis propria without nodal involvement (T1 or T2)	**Stage II** Tumor extension to the adventitia (T3) without nodal involvement or earlier stage primary tumor (T1–T2) with involvement of two or fewer nodes	**Stage III** Tumor invasion to adjacent structures (T4) without nodal involvement or earlier stage primary tumor with nodal involvement	**Stage IV** Distant metastases
Treatment	Resection without radiotherapy or systemic therapy	Combination of radiotherapy, systemic therapy, and resection	Combination of radiotherapy, systemic therapy, and resection	Systemic therapy (chemotherapy, immunotherapy, HER2-targeted therapy)
Prognosis	5-year survival >80%	5-year survival 50%–60%	5-year survival 40%–50%	5-year survival <10%
Potential CV toxicities	**Radiation:** radiation-induced cardiovascular disease **Fluorouracil (5-FU):** vasospasm, chest pain, arrhythmia, cardiac failure **HER2-directed therapy:** cardiomyopathy/heart failure **VEGF inhibitors:** hypertension, arterial and venous thrombotic events, bleeding, cardiomyopathy **Immune checkpoint inhibitors:** myocarditis, cardiomyopathy, pericarditis, arrhythmias, vasculitis, ischemic events			

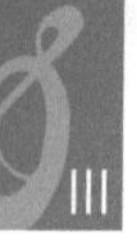

Gastric cancer Stages	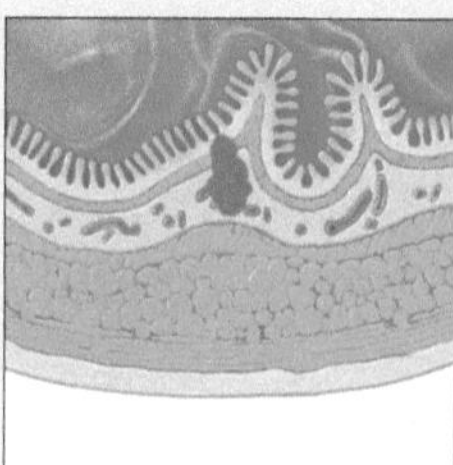 **Stage I**	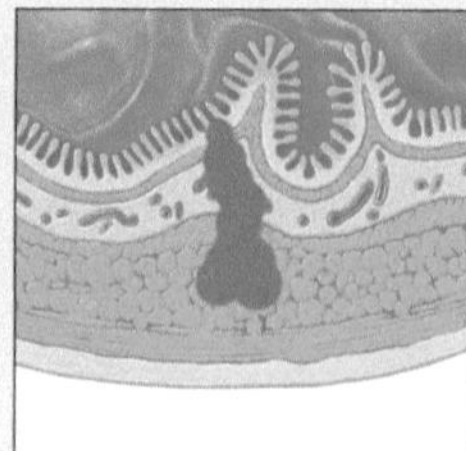 **Stage II**	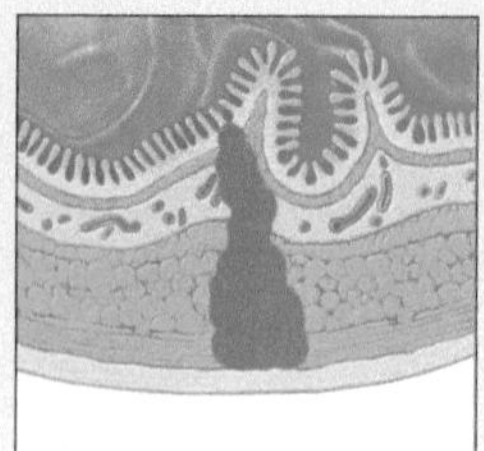 **Stage III**	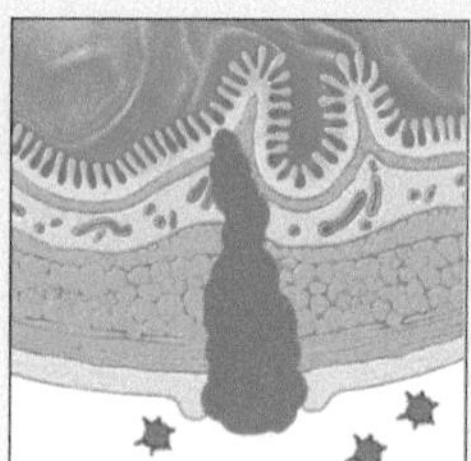 **Stage IV**
	Tumor extension no more than to the muscularis propria without nodal involvement (T1 or T2)	Tumor extension to the adventitia (T3) without nodal involvement or earlier stage primary tumor (T1–T2) with involvement nodes	Tumor invasion to adjacent structures (T4) without nodal involvement or earlier stage primary tumor with nodal involvement	Distant metastases or very locally advanced and invasive primary tumor
Treatment	Resection without radiotherapy or systemic therapy	Perioperative chemotherapy and resection Chemoradiotherapy for unresectable disease	Perioperative chemotherapy and resection Chemoradiotherapy for unresectable disease	Systemic therapy (chemotherapy, immunotherapy, HER2-targeted therapy)
Prognosis	5-year survival >80%	5-year survival 50%–60%	5-year survival 40%–50%	5-year survival <10%

Potential CV toxicities

Fluoropyrimidine: vasospasm, ischemia, arrhythmia, cardiac dysfunction
HER2-directed therapy: cardiomyopathy and heart failure
VEGF inhibitors: hypertension, arterial and venous thromboembolic events, bleeding
Immune checkpoint inhibitors: myocarditis, arrhythmias, cardiomyopathy, vasculitis, pericarditis

CHAPTER OUTLINE

ESOPHAGEAL CANCER

KEY POINTS ABOUT ESOPHAGEAL CANCER

- Relatively uncommon cancer (annual incidence 4.3/100,000)
- The median age at diagnosis is 68 years.
- The incidence of squamous cell cancer of the esophagus has declined substantially, whereas the incidence of adenocarcinoma of the distal esophagus and especially the gastroesophageal junction has increased in recent decades.
- The most common risk factors for squamous cell esophageal cancer are alcohol use and tobacco smoking and for esophageal adenocarcinoma obesity and chronic gastroesophageal reflux disease (GERD).
- 5-year survival prognosis is approximately 20% overall; survival beyond 2 years is uncommon in metastatic disease.
- Esophageal cancer limited to the mucosa can often be endoscopically resected.
- Patients with more advanced, but localized tumors, T3, T4, or node-positive, are usually treated with multimodality therapy, most commonly, neoadjuvant chemoradiotherapy followed by resection.
- Systemic therapy is the primary treatment for metastatic disease, historically, with fluoropyrimidines and platinum drugs, and more recently, with the addition of immune checkpoint inhibitors.
- Both systemic therapy and radiotherapy for esophageal cancer have the potential to result in cardiotoxicity in patients undergoing treatment, but cardiotoxicity for localized disease is rare.

Incidence

According to the Surveillance, Epidemiology, and End Results (SEERs) registry, the estimated number of new cases of esophageal cancer in the United States in 2019 was 17,650. The annual incidence is 4.3/100,000. Esophageal cancer is more common in males than females, and the difference is more prominent in cases of adenocarcinoma. Worldwide, esophageal cancer is estimated to affect almost 600,000 patients, with the majority of them dying as a result of the cancer.

Risk Factors

Established risk factors for squamous cell carcinoma of the esophagus include tobacco smoking and alcohol use, especially when used in combination.[1] Less-common causes include achalasia, prior thoracic radiation therapy, and ingestion of caustic chemicals resulting in tissue injury. Intake of fruits and vegetables appears protective and some studies have suggested an increased risk related to red meat consumption and drinking of very hot beverages. Although the incidence of squamous cell carcinoma has decreased markedly in the United States and Europe, squamous cell cancer remains the most common esophageal cancer histology worldwide. The decrease in the incidence of esophageal squamous cell cancer is likely in large part explained by a decrease in tobacco smoking.[2] On the other hand, the incidence of esophageal adenocarcinoma has increased substantially in the United States and Europe, largely owing to increased rates of obesity and chronic gastrointestinal reflux disease (GERD). The development of adenocarcinoma in patients with GERD is thought to be secondary metaplasia of the squamous epithelium or Barrett's esophagus. Consequently, patients with chronic GERD are at an increased risk of developing esophageal adnocarcinoma.[3] Other risk factors associated with esophageal adenocarcinoma include smoking[4] and obesity.[5]

Prognosis

Overall, the prognosis of esophageal cancer remains poor, and survival highly depends on stage. Among all patients diagnosed with esophageal cancer, approximately 20% are expected to be alive 5 years from diagnosis. Survival beyond 2 years is uncommon in metastatic disease. With the exception of the earliest stages (T1N0) esophageal tumors, almost half of patients with locoregional esophageal cancer will experience recurrence of the malignancy and eventually die of metastatic disease.[6] Overall, the prognosis for patients with esophageal cancer has improved over the last few decades, and the improvement in survival is seen across all stages of the disease.

Treatment Overview

Very Early Stage Disease (T1a)

In cases of early-stage esophageal cancer, endoscopic therapy can be very effective and even curative, but such therapy is generally limited to the earliest stages of the cancer (T1a), where there is minimal invasion limited to the mucosa or for cancer *in situ*.[1] Endoscopic mucosal resection, endoscopic submucosal dissection, and radiofrequency ablation are among the endoscopic techniques used.

Localized Disease

The management of more advanced, but localized, esophageal cancer is best done in a multidisciplinary setting. Patients with node-negative T1b and T2 tumors are typically treated with esophagectomy alone. In cases of nodal involvement and/or more advanced primary tumors (T3 and T4), multimodality therapy is required for optimal outcomes. The role of neoadjuvant chemoradiation therapy for resectable T2N0 esophageal cancer is unclear. For patients with squamous cell carcinoma, neoadjuvant chemoradiotherapy, typically combining external beam radiotherapy with weekly carboplatin and paclitaxel, is preferred, and results in outcomes better than observed with surgery alone.[7,8] In patients where radiotherapy is contraindicated, neoadjuvant chemotherapy followed by resection yields better outcomes than surgery alone.[9] The additional benefit of resection following chemoradiotherapy has been questioned in patients with squamous cell carcinoma because of the exceptional responses seen with chemoradiotherapy, with pathologic complete response rates approaching 50%. However, given the lack of definitive data for chemoradiotherapy alone, surgery is recommended following neoadjuvant therapy (trimodality therapy) with definitive chemoradiotherapy alone (bimodality therapy) reserved for patients either unfit for surgery or unwilling to undergo surgery. A similar treatment paradigm is used for patients with adenocarcinoma of the esophagus, although resection is considered an essential component of the treatment unless contraindicated owing to comorbidities. Data do support neoadjuvant and adjuvant chemotherapy (with omission of chemoradiotherapy), particularly for Siewert type III disease, and chemotherapy with FLOT (5-*f*luorouracil, *l*eucovorin, *o*xaliplatin and docetaxel [*T*axotere]).[10]

Patients with nonmetastatic, but inoperable esophageal cancer, including cervical esophageal cancer, but fit for combined modality therapy, should be considered for definitive chemoradiotherapy. Patients with squamous cell carcinoma can be considered for cisplatin and 5-fluorouracil (5-FU) given concurrently with radiation therapy.[11] Carboplatin and paclitaxel is also a reasonable combination with radiation therapy, especially for adenocarcinoma.[7]

Metastatic Disease

In patients with metastatic disease, chemotherapy is the mainstay of therapy with radiotherapy reserved as palliative therapy for lesions causing pain or mechanical complications, such as dysphagia or hemorrhage. In general, the chemotherapy for esophageal adenocarcinoma follows the treatment paradigms used for gastric cancer. The therapy for advanced squamous cell cancer of the esophagus is less well-defined than for adenocarcinoma but practically very similar. Fluoropyrimidines are commonly used for esophageal cancer, typically in combinations with other agents, such as oxaliplatin and cisplatin.[12] Doublet cytotoxic therapy is preferred over triplet therapy, given higher toxicity and lack of data supporting overall survival benefit of triplet therapy compared with doublet therapy. In younger and more fit patients, triplet therapy may be considered, especially if a radiologic response is needed, but such therapy may have substantial toxicity.[13]

Patients with human epidermal growth factor 2 (HER2) overexpressing metastatic adenocarcinoma of the esophagus may benefit from the addition of trastuzumab, a monoclonal antibody targeting HER2.[14] Currently, no data suggest continuing trastuzumab beyond first line and, thus far, other HER2-targeted drugs, such as lapatinib and ado-trastuzumab emtansine, have not been shown to be effective in HER2-positive gastroesophageal cancer.[15,16]

Anthracyclines have been used frequently for both localized and metastatic esophageal cancer, but recent studies do not support their use,[17] and, therefore, anthracyclines should not be used. Second-line therapy of metastatic disease should be considered for fit patients, but, unfortunately, the response duration is relatively short.

Commonly used second-line agents include taxanes, such as paclitaxel (often in combination with the vascular endothelial growth factor [VEGF] receptor-2 monoclonal antibody, ramucirumab in cases of adenocarcinoma) and docetaxel, as well as irinotecan.[18,19] A more commonly used VEGF inhibitor, bevacizumab, was not shown to have activity in metastatic gastric cancer. Recently, an oral cytotoxic therapy, trifluridine/tipiracil (TAS-102) was shown to modestly improve survival over placebo in patients with heavily pretreated metastatic gastric cancer.[20]

In patients with mismatch repair deficient (high microsatellite instability) cancers, immunotherapy with immune checkpoint inhibitors, such as pembrolizumab, can be very effective, even in the first-line setting.[21] Immunotherapy also does have activity in programmed death ligand-1 (PD-L1) positive, mismatch repair proficient gastric and esophageal cancer, both upfront and in later lines of therapy. Recently, pembrolizumab was shown to be noninferior to cytotoxic chemotherapy in the first-line setting in patients with a PD-L1 combined positive score (CPS) of 1% or more. Further, there was a trend toward improvement in overall survival in patients with a PD-L1 CPS of 10% or more.[22] Immunotherapy is also effective in patients progressing on cytotoxic chemotherapy.[23] Currently, the United States (US) Food and Drug Administration approval for pembrolizumab is in the third-line setting in patients with PD-L1 CPS 1 or greater. In patients with PD-L1 positive esophageal cancer (PD-L1 combined positive score ≥10%) progressing on first-line chemotherapy, pembrolizumab yields better survival than second-line cytotoxic chemotherapy.[24]

Cardiovascular Risk

Systemic therapy for esophageal cancer rarely results in cardiotoxicity. Although several of the drugs used for treatment of patients with esophageal cancer are associated with cardiotoxicity, clinical cardiac complications seem rare. Drugs associated with cardiotoxicity include the HER2-directed monoclonal antibody trastuzumab, the VEGF- and VEGF-R2 directed monoclonal antibodies bevacizumab and ramucirumab, and checkpoint inhibitors, such as pembrolizumab. Other drugs that are commonly used for esophageal cancer and are occasionally associated with cardiotoxicity include fluoropyrimidines (5-fluorouracil and capecitabine) and taxanes (e.g., paclitaxel and docetaxel). Anthracyclines have a well-documented risk of cardiotoxicity and were commonly used in the treatment of esophageal cancer in the past but should rarely, if ever, be used given lack of efficacy.

External beam radiotherapy is considered standard therapy in patients with locally advanced disease, as either definitive or neoadjuvant therapy. For tumors involving the middle and distal esophagus, radiation dose to the heart may be substantial. A recent SEER analysis suggested there was a higher rate of cardiac mortality in patients with localized esophageal cancer who received radiotherapy as part of the treatment course, although this analysis has some limitations.[25] Data derived from the use of radiotherapy for other thoracic malignancies, including breast cancer, lung cancer, and mediastinal Hodgkin lymphoma, more clearly demonstrate a dose-dependent risk of cardiac morbidity associated with radiation exposure to the heart. Modern external beam radiation techniques, such as intensity-modulated radiotherapy (IMRT) and proton beam radiotherapy, are capable of reducing radiation exposure to the heart, compared with older techniques, with recent evidence suggesting a reduction in cardiac morbidity.[26] Proton beam radiotherapy substantially reduces radiation exposure to the heart compared to photon-based techniques (including IMRT),[27] although there are currently only a limited number of proton beam facilities worldwide. An ongoing National Cancer Institute funded multicenter phase III randomized controlled trial (NCT03801876) is comparing IMRT versus proton beam radiotherapy for the treatment of esophageal cancer, with the coprimary endpoints of survival and cardiopulmonary morbidity.

GASTRIC CANCER

KEY POINTS ABOUT GASTRIC CANCER

- Relatively uncommon cancer with declining incidence (annual incidence in the United States is 7.4/100,000).
- The median age at diagnosis is 68 years.
- The vast majority of gastric cancers are of the adenocarcinoma type, and there are two histologic variants, intestinal type (more common) and diffuse type (less common).
- Risk factors for gastric cancer include *Helicobacter pylori*, obesity, consumption of salt and nitrates, and smoking.

KEY POINTS ABOUT GASTRIC CANCER—cont'd

- Early-stage (intramucosal) gastric cancer can be resected endoscopically.
- Patients with more advanced gastric cancer, such as T2 to T4, and/or node positive cancers, should be given perioperative chemotherapy.
- Radiation therapy should be considered for: (1) resectable gastric cancer if the surgical margin is positive or if macroscopic disease was left behind, or (2) if not resectable, but localized disease, and for palliative purposes, such as for bleeding tumors or tumors resulting in localized pain or obstruction.
- Patients with metastatic gastric cancers and good performance status should be treated with combination chemotherapy, the most common being fluoropyrimidines, platinum drugs, HER2-directed drugs, such as trastuzumab, and immune checkpoint inhibitors.
- Immunotherapy as upfront therapy can be considered for patients with mismatch repair-deficient gastric cancer, otherwise, it is typically considered in the third-line setting and beyond based on PD-L1 combined positive score (CPS).
- Cardiotoxicity related to gastric cancer therapy is most commonly seen as fluoropyrimidine-induced vasospasm, HER2-targeted cardiomyopathy or complications of checkpoint inhibitor therapy resulting in myocarditis.

Incidence

The annual incidence of gastric cancer in the United States is 7.4/100,000, and 27,510 new cases were expected in the United States in 2019. The annual incidence in the United States has steadily decreased over the last several decades. Although a similar decrease in the incidence has been seen worldwide, gastric cancer remains a large problem and a common cause of cancer death, and more than a million new cases and more than 700,000 deaths had been estimated worldwide in 2018. The median age at diagnosis in the United States is 68 years. Although an uncommon cancer in the United States and Europe, gastric cancer is common worldwide and is estimated to be the second most common cancer and the fourth leading cause of cancer death.[28] The burden of gastric cancer remains very high in Asia, Latin America, and eastern Europe.[29]

Risk Factors

The risk factors of gastric cancer are well established. Chronic infection with *Helicobacter pylori* is the most common cause of sporadic distal gastric cancer.[28] Other reported risk factors for gastric cancer include Epstein-Barr virus and various environmental factors, such as low consumption of fruits and vegetables, consumption of salt and nitrates, obesity, smoking, and chronic atrophic gastritis.[3,5,30] A small minority of gastric cancer cases is considered hereditary, most commonly secondary to mutations in *CDH1* (hereditary diffuse gastric cancer).[31]

Prognosis

Early-stage, resected gastric cancer has a relatively good prognosis with almost 50% of patients being cured. More advanced, but nonmetastatic, gastric cancer (either more advanced T-stage or node-positive cancer) is associated with a substantially higher risk of recurrence and death, even with perioperative therapy. The prognosis of metastatic gastric cancer remains relatively poor with the majority of patients dying within 2 years of diagnosis of metastatic disease.[13]

Treatment Overview

The only curative treatment for gastric cancer is resection. For the earliest stages of gastric cancer limited to the mucosa (T1a), endoscopic resection is appropriate, but it requires considerable experience and specialized equipment. For more advanced gastric cancer, a partial or total gastrectomy is usually required. Given the risk of lymph node metastases in patients with stage T2 or higher, surgery alone is considered inadequate. Therefore, perioperative therapy is considered standard for all patients deemed to be fit enough for such therapy.

On the basis of a National Cancer Institute funded multicenter phase III randomized trial published in 2001, external beam radiation therapy was considered an essential component of adjuvant therapy given superior results of adjuvant chemoradiotherapy compared with surgery alone.[32] With improved surgical techniques, especially more aggressive nodal dissection, patient survival has improved.[33] Radiation therapy is no longer considered mandatory for patients who have undergone adequate nodal dissection (D2), especially as trials have failed to show improvement in survival over chemotherapy alone.[34,35] Radiation therapy should be considered in patients with microscopically (R1) or macroscopically (R2) positive margin following resection. Radiation therapy can also be effective in relieving symptoms and complications of locally advanced gastric cancer and as a component of therapy in patients unable or unwilling to undergo resection.

In 2006, perioperative therapy with epirubicin, cisplatin, and 5-FU was shown to result in superior survival compared with resection alone.[36] Since then, the role of the epirubicin has been called into question, and a recent randomized trial showed that the addition of epirubicin to 5-FU and cisplatin did not improve outcomes.[37] More recently, a randomized phase III trial confirmed that FLOT was superior to epirubicin, cisplatin, and 5-FU as perioperative therapy.[10] Anthracyclines, therefore, are no longer considered to have a role in the perioperative management of gastric cancer.

Therapy for metastatic gastric cancer, metastatic gastroesophageal junction cancer, and metastatic esophageal cancer is very similar and has been described in more detail in the section on esophageal cancer.

Cardiovascular Risk

As with esophageal cancer, there is risk of cardiovascular toxicity, mostly related to the systemic therapy used, and that risk is discussed in greater detail above in the section on esophageal cancer, as well as in subsequent sections on individual systemic therapy agents.

Cancer Treatments With Potential Cardiovascular Side Effects

Fluoropyrimidines

Cardiotoxicity is a well-known complication of fluoropyrimidines, including 5-fluorouracil and its oral prodrug, capecitabine.[38,39] In fact, fluoropyrimidines are second only to anthracyclines in terms of historic association with cardiotoxicity.[40] The risk of cardiotoxicity is reported to be increased in patients with concurrent thoracic radiation therapy, multiagent chemotherapy, and along with preexisting cardiac disease. Cardiotoxicity occurs in up to 18% of patients exposed to fluoropyrimidines[38,39] In practice, however, cardiotoxicity seems to be less common than reported.

Bolus administration of 5-FU is associated with a much lower rate of cardiotoxicity (~2% to 5%).[41] This is likely secondary to the short half-life of 5-FU (15 to 20 minutes) and the rapid clearance when given in bolus fashion.[41] Capecitabine, an oral prodrug of 5-FU, can also result in cardiotoxicity and the incidence appears similar to or slightly less than that of 5-FU given as continuous infusion.[42]

The most common 5-fluorouracil cardiotoxicity results from coronary vasospasms, which can result in chest pain and, in extreme cases, myocardial infarction. Silent ischemia, congestive heart failure, dilated cardiomyopathy, tachyarrhythmias, and sudden death have also been reported as a consequence of fluoropyrimidine therapy.[43] Cerebral artery vasospasms are less common and can result in transient ischemic attacks and stroke. In cases of vasospasms on infusional therapy, bolus therapy appears to be a safer alternative. Vasodilator therapy is advocated, but may not prevent all cases of fluoropyrimidine cardiotoxicity.[44]

Anthracyclines

Severe and irreversible cardiomyopathy is a well-established complication of anthracycline therapy.[40] Although anthracyclines were frequently used in the treatment of gastroesophageal cancer in the past, recent trials and meta-analyses have suggested limited benefit when compared with nonanthracycline regimens. Therefore, the role of anthracyclines in therapy has diminished, and this group of cytotoxic drugs should be avoided.[45]

Taxanes

Paclitaxel and docetaxel have both been associated with cardiovascular toxicity.[46] Bradyarrhythmia has been reported secondary to paclitaxel use along with rare cases of myocardial ischemia and even infarction, especially in patients with underlying cardiac disease.[46] Docetaxel has also been reported to be associated with myocardial ischemia, but that seems to be a rare complication.[47]

Platinum Drugs

Oxaliplatin and cisplatin are commonly used in the treatment of gastroesophageal cancer, and both drugs have been associated with cardiotoxicity and vascular toxicity (esp., thrombotic events). Cisplatin use frequently results in electrolyte disturbances,

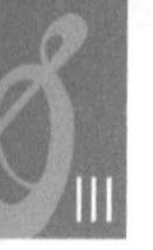

most commonly, hypomagnesemia and hypokalemia, which in turn may result in arrhythmias. Cisplatin has also been reported to result in hypertension.

Trastuzumab

Cardiotoxicity of trastuzumab is well-established and usually in the form of left ventricular dysfunction. Nearly half of all patients on trastuzumab therapy for breast cancer develop a drop in left ventricular ejection fraction of more than 10%.[48] Symptomatic heart failure, on the other hand, is much less common (<5%).[49] Left ventricular dysfunction with trastuzumab has been considered to be reversible, but this may be only partial and is not seen in all patients. These patients may require longer follow up than originally thought. Reexposure can be tried in those with complete reversibility upon cessation of trastuzumab therapy. Cardiovascular medications seem to be of benefit for cardiac function recovery.[49]

Inhibitors of Vascular Endothelial Growth Factor (VEGF) Signaling

The VEGF-R2 inhibiting monoclonal antibody, ramucirumab, is commonly used in the treatment of advanced gastroesophageal adenocarcinoma.[19] VEGF inhibitors have a well-established risk of cardiovascular toxicity, especially hypertension, which generally is manageable with antihypertensive therapy. Hemorrhage and venous and arterial thromboembolic complications are more likely to occur in patients treated with ramucirumab than placebo, but the overall risk of such severe complications is low.[19]

Immune Checkpoint Inhibitor Therapy

Cardiotoxicity is now well-established but is an uncommon adverse effect of immune checkpoint inhibitor (ICI) therapy.[50] The precise incidence of ICI-induced cardiotoxicity remains to be defined. ICI therapy elicits an immune response, even in the cardiovascular system and even to the point of fulminant myocarditis. The latter can be seen as early as 1 to 2 weeks after therapy is begun. Pericarditis is also a known complication of ICI therapy. Decrease in cardiac function and Takotsubo cardiomyopathy has also been reported, as well as myocardial infarction and vasculitis. With increasing use of ICI for upper gastrointestinal malignancies, cardiotoxicity likely will be increasingly recognized in this population.

REFERENCES

1. Lagergren J, Smyth E, Cunningham D, et al. Oesophageal cancer. *Lancet*. 2017;390:2383–2396.
2. Engel LS, Chow WH, Vaughan TL, et al. Population attributable risks of esophageal and gastric cancers. *J Natl Cancer Inst*. 2003;95:1404–1413.
3. Spechler SJ. Barrett esophagus and risk of esophageal cancer: a clinical review. *JAMA*. 2013;310:627–636.
4. Cook MB, Kamangar F, Whiteman DC, et al. Cigarette smoking and adenocarcinomas of the esophagus and esophagogastric junction: a pooled analysis from the international BEACON consortium. *J Natl Cancer Inst*. 2010;102:1344–1353.
5. Turati F, Tramacere I, La Vecchia C, et al. A meta-analysis of body mass index and esophageal and gastric cardia adenocarcinoma. *Ann Oncol*. 2013;24:609–617.
6. Shapiro J, van Lanschot JJB, Hulshof M, et al. Neoadjuvant chemoradiotherapy plus surgery versus surgery alone for oesophageal or junctional cancer (CROSS): long-term results of a randomised controlled trial. *Lancet Oncol*. 2015;16:1090–1098.
7. van Hagen P, Hulshof MC, van Lanschot JJ, et al. Preoperative chemoradiotherapy for esophageal or junctional cancer. *N Engl J Med*. 2012;366:2074–2084.
8. Chan KKW, Saluja R, Delos Santos K, et al. Neoadjuvant treatments for locally advanced, resectable esophageal cancer: a network meta-analysis. *Int J Cancer*. 2018;143:430–437.
9. Kidane B, Coughlin S, Vogt K, et al. Preoperative chemotherapy for resectable thoracic esophageal cancer. *Cochrane Database Syst Rev*. 2015;CD001556.
10. Al-Batran SE, Homann N, Pauligk C, et al. Perioperative chemotherapy with fluorouracil plus leucovorin, oxaliplatin, and docetaxel versus fluorouracil or capecitabine plus cisplatin and epirubicin for locally advanced, resectable gastric or gastro-oesophageal junction adenocarcinoma (FLOT4): a randomised, phase 2/3 trial. *Lancet*. 2019;393:1948–1957.
11. Minsky BD, Pajak TF, Ginsberg RJ, et al. INT 0123 (Radiation Therapy Oncology Group 94-05) phase III trial of combined-modality therapy for esophageal cancer: high-dose versus standard-dose radiation therapy. *J Clin Oncol*. 2002;20:1167–1174.
12. Cunningham D, Starling N, Rao S, et al. Capecitabine and oxaliplatin for advanced esophagogastric cancer. *N Engl J Med*. 2008;358:36–46.
13. Van Cutsem E, Moiseyenko VM, Tjulandin S, et al. Phase III study of docetaxel and cisplatin plus fluorouracil compared with cisplatin and fluorouracil as first-line therapy for advanced gastric cancer: a report of the V325 Study Group. *J Clin Oncol*. 2006;24:4991–4997.
14. Bang YJ, Van Cutsem E, Feyereislova A, et al. Trastuzumab in combination with chemotherapy versus chemotherapy alone for treatment of HER2-positive advanced gastric or gastro-oesophageal junction cancer (ToGA): a phase 3, open-label, randomised controlled trial. *Lancet*. 2010;376:687–697.
15. Satoh T, Xu RH, Chung HC, et al. Lapatinib plus paclitaxel versus paclitaxel alone in the second-line treatment of HER2-amplified advanced gastric cancer in Asian populations: TyTAN—a randomized, phase III study. *J Clin Oncol*. 2014;32:2039–2049.
16. Thuss-Patience PC, Shah MA, Ohtsu A, et al. Trastuzumab emtansine versus taxane use for previously treated HER2-positive locally advanced or metastatic gastric or gastro-oesophageal junction adenocarcinoma (GATSBY): an international randomised, open-label, adaptive, phase 2/3 study. *Lancet Oncol*. 2017;18:640–653.
17. Ter Veer E, Haj Mohammad N, van Valkenhoef G, et al. The Efficacy and Safety of First-line Chemotherapy in Advanced Esophagogastric Cancer: A Network Meta-analysis. *J Natl Cancer Inst*. 2016;108.
18. Hironaka S, Ueda S, Yasui H, et al. Randomized, open-label, phase III study comparing irinotecan with paclitaxel in patients with advanced gastric cancer without severe peritoneal metastasis after failure of prior combination chemotherapy using fluoropyrimidine plus platinum: WJOG 4007 trial. *J Clin Oncol*. 2013;31:4438–4444.
19. Wilke H, Muro K, Van Cutsem E, et al. Ramucirumab plus paclitaxel versus placebo plus paclitaxel in patients with previously treated advanced gastric or gastro-oesophageal junction adenocarcinoma (RAINBOW): a double-blind, randomised phase 3 trial. *Lancet Oncol*. 2014;15:1224–1235.

20. Shitara K, Doi T, Dvorkin M, et al. Trifluridine/tipiracil versus placebo in patients with heavily pretreated metastatic gastric cancer (TAGS): a randomised, double-blind, placebo-controlled, phase 3 trial. *Lancet Oncol.* 2018;19:1437–1448.
21. Marabelle A, Le DT, Ascierto PA, et al. Efficacy of Pembrolizumab in patients with noncolorectal high microsatellite instability/mismatch repair-deficient cancer: Results from the phase II KEYNOTE-158 Study. *J Clin Oncol.* 2019;JCO1902105.
22. Tabernero J, Van Cutsem E, Bang YJ, et al. Pembrolizumab with or without chemotherapy versus chemotherapy for advanced gastric or gastroesophageal junction (G/GEJ) adenocarcinoma: The phase III KEYNOTE-062 study. *J Clin Oncol.* 2019;(suppl; abstr LBA4007):37.
23. Kato K, Cho BC, Takahashi M, et al. Nivolumab versus chemotherapy in patients with advanced oesophageal squamous cell carcinoma refractory or intolerant to previous chemotherapy (ATTRACTION-3): a multicentre, randomised, open-label, phase 3 trial. *Lancet Oncol.* 2019;20:1506–1517.
24. Kojima T, Muro K, Francois E, et al. Pembrolizumab versus chemotherapy as second-line therapy for advanced esophageal cancer: phase III KEYNOTE-181 study. *J Clin Oncol.* 2019;37:4010.
25. Frandsen J, Boothe D, Gaffney DK, et al. Increased risk of death due to heart disease after radiotherapy for esophageal cancer. *J Gastrointest Oncol.* 2015;6:516–523.
26. Lin SH, Merrell KW, Shen J, et al. Multi-institutional analysis of radiation modality use and postoperative outcomes of neoadjuvant chemoradiation for esophageal cancer. *Radiother Oncol.* 2017;123:376–381.
27. Shiraishi Y, Xu C, Yang J, et al. Dosimetric comparison to the heart and cardiac substructure in a large cohort of esophageal patients with cancer treated with proton beam therapy or Intensity-modulated radiation therapy. *Radiother Oncol.* 2017;125:48–54.
28. Van Cutsem E, Sagaert X, Topal B, et al. Gastric cancer. *Lancet.* 2016;388:2654–2664.
29. Ferro A, Peleteiro B, Malvezzi M, et al. Worldwide trends in gastric cancer mortality (1980-2011), with predictions to 2015, and incidence by subtype. *Eur J Cancer.* 2014;50:1330–1344.
30. Yang P, Zhou Y, Chen B, et al. Overweight, obesity and gastric cancer risk: results from a meta-analysis of cohort studies. *Eur J Cancer.* 2009;45:2867–2873.
31. Oliveira C, Pinheiro H, Figueiredo J, et al. Familial gastric cancer: genetic susceptibility, pathology, and implications for management. *Lancet Oncol.* 2015;16:e60–e70.
32. Macdonald JS, Smalley SR, Benedetti J, et al. Chemoradiotherapy after surgery compared with surgery alone for adenocarcinoma of the stomach or gastroesophageal junction. *N Engl J Med.* 2001;345:725–730.
33. Songun I, Putter H, Kranenbarg EM, et al. Surgical treatment of gastric cancer: 15-year follow-up results of the randomised nationwide Dutch D1D2 trial. *Lancet Oncol.* 2010;11:439–449.
34. Park SH, Sohn TS, Lee J, et al. Phase III trial to compare adjuvant chemotherapy with Capecitabine and Cisplatin versus concurrent chemoradiotherapy in gastric cancer: Final report of the adjuvant chemoradiotherapy in stomach tumors trial, including survival and subset analyses. *J Clin Oncol.* 2015;33:3130–3136.
35. Cats A, Jansen EPM, van Grieken NCT, et al. Chemotherapy versus chemoradiotherapy after surgery and preoperative chemotherapy for resectable gastric cancer (CRITICS): an international, open-label, randomised phase 3 trial. *Lancet Oncol.* 2018;19:616–628.
36. Cunningham D, Allum WH, Stenning SP, et al. Perioperative chemotherapy versus surgery alone for resectable gastroesophageal cancer. *N Engl J Med.* 2006;355:11–20.
37. Fuchs CS, Niedzwiecki D, Mamon HJ, et al. Adjuvant chemoradiotherapy with Epirubicin, Cisplatin, and Fluorouracil compared with adjuvant chemoradiotherapy with Fluorouracil and Leucovorin after curative resection of gastric Cancer: Results from CALGB 80101 (Alliance). *J Clin Oncol.* 2017;35:3671–3677.
38. Kwakman JJ, Simkens LH, Mol L, et al. Incidence of capecitabine-related cardiotoxicity in different treatment schedules of metastatic colorectal cancer: a retrospective analysis of the CAIRO studies of the Dutch Colorectal Cancer Group. *Eur J Cancer.* 2017; 76:93–99.
39. Abdel-Rahman O. 5-Fluorouracil-related cardiotoxicity; findings from five randomized studies of 5-Fluorouracil-based regimens in metastatic colorectal cancer. *Clin Colorectal Cancer.* 2019;18:58–63.
40. Levis BE, Binkley PF, Shapiro CL. Cardiotoxic effects of anthracycline-based therapy: what is the evidence and what are the potential harms? *Lancet Oncol.* 2017;18:e445–e456.
41. Sara JD, Kaur J, Khodadadi R, et al. 5-fluorouracil and cardiotoxicity: a review. *Ther Adv Med Oncol.* 2018;10:1758835918780140.
42. Polk A, Shahmarvand N, Vistisen K, et al. Incidence and risk factors for capecitabine-induced symptomatic cardiotoxicity: a retrospective study of 452 consecutive patients with metastatic breast cancer. *BMJ Open.* 2016;6:e012798.
43. Polk A, Vaage-Nilsen M, Vistisen K, et al. Cardiotoxicity in patients with cancer treated with 5-fluorouracil or capecitabine: a systematic review of incidence, manifestations and predisposing factors. *Cancer Treat Rev.* 2013;39:974–984.
44. Eskilsson J, Albertsson M. Failure of preventing 5-fluorouracil cardiotoxicity by prophylactic treatment with verapamil. *Acta Oncol.* 1990;29:1001–1003.
45. Ashraf N, Kim R. Treatment of gastric and gastroesophageal cancers-do we really need anthracyclines? *JAMA Oncol.* 2017;3:1172–1173.
46. Rowinsky EK, McGuire WP, Guarnieri T, et al. Cardiac disturbances during the administration of taxol. *J Clin Oncol.* 1991;9:1704–1712.
47. Yeh ET, Bickford CL. Cardiovascular complications of cancer therapy: incidence, pathogenesis, diagnosis, and management. *J Am Coll Cardiol.* 2009;53:2231–2247.
48. Guarneri V, Lenihan DJ, Valero V, et al. Long-term cardiac tolerability of trastuzumab in metastatic breast cancer: the M.D. Anderson Cancer Center experience. *J Clin Oncol.* 2006;24:4107–4115.
49. Moslehi JJ. Cardiovascular toxic effects of targeted cancer therapies. *N Engl J Med.* 2016;375:1457–1467.
50. Lyon AR, Yousaf N, Battisti NML, et al. Immune checkpoint inhibitors and cardiovascular toxicity. *Lancet Oncol.* 2018;19:e447–e458.

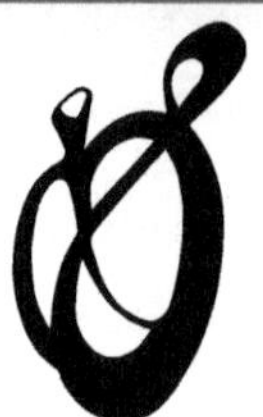

42 Hepatobiliary Carcinomas

THORVARDUR R. HALFDANARSON, MOHAMED BASSAM SONBOL, AND JASON S. STARR

Hepatocellular Carcinoma Stages	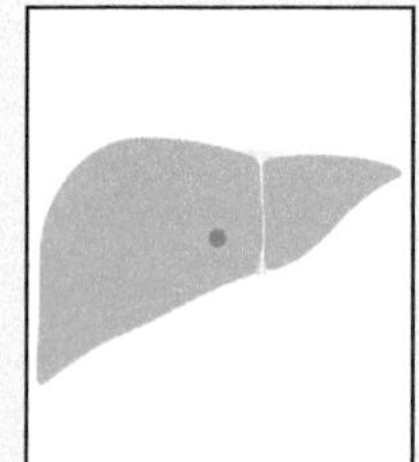 **Very early stage**	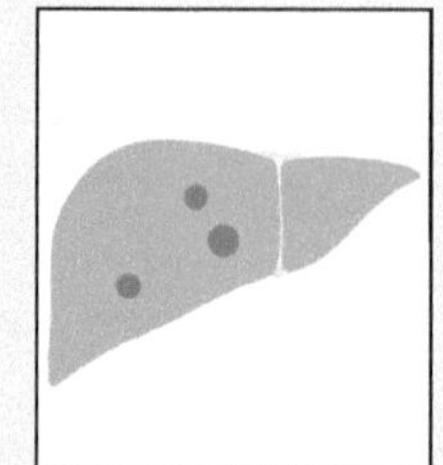 **Early stage**	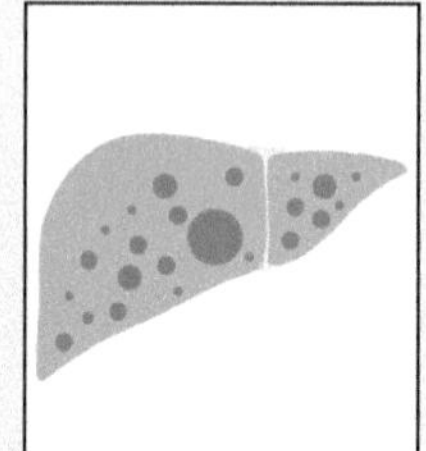 **Intermediate stage**	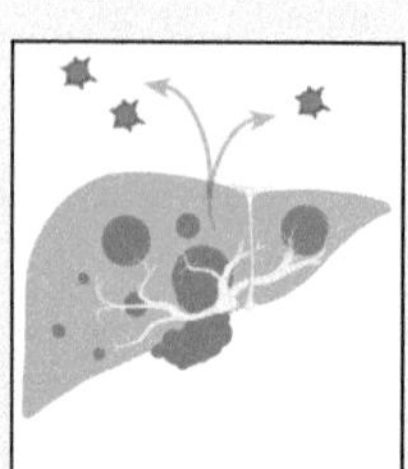 **Advanced stage**
	Single tumor ≤2 cm, preserved liver function, good performance status	Single tumor or up to three tumors ≤3 cm, preserved liver function, good performance status	Multiple tumor nodules, preserved liver function, good performance status	Extrahepatic metastases, portal invasion, preserved liver function, good performance status
Treatment	Ablation, resection, or stereotactic radiotherapy	Ablation, resection, or stereotactic radiotherapy Liver transplant in select cases	Chemoembolization	Systemic therapy (chemotherapy, immunotherapy, targeted therapy [VEGF-TKIs])
Prognosis	5-year survival >75%	5-year survival >50%	5-year survival <30%	5-year survival <10%
Potential CV toxicities				**VEGF inhibitors:** hypertension, arterial and venous thromboembolic events, bleeding **Immune checkpoint inhibitors:** myocarditis, arrhythmias, cardiomyopathy, vasculitis, pericarditis, pericardial effusion

CHAPTER OUTLINE

HEPATOCELLULAR CARCINOMA

KEY POINTS ABOUT HEPATOCELLULAR CARCINOMA (HCC)

- HCC is a relatively uncommon cancer in the United States (annual incidence 6/100,000), but the incidence is rising; it is the fourth leading cause of cancer-related death worldwide.
- Common risk factors include viral hepatitis, excessive alcohol consumption, environmental toxins (e.g., aflatoxin), nonalcoholic fatty liver disease, and iron overload (e.g., hemochromatosis).
- 5-year survival prognosis is very variable and highly dependent on stage and underlying liver disease.
- Localized HCC can often be treated with resection or ablative therapy, and locally advanced (i.e., nonmetastatic) HCC can be treated with hepatic artery embolization therapy.
- Liver transplantation is an option for select patients fulfilling transplant criteria.
- Systemic therapy is indicated for patients with metastatic disease, which includes tyrosine kinase inhibitors (sorafenib, lenvatinib, cabozantinib, regorafenib), immune checkpoint inhibitors (nivolumab, atezolizumab), and monoclonal antibody against vascular endothelial growth (VEGF) and VEGF-R2 inhibitors (bevacizumab, ramucirumab).
- Cardiovascular risks seen in patients with HCC is primarily secondary to therapy with multikinase inhibitors (hypertension, arterial thromboembolic events) and immune checkpoint inhibitors (myocarditis).

Incidence

There is considerable variability in the incidence of hepatocellular carcinoma (HCC) worldwide.[1,2] Overall, it is the fifth most common cancer diagnosed in men and the ninth most commonly diagnosed cancer in women. The incidence is more than two-fold higher in men compared with women.[3] HCC is the fourth leading cause of cancer death in the world. The estimated annual incidence of HCC is rising in the United States and is currently 6/100,000. HCC incidence is also rising in Latin America and Europe.[4]

Risk Factors

The risk factors for HCC are well-established. They include chronic viral hepatitis (hepatitis B and C), excessive alcohol consumption, environmental toxins (e.g., aflatoxin), nonalcoholic fatty liver disease, diabetes, and iron overload disorders (e.g., hemochromatosis).[1,2] There is substantial variation in risk factors across the world. The majority of HCC cases occur in sub-Saharan African and Eastern Asia, mostly secondary to chronic hepatitis B and aflatoxin exposure.[1] Nonalcoholic fatty liver disease, often associated with metabolic syndrome, is an increasingly recognized and important cause of HCC in the developed world.

Prognosis

The prognosis for patients with HCC is determined by the malignancy itself, as well as the underlying liver disease. Therefore, the prognostic evaluation of patients with HCC needs to take into consideration the stage of the malignancy itself, as well as the severity of the liver disease and the patient's performance status. Several prognostic and staging

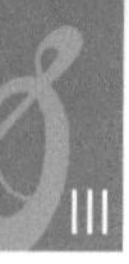

systems have been proposed. One of the more commonly used systems is the Barcelona Clinic Liver Cancer, which has been extensively validated. No single system prognostic algorithm has been shown to be superior; however, some algorithms may perform better than others in predicting outcomes.[1] The prognosis for patients with advanced disease is poor, with an average survival approaching 1 year. On the other hand, the prognosis for patients with localized disease varies greatly based on patient characteristics and underlying liver disease. In patients with resected tumors smaller than 5 cm, the 5-year overall survival can exceed 70%.[1] In appropriately selected patients with HCC treated with liver transplantation, 5-year overall survival may exceed 70% as well, but multiple factors can influence outcomes following regional therapy, including tumor size, presence or absence of vascular invasion, alpha-fetoprotein level, and the treatment utilized.[5] In patients not eligible for resection and/or transplantation and treated with catheter-based transarterial therapy, such as chemoembolization, radioembolization, or drug-eluting bead embolization, 5-year survival is generally less than 30%.[6]

Treatment Overview

The treatment of patients with HCC differs from the treatment of patients with other solid tumors given the high frequency of underlying liver disease, which can limit treatment options. As such, many patients with advanced HCC have advanced hepatic dysfunction at the time of diagnosis and may not be eligible for systemic therapy. Patients with Child-Pugh B and C liver disease are typically excluded from clinical trials; thus, limited data are available for treating these patients. For many of these patients, the prognosis is driven more by the end-stage liver disease than by the malignancy itself. Therefore, the optimal treatment is best done in a multidisciplinary setting involving multiple specialties, including gastroenterology/hepatology, surgery, interventional radiology, medical oncology, and radiation oncology.[1,7]

In patients with localized HCC without cirrhosis, hepatic resection is the treatment of choice if the tumor is considered resectable, and resection is favored over ablative therapy. For patients with HCC without cirrhosis, and who are candidates for resection, the 5-year survival rate can approach 90%. The prognosis (as mentioned above) is dictated by whether the tumor is a solitary lesion, the presence or absence of vascular invasion, and whether a negative margin was achieved on surgical resection. To date, no studies have shown that adjuvant therapy reduces the risk of recurrence. A trial of adjuvant sorafenib therapy showed no survival advantage. Liver transplantation may offer the best chances of long-term survival, but unfortunately, most patients are not eligible for transplantation.[8] Several criteria are used to select patients for transplantation, with Milan criteria being the most commonly used (a single mass 5 cm or less or up to three masses 3 cm or less). Patients fulfilling these criteria have less than 15% chance of recurrence, and 5-year overall survival rates exceed 70% following liver transplantation.

In patients with localized HCC, who are not candidates for liver transplantation are awaiting transplantation, locoregional therapy, such as tumor ablation, is an option. Multiple ablative modalities exist, including radiofrequency ablation, microwave ablation, percutaneous injection therapy, and stereotactic body radiation therapy, but clinical trials comparing these different modalities have not been done.[9,10] The selection of the treatment modality depends on patient and tumor characteristics, equipment availability, and the experience of the treating physicians. Transcatheter embolization therapy (hepatic artery embolization therapy) has been extensively evaluated in patients with HCC who are not candidates for resection or transplantation, and as a bridge therapy in patients awaiting transplantation. Multiple different options exist, but transarterial chemoembolization is the one most commonly used, and it has been shown to improve survival.[11] Transcatheter radioembolization with Yttrium-90-coated beads has also been studied in HCC, but few comparative studies exist.[6,7] Current guidelines recommend locoregional therapy over no therapy in patients with HCC who are not candidates for resection or transplantation.[7]

For patients with metastatic HCC or locally advanced HCC not suitable for regional therapy, systemic therapy has been shown to be effective in prolonging survival when compared with placebo. A landmark, randomized clinical trial of tyrosine kinase inhibitor (TKI) sorafenib versus placebo in patients with advanced HCC confirmed survival advantage of sorafenib over placebo. In this trial, patients on sorafenib had a longer median overall survival than patients on placebo, 10.7 months versus 7.9 months, respectively.[12] Sorafenib was the treatment of choice and the only systemic therapy with proven survival benefit for over a decade until a randomized trial of another TKI, lenvatinib, compared with sorafenib was published in 2018.[13] In this trial, median overall survival was noninferior in the lenvatinib group compared with the sorafenib group (13.6 months for lenvatinib, 12.3 months for sorafenib, [HR 0.92 to 95% CI 0.79 to 1.06]). The adverse event profile of sorafenib and lenvatinib differs, with sorafenib causing more palmar-plantar erythrodysesthesia (also known as hand-foot syndrome) and lenvatinib more likely to result in hypertension. Lenvatinib is a reasonable option as first-line TKI therapy, especially in patients where a radiographic response is desired, as lenvatinib was associated with a higher response rate compared with sorafenib, 40.6% versus 12.4% ($P \leq .0001$), respectively. In late 2019, the results of the IMbrave150 were presented (in abstract form), suggesting a potentially new standard of therapy for advanced HCC with the combination of atezolizumab, an immune checkpoint inhibitor (ICI) targeting programmed death-ligand 1 (PD-L1) and bevacizumab. In this trial, 501 patients were randomized to the combination of atezolizumab plus bevacizumab versus sorafenib. The atezolizumab and bevacizumab combination resulted in a longer median overall survival (not estimable for atezolizumab/bevacizumab, 13.2 months for sorafenib [HR 0.58, 95% CI 0.42 to 0.79]). Six-month overall survival was superior for atezolizumab/bevacizumab, 85%, versus 72% for sorafenib. The combination of atezolizumab and bevacizumab was also superior in terms of median progression-free survival and response rate.

For patients with progressive HCC following sorafenib, there are several treatment options. To date, no data are available regarding systemic therapy following progression of first-line therapy with atezolizumab and bevacizumab because most trials have evaluated patients who have previously progressed on sorafenib as first-line therapy. These options include checkpoint inhibitor, TKIs targeting vascular endothelial growth factor (VEGF), and ramucirumab (a monoclonal antibody against VEGF receptor 2). Regorafenib, a VEGF TKI, was shown to be superior to placebo in a randomized phase 3 clinical trial improving median overall survival (10.7 months for regorafenib, 7.8 months for placebo).[14] Similarly, cabozantinib was shown to improve median overall survival compared with placebo in a phase 3 randomized clinical trial.[15] In this trial, the median overall survival of patients treated with cabozantinib was 10.2 months compared with 8.0 months for placebo. Ramucirumab was also shown to have modest activity in patients with HCC and elevated alpha fetoprotein defined as 400 ng/mL or more and improved overall survival compared with placebo (8.5 months vs. 7.3 months).[16] Earlier data were showing promising activity of immune checkpoint inhibitors based on a phase 1/2 clinical trial studying nivolumab in the second-line setting. This study showed an overall response rate of 15% to 20% and a 6-month progression-free survival and overall survival rate of 37% and 83%, resepcitvely.[17] However, the role of ICIs as monotherapy in the second-line setting is now being called into question, with the negative results of a randomized trial showing lack of superiority of pembrolizumab compared with best supportive care (BSC) in the second-line setting.[18]

Cardiovascular Risk

Systemic therapy for HCC can result in cardiovascular complications, mostly owing to the cardiotoxicity of the drugs used to target the VEGF pathway and, more rarely, related to immune checkpoint inhibitor therapy. The locoregional therapy used in treating patients with HCC is unlikely to result in cardiovascular complications, although it is conceivable that transarterial embolization therapy could result in arterial embolic events. Patients with HCC frequently have substantial liver dysfunction, which could potentially affect drug metabolism, resulting in cardiotoxicity and other noncardiac adverse events. Care must be taken in patients with liver dysfunction when prescribing drugs other than antitumor-directed therapy out of concerns for impaired metabolism and elimination of drugs in these patients.

Cancer Treatments With Potential Cardiovascular Side effects

Tyrosine Kinase Inhibitors

Tyrosine kinase inhibitors targeting VEGF are known to cause hypertension, which can be severe, as well as cardiac ischemia and left ventricular systolic dysfunction.[19,20] Lenvatinib seems more likely to result in severe hypertension than sorafenib.[13] A large meta-analysis reported an increased risk of arterial thrombotic events with sorafenib, a finding also observed in a large trial of patients with renal cell carcinoma.[21] Unlike the risk of arterial thrombotic events, the risk of venous thrombotic events does not seem to be increased with the use of kinase inhibitors. Despite the above, a population-based study from Canada did not corroborate the finding that kinase inhibitors increase cause-specific risk of ischemic heart disease and cerebrovascular accidents compared with age- and gender-matched individuals without cancer.[22] Cardiac arrhythmias and QT interval prolongation is a class effect of TKIs targeting the VEGF pathway, but the clinical significance of the QT prolongation remains uncertain.[19,23]

Monoclonal Antibody Inhibitors of Vascular Endothelial Growth Factor

The monoclonal and VEGF-R2-directed antibodies bevacizumab and ramucirumab have been associated with hypertension and arterial thrombotic events, and a meta-analysis has suggested that the cardiovascular risk related to monoclonal antibodies and kinase inhibitors is similar.[24,25] The cardiovascular risk of bevacizumab may be associated with the use of concurrent chemotherapy and may differ among patients with different tumor types.[26] Ramucirumab has similarly been associated with an increased risk of hypertension and bleeding.[27]

Immune Checkpoint Inhibitors

The cardiotoxicity of ICIs is well-establish but fortunately uncommon.[28] ICIs have been reported to cause myocarditis, which can be fatal and may occur shortly after therapy is begun.[28,29] Other manifestations of cardiotoxicity can include ventricular systolic dysfunction (with occasional Takotsubo syndrome appearance of the left ventricle), pericardial effusion, atrial fibrillation, ventricular arrhythmia, and conduction abnormalities. Given the increasing utilization of these therapies, clinical vigilance is required to recognize these immune-related adverse events early in their course.

BILIARY TRACT CANCERS

KEY POINTS ABOUT BILIARY TRACT CANCER

- Relatively uncommon malignancy in the United States, but the incidence of biliary tract cancer is rising, particularly intrahepatic cholangiocarcinoma.
- Risk factors for different anatomic locations of the primary tumor are different (can arise anywhere along the biliary drainage system).
- Primary sclerosing cholangitis is strongly associated with biliary tract cancer (BTC), but other risk factors include liver flukes, viral hepatitis, chronic liver disease (e.g., nonalcoholic steatohepatitis [NASH]), and in the case of gallbladder cancer, gallstone disease and chronic cholecystitis
- Survival prognosis: 5 years.
- Resection is the only curative option for the minority of patients with localized disease.
- For the majority of patients, systemic therapy is the mainstay of treatment; it commonly includes gemcitabine, cisplatin, 5-fluorouracil, oxaliplatin, and paclitaxel/nab-paclitaxel.
- Targeted therapies (i.e., FGFR2, IDH1, HER-2) are on the horizon for the treatment of BTC.
- Cardiovascular risk of therapy in patients with biliary malignancies is low and mostly related to the use of fluoropyrimidines; increasing use of targeted therapy may result in cardiotoxicity in some patients.

Incidence

Biliary tract cancer (BTC) can arise anywhere along the biliary ductal system from the intrahepatic ducts to the extrahepatic biliary system, including the gall bladder and the ampulla of Vater. There are substantial differences in the biology, genetics, presentation, and outcomes, depending on the anatomic origin of the malignancy.[30] Moreover, there are substantial regional differences in the incidence of biliary tract cancer. Extrahepatic cholangiocarcinoma and gallbladder carcinoma are particularly common in Asia and South America.[31] The incidence in the United

States has increased by almost 65% in recent decades from 1.7/100,000 in 1973 through 1975 to 2.8/100,000 in 2011 through 2012.[32] In 2020, almost 12,000 new cases of extrahepatic cholangiocarcinoma are expected, with two thirds being of gallbladder origin.[3] Of interest, the incidence of intrahepatic cholangiocarcinoma has been rising in North America, and internationally, over the past two decades. The median age of diagnosis in the United States is around 70 years, but patients with underlying conditions predisposing them to biliary tract cancer, such as primary sclerosing cholangitis, are often diagnosed at a much earlier age.[32]

Risk Factors

Several factors are known to predispose individuals to biliary tract cancer. The risk factors are different based on the anatomic origin of the tumor, but there is also substantial geographic variability in risk. Primary sclerosing cholangitis is strongly associated with a risk of developing BTC, with up to 15% lifetime risk.[33] Fibropolycystic liver disease, such as Caroli disease, and choledochal cysts increase the risk, and patients are often diagnosed at an early age with BTC.[34] Hereditary disorders, such as Lynch syndrome and cystic fibrosis, are associated with an increased risk of BTC. Established risk factors for intrahepatic biliary carcinoma are liver flukes (East Asia), viral hepatitis, chronic nonviral liver disease, particularly obesity, and metabolic syndrome causing nonalcoholic steatohepatitis (NASH).[34] Risk factors for gallbladder carcinoma include gallstone disease, chronic cholecystitis, gallbladder polyps, diabetes, obesity, environmental toxins, primary sclerosing cholangitis, and infections.

Prognosis

The prognosis of metastatic BTC is poor. According to a recent population-based study using surveillance, epidemiology, and end results (SEER). The median overall survival of all patients with BTC was only 7 months.[32] The majority of patients present with advanced disease and are not candidates for therapy with curative intent and, therefore, the goal of the treatment is palliative. Recurrences are common following resection, even when adjuvant therapy is utilized, and the majority of patients who undergo resection will experience recurrence and die within 5 years.[35]

Treatment Overview

Resection is the treatment of choice of localized BTC and is the only curative therapy. Resection of BTC should follow surgical oncology principles with regional lymphadenectomy when appropriate.[36] Adjuvant therapy is recommended in most patients following curative resection.[37] In most instances, chemotherapy (i.e., capecitabine) is considered the adjuvant therapy of choice, with radiation therapy reserved for patients with involved or close surgical margins. The benefits of adjuvant therapy are modest, seen in meta-analyses and prospective trials, but not all trials have confirmed a survival benefit.[35, 37] Selected patients with localized but unresectable hilar cholangiocarcinoma may be candidates for liver transplantation following neoadjuvant chemoradiation therapy.[38] Such patients usually are maintained on oral capecitabine after chemoradiation therapy until a liver becomes available.

For localized but nonresectable BTC, a combination of chemotherapy and radiotherapy can provide a meaningful benefit in terms of survival prolongation and symptom palliation.[39] Patients with nonresectable BTC frequently suffer from biliary obstruction, and biliary drainage interventions are frequently needed, usually in the form of placement of internal biliary stents or external drains.

In patients with metastatic biliary carcinoma, systemic therapy is the treatment of choice. Cytotoxic chemotherapy has been shown to prolong survival and improve quality of life in patients with advanced BTC.[40] Gemcitabine had been commonly used as monotherapy until the combination of gemcitabine with cisplatin was shown to be superior to gemcitabine alone. Thus, gemcitabine with cisplatin became the first-line therapy of choice.[41] Other first-line systemic therapy combinations exist, such as gemcitabine with oxaliplatin, gemcitabine with capecitabine, gemcitabine with nab-paclitaxel, as well as gemcitabine with nab-paclitaxel and cisplatin.[42,43] Until recently, no standard existed for second-line therapy and beyond and fluoropyrimidine-containing therapy was commonly used. A recent randomized phase 3 clinical trial compared therapy with 5-fluorouracil, oxaliplatin, and leucovorin combined with BSC without systemic therapy to BSC alone in patients who progressed on gemcitabine with cisplatin. Patients receiving 5-fluorouracil, oxaliplatin, and leucovorin with BSC had a longer overall survival compared with those on BSC alone. Biliary tract cancer, especially intrahepatic cholangiocarcinoma, frequently has potentially targetable molecular alterations. In the case of intrahepatic cholangiocarcinoma, mutations in isocitrate dehydrogenase (IDH, 20% incidence) and fusions of fibroblast growth factor receptor-2 (FGFR2, 15% to 20% incidence) can be detected with next generation sequencing. Targeted therapy for both alterations is being evaluated in multiple clinical trials.[44] Recently, tropomyosin receptor kinase (TRK) inhibitors have been found to be highly active in patients with malignancies harboring a fusion in TRK (<1% incidence).[45] Human epidermal growth factor receptor (HER)-2 amplification is occasionally found in patients with gallbladder carcinoma and is potentially targetable. Therapy with immune checkpoint inhibitor is appropriate for patients with mismatch repair deficient/microsatellite instability high (2% incidence) biliary tract cancer but have not yet been shown to have substantial efficacy in patients without mismatch repair deficiency.

Cardiovascular Risk

The cardiovascular risk associated with therapy of BTC is minimal. Most of the systemic agents have a low risk of cardiotoxicity, with the exception of the fluoropyrimidines, 5-fluorouracil, and capecitabine, which can occasionally result in cardiotoxicity. Because BTCs are relatively rich in targetable molecular alterations, therapy targeting specific alterations is expected to become a significant component of the systemic therapy in the future, likely associated with some cardiovascular toxicity.

Cancer Treatments With Potential Cardiovascular Side Effects

Fluoropyrimidines

Coronary vasospasm is a well-known complication of therapy with fluoropyrimidines, both 5-fluorouracil and capecitabine.[46] Cardiotoxicity has been reported to occur in up to 18% of patients exposed to fluoropyrimidines. The cardiotoxicity is discussed in greater detail in other chapters, including the section on esophageal and gastric cancer.

Platinum Drugs

Both oxaliplatin and cisplatin have been associated with cardiotoxicity. Cisplatin frequently results in electrolyte disturbances, including hypomagnesemia, which can result in cardiac arrhythmia. Arrhythmias may occur in the absence of electrolyte abnormalities.[47] Other complications include arterial and venous thrombotic events and hypertension, less commonly declines in cardiac function.

Paclitaxel

Paclitaxel is an uncommon cause of cardiotoxicity; arrhythmias are the most commonly recognized cardiac adverse events.[48] This is discussed in greater detail in other chapters, including the section on esophageal and gastric cancer.

Gemcitabine

Rarely has gemcitabine been associated with cardiotoxicity, including cardiomyopathy.[49]

REFERENCES

1. Forner A, Reig M, Bruix J. Hepatocellular carcinoma. *Lancet*. 2018;391:1301–1314.
2. Yang JD, Hainaut P, Gores GJ, et al. A global view of hepatocellular carcinoma: trends, risk, prevention and management. *Nat Rev Gastroenterol Hepatol*. 2019;16:589–604.
3. Siegel RL, Miller KD, Jemal A. Cancer statistics, 2020. *CA Cancer J Clin*. 2020;70:7–30.
4. Bertuccio P, Turati F, Carioli G, et al. Global trends and predictions in hepatocellular carcinoma mortality. *J Hepatol*. 2017;67:302–309.
5. She WH, Chan ACY, Cheung TT, et al. Survival outcomes of liver transplantation for hepatocellular carcinoma in patients with normal, high and very high preoperative alpha-fetoprotein levels. *World J Hepatol*. 2018;10:308–318.
6. Katsanos K, Kitrou P, Spiliopoulos S, et al. Comparative effectiveness of different transarterial embolization therapies alone or in combination with local ablative or adjuvant systemic treatments for unresectable hepatocellular carcinoma: a network meta-analysis of randomized controlled trials. *PLoS One*. 2017;12:e0184597.
7. Heimbach JK, Kulik LM, Finn RS, et al. AASLD guidelines for the treatment of hepatocellular carcinoma. *Hepatology*. 2018;67:358–380.
8. Sapisochin G, Bruix J. Liver transplantation for hepatocellular carcinoma: outcomes and novel surgical approaches. *Nat Rev Gastroenterol Hepatol*. 2017;14:203–217.
9. Rim CH, Kim HJ, Seong J. Clinical feasibility and efficacy of stereotactic body radiotherapy for hepatocellular carcinoma: a systematic review and meta-analysis of observational studies. *Radiother Oncol*. 2019;131:135–144.
10. Zhu GQ, Sun M, Liao WT, et al. Comparative efficacy and safety between ablative therapies or surgery for small hepatocellular carcinoma: a network meta-analysis. *Expert Rev Gastroenterol Hepatol*. 2018;12:935–945.
11. Llovet JM, Bruix J. Systematic review of randomized trials for unresectable hepatocellular carcinoma: chemoembolization improves survival. *Hepatology*. 2003;37:429–442.
12. Llovet JM, Ricci S, Mazzaferro V, et al. Sorafenib in advanced hepatocellular carcinoma. *N Engl J Med*. 2008;359:378–390.
13. Kudo M, Finn RS, Qin S, et al. Lenvatinib versus sorafenib in first-line treatment of patients with unresectable hepatocellular carcinoma: a randomised phase 3 non-inferiority trial. *Lancet*. 2018;391:1163–1173.
14. Bruix J, Qin S, Merle P, et al. Regorafenib for patients with hepatocellular carcinoma who progressed on sorafenib treatment (RESORCE): a randomised, double-blind, placebo-controlled, phase 3 trial. *Lancet*. 2017;389:56–66.

15. Abou-Alfa GK, Meyer T, Cheng AL, et al. Cabozantinib in patients with advanced and progressing hepatocellular carcinoma. *N Engl J Med*. 2018;379:54–63.
16. Zhu AX, Kang YK, Yen CJ, et al. Ramucirumab after sorafenib in patients with advanced hepatocellular carcinoma and increased alpha-fetoprotein concentrations (REACH-2): a randomised, double-blind, placebo-controlled, phase 3 trial. *Lancet Oncol*. 2019;20:282–296.
17. El-Khoueiry AB, Sangro B, Yau T, et al. Nivolumab in patients with advanced hepatocellular carcinoma (CheckMate 040): an open-label, non-comparative, phase 1/2 dose escalation and expansion trial. *Lancet*. 2017;389:2492–2502.
18. Finn RS, Ryoo BY, Merle P, et al. Pembrolizumab as second-line therapy in patients with advanced hepatocellular carcinoma in KEYNOTE-240: a randomized, double-blind, phase III trial. *J Clin Oncol*. 2020;8:193–202.
19. Totzeck M, Mincu RI, Mrotzek S, et al. Cardiovascular diseases in patients receiving small molecules with anti-vascular endothelial growth factor activity: a meta-analysis of approximately 29,000 patients with cancer. *Eur J Prev Cardiol*. 2018;25:482–494.
20. Touyz RM, Herrmann J. Cardiotoxicity with vascular endothelial growth factor inhibitor therapy. *NPJ Precis Oncol*. 2018;2:13.
21. Choueiri TK, Schutz FA, Je Y, et al. Risk of arterial thromboembolic events with sunitinib and sorafenib: a systematic review and meta-analysis of clinical trials. *J Clin Oncol*. 2010;28:2280–2285.
22. Srikanthan A, Ethier JL, Ocana A, et al. Cardiovascular toxicity of multi-tyrosine kinase inhibitors in advanced solid tumors: a population-based observational study. *PLoS One*. 2015;10:e0122735.
23. Shah RR, Morganroth J. Update on cardiovascular safety of tyrosine kinase inhibitors: with a special focus on QT interval, left ventricular dysfunction and overall risk/benefit. *Drug Saf*. 2015;38:693–710.
24. Abdel-Qadir H, Ethier JL, Lee DS, et al. Cardiovascular toxicity of angiogenesis inhibitors in treatment of malignancy: a systematic review and meta-analysis. *Cancer Treat Rev*. 2017;53:120–127.
25. Totzeck M, Mincu RI, Rassaf T. Cardiovascular adverse events in patients with cancer treated with bevacizumab: a meta-analysis of more than 20 000 patients. *J Am Heart Assoc*. 2017;6:e006278.
26. Schutz FA, Je Y, Azzi GR, et al. Bevacizumab increases the risk of arterial ischemia: a large study in patients with cancer with a focus on different subgroup outcomes. *Ann Oncol*. 2011;22:1404–1412.
27. Abdel-Rahman O, ElHalawani H. Risk of cardiovascular adverse events in patients with solid tumors treated with ramucirumab: a meta analysis and summary of other VEGF targeted agents. *Crit Rev Oncol Hematol*. 2016;102:89–100.
28. Salem JE, Manouchehri A, Moey M, et al. Cardiovascular toxicities associated with immune checkpoint inhibitors: an observational, retrospective, pharmacovigilance study. *Lancet Oncol*. 2018;19:1579–1589.
29. Johnson DB, Balko JM, Compton ML, et al. Fulminant myocarditis with combination immune checkpoint blockade. *N Engl J Med*. 2016;375:1749–1755.
30. Hang H, Jeong S, Sha M, et al. Cholangiocarcinoma: anatomical location-dependent clinical, prognostic, and genetic disparities. *Ann Transl Med*. 2019;7:744.
31. Miranda-Filho A, Pineros M, Ferreccio C, et al. Gallbladder and extrahepatic bile duct cancers in the Americas: incidence and mortality patterns and trends. *Int J Cancer*. 2020;147:978–989.
32. Mukkamalla SKR, Naseri HM, Kim BM, et al. Trends in incidence and factors affecting survival of patients with cholangiocarcinoma in the United States. *J Natl Compr Canc Netw*. 2018;16:370–376.
33. Bergquist A, Ekbom A, Olsson R, et al. Hepatic and extrahepatic malignancies in primary sclerosing cholangitis. *J Hepatol*. 2002;36:321–327.
34. Gupta A, Dixon E. Epidemiology and risk factors: intrahepatic cholangiocarcinoma. *Hepatobiliary Surg Nutr*. 2017;6:101–104.
35. Rangarajan K, Simmons G, Manas D, et al. Systemic adjuvant chemotherapy for cholangiocarcinoma surgery: a systematic review and meta-analysis. *Eur J Surg Oncol*. 2019;46:684–693.
36. Ejaz A, Cloyd JM, Pawlik TM. Advances in the diagnosis and treatment of patients with intrahepatic cholangiocarcinoma. *Ann Surg Oncol*. 2020;27:552–560.
37. Shroff RT, Kennedy EB, Bachini M, et al. Adjuvant therapy for resected biliary tract cancer: ASCO Clinical Practice Guideline. *J Clin Oncol*. 2019;37:1015–1027.
38. Rea DJ, Heimbach JK, Rosen CB, et al. Liver transplantation with neoadjuvant chemoradiation is more effective than resection for hilar cholangiocarcinoma. *Ann Surg*. 2005;242:451–458; discussion 458–461.
39. Green BL, House MG. Nonsurgical approaches to treat biliary tract and liver tumors. *Surg Oncol Clin N Am*. 2019;28:573–586.
40. Sharma A, Dwary AD, Mohanti BK, et al. Best supportive care compared with chemotherapy for unresectable gall bladder cancer: a randomized controlled study. *J Clin Oncol*. 2010;28:4581–4586.
41. Valle J, Wasan H, Palmer DH, et al. Cisplatin plus gemcitabine versus gemcitabine for biliary tract cancer. *N Engl J Med*. 2010;362:1273–1281.
42. Kim ST, Kang JH, Lee J, et al. Capecitabine plus oxaliplatin versus gemcitabine plus oxaliplatin as first-line therapy for advanced biliary tract cancers: a multicenter, open-label, randomized, phase III, noninferiority trial. *Ann Oncol*. 2019;30:788–795.
43. Shroff RT, Javle MM, Xiao L, et al. Gemcitabine, cisplatin, and nab-paclitaxel for the treatment of advanced biliary tract cancers: a phase 2 clinical trial. *JAMA Oncol*. 2019;5:824–830.
44. Kelley RK, Bridgewater J, Gores GJ, et al. Systemic therapies for intrahepatic cholangiocarcinoma. *J Hepatol*. 2020;72:353–363.
45. Drilon A, Laetsch TW, Kummar S, et al. Efficacy of larotrectinib in TRK fusion-positive cancers in adults and children. *N Engl J Med*. 2018;378:731–739.
46. Sara JD, Kaur J, Khodadadi R, et al. 5-fluorouracil and cardiotoxicity: a review. *Ther Adv Med Oncol*. 2018;10:1758835918780140.
47. Demkow U, Stelmaszczyk-Emmel A. Cardiotoxicity of cisplatin-based chemotherapy in advanced non-small cell lung patients with cancer. *Respir Physiol Neurobiol*. 2013;187:64–67.
48. Arbuck SG, Strauss H, Rowinsky E, et al. A reassessment of cardiac toxicity associated with Taxol. *J Natl Cancer Inst Monogr*. 1993:117–130.
49. Khan MF, Gottesman S, Boyella R, et al. Gemcitabine-induced cardiomyopathy: a case report and review of the literature. *J Med Case Rep*. 2014;8:220.

43 Pancreatic Cancer

IBRAHIM BÜDEYRI, CHRISTOPH W. MICHALSKI, AND JÖRG KLEEFF

Stages	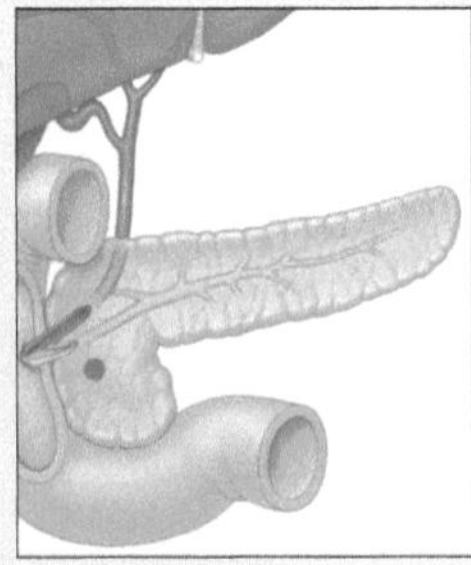 **Stage I** <4 cm, limited to pancreas, no LN involvement	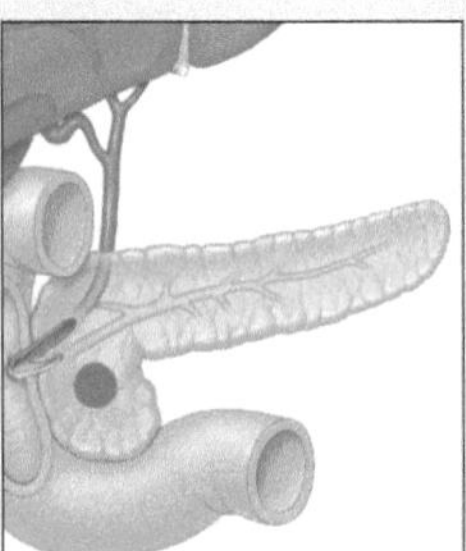 **Stage II** >4 cm (IIA) or any regional LN involvement (IIB)	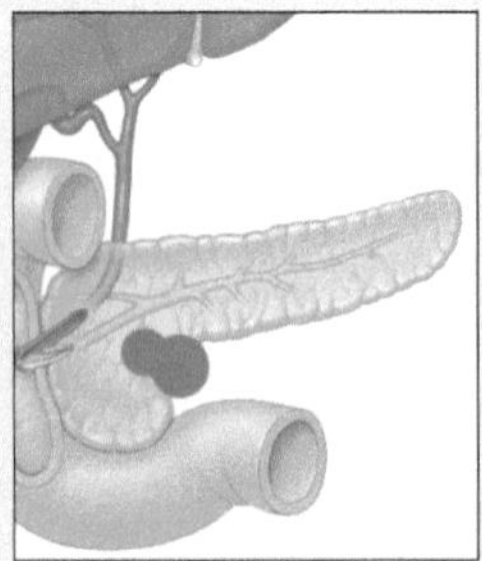 **Stage III** Involves the superior mesenteric artery or celiac axis ± LN involvement	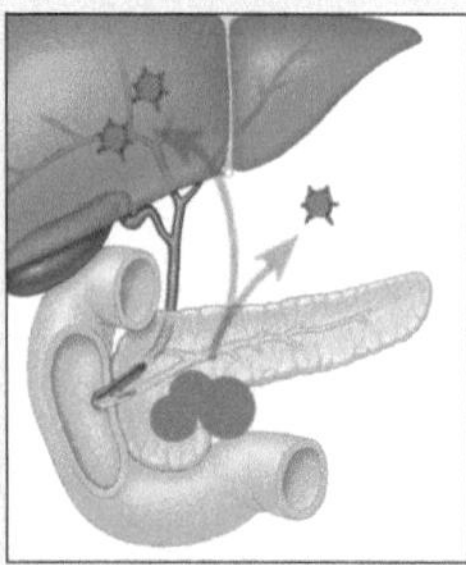 **Stage IV** Metastasis to distant organs ± LN involvement
Treatment	Surgery adjuvant chemotherapy (FOLFIRINOX or gemcitabine/capecitabine or gemcitabine)	Surgery adjuvant chemotherapy (FOLFIRINOX or gemcitabine/capecitabine or gemcitabine)	Neoadjuvant chemotherapy (FOLFIRINOX or gemcitabine + albumin-bound paclitaxel) ± radiotherapy Surgery ± adjuvant chemotherapy	Palliative chemotherapy (FOLFIRINOX or gemcitabine + albumin-bound paclitaxel or gemcitabine monotherapy)
Prognosis	5-year survival up tp 50%	5-year survival 20%	5-year survival <20%	5-year survival <5%

Potential CV toxicities

FOLFIRINOX:
Fluorouracil (5-FU): cardiac ischemia/ infarction, coronary vasospasm, thrombosis, arrhythmias, sudden death
Gemcitabine: thromboembolism, arrhythmias
Oxaliplatin: QTc prolongation and Torsades
Paclitaxel (albumin-bound): hypotension, bradycardia, supraventricular tachycardia, QTc prolongation, cardiac arrest, chest pain, cardiac ischemia/infarction, pulmonary embolism, cardiac dysfunction, heart failure

CHAPTER OUTLINE

KEY POINTS ABOUT PANCREATIC CANCER

- Pancreatic cancer has the lowest survival rate among any solid tumors.[1,2]
- Median age at diagnosis is 70 years.[1]
- Risk factors include smoking and obesity.[3]
- Most patients are diagnosed at an advanced stage.[1,2]
- Prognosis and treatment options vary based on stage at diagnosis.
- Perioperative precautions must be taken for thromboembolic events after extended surgeries.

INCIDENCE

As the fourth leading cause of cancer-related deaths in the United States, pancreatic ductal adenocarcinoma is a lethal disease with an overall 5-year survival rate of less than 10%.[1] Approximately 56,770 new cases of pancreatic cancer and 45,750 pancreatic cancer deaths are predicted in 2019 in the United States,[1,2] and incidence and mortality rates continue to increase.[1,2] More than one half of the cases are diagnosed at an advanced stage.[1,2] Pancreatic cancer is slightly more common in men than in women and is most often diagnosed between 65 and 74 years of age.[1] The median age at diagnosis is 70 years.[1]

RISK FACTORS

The incidence of pancreatic cancer increases with age.[1] Generally, smoking and obesity are important factors that increase the risk of developing pancreatic cancer.[3,4] Other risk factors include a personal history of diabetes or chronic pancreatitis, a family history of pancreatic cancer or pancreatitis, and hereditary conditions, such as hereditary nonpolyposis colon cancer (also known as Lynch syndrome), von Hippel-Lindau syndrome, Peutz-Jeghers syndrome, hereditary breast and ovarian cancer syndrome, and familial atypical multiple mole melanoma syndrome.[1] Diabetes mellitus is both a risk factor for pancreatic cancer, and, especially if newly diagnosed in people over the age of 50 years, an early marker for pancreatic cancer.[5–8]

PROGNOSIS

Patients with localized pancreatic cancer have a 37.4% 5-year survival.[1] However, 5-year survival rates of patients with regionally advanced disease decrease to 12.4%.[1] For those presenting with metastatic disease, 5-year survival is estimated to be only 2.9%.[1] Current 5-year survival with surgery and adjuvant combination of gemcitabine and capecitabine is 28.8%.[9] Most recently, excellent median survival rates of more than 50 months and a 3-year survival rate of 63.4% have been shown when combining surgery with FOLFIRINOX (**fol**inic acid, 5-**f**luorouracil, **irin**otecan, **ox**aliplatin) chemotherapy, albeit at the expense of considerable but manageable toxicity.[10]

TREATMENT OVERVIEW

Treatment of pancreatic cancer varies depending on stage,[11] surgical resectability, and patient's general performance status. Pancreatic ductal adenocarcinoma is the most common histologic subtype of pancreatic cancer.[4] Tumors of the pancreatic head are removed via a partial pancreaticoduodenectomy with or without resection of the distal stomach, whereas those in the body or tail of the pancreas are removed by distal pancreatectomy with splenectomy.[12] Pancreatic cancer surgeries are increasingly performed through minimal invasive approaches using laparoscopy and robotically assisted techniques, reducing intraoperative blood loss and hospital stay.[13]

Localized cancer is treated with surgery and adjuvant chemotherapy, whereas patients with borderline resectable or locally advanced disease may require neoadjuvant chemotherapy with FOLFIRINOX or gemcitabine plus albumin-bound paclitaxel (and/or radiochemotherapy), followed by surgery and possibly adjuvant chemotherapy.[12,13] Patients with metastatic disease are often treated with FOLFIRINOX,[14] combination chemotherapy with gemcitabine plus albumin-bound paclitaxel or gemcitabine monotherapies depending on Eastern Cooperative Oncology Group (ECOG) performance status.[15] Absence of specific tumor markers and difficulties in imaging early-stage tumors limit early intervention and, thus, options for cure.[4,12] Yet, with a wider use of new combination chemotherapies and extended surgical resections, longer survival times have been achieved over the last years. A median overall survival of 28 months following surgical resection is reported for the adjuvant combination of gemcitabine and capecitabine[9] and 54 months for adjuvant FOLFIRINOX chemotherapy.[10]

CARDIOVASCULAR RISK

From a cardiovascular perspective, systemic treatments for pancreatic cancer are usually well tolerated by the patients. Yet, a high degree of vigilance is required while using capecitabine and albumin-bound paclitaxel, especially in patients with comorbid cardiovascular disorders (Table 43.1).[9,10,14,16–24] Pancreatic cancer has been associated with a 16-fold increased risk of venous thromboembolism compared with the general population.[25] Although the exact pathophysiology is still unknown, it is assumed that pancreatic cancer induces a prothrombotic and hypercoagulable state through production of cytokines, mucins, procoagulant, and proinflammatory factors.[26] Longer hospital stays owing to extended surgery, intraoperative vascular injury, or portal vein reconstruction can also increase the risk of thromboembolic events.

Routine preoperative cardiovascular workup should include blood pressure control in both arms and a chest X-ray or chest computerized tomography. An electrocardiogram (ECG) should be done in any patient, especially in those with risk factors for coronary artery disease, particularly, as it helps to diagnose an existing abnormal rhythm preoperatively and helps create a baseline for follow-up ECGs postoperatively. A cardiologic consultation is required in patients with known cardiac diseases, abnormal ECGs, a history of diabetes mellitus, hypertension, obesity,

TABLE 43.1 Systemic Cancer Treatments in Pancreatic Cancer With Potential CV Side Effects

SYSTEMIC CANCER TREATMENTS	POTENTIAL CV SIDE EFFECTS
Gemcitabine[16]	Thromboembolism,[9,10,14] Cardiac Rhythm Problems[17]
Capecitabine[18]	Cardiac Ischemia/Infarction Sudden Death Coronary Artery Thrombosis Coronary Vasospasm Ventricular Extrasystoles Tachycardia Conduction Disturbances (Complete AVB)[19,20]
Paclitaxel (albumin-bound)[21]	Hypotension Sinus Bradycardia Cardiac Ischemia/Infarction Chest Pain Cardiac Arrest QTc Prolongation Supraventricular Tachycardia CHF LVD Pulmonary Embolism[20–24]
FOLFIRINOX	Thromboembolism[10,14] Cardiac Ischemia[20]

CV, Cardiovascular; AVB, atrioventricular block; CHF, congestive heart failure; LVD, left ventricular dysfunction.

alcohol or drug abuse, syncope, or chronic respiratory lung disease. Those patients with a heart murmur and symptoms, such as syncope or chest pain, or signs or symptoms of heart failure should undergo an ECG. The Canadian Cardiovascular Society Guidelines Committee suggests measuring preoperative N-terminal pro-B-type natriuretic peptide (NT-pro-BNP) in patients undergoing noncardiac surgery who are 65 years of age or older, are 45 to 64 years of age but with significant cardiovascular disease, or have a Revised Cardiac Risk Index score equal to or greater than 1.[27] Intraoperatively, standard cardiovascular surveillance under general anesthesia comprises pulse oximetry, capnography, and BP and ECG monitoring. Pivotal for pancreatic surgeries is invasive arterial pressure monitoring and a central venous access.[28,29]

REFERENCES

1. National Institute of Cancer Surveillance Epidemeology, and End Results Program. *Cancer Stat Facts: Pancreatic Cancer.* Available at: https://seer.cancer.gov/statfacts/html/pancreas.html. Accessed May 12, 2019.
2. Siegel RL, Miller KD, Jemal A. Cancer statistics, 2019. *CA Cancer J Clin.* 2019;69(1):7–34.
3. Islami F, Goding Sauer A, Miller KD, et al. Proportion and number of cancer cases and deaths attributable to potentially modifiable risk factors in the United States. *CA Cancer J Clin.* 2018;68(1):31–54.

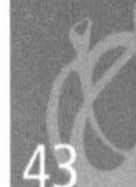

4. Aier I, Semwal R, Sharma A, Varadwaj PK. A systematic assessment of statistics, risk factors, and underlying features involved in pancreatic cancer. *Cancer Epidemiol.* 2019;58:104–110.
5. Chari ST, Leibson CL, Rabe KG, Ransom J, DE Andrade M, Petersen GM. Probability of pancreatic cancer following diabetes: a population-based study. *Gastroenterology.* 2005;129(2):504–511.
6. Ben Q, Xu M, Ning X, et al. Diabetes mellitus and risk of pancreatic cancer: a meta-analysis of cohort studies. *Eur J Cancer.* 2011;47(13):1928–1937.
7. Hart PA, Bellin MD, Andersen DK, et al. Type 3c (pancreatogenic) diabetes mellitus secondary to chronic pancreatitis and pancreatic cancer. *Lancet Gastroenterol Hepatol.* 2016;1(3):226–237.
8. Andersen DK, Korc M, Petersen GM, et al. Diabetes, pancreatogenic diabetes, and pancreatic cancer. *Diabetes.* 2017;66(5):1103–1110.
9. Neoptolemos JP, Palmer DH, Ghaneh P, et al. Comparison of adjuvant gemcitabine and capecitabine with gemcitabine monotherapy in patients with resected pancreatic cancer (ESPAC-4): a multicentre, open-label, randomised, phase 3 trial. *Lancet.* 2017;389(10073):1011–1024.
10. Conroy T, Hammel P, Hebbar M, et al. FOLFIRINOX or gemcitabine as adjuvant therapy for pancreatic cancer. *N Engl J Med.* 2018;379(25):2395–2406.
11. Gress DM, Edge SB, Greene FL, et al. Principles of cancer staging. In: *AJCC Cancer Staging Manual,* 8th ed. New York, NY: Springer; 2017.
12. Kleeff J, Korc M, Apte M, et al. Pancreatic cancer. *Nat Rev Dis Primers.* 2016;2:16022.
13. Michalski CW, Liu B, Büchler MW, Hackert T. Evolution of pancreatic cancer surgery. *Pancreat Cancer.* 2017;1–15.
14. Conroy T, Desseigne F, Ychou M, et al. FOLFIRINOX versus gemcitabine for metastatic pancreatic cancer. *N Engl J Med.* 2011;364(19):1817–1825.
15. Von Hoff DD, Ervin T, Arena FP, et al. Increased survival in pancreatic cancer with nab-paclitaxel plus gemcitabine. *N Engl J Med.* 2013;369(18):1691–1703.
16. GEMZAR [Package Insert]. *FDA-approved manufacturer's package insert for gemzar.*
Available at: https://www.accessdata.fda.gov/drugsatfda_docs/label/1998/20509lbl.pdf.
17. Burris H III, Moore MJ, Andersen J, et al. Improvements in survival and clinical benefit with gemcitabine as first-line therapy for patients with advanced pancreas cancer: a randomized trial. *J Clin Oncol.* 1997;15(6):2403–2413.
18. XELODA [Package Insert]. *FDA-approved manufacturer's package insert for xeloda.*
Available at: https://www.accessdata.fda.gov/drugsatfda_docs/label/2015/020896s037lbl.pdf.
19. Kosmas C, Kallistratos MS, Kopterides P, et al. Cardiotoxicity of fluoropyrimidines in different schedules of administration: a prospective study. *J Cancer Res Clin Oncol.* 2008;134(1):75–82.
20. Curigliano G, Mayer EL, Burstein HJ, Winer EP, Goldhirsch A. Cardiac toxicity from systemic cancer therapy: a comprehensive review. *Prog Cardiovasc Dis.* 2010;53(2):94–104.
21. ABRAXANE [Package Insert]. *FDA-approved manufacturer's package insert for abraxane.*
Available at: https://www.accessdata.fda.gov/drugsatfda_docs/label/2013/021660s037lbl.pdf.
22. Rowinsky EK, Mcguire WP, Guarnieri T, et al. Cardiac disturbances during the administration of taxol. *J Clin Oncol.* 1991;*9*(9):1704–1712.
23. Arbuck SG, Strauss H, Rowinsky E, et al. A reassessment of cardiac toxicity associated with taxol. *J Natl Cancer Inst Monogr.* 1993;(15):117–130.
24. Del Mastro L, Perrone F, Repetto L, et al. Weekly paclitaxel as first-line chemotherapy in elderly advanced breast patients with cancer: a phase II study of the Gruppo Italiano di Oncologia Geriatrica (GIOGer). *Ann Oncol.* 2005;16(2):253–258.
25. Cronin-Fenton DP, Søndergaard F, Pedersen LA, et al. Hospitalisation for venous thromboembolism in patients with cancer and the general population: a population-based cohort study in Denmark, 1997–2006. *Br J Cancer.* 2010;*103*(7):947.
26. Ansari D, Ansari D, Andersson R, Andrén-Sandberg Å. Pancreatic cancer and thromboembolic disease, 150 years after Trousseau. *Hepatobiliary Surg Nutr.* 2015;4(5):325.
27. Duceppe E, Parlow J, Macdonald P, et al. Canadian Cardiovascular Society guidelines on perioperative cardiac risk assessment and management for patients who undergo noncardiac surgery. *Can J Cardiol.* 2017;33(1):17–32.
28. Marandola M, Albante A. Anaesthesia and pancreatic surgery: techniques, clinical practice and pain management. *World J Anesthesiol.* 2014;3(1):1–11.
29. Amorese G. Preoperative evaluation and anesthesia in minimally invasive surgery of the pancreas. In: Boggi U, Ed. *Minimally Invasive Surgery of the Pancreas.* Milano: Springer; 2018:49–63.

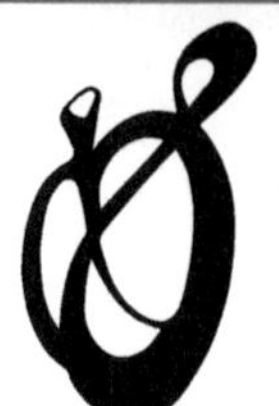

44 Cutaneous Melanoma

TIENUSH RASSAF AND DIRK SCHADENDORF

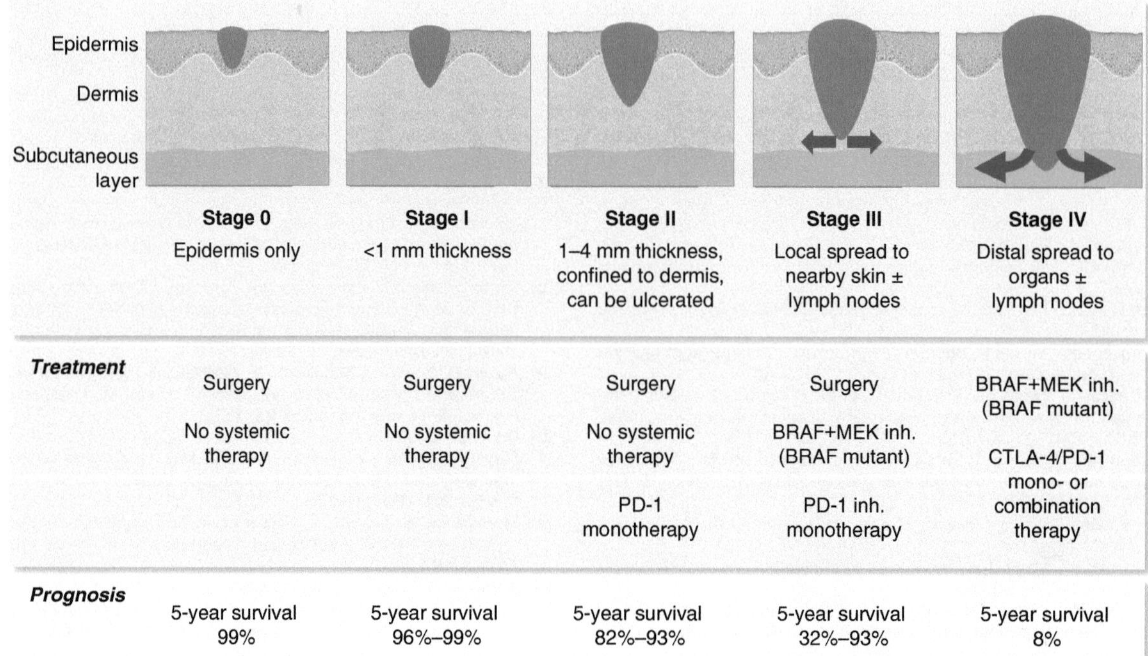

	Stage 0	Stage I	Stage II	Stage III	Stage IV
	Epidermis only	<1 mm thickness	1–4 mm thickness, confined to dermis, can be ulcerated	Local spread to nearby skin ± lymph nodes	Distal spread to organs ± lymph nodes
Treatment	Surgery No systemic therapy	Surgery No systemic therapy	Surgery No systemic therapy PD-1 monotherapy	Surgery BRAF+MEK inh. (BRAF mutant) PD-1 inh. monotherapy	BRAF+MEK inh. (BRAF mutant) CTLA-4/PD-1 mono- or combination therapy
Prognosis	5-year survival 99%	5-year survival 96%–99%	5-year survival 82%–93%	5-year survival 32%–93%	5-year survival 8%

Potential CV toxicities

BRAF inhibitors:
Vemurafenib: QTc prolongation, hypertension, edema, atrial fibrillation,
Dabrafenib: hypertension, edema, cardiomyopathy (esp., in combination with trametinib)
Encorafenib: QTc prolongation

MEK inhibitors:
Trametinib: hypertension, bradycardia, cardiomyopathy, heart failure
Cobimetinib: hypertension, cardiomyopathy
Binimetinib: hypertension, edema, cardiomyopathy, venous thromboembolism

Immune checkpoint inhibitors:
myocarditis, arrhythmias, cardiomyopathy, vasculitis, pericarditis

CHAPTER OUTLINE

CUTANEOUS MELANOMA

KEY POINTS ABOUT MELANOMA

- The incidence of melanoma is rising faster than for any other malignancy and shows regional variation (4% to 5% of women and men in the United States and 1% to 2% in Europe).
- The median age at diagnosis is around 50 years, but melanoma is not uncommon in young adults.
- The strongest risk factors are exposure to ultraviolet radiation (sunburns, indoor tanning) at less than 35 years of age, previous melanoma, and positive family history.
- The majority of patients have early stage (stage I and II) disease at diagnosis.
- The treatment strategy and prognosis vary based on stage at presentation.
- Targeted (BRAF/MEK [mitogen-activated protein kinase] inhibitors) and immune therapies (immune checkpoint inhibitors) comprise the new cornerstone of systemic therapy in stage III and IV but bear the risk of heart failure, arrhythmia, hypertension, and myocarditis.

Incidence

Worldwide, about 232,100 cancer cases (1.7%) of all newly diagnosed primary malignant cancers are cutaneous melanoma, and about 55,500 cancer deaths (0.7% of all cancer deaths) are due to cutaneous melanoma annually.

Risk Factors

The incidence and mortality rates of cutaneous melanoma differ widely. Incidence rates have increased since the early 1970s in predominantly fair-skinned populations.

Prognosis

Five-year age-standardized relative survival for cutaneous melanoma diagnosed in 2000–2007 in Europe range from 74.3% (Eastern Europe) to 87.7% (Northern Europe).[1] In the United States, 5-year relative survival (without age standardization) is 92%. For primary melanoma without lymph node involvement, the relative 5-year relative survival in stage I is 98% and 90% in stage II.[2] Mortality rates differ widely across the globe, depending on access to early detection and primary care.

Once melanoma has spread, it rapidly becomes life-threatening. For decades treatment options were limited and not successful. Over the last 10 years increased biological understanding and access to innovative therapeutic substances have transformed advanced melanoma into a new oncologic model for treating solid cancers.[3] Based on immune checkpoint inhibition or targeting BRAFV600E mutations using selected BRAF-inhibitors combined with MEK-inhibitors, response and overall survival rates have improved significantly.

Treatment Overview

Melanoma is diagnosed histopathologically, and subsequent treatment decisions are mainly based on histologic classification and risk calculation. Classification refers to tumor thickness according to Breslow[4] (T stage), lymph node involvement (N stage), and presence of metastasis (M stage). The majority of melanomas are diagnosed before lymph node or distant metastases occur (a N0, M0 stage).[5,6]

The majority of high-risk melanomas are readily detected and diagnosed by visual inspection by an experienced physician owing to their prominent pigmentation and morphologic pattern. The primary treatment of cutaneous melanomas consists of wide local excision with different safety margins, depending on the tumor thickness of the melanoma ranging up to 2 cm. Sentinel lymph node biopsy is recommended for melanomas starting from primary melanomas with tumor thickness 1.0 mm or greater.

A substantial risk of recurrence exists for patients with melanoma after definitive surgery in stage IIB/C, III, and resectable stage IV. In these tumor stages, adjuvant treatment, with agents already approved or in clinical trials, is aiming at preventing disease relapse and spread to distant organ sites, thereby improving overall survival. For stage II-IV melanoma, ICI therapy for all patients and BRAF/MEK inhibitor therapy for BRAF-mutated tumors has been established as the standard of care. For stage IV melanoma, combination immune checkpoint inhibitor (ICI) therapy with ipilimumab and nivolumab shows increased antitumor activity, but patients are at an increased risk for immune-related adverse events. Lately, anti-PD1 ICI monotherapy with nivolumab was approved for adjuvant therapy in patients after total resection.[3]

Cardiovascular Risk

The clinical benefit of novel therapeutics for cancer treatment may be significantly impaired by concomitant cardiotoxicity. Targeted and immune therapies may induce heart failure, myocarditis, arrhythmia, and hypertension. The underlying mechanisms, a timely diagnosis, and treatment are relevant to cardio-oncology, which has emerged as the optimal treatment approach to prevent and mitigate cardiotoxicity.

CARDIOVASCULAR SIDE EFFECTS OF SYSTEMIC CANCER TREATMENTS IN METASTATIC MELANOMA

Cancer Treatments With Potential Cardiovascular Side Effects

Therapy With BRAF/MEK Inhibitors

Targeted cancer therapies are promising new treatment options. In this context, mutation of rapidly accelerated fibrosarcoma kinase B (BRAF) was found in around 40% of the entire melanoma population and is therefore predestined as a possible therapy target.[3,7] The most common mutation is the substitution of valine to glutamine at codon 600 in exon 15 (V600E).[8,9] Oral small molecule kinase inhibitors are approved as first-line therapy of locally advanced and metastatic disease for BRAFv600-mutated melanoma.[3] Cardiotoxicity is described as a critical safety issue for the use of this class of drugs in the treatment of melanoma.[9] Several phase 3 clinical trials have identified cardiovascular adverse events to be important for therapy management showing an increased incidence of left ventricular ejection fraction (LVEF) reduction, arterial hypertension, and prolongation of QTc interval.[10]

BRAFv600-mutation leads to a subsequent upregulation of the canonic mitogen-activated phosphokinase (MAPK) pathway responsible for tumor growth and proliferation.[7,11] In some patients, therapy with BRAF inhibitors induces a paradoxical hyperactivation of the downstream MAPK pathway through MEK, thereby bypassing BRAF inhibition.[13,14] Therefore, a combination of BRAF and MEK inhibitors has emerged as optimal treatment of metastatic BRAF-mutated melanoma with improved survival rates compared with monotherapy. Vemurafenib/cobimetinib,[15] dabrafenib/trametinib,[16] and encorafenib/binimetinib[17] are available treatment options. Median overall survival in BRAF- plus MEK-inhibitor-treated and previously untreated patients with stage IV melanoma ranges between 22 and 33 months and 3- to 5-year overall survival has reached 40%.[3] With this huge improvement of survival, treatment and management of adverse events, especially cardiovascular toxicity, has become more important.

Cardiotoxicity through BRAF/MEK inhibition is most likely a result of direct interference with the cardiovascular MAPK signaling. Activation of ERK (extracellular signal-regulated kinases) is important for maintaining myocardial integrity.[18] ERK1/2 has multiple cardioprotective capacities, protecting cardiomyocytes from oxidative stress, hypertrophy, and apoptosis.[18] Therefore, inhibition of MAPK signaling can lead to a clinically relevant cardiomyopathy.[18–21] Heart failure is seen in 5% to 12% of all patients on BRAF/MEK inhibitors across all CTCAE (Common Terminology Criteria for Adverse Events) grades.[17,22] This holds particularly true in the presence of a "second hit," such as preexisting hypertension, coronary artery disease, or exposure to other cardiotoxic drugs.[23]

Arterial hypertension occurred in 10% to 15% of patients treated with BRAF/MEK inhibitors.[17,22] One possible pathomechanism is the interference with the renin-angiotensin system by BRAF and MEK signal inhibition.[24] Another mechanism is related to the impairment of the vascular endothelial growth factor pathway, which is mediated through the MAPK pathway contributing to a reduced bioavailability of vasodilatory nitric oxide (NO).[24] Furthermore, an upregulation of CD47 expression on cell surfaces induced by BRAF/MEK inhibitor has recently been described, which, in turn, can further reduce NO/cyclic guanosine monophosphate levels.[9,20] Taken together, these mechanisms contribute to recurrent vasoconstriction, hypertension, and an imbalance between thrombotic and antithrombotic states.[25] Additionally, these changes promote thrombosis and therefore help to explain the occurrence of pulmonary embolism and myocardial infarction in relation to BRAF/MEK inhibitor therapy.

In the clinical setting, patients on therapy should be evaluated carefully by cardio-oncology teams. To detect adverse cardiovascular events, echocardiographic assessment of baseline and follow-up ejection fraction is recommended.[26] Occurrence of a relevant, moderate-to-severe reduction in ejection fraction (from baseline) should lead to a consideration of alternative therapies for melanoma. Currently, efficacy of established heart failure therapies (i.e., angiotensin-converting enzyme inhibitors and beta-blockers) is not proven for these patients. In addition to ejection fraction, the QTc interval should be evaluated at baseline and follow up as QTc prolongation is the second most frequent adverse cardiovascular event in patients with BRAF/MEK inhibition. Consideration should be given to terminate therapy whenever QTc increases by more than 60 msec to a level above 500 msec.[26]

To optimize the outcome for each patient, it is important to balance the clinical impact of therapy disruption against the clinical impact of adverse events. Because of shown improvement of survival of patients with end-stage melanoma under BRAF/MEK therapy, treating doctors must ask themselves if a therapy disruption or termination is also ethical reasonable.

Immune Checkpoint Inhibitor Therapy

The improvement of systemic therapy in advanced melanoma was further driven by immune checkpoint inhibitors against CTLA-4 (ipilimumab) and PD-1 (pembrolizumab, nivolumab). Melanoma became the lead indication for the approval of ICI across oncology.[3]

Immune checkpoint therapy induces an enhanced activity of the adaptive immune system. Therefore, patients receiving ICI therapy are susceptible to autoimmune adverse events.[27] More than 90% of patients receiving combination ICI therapy with ipilimumab and nivolumab develop immune-related adverse events and 50% serious (grade 3 to 4) adverse events defined as causing or prolonging hospitalization, disabling, or life threatening.[28,29] The most frequent side effects are colitis and pneumonitis.[29] Cardiac adverse events, particularly autoimmune myocarditis, are increasingly reported and can be found in up to 1.14% of patients.[29,30] Despite the low reported prevalence, ICI-related myocarditis has the highest mortality rate of 40% to 50% and is the second most frequent ICI-related fatality.[29,31–33]

Myocarditis related to ICI typically occurs within the early phase of ICI treatment—17 to 65 days after initiation of therapy.[28,34,35] Dual immunotherapy (e.g., ipilimumab and nivolumab) serves as an important risk factor for the onset of myocarditis and mortality.[28,29,32] Additional risk factors include concurrent cardiotoxic tumor therapy, preexisting cardiovascular disease, and previous autoimmune disease.[28,31] Myocarditis can be associated with other autoimmune disorders, particularly myositis or a myasthenia-like disorder.[28,34] ICI-related myocarditis typically manifests with heart failure symptoms, such as dyspnea, pulmonary edema, and chest pain.[28,32] Myocardial effusion with the risk for cardiac tamponade is commonly observerd.[28,32] Arrhythmia is common in patients with ICI-related myocarditis and can be life-threatening. A reduced LVEF is found in approximately 50% of patients. An oligo- or asymptomatic presentation of ICI-related myocarditis can occur and may have been underdiagnosed in the past.[28,32,36,37] Elevated brain natriuretic peptides and troponin was found to be predictive for ICI-related myocarditis in 46% to 100%.[28,30,32] Cardiac imaging, such as magnetic resonance imaging and positron emission tomography, might serve as additional tools for the detection of ICI-related myocarditis.[28,30]

Baseline cardiac assessment and surveillance during ICI therapy, including electrocardiogram, echocardiogram, and cardiac biomarkers is recommended.[28,38] In case of suspected ICI-related myocarditis, interdisciplinary management by the treating oncologist and a cardio-oncology specialist is necessary.[30] ICI therapy should be immediately withdrawn and cardiac status including LVEF and cardiac biomarkers should be assessed as mentioned before. Intensive care treatment may be necessary for severe myocarditis.[28,38] Initially, 1 to 2 mg/kg prednisone should be administered. In the absence of an immediate response, immunosuppressive therapy with mycophenolate, infliximab, or antithymocyte globulin should be considered. Symptoms and complications of heart failure should be managed according to established guidelines and cardiac medication, such as angiotensin converting enzyme inhibitors or betablockers, can be administered.[28] In case of troponin elevation and signs for myocardial ischemia, coronary angiography should be performed according to current guidelines for non ST-segment elevation myocardial infarction.[28,38]

In case of severe myocarditis, ICI therapy should be permanently discontinued. In case of mild cardiotoxicity (e.g., subclinical left ventricular dysfunction or pericardial effusion), an ICI rechallenge might be appropriate after the symptoms resolve, particularly if a beneficial tumor response to ICI therapy was observed but requires intensive cardiovascular surveillance for recurrence.[28]

SUMMARY

Novel adjuvant cancer treatments in stage III and stage IV melanoma will likely increase overall survival rates of patients with melanoma. Using a PD1-based treatment algorithms and targeted agents in BRAFv600 mutant melanoma 5-year overall survival rates of metastatic melanoma have increased substantially from below 10% to up to 40% to 50% today in countries with access to these innovations.[39] Monitoring and management strategies must be established to detect and treat early stages of cardiotoxicity,[40] which may have an impact on the quality of life of these survivors.

REFERENCES

1. Crocetti E, Mallone S, Robsahm TE, et al. Survival of patients with skin melanoma in Europe increases further: results of the EUROCARE-5 study. *Eur J Cancer.* 2015;51(15):2179–2190.
2. Miller KD, Siegel RL, Lin CC, et al. Cancer treatment and survivorship statistics, 2016. *CA Cancer J Clin.* 2016;66(4):271–289.
3. Schadendorf D, Berking C, Gutzmer R, et al. Melanoma. *Lancet.* 2018; 392(10151):971–984.
4. Breslow A. Thickness, cross-sectional areas and depth of invasion in the prognosis of cutaneous melanoma. *Ann Surg.* 1970;172(5): 902–908.
5. Balch CM, Gershenwald JE, Soong SJ, et al. Final version of 2009 AJCC melanoma staging and classification. *J Clin Oncol.* 2009; 27(36):6199–6206.
6. Gershenwald JE, Scolyer RA, Hess KR, et al. Melanoma staging: evidence-based changes in the American Joint Committee on Cancer eighth edition cancer staging manual. *CA Cancer J Clin.* 2017; 67(6):472–492.
7. Davies H, Bignell GR, Cox C, et al. Mutations of the BRAF gene in human cancer. *Nature.* 2002;417(6892):949–954.
8. Alsina J, Gorsk DH, Germino FJ, et al. Detection of mutations in the mitogen-activated protein kinase pathway in human melanoma. *Clin Cancer Res.* 2003;9(17):6419–6425.
9. Bronte E, Bronte G, Novo G, et al. Cardiotoxicity mechanisms of the combination of BRAF-inhibitors and MEK-inhibitors. *Pharmacol Ther.* 2018;192:65–73.
10. Livingstone E, Zimmer L, Vaubel J, Schadendorf D. BRAF, MEK and KIT inhibitors for melanoma: adverse events and their management. *Chin Clin Oncol.* 2014;3(3):29.
11. Bronte E, Bronte G, Novo G, et al. What links BRAF to the heart function? New insights from the cardiotoxicity of BRAF inhibitors in cancer treatment. *Oncotarget.* 2015;6(34):35589–35601.
12. Solit DB, Rosen N. Resistance to BRAF inhibition in melanomas. *N Engl J Med.* 2011;364(8):772–774.
13. Wagle N, Van Allen EM, Treacy DJ, et al. MAP kinase pathway alterations in BRAF-mutant melanoma patients with acquired resistance to combined RAF/MEK inhibition. *Cancer Discov.* 2014;4(1):61–68.
14. Larkin J, Ascierto PA, Dréno B, et al. Combined vemurafenib and cobimetinib in BRAF-mutated melanoma. *N Engl J Med.* 2014;371(20): 1867–1876.
15. Long GV, Stroyakovskiy D, Gogas H, et al. Dabrafenib and trametinib versus dabrafenib and placebo for Val600 BRAF-mutant melanoma: a multicentre, double-blind, phase 3 randomised controlled trial. *Lancet.* 2015;386(9992):444–451.
16. Dummer R, Ascierto PA, Gogas HJ, et al. Encorafenib plus binimetinib versus vemurafenib or encorafenib in patients with BRAF-mutant melanoma (COLUMBUS): a multicentre, open-label, randomised phase 3 trial. *Lancet Oncol.* 2018;19(5):603–615.
17. Banks M, Crowell K, Proctor A, Jensen BC. Cardiovascular effects of the MEK inhibitor, trametinib: a case report, literature review, and consideration of mechanism. *Cardiovasc Toxicol.* 2017;17(4):487–493.
18. Kubin T, Cetinkaya A, Schönburg M, et al. The MEK1 inhibitors UO126 and PD98059 block PDGF-AB induced phosphorylation of threonine 292 in porcine smooth muscle cells. *Cytokine.* 2017;95:51–54.
19. Liu F, Jiang CC, Yan XG, et al. BRAF/MEK inhibitors promote CD47 expression that is reversible by ERK inhibition in melanoma. *Oncotarget.* 2017;8(41):69477–69492.
20. Rose BA, Force T, Wang Y. Mitogen-activated protein kinase signaling in the heart: angels versus demons in a heart-breaking tale. *Physiol Rev.* 2010;90(4):1507–1546.
21. Ascierto PA, McArthur GA, Dréno B, et al. Cobimetinib combined with vemurafenib in advanced BRAF(V600)-mutant melanoma (coBRIM): updated efficacy results from a randomised, double-blind, phase 3 trial. *Lancet Oncol.* 2016;17(9):1248–1260.
22. Knispel S, Zimmer L, Kanaki T, et al. The safety and efficacy of dabrafenib and trametinib for the treatment of melanoma. *Expert Opin Drug Saf.* 2018;17(1):73–87.
23. Zhu H, Tan L, Li Y, et al. Increased apoptosis in the paraventricular nucleus mediated by AT1R/Ras/ERK1/2 signaling results in sympathetic hyperactivity and renovascular hypertension in rats after kidney injury. *Front Physiol.* 2017;8:41.
24. Bronte G, Bronte E, Novo G, et al. Conquests and perspectives of cardio-oncology in the field of tumor angiogenesis-targeting tyrosine kinase inhibitor-based therapy. *Expert Opin Drug Saf.* 2015; 14(2):253–267.
25. Totzeck M, Hendgen-Cotta UB, Luedike P, et al. Nitrite regulates hypoxic vasodilation via myoglobin-dependent nitric oxide generation. *Circulation.* 2012;126(3):325–334.
26. Totzeck M, Schuler M, Stuschke M, Heusch G, Rassaf T. Cardio-oncology—strategies for management of cancer-therapy related cardiovascular disease. *Int J Cardiol.* 2019;280:163–175.
27. Ascierto PA, Del Vecchio M, Robert C, et al. Ipilimumab 10 mg/kg versus ipilimumab 3 mg/kg in patients with unresectable or metastatic melanoma: a randomised, double-blind, multicentre, phase 3 trial. *Lancet Oncol.* 2017;18(5):611–622.
28. Lyon AR, Yousaf N, Battisti NML, Moslehi J, Larkin J. Immune checkpoint inhibitors and cardiovascular toxicity. *Lancet Oncol.* 2018; 19(9):e447–e458.
29. Wang DY, Salem JE, Cohen JV, et al. Fatal toxic effects associated with immune checkpoint inhibitors: a systematic review and meta-analysis. *JAMA Oncol.* 2018;4(12):1721–1728.

30. Michel L, Rassaf T. Cardio-oncology: need for novel structures. *Eur J Med Res*. 2019;24(1):1.
31. Ganatra S, Neilan TG. Immune checkpoint inhibitor-associated myocarditis. *Oncologist*. 2018;23(8):879–886.
32. Mahmood SS, Fradley MG, Cohen JV, et al. Myocarditis in patients treated with immune checkpoint inhibitors. *J Am Coll Cardiol*. 2018;71(16):1755–1764.
33. Moslehi JJ, Salem JE, Sosman JA, Lebrun-Vignes B, Johnson DB. Increased reporting of fatal immune checkpoint inhibitor-associated myocarditis. *Lancet*. 2018;391(10124):933.
34. Anquetil C, Salem JE, Lebrun-Vignes B, et al. Immune checkpoint inhibitor-associated myositis. *Circulation*. 2018;138(7):743–745.
35. Michel L, Rassaf T, Totzeck M. Biomarkers for the detection of apparent and subclinical cancer therapy-related cardiotoxicity. *J Thorac Dis*. 2018;10:S4282–S4295.
36. Norwood TG, Westbrook BC, Johnson DB, et al. Smoldering myocarditis following immune checkpoint blockade. *J Immunother Cancer*. 2017;5(1):91.
37. Thibault C, Vano Y, Soulat G, Mirabel M. Immune checkpoint inhibitors myocarditis: not all cases are clinically patent. *Eur Heart J*. 2018;39(38):3553.
38. Brahmer JR, Lacchetti C, Thompson JA. Management of immune-related adverse events in patients treated with immune checkpoint inhibitor therapy: American Society of Clinical Oncology Clinical Practice Guideline Summary. *J Oncol Pract*. 2018;14(4): 247–249.
39. Kandolf Sekulovic L, Peris K, Hauschild A, et al. More than 5000 patients with metastatic melanoma in Europe per year do not have access to recommended first-line innovative treatments. *Eur J Cancer*. 2017;75:313–322.
40. Michel L, Helfrich I, Hendgen-Cotta UB, et al. Targeting early stages of cardiotoxicity from anti-PD1 immune checkpoint inhibitor therapy. *Eur Heart J*. 2021. doi: 10.1093/eurheartj/ehab430. [Online ahead of print.]

45 Head and Neck Cancers

LACHELLE D. WEEKS AND ROBERT I. HADDAD

T Category[a]	Criteria
T0	No primary tumor identified
T1	Tumor size ≤ 2 cm in greatest dimension
T2	Tumor size > 2 cm but ≤ 4 cm in greatest dimension
T3	Tumor size > 4 cm in greatest dimension or extension to lingual surface of epiglottis
T4	Moderately advanced tumor invading larynx, extrinsic tongue muscles, medial pterygoid, hard palate, or mandible or beyond
Clinical N category	**Criteria**
Nx	Regional nodes cannot be assessed
N0	No regional nodal metastasis
N1	Metastasis to one or more ipsilateral nodes, ≤ 6 cm
N2	Metastasis to contralateral or bilateral lymph nodes, ≤ 6 cm
N3	Metastasis in any cervical lymph node > 6 cm
Pathologic N category	**Criteria**
Nx	Regional nodes cannot be assessed
pN0	No regional nodal metastasis identified
pN1	Metastasis to 4 or fewer lymph nodes
pN2	Metastasis to 5 or more lymph nodes
M category	**Criteria**
M0	Absence of distant metastasis
M1	Presence of distant metastasis

T1 T2 T3 T4

N1 N2a N2b N2c N3

T category	N category	M category	Stage group
T0, T1, or T2	N0 or N1	M0	I
T0, T1, or T2	N2	M0	II
T3	N0, N1, or N2	M0	II
T0, T1, T2 T3, or T4	N3	M0	III
T4	N0, N1, N2, or N3	M0	III
Any T	Any N	M1	IV

Stages	Stage I	Stage II	Stage III	Stage IV	Metastatic
Treatment	Surgery and/or radiation therapy (Intensity modulated radiation therapy [IMRT], if upstaging or high-risk features, adjuvant treatment		Non-metastatic (Surgery, single modality radiation therapy), usual standard chemo-radiation therapy with cisplatin or cetuximab, or TPF (docetaxel, cisplatin, and 5-FU)		Metastatic, recurrent or unresectable: platinum-based chemotherapy, preferably in combination with 5-FU and cetuximab, or gemcitabine; Second line if progression, immune checkpoint inhibitors (ICI): nivolumab or pembrolizumab
Prognosis	90%	70%	60%	40%	
Potential CV toxicities	Radiation-induced vascular disease, autonomic dysfunction		**Cisplatin:** hypertension, arterial and venous thrombosis, arrhythmias **Gemcitabine:** edema, vascular events/ischemia **Doxetaxel:** hypotension, arrhythmias **5-FU:** vasospasm, chest pain, arrhythmia, cardiac failure **Cetuximab:** thrombotic events (US black box warning for cardiopulmonary arrest) **Immune checkpoint inhibitors:** myocarditis, cardiomyopathy, pericarditis, arteritis, arrhythmias		

CHAPTER OUTLINE

KEY POINTS ABOUT HEAD AND NECK CANCER

- Worldwide, head and neck cancer accounts for 380,000 deaths annually.
- Major risk factors for head and neck cancers include smoking, heavy alcohol use, and infection with human papilloma virus (HPV).
- With treatment, 5-year survival rates are 70% to 90% for early stage disease (stages I and II) and 40% to 60% for advanced disease (stages III and IV).
- Early stage head and neck cancer is managed with local treatment that is, either surgery, radiation, or both. Systemic treatment with chemotherapy or immunotherapy is used for advanced, recurrent, or metastatic disease.
- Treatment-related cardiovascular toxicities include carotid artery stenosis, electrolyte loss, coronary vasospasm, pericardial effusion, and myocarditis.

INCIDENCE

Head and neck cancers are a heterogenous group of malignancies arising in the oral cavity, oropharynx, nasopharynx, larynx, nasal cavity, paranasal sinuses, and salivary glands. Worldwide, head and neck cancer accounts for approximately 380,000 deaths annually. In the United States, head and neck cancers account for 3% of all malignancies; an estimated 63,000 individuals develop head and neck cancer and 13,000 die from it each year.[1] Head and neck cancers of the oral cavity, oropharynx, and larynx are more common in North America and Europe, whereas nasopharyngeal cancer is more common in the Mediterranean and Far East.

RISK FACTORS

Head and neck cancers arise more often in men than in women and in patients of lower socioeconomic status.[2] Smoking is one of the most important risk factors, and risk of head and neck cancer increases with smoking duration and declines with smoking cessation.[3] Alcohol is another independent risk factor and the combination of alcohol use and smoking further increases the risk of head and neck cancer.[4] Viral infections have also been associated with increased risk of head and neck cancer. Epstein-Barr virus has been implicated as the primary etiologic agent in the pathogenesis of nasopharyngeal carcinoma, particularly in South East Asia and other regions where nasopharyngeal cancer is endemic.[5] Finally, human papilloma virus (HPV), the most commonly diagnosed sexually transmitted infection in the United States has been etiologically linked with oropharyngeal squamous cell carcinomas. HPV 16 is the viral subtype detected in most patients. Over 50% of all oropharyngeal cancers are HPV 16 positive. The proportion of HPV associated head and neck cancer is rising in the United States.[6] HPV positive head and neck cancers have a better prognosis and are as shown in Table 45.1 are clinically distinct from HPV negative cancers.[7]

DIAGNOSIS AND STAGING

The workup of head and neck cancers involves a detailed head and neck physical examination with direct visualization of the primary tumor by fiberoptic flexible laryngopharyngoscopy. An examination under anesthesia may be required to assess the deeper structures or for patients who cannot tolerate an awake examination in the outpatient setting. Subsequently, fine-needle aspiration, core

TABLE 45.1 **Characteristics of HPV Positive Versus HPV Negative Head and Neck Cancers**

	HPV POSITIVE	HPV NEGATIVE
Demographic features	Younger age Linked to sexual behavior Nonsmokers Nondrinkers Higher socioeconomic status	Older age Not linked to sexual behavior Smokers· Drinkers Lower socioeconomic status
Primary site	Oropharynx	Any
Presentation	Painless neck mass	Sore throat Dysphagia Otalgia

HPV, Human papilloma virus.

biopsy, or excisional biopsy of a neck node or primary tumor should be performed to obtain a pathologic diagnosis. A contrast-enhanced computed tomography (CT) scan of the head and neck or magnetic resonance image of the head and neck should be obtained to assess the extent of local and regional disease. A CT-positron emission tomography fusion is useful for identifying involved lymph nodes and distant metastases.

The data obtained from these clinical assessments derive the clinical stage of the cancer. The TNM (tumor, node, metastasis) staging system is used and the new American Joint Committee on Cancer 8 classification system incorporates HPV status into staging to better reflect the prognosis of these two groups.[8]

TREATMENT OVERVIEW

For many head and neck sites, primary surgery and definitive radiation offer similar rates of local control and cure for localized, early stage disease (stage I–II). Thus, the initial choice of surgery or radiation depends on the surgical accessibility of the tumor, the anticipated functional outcome with resection, and the morbidity associated with surgery versus radiation. After surgical resection of the primary tumor there may be an indication for postoperative radiation or concurrent chemotherapy and radiation (chemoRT) if high-risk pathologic features, such as positive margins, perineural invasion, lymphovascular invasion, and extra nodal extension, are identified in the resected specimen. The finding of multiple positive lymph nodes on elective lymph node dissection at the time of surgery is also an indication for postoperative radiation therapy. For patients receiving primary chemotherapy or chemoRT, neck dissection following systemic treatment is often indicated for lymph node positive disease based on response to chemotherapy.

Intensity modulated radiation therapy (IMRT) is the major modality of radiation used in the treatment of cancers of the head and neck. IMRT allows for modulation of the intensity of radiation such that a higher radiation dose can be delivered to a target (i.e., tumor or involved lymph node region) with a marked reduction in the amount of radiation delivered to surrounding uninvolved tissues. The radiation dose used depends on the size and location of the primary tumor and the neck lymph nodes. For definitive radiation, primary tumors and gross lymphadenopathy are managed with treatment doses greater than or equal to 70 Gy in 2 Gy fractions. Low-risk neck nodal regions are treated with doses at or exceeding 50 Gy. In the postoperative setting doses of radiation from 60 to 66 Gy are required for treatment of microscopic disease. A lower dose of postoperative radiation (e.g., 54 Gy) is currently under investigation for HPV positive disease with equivalent survival statistics.[9]

More advanced stage disease has higher rates of local recurrence and distant metastases and requires combined modality approaches to increase the chance of long-term disease control and cure. Optimal sequencing of therapeutic interventions requires multidisciplinary input and is dictated by the site of the primary tumor, the disease extent, patient comorbid conditions, and patient preferences based on functional preservation and cosmetic outcome. In nonmetastatic disease, cisplatin, given at 100 mg/m^2 every 3 weeks in combination with radiation is the current standard of care chemotherapeutic agent for chemoRT for patients (age < 70 and performance status 0-1).[9,10] In less-fit patients (those with cardiovascular or renal comorbidity, age > 70, or performance status > 1), 40 mg/m^2 weekly is used. This weekly regimen has lower renal toxicity and less potential for severe nausea and vomiting.[10,11] As an alternative, cetuximab, an inhibitor of the epidermal growth factor receptor, can be used for stage III or IV nonmetastatic head and neck cancer. Patients receive this medication as an initial loading dose of 400 mg/m^2 followed by weekly 250 mg/m^2 in combination with radiation.[12] Another option is the taxotere platinol 5-fluorouracil (TPF) regimen, which involves sequential combined modality therapy with docetaxel (75 mg/m^2), cisplatin (100 mg/m^2), and 5-fluorouracil (5-FU, 1000 mg/m^2) given every 3 weeks for 3 cycles followed by carboplatin (area under the curve [AUC] of 1.5) weekly with daily radiation.[13]

For metastatic disease, recurrent disease, or nonresectable cancers, first-line systemic therapy involves the use of a platinum-based chemotherapy regimen. The combination of platinum agent (cisplatin or carboplatin), 5-FU and cetuximab has been shown to have improved overall survival as compared with platinum and 5-FU alone.[14] An alternative combination of carboplatin and gemcitabine is favored specifically for nasopharyngeal cancers.[15,16] More recently, the PD-1 inhibitors, nivolumab and pembrolizumab, were approved for use in patients with recurrent head and neck cancer whose disease has progressed after treatment with platinum-containing therapy.[17–19]

CARDIOVASCULAR RISK

Patients with head and neck cancer have an increased noncancer mortality with cardiovascular disease comprising a significant portion of noncancer mortality in this population.[20–22] Importantly, patients with head and neck cancer have a high baseline risk for cardiovascular disease based on common risk factors for malignancy and cardiovascular disease in this population, such as smoking and alcohol use.[22] However, cardiovascular disease risk is increased even in patients without a significant smoking history[23] owing to potential cardiovascular effects of local (e.g., radiation) or systemic head and neck cancer therapies. The cardiovascular risks of head and neck cancer therapies are summarized in Table 45.2.

TABLE 45.2 Cardiovascular Risks of Head and Neck Cancer Therapy

LOCAL CANCER THERAPY	POTENTIAL CARDIOVASCULAR SIDE EFFECTS
Surgery	Perioperative complications related to anesthesia and preexisting cardiac comorbidity
Radiation therapy	Accelerated atherosclerosis leading to carotid artery stenosis, increased risk of TIA/stroke Carotid sinus damage leading to dysautonomia (blood pressure lability, orthostatic hypotension, tachyarrhythmias, bradyarrhythmias) Hypothalamic-pituitary axis damage leading to hormone dysregulation leading to metabolic syndrome
Systemic Cancer Therapy	**Potential Cardiovascular Side Effects**
Cisplatin	Arterial and venous thromboembolic events Volume overload from renal impairment Electrolyte disturbance and cation wasting
Docetaxel	Chest pain Increased capillary permeability Volume overload (pleural and pericardial infusion)
5-Fluorouracil	Chest pain Arrhythmia Coronary vasospasm
Cetuximab	Cardiopulmonary arrest
Gemcitabine	Thrombotic microangiopathy
Immunotherapy Nivolumab and Pembrolizumab	Myocarditis

TIA, Transient ischemic attack.

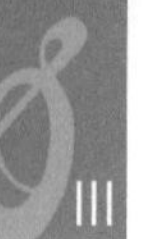

CARDIOVASCULAR SIDE EFFECTS OF HEAD AND NECK CANCER THERAPY

Cardiovascular Side Effects of Local Therapy

Surgery

In the hands of a skilled surgeon, the major risks of surgical management of head and neck surgery arise from general anesthesia. The individual risk is related to patient characteristics and is not specific to patients with head and neck cancer. Patients with underlying cardiovascular disease, including peripheral artery disease or prior stroke, have an increased risk of perioperative cardiac complications compared with patients without atherosclerosis. Patients should undergo a presurgical cardiovascular risk assessment prior to surgery to estimate risk of perioperative cardiovascular events[7] (see Chapter 6).

Radiation

Radiation of the head and neck is associated with cardiovascular toxicity arising from radiation-induced accelerated atherosclerosis, dysautonomia, and hormone dysregulation from damage to the thyroid gland and the hypothalamic-pituitary axis.[24] With the advancement of IMRT and proton beam therapy, skilled radiation oncologists can target the tumor and spare the surrounding tissues thereby reducing the outlined toxicities. Radiation-induced accelerated atherosclerosis leads to a significantly increased incidence of radiation-induced carotid artery stenosis in patients with head and neck cancer.[25] In one prospective study carotid artery stenosis greater than 70% was observed in 11.7% of patients who had undergone cervical irradiation.[26] The increased risk of carotid artery stenosis confers an increased risk of stroke and transient ischemic attack (TIA) in this population.[27–31] Studies have suggested the risk of stroke and TIA are at least doubled in the setting of neck radiation therapy,[32] with an 11-year mean interval time of development of stroke.[31] Currently, no specific guidelines govern surveillance and management of asymptomatic carotid artery disease, though consensus recommendations have been published (see Chapter 26, Table 26.2). Patients who have received cervical radiation require lifelong follow up to control aggressively cardiovascular risk factors, such as hypertension, diabetes, and hyperlipidemia, and should be regularly assessed for carotid bruits and neurologic symptoms owing to an increased risk of stroke and TIA.[24] When suspected or as a surveillance strategy for carotid artery disease, carotid ultrasound with Doppler is the modality of choice, Carotid stenosis greater than 70% should be referred for specialist consultation whether revascularization via carotid angioplasty and stenting or carotid endarterectomy is recommended. Carotid artery stenosis arising in patients who have previously been irradiated has an increased risk of progression and has a significantly higher risk of restenosis after stenting compared with the general population (88% vs. 22% chance of restenosis after 2 years).[33] Additionally, carotid endarterectomy can be technically difficult to perform owing to bilateral disease and scarring after radiation.[24]

Cervical radiation also confers a risk of dysautonomia owing to damage to the carotid sinus and baroreceptor reflex resulting in blood pressure lability, orthostatic symptoms, sinus tachycardia and sinus dysfunction with bradyarrythmias.[34] Lastly, damage to the thyroid gland can lead to hypothyroidism with its well-known cardiovascular consequences (i.e., reduced cardiac output and increased peripheral vascular resistance). Furthermore, damage to the hypothalamic-pituitary axis with radiation of head and neck malignancies can lead to central hormone dysregulation and the metabolic syndrome, which further emphasizes the importance of therapy for hyperlipidemia, hypertension, and hyperglycemia in this population to reduce the risk of adverse cardiovascular and cerebrovascular outcomes.[24,35]

Systemic Head and Neck Cancer Treatments With Potential Cardiovascular Side Effects

Platinum-Based Agents

Platinum drugs can cause endothelial dysfunction and injury as well as arterial and venous thromboembolic events (see Chapters 8 and 17). Furthermore, cisplatin and, to a lesser degree, carboplatin can cause renal impairment and cation wasting[36] (see Chapters 11 and 20). Loss of magnesium and calcium in the urine, a common result of platinum-related toxicity, can cause symptomatic hypomagnesemia and hypocalcemia. Electrolyte loss is exacerbated in the patient with uncontrolled vomiting, although this is generally well managed with current antiemetic regimens. Careful electrolyte monitoring is mandatory during cisplatin therapy and appropriate hydration and repletion should be undertaken to avoid serious toxicities. Electrocardiographic monitoring may be required for certain patients based on their individual risk and symptoms. Special attention should be given for patients with baseline renal dysfunction and patients on diuretics and other nephrotoxic medications. Cardiology input is necessary to adjust medication regimens (e.g., furosemide, angiotensin-converting enzyme inhibitors) based on individual risk. Patients who receive high-dose cisplatin require significant intravenous fluid support, and especially those with a history of congestive heart failure, should be monitored for the development of fluid overload and pulmonary edema during therapy.

Docetaxel

Treatment with docetaxel can cause fluid retention manifesting as peripheral edema of the extremities, pericardial effusions, and pleural effusions. It is believed that this phenomenon is caused by increased capillary permeability and insufficient lymphatic drainage and is unrelated to hypoalbuminemia or docetaxel-induced cardiac, renal, or hepatic dysfunction.[37] The severity of fluid retention is dose dependent and risk accumulates with each administration. However, this fluid retention syndrome is prevented with pretreatment using systemic corticosteroids, which also are utilized to prevent docetaxel hypersensitivity. Steroid use decreases the risk of fluid retention from 20% to 6%[38] Acute ischemic presentations (e.g., chest pain) are not as common with docetaxel as they are with paclitaxel.

5-Fluorouracil

The cardiotoxicity of 5-FU manifests as chest pain and arrhythmia. This typically occurs around the time of infusion and can be associated with elevated cardiac enzymes and electrocardiographic changes.[39,40] Cardiogenic shock and sudden death have been reported, but they are uncommon. The suspected etiology of this is coronary vasospasm. Patients who have a history of coronary artery disease, prior myocardial infarction, or prior chest irradiation are at higher risk for this side effect. Symptoms are usually reversed with drug discontinuation and vasodilator therapy but may recur with drug reexposure even on vasodilator therapy.

Cetuximab

Cardiotoxicity with cetuximab is rare but can be severe. Cardiopulmonary arrest has been reported in 2% of patients treated with cetuximab and concurrent radiation in head and neck cancer.[41] The mechanism of cardiopulmonary arrest is thought to be caused by electrolyte abnormalities, but is not well defined.[12]

Gemcitabine

The toxicity profile of gemcitabine is primarily hematologic, involving myelosuppression and consequent cytopenias. Thrombotic microangiopathy resulting in renal failure is a rare late complication of gemcitabine therapy, occurring with an estimated overall incidence of 0.015%.[42] Resolution of thrombotic microangiopathy is observed with gemcitabine discontinuation in most patients. Peripheral edema can be noted during treatment, but is rarely owing to cardiotoxicity-induced heart failure.

Immunotherapy: Nivolumab and Pembrolizumab

Cardiotoxicity of immunotherapy manifesting as severe myocarditis has been reported with both pembrolizumab[47] and nivolumab.[48] This is thought to be due to the induction of autoreactive T cells targeting cardiac myocytes in patients receiving these agents. The presentation of immune checkpoint inhibitor myocarditis is that of a clinical syndrome with chest pain; shortness of breath; presyncope and syncope; bradycardia; heart block; ventricular ectopy; and arrhythmias. The incidence of severe myocarditis is increased when pembrolizumab or nivolumab is used in combination with the checkpoint inhibitor ipilimumab but still remains at $<1\%$. Prompt initiation of steroids is recommended upon suspicion of immune checkpoint inhibitor myocarditis while confirming the diagnosis by endomyocardial biopsy or cardiac MRI. However, the incidence rate of severe myocarditis when ipilimumab combinations are used is still low, approximately 0.3%.[43,48]

REFERENCES

1. Seigel RL, Miller KD, Jemal A. Cancer statistics. 2017. *CA Cancer J Clin.* 2017;67(1):7.
2. Wyss A, Hashibe M, Chuang SC, et al. Cigarette, cigar and pipe smoking and the risk of head and neck cancers: pooled analysis in the International Head and Neck Cancer Epidemiology Consortium. *Am J Epidemiol.* 2013;178(5):679.
3. Lewin F, Norell SE, Johansson H, et al. Smoking tobacco, oral snuff and alcohol in the etiology of squamous cell carcinoma of the head and neck: a population-based case referent study in Sweden. *Cancer.* 1998;82(7):1367.
4. Hashibe M, Brennan P, Benhamou S, et al, Alcohol drinking in never users of tobacco, cigarette smoking in never drinkers, and the risk of head and neck cancer: pooled analysis in the International Head and Neck Cancer Epidemiology Consortium. *J Natl Cancer Inst.* 2007;99(10):777.

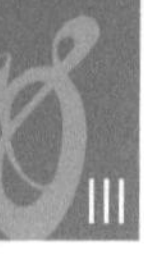

5. Nakanishi Y, Wakisaka N, Kondo S, et al. Progression of understanding for the role of Epstein-Barr virus and management of nasopharyngeal carcinoma. *Cancer Metastasis Rev.* 2017;36(3):435.
6. Chaturvedi AK, Engels EA, Anderson WF, Gillison ML. Incidence trends for human papillomavirus-related and -unrelated oral squamous cell carcinomas in the United States. *J Clin Oncol.* 2008;26(4):612.
7. Ang KK, Harris J, Wheeler R, et al. Human papillomavirus and survival of patients with oropharyngeal cancer. *N Engl J Med.* 2010;363:24.
8. Amin M, Edge S, Greene F, et al. *AJCC Cancer Staging Manual.* ed 8. New York: Springer; 2017.
9. Marur S, Li S, Cmelak AJ, et al. E1308: phase II trial of induction chemotherapy followed by reduced-dose radiation and weekly cetuximab in patients with HPV-associated resectable squamous cell carcinoma of the oropharynx—ECOG-ACRIN Cancer Research Group. *J Clin Oncol.* 2016;35(5):490.
10. Noronha V, Joshi A, Patil VM, et al. Once-a-week versus once-every-3-weeks cisplatin chemoradiation for locally advanced head and neck cancer: a phase III randomized noninferiority trial. *J Clin Oncol.* 2018;36(11):1064.
11. Beckmann GK, Hoppe F, Pfreunder L, et al. Hyperfractionated accelerated radiotherapy in combination with weekly cisplatin for locally advanced head and neck cancer. *Head Neck.* 2005;27:36–43.
12. Bonner JA, Harari PM, Giralt J, et al. Radiotherapy plus cetuximab for squamous-cell carcinoma of the head and neck. *N Engl J Med.* 2006;354:567–578.
13. Forastiere AA, Goepfert H, Maor M, et al. Concurrent chemotherapy and radiotherapy for organ preservation in advanced laryngeal cancer. *N Engl J Med.* 2003;349(22):2091.
14. Posner MR, Hershock DM, Blajman CR, et al. Cisplatin and fluorouracil alone or with docetaxel in head and neck cancer. *N Engl J Med.* 2007;357:1705–1715.
15. Vermorken JB, Mesia R, Rivera F, Remenar E. Platinum based chemotherapy plus cetuximab in head and neck cancer. *N Engl J Med.* 2008;359(11):1116.
16. Jin Y, Cai XY, Shi YX, et al. Comparison of five cisplatin-based regimens frequently used as the first line protocols in metastatic nasopharyngeal carcinoma. *J Cancer Res Clin Oncol.* 2012;138(10):1717.
17. Zhang L, Huang T, Hong S, et al. Gemcitabine plus cisplatin versus fluorouracil plus cisplatin in recurrent or metastatic nasopharyngeal carcinoma: a multicenter randomized, open-label, phase 3 trial. *Lancet.* 2016;388:1883.
18. Harrington KJ, Ferris RL, Blumenschein G, et al. Nivolumab versus standard, single-agent therapy of investigator's choice in recurrent or metastatic squamous cell carcinoma of the head and neck (Checkmate 141): health-related quality of life results from a randomized, phase 3 trial. *Lancet Oncol.* 2017;18(8):1104.
19. Ferris RL, Blumenschein G, Fayette J, et al. Nivolumab for recurrent squamous cell carcinoma of the head and neck. *N Engl J Med.* 2016;375(19):1856.
20. van der Schroeff, van de Schans SA, Piccirillo JF, et al. Conditional relative survival in head and neck squamous cell carcinoma: permanent excess mortality risk for long-term survivors. *Head Neck.* 2010;32(12):1613.
21. Baxi SS, Pinheiro LC, Patil SM, et al. Causes of death in long term survivors of head and neck cancer. *Cancer.* 2014;120(10):1507.
22. Rose BS, Jeong JH, Nath SK, et al. Population based study of competing mortality in head and neck cancer. *J Clin Oncol.* 2011;29(26):3503.
23. Okoye C, Bucher J, Tatsuoka C, et al. Cardiovascular risk and prevention in head and neck patients treated with radiotherapy. *Head Neck.* 2017;39(3):527.
24. Mahmood S, Nohria A. Cardiovascular complications of cranial and neck radiation. *Curr Treat Options Cardiovasc Med.* 2016; 18:45.
25. Elerding SC, Fernandez RN, Grotta JC et al. Carotid artery disease following external cervical irradiation. *Ann Surg.* 1984;194:609.
26. Cheng SW, Wu LL, Ting AC et al. Irradiation-induced extracranial carotid stenosis in patients with head and neck malignancies. *Am J Surg.* 1999;178:323.
27. Fleisher LA, Fleischmann KE, Auerbach AD, et al. 2014 ACC/AHA guideline on perioperative cardiovascular evaluation and management of patients undergoing noncardiac surgery: executive summary: a report of the American College of Cardiology/American Heart Association Task Force on practice guidelines. *Circulation.* 2014;13(24):2215.
28. Dorth JA, Broadwater G, Brizel DM. Incidence and risk factors of significant carotid artery stenosis in asymptomatic survivors of head and neck cancer after radiotherapy. *Head Neck.* 2014;36(2):215.
29. Chang YJ, Chang TC, Lee TH, Ryu SJ. Predictors of carotid artery stenosis after radiotherapy for head and neck cancers. *J Vasc Surg.* 2009;550(2):280.
30. Smith, GL, Smith BD, Buchholz TA, et al. Cerebrovascular disease risk in older head and neck patients with cancer after radiotherapy. *J Clin Oncol.* 2008;26(31):5119.
31. Dorresteijn LD, Kappelle AC, Boogerd W et al. Increased risk of ischemic stroke after radiotherapy on the neck in patients younger than 60 years. *J Clin Oncol.* 2002;20(1):282.
32. Plummer C, Henderson RD, O'Sullivan JD, et al. Ischemic stroke and transient ischemic attack after head and neck radiotherapy: a review. *Stroke.* 2011;42:2410-2418.
33. Protack CD, Bakken AM, Saad WE, et al. Radiation arteritis a contraindication to carotid stenting? *J Vasc Surg.* 2007;45(1):110.
34. Timmers HJ, Karemaker JM, Lenders JW, et al. Baroreflex failure following radiation therapy for nasopharyngeal carcinoma. *Clin Auton Res.* 1999;9:317–324.
35. Appleman-Dijkstra NM, Malgo F, Neelis KJ. Pituitary dysfunction in adult patients after cranial irradiation for head and nasopharyngeal tumors. *Radiother Oncol.* 2014;113:102.
36. Schilsky RL, Anderson T. Hypomagnesemia and renal magnesium wasting in patients receiving cisplatin. *Ann Intern Med.* 1979;90(6): 929.
37. Semb KA, Aamdal S, Oian P. Capillary protein leak syndrome appears to explain fluid retention in patients with cancer who receive docetaxel treatment. *J Clin Oncol.* 1998;16:3426.
38. Piccart MJ, Klijin J, Paridaens R, et al. Corticosteroids significantly delay the onset of docetaxel-induced fluid retention: final results of a randomized study of the EORTC investigational drug branch for breast cancer. *J Clin Oncol.* 1997;15(9):3149.
39. Tsavaris N, Kosmas C, Vadiaka M, et al. Cardiotoxicity following different doses and schedules of 5-fluorouracil administration for malignancy—a survey of 427 patients. *Med Sci Monit.* 2002; 8:151.
40. Meyer CC, Calis KA, Burke LB, et al. Symptomatic cardiotoxicity associated with 5-fluorouracil. *Pharmacotherapy.* 1997;17:729.
41. Yeh ET. Cardiotoxicity induced by chemotherapy and antibody therapy. *Annu Rev Med.* 2006;57:485–498.
42. Humphreys BD, Sharman JP, Hendersn JM, et al. Gemcitabine-associated thrombotic microangiopathy. *Cancer.* 2004;100:2664.
43. Johnson DB, Balko JM, Compton ML, et al. Fulminant myocarditis with combination immune checkpoint blockage. *N Engl J Med.* 2016;375:1749.

46 Thyroid Cancer

JEENA VARGHESE AND MOHAMED S. ALI

Papillary/follicular (and anaplastic) thyroid cancer

Stages	**Stage I**	**Stage II**	**Stage III**	**Stage IV**
Age younger than 55 years	Any size tumor, confined to thyroid or spread to local LNs	Any size tumor and nodal status, positive metastatic state		
Age older than 55 years	Tumor ≤4 cm in greatest dimension limited to the thyroid	Tumor >4 cm limited to the thyroid, or gross extrathyroidal extension invading only strap muscles or metastasis to regional LNs	Includes gross extrathyroidal extension beyond the strap muscles	Any size tumor and nodal status, positive metastatic state
Treatment	Surgery Radioactive iodine TSH suppression	Surgery Radioactive iodine, TSH suppression Tyrosine kinase inhibitors (Lenvatinib, Sorafenib)		
Prognosis	5-year survival 99%	5-year survival 99%	5-year survival 70%–90%	5-year survival near 50%
Potential CV toxicities	Atrial fibrillation	Atrial fibrillation **Lenvatinib:** hypertension, cardiomyopathy/heart failure, prolonged QT interval, arterial and venous thromboembolism, peripheral edema **Sorafenib:** hypertension, cardiomyopathy/heart failure, ischemic heart disease **Anaplastic with BRAF V600E mutation:** Trametinib ± Dabrafenib: hypertension, cardiomyopathy/heart failure		

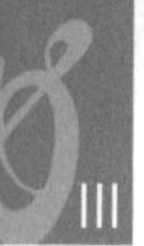

Medullary thyroid cancer

	Stage I	Stage II	Stage III	Stage IV
Stages	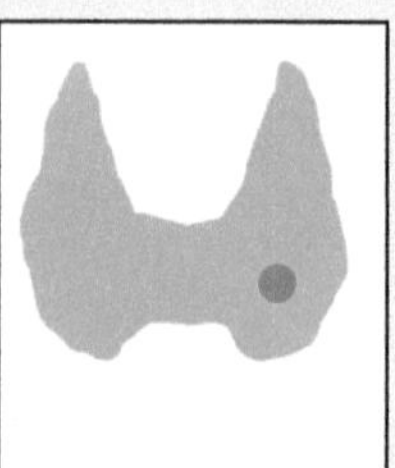	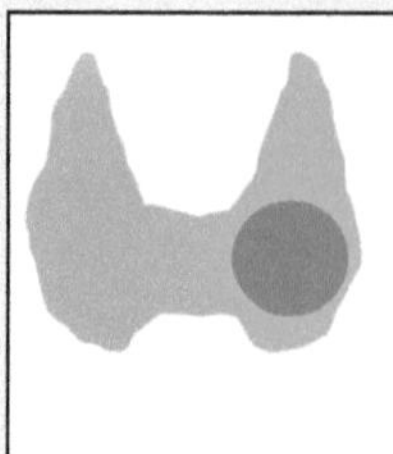	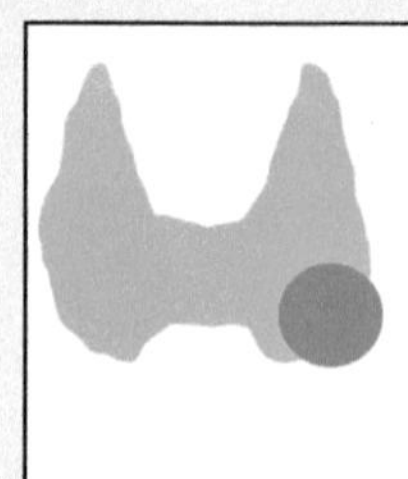	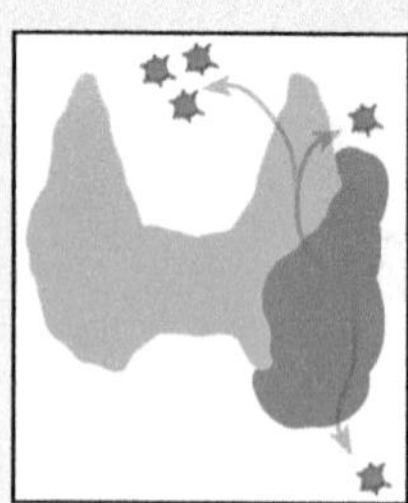
	Tumor ≤2 cm in greatest dimension limited to the thyroid	Tumors >2 cm confined to the thyroid or tumors of any size without lymph node metastasis that demonstrate gross extrathyroidal extension invading only the strap muscles (sternohyoid, sternothyroid, thyrohyoid, or omohyoid muscles)	Tumors of any size, metastatic lymph node involvement in the central neck (levels VI or VII; pretracheal, paratracheal, or prelaryngeal/Delphian, or upper mediastinal lymph nodes) with or without gross invasion into the strap muscles (sternohyoid, sternothyroid, thyrohyoid, or omohyoid muscles)	Any distant metastases, or lymph node involvement outside of the central neck (level VI/VII), or gross invasion into other structures of the neck (beyond just strap muscle involvement)
Treatment	Surgery	Surgery	Surgery Tyrosine kinase inhibitors (Vandetenib, Cobaznatinib)	
Prognosis	5-year survival 99%	5-year survival 98%	5-year survival 80%	5-year survival near 28%
Potential CV toxicities	Atrial fibrillation		**Vandetanib:** hypertension, QT prolongation/ sudden cardiac death (black box warning) **Cabozantinib:** hypertension, arterial and venous thromboembolism, syncope	

CHAPTER OUTLINE

INCIDENCE
RISK FACTORS
PROGNOSIS
STAGING OF THYROID CANCER
TREATMENT
SURGERY
CARDIOVASCULAR RISKS
TSH SUPPRESSION THERAPY (IATROGENIC SUBCLINICAL HYPERTHYROIDISM)
CHEMOTHERAPY
TYROSINE KINASE INHIBITOR AND IMMUNOTHERAPY
IMMUNOTHERAPY

KEY POINTS

- Thyroid cancer is the most common endocrine malignancy accounting for 3% of all newly diagnosed cancers in the United States.
- The median age of diagnosis is 51 years (SEER statistics).
- Risk factors for thyroid cancer include genetics (MEN2-mutation of the RET protooncogene, Cowden syndrome, familial polyposis), gender (higher incidence in women), age (most cases occur at age >40), and prior exposure of the thyroid to radiation.
- Seventy percent of thryoid cancers are diagnosed at an early stage where the cancer is localized to the thyroid gland.
- Surgery is the primary mode of treatment followed by radioactive iodine therapy in patients with differentiated thyroid cancer.
- Thyroid cancer treatment is generally well tolerated from a cardiovascular disease standpoint, although tyrosine kinase inhibitor toxicities can be seen.

INCIDENCE

Endocrine cancers are relatively uncommon. Thyroid cancer is the most common of endocrine malignancies. Differentiated thyroid cancer (DTC), which includes papillary thyroid cancer and follicular thyroid cancer, comprises the vast majority (>90%) of all thyroid cancers. The yearly incidence of DTC has continued to rise over the past decade. Other types of thyroid cancer include medullary thyroid cancer (MTC), which comprises 5% to 10% of all thyroid cancer and, very rarely (1% to 2%), anaplastic thyroid cancer.

RISK FACTORS

Risk factors include gender, family history, and exposure to ionizing radiation. Women have a three- to four-fold higher incidence of thyroid cancer. About 25% of MTC are familial and inherited. Thyroid cancers can be seen with other inherited conditions, such as Cowden disease and familial adenomatous polyposis. Exposure to ionizing radiation, either environmental (nuclear disasters) or as a part of treatment for tonsillitis, acne, head/neck malignancies, or lymphoma, is a risk factor for developing thyroid cancer.[1–3]

PROGNOSIS

Despite the increase in incidence, the prognosis is generally excellent with 5-year survival exceeding 95%. The (rare) exception is anaplastic thyroid cancer, which is the most aggressive form of thyroid cancer. All anaplastic thyroid cancers are considered stage IV with poor prognosis with 5-year survival being around 7%.[3,4]

STAGING OF THYROID CANCER

Multiple staging systems have been developed to predict the risk of mortality in cases of thyroid cancer and use a combination of histology, size of the tumor, and extra thyroidal extension (lymph nodes and distant disease) to stratify patients. The American Joint Committee on Cancer (AJCC) uses the combination of TNM Classification and an age of more than 55 years at diagnosis as a risk factor for staging cases of DTC.

TREATMENT

Thyroid cancer is generally treated with surgery, thyrotropin (TSH) suppression with levothyroxine (iatrogenic subclinical hyperthyroidism), chemotherapy, radiotherapy, tyrosine kinase inhibitors (TKIs), and immunotherapy.[5]

SURGERY

Surgery is often curative in patients with localized disease. Surgery is followed by radioactive iodine treatment in patients at higher risk with DTC. External beam radiation is used very rarely in patients with advanced disease.

CARDIOVASCULAR RISKS

Thyroid cancer treatment is generally well tolerated from a cardiovascular point of view. More recently there have been reports of increased cardiovascular risk in thyroid cancer survivors likely because of TSH suppressive therapy needed for treatment of papillary thyroid cancer (PTC). TKIs, which target angiogenesis, are approved for treatment in patients with progressive metastatic disease and the most common side effect is hypertension and rarely develop heart failure.

TSH SUPPRESSION THERAPY (IATROGENIC SUBCLINICAL HYPERTHYROIDISM)

TSH suppressive therapy used in patients with DTC can be associated with an increased risk of cardiovascular disease, particularly atrial fibrillation. The risk increases with a higher degree of TSH suppression. Because TSH suppression is an integral part of thyroid cancer management, these patients will benefit from regular assessment and modification of cardiovascular risk factors.[5–9]

CHEMOTHERAPY

Medullary thyroid cancer, anaplastic and advanced PTC can be treated with chemotherapy, which includes cytotoxic therapy, TKIs, and immunotherapy.

The most effective cytotoxic therapy the combination of doxorubicin with another agent, or 5-fluorouracil and dacarbazine. Doxorubicin causes dose-dependent cardiotoxicity and may precipitate irreversible left ventricular dysfunction and heart failure. An echocardiogram should be done for early detection of a decrease in ejection fraction. Less frequently doxorubicin may precipitate pericarditis and arrhythmias. Stress-induced (Takotsubo) cardiomyopathy has also been reported with doxorubicin.[10] However, owing to the high toxicity and poor response rates, cytotoxic chemotherapy is not routinely used.

TYROSINE KINASE INHIBITOR AND IMMUNOTHERAPY

Target therapy with TKIs has revolutionized the treatment of advanced thyroid cancers. They have been increasingly used in practice, for example, sorafenib and lenvatinib for DTC, vandetanib and cabozantinib for MTC. TKIs work via inhibition vascular endothelial growth factor receptors (VEGFR)-mediated angiogenesis inhibition. TKIs also target several other mutations involved in the pathogenesis of thyroid cancer, such as *BRAFV600E* mutation, which was found in 40% of PTC, and *RAS* mutation which is the most frequent mutation in follicular thyroid cancer (FTC).[11,12]

Angiogenesis inhibitors increase the risk of hypertension, proteinuria, hypothyroidism, arterial thromboembolism, cardiac ischemia, and heart failure. Hypertension, the most common side effect of VEGF inhibitors, occurs in at least 20% to 30% of patients. These agents can also cause QTc prolongation and *Torsades de Pointes*, especially in patients on vandetanib and cabozantinib.[13–16] VEGFR TKIs are also associated with increased risk of all grades of congestive heart failure (CHF). In a meta-analysis by Schutz and colleagues evaluating sunitinib and sorafenib, cardiac ischemia and CHF were the second most common causes of mortality. They reported two fatal CHF events and 15% of deaths were caused by myocardial ischemia.[17]

Patients on VEGF inhibitors should be followed with blood pressure screening, urine analysis for proteinuria and renal functions before and during the treatment. Routine electrocardiogram and echocardiogram are recommended for all patients on VEGFR TKIs. However, closer periodic monitoring is reserved for selected elderly patients or patients at high risk with cardiovascular comorbidities.[17]

Angiotensin-converting enzyme inhibitors, angiotensin II receptor blockers, and calcium channel blockers are used as first-line therapy for hypertension. Angiotensin-converting enzyme inhibitors, angiotensin II receptor blockers, and beta blockers are preferred for those with heart failure. Because many calcium channel blockers are metabolized by CYP3A4, which also metabolizes most of the TKIs, caution is required to prevent the risk of drug interactions. Diuretics should not be first-line owing to increased risk of dehydration and QTc prolongation related to electrolytes disturbance. If hypertension is refractory, VEGF inhibitors should be stopped and resumed at a lower dose after control of blood pressure.[15,18,19]

IMMUNOTHERAPY

Immune checkpoint inhibitors recently have been introduced in the management of different advanced cancers, including thyroid cancer. A number of cardiovascular disease manifestations have been recognized with this class of agents including decline in cardiac function, Takotsubo's, acute coronary syndrome, pericarditis, and myocarditis. The latter has been of greatest concern as a fulminant course can develop with a 40% to 60% fatality rate. Clinical suspicion needs to be high and prompt recognition and initiation of steroid therapy is critical (see Chapter 54).[20,21]

REFERENCES

1. Haugen BR, et al. 2015 American Thyroid Association Management guidelines for adult patients with thyroid nodules and differentiated thyroid cancer: The American Thyroid Association Guidelines Task Force on thyroid nodules and differentiated thyroid cancer. *Thyroid.* 2016;26(1):1–133.
2. Wells SA, Jr, et al. Revised American Thyroid Association guidelines for the management of medullary thyroid carcinoma. *Thyroid.* 2015;25(6):567–610.
3. Smallridge RC, et al. American Thyroid Association guidelines for management of patients with anaplastic thyroid cancer. *Thyroid.* 2012;22(11):1104–1139.
4. Park J, et al. Risk factors for cardiovascular disease among thyroid cancer survivors: findings from the Utah Cancer Survivors Study. *J Clin Endocrinol Metab.* 2018;103(7):2468–2477.
5. Klein Hesselink EN, et al. Long-term cardiovascular mortality in patients with differentiated thyroid carcinoma: an observational study. *J Clin Oncol.* 2013;31(32):4046–4053.
6. Klein Hesselink EN, et al. NT-proBNP is increased in differentiated thyroid carcinoma patients and may predict cardiovascular risk. *Clin Biochem.* 2017;50(12):696–702.
7. Miyakawa M. [Effects of thyrotropin-suppressive therapy in patients with well-differentiated thyroid carcinoma]. *Nihon Rinsho.* 2007;65(11):2073–2077.
8. Danzi S, Klein I. Thyroid hormone and the cardiovascular system. *Med Clin North Am.* 2012;96(2):257–268.
9. Abonowara A, et al. Prevalence of atrial fibrillation in patients taking TSH suppression therapy for management of thyroid cancer. *Clin Invest Med.* 2012;35(3):E152–E156.
10. Volkova M, Russell R, 3rd. Anthracycline cardiotoxicity: prevalence, pathogenesis and treatment. *Curr Cardiol Rev.* 2011;7(4): 214–220.
11. Viola D, et al. Treatment of advanced thyroid cancer with targeted therapies: ten years of experience. *Endocr Relat Cancer.* 2016;23(4):R185–R205.
12. Valerio, et al. Targeted therapy in thyroid cancer: state of the art. *Clin Oncol (R Coll Radiol).* 2017;29(5):316–324.
13. Abdel-Qadir H, et al. Cardiovascular toxicity of angiogenesis inhibitors in treatment of malignancy: a systematic review and meta-analysis. *Cancer Treat Rev.* 2017;53:120–127.
14. Ghatalia P, et al. QTc interval prolongation with vascular endothelial growth factor receptor tyrosine kinase inhibitors. *Br J Cancer.* 2015;112(2):296–305.
15. Resteghini C, et al. Management of tyrosine kinase inhibitors (TKI) side effects in differentiated and medullary thyroid patients with cancer. *Best Pract Res Clin Endocrinol Metab.* 2017;31(3):349–361.
16. Shah RR, Morganroth L. Update on cardiovascular safety of tyrosine kinase inhibitors: with a special focus on QT interval, left ventricular dysfunction and overall risk/benefit. *Drug Saf.* 2015;38(8):693–710.
17. Ghatalia P, et al. Congestive heart failure with vascular endothelial growth factor receptor tyrosine kinase inhibitors. *Crit Rev Oncol Hematol.* 2015;94(2):228–237.
18. Imran TF, et al. Heart failure associated with small molecule tyrosine kinase inhibitors. *Int J Cardiol.* 2016;206:110–111.
19. Copur MS, Obermiller A. An algorithm for the management of hypertension in the setting of vascular endothelial growth factor signaling inhibition. *Clin Colorectal Cancer.* 2011;10(3):151–156.
20. Varricchi G, et al. Cardiotoxicity of immune checkpoint inhibitors. *ESMO Open.* 2017;2(4):e000247.
21. Puzanov I, et al. Managing toxicities associated with immune checkpoint inhibitors: consensus recommendations from the Society for Immunotherapy of Cancer (SITC) Toxicity Management Working Group. *J Immunother Cancer.* 2017;5(1):95.

47 Glioblastoma

THOMAS J. KALEY

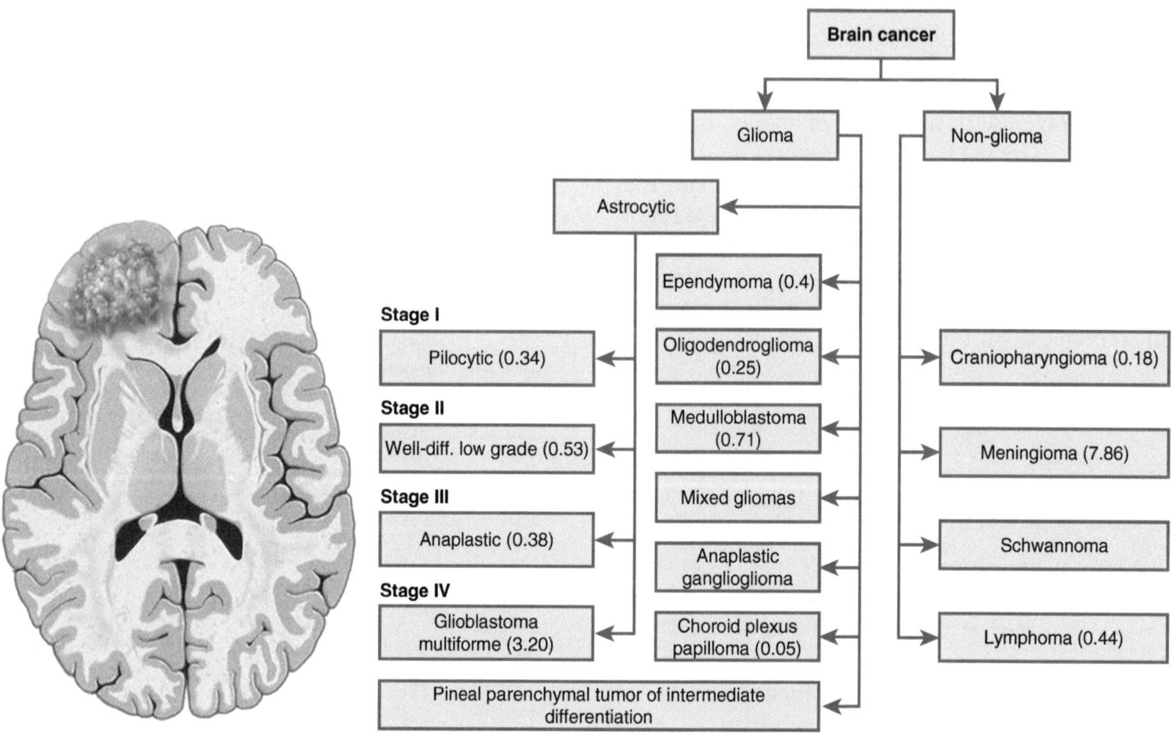

WHO Grade	*Tumor type*	*Treatment*	*Prognosis*	*Potential CV complications*
1	Pilocytic astrocytoma	Total resection ideal	5-year survival rate: 100%	None expected
2	Astrocytoma Oligodendroglioma Oligoastocytoma	Total resection Subtotal resection (plus radiation and temzolomide or procarbazine/lomustine/ vincristine chemotherapy)	5-year survival rate: 40%–80%	**Procarbazine:** edema, flushing, hypotension, syncope, tachycardia **Vincristine:** hypertension, hypotension, ischemic heart disease, myocardial infarction **Temozolomide:** peripheral edema
3	Anaplastistic astrocytoma Anaplastic oligodendroglioma Anaplastic oligoastocytoma	Resection (plus radiation and temzolomide or procarbazine/lomustine/ vincristine chemotherapy)	5-year survival rate: 30%–60%	As above
4	Glioblastoma multiforme	Surgery Radiation (involved field) *plus* temozolomide (and lomustine [carmustine]) bevacizumab	5-year survival rate: 10%	As above, plus **Carmustine:** chest pain, occlusive arterial disease (rare) **Bevacizumab:** hypertension, peripheral edema, venous and arterial thromboembolism, cardiomyopathy, syncope

CHAPTER OUTLINE

KEY POINTS

- Primary malignant brain tumors are rare, but glioblastoma is the most common type.
- Glioblastoma remains one of the deadliest malignancies, with a median overall survival of only 15 to 20 months.
- Standard treatment includes maximum surgical resection followed by radiation and concomitant temozolomide followed by adjuvant temozolomide with or without Optune therapy, and bevacizumab at the time of recurrence.
- Optune is a wearable device that delivers electric tumor-treating fields to the tumor via transducer arrays placed on the patients scalp.
- Implanted devices, such as pacemakers, are a contraindication to Optune therapy.
- The main treatment-related cardiovascular risks involve bevacizumab therapy.
- Patients with glioblastoma have the additional risk of intracranial hemorrhage, which complicates the treatment of arterial and venous thromboembolism in these patients.
- Patients with glioblastoma who develop thromboembolic disease and have no imaging evidence of acute hemorrhage, in general, should be recommended for anticoagulation similar to other patients with cancer.

INCIDENCE

According to the Central Brain Tumor Registry, the 2019 estimated incidence of new primary malignant brain tumors diagnosed in the United States is 26,170, of which glioblastoma is the most common type representing approximately half of those patients.[1] Despite ongoing research and novel therapeutics, the median overall survival remains dismal. Incidence increases with age with a median age at diagnosis of 65 years.

RISK FACTORS

The overwhelming majority of glioblastomas (and all primary brain tumors for that matter) are sporadic with no clear identifiable cause except in the exceptionally rare cases of genetic predisposition syndromes, such as neurofibromatosis or *Li Fraumeni* syndrome. The only clear environmental risk factor for the development of brain tumors is a history of exposure to high doses of ionizing radiation such as is administered for the treatment of childhood cancers (i.e., some leukemias or meduloblastoma) where cranial radiation is part of the treatment plan. Recently much attention has been given to radiofrequency radiation associated with cell phone use. However, the data are limited, conflicting, and overall inconclusive and no clear biologic mechanism of carcinogenesis has been confirmed.

BACKGROUND

Gliomas are a group of primary brain tumors that are graded 1 to 4.[2] Grade 1 tumors (i.e., pilocytic astrocytoma) are typically benign and curable with surgery. Grade 2 tumors are the "low-grade" astrocytoma and oligodendroglioma, which get the misnomer of being "benign" because of their histologic appearance, even though they are universally fatal. Grade 3 tumors are the anaplastic astrocytoma and oligodendroglioma and grade 4 tumors are glioblastoma, which are classified together as malignant gliomas. The treatment for malignant gliomas, with the exception of the rare anaplastic oligodendrogliomas, is virtually the same. The rest of this chapter will focus on glioblastoma. Most commonly glioblastomas arise as a *de novo* grade 4 tumor and, much less commonly, as a progression from a previous lower grade astrocytoma. Glioblastomas are unique in that they are not staged according to the usual TMN system. One reason is the extremely low likelihood of their spread outside the central nervous system.

PROGNOSIS

Glioblastoma is universally fatal and can lead to substantial neurologic morbidity, with symptoms depending on where in the brain they arise. Even with the best available therapies, the overall survival with glioblastoma remains dismal, with a median overall survival of 15 to 20 months.[3,4] Certain subgroups tend to fare better, in particular those harboring methylation of the *MGMT* promoter, but the disease still remains incurable.[5]

TREATMENT OVERVIEW

The best conventional treatment for a newly diagnosed glioblastoma consists of maximum surgical resection followed by focal radiation with concomitant temozolomide chemotherapy followed by adjuvant temozolomide with or without addition of the Optune device. At the time of recurrence, approved therapies include bevacizumab and the Optune device. Additional therapies included in the National Comprehensive Cancer Network (NCCN) guidelines at a level 2a recommendation or higher include carmustine, lomustine, and temozolomide (for recurrence). Across all timepoints of the disease, the top recommendation is enrollment in a clinical trial.

Radiation therapy is typically standard external beam radiotherapy delivered to the focal site of disease to a dose of 60 Gy. Temozolomide, an alkylator chemotherapy, is administered at 75 mg/m^2 daily during radiation (42 days) followed by adjuvant therapy at 150 to 200 mg/m^2 on days 1 through 5 of a 28-day cycle for at least 6 cycles unless toxicity or disease progression occurs prior. With this approach, median overall survival is approximately 15 months.[3] Tumor-treating fields (Optune device) are a more recently approved strategy where external local fields are applied through arrays placed on the scalp that deliver alternating fields to the tumor in hopes of arresting cell growth and causing cancer cell death. The device initially was approved for recurrent disease and more recently for upfront therapy after radiation in combination with temozolomide based on a randomized phase III trial demonstrating an improvement in median overall survival from 15.6 months with temozolomide alone to 20.5 months with temozolomide plus the Optune device.[4,6]

Bevacizumab has had a complicated relationship with glioblastoma. Bevacizumab was initially approved for recurrent glioblastoma after showing improvement in 6-month progression-free survival rates compared with historic controls. In addition, the drug provides symptomatic benefit in patients with large or unresectable tumors and significant peritumoral edema and neurologic dysfunction.[7] Subsequently, two large randomized phase III trials investigating the addition of bevacizumab to radiation and temozolomide in newly diagnosed glioblastoma failed to demonstrate an overall survival advantage with bevacizumab.[8,9] Recently, a randomized phase III trial comparing lomustine alone with lomustine with bevacizumab also failed to demonstrate an overall survival advantage with bevacizumab, but did demonstrate a progression-free survival advantage that may have implications for quality of life and prevention of functional disability in some patients.[10]

CARDIOVASCULAR RISK

Overall, local and systemic treatments for glioblastoma are well tolerated from a cardiovascular perspective. Cardiovascular concerns can be broken down into two groups: toxicities of the therapies themselves and disease-specific cardiovascular complications.

Cardiovascular Toxicity of Glioblastoma Therapies

In general, therapy is well tolerated without much cardiovascular toxicity for most glioblastoma therapies. The mainstay of treatment, whether or not the patient receives any systemic chemotherapy, has been radiation. Although radiation is focal and delivered only to the tumor area, there is the chronic risk of vascular breakdown and subsequent stroke. This likely relates to the volume of radiation administered, but is rather unavoidable as clearly patients treated with radiation fair better than those with just supportive care. However, in patients with glioblastoma who have a stroke, evaluation of vessels to investigate for widespread atherosclerotic disease is important because in the absence of diffuse atherosclerosis and/or other cardiovascular risk factors, if the stroke is in the field of radiation then radiation-induced vasculopathy should be considered as a possible mechanism of stroke.

The rationale for approval of the locally delivered Optune device for recurrent glioblastoma was its safety and lack of substantial toxicity. However, patients were excluded from the trials if they had an implanted electronic medical device, such as a pacemaker or defibrillator. The presence of a pacemaker or defibrillator is a contraindication to the administration of Optune therapy owing to the theoretic concern of the tumor treating fields creating an electrophysiologic disturbance for cardiac conduction. In patients who were treated in the recurrent glioblastoma study where they received only the device therapy, the reported grade 2 or greater toxicities did not include any arrhythmias.[6]

Temozolomide, along with carmustine and lomustine, are traditional cytotoxic chemotherapies that fall into the alkylator therapy category. None of these three drugs has been associated with any substantial cardiovascular toxicity. Trial data that demonstrated benefit in newly diagnosed glioblastoma failed to show any grade 3 or higher cardiovascular toxicities.[3]

Bevacizumab, approved for recurrent glioblastoma is typically administered in the United States to most patients with glioblastoma at some point in their disease course, including earlier on in order to control edema and provide symptomatic benefit. The cardiovascular toxicities with bevacizumab have been well described. The most common toxicity seen with bevacizumab administration is the development of hypertension. This is illustrated in the BRAIN trial, a randomized noncomparative phase II trial of bevacizumab alone and in combination with irinotecan for recurrent glioblastoma, enrolled a total of 163 patients.[7] The most common cardiovascular toxicity, hypertension, was seen in 31% of patients, with 5% of patients developing grade 3 or greater hypertension. Additional cardiovascular toxicities included venous thromboembolism (VTE, 7%), arterial thromboembolism (6%), one patient developed reversible posterior leukoencephalopathy syndrome, and five patients experienced intracranial hemorrhage. Two of the patients with intracranial hemorrhages (both grade 1) and one of the patients with VTE were on anticoagulation prior to the events.

The Investigational Drug Steering Committee of the National Cancer Institute has published recommendations on the management of cardiovascular toxicities with vascular endothelial growth factor pathway inhibitors.[11] The key points to managing hypertension in these patients involve early identification of hypertension and aggressive management of preexisting hypertension as well as active monitoring of blood pressure during treatment, more frequently in the first month of therapy. The goal blood pressure should be less than 140/90 for most patients and lower in those patients with preexisting cardiovascular risk factors.

Glioblastoma Specific Cardiovascular Concerns

Two additional cardiovascular concerns in patients with glioblastoma are venous thromboembolic disease and treatment with anticoagulation and intracranial hemorrhage.

As with all patients with cancer, patients with glioblastoma are at higher risk of VTE because of the hypercoagulable state associated with the disease itself. This may be increased even further in patients with glioblastoma because symptomatic tumors may cause substantial difficulties with mobility and gait dysfunction owing to the specific location of the brain impacted by the malignant process. In the pre-bevacizumab era, a study looking at VTE risk in patients with malignant glioma undergoing treatment found a 26% risk of deep vein thrombosis, with a maximum incidence in the first 7 months after surgical resection while chemotherapy was being administered.[12]

Patients with glioblastoma who develop VTE have the additional concern of intracranial hemorrhage with anticoagulation therapy. In general, anticoagulation with a low-molecular weight heparin (LMWH) is preferred to placement of a filter in these patients because of the improved benefit of LMWH and lower complication rate. There have been no prospective randomized trials to answer these questions. In a large retrospective study, VTE treatment with LMWH was compared in patients with brain tumors versus patients with systemic cancers without known brain disease.[13] In this study, the incidence of major bleeding was similar in both groups (8.6 vs. 5.0 per 100 patient-years) and the intracranial hemorrhage rate in patients with brain tumors was 4.4%, none of which were fatal. It is unclear what the true incidence of intracranial hemorrhage is in patients with glioblastoma; however, most estimates hover around that same number.

REFERENCES

1. Ostrom QT, Gittleman H, Truitt G, Boscia A, Kruchko C, Barnholtz-Sloan JS. CBTRUS Statistical Report: Primary Brain and Other Central Nervous System Tumors Diagnosed in the United States in 2011–2015. *Neuro Oncol*. 2018;20:iv1–iv86.
2. Louis DN, Perry A, Reifenberger G, et al. The 2016 World Health Organization Classification of Tumors of the Central Nervous System: a summary. *Acta Neuropathol*. 2016;131:803–820.
3. Stupp R, Mason WP, van den Bent MJ, et al. Radiotherapy plus concomitant and adjuvant temozolomide for glioblastoma. *N Engl J Med*. 2005;352:987–996.
4. Stupp R, Taillibert S, Kanner AA, et al. Mintenance therapy with tumor-treating fields plus temozolomide vs temozolomide alone for glioblastoma: a randomized clinical trial. *JAMA*. 2015;314:2535–2543.
5. Hegi ME, Diserens AC, Gorlia T, et al. MGMT gene silencing and benefit from temozolomide in glioblastoma. *N Engl J Med*. 2005;352:997–1003.
6. Stupp R, Wong ET, Kanner AA, et al. NovoTTF-100A versus physician's choice chemotherapy in recurrent glioblastoma: a randomised phase III trial of a novel treatment modality. *Eur J Cancer*. 2012;48:2192–2202.
7. Friedman HS, Prados MD, Wen PY, et al. Bevacizumab alone and in combination with irinotecan in recurrent glioblastoma. *J Clin Oncol*. 2009;27:4733–4740.
8. Chinot OL, Wick W, Mason W, et al. Bevacizumab plus radiotherapy-temozolomide for newly diagnosed glioblastoma. *N Engl J Med*. 2014;370:709–722.
9. Gilbert MR, Dignam JJ, Armstrong TS, et al. A randomized trial of bevacizumab for newly diagnosed glioblastoma. *N Engl J Med*. 2014;370:699–708.
10. Wick W, Gorlia T, Bendszus M, et al. Lomustine and bevacizumab in progressive glioblastoma. *N Engl J Med*. 2017;377:1954–1963.
11. Maitland ML, Bakris GL, Black HR, et al. Initial assessment, surveillance, and management of blood pressure in patients receiving vascular endothelial growth factor signaling pathway inhibitors. *J Natl Cancer Inst*. 2010;102:596–604.
12. Brandes AA, Scelzi E, Salmistraro G, et al. Incidence of risk of thromboembolism during treatment high-grade gliomas: a prospective study. *Eur J Cancer*. 1997;33:1592–1596.
13. Chai-Adisaksopha C, Linkins LA, ALKindi SY, Cheah M, Crowther MA, Iorio A. Outcomes of low-molecular-weight heparin treatment for venous thromboembolism in patients with primary and metastatic brain tumours. *Thromb Haemost*. 2017;117:589–594.

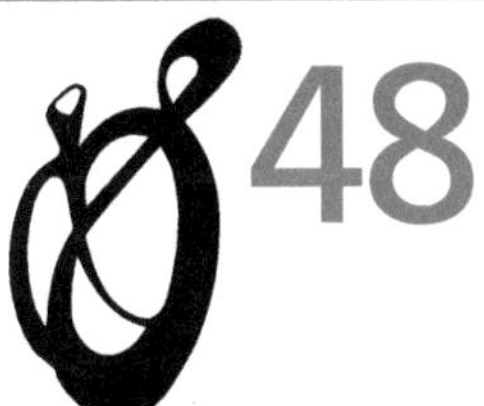

48 Introduction to the Management of Soft Tissue Sarcomas

ZOLTAN SZUCS AND ROBIN L. JONES

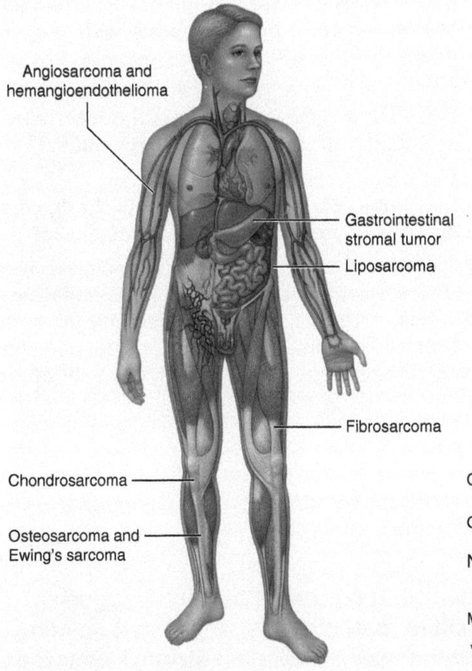

Angiosarcoma and hemangioendothelioma

Gastrointestinal stromal tumor

Liposarcoma

Fibrosarcoma

Chondrosarcoma

Osteosarcoma and Ewing's sarcoma

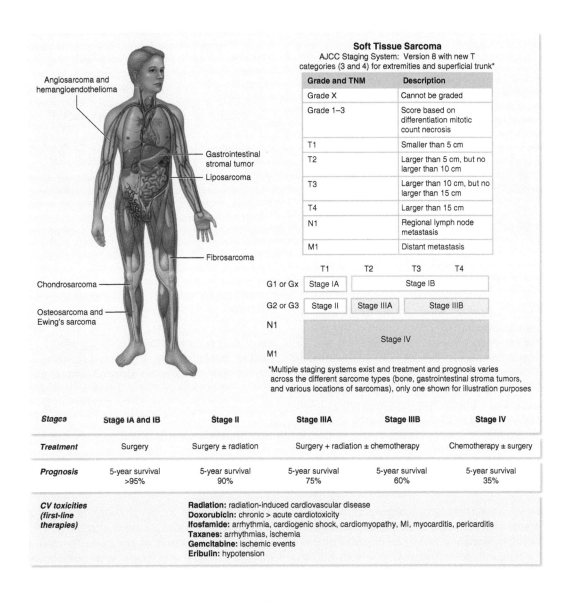

Soft Tissue Sarcoma

AJCC Staging System: Version 8 with new T categories (3 and 4) for extremities and superficial trunk*

Grade and TNM	Description
Grade X	Cannot be graded
Grade 1–3	Score based on differentiation mitotic count necrosis
T1	Smaller than 5 cm
T2	Larger than 5 cm, but no larger than 10 cm
T3	Larger than 10 cm, but no larger than 15 cm
T4	Larger than 15 cm
N1	Regional lymph node metastasis
M1	Distant metastasis

	T1	T2	T3	T4
G1 or Gx	Stage IA	Stage IB		
G2 or G3	Stage II	Stage IIIA	Stage IIIB	
N1	Stage IV			
M1				

*Multiple staging systems exist and treatment and prognosis varies across the different sarcome types (bone, gastrointestinal stroma tumors, and various locations of sarcomas), only one shown for illustration purposes

Stages	**Stage IA and IB**	**Stage II**	**Stage IIIA**	**Stage IIIB**	**Stage IV**
Treatment	Surgery	Surgery ± radiation	Surgery + radiation ± chemotherapy		Chemotherapy ± surgery
Prognosis	5-year survival >95%	5-year survival 90%	5-year survival 75%	5-year survival 60%	5-year survival 35%

CV toxicities (first-line therapies)

Radiation: radiation-induced cardiovascular disease
Doxorubicin: chronic > acute cardiotoxicity
Ifosfamide: arrhythmia, cardiogenic shock, cardiomyopathy, MI, myocarditis, pericarditis
Taxanes: arrhythmias, ischemia
Gemcitabine: ischemic events
Eribulin: hypotension

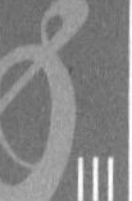

CHAPTER OUTLINE

KEY POINTS

- Sarcomas are an extremely heterogeneous group of mesenchymal cancers accounting for approximately 1% of all adult malignancies.
- Pathologic diagnosis should rely on specialized expertise of highly skilled pathologists in referral centers.
- Molecular pathology, including individual genetic profiling, is becoming an integral part of diagnosis and is a platform for future research to find new therapeutic options.
- A prevalent nihilistic approach of treating advanced/metastatic soft tissue sarcomas (STS) cannot be accepted; median survival after the development of distant metastases is up to 14.3 to 19 months, not any worse than figures seen in some of the more frequent solid tumor types.
- Auxiliary local interventions, such as metastasectomy, radiofrequency ablation/microwave ablation should always be considered in cases with oligometastatic disease.
- One of the most important factors to consider in therapeutic decision-making is the ascertained chemosensitivity of the specific sarcoma subtype to be treated.
- Doxorubicin-based therapy is still the "gold standard" first-line choice in the palliation of all STS.
- The introduction of novel antineoplastic agents, such as pazopanib, trabectedin, and eribulin have further exposed the differential sensitivity of various subtypes of sarcomas to specific agents, and challenges a rigid "one therapeutic sequence fits all" approach.

INTRODUCTION

Owing to the extreme histologic heterogeneity of soft tissue sarcomas (STS), their management is an art of its own. More recently the treatment of STS has been slowly shifting toward a more individualized, histology driven approach. The introduction of novel antineoplastic agents, such as pazopanib, trabectedin, and eribulin has further exposed the differential sensitivity of various sarcoma subtypes to specific agents.

The latest World Health Organization classification lists around 100 sarcoma subtypes; thus, the pathologic diagnostic process often relies (and should rely) on specialized expertise of highly skilled pathologists in referral centers.[2] Among adults, gastrointestinal stromal tumors (GIST) are the most common STS (~18%), followed by pleomorphic/unclassified STS (~16%), liposarcomas (~15%), leiomyosarcomas (~11%), and dermatofibrosarcoma (~5%).[3]

EPIDEMIOLOGY

Sarcomas are an extremely heterogeneous group of mesenchymal cancers accounting for approximately 1% of all adult malignancies and 12% of pediatric cancers. With an incidence of approximately 45 million population per year, approximately every fifth sarcoma originates from the bone, whereas the remaining 80% to 85% of cases arise from soft tissues.[1] Although most STS arise from the extremities, they can originate from any part of the body, necessitating complex multidisciplinary management.

RISK FACTORS AND SCREENING

In the majority of cases there is no known ris factor. Radiation-associated sarcomas are a well known complication of previous therapy for lym phoma, breast, cervical, and testicular cance Radiation-associated sarcomas occur in less tha 1% of treated patients. Pleomorphic and angiosar coma are common radiation-associated sarcom subtypes.

A number of genetic conditions predispose to th development of sarcomas and soft tissue tumor including neurofibromatosis 1, retinoblastoma, Li-Fraumeni, and Gardener's syndrome.

Chronic lymphoedema can result in angiosarcoma, which was first described by Stewart and Treves after mastectomy in patients with breast cancer.

Immunodeficiency and human herpes virus 8 infection cause Kaposi's sarcoma. Furthermore, Epstein-Barr virus infection has been associated with smooth muscle tumors, including leiomyosarcoma.

Currently, there is no screening for sarcomas. However, patients with any of the hereditary syndromes described above should undergo appropriate surveillance and follow up in experienced clinics.

DIAGNOSIS AND STAGING

The diagnosis of STS is often delayed owing to the rarity of STS, the lack of unique sarcoma-specific symptoms, and a series of challenging obstacles.[4] STS mainly metastasize through the hematogenic route, with a strong tropism to the lungs in 70% to 80% of cases. Approximately 10% of patients have metastatic disease at presentation, with an additional 20% to 25% developing distant spread despite having received primary treatment of curative intent.[5] The incidence of metastases in large (>5 cm), deeply seated, intermediate or high-grade STS increases to 40% to 50%.[6] Lymph node spread is rare in the majority of sarcoma subtypes. Consequently, owing to the rarity, the majority of clinicians, radiologists, and pathologists have very limited experience diagnosing and treating sarcomas. This is further compounded by the wide variability in anatomic presentation of these tumors.

Magnetic resonance imaging is the imaging modality of choice for STS of the extremities, trunk, head, and neck. It can distinguish tumor from adjacent muscle and fat. Computed tomographic (CT) imaging can be used for primary sarcomas of the abdomen and pelvis. In addition, CT can detect lung metastases (the most common site of initial metastatic spread). Plain radiographs, magnetic resonance imaging, and CT can be used to image primary bone tumors.

Early recognition and biopsy are critical. In an adult patient, any soft tissue mass that is symptomatic or enlarging, any mass more than 5 cm or any new mass persisting beyond 4 weeks should be biopsied. Usually a core biopsy is performed and the entire biopsy tract is removed at the time of surgical resection.

Developing an all-encompassing staging system for such a diverse group of histologic subtypes and widespread anatomic primary sites is challenging. The most recent American Joint Committee on Cancer staging system (version 8), has been developed with specific staging systems for different anatomic primary sites. Further work is required to refine this system.

PROGNOSIS

The overall 5-year survival of STS is around 55%, with extreme variations depending on the anatomic location of the primary tumor. Whereas the 5-year overall survival (OS) figures for STS arising in the mediastinum or the heart is a dismal 10% to 15%, for those affecting the limbs it is around 70% and survival is above 90% for skin sarcomas.[7]

TREATMENT

The management of such a diverse pool of distinct diseases puts the responsible oncologist in a difficult position when it comes to therapeutic decision-making.

Standard management for localized STS consists of complete surgical resection with or without pre-and/or postoperative radiation.[8] A large study from the French Sarcoma Group has highlighted the importance of management by specialist sarcoma teams, particularly the importance of pretreatment imaging/biopsy and the importance of planned initial intervention.[9]

BASIC PRINCIPLES OF TREATING ADVANCED/METASTATIC STS

Until recently, most adult STS were lumped into the same basket and treated very similarly. With the advancements seen in molecular pathologic classification of sarcomas and the increasing availability of molecular targeted agents and novel chemotherapeutics, a growing consensus among sarcoma specialists is that the selection and sequencing of treatment should be individualized and histology driven. The overwhelming majority of patients who develop metastatic STS are incurable and the common perception, even among nonsarcoma specialist oncologists is that very little help can be offered to these patients. We contest this approach, as the median survival after development of distant metastases is up to 14.3 to 19 months, similar to figures seen with some of the more frequent solid tumor types (e.g., lung and pancreatic cancer). Moreover, 20% to 25% of patients are still alive at 2 to 3 years after the diagnosis of metastatic disease, which is better than that for some other solid tumors.[10]

Patients with oligometastatic disease confined to a single organ may be considered for metastasectomy. With a careful appropriate work-up and patient selection, pulmonary metastasectomy can yield 5-year survival figures of up to 40%.[11] In addition, targeted ablative therapies, including radiofrequency ablation can be meaningful palliative interventions, potentially even improving OS in patients with oligometastatic disease.[12] Most of the studies of local therapy in metastatic sarcoma have been limited by selection bias, small patient numbers, and limited follow up. Nevertheless, local therapies are carefully considered and debated within a multidisciplinary team setting throughout the patient's journey, especially if systemic therapy results in durable control of metastatic disease.

For patients with nonresectable advanced/metastatic STS, systemic antineoplastic treatment is given with palliative intent, that is, to decrease tumor burden in order to alleviate symptoms and improve quality of life. It must be noted that unlike most solid tumors, some untreated metastatic STS patients can remain asymptomatic for long periods, even several years. Once the biological behavior of the disease is ascertained with serial imaging, for patients with slowly growing asymptomatic, low-grade STS a "watchful wait" strategy can be pursued. In contrast, for patients with quickly expanding high-grade tumors and especially in those with chemotherapy-sensitive subtypes (i.e., synovial sarcoma, myxoid liposarcoma, and uterine leiomyosarcoma) upfront chemotherapy may offer the best results.

For nonresectable metastatic STS, chemotherapy is the mainstay of treatment, but very careful evaluation is required before initiating therapy. One of the most important factors to consider is the ascertained chemosensitivity of the sarcoma subtype. Based on our own institutional experience and national consensus statements, chemotherapy should not be recommended for certain pathologies, including, but not limited to alveolar soft part sarcoma, clear cell sarcoma, low-grade fibromyxoid sarcoma, and extraskeletal myxoid chondrosarcoma owing to their limited response rates to standard chemotherapeutic agents.[13] Extremely modest outcomes have been observed with systemic chemotherapy in the treatment of malignant peripheral nerve sheath tumor, myxofibrosarcoma, solitary fibrous tumor, and endometrial stromal sarcoma (ESS).[13] Patients affected by these relatively chemotherapy-insensitive sarcomas need to be thoroughly informed about the pros and cons of chemotherapy and closely involved in the decision-making process. It could be argued that patients with these tumors should be offered participation in early stage clinical trials, rather than exposure to the toxicity of conventional chemotherapy.

Anthracycline-based treatment remains standard first-line therapy in the palliation of advanced/metastatic STS. Doxorubicin was first introduced in the early 1970s for the treatment of STS and subsequently a clear dose-response relationship has been established. 75 mg/m^2 per cycle has become the standard monotherapy dose, with objective response rates ranging from 10% to 25%.[14]

Several attempts have been made to explore whether multiagent chemotherapy could improve response rates and OS. The landmark EORTC 62012 trial, however, failed to show an OS benefit with the addition of ifosfamide to doxorubicin.[8] Nevertheless, under special circumstances where more robust immediate objective response is needed (imminent risk of obstruction of any sort, close proximity of the tumor to vital organs/structures) the use of combination chemotherapy can be justified.

With the heterogeneity of STS diagnoses it is not surprising that some subtypes fare better than others. Younger age (<40 years), liposarcoma or synovial sarcoma histology, lack of bone metastases, and combination therapy were associated with a better outcome in a retrospective analysis of almost 500 patients.[15] Among liposarcomas, the myxoid subtype shows an increased sensitivity to doxorubicin-based chemotherapy.[16] Synovial sarcomas are exquisitely sensitive to alkylating agents, thus the use of upfront ifosfamide (in sequence or in conjunction with doxorubicin) is highly encouraged.[17] Mounting evidence indicates that, although taxanes (as single agent) play very little role in the management of STS in general, their use led to impressive results in the treatment of advanced angiosarcomas.[18] Nevertheless, doxorubicin and pegylated liposomal doxorubicin are also active agents against angiosarcoma, thus offering a plethora of treatment options in the first-line setting.[19]

TREATMENT BEYOND FAILURE OF FIRST-LINE CHEMOTHERAPY

Sequential administration of active, single agent chemotherapy may maximize the duration of disease control and minimize treatment-associated toxicities. When a sequential treatment approach is followed, ifosfamide is one of the obvious second-line choices after anthracycline failure. Within the second-line setting single agent ifosfamide has similar antitumor activity to that of first-line doxorubicin, with objective response rates of up to 25%.[20] A dose-response relationship has been established for ifosfamide in metastatic STS, with a minimum required dose of 6 g/m^2 per cycle and additional responses demonstrated at 10 g/m^2 or greater per cycle doses.[21,22] The well-known severe ifosfamide-related toxicities (e.g., hemorrhagic cystitis, renal tubular acidosis, salt-wasting nephropathy, and central nervous system toxicity) make the administration and side effect monitoring of high-dose treatment quite challenging. Toxicity can be reduced by protracted infusional, rather than bolus administration of the drug.

The DNA minor groove binder trabectedin has shown antitumor activity against STS, particularly in anthracycline pretreated advanced liposarcoma and leiomyosarcoma.[23] Physicians should be aware of the rare (but potentially life-threatening) toxicity of trabectedin, including neutropenic sepsis, rhabdomyolysis, hepatotoxicity, and skin and soft tissue necrosis following extravasation.[24]

Based on the results of the international, randomized, double-blinded, phase III PALETTE trial, the orally bioavailable antiangiogenic, multitarget tyrosine kinase inhibitor (TKI) pazopanib is a reasonable treatment choice for patients with advanced or metastatic nonadipocytic STS who progress after an anthracycline-containing regimen.[25] Pazopanib is the first molecular targeted agent approved by regulatory authorities for advanced adult STS who had received prior chemotherapy (excluding GISTs and liposarcomas).

The microtubules dynamics inhibitor eribulin has emerged as a potent treatment option for the management of anthracycline pretreated liposarcoma.[26]

Gemcitabine, with or without docetaxel, is commonly used in some specific sarcoma subtypes, even though neither of these drugs were *per se* approved for this indication.[27]

No clear guidance indicates how to sequence different chemotherapy options in the palliative treatment of advanced/metastatic STS; however, the histologic subtype and patient preference should guide the clinician in the everyday practice (Table 48.1).

EMERGING NONCHEMOTHERAPEUTIC TREATMENT OPTIONS IN THE MANAGEMENT OF STS

The most dramatic example of translating molecular understanding to novel therapies is seen for GIST with the use of the selective TKI imatinib (followed by the introduction of a number of other molecular targeted agents)[28] (Table 48.2). Unfortunately, imatinib is of limited utility for treatment of nonGIST STS, with the exception of dermatofibrosarcoma protuberans and tenosynovial giant cell tumor/pigmented villonodular synovitis where it has some documented activity.[29,30] The armamentarium of nonchemotherapeutic treatment options is quickly expanding in the treatment of different STS subtypes (see Table 48.2).

Advanced neoplasms with perivascular epithelioid cell differentiation (PEComa), such as recurrent angiomyolipoma/lymphangioleiomyomatosis, showed encouraging responses to the mammalian target of rapamycin (mTOR) inhibitor, sirolimus, which can be considered as a first-line treatment choice in progressive/symptomatic disease.[31,32]

The multitarget antiangiogenic TKI sunitinib appears active against the rare and chemotherapy-refractory alveolar soft part sarcoma and has anecdotal activity against solitary fibrous tumor/hemangiopericytoma and clear cell sarcoma.[33] The commercially not as yet available TKI cediranib is a potent oral inhibitor of all three vascular endothelial growth factor receptors (VEGFR). Activity in

TABLE 48.1 **Histotype Tailored Systemic Treatment of Soft Tissue Sarcomas (STS)**

HISTOLOGIC SUBTYPE	1ST LINE	FURTHER LINE	SPECIAL CONSIDERATIONS
Leiomyosarcomas (LMS)	Doxorubicin (± ifosfamide)	Gemcitabine/docetaxel Trabectedin Gemcitabine Liposomal doxorubicin Dacarbazine	Uterine LMS exquisitely chemotherapy sensitive
Angiosarcoma	(weekly) Paclitaxel Doxorubicin	Doxorubicin (weekly) Paclitaxel Liposomal doxorubicin Gemcitabine/docetaxel Dacarbazine (± gemcitabine) Trabectedin	Particularly radiation induced angiosarcomas of the breast/chest wall and those of the scalp respond visibly well to weekly paclitaxel
Liposarcomas	Doxorubicin (± ifosfamide)	Eribulin Trabectedin Ifosfamide	Myxoid/round cell liposarcomas are exquisitely chemosensitive. Dedifferentiated liposarcomas are relatively chemotherapy insensitive
Synovial sarcoma	Doxorubicin (± ifosfamide; with maintenance ifosfamide after cumulative dose of anthracycline is reached)	Ifosfamide (re-challenge) Trabectedin	Exquisite sensitivity to ifosfamide, thus upfront use of this agent is strongly recommended
Undifferentiated pleomorphic sarcomas	Doxorubicin (± ifosfamide)	Gemcitabine/docetaxel Trabectedin Liposomal doxorubicin Dacarbazine	

TABLE 48.2 **Molecular Targeted Soft Tissue Sarcomas (STS) Treatment Options**

AGENT	TARGET	HISTIOTYPE	SPECIAL CONSIDERATIONS
Pazopanib	KIT, PDGFRA, and PDGFRB	All nonlipogenic STS hemangiopericytoma malignant solitary fibrous tumor DT/AF	PFS gain in the "beyond anthracycline failure" setting for all nonlipogenic STS Might become first-line choice agent in the treatment of DT/AF
Sunitinib	KIT, PDGFRA, and VEGFR	Hemangiopericytoma malignant solitary fibrous tumor clear cell sarcoma, alveolar soft part sarcoma	
Cediranib	VEGFR	Alveolar soft part sarcoma	Agent is not commercially available
Imatinib	KIT and PDGFRA	Dermatofibrosarcoma protuberans PVNS DT/AF	
Crizotinib	ALK	Inflammatory myofibroblastic tumor	Presence of ALK translocation is prerequisite of treatment
larotrectinib	NTRK	STS	NTRK fusion
Sirolimus (and its' analogues)	mTOR	PEComas: angiomyolipomas lymphangioleiomyomatosis ESS (+hormonal treatment)	Can reverse endocrine resistance in addition to hormonal treatment
Palbociclib	CDK4/CDK6	Liposarcomas	For CDK4 amplified tumors. Mostly disease stabilization as best response to treatment
Aromatase inhibitors	ER/PR	Uterine leiomyosarcoma ESS	ER/PR receptor positivity is a prerequisite for the initiation of endocrine treatment, with a tendency of more pronounced response in strong (>90%) hormone receptor expression. Special consideration of hormonal manipulation in indolent low/intermediate grade tumors

alveolar soft part sarcoma was suggested in a phase II trial of 46 patients with nonresectable disease. The objective response rate was 35%, and 60% had stable disease; the 6-month disease control rate was 84%.[34]

Inflammatory myofibroblastic tumor (IMT) is a distinctive mesenchymal neoplasm characterized by spindle-cell proliferation with an inflammatory infiltrate. Approximately half of IMTs carry rearrangements of the anaplastic lymphoma kinase (ALK) locus on chromosome 2p23, causing aberrant ALK expression. A sustained partial response to the ALK inhibitor crizotinib was reported in a patient with ALK-translocated IMT, as compared with no observed activity in another patient without the ALK translocation.[35]

The platelet-derived growth factor (PDGF) signaling pathways have been implicated in tumorigenesis and angiogenesis in a VEGF-independent manner in STS. Olaratumab is a human immunoglobulin G subclass 1 (IgG1) monoclonal antibody that binds to platelet-derived growth factor receptor alpha (PDGF-α) and thus blocks PDGF ligands from binding. Olaratumab showed antitumor efficacy against a variety of histologic STS subtypes in an open-label randomized phase II study comparing doxorubicin with and without olaratumab.[36] The reason for the discrepancy seen between the degree of progression free survival (PFS) and OS gain requires further elucidation.[37] Nevertheless, in October 2016 the US Food and Drug Administration granted accelerated approval to olaratumab for the treatment of patients with STS not amenable to curative treatment with radiotherapy or surgery and with a histologic subtype for which an anthracycline-containing regimen is appropriate. A phase III trial comparing doxorubicin with either olaratumab or placebo (the ANNOUNCE trial) has failed to confirm a survival advantage with the addition of olaratumab.[38]

More than 90% of well-differentiated or dedifferentiated liposarcomas have amplification of *cyclin-dependent kinase 4* (*CDK4*). A phase II open-label trial of 35 assessable patients showed a modest benefit of the selective CDK4/CDK6 inhibitor palbociclib in this patient population.[39] With new licensed treatment options, such as eribulin in the management of liposarcomas, randomized trials are needed to confirm the relative benefits of CDK4 inhibitors in this histological subtype.

Multi-targeted TKIs, such as imatinib, sorafenib, and more recently pazopanib, have all been found to be effective nonchemotherapeutic options to control desmoid tumors/aggressive fibromatosis (DT/AF).[40–42] Although the most mature and encouraging clinical data are available for the use of sorafenib in DT/AF, it is not a licensed agent for the treatment of STS. So far, pazopanib is the only licensed TKI for the treatment of STS and, over the last few years, significant expertise has built up with its use and toxicity management. Pazopanib demonstrated important activity against DT/AF, both in terms of symptom control and radiologic response, according to a bi-institutional series of eight patients.[42] The DESMOPAZ multicenter noncomparative randomized phase II trial furthermore confirmed meaningful clinical activity of pazopanib in patients with progressive DT.[43]

The aromatase inhibitor letrozole can be an effective nonchemotherapeutic option to control advanced uterine leiomyosarcoma.[44,45]

Endocrine therapy, including several aromatase inhibitors (aminoglutethimide, letrozole, anastrazole), has been used with some modest success in the treatment of hormone receptor expressing low-grade ESS.[46] Most interestingly, endocrine resistance developing on hormonal treatment can be reversed by the addition of an mTOR inhibitor. In a single patient case report of a medroxyprogesterone acetate pretreated, progressing low-grade metastatic ESS, a partial response was achieved following the addition of sirolimus to the hormone treatment. The reinstated response to medroxyprogesterone acetate has been maintained for more than 2 years with minimal toxicity.[47] This observation is highly encouraging and undoubtedly deserves further investigation.

Immunotherapy may have a role in the treatment of metastatic STS. In the phase II SARC028 trial with single agent use of the anti-PD-1 antibody pembrolizumab in 80 patients with bone or soft tissue sarcomas, no objective responses were seen in leiomyosarcomas or synovial sarcomas, but a 33.3% ORR (3/9) was seen in patients with undifferentiated pleomorphic sarcomas.[48] Future studies will need to further evaluate the role of immunotherapy in STS treatment.

NTRK inhibitors have also emerged as an effective systemic therapy option in a small number of sarcomas harboring NTRK fusions.[49]

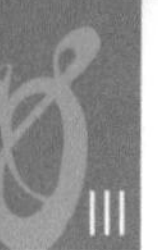

CARDIOVASCULAR RISK

Consideration must be given to the anatomic location of primary tumors and the administration of pre- and/or postoperative radiation, particularly in the chest.[50] This applies to other local treatment modalities.

Given the central role of anthracyclines in the treatment of sarcomas, consideration for cardiotoxicity is a must.[50] A recent analysis of over 500 patients treated with doxorubicin within a prospective randomized phase III trial has reported that approximately 50% of patients develop an asymptomatic decrease in left ventricular ejection fraction, but symptomatic cardiotoxicity was observed in only 1% of patients. Notably, this trial of doxorubicin with either olaratumab or placebo allowed up to eight cycles of doxorubicin with dexrazoxane cardioprotection. These data highlight the continued importance of anthracyclines in the management of sarcomas, and the need for greater collaboration across disciplines and the utility of cardioprotection. The higher anthracycline dose spectrum used in patients with sarcoma increases their risk of cardiotoxicity significantly.

Cardiovascular (CV) toxicity with ifosfamide is rare; greater toxicity concerns relate to hemorrhagic cystitis, renal tubular acidosis, salt-wasting nephropathy, and central nervous system toxicity.[50]

Eribulin can lead to peripheral edema, hypotension, and QTc prolongation.

Trabectedin has a low CV risk profile, although a recent study has highlighted that patients with sarcoma receiving this drug after previous anthracycline-based therapy are at risk of cardiotoxicity. This again highlights the importance of cardio-oncology in the treatment of patients with advanced sarcomas.

Pazopanib and other VEGF and TKIs do result in CV toxicity; this is particularly relevant in the treatment of patients with advanced sarcoma because most of them will have received prior anthracycline-based therapy.

SUMMARY

Considering that doxorubicin monotherapy is still the "gold standard" first-line treatment for most STS more than 40 years since its introduction, there is significant room for improvement in how we manage this group of diseases. Nevertheless, clinical research and hands-on experience has helped us to better rationalize and sequence different treatment options. One cannot possibly expect that with the heterogeneity and extremely low incidence of STS we would ever have unequivocal clinical trial evidence supporting the differential treatment of each subtype. Advancements in molecular pathology have had a leading role in guiding the clinician to better tailor treatment according to tissue diagnosis. We expect that molecular profiling of STS will become more and more important in therapeutic decision-making. Auxiliary local treatment modalities, such as radiofrequency ablation, will have a more integral role in the palliation of advanced STS.

The management of STS is an extremely complex task and patients with sarcoma should be treated or at least discussed in high-volume centers with specialized expertise in the field. However, owing to geographic and logistic reasons, patients may wish to receive treatment close to home; for this reason, it is important that practicing oncologists are aware of the recent developments in the management of these rare diseases. In this chapter, we provide a concise overview of current systemic treatment principles for advanced STS, without exhausting all the finer details and nuances of clinical decision-making.

REFERENCES

1. Siegel RL, Miller KD, Jemal A. Cancer statistics, 2016. *CA Cancer J Clin*. 2016;66:7.
2. Fletcher CDM, Bridge JA, Hogendoorn PCW, et al. *World Health Organization Classification of Tumours of Soft Tissue and Bone*. 4th ed. Lyon: IARC Press; 2013.
3. Ducimetière F, Lurkin A, Ranchère-Vince D, et al. Incidence of sarcoma histotypes and molecular subtypes in a prospective epidemiological study with central pathology review and molecular testing. *PLoS One*. 2011;6(8):e20294.
4. Szucs Z, Davidson D, Wong HH, et al. A comprehensive single institutional review of 2 years in a designated fast-track sarcoma diagnostic clinic linked with a sarcoma specialist advisory group: meeting the target but failing the task? *Sarcoma*. 2016;2016:6032606.
5. Zagars GK, Ballo MT, Pisters PW, et al. Prognostic factors for patients with localized soft-tissue sarcoma treated with conservation surgery and radiation therapy: an analysis of 1225 patients. *Cancer*. 2003;97:2530.
6. Coindre JM, Terrier P, Guillou L, et al. Predictive value of grade fo metastasis development in the main histologic types of adult sof tissue sarcomas: a study of 1240 patients from the French Federa tion of Cancer Centers Sarcoma Group. *Cancer*. 2001;91:1914.
7. Stiller CA, Trama A, Serraino D, et al; RARECARE Working Grou Descriptive epidemiology of sarcomas in Europe: report from th RARECARE project. *Eur J Cancer*. 2013;49(3):684–695.

8. O'Sullivan B, Davis AM, Turcotte R, et al. Preoperative versus postoperative radiotherapy in soft-tissue sarcoma of the limbs: a randomised trial. *Lancet.* 2002;359(9325):2235–2241.
9. Blay JY, NETSARC/REPPS/RESOS and French Sarcoma Group–Groupe d'Etude des Tumeurs Osseuses (GSF-GETO) Networks. Surgery in reference centers improves survival of sarcoma patients: a nationwide study. *Ann Oncol.* 2019;30(7):1143–1153.
10. Judson I, Verweij J, Gelderblom H, et al. European Organisation and Treatment of Cancer Soft Tissue and Bone Sarcoma Group. Doxorubicin alone versus intensified doxorubicin plus ifosfamide for first- of advanced or metastatic soft-tissue sarcoma: a randomised controlled phase 3 trial. *Lancet Oncol.* 2014;15(4):415–423.
11. Dossett LA, Toloza EM, Fontaine J, et al. Outcomes and clinical predictors of improved survival in patients undergoing pulmonary metastasectomy for sarcoma. *J Surg Oncol.* 20151;112(1):103–106.
12. Jones RL, McCall J, Adam A, et al. Radiofrequency ablation is a feasible therapeutic option in the multi-modality management of sarcoma. *Eur J Surg Oncol.* 2010;36(5):477–482.
13. Dangoor A, Seddon B, Gerrand C, Grimer R, Whelan J, Judson I. UK guidelines for the management of soft tissue sarcomas. *Clin Sarcoma Res.* 2016;6:20.
14. Demetri GD, Elias AD. Results of single-agent and combination chemotherapy for advanced soft tissue sarcomas. Implications for decision making in the clinic. *Hematol Oncol Clin North Am.* 1995; 9:765.
15. Karavasilis V, Seddon BM, Ashley S, et al. Significant clinical benefit of first-line palliative chemotherapy in advanced soft-tissue sarcoma: retrospective analysis and identification of prognostic factors in 488 patients. *Cancer.* 2008;112:1585.
16. Jones RL, Fisher C, Al-Muderis O, Judson IR. Differential sensitivity of liposarcoma subtypes to chemotherapy. *Eur J Cancer.* 2005; 41:2853.
17. Vlenterie M, Litière S, Rizzo E, et al. Outcome of chemotherapy in advanced synovial sarcoma patients: review of 15 clinical trials from the European Organisation for Research and Treatment of Cancer Soft Tissue and Bone Sarcoma Group; setting a new landmark for studies in this entity. *Eur J Cancer.* 2016;58:62.
18. Schlemmer M, Reichardt P, Verweij J, et al. Paclitaxel in patients with advanced angiosarcomas of soft tissue: a retrospective study of the EORTC soft tissue and bone sarcoma group. *Eur J Cancer.* 2008;44:2433.
19. Young RJ, Natukunda A, Litière S, et al. First-line anthracycline-based chemotherapy for angiosarcoma and other soft tissue sarcoma subtypes: pooled analysis of eleven European Organisation for Research and Treatment of Cancer Soft Tissue and Bone Sarcoma Group trials. *Eur J Cancer.* 2014;50:3178.
20. van Oosterom AT, Mouridsen HT, Nielsen OS, et al. Results of randomised studies of the EORTC Soft Tissue and Bone Sarcoma Group (STBSG) with two different ifosfamide regimens in first- and second-line chemotherapy in advanced soft tissue sarcoma patients. *Eur J Cancer.* 2002;38:2397.
21. Patel SR, Vadhan-Raj S, Papadopolous N, et al. High-dose ifosfamide in bone and soft tissue sarcomas: results of phase II and pilot studies—dose-response and schedule dependence. *J Clin Oncol.* 1997;15:2378.
22. Rahal AS, Cioffi A, Rahal C, et al. High-dose ifosfamide (HDI) in metastatic synovial sarcoma: the Institut Gustave Roussy experience. *J Clin Oncol.* 2012;30:10044.
23. Demetri GD, von Mehren M, Jones RL, et al. Efficacy and safety of trabectedin or dacarbazine for metastatic liposarcoma or leiomyosarcoma after failure of conventional chemotherapy: results of a phase III randomized multicenter clinical trial. *J Clin Oncol.* 2016;34:786.
24. Jordan K, Jahn F, Jordan B, et al. Trabectedin: supportive care strategies and safety profile. *Crit Rev Oncol Hematol.* 2015;94:279.
25. van der Graaf WT, Blay JY, Chawla SP, et al. EORTC Soft Tissue and Bone Sarcoma Group; PALETTE study group. Pazopanib for metastatic soft-tissue sarcoma (PALETTE): a randomised, double-blind, placebo-controlled phase 3 trial. *Lancet.* 2012;379(9829): 1879–1886.
26. Schöffski P, Chawla S, Maki RG, et al. Eribulin versus dacarbazine in previously treated patients with advanced liposarcoma or leiomyosarcoma: a randomised, open-label, multicentre, phase 3 trial. *Lancet.* 2016;387:1629.
27. Pautier P, Floquet A, Penel N, et al. Randomized multicenter and stratified phase II study of gemcitabine and docetaxel versus gemcitabine in patients with metastatic or relapsed leiomyosarcomas: a federation National des Centres de Lutte contre le Cancer (FNCLCC) French Sarcoma Group study (TAXOGEM study). *Oncologist.* 2012;17:1213–1220.
28. Szucs Z, Thway K, Fisher C, et al. Molecular subtypes of gastrointestinal stromal tumors and their prognostic and therapeutic implications. *Future Oncol.* 2017;13:93–107.
29. Cassier PA, Gelderblom H, Stacchiotti S, et al. Efficacy of imatinib mesylate for the treatment of locally advanced and/or metastatic tenosynovial giant cell tumor/pigmented villonodular synovitis. *Cancer.* 2012;118(6):1649–1655.
30. Stacchiotti S, Pantaleo MA, Negri T, et al. Efficacy and biological activity of imatinib in metastatic dermatofibrosarcoma protuberans (DFSP). *Clin Cancer Res.* 2016;22(4):837–846.
31. Wagner AJ, Malinowska-Kolodziej I, Morgan JA, et al. Clinical activity of mTOR inhibition with sirolimus in malignant perivascular epithelioid cell tumors: targeting the pathogenic activation of mTORC1 in tumors. *J Clin Oncol.* 2010;28:835.
32. Dickson MA, Schwartz GK, Antonescu CR, et al. Extrarenal perivascular epithelioid cell tumors (PEComas) respond to mTOR inhibition: clinical and molecular correlates. *Int J Cancer.* 2013;132:1711.
33. Stacchiotti S, Negri T, Libertini M, et al. Sunitinib malate in solitary fibrous tumor (SFT). *Ann Oncol.* 2012;23:3171.
34. Judson I, Leahy M, Bhadri V, et al. On behalf of the CASPS Trial Management Group and Investigators. Activity of cediranib in alveolar soft part sarcoma (ASPS) confirmed by CASPS (cediranib in ASPS), an international, randomised phase II trial (C2130/A12118). *J Clin Oncol.* 2017;35(suppl 15):11004–11004.
35. Schöffski P, Wozniak A, Stacchiotti S, et al. Activity and safety of crizotinib in patients with advanced clear-cell sarcoma with MET alterations: European Organization for Research and Treatment of Cancer phase II trial 90101 'CREATE.' *Ann Oncol.* 2017;28:3000–3008.
36. Tap WD, Jones RL, Van Tine BA, et al. Olaratumab and doxorubicin versus doxorubicin alone for treatment of soft-tissue sarcoma: an open-label phase 1b and randomised phase 2 trial. *Lancet.* 2016; 388:488.
37. Judson I, van der Graaf WT. Sarcoma: Olaratumab—really a breakthrough for soft-tissue sarcomas? *Nat Rev Clin Oncol.* 2016;13(9): 534–536.
38. Tap WD, Wagner AJ, Papai ZS, et al. ANNOUNCE: A randomized, placebo (PBO)-controlled, double-blind, phase (Ph) III trial of doxorubicin (dox) + olaratumab versus dox + PBO in patients (pts) with advanced soft tissue sarcomas (STS). *J Clin Oncol.* 2019; 37(suppl 18):LBA3–LBA3.
39. Dickson MA, Schwartz GK, Keohan ML, et al. Progression-free survival among patients with well-differentiated or dedifferentiated liposarcoma treated with CDK4 inhibitor palbociclib: a phase 2 clinical trial. *JAMA Oncol.* 2016;2:937.
40. Kasper B, Grünwald V, Reichardt P, et al. Phase II study evaluating imatinib to induce progression arrest in RECIST progressive desmoid tumors not amenable to surgical resection with R0 intent or accompanied by unacceptable function loss—a study of the German Interdisciplinary Sarcoma Group (GISG) *Ann Oncol.* 2014;25:494.
41. Munhoz RR, Lefkowitz RA, Kuk D, et al. Efficacy of sorafenib in patients with desmoid-type fibromatosis. *J Clin Oncol.* 2016;34 (suppl; abstr 11065).
42. Szucs Z, Messiou C, Wong HH, et al. Pazopanib, a promising option for the treatment of aggressive fibromatosis. *Anticancer Drugs.* 2017;28:421–426.
43. Toulmonde M, Ray-Coquard I, Pulido M, et al. DESMOPAZ pazopanib (PZ) versus IV methotrexate/vinblastine (MV) in adult patients with progressive desmoid tumors (DT) a randomized phase II study from the French Sarcoma Group. *J Clin Oncol.* 2018;36(suppl 15):11501–11501.
44. George S, Feng Y, Manola J, et al. Phase 2 trial of aromatase inhibition with letrozole in patients with uterine leiomyosarcomas expressing estrogen and/or progesterone receptors. *Cancer.* 2014; 120(5):738–743.

45. Thanopoulou E, Thway K, Khabra K, Judson I. Treatment of hormone positive uterine leiomyosarcoma with aromatase inhibitors. *Clin Sarcoma Res*. 2014;4:5.
46. Nakamura K, Nakayama K, Ishikawa M, et al. Letrozole as second-line hormonal treatment for recurrent low-grade endometrial stromal sarcoma: a case report and review of the literature. *Oncol Lett*. 2016;12(5):3856–3860.
47. Martin-Liberal J, Benson C, Messiou C, et al. Reversion of hormone treatment resistance with the addition of an mTOR inhibitor in endometrial stromal sarcoma. *Case Rep Med*. 2014;2014:612496.
48. Tawbi AH, Burgess MA, Crowley J, et al. Safety and efficacy of PD-1 blockade using pembrolizumab in patients with advanced soft tissue (STS) and bone sarcomas (BS): results of SARC028—a multicenter phase II study. *J Clin Oncol*. 2016;34(suppl 15):11006.
49. Miettinen M, Felisiak-Golabek A, Luiña Contreras A, et al. New fusion sarcomas: histopathology and clinical significance of selected entities. *Hum Pathol*. 2019;86:57–65.
50. Jones RL, Ewer MS. Cardiac and cardiovascular toxicity of nonanthracycline anticancer drugs. *Expert Rev Anticancer Ther*. 2006;6(9):1249–1269.

49 Acute and Chronic Leukemias

KRISTEN B. McCULLOUGH AND MRINAL M. PATNAIK

Disease state	**Acute myeloid leukemia**	**Acute lymphoblastic leukemia**	**Chronic myeloid leukemia**	**Chronic lymphocytic leukemia**
	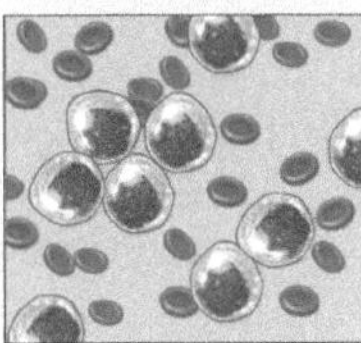	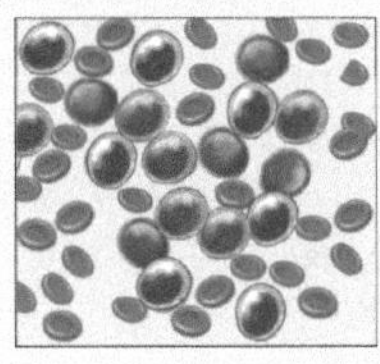	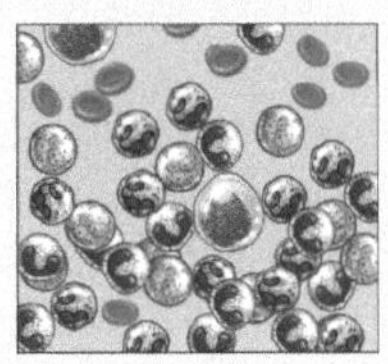	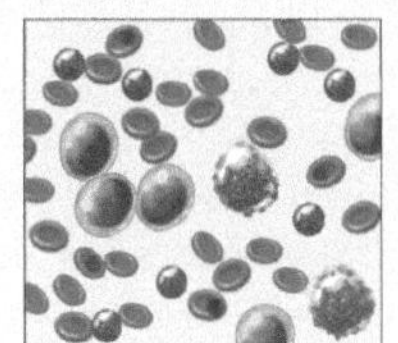
Median age	65–74 years	<20 years and 55–64 years	65–74 years	65–74 years
Classification/ diagnostic criteria	2016 WHO Classification of myeloid neoplasms and acute leukemia			2016 WHO classification of lymphoid neoplasms
Prognostic index/ risk stratification	ELN-2017 risk stratification	Based on age, WBC, organ involvement, immunophenotype, cytogenetics, and (early) response to treatment	EUTOS score ELTS score	CLL – IPI
Treatment	**Induction:** Cytarabine + anthracycline (7 + 3) **Consolidation:** High-dose cytarabine consolidation (HiDAC)	**Adolescents and young adults:** C10403 or Berlin-Frankfurt-Münster **Adults (age ~ 40+):** Hyper-CVAD alternating with high methotrexate and cytarabine ± rituximab Hyper-CVAD alternating with high methotrexate and cytarabine ± TKI	**First line:** Imatinib **Subsequent options:** Dasatinib Nilotinib Bosutinib Ponatinib	Ibrutinib Venetoclax + obinutuzumab Acalabrutinib ± obinutuzumab
Main CV side effects of therapy	**Anthracyclines:** Heart failure	**Anthracyclines:** Heart failure **Pegasparagase:** Hypertriglyceridemia, thrombosis	**First line:** No CV effects **Subsequent options:** QTc prolongation Pericardial effusions Arterial occlusive events Hypertension Ischemic heart disease	**Ibrutinib and acalabrutinib:** Hypertension Atrial fibrillation Bleeding

CHAPTER OUTLINE

KEY POINTS

- Leukemias account for 0.3% to 1.2% of all malignancies with chronic lymphocytic leukemia (CLL) and acute myeloid leukemia (AML) being the most common (one-third of all leukemia cases each).
- Risk factors for leukemias are ill-defined, with the exception of a few well-documented risks, including exposure to alkylating agents or topoisomerase II inhibitors (AML) and ionizing radiation.
- Prognosis differs for each of the four leukemia types based on age, cytogenetics, and molecular aberrations.
- Treatment is disease-specific; for AML: cytarabine + anthracycline (7 + 3), with the addition of targeted agents, such as midostaurin (*FLT3*) and gemtuzumab ozogamicin (CD33); for ALL multiagent cytotoxic chemotherapy regimens plus or minus *BCR-ABL1* tyrosine kinase inhibitors (TKIs) or rituximab (CD20); for CLL Bruton tyrosine kinase (BTK) inhibitors, BCL2 inhibitors, and CD20-targeted monoclonal antibodies; and for chronic myeloid leukemia, *BCR-ABL1* TKIs.
- Cardiovascular risks include those of anthracycline exposure with the need for lifetime dose monitoring for acute lymphoblastic leukemia and AML.
- QTc prolongation, pericardial effusions, and arterial occlusive events are the main concerns for *BCR-ABL1* TKIs.
- Atrial fibrillation and hypertension are the main CV concerns for BTK inhibitors.
- Myelodysplastic syndromes and myeloproliferative neoplasms are unique myeloid entities that may have either treatment-related or disease-related risk for thrombosis necessitating antiplatelet and anticoagulation therapy.
- Patients with clonal hematopoiesis of indeterminate potential have presumptive cancer related driver mutations increasing their risk for hematologic malignancy and all-cause mortality owing to accelerated cardiovascular disease (inflammatory milieu and endothelial dysfunction).

INTRODUCTION

Acute and chronic leukemias are characterized by unregulated cellular differentiation and proliferation occurring during specific phases in canonic hematopoiesis. Acute leukemias are caused by differentiation arrests occurring early during hematopoiesis, resulting in immature myeloid or lymphoid precursors, often called blasts, proliferating in an uncontrolled fashion. In contrast, chronic leukemias, in general, are a consequence of malignant cells developing later in hematopoiesis, resulting in relatively mature myeloid or lymphoid lineage cells that are unable to undergo routine cell death or apoptosis (Fig. 49.1).

In 2020, 60,530 new cases of leukemia were estimated in the U.S., compromising approximately 3.5% of new cancer diagnoses.[1] Of those, the incidence of acute and chronic leukemias is anticipated to be nearly equivalent, with the most prominent types being acute myeloid leukemia (AML; 34%) and chronic lymphocytic leukemia (CLL; 33%). More than 50% of acute lymphoblastic leukemia (ALL) cases are diagnosed in patients less than 20 years of age, making it the most common cancer in children. In contrast, AML, chronic myeloid leukemia (CML), and CLL occur most frequently in patients 65 to 74 years of age.

PROGNOSIS

Prognosis in acute and chronic leukemias is highly dependent on the cytogenetic and molecular aberrations encountered. Cytogenetic aberrations can be analysed using metaphase cytogenetics, interphase fluorescence *in situ* hybridization and array-based genomic hybridization assays, whereas molecular abnormalities are identified using targeted next generation sequencing assays, including whole

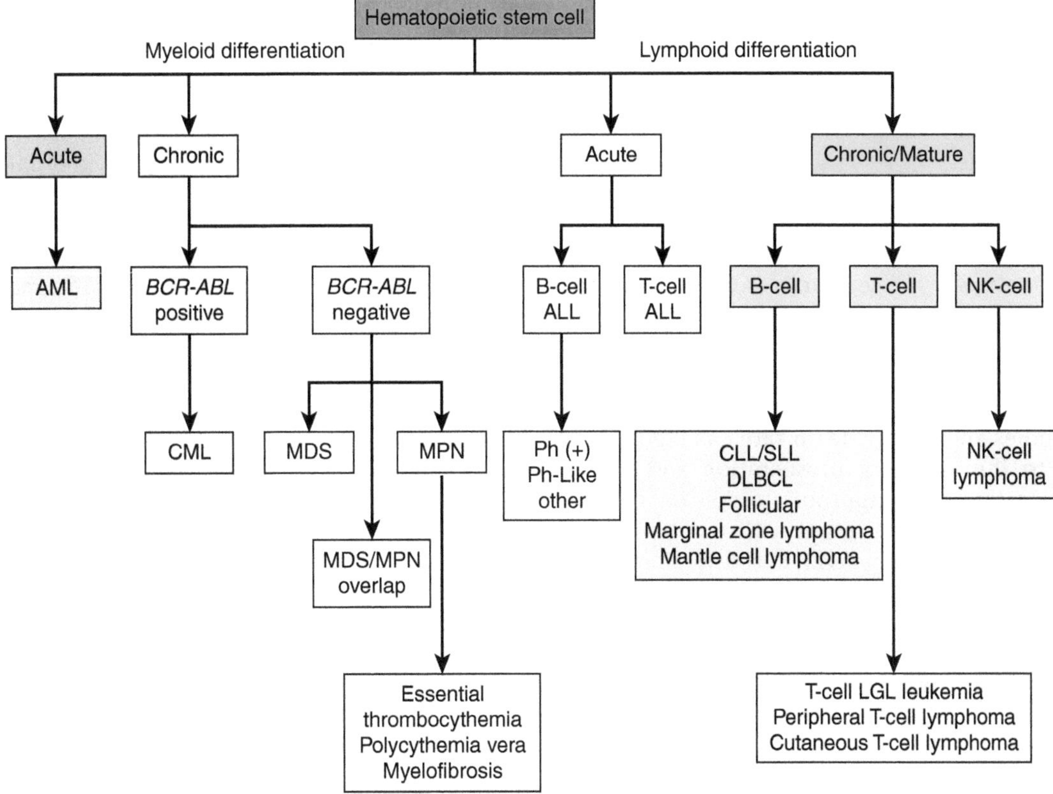

FIG 49.1 Overview of hematopoietic stem cell differentiation and the most frequently occurring disease states. *ALL*, Acute lymphoblastic leukemia; *AML*, acute myeloid leukemia; *CLL*, chronic lymphocytic leukemia; *CML*, chronic myeloid leukemia; *DLBCL*, diffuse large B-cell lymphoma; *LGL*, large granular lymphocyte; *MDS*, myelodysplastic syndrome; *MPN*, myeloproliferative neoplasms; *NK*, natural killer; *Ph*, Philadelphia chromosome (*BCR-ABL1*); *SLL*, small lymphocytic leukemia.

exome sequencing and in some cases fusion detection using fluorescence *in situ* hybridization and/or transcriptomic analysis (Q-PCR or RNA-seq). When appropriate, specific key cytogenetic features will be highlighted throughout the chapter.

TREATMENT STRATEGIES FOR ACUTE MYELOID AND LYMPHOID MALIGNANCIES

Acute Myeloid Leukemia

The mainstay of treatment in patients with minimal comorbidities remains aggressive chemotherapy with the goal of complete remission (CR), which is achieved in 60% to 70% of patients.[2] Standard risk treatment includes a combination of anthracycline for 3 days and cytarabine continuous infusion for 7 days (7 + 3). Pretreatment evaluation with an echocardiogram is encouraged for baseline cardiac assessment, owing to the age of the population and cumulative anthracycline administration. In patients who achieve a CR, consolidation chemotherapy is generally with high-dose cytarabine over 3 to 5 days.[3] Patients at intermediate or high risk are treated similarly, but should be evaluated early for allogeneic hematopoietic stem cell transplant (HSCT).

Some evidence suggests that patients with a favorable prognosis, such as core binding factor AML [(t8;21)(q22;22), inv(16)(p13q22)/t(6;16)(p13q22)], may benefit from the addition of gemtuzumab ozogamicin, a humanized CD33-directed monoclonal antibody-drug conjugate linked to a cytotoxic calicheamicin derivative.[4] This is not thought to contribute to cardiotoxicity of traditional therapy, but does increase the risk for hepatic venoocclusive disease, especially in the context of planned allogeneic HSCT. In patients with *FLT3*-mutated AML, midostaurin, a *FLT3* inhibitor, is added on days 8 through 21 to induction and consolidation therapy with improvement in disease-free and overall survival (OS).[5] Midostaurin

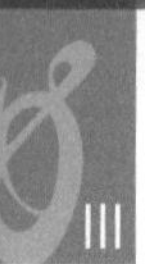

is associated with moderate emetogenic potential and may cause nausea, vomiting, diarrhea and subsequent electrolyte derangements. Although evaluation of QTc in healthy individuals was unrevealing, QTc prolongation has occurred in more than 18% of patients with AML.

Acute Promyelocytic Leukemia

Acute promyelocytic leukemia (APL), a rare subtype of AML, is characterized by t(15;17)(q24;21) and creation of a fusion oncogene, *PML-RARA*. In the context of clinical trials, APL is curable in more than 90% of patients; however, real-world population studies show early death rates as high as 24% owing to the acuity of presentation and lack of knowledge regarding appropriate disease management.[6] Patients often present with a complex consumptive coagulopathy and fibrinolysis resulting in a significantly elevated hemorrhagic risk, therefore emergent hospitalization and treatment are required.[7]

Low risk APL (white blood cells $< 10 \times 10^9$/L and platelets $< 40 \times 10^9$/L) is managed without cytotoxic chemotherapy. All-*trans* retinoic acid (ATRA) plus arsenic trioxide (ATO) are continued daily until hematologic remission and are again utilized in an on/off strategy for consolidation.[8] Both agents are capable of inducing promyelocyte differentiation. The absence of cytotoxic chemotherapy to manage the influx of mature myelocytes increases the risk of differentiation syndrome. This syndrome is characterized by dyspnea, fever, weight gain, edema, hypotension, pleuropericardial effusion, and acute renal failure. Patients are treated preemptively with prednisone 0.5 mg/kg/day throughout induction. If differentiation syndrome presents, prophylactic prednisone is escalated to dexamethasone 10 mg every 12 hours for at least three days. The decision to hold ATRA/ATO is dependent on the severity of differentiation syndrome. Hydroxyurea may also be added to control leukocytosis.[8]

ATO prolongs the QT interval through inhibition of the potassium efflux channel which slows ventricular repolarization. It is recommended to monitor an electrocardiogram and electrolytes at least one to two times per week during active therapy and to correct any electrolyte abnormalities aggressively (K > 4 mmol/L and Mg > 2 mg/dL). Concomitant medications that can prolong the QT interval should be avoided, discontinued, or switched to alternatives if able, before consideration is given to hold ATO or reduce its dose.

Acute Lymphoblastic Leukemia

ALL are either B-cell or T-cell lineage in origin. B-cell lineage disease may be Philadelphia chromosome positive (Ph(+)), Philadelphia chromosome-like (Ph-like), or otherwise classified. Ph(+) ALL demonstrates t(9;22)(q31;q11) (*BCR-ABL1*) and is responsive to incorporation of TKIs in multiagent chemotherapy.[9] TKIs will be explored in the context of CML (see below). Ph-like ALL is characterized by mutations and translocations that activate tyrosine kinase (*ABL1*, *ABL2*, *CSF1R*, *PDGFRB*) or cytokine receptor signaling (*JAK2*, *CRLF2*, and *EPOR*), and are potentially amenable to therapeutic targeting with TKIs. High risk B-ALL subtypes associated with a high rate of disease relapse include t(4;11)(q21;q23) and t(8;14)(q24;q32). T-cell ALLs most often present in young males (2:1 predominance) and genetic abnormalities in childhood include T-cell receptor gene rearrangements, such as t(11;14)(p13;q11) and t(7;11)(q35;p13). In adults, deletion of tumor suppressor gene *CDKN2A* or activation of *NOTCH1* are more common.

The mainstay of treatment in adult ALL, whether B-cell or T-cell in origin, is multiagent chemotherapy in a sequential fashion, including induction, consolidation, intensification, and maintenance for total treatment duration of 2 to 3 years, unless allogeneic HSCT is contemplated once CR is achieved. Regimen selection in adults depends on age and performance status. Patients up to the age of 39 years should be treated as adolescents and young adults with regimens such as C10403 or the Berlin-Frankfurt-Münster regimen owing to better relapse-free and OS.[10] These regimens rely heavily on the use of pegasparagase in addition to cytotoxic chemotherapy with agents such as daunorubicin, vincristine, corticosteroids, cytarabine, methotrexate, and mercaptopurine. In patients 40 years of age and older, pegasparagase is often omitted in favor of conventional cytotoxic therapies, such as Hyper-CVAD with or without rituximab, including Hyperfractionated cyclophosphamide, vincristine, doxorubicin and dexamethasone, alternating with high-dose methotrexate and cytarabine.

Pegasparagase, an agent targeted at depletin asparagine stores for dependent leukemia cells, well known to cause hepatotoxicity, thrombosi hypertriglyceridemia, and pancreatitis, the latter of which are more common in adults than in pediatric patients and require close follow up and management.[11] Additionally, long-term follow up of childhood ALL survivors demonstrates an increased risk for hypertension, heart failure, coronary artery disease, atherosclerosis, arterial hypertension, and stroke, suggesting that the cumulative effects of multi-year therapy are not benign.[12,13]

Special Circumstances in Acute Lymphoblastic Leukemia

Targeted therapy in relapsed/refractory ALL has expanded to include monoclonal antibody therapy, bispecific T-cell engager (BiTE) therapy, and chimeric antigen receptor (CAR) T-cell therapy. Inotuzumab ozogamicin, a humanized CD22-directed monoclonal antibody-drug conjugate, has shown excellent response rates in the relapsed refractory setting (CR rates of 80% vs. chemotherapy alone 29%), but is associated with a risk of hepatic veno-occlusive disease (11%) in the context of allogeneic HSCT.[14] Blinatumomab is a BiTE therapy with dual binding to CD19 on malignant B-cells and CD3 on endogenous T-cells allowing activation of the host immune system. Blinatumomab is indicated in relapsed/refractory disease or in those with minimal residual disease (MRD).[15] When compared with salvage chemotherapy the median OS for blinatumomab was 7.7 months versus 4 months and among patients who achieved CR, the rate of MRD negativity was 75% in the blinatumomab group versus 48% for chemotherapy.[15] When blinatumomab was assessed for treatment of patients who were MRD positive, 78% achieved MRD negativity with substantially longer OS in responders (38.9 vs. 12.5 months). Patients should be monitored closely for cytokine release syndrome (fever, hypothermia, hypotension, hypoxia, and renal failure) and neurotoxicity (confusion, word-finding difficulty, somnolence, ataxia, tremor, seizure). Side effect management for blinatumomab includes corticosteroids and tocilizumab, an IL-6 receptor blocking monoclonal antibody. Lastly, tisagenlecleucel, an autologous anti-CD19 chimeric antigen receptor T-cell therapy, identify and eliminate CD19 expressing malignant cells and is indicated for those 18 years of age and older.[16] OS at 6 months and 12 months was 90% and 76%, respectively in pediatric and young adults up to 25 years of age. Results in adults demonstrate 69% complete remission and median duration of remission 17.6 months.[17] Common toxicities include CRS and neurotoxicity, similar to BiTE therapy and are managed with corticosteroids and tocilizumab.

TREATMENT STRATEGIES FOR CHRONIC MYELOID AND LYMPHOID MALIGNANCIES

Chronic Myeloid Leukemia

CML is characterized by a balanced translocation, t(9;22)(q31;q11), creating a truncated chromosome 22 also known as the Philadelphia (Ph) chromosome. This balanced translocation produces a fusion oncogene, *BCR-ABL1*, resulting in a constitutively active tyrosine kinase that drives unregulated cell growth and proliferation. CML can present in chronic, accelerated, or blast phase. Treatment outlined here reflects management of chronic phase CML, the most common state at diagnosis. TKIs used for CML directly target the molecular fingerprint of the disease, that is, the *BCR-ABL1* fusion oncogene product by blocking the adenosine triphosphate binding site domain, critical for its function and role in proliferation and survival pathways. Available TKIs include imatinib, dasatinib, nilotinib, bosutinib, and ponatinib. With limited exceptions, first-line treatment is generally with imatinib, although several agents carry indications for first-line use.

Imatinib is a first generation TKI and as of early 2020 the only agent available generically. It is effective in a majority of patients, but can be difficult to tolerate owing to the development of significant peripheral and periorbital edema, muscle cramping, and gastrointestinal disturbances.[18] Importantly, it is the only TKI with almost two decades of follow up and has not been associated with significant cardiovascular or peripheral vascular toxicity.

Dasatinib, a second generation TKI with significantly higher potency compared with imatinib, is often reserved for accelerated phase CML, failure or intolerance to imatinib, or in the presence of a known kinase domain mutation with imatinib resistance. In front-line therapy, patients on dasatinib achieved a more rapid and deeper reduction in their *BCR-ABL1* transcripts than those on imatinib, although progression-free survival (PFS) at 4 years was 90% in both groups and OS was 93% for dasatinib and 92% for imatinib.[19] Common toxicities included fluid retention (pleural effusion), pulmonary hypertension, thrombocytopenia, diarrhea, headache, myalgias, rash, and nausea. There are reports of pulmonary arterial hypertension and arterial ischemic events, although the incidence of both is low at less than 4%. QTc prolongation occurs in approximately 8% of patients.[20]

Nilotinib, a second generation TKI, produced similar results to dasatinib with early deep responses, but limited clinically significant differences in overall or PFS compared with imatinib.[21] When compared in front-line therapy with imatinib, at 5-year follow up, OS and PFS were all greater than 90% for both dosing cohorts of nilotinib and imatinib. Numerically more cardiovascular events of any grade occurred with nilotinib at 300 or 400 mg versus imatinib, including hypertension (10.4% vs. 8.3% vs. 4.3%), ischemic heart disease (3.9% vs. 8.7% vs. 1.8%), stroke (1.4% vs. 3.2% vs. 0.4%), peripheral artery disease (2.5% vs. 2.5% vs. 0%), hypercholesterolemia (27.6% vs. 26.7% vs. 3.9%), and hyperglycemia (49.8% vs. 52.7% vs. 30.7%), which frequency occurred linearly with time on treatment.[21]

Bosutinib, the last second generation TKI, is reserved for use in patients with CML refractory or intolerant to up-front therapy. Data on survival remain immature and dosing somewhat controversial as randomized trials have utilized different doses.[22] The primary toxicity is diarrhea in greater than 70% of patients, and cardiovascular events being infrequent with hypertension in 6% and palpitations in 2%.[22]

Ponatinib, a third generation TKI, is utilized in patients who harbor the *T315I* gate-keeper mutation conferring resistance to all other TKI therapy. Ponatinib has a significant incidence of arterial occlusive events, which initially were reported in 9% of patients, but subsequent follow up has documented an incidence closer to 35% with heart failure occurring in up to 9% of patients.[23] A dose reduction from the initial treatment strategy of 45 mg/day to 30 mg/day corresponded to a 33% reduction in arterial occlusive events.[23] Patients with at least two preexisting risk factors (hypertension, hypercholesterolemia, diabetes, obesity, a history of ischemic disease, nonischemic cardiac disease, or venous thromboembolism) are twice as likely to develop an arterial occlusive event and serious consideration should be given to aggressively managing risk or utilizing alternative therapy, if able.[23]

Myelodysplastic Syndromes

Myelodysplastic syndromes (MDS) are a heterogeneous group of clonal hematopoietic stem cell disorders characterized by marrow dysplasia and variable risk of transformation to AML. Prognosis in MDS is predicated on cytogenetics, baseline cytopenias, and bone marrow blasts at diagnosis.[24] Treatment of MDS includes use of supportive cares with erythropoietin stimulating agents (epoetin alfa, darbepoetin alfa), thrombopoietin stimulating agents (eltrombopag, romiplostim), granulocyte stimulating factor (filgrastim), and iron-chelating agents (deferoxamine, deferiprone, and deferasirox). Management of iron overload in heavily transfused patients at lower risk MDS is recommended to reduce the incidence of cardiac iron deposition leading to heart failure. Epigenetic therapies with hypomethylating agents, azacitidine and decitabine, are generally well tolerated and complications are largely myelosuppressive in nature though response rates are poor with combination CR or partial response of less than 40%.[25,26] Use of lenalidomide in patients with MDS and isolated del5q has markedly better response rates (80%) with up to 75% showing complete or partial cytogenetic response in low risk disease.[27] Cardiovascular complications are not routinely noted with hypomethylating agents. Lenalidomide is associated with venous thromboembolism and primary prophylaxis proves challenging with thrombocytopenia but it is encouraged.

Myeloproliferative Neoplasms

Myeloproliferative neoplasms (MPN) include, but are not limited to, polycythemia vera (PV), essential thrombocytosis (ET), and primary myelofibrosis (PMF), and they arise from clonal mutations resulting in constitutively active hematopoiesis. PV demonstrates approximately 99% *JAK2* V617F mutation frequency. In ET and PMF, approximately 55% and 65% of cases harbor mutant *JAK2* V617F, 15% to 24% and 25% to 35% harbor mutant *CALR*; and 4% and 8% harbor mutant *MPL*, respectively.[28] A known driver mutation is not found in 10% to 20% of patients (triple negative patients). Although PV is characterized by erythrocytosis and ET by thrombocytosis, both diseases can have overlapping features of leucocytosis, splenomegaly, thrombosis, and pruritus. Many of these symptoms are present in PMF as well, except patients characteristically have bone marrow fibrosis and extramedullary hematopoiesis. These diseases are largely managed with supportive care, but require routine follow up owing to their proclivity for transformation to a fibrotic or acute leukemic state.

Thrombosis is the greatest risk for patients with PV and ET and it remains a poor prognostic risk factor. Recent retrospective reviews noted a history of thrombosis in 23% of patients with PV and 22% in those with ET.[29] Risk factors for arterial thrombosis in ET, besides a prior history of thrombosis, include age more than 60 years, hypertension, tobacco use, *JAK2* V617F mutation, and leukocyte count greater than 11 $\times$ 10^9/L.[30] In PV, the historic presence of thrombosis predicts recurrence and a history of hypertension increases the risk for arterial thrombosis and advanced age for venous thrombosis.[30]

The primary treatment modality in ET and PV is aspirin 81 to 100 mg/day with the addition of phlebotomy targeting a hematocrit of 45% in patients with PV.[31] Twice daily aspirin dosing can be considered in patients whose vasomotor symptoms are poorly controlled, are at high risk for arterial thrombosis, have hypertension, or leukocytosis.[32] Cytoreductive therapy with first-line hydroxyurea, or second-line busulfan or pegylated interferon alfa, is primarily reserved for high risk disease in PV (age $>$ 60, history of thrombosis, symptomatic splenomegaly, uncontrolled cardiovascular risk factors, thrombocytosis) and ET (age $>$ 60 and presence of *JAK2* V617F mutation). Recent evidence suggests that pegylated interferon alfa could be considered as first-line therapy, although it carries more toxicities (depression 12.2%, hypertension 11%, flu-like symptoms, 24.3%).

Symptomatic management is also the most common strategy in PMF. Anemia is most often managed with androgens, danazol, thalidomide with prednisone, or erythropoetin stimulating agents; with response rates in general being in the vicinity of 15% to 25% for any given therapy.[33] Symptomatic splenomegaly can be treated with hydroxyurea or, in extreme cases, splenic radiation or surgical splenectomy. Ruxolitinib, a *JAK* inhibitor, has shown benefit for the management of splenomegaly in up to 44% and constitutional symptoms in up to 46% of patients, but has been associated with side effects that include myelosuppression and opportunistic infections.[34] The only curative strategy for PMF, allogeneic HSCT, is reserved for younger patients with high risk disease and is associated with significant morbidity and mortality.[35]

Chronic Lymphocytic Leukemia

CLL is a diverse disease entity in which some patients can be observed for many years without intervention whereas others need immediate and continuous therapy. Patients with del(17p13.1), associated with the loss of *TP53*, a prominent tumor suppressor gene, have a particularly poor prognosis.[36] The acquisition of additional mutations over time and an increase in karyotype complexity, also known as clonal evolution, is common.[37] In contrast, a somatic hypermutation in the variable region of *IGHV* is static throughout the disease course and confers a favorable prognosis and prolonged survival.[38] The CLL International Prognostic Index utilizes major prognostic factors, including age, clinical stage, *IGHV* mutational status, *TP53* abnormalities, and beta-2 microglobulin to predict OS and time to first treatment.[39] Initial treatment options for CLL are diverse and rapidly changing, but may include monotherapy or combinations of the following: ibrutinib, acalabrutinib with or without obinutuzumab, or venetoclax plus obinutuzumab.

The first generation Bruton tyrosine kinase (BTK) inhibitor ibrutinib is appropriate for frontline CLL in all patient categories and has demonstrated superiority versus chlorambucil, FCR (fludarabine, cyclophosphamide, rituximab), and bendamustine/rituximab with overall response rates and 2-year OS in excess of 90%.[40] Although ibrutinib is indicated in all age groups, patients older than 80 years of age have a higher discontinuation rate for toxicities. Atrial fibrillation is a common cardiovascular toxicity occurring in approximately 9% to 15% of patients; the risk is higher in patients greater than 65 years of age or with a history of atrial fibrillation.[41] Ibrutinib is metabolized primarily via CYP3A4 and is also a P-glycoprotein inhibitor. If a drug that is a potential P-glycoprotein substrate is required for therapy, it is advised that its administration be separated from ibrutinib by at least 6 hours. Rate control presents a challenge owing to ibrutinib metabolism via CYP3A4 being inhibited by agents such as diltiazem and verapamil, necessitating a dose reduction of ibrutinib of at least 33%. Anticoagulation with ibrutinib is also challenging owing to the role of BTK in platelet activation. Patients on warfarin have been excluded from clinical trials owing to early reports of major hemorrhage with concomitant ibrutinib. Therefore, practice has favored use of direct oral anticoagulants, such as apixaban or rivaroxaban, recognizing that they are also P-glycoprotein substrates, thus risk is not completely absent.[42] If anticoagulation or antiplatelet therapy is required, it is advisable to limit the use of dual therapy and CYP3A4-interacting medications, high dose vitamin E, nonsteroidal anti-inflammatories, and herbal products with anticoagulant or antiplatelet properties.[43] New or worsening hypertension occurs in up to 78% of patients and it is associated with an increased risk of additional cardiovascular comorbidities including heart failure, stroke, myocardial infarction, and ventricular arrhythmia.[44]

The second generation BTK inhibitor, acalabrutinib, has fewer off-target kinase effects and is indicated as monotherapy or in combination with obinutuzumab.[45] The most common grade 1 to 2 adverse events are headache and diarrhea occurring in approximately 40% of patients. Cardiovascular toxicities are less commonly seen, atrial fibrillation in 3% to 5% and hypertension in 11% to 14%.

Venetoclax, a BCL2 inhibitor, is also approved in multiple treatment settings. In relapsed refractory disease, response rates of 79% with 20% CR were observed.[46] Newly diagnosed patients treated with venetoclax and obinutuzumab achieved an overall response rate of 85%, with CR 46%.[47] Owing to the high risk of tumor lysis syndrome, venetoclax is administered in a 5-week ramp-up schedule with vigilant monitoring of electrolytes, renal function, and fluid status. Additional side effects include myelosuppression, nausea, diarrhea, fatigue, and liver function abnormalities.

Clonal Hematopoiesis

Clonal hematopoiesis (CH) refers to the accumulation of somatic mutations in hematopoietic stem cells and the subsequent expansion of these mutant clones over time.[48] Although generally a function of aging, acquisition of presumptive leukemia driver mutations with a variant allele frequency of 2% or greater (defined as CHIP or CH-PD) leads to an increased risk of subsequent hematologic malignancies (0.5% to 1% per year) and an increase in all-cause mortality largely from accelerated vascular and cardiovascular disease.[49] The most common variants are seen in *DNMT3A* (50%), *TET2* (9%), and *ASXL1* (8%).[50] The presence of CHIP creates vascular inflammation from clonally derived monocytes and macrophages generating a milieu favorable for atherosclerosis and increasing the risk for stroke, myocardial infarction, and all-cause mortality.[50,51] Management strategies remain to be defined, but patients with preexisting risk factors appear to be at greater risk, so management of concomitant hypertension, hyperlipidemia, diabetes mellitus, obesity, and smoking status are reasonable advisable interventions.

CONCLUSION

Significant advances have been made in the diagnosis, prognosis, and management of acute and chronic leukemias over the past two decades. Disease states that were originally treated almost entirely with cytotoxic chemotherapy in a cyclic nature are transitioning to combination or full oral therapies. This creates an element of chronicity to these disease states, treatment side effects, and long-term complications. Cardiac side effects, including effusions, heart failure, arterial or venous occlusive events, atrial fibrillation, hypertension, hyperlipidemia, and many others, require vigilant monitoring and a team-based approach for comprehensive and timely management.

REFERENCES

1. Siegel RL, Miller KD, Jemal A. Cancer statistics, 2020. *CA Cancer J Clin.* 2020;70(1):7–30.
2. Fernandez HF, Sun Z, Yao X, et al. Anthracycline dose intensification in acute myeloid leukemia. *N Engl J Med.* 2009;361(13):1249–1259.
3. Mayer RJ, Davis RB, Schiffer CA, et al. Intensive postremission chemotherapy in adults with acute myeloid leukemia. Cancer and leukemia group B. *N Engl J Med.* 1994;331(14):896–903.
4. Burnett AK, Hills RK, Milligan D, et al. Identification of patients with acute myeloblastic leukemia who benefit from the addition of gemtuzumab ozogamicin: results of the MRC AML15 trial. *J Clin Oncol.* 2011;29(4):369–377.
5. Stone RM, Mandrekar SJ, Sanford BL, et al. Midostaurin plus chemotherapy for acute myeloid leukemia with a *FLT3* mutation. *N Engl J Med.* 2017;377(5):454–464.
6. McClellan JS, Kohrt HE, Coutre S, et al. Treatment advances have not improved the early death rate in acute promyelocytic leukemia. *Haematologica.* 2012;97(1):133–136.
7. Sanz MA, Fenaux P, Tallman MS, et al. Management of acute promyelocytic leukemia: updated recommendations from an expert panel of the European LeukemiaNet. *Blood.* 2019;133(15):1630–1643.

8. Lo-Coco F, Avvisati G, Vignetti M, et al. Retinoic acid and arsenic trioxide for acute promyelocytic leukemia. *N Engl J Med.* 2013;369(2):111–121.
9. Ravandi F, Othus M, O'Brien SM, et al. US Intergroup study of chemotherapy plus dasatinib and allogeneic stem cell transplant in philadelphia chromosome positive ALL. *Blood Adv.* 2016;1(3):250–259.
10. Stock W, Luger SM, Advani AS, et al. A pediatric regimen for older adolescents and young adults with acute lymphoblastic leukemia: results of CALGB 10403. *Blood.* 2019;133(14):1548–1559.
11. Christ TN, Stock W, Knoebel RW. Incidence of asparaginase-related hepatotoxicity, pancreatitis, and thrombotic events in adults with acute lymphoblastic leukemia treated with a pediatric-inspired regimen. *J Oncol Pharm Pract.* 2018;24(4):299–308.
12. Nottage KA, Ness KK, Li C, et al. Metabolic syndrome and cardiovascular risk among long-term survivors of acute lymphoblastic leukaemia—From the St. Jude Lifetime Cohort. *Br J Haematol.* 2014;165(3):364–374.
13. Ociepa T, Bartnik M, Zielezinska K, et al. Prevalence and risk factors for arterial hypertension development in childhood acute lymphoblastic leukemia survivors. *J Pediatr Hematol Oncol.* 2019;41(3):175–180.
14. Kantarjian HM, DeAngelo DJ, Stelljes M, et al. Inotuzumab ozogamicin versus standard therapy for acute lymphoblastic leukemia. *N Engl J Med.* 2016;375(8):740–753.
15. Kantarjian H, Stein A, Gokbuget N, et al. Blinatumomab versus chemotherapy for advanced acute lymphoblastic leukemia. *N Engl J Med.* 2017;376(9):836–847.
16. Maude SL, Laetsch TW, Buechner J, et al. Tisagenlecleucel in children and young adults with B-cell lymphoblastic leukemia. *N Engl J Med.* 2018;378(5):439–448.
17. Shah BD, Bishop MR, Oluwole OO, et al. KTE-X19 anti-CD19 CAR T-cell therapy in adult relapsed/refractory acute lymphoblastic leukemia: ZUMA-3 phase 1 results. *Blood.* 2021;138(1):11–22.
18. Hochhaus A, Larson RA, Guilhot F, et al. Long-term outcomes of imatinib treatment for chronic myeloid leukemia. *N Engl J Med.* 2017;376(10):917–927.
19. Cortes JE, Saglio G, Kantarjian HM, et al. Final 5-year study results of DASISION: the dasatinib versus imatinib study in treatment-naive chronic myeloid leukemia patients trial. *J Clin Oncol.* 2016;34(20):2333–2340.
20. Porta-Sanchez A, Gilbert C, Spears D, et al. Incidence, diagnosis, and management of Qt prolongation induced by cancer therapies: a systematic review. *J Am Heart Assoc.* 2017;6(12):e007724.
21. Hochhaus A, Saglio G, Hughes TP, et al. Long-term benefits and risks of frontline nilotinib vs imatinib for chronic myeloid leukemia in chronic phase: 5-year update of the randomized ENESTnd trial. *Leukemia.* 2016;30(5):1044–1054.
22. Brummendorf TH, Cortes JE, de Souza CA, et al. Bosutinib versus imatinib in newly diagnosed chronic-phase chronic myeloid leukaemia: results from the 24-month follow-up of the BELA trial. *Br J Haematol.* 2015;168(1):69–81.
23. Cortes JE, Kim DW, Pinilla-Ibarz J, et al. Ponatinib efficacy and safety in Philadelphia chromosome-positive leukemia: final 5-year results of the phase 2 PACE trial. *Blood.* 2018;132(4):393–404.
24. Greenberg PL, Tuechler H, Schanz J, et al. Revised international prognostic scoring system for myelodysplastic syndromes. *Blood.* 2012;120(12):2454–2465.
25. Fenaux P, Mufti GJ, Hellstrom-Lindberg E, et al. Efficacy of azacitidine compared with that of conventional care regimens in the treatment of higher-risk myelodysplastic syndromes: a randomised, open-label, phase III study. *Lancet Oncol.* 2009;10(3):223–232.
26. Steensma DP, Baer MR, Slack JL, et al. Multicenter study of decitabine administered daily for 5 days every 4 weeks to adults with myelodysplastic syndromes: the alternative dosing for outpatient treatment (ADOPT) trial. *J Clin Oncol.* 2009;27(23):3842–3848.
27. List A, Dewald G, Bennett J, et al. Lenalidomide in the myelodysplastic syndrome with chromosome 5q deletion. *N Engl J Med.* 2006;355(14):1456–1465.
28. Tefferi A, Barbui T. Polycythemia vera and essential thrombocythemia: 2019 update on diagnosis, risk-stratification and management. *Am J Hematol.* 2019;94(1):133–143.
29. Szuber N, Mudireddy M, Nicolosi M, et al. 3023 Mayo Clinic patients with myeloproliferative neoplasms: risk-stratified comparison of survival and outcomes data among disease subgroups. *Mayo Clin Proc.* 2019;94(4):599–610.
30. Carobbio A, Thiele J, Passamonti F, et al. Risk factors for arterial and venous thrombosis in WHO-defined essential thrombocythemia: an international study of 891 patients. *Blood.* 2011;117(22):5857–5859.
31. Landolfi R, Marchioli R, Kutti J, et al. Efficacy and safety of low-dose aspirin in polycythemia vera. *N Engl J Med.* 2004;350(2):114–124.
32. Tefferi A, Vannucchi AM, Barbui T. Polycythemia vera treatment algorithm 2018. *Blood Cancer J.* 2018;8(1):3.
33. Tefferi A. Primary myelofibrosis: 2019 update on diagnosis, risk-stratification and management. *Am J Hematol.* 2018;93(12):1551–1560.
34. Verstovsek S, Mesa RA, Gotlib J, et al. A double-blind, placebo-controlled trial of ruxolitinib for myelofibrosis. *N Engl J Med.* 2012;366(9):799–807.
35. Ballen KK, Shrestha S, Sobocinski KA, et al. Outcome of transplantation for myelofibrosis. *Biol Blood Marrow Transplant.* 2010;16(3):358–367.
36. Dohner H, Stilgenbauer S, Benner A, et al. Genomic aberrations and survival in chronic lymphocytic leukemia. *N Engl J Med.* 2000;343(26):1910–1916.
37. Shanafelt TD, Witzig TE, Fink SR, et al. Prospective evaluation of clonal evolution during long-term follow-up of patients with untreated early-stage chronic lymphocytic leukemia. *J Clin Oncol.* 2006;24(28):4634–4641.
38. Damle RN, Wasil T, Fais F, et al. Ig V gene mutation status and CD38 expression as novel prognostic indicators in chronic lymphocytic leukemia. *Blood.* 1999;94(6):1840–1847.
39. Gentile M, Shanafelt TD, Rossi D, et al. Validation of the CLL-IPI and comparison with the MDACC prognostic index in newly diagnosed patients. *Blood.* 2016;128(16):2093–2095.
40. Shanafelt TD, Wang XV, Kay NE, et al. Ibrutinib-rituximab or chemoimmunotherapy for chronic lymphocytic leukemia. *N Engl J Med.* 2019;381(5):432–443.
41. Leong DP, Caron F, Hillis C, et al. The risk of atrial fibrillation with ibrutinib use: a systematic review and meta-analysis. *Blood.* 2016;128(1):138–140.
42. Chai KL, Rowan G, Seymour JF, et al. Practical recommendations for the choice of anticoagulants in the management of patients with atrial fibrillation on ibrutinib. *Leuk Lymphoma.* 2017;58(12):2811–2814.
43. Boriani G, Corradini P, Cuneo A, et al. Practical management of ibrutinib in the real life: focus on atrial fibrillation and bleeding. *Hematol Oncol.* 2018;36(4):624–632.
44. Dickerson T, Wiczer T, Waller A, et al. Hypertension and incident cardiovascular events following ibrutinib initiation. *Blood.* 2019;134(22):1919–1928.
45. Byrd JC, Harrington B, O'Brien S, et al. Acalabrutinib (ACP-196) in relapsed chronic lymphocytic leukemia. *N Engl J Med.* 2016;374(4):323–332.
46. Roberts AW, Davids MS, Pagel JM, et al. Targeting BCL2 with venetoclax in relapsed chronic lymphocytic leukemia. *N Engl J Med.* 2016;374(4):311–322.
47. Fischer K, Al-Sawaf O, Bahlo J, et al. Venetoclax and obinutuzumab in patients with CLL and coexisting conditions. *N Engl J Med.* 2019;380(23):2225–2236.
48. Bowman RL, Busque L, Levine RL. Clonal hematopoiesis and evolution to hematopoietic malignancies. *Cell Stem Cell.* 2018;22(2):157–170.
49. Coombs CC, Zehir A, Devlin SM, et al. Therapy-related clonal hematopoiesis in patients with non-hematologic cancers is common and associated with adverse clinical outcomes. *Cell Stem Cell.* 2017;21(3):374–382.e374.
50. Jaiswal S, Fontanillas P, Flannick J, et al. Age-related clonal hematopoiesis associated with adverse outcomes. *N Engl J Med.* 2014;371(26):2488–2498.
51. Jaiswal S, Natarajan P, Silver AJ, et al. Clonal hematopoiesis and risk of atherosclerotic cardiovascular disease. *N Engl J Med.* 2017;377(2):111–121.

50 Lymphomas

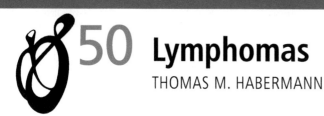

THOMAS M. HABERMANN

Stages

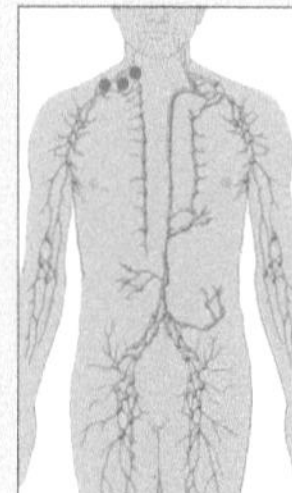

Stage I
Localized disease; single LN region or single organ

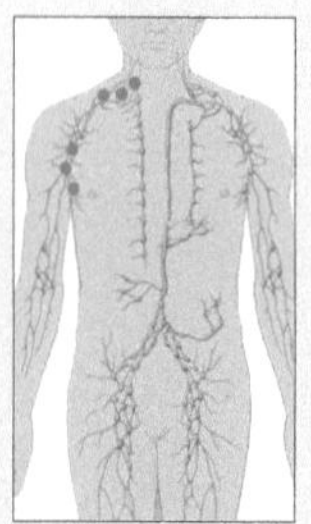

Stage II
Two or more LN regions on the same side of the diaphragm

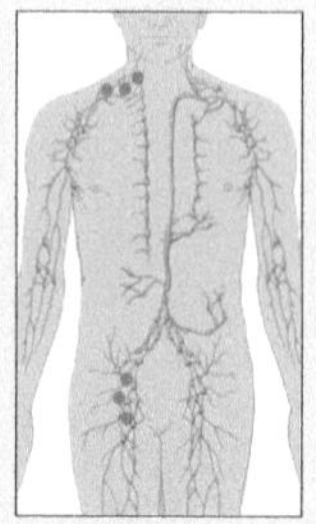

Stage III
Two or more LN regions above and below the diaphragm

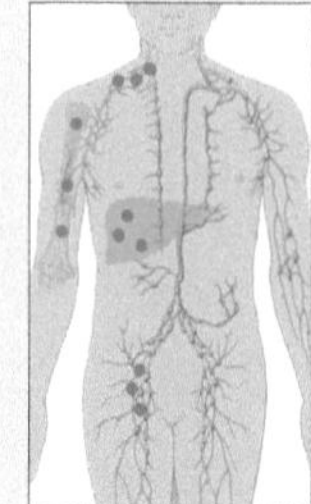

Stage IV
Widespread disease, multiple organs with or without LN involvement

Prognosis

Non-hodgkin lymphoma -
International prognostic index*
- Age >60
- LDH >1x ULN
- ECOG >1
- Stage III or IV
- Extranodal sites >1

Score	Risk group	5-year survival
0–1	Low	70%
2	Low-intermediate	50%
3	High-intermediate	40%
4–5	High	30%

*1 score point for each of the following

Hodgkin lymphoma -
International prognostic score*
- Age >45 years
- Male gender
- Stage IV
- Serum albumin <4 g/dL
- Hemoglobin <10.5 g/dL
- White blood cell count
- Absolute lymphocyte count <600/μL and/or <8%

Score	5-year survival
0	88%
1	84%
2	80%
3	74%
4	67%
5–7	62%

Treatment

	Indolent	Aggressive
Stage I:	Radiation	Radiation ± chemotherapy (e.g. R-CHOP)
Stage II–IV:	Chemotherapy ± immunotherapy	Chemotherapy ± immunotherapy Stem cell transplantation

	Favorable **	Unfavorable**
Stage I–II:	ABVD (3 or 6 cycles) + IFRT	
Stage III–IV:	ABVD (6-8 cycles)	BEACOPP (6-8) Stem cell transplantation

**For definition see text, page 50–90

Potential CV toxicities

Bendamustine	Tachycardia, chest pain, hypotension, hypertension
Busulfan	Arrhythmias, hypertension, hypotension, thrombosis, chest pain, cardiomyopathy (endocardial fibrosis)
Carmustine	Chest pain, arterial occlusive disease, tachycardia
Cyclophosphamide	Arrhythmias, hemorrhagic myocarditis, pericarditis, pericardial effusion, tamponade, arterial and venous thrombosis
Doxorubicin	Chronic > acute cardiotoxicity
Etoposide	Hypotension with rapid infusion
Fludarabine	Angina pectoris, cardiac arrhythmia, cardiac failure, stroke, myocardial infarction, deep vein thrombosis
Melphalan	Atrial fibrillation, peripheral edema, vasculitis
Mitoxantrone	Arrhythmia, cardiomyopathy, ischemia, hypertension
Rituximab	Hypertension, chest tightness, hypotension
Vincristine	Hypertension, hypotension, ischemic heart disease

Bleomycin	Ischemic heart disease, Raynaud's phenomenon
Busulfan	See NHL
Carboplatin	Arterial and venous thrombotic events, ischemic events, hypertension
Carmustine	Chest pain, arterial occlusive disease, tachycardia
Cisplatin	Arterial and venous thrombotic events, arrhythmias, hypertension, vasospasm
Cyclophosphamide	See NHL
Cytarabine	Angina pectoris, chest pain, local thrombophlebitis, pericarditis
Doxorubicin	See NHL
Etoposide	See NHL
Fludarabine	See NHL
Ifosfamide	Arrhythmia, cardiogenic shock, cardiomyopathy, MI, myocarditis, pericarditis
Melphalan	Atrial fibrillation, peripheral edema, vasculitis
Nivolumab	Hypertension, pulmonary embolism, myocarditis
Oxaliplatin	Chest pain, thromboembolism, prolonged QT, torsades, hypertension
Pembrolizumab	Arrhythmia, pericarditis, myocarditis, MI, tamponade, pulmonary embolism
Procarbazine	Hypertension, hypotension, ischemic heart disease, myocardial infarction
Vinblastine	Hypertension, ischemic heart disease, limb ischemia, Raynaud's phenomenon
Vincristine	Hypertension, stroke, ischemic heart disease, myocardial infarction

CHAPTER OUTLINE

INTRODUCTION

The lymphomas represent 4% of all malignancies. In the 2017 World Health Organization (WHO) classification, there are approximately 106 subtypes of lymphoma[1]; a simplified overview is presented in Fig. 50.1. The biology, natural history, management strategies, and outcomes of the histologic subtypes show notable differences. Diffuse large B-cell lymphoma (DLBCL), high-grade B-cell lymphoma with MYC and/or BCL2 and BCL6 rearrangements, Burkitt lymphoma, and other aggressive lymphomas are potentially curable. In contrast, follicular lymphoma (FL), marginal zone lymphoma (MZL), mantle cell lymphoma (MCL) and other low-grade small cell lymphomas have a long survival time, are not curable, and respond to different therapies over time. This in this chapter we will focus on those subtypes of lymphoma that are clinically most relevant for cardio-onco-hematology.

DIFFUSE LARGE B-CELL NON-HODGKIN LYMPHOMA AND OTHER AGGRESSIVE LYMPHOMAS

KEY POINTS ABOUT DIFFUSE LARGE B-CELL NON-HODGKIN LYMPHOMA

- Most common lymphoma subtype
- Median age at diagnosis 62 years
- Risk factors include HIV infection, seropositivity for hepatitis C, B-cell activating autoimmune diseases, and any atopic disorder
- The treatment strategy is based on curative intent.
- Anthracyclines are the mainstay of treatment, posing a cardiomyopathy risk

Incidence

DLBCL has the highest incidence and prevalence among all lymphomas (25% and 32.5%) and incidence of 6 to 7 per 100,000 men and women, age adjusted to the US standard population, per year.[2,3]

Risk Factors

The associations with DLBCL include HIV infection, seropositive for hepatitis C virus (HCV), B-cell activating autoimmune disorders, and a family history of non-Hodgkin lymphoma (NHL).

Prognosis

The International Prognostic Factor Index score, integrates the primary survival factors (1 point each): age (>60 years), performance score (ECOG >1) serum lactate dehydrogenase (above normal), Ann arbor stage (III or IV), and more than one extranodal disease site.[4] In 2020, molecular subtype analysis of the lymphomas is not incorporated into routine clinical practice although in DLBCL molecular subtypes are associated with distinct pathogenic mechanisms and outcomes.[5]

Lymphomas
Normal immunophenotypes:
B cells: CD19, CD20, CD22, Kappa/lambda
T cells: CD3, CD5, CD4 or CD8
~40%
Hodgkin lymphoma
(+) CD30 and (+) CD 15
(-) for B-cell antigen expression
Characteristic for
Reed-Sternberg (RS) cells
• usually at a singal site in lymphatic system (node) with progression contiguously with lymphatic system.
• Bimodal age distribution
• Better prognosis
~60%
Non-Hodgkin lymphomas (NHL)
• Lymphadenopathy more diffuse, can have extra nodal involvement, irregular pattern of spread, B symptoms not as common
Multiple myeloma
Monoclonal tumor of plasma cells, too much Ig, high serum free light chain
(CRAB)
Hyper**C**alemia
Renal insufficieny (measure creatinine)
Anemia
Bone lesions
Lymphoproliferative disorders
Others
Classic
Histologic sub-type not as important to treatment as stage
Nodular lymphocyte
5% RS cells abent, lymphocyte predominant (LP) tumour B cell are present
Most common
Nodular sclerosis
Collagen bands extend from the node capsule to encircle nodules of abnormal tissue. Characteristic lacunar cell variant of the RS. Cellular infiltrate.
Mixed cellularity
RS are numerous and lymphocyte numbers are intermediate
Lymphocyte rich
Scanty RS; multiple small lymphocytes with few eosinophils and plasma cells; nodular and diffuse types
Lymphocyte depletion
Reticular pattern with dominance of RS + sparse numbers of lymphocytes or a diffuse fibrosis pattern lymph node is replaced
B-cell
~90%
T-cell
~10%
Histologic sub-type correlates with behavior and treatment
Low grade
Slow growing
Poorly responsive to treatment
Includes
• Lymphomas of small lymphocytes (similar to CLL)
• **"Folicular" Lymphoma** t(14:18), CD20 (+), CD10(+), Bcl-2(+)
• **Marginal zone lymphoma**
Aggressive/ intermediate
Faster growing
Potential for cure
Most common wide age range
Includes
• Most T-cell lymphomas
• **Diffuse large B-cell lymphoma** CD20(+)
High grade
Very lethal if untreated
Behave and treated like acute leukemias, very high mitotic rate correlated with rapid growth, response to treatment and relapse
Includes:
• Lymphoblastic
• **Burkitt lymphomas** t(8;14), Myc + immunoglobulin translocation
Ann arbor criteria (Hodgkin and Non-Hodgkin lymphoma)
I single node, single region
II two regions
III crossed the diaphragm
IV involves extra lymphatic organs
A = absence of constitutional symptoms
B = presence of constitutional symptoms (B symptoms)
E = extra nodal
X = "Bulky disease." Deposit > 10 cm or mediastinum wider than 1/3 chest
S = Spread to spleen
The international staging system (ISS) for multiple myeloma
I: β2M < 3.5 mg/L albumin ≥ 35 g/L (median survival 62 months)
II: β2M < 3.5 mg/L and albumin < 35 g/L; or β2M 3.5 mg/L - 5.5 mg/L irrespective of the serum albumin (median survival 45 months)
III: β2M ≥ 5.5 mg/L (median survival 29 months)
(other staging system is duriesalmon)

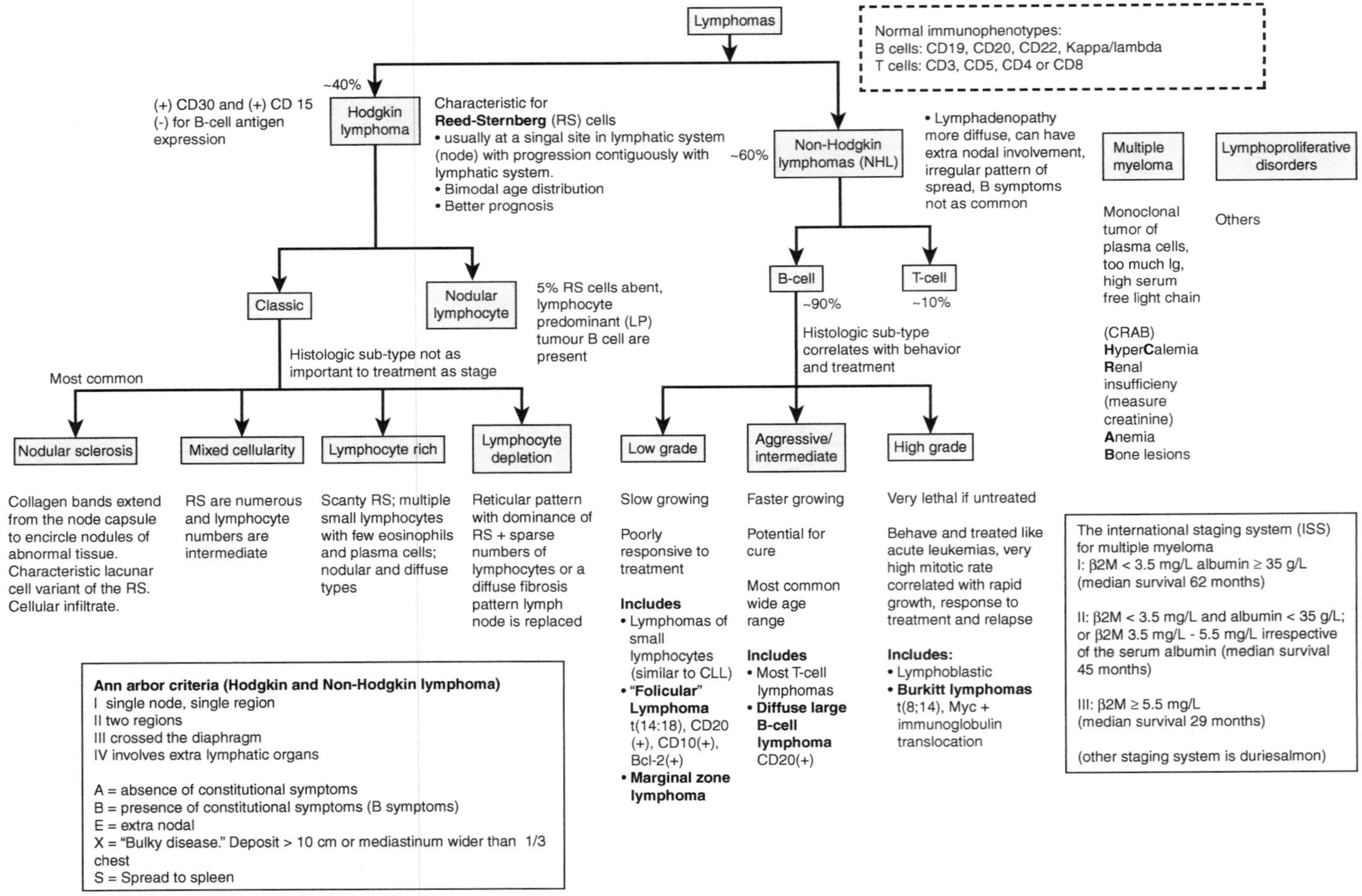

FIG.50.1 Overview of the classification of lymphomas. (Amy Margaret Chung, MD)

Treatment Overview

Of patients with DLBCL, 65% to 75% are cured with immunochemotherapy, and R-CHOP (*r*ituximab, *c*yclophosphamide, *h*ydroxylated doxorubicin [Adriamycin], *O*ncovin [vincristine], and *p*rednisone) is the standard of care.[6] Outcomes are variable and can be predicted based on clinical factors.[7] Less than 10% of patients with primary refractory disease have a prolonged disease-free survival.[8] Patients after 24 months who have not relapsed, have not progressed, and have not been retreated, have a survival at 5 years similar to an age- and sex-matched population, referred to as EFS24 (event-free survival at 24 months).[9] In an analysis of 13 randomized clinical trials that included 5853 patients followed with radiology scans at defined intervals, the PFS24 (progression-free survival at 24 months) was also similar to age- and sex-matched population with a 93% overall survival (OS) at 3 years (vs. 20% without PFS24).[10] The risk of late relapse is higher for DLBCL patients with concurrent indolent lymphoma.[11] In patients with relapsed or refractory disease, autologous peripheral blood stem cell transplantation (ASCT) and chimeric antigen receptor T-cell therapy are effective approaches. In one series, 50% of patients treated with ASCT were alive and disease free long-term. In early 2020, there were three approved therapies.

Posttransplant lymphomas (PTLD) are a diverse group of lymphomas.[12] In a series of 225 cases where the tissue was reviewed and classified according to the 2017 WHO classification, 74% were DLBCL[13], and the 2-year OS after EFS24 was 87%.[13] The management of PTLD is complex and involves decreasing immunosuppression, single agent rituximab, and in patients who do not respond to these approaches or who have advanced disease, R-CHOP.

High-grade B-cell lymphoma with MYC and BCL2 and/or BCL6 gene rearrangements is an aggressive disease.[14] Patients aged 60 or less are given more aggressive treatment regimens.

Patients with Burkitt lymphoma are treated with aggressive regimens including R-CDOX-M/IVAC (rituximab, cyclophosphamide, vincristine, doxorubicin, intrathecal [IT] methotrexate and cytarabine, high-dose methotrexate intrathecal methotrexate, etoposide, ifosfamide, cytrabine, and IT methotrexate) have a 2-year OS rate of 84% and event-free survival rate of 80%.[15]

The T-cell lymphoproliferative disorders are a complex group of diseases. Their natural history is quite complex. The EFS24 is predictive in some subsets.[16]

Cardiovascular Risk

Anthracyclines are incorporated into the frontline management of DLBCL. Anthracycline cardiotoxicity is a significant complication in DLBCL and other aggressive lymphomas. Cardiac toxicity includes an uncommon acute pericarditis-myocarditis syndrome and congestive heart failure that is best documented for doxorubicin administered as a bolus of 45 to 60 mg/m^2 every 21 days on a cumulative dose exceeding at 250 to 300 mg/m^2.[17] The risk for cardiomyopathy, however, can emerge at lower doses and inter-individual variability is noteworthy. Screening and recognition are important, for early intervention and stabilization and recovery of cardiac function.[18]

Indolent Lymphomas

NHL may be aggressive or indolent ("low-grade"). The paradox of lymphoma is that aggressive lymphomas are potentially curable, and patients who do not respond to initial therapy have a worse prognosis and shorter survival time. In contrast, the majority of patients with indolent lymphoma are not curable, respond to many different therapeutic interventions, and live a long period of time. Indolent FL arise from cells that populate lymph nodes and the bone marrow but may also involve extranodal sites. The WHO Classification does not divide lymphomas by grade and, because they are not indolent, the preferred name used is "small B-cell lymphomas" in the most recent classification.[1] The small B-cell lymphomas discussed in this section include FL, nodal MZL, splenic MZL, extranodal MZL of mucosa-associated lymphoid tissue lymphoma, and lymphoplasmacytic lymphoma/Waldenström acroglobulinemia (LPL/WM).

FOLLICULAR LYMPHOMA

KEY POINTS ABOUT FOLLICULAR LYMPHOMA

- Follicular lymphoma is the second most common non-Hodgkin lymphoma.
- Follicular grades 1, 2, and 3A are considered nonaggressive.
- Follicular grade 3B should be treated as diffuse large B-cell lymphoma.

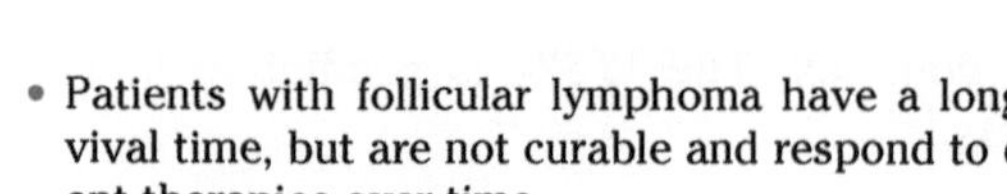

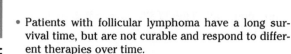

- Patients with follicular lymphoma have a long survival time, but are not curable and respond to different therapies over time.
- In the immunochemotherapy era, 77% to 80% of patients are alive at 10 years.

Incidence

The prevalence of FL among all lymphomas is 17%, with an incidence of 3.3 per 100,000/year, age adjusted to the general population in the United States.[2,3]

Risk Factors

In contrast to other NHL subtypes, there is not a male dominance in FL or MZL. With regard to etiology, Sjögren syndrome is a risk factor in FL. The risk of FL is increased with a first-degree relative with NHL. The incidence rate for FL is lower among African-Americans and Hispanics.

Prognosis

The natural history of FL is based on a number of factors. Rituximab combined with chemotherapy has improved the OS. A simplified scoring system incorporating beta-2 microglobulin and bone marrow involvement predicts outcomes.[19] The EFS24 offers more prognostic clarity than event-free survival at 12 months (EFS12) in patients treated with immunochemotherapy. Patients who fail EFS24 have an inferior OS compared with those who achieve EFS24.[20] In a pooled analysis of 1654 patients with FL grade 1 to 3A in the immunochemotherapy era, the 10-year OS was 80% in the French cohort and 77% in the US cohort.[21] In an analysis of the competing risks of death, 56.5% of patients died of lymphoma, one half secondary to histologic transformation. There were 16.9% of deaths that were treatment related. Positron emission tomography (PET) scans have been reported to predict outcome in FL.[22]

Treatment Overview

The management of FL includes observation, single-agent rituximab, immunochemotherapy, immunotherapy, ASCT, and other approaches. FL, grade 1, 2, and 3A management includes the following. For limited stage IA disease, radiation therapy is potentially curable. For all other patients, the following approaches apply.

Asymptomatic patients with nonbulky disease, with no threatened end-organ function, not steadily progressing or cytopenias may be observed (observation or “watch and wait”). The most commonly employed criteria for treatment are the GELF (Groupe D’Etude des Lymphomes Folliuculares), which are low tumor burden as defined as no mass greater than 7 cm, fewer than three masses greater than 3 cm, no systemic or B symptoms, no splenomegaly greater than 16 cm by computed tomography (CT) scan, no risk of vital organ compression, no leukemic phase greater than 5000/μL circulating lymphocytes, and no cytopenias (defined as platelets <100,000/μL, hemoglobin <10 g/dL, or absolute neutrophil count >1500/μL).[23] Initial observation is supported by the National Comprehensive Cancer Network (NCCN) guidelines, the British Society of Hematology, and the Lymphoma Canadian Scientific Advisory Committee. Patients who progress, relapse, or are retreated within 12 months from the time of diagnosis have a modest increase in mortality compared to the general population while those that achieve an EFS12 after initial observation have an excellent subsequent prognosis as related to sex- and age-matched population data.[20]

Single-agent rituximab is the initial treatment of choice in patients with low-tumor burden. The majority of patients with FL present with low-tumor burden. In a trial comparing observation versus four weekly doses of rituximab versus four weekly doses of rituximab followed by maintenance therapy every 2 months for 2 years, 60% of patients with four doses of rituximab remained progression-free at 3 years with a 3-year OS of 94% in the observation arm and 97% in the maintenance arm.[24] In the RESORT trial, patients were initially treated with single-agent rituximab at a dose of 375 mg/m^2 for four doses and then randomized to maintenance rituximab or observation with retreatment at each disease progression; there was no improvement in outcome with maintenance rituximab.[25]

The most common immunochemotherapy regimens employed internationally are R-CVP (*r*ituximab, *c*yclophosphamide, doxorubicin, *v*incristine, and *p*rednisone), R-CHOP, and BR (*b*endamustine/*r*ituximab). BR has been more commonly utilized in recent years with less alopecia, and fewer infections and peripheral neuropathy than R-CHOP therapy and an improved progression-free survival. The OS in FL has improved in the immunochemotherapy era with estimates from the National Lympho Care study describing 70% to 80% OS rates at 8 years.[26] Early event status, as defined as time from diagnosis to progression, relapse, retreatment, or death from any cause, is predictive of outcome in FL.[20] Patients who fail to achieve an EFS12 and EFS24 have an inferior OS. In contrast, patients achieving EFS12 have no added mortality beyond the age- and sex-matched population. Patients with early events after immunochemotherapy have especially poor outcomes. Reassessment of patient status at 12 months from diagnosis in those with FL or at 24 months in patients treated with immunochemotherapy is a strong predictor of subsequent OS in FL. The 2-year OS rates of the EFS12 failures was in the range of 78% versus 98% in those patients who achieved EFS12. The median survival of these EFS12 failures was approximately 3 years versus 97% in those patients who were event free.

FL may transform into DLBCL. Historically the rates of transformation were 3% to 4%/year with 5-year survival rates of 17% to 21%. The risk of transformation in a population-based study by Link and colleagues was 10.7% at 5 years, with an estimated rate of transformation of 2%/year.[27] The transformation rate was highest in patients who were initially observed and lowest in patients who initially received rituximab monotherapy (14.4% vs. 3.2%; $P = .021$). The median OS following transformation was 50 months and was superior in patients with transformation greater than 18 months after FL diagnosis compared with earlier transformation (5-year OS 66% vs. 22%; $P < .001$). Previously patients who were anthracycline-naïve who receive R-CHOP after transformation had outcomes indistinguishable from patients with *de novo* DLBCL. Autologous stem cell transplantation is a consideration in these patients. In a multicenter analysis of 172 patients with transformed FL, improved outcomes were seen in patients treated with autologous stem cell transplantation.[28] The use of high-dose therapy with ASCT in the treatment of FL has not been fully established. A meta-analysis reported that high-dose therapy and ASCT does not improve OS in FL.[29] The International Bone Marrow Transplant Registry reported on 904 patients with FL. In 176 allogeneic SCT, 131 purged ASCT, and 597 unpurged transplants, the recurrence rates were 21%, 43%, and 58% with 5-year OS rates of 51%, 62%, and 55%.[30]

Second-generation anti-CD20 antibodies are active. Obinutuzumab, a second-generation type 2 anti-CD20 antibody, has a 50% overall response rate. With combination chemotherapy, progression-free survival rates are superior. In the GADOLIN study, patients refractory to rituximab were randomized to obinutozumab plus bendamustine or bendamustine monotherapy with patients non-progressing in the obinutuzumab group going on the maintenance obinutuzumab.[31] The progression-free survival was improved in patients treated with bendamustine and obinutuzumab. Reported overall response rate (ORR) with lenalidomide in the relapsed/refractory setting were approximately 30%.[32] When combined with rituximab, the complete remission (CR) rate was 87%, which has led to a multicenter phase III open-label, randomized study comparing lenalidomide and rituximab versus rituximab chemotherapy followed by rituximab maintenance in previously untreated patients (the "RELEVANCE" [Rituximab Lenalidomide versus Any Chemotherapy] trial).[33]

Cardiovascular Risk

The major cardiovascular risks are associated with anthracyclines (see above) and rituximab. Severe cardiovascular complications can be encountered during an infusion reaction, including hypotension, hypoxia, acute myocardial infarction, Takotsubo's arrhythmias, and cardiogenic shock. Otherwise, hypertension has been reported as well as minor hypotensive episodes. The risk of cardiotoxicity is not higher with the combination of anthracyclines with rituximab than with anthracyclines alone. There are no severe cardiovascular complications with bendamustine or obinutozumab limiting their use.

MARGINAL ZONE LYMPHOMA

KEY POINTS ABOUT MARGINAL ZONE LYMPHOMA

- The three types of marginal zone lymphoma (MZL) are nodal, splenic, and extranodal.
- The approaches to treatment are diverse.

Incidence

The prevalence among all lymphomas of MZL is 8.3%, and 1.1% for lymphoplasmacytic lymphoma, with an annual incidence rate of 1.8 per 100,000.[2]

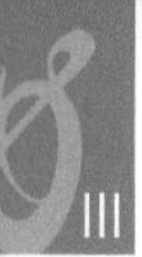

Risk Factors

In contrast to other NHL subtypes, there is not a male dominance in MZL. With regard to etiology, Sjögren syndrome is a risk factor in MZL. In MZL, *Helicobacter pylori* is associated with gastric lymphoma. HCV plays a role in some types of MZL. Decreased risk was associated with alcohol consumption in MZL and LPL/WM in a study of 17,471 cases and 23,096 controls. Incidence rates for MZL are lower in among African-Americans and Hispanics.

Prognosis

In contrast to aggressive lymphomas, the 2-year survival rates range from 89% to 95% in MZL and 88% to 93% in FL.

TREATMENT OVERVIEW

Extranodal Marginal Zone Lymphoma

Exranodal MZL involve many organs, including gastric, lung, parotid gland, and various other sites. Radiation therapy is utilized in many patients.

The National Comprehensive Cancer Network and the European Society of Medical Oncology (ESMO) have published practice guidelines for diagnosis, treatment, and follow up of gastric MZL.[34] *H. pylori* eradication with triple therapy (proton pump inhibitor, amoxicillin, and clarithromycin) or quadruple therapy (proton pump inhibitor, bismuth, tetracycline, and metronidazole) are the standard therapies for gastric MALT, irrespective of stage. Of patients, 75% to 85% respond to the antimicrobial therapy. With long-term follow up, 30% of patients are in CR, and 60% of patients remain stable for years. In a meta-analysis of 1408 patients, the ORR for stage IE disease was 78%.[35] The CR rate with radiation therapy was 100% with an event-free survival of 100%.[36] This is the treatment of choice in patients who have relapsed after antibiotic therapy. The ORR after HPE therapy with single agent rituximab was 77% with a CR rate of 46% and with 54% of patients disease free.[37] The approaches to FL are the same approaches in advanced MZL and are supported by the NCCN guidelines.

Pulmonary MZL is most commonly limited in stage, with only 14% of patients in the largest published series having stage III/IV disease.[38] The 10-year OS was about 75%. Treatment approaches include observation, surgery to remove the lesion if a single site, single-agent rituximab, and systemic chemotherapy. Observation or a "watch and wait" approach may be incorporated at the time of initial diagnosis or in asymptomatic patients who have relapsed. In patients treated with a local approach, mainly surgical resection, there was an improved progression-free survival versus those receiving systemic treatment in the International Extranodal Lymphoma Study Group (IELSG) study where 63 (30%) of patients underwent surgical resection of the disease and experienced an improved PFS (P = .003). Systemic treatment approaches include single-agent rituximab or immunochemotherapy which would include BR, R-CVP, or R-CHOP as in the FL treatment. The PFS at 5-years in the IELSG study was 65%. Systemic treatment is reserved for patients with advanced disease, patients who are in relapse after incomplete surgical resection, and for patients who have relapsed. Patients who relapse with nonbulky disease and who are asymptomatic may be observed.

The majority of patients with parotid MZL present with limited-stage disease (76% in IELSG 41).[39] Patients with parotid gland MZL have a long survival. The median survival was 18.3 years in the IELSG 41 study, and the median time to progression was 9.3 years. Patients with salivary gland MALT lymphoma have an excellent prognosis regardless of initial treatment.

Splenic Marginal Zone Lymphoma

Splenic MZL accounts for 20% of MZL cases. In patients with significant splenomegaly, splenectomy is a treatment option and patients experience a prolonged disease-free survival. Rituximab as a single agent has significant activity. This can be performed safely and offers durable long-term remissions in a number of patients. Anti-HCV therapy is efficacious i seropositive.

Nodal Marginal Zone Lymphoma

Nodal MZL accounts for 10% of MZL cases. Th 5-year OS was 56% in nodal MZL as opposed to 81 in MALT lymphoma, with a respective 5-year failure free survival rates of 28% and 56%. The treatment o nodal MZL is according to FL algorithms, which i the current recommendation of the NCCN guide lines. Initial management strategies include observa tion, single-agent rituximab, and immunochemothe apy. In a study that randomized patients after fou weekly doses of rituximab to maintenance rituxima versus observation in the ECOG trial E4402, an improvement was found in the time to treatment failure in patients who were treated with rituximab 375 mg/m^2 weekly four times followed by maintenance rituximab every 3 months until treatment failure.[40] In patients with advanced disease, immunochemotherapy is the treatment of choice. The transformation rates are 12.5% to 18%, and these patients should be treated in similar treatment patterns as DLBCL.

Cardiovascular Risk

Anthracycline and rituximab therapies are associated with cardiotoxicity as above.

LYMPHOPLASMACTYTIC LYMPHOMA/ WALDENSTRÖM'S MACROGLOBULINEMIA

KEY POINTS ABOUT WALDENSTRÖM'S MACROGLOBULINEMIA

- Spike on serum protein electrophoresis secondary to monoclonal protein in WM
- Ibrutinib is an active targeted agent in this disease.

Incidence

The prevalence among all lymphomas is 1.1% for the lymphoplasmacytic lymphoma and incidence is 0.6 per 100,000.[2,3]

Risk Factors

Sjögren syndrome is a risk factor for LPL/WM. There is an association of hepatitis C in LPL/WM. Decreased risk was associated with alcohol consumption in LPL/WM in a study of 17,471 cases and 23,096 controls. Incidence rates for LP lymphomas are lower among African-Americans and Hispanics.

Treatment Overview

LPL/WM is not curable and it has a heterogeneous course. Waldenström macoglobulinemia must be differentiated from an IgM monoclonal protein of undetermined significance (MGUS) and smoldering LPL/WM. Greater than 90% of LPL/WM harbor the *MYD88* L265P genetic mutation. This mutation is not specific to LPL/WM because 50% of IgM MGUS, 30% of DLBCL of nongerminal center type, 50% of primary cutaneous DLBCL, leg type, and some cases of nodal and splenic marginal zone harbor the mutation.

Treatment approaches are as follows.[41] Patients with IgM MGUS or smoldering LPL/WM with preserved marrow function should be observed with follow up. When treatment is indicated, different options exist. Single-agent rituximab results in a median PFS of 16 to 29 months with an ORR of 25% to 40%. Rituximab monotherapy is contraindicated in patients with symptomatic hyperviscosity and is best avoided in patients with very high serum IgM levels. Plasma exchange should be urgently initiated before immunochemotherapy for hyperviscosity-related symptoms, which include spontaneous bleeding from mucous membranes, visual changes from retinopathy, and neurologic symptoms (ranging from headache and vertigo to seizures and coma).

Immunochemotherapy: Bendamustine rituximab is recommended for bulky disease, significant cytopenias, and constitutional symptoms. Dexamethasone-rituximab-cyclophosphamide is an alternative for nonbulky disease. Stem cell harvest should be considered for future use in patients aged 70 and younger who are potential candidates for ASCT.

In patients who have relapsed, the original therapy may be considered if the time to next therapy is 3 years or more. In patients harboring *MYD88* L265P mutation, ibrutinib is efficacious.[42]

Cardiovascular Risk

Ibrutinib is associated with atrial arrhythmias as well as ventricular arrhythmias and, most commonly, hypertension; bradycardia is rare.

HODGKIN LYMPHOMA

KEY POINTS ABOUT HODGKIN LYMPHOMA

- The histologies of Hodgkin lymphoma (HL) include nodular sclerosis classic, mixed cellularity HL, lymphocytic-rich HL, lymphocyte-depleted HL, and nodular lymphocyte predominant HL.
- HL is the model of therapy for potentially curing a malignant disease with radiation therapy, combination

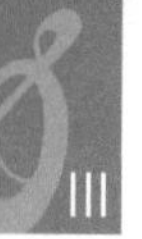

chemotherapy, autologous peripheral blood stem cell transplantation, and immunotherapy. Initial treatment is based on stage.

- ABVD (Adriamycin, bleomycin, vinblastine, and dacarbazine) is the backbone of treatment for HL in North America.
- Prognosis is excellent, with overall survival exceeding 90% in patients with limited stage disease and 75% with advanced disease.
- Therapeutic approaches have decreased the risks of long-term toxicities, including cardiomyopathy secondary to radiation therapy and anthracyclines, pulmonary fibrosis secondary to bleomycin and radiation therapy, secondary cancers (breast, lung, esophageal, skin, and others), acute leukemia, and non-Hodgkin lymphoma (4% risk at 10 years).

Incidence

One in ten lymphomas are Hodgkin lymphoma (HL) in the recent decades. In the last decade the annual estimated number of new cases was 8500.

Risk Factors

HL is associated with the Epstein Barr virus.

Prognosis

In the phase III North American Intergroup E2496 trial in patients with advanced disease, the CR rates were 73% and, at a median follow up of 6.4 years, the failure-free survival was 74% for patients treated with ABVD.[43] The majority of relapses occurred in the first 2 years in the ABVD arm, which is the current standard of care internationally. A prognostic scoring system was developed in the study of 854 patients.[44] Age greater than or equal to 45, hemoglobin of less than 10.5 g/dL in stage IV disease were adverse prognostic factors. The 5-year progression-free survival was 83 % with 0 factors, 74% with 1 factor, and 63% with 3 factors.

Treatment Overview

Initial treatment is based on stage. Of patients, 30% present with a favorable stage HL (stage IA, IB, and IIA; mediastinal mass <7 cm; no extranodal disease; erythrocyte sedimentation rate (ESR) <30 mm/h; and fewer than 3 nodal sites). In the German Hodgkin Lymphoma Study Group trial HD10 four-arm randomized clinical trial with 287 to 288 patients in each arm, patients treated with 2 cycles of ABVD followed by 20 Gy of radiation therapy had an OS of 95.1% at 8 years.[45] In patients with a negative PET scan, radiation therapy can be omitted with the results from the UK RAPID trial where the patients were randomized to 30 Gy radiation therapy versus observation and the 3-year progression-free survival was 94.6% and 90.8%, respectively.[46] Patients with early unfavorable HL disease (large mediastinal mass (>7 cm) [a]; extanodal disease [b], increased ESR (>30 mm/h) [c]; 3 or more nodal areas; IIB with c or d) are treated with ABVD for 4 cycles and 30 Gy radiation therapy as per the HD 14 trial.[47] In the phase III North American Intergroup E2496 trial in patients with advanced disease where patients were treated with 6 cycles of ABVD chemotherapy and 36 Gy of modified involved field radiation therapy to the mediastinum, hila, and supraclavicular nodes for a mass greater than 10 cm, the CR rates were 73% and at a median follow up of 6.4 years the failure-free survival was 74% for patients treated with ABVD.[43] For those who received radiation therapy, the 5-year failure-free survival was 85%.[43] In the ECHELON-1 trial, the substitution of brentuximab vedotin for bleomycin resulted in an improvement in progression-free survival.[48]

In patients who relapse, ASCT results in long-term remission in 30% to 60% of patients. Brentuximab vedotin, and anti-CD30 conjugate, resulted in a 5-year PFS rate of 22% in 102 patients treated.[49] Nivolumab, an IgG4 anti-PD-1 antibody, selectively blocks PD-1 and PD-L1/PD-L2 interactions. In the initial trial, the overall response rate was 87% with a CR rate of 17%.[50] These two biologic agents are now main therapies in the relapsed setting in patients with relapsed refractory HL.

Cardiovascular Risk

Patients are at significant risk of cardiovascular disease when treated with doxorubicin or radiation therapy. The doses utilized in the 1980s, 44 Gy with a boost, are no longer employed, significantly reducing the risk of coronary artery disease and heart valve disease (see corresponding chapters).

CONCLUSION

Remarkable advances have been made in the diagnosis and management of lymphoid neoplasms. Radiation management strategies have changed remarkably in the last decade in HL. Cardiac side effects, including anthracycline-induced cardiomyopathy and cardiac arrhythmias, with biologic agents, such as rituximab and ibrutinib, require future research, monitoring, and a team-based approach.

REFERENCES

1. Swerdlow SH, Campo E, Harris NL, et al., eds. *WHO Classification of Tumours of Haematopoietic and Lymphoid Tissues*. Revised 4th ed. Lyon: IARC; 2017.
2. Al-Hamadani M, Habermann TM, Cerhan JR, et al. Non-Hodgkin lymphoma subtype distribution, geodemographic patterns, and survival in the US: a longitudinal analysis of the National Cancer Data Base from 1998 to 2011. *Am J Hematol*. 2015;90(9):790–795.
3. Teras LR, DeSantis CE, Cerhan JR, et al. 2016 US lymphoid malignancy statistics by World Health Organization subtypes. *CA Cancer J Clin*. 2016;66:(6)443–459.
4. The International Non-Hodgkin's Lymphoma Prognostic Factors Project. A predictive model for aggressive non-Hodgkin's lymphoma. *N Engl J Med*. 1993;329:987–994.
5. Chapuy B, Stewart C, Dunford AJ, et al. Molecular subtypes of diffuse large B cell lymphoma are associated with distinct pathogenic mechanisms and outcomes. *Nat Med*. 2018;24(5):679–690.
6. Zelenetz AD, Gordon LI, Abramson JS, et al. B-cell lymphomas, version 3.2019 featured updates to the NCCN guidelines. *J Natl Compr Canc Netw*. 2019:651–661.
7. Maurer MJ, Jais JP, Ghesquieres H, et al. Personalized risk prediction for event-free survival at 24 months in patients with diffuse large B-cell lymphoma. *Am J Hematol*. 2016;91:179–184.
8. Farooq U, Maurer MJ, Thompson CA, et al. Clinical heterogeneity of diffuse large B cell lymphoma following failure of front-line immunochemotherapy. *Br J Haematol*. 2017;179:50–60.
9. Maurer MJ, Ghesquieres H, Jais JP, et al. Event-free survival at 24 months is a robust end point for disease-related outcome in diffuse large B-cell lymphoma treated with immunochemotherapy. *J Clin Oncol*. 2014;32:1066–1073.
10. Maurer MJ, Habermann TM, Shi Q, et al. Progression-free survival at 24 months (PFS24) and subsequent outcome for patients with diffuse large B-cell lymphoma (DLBCL) enrolled on randomized clinical trials. *Ann Oncol*. 2018;29:1822–1827.
11. Wang Y, Farooq U, Link BK, et al. Late relapses in patients with diffuse large B-cell lymphoma treated with immunochemotherapy. *J Clin Oncol*. 2019;37:1819–1827.
12. Dierickx D, Habermann TM. Post-transplantation lymphoproliferative disorders in adults. *N Engl J Med*. 2018;378:549–562.
13. Habermann TM, Fama A, Ristow, KM, et al. Clinical characteristics and outcomes of an analysis of a single institution experience of the 2017 World Health Organization (WHO) Classification of post-transplant lymphoproliferative disorders (PTLD). *Blood*. 2018; 132(suppl 1):456.
14. McPhail ED, Maurer MJ, Macon WR, et al. Inferior survival in high-grade B-cell lymphoma with MYC and BCL2 and/or BCL6 rearrangements is not associated with MYC/IG gene rearrangements. *Haematologica*. 2018;103:1899–1907.
15. King RL, Khurana A, Mwangi R, Fama A, Ristow KM, Maurer MJ, Macon WR, Ansell SM, Bennani NN, Kudva YC, Walker RC, Watt KD, Schwab TR, Kushwaha SS, Cerhan JR, Habermann TM. Clinicopathologic Characteristics, Treatment, and Outcomes of Post-transplant Lymphoproliferative Disorders: A Single-institution Experience Using 2017 WHO Diagnostic Criteria. *Hemasphere*. 2021 Oct; 5 (10):e640 Epub 2021 Sept 06.
16. Maurer MJ, Ellin F, Srour L, et al. International assessment of event-free survival at 24 months and subsequent survival in peripheral T-cell lymphoma. *J Clin Oncol*. 2017;35:4019–4026.
17. Von Hoff DD, Layard MW, Basa P, et al. Risk factors for doxorubicin-induced congestive heart failure. *Ann Int Med*. 1979;91:710–717.
18. Hershman DL, McBride RB, Eisenberger A, et al. Doxorubicin, cardiac risk factors, and cardiac toxicity in elderly patients with diffuse large B-cell non-Hodgkin's lymphoma. *J Clin Oncol*. 2008; 26:3159–3165.
19. Bachy E, Maurer MJ, Habermann TM, et al. A simplified scoring system in de novo follicular lymphoma treated initially with immunochemotherapy. *Blood*. 2018;132:49–58.
20. Maurer MJ, Bachy E, Ghesquiéres H, et al. Early event status informs subsequent outcome in newly diagnosed follicular lymphoma. *Am J Hematol*. 2016;91:1096–1101.
21. Sarkozy C, Maurer MJ, Link BK, et al. Cause of death in follicular lymphoma in the first decade of the rituximab era: a pooled analysis of French and US cohorts. *J Clin Oncol*. 2019;37:144–152.
22. St-Pierre F, Broski SM, LaPlant BR, et al. Detection of extranodal and spleen involvement by FDG-PET imaging predicts adverse survival in untreated follicular lymphoma. *Am J Hematol*. 2019; 94(7):786–793.
23. Brice P, Bastion Y, Lepage E, et al. Comparison in low-tumor-burden follicular lymphomas between and initial no treatment policy, prednimustine, and interferon alfa: a randomized study from the Groupe d'Edude des Lymphomes Folliculares-Groupe d'Etude des Lymphomes de l'Adulte. *J Clin Oncol*. 1997;15:1110–1117.
24. Ardeshna KM, Qian W, Smith P, et al. Rituximab versus a watch-and-wait approach in patients with advanced-stage, asymptomatic, non-bulky follicular lymphoma: an open-label randomized phase 3 trial. *Lancet Oncol*. 2014;15:424–435.
25. Kahl BS, Hong F, Williams ME, et al. Rituximab extended schedule or re-treatment trial for low-tumor burden follicular lymphoma: Eastern Cooperative Oncology Group protocol E4402. *J Clin Oncol*. 2014;32:3096–3102.
26. Nooka AK, Nabhan C, Zhou X, et al. Examination of the follicular lymphoma international prognostic index (FLIPI) in the National Lympho Care study (NLCS): a prospective US patient cohort treated predominantly in community practices. *Ann Oncol*. 2013; 24:441–448.
27. Link BK, Maurer MJ, Nowakowski G, et al. Rates and outcomes of follicular lymphoma transformation in the immunochemotherapy era: a report from the University of Iowa/Mayo Clinic Specialized Program of Research Excellence Molecular Epidemiology Resource. *J Clin Oncol*. 2013;31:3272–3278.
28. Villa D, Crump M, Panzarella T, et al. Autologous and allogeneic stem-cell transplantation for transformed follicular lymphoma: a report of the Canadian blood and marrow transplant group. *J Clin Oncol*. 2013;31:1164–1171.
29. Al Khabori M, de Almeida JR, Guyatt GH, et al. Autologous stem cell transplantation in follicular lymphoma: a systemic review and meta-analysis. *J Natl Cancer Inst*. 2012;104:18–28.
30. van Besien K, Loberiza FR Jr, Bajorunaite R, et al. Comparison of autologous and allogenic stem cell transplantation for follicular lymphoma. *Blood*. 2003;102:3521–3529.
31. Sehn LH, Chua N, Mayer J, et al. Obinutuzumab plus bendamustine versus bendamustine monotherapy in patients with rituximab-refractory indolent non-Hodgkin lymphoma (GADOLIN): a randomized, open-label, multicenter, phase 3 trial. *Lancet Oncol*. 2016; 17:1081–1088.
32. Witzig TE, Nowakowski GS, Habermann TM, et al. A comprehensive review of lenalidomide therapy for B-cell non-Hodgkin lymphoma. *Ann Oncol*. 2015;26:1667–1677.
33. Morschhauser F, Fowler NH, Feugier P, et al. Rituximab plus lenalidomide in advanced untreated follicular lymphoma. *N Engl J Med*. 2018;379:934–947.
34. Zucca E, Copie-Bergman C, Ricardi U, et al. Gastric marginal zone lymphoma of MALT type: ESMO clinical practice guidelines for diagnosis, treatment, and follow-up. *Ann Oncol*. 2013;24(suppl 6): vi144–vi148.
35. Zullo A, Hassan C, Cristofari F, et al. Effects of *Helicobacter pylori* eradication on early stage gastric mucosa-associated lymphoid tissue lymphoma. *Clin Gastroenterol Hepatol*. 2010;8:105–110.
36. Schechter NR, Portlock CS, Yahalom J, et al. Treatment of mucosa-associated lymphoid tissue lymphoma of the stomach with radiation alone. *J Clin Oncol*. 1998;16:1916–1921.
37. Martinelli G, Laszlo D, Ferreri AJ, et al. Clinical activity of rituximab in gastric marginal zone non-Hodgkin lymphoma resistant to

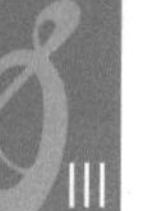

or not eligible for anti-*Helicobacter pylori* therapy. *J Clin Oncol.* 2005;23:1979–1983.

38. Sammassimo S, Pruneri G, Andreola G, et al. A retrospective international study on primary extranodal marginal zone lymphoma of the lung (BALT lymphoma) on behalf of International Extranodal Lymphoma Study Group (IELSG). *Hematol Oncol.* 2016;34:177–183.
39. Jackson ME, Mian M, Kalpakais CH, et al. Extranodal marginal zone lymphoma of mucosa-associated lymphoid tissue of the salivary glands: a multicenter, international experience of 248 patients (IELSG 41). *Oncologist.* 2015;20:1149–1153.
40. Williams ME, Hong F, Gascoyne RD, et al. Rituximab extended schedule or retreatment trial for low tumour burden non-follicular indolent B-cell non-Hodgkin lymphomas: Eastern Cooperative Oncology Group Protocol E4402. *Br J Haematol.* 2016;173:867–875.
41. Kapoor P, Ansell SM, Fonseca R, et al. Diagnosis and management of Waldenström macroglobulinemia Mayo stratification of macroglobulinemia and risk-adapted therapy (mSMART) guidelines 2016. *JAMA Oncol.* 2017;3:1257–1265.
42. Treon SP, Tripas CK, Meid K, et al. Ibrutinib in previously treated Waldenström's macroglobulinemia. *N Engl J Med.* 2015;372:1430–1440.
43. Advani RH, Hong F, Fisher RI, et al. Randomized phase III trial comparing ABVD plus radiotherapy with the Stanford V Regimen in patients with stages I or II locally extensive, bulky mediastinal Hodgkin lymphoma: a subset analysis of the North American Intergroup E2496 trial. *J Clin Oncol.* 2015;33(17):1936–1942.
44. Diefenbach CS, Li H, Hong F, et al. Evaluation of the International Prognostic Score (IPS-7) and a Simpler Prognostic Score (IPS-3) for advanced Hodgkin lymphoma in the modern era. *Br J Haematol.* 2015;171(4):530–538.
45. Engert A, Plütschow A, Eich HT, et al. Reduced treatment intensity in patients with early-stage Hodgkin's lymphoma. *N Engl J Med.* 2010;363:640–652.
46. Johnson P, Federico M, Kirkwood A, et al. Adapted treatment guided by interim PET-CT scan in advanced Hodgkin's lymphoma. *N Engl J Med.* 2016;374:2419–2429.
47. Eich HT, Diehl V, Görgen H, et al. Intensified chemotherapy and dose-reduced involved-field radiotherapy in patients with early unfavorable Hodgkin's lymphoma: final analysis of the German Hodgkin Study Group HD11 trial. *N Engl J Med.* 2010;28: 4199–4206.
48. Connors JM, Jurczak W, Straus DJ, et al. Brentuximab vedotin with chemotherapy for stage III or IV Hodgkin's lymphoma. *N Engl J Med.* 2018;378:331–344.
49. Chen R, Gopal A, Smith SE, et al. Five-year survival and durability results of brentuximab vedotin in patients with relapsed or refractory Hodgkin lymphoma. *Blood.* 2016;128:1562–1566.
50. Ansell SM, Lesokhim AM, Borrello I, et al. PD-1 blockade with nivolumab in relapsed or refractory Hodgkin's lymphoma. *N Engl J Med.* 2015;372:311–319.

51 Multiple Myeloma and Cardiac Amyloidosis

ANGELA DISPENZIERI

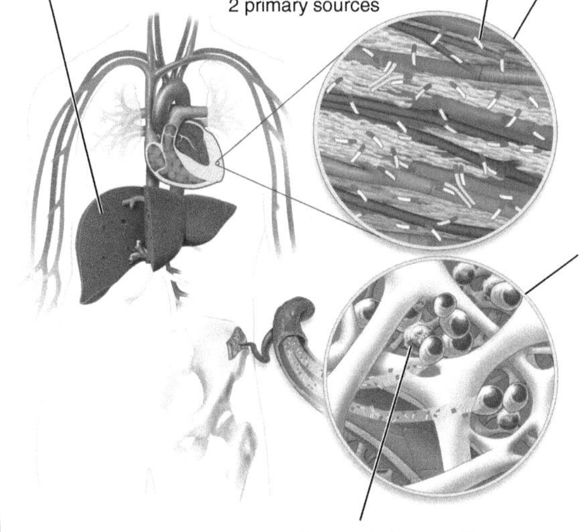

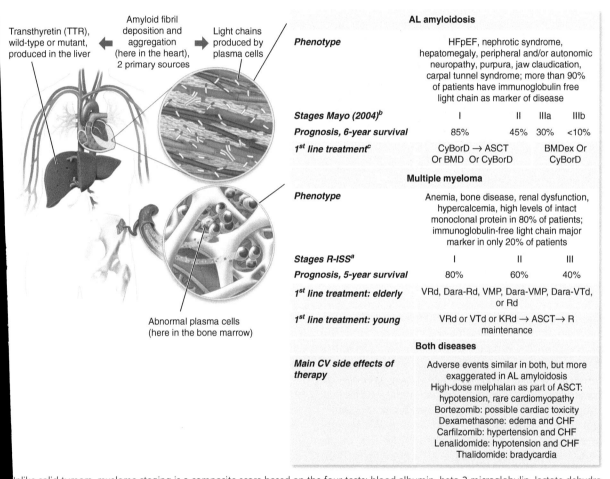

Transthyretin (TTR), wild-type or mutant, produced in the liver

Amyloid fibril deposition and aggregation (here in the heart), 2 primary sources

Light chains produced by plasma cells

Abnormal plasma cells (here in the bone marrow)

	AL amyloidosis			
Phenotype	HFpEF, nephrotic syndrome, hepatomegaly, peripheral and/or autonomic neuropathy, purpura, jaw claudication, carpal tunnel syndrome; more than 90% of patients have immunoglobulin free light chain as marker of disease			
Stages Mayo (2004)[b]	I	II	IIIa	IIIb
Prognosis, 6-year survival	85%	45%	30%	<10%
1st line treatment[c]	CyBorD → ASCT Or BMD Or CyBorD		BMDex Or CyBorD	
	Multiple myeloma			
Phenotype	Anemia, bone disease, renal dysfunction, hypercalcemia, high levels of intact monoclonal protein in 80% of patients; immunoglobulin-free light chain major marker in only 20% of patients			
Stages R-ISS[a]	I	II	III	
Prognosis, 5-year survival	80%	60%	40%	
1st line treatment: elderly	VRd, Dara-Rd, VMP, Dara-VMP, Dara-VTd, or Rd			
1st line treatment: young	VRd or VTd or KRd → ASCT→ R maintenance			
	Both diseases			
Main CV side effects of therapy	Adverse events similar in both, but more exaggerated in AL amyloidosis High-dose melphalan as part of ASCT: hypotension, rare cardiomyopathy Bortezomib: possible cardiac toxicity Dexamethasone: edema and CHF Carfilzomib: hypertension and CHF Lenalidomide: hypotension and CHF Thalidomide: bradycardia			

Jnlike solid tumors, myeloma staging is a composite score based on the four tests: blood albumin, beta-2 microglobulin, lactate dehydro- enate (LDH), and bone marrow Fluorescent *in situ* hybridization (FISH). Stage I is albumin 3.5 g/dL or greater, beta-2 microglobulin is less han 3.5 mg/L, normal LDH, and no high-risk FISH. Stage III is beta-2 microglobulin 5.5 mg/L or greater and either high LDH or high-risk SH. Stage II is neither stage I nor III. T two amyloid staging systems are commonly used. Both are from the Mayo Clinic. The first is purely ased on troponin and NT-proBNP (above), and the second is the Mayo (2012) system, which also includes the immunoglobulin free light hain, a measure of tumor burden. The Mayo (2004) system uses the following cut-offs: Stage I, troponin T less than 0.035 mcg/L and T-proBNP less than 332 ng/L; stage II, either troponin T 0.035 μg/L or greater or NT-proBNP greater than 332 ng/L; stage IIIa, both tro- pnin T 0.035 μg/L or greater, and NT-proBNP greater than 332 ng/L, but NT-proBNP less than 8500 ng/L; stage IIIa, both troponin T 0.035 g/L or greater and NT-proBNP greater than 8500 ng/L. See Table 51.2 for conversion factors when troponin I, high-sensitivity troponin T BNP are the only available assays. A hard cut-off for ASCT is a troponin T greater than 0.06 μg/L ASCT, autologous stem cell transplant ter high-dose melphalan; B, bor, or V, bortezomib (Velcade); C or Cy, cyclophosphamide; CHF, congestive heart failure; D or d, dexa- ethasone; Dara, daratumumab (Darzylex); HFpEF, heart failure with preserved ejection fraction; K, carfilzomib (Kyprolis); M, melphalan; prednisone; R, lenalidomide (Revlimid); R-ISS, revised international staging system; T, thalidomide.

CHAPTER OUTLINE

KEY POINTS

- In the United States the 2018 annual estimate for new cases of multiple myeloma (MM) is 30,770 and of deaths is 12,770.[1]
- The incidence of immunoglobulin light-chain (AL) amyloidosis is 12 cases per million per year.[2] It is imperative that AL amyloidosis be distinguished from both the inherited and the acquired form of transthyretin (ATTR) amyloidosis.
- Neither disease is thought to be curable, although young patients with Revised International Staging System (R-ISS) stage I myeloma are expected to have a median overall survival of 8 to 10 years. More than 20% of patients with AL amyloidosis are alive at 10 years.
- For fit patients with AL amyloidosis, autologous stem cell transplant (ASCT) is considered to an important part of therapy, although there are differing interpretations of the data in terms of the relative importance of ASCT for this disease.
- Treatment of amyloidosis is directed to the cause of fibril production.
- Cardiovascular aspects with therapy pertain to the use of immune modulatory drugs in MM, which require consideration for thrombo prophylaxis, and proteasome inhibitor in both MM and AL amyloidosis, which can lead to heart failure presentations (esp., carfilzomib).

INTRODUCTION

Multiple myeloma (MM) and immunoglobulin light chain amyloidosis are plasma cell disorders. Both are characterized by increased clonal plasma cells in the bone marrow and detectable monoclonal proteins in the serum and/or urine. After lymphoma, myeloma is the second most common hematologic malignancy, comprising 1.8% of all malignancies. Immunoglobulin light chain (AL) amyloidosis is about one-fifth as common as MM, and approximately 10% to 15% of patients with myeloma will have AL amyloidosis. Both are diseases of the elderly, with median ages at diagnosis of approximately 70 years.[1,2] Men are 1.6 times more likely to develop MM, and African-Americans are twice as likely to develop MM than whites.

DIAGNOSIS AND DIFFERENTIAL DIAGNOSIS

As shown in the Central Illustration, clinical manifestations are dissimilar for the two diseases. In myeloma, the defining symptoms and signs are anemia, bone pain (or asymptomatic lesions), hypercalcemia, renal dysfunction, and high levels of serum monoclonal proteins (most commonly found on serum protein electrophoresis), and bone marrow plasma cells. When present, fatigue is a function of anemia, renal failure, or hypercalcemia. Occasionally, significant abnormalities are incidentally found even before patients are symptomatic. One must distinguish MM from its truly asymptomatic form (smoldering myeloma) and from its precancerous form (monoclonal gammopathy of undetermined significance).

The diagnosis of AL amyloidosis is often more challenging than that of MM. Fatigue and edema are the most common presenting symptoms. Fatigue often relates to heart failure with preserved ejection fraction (HFpEF) and edema to either cardiomyopathy and/or nephrotic syndrome. The cardiomyopathy of AL amyloidosis is frequently overlooked in part owing to the preserved ejection fraction, and there are significant delays before a diagnosis is made.[3] Patients may have hepatomegaly with a cholestatic picture, a small fiber peripheral neuropathy, autonomic dysfunction, signs of microvascula involvement (periorbital purpura, jaw claudication), early satiety, or changes in their bowel patterns. The diagnosis is made by a tissue biopsy with (sub-) typing of the amyloid to prove that it is indeed AL amyloidosis rather than another form of inherited or acquired amyloidosis (Table 51.1). Elevated serum immunoglobulin free light chains and/or the presence of a monoclonal protein by immunofixation are supportive of a diagnosis of AL amyloidosis, but not definitive. The differential diagnosis for AL amyloidosis includes monoclonal gammopathy of undetermined significance, MM, and other types of amyloidosis, especially wild type transthyretin ($ATTR_{wt}$) amyloidosis. The diagnosis of acquired form of transthyretin (ATTR) amyloidosis can be made with a positive 99m-technetium pyrophosphate (PYP) or 99m-technetium (99mTc) and 3,3-diphosphono-1,2-propanodicarboxylic acid (DPD) scan in the ABSENCE of a monoclonal protein by immunofixation or by serum immunoglobulin free light chain assay (Fig. 51.1).[4] Cardiac imaging with echocardiography and magnetic resonance imaging can help support a diagnosis of AL amyloidosis, but neither is diagnostic nor can either distinguish AL from ATTR. This holds true also for echo strain imaging, although apical sparring on the bull's eye view of global longitudinal strain ("cherry on top" appearance) should prompt further investigation into amyloidosis (sensitivity 96%, specificity 88% in patients without coronary artery disease). Increased left ventricular wall thickness, septal hypertrophy with granular sparking myocardium, and pericardial and pleural effusions are other echocardiographic features of amyloidosis. Lack of R-wave progression in the precordial leads (pseudoinfarction pattern) and low voltage are the classic electrocardiographic features, but have low sensitivity. A QTc greater than 440 ms and a Sokolow-Lyon index equal to or less than 1.5 mV have a sensitivity of 85% and a specificity of 100% for cardiac amyloidosis, mainly the AL subtype. The diagnosis of AL always requires a Congo red positive tissue biopsy that has been typed to be composed of immunoglobulins.

PROGNOSIS

For patients with MM, staging is not directly related to tumor burden, but rather the genetics of the tumor (i.e., plasma cells), which is most commonly determined by fluorescent *in situ* hybridization (FISH). Certain cytogenetics, such as deletion 17p, translocation t(4;14), and t(14;20), are considered high-risk features. These bone marrow plasma cell abnormalities, along with serum albumin, serum beta-2 microglobulin, and lactate dehydrogenase (LDH) are the components of the Revised International Staging System (R-ISS), and patients are placed into three groups with discrete outcomes (Table 51.2).[5] The relative risk of death between each of the stages is approximately 3, yielding approximate 5-year overall survival rates of 80%, 60%, and 40%, respectively.

The greatest risk of death for patients with AL amyloidosis is during the first 6 to 12 months after diagnosis. It is during this period that approximately 30% of patients die.[6] After the first year, the slope of the survival curves, especially for those with stage III disease, becomes less steep. Overall, for patients with AL amyloidosis, 6-year survival

TABLE 51.1 Nomenclature of Most Common Forms of Amyloidosis Affecting the Heart

AMYLOID TYPE	PRECURSOR PROTEIN	CLINICAL
AL or AH	Immunoglobulin (light or heavy chain)	Immunoglobulin amyloidosis (formerly known as primary) Systemic or localized amyloidosis
$ATTR_{wt}$	Transthyretin	Age-related (formerly known as senile) amyloidosis; heart and ligaments
$ATTR_v$	Transthyretin, mutants	Familial amyloidosis; most often heart and/or nerve
AApoAI	Apolipoprotein AI, mutant	Kidney, liver, rarely heart, larynx, skin
AApoAII	Apolipoprotein AII, mutant	Kidney, heart
AApoAIV	Apolipoprotein AIV, no mutation recognized	Heart, kidney
AA	Serum amyloid A (SAA)	Secondary or familial Mediterranean fever; familial periodic fever syndromes associated with mutated tumor necrosis factor receptor; most often kidney; rarely heart

A, Secondary amyloid; *AH*, immunoglobulin heavy chain amyloid; *AL*, immunoglobulin light chain; *AApo*, apolipoprotein amyloid; *ATTR*, acquired form of transthyretin.

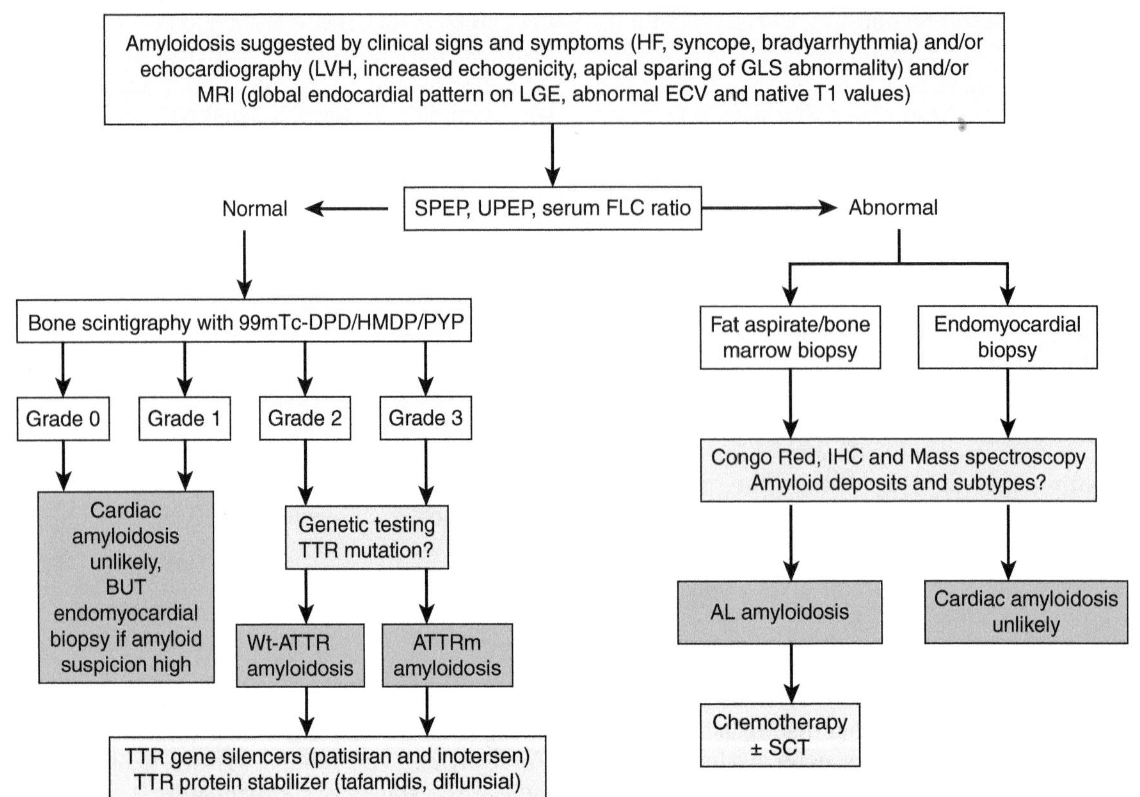

FIG. 51.1 Approach to a patient with suspected cardiac amyloidosis. *ECV,* Extracellular volume; *FLC,* free light chain ratio; *GLS,* global longitudinal strain; *HF,* heart failure; *HC,* immunohistochemistry; *LGE,* late gadolinium enhancement; *LVH,* left ventricular hypertrophy; *SCT,* stem cell transplantation; *TTR,* transthyretin.

rates are 85%, 45%, 30%, and less than 10% for patients with stage I, II, IIIa and IIIb, respectively.[7] Among those patients who achieve a deep hematologic response (a very good partial response or better), more than 80% of them are alive at 6 years. Staging for patients with AL amyloidosis is done using serum troponin, N-terminal pro-brain natriuretic peptide (NT-proBNP), and immunoglobulin free light chain (Tables 51.3 and 51.4).[8–12]

TREATMENT AND SIDE EFFECTS

Many of the drugs to treat these two conditions are the same as are the side effects but typically more severe in AL amyloidosis. Over the course of 15 years, nine drugs have been approved for MM, several of which are shown in Central Illustration. Other drugs used to treat myeloma not shown in the Central Illustration include pomalidomide (another immune modulatory drug [IMiD]), ixazomib (another proteasome inhibitor), daratumumab (an antibody directed at CD38), elotuzumab (an antibody directed at SLAMF7), and panobinostat (a histone deacetylase inhibitor). Additional promising drugs for the treatment of myeloma are in clinical trials (discussed below). Although there are no US Food and Drug Administration (FDA) approved drugs for the treatment of AL amyloidosis, many myeloma drugs are employed to treat this otherwise progressive and lethal disease. Such pharmacologic advances have resulted in approximately a doubling of overall survival for both MM and AL amyloidosis in the past two decades.[6,13,14]

Among patients with MM, treatment strategies are aligned with age (and functional status) and

TABLE 51.2 Prognostic Staging Systems in Multiple Myeloma

	DURIE-SALMON		INTERNATIONAL STAGING SYSTEM		REVISED INTERNATIONAL STAGING SYSTEM	
Stage I	Low cell mass: < 0.6 × 10^{12} cells/m^2 PLUS all of the following: Hgb > 10 g/dL Serum IgG <5 g/dL Serum IgA < 3 g/dL Normal serum calcium Urine monoclonal protein excretion < 4 g/day No generalized lytic bone lesions	62 months	β2M < 3.5 mg/L and serum albumin ≥3.5 g/dL	62 months	β2M < 3.5 mg/L and serum albumin ≥ 3.5 g/dL No high-risk cytogenetics (FISH) Normal LDH	82 months
Stage II	Neither stage I nor stage III	44 months	Neither stage I nor stage III	44 months	Neither stage I nor stage III	62 months
Stage III	High cell mass: > 1.2 × 10^{12} cells/m^2 PLUS ≥ 1 of the following: Hgb < 8.5 g/dL Serum IgG >7 g/dL Serum IgA > 5 g/dL Serum calcium > 12 mg/dL (3 μmol/L) Urine monoclonal protein excretion > 12 g/day Advanced lytic bone lesions	29 months	β2M ≥ 5.5 mg/L	29 months	β2M ≥ 5.5 mg/L PLUS ≥ 1 of the following: High-risk cytogenetics (FISH) T(4;14) T(14;16) Del(17p) LDH > ULN	40 months
Subclass	A: Serum creatinine < 2 mg/dL B: Serum creatinine ≥ 2 mg/dL					

FISH, fluorescent in situ hybridization; *LDH,* lactate dehydrogenase; *ULN,* upper limit of normal.

TABLE 51.3 Prognostic Biomarker-Based Staging Systems in Amyloidosis

	AL AMYLOIDOSIS	MODEL	MEDIAN OVERALL SURVIVAL
Revised Mayo Model[a]	cTnT ≥ 0.025 ug/L	Stage I = all negative	94.1 months
	NT-pro BNP ≥ 1800 ng/L	Stage II = 1 positive	40.3 months
	Difference between involved and uninvolved light chain > 180 mg/L	Stage III = 2 positive	14.0 months
		Stage IV = all positive	5.8 months
ATTR Amyloidosis			**Median Overall Survival**
National Amyloidosis Center[b]	NT-pro BNP > 3000 ng/L	Stage I = all negative	62.9 months
	eGFR < 45 mL/min/1.73 m^2	Stage II = 1 positive	46.7 months
		Stage III = all positive	24.1 months

[a]Kumar S, Dispenzieri A, Lacy MQ, et al. Revised prognostic staging system for light chain amyloidosis incorporating cardiac biomarkers and serum free light chain measurements. *J Clin Oncol.* 2012;30:989–995.
[b]Gillmore JD, Damy T, Fontana M, et al. A new staging system for cardiac transthyretin amyloidosis. *Eur Heart J.* 2018;39(30):2799–2806.
ATTR, Acquired form of transthyretin; *NT*-proBNP, N-terminal pro-brain natriuretic peptide.

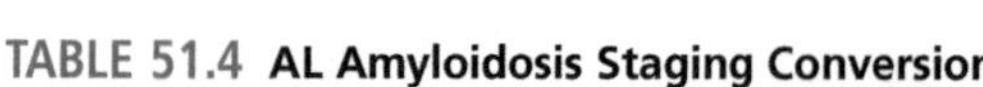

TABLE 51.4 AL Amyloidosis Staging Conversions

Model	cTnT, µg/L	cTnI, µg/L	Hs-cTnT, ng/L	NT-proBNP, ng/L	BNP, ng/L
Mayo 2004 model[a]	≥ 0.035	≥ 0.1	≥ 50[e]	≥ 332	81[g]
Euro 2015 modification of Mayo 2004 model[b]	≥ 0.035	≥ 0.1[f]	≥ 50 ng/L[e,f]	≥ 332 ≥ 8500	81[g] > 700[g]
Mayo 2012 model[c]	≥ 0.025	ND	>40f	≥ 1800	≥ 400[h]
Mayo ASCT troponin risk marker[d]	≥ 0.06	ND	≥75f	NA	NA

[a]Original three-stage model using cTnT and NT-proBNP cut-points as listed. cTnI also tested in same paper.
[b]Original three-stage model using cTnT and NT-proBNP cut-points as listed, but separate stage III into IIIa and IIIb based on whether or not NT-proBNP is higher than 8500 ng/L.
[c]A four-stage model using cTnT and NT-proBNP cut-points as listed along with difference of involved free light chain ≥ 18 mg/dL.
[d]Simple binary troponin T threshold predicting for transplant-related mortality 25% vs. 4%.
[e]In separate study, Hs-cTnT 54 found to be comparable to cTnT cut-point of 0.035, but reanalysis using quartic formula yielded 51 ng/L.
[f]Extrapolated numbers are based on quartic formula applied to a dataset of 224 newly diagnosed AL amyloidosis cases.[12]
[g]Separate study demonstrated similarity between original troponin T cut-offs and troponin I and BNP cut-offs.
[h]In Mayo 2012 study, this BNP threshold was found to be comparable to NT-proBNP.
ASCT, Autologous stem cell transplantation; *NA,* not applicable; *ND,* no data.
Modified from Muchtar E, Kumar SK, Gertz MA, et al. Staging systems use for risk stratification of systemic amyloidosis in the era of high-sensitivity troponin T assay. *Blood.* 2019;133:763–766.

cytogenetic risk more so than tumor burden or R-ISS stage. The general MM treatment plan is induction (typically the first 4 months of therapy), followed by consolidation (ASCT in those eligible or continuation of induction for non-ASCT candidates), and maintenance (most often lenalidomide, but in certain cases bortezomib, ixazomib, or carfilzomib).

The general strategy to treat AL amyloidosis is based on the extent of cardiac involvement (dysfunction) followed in part by tumor burden as measured by serum free light chains. The distinction between amyloid with and without myeloma is in part semantics because so much of the prognosis is dependent on cardiac involvement. Early death relates predominantly to the severity of cardiac impairment (Central Illustration). That said, clonal burden has an impact on both presentation and long-term outcomes. A patient with AL amyloidosis who has fewer than 10% bone marrow plasma cells at diagnosis is (1) less likely to have cardiac involvement, (2) more likely to have a very deep response to chemotherapy, that is a complete response; and (3) very likely to expect a median overall survival of greater than 10 to 15 years assuming they survive the first year after diagnosis. In contrast, those patients with AL amyloidosis with more than 10% to 20% bone marrow plasma cells, whether or not they have classic myeloma bone lesions or classic myeloma kidney, are (1) more likely to have cardiac involvement, (2) less likely to have a deep response to chemotherapy, and (3) in general have shorter long- term survival, even if they survive past the first year.[15,16]

TOXICITY OF THERAPY

Each of the different chemotherapeutic agents used to kill bone marrow plasma cells have their own cardiac toxicities, but a few additional general principles need to be considered as well. Virtually all chemotherapy is myelosuppressive, which increases a patient's risk of sepsis syndrome and all the cytokine-mediated toxicities that accompany it. Practically every regimen incorporates corticosteroids into the treatment plan—most often as a potent killer of plasma cells, but also sometimes as a knee-jerk antiemetic. The fluid retention that accompanies high-doses of weekly—and even sometimes daily—corticosteroids can aggravate hypertension, diastolic dysfunction, and systolic dysfunction, resulting in congestive heart failure (CHF). In addition, chronic steroid use can result in reduced adrenal reserve or frank adrenal insufficiency, resulting in cardiovascular collapse when stressed. The use of beta-blockers in patients with myeloma has been associated with a better overall survival in a retrospective study.[17] In contrast, beta-blockers and calcium channel blockers (anything that slows the heart rate) can precipitate worsening functional status and even CHF among patients with AL amyloidosis.

Monitoring and Management of Cardiotoxicity

Understanding a patient's baseline cardiac risk factors is a first step. Next realizing which drugs put patients at risk is essential. To best monitor patients receiving myeloma and especially AL amyloidosis therapies, attention to weight and fluid status, blood pressure (low in the case of lenalidomide and high in the case of carfilzomib), heart rate (thalidomide, lenalidomide and pomalidomide), and NT-proBNP in the case of patients with high-risk baseline factors or high-risk medications. Progressive elevation of NT-proBNP during chemotherapy for MM is related to asymptomatic cardiovascular events.[18] In a prospective observational study of 93 patients treated with either bortezomib or carfilzomib, patients with a baseline elevated BNP level higher than 100 pg/mL or N-terminal proBNP level higher than 125 pg/mL had an increased risk for cardiovascular adverse events (OR, 10.8; $P < .001$). Elevated natriuretic peptides mid first cycle of treatment with carfilzomib were also associated with a substantially higher risk of cardiovascular adverse events (OR, 36.0; $P < .001$).[19] Serial echocardiograms are not likely helpful because of their low sensitivity. Serial global longitudinal strain may be useful, but more data are required.[20]

In case of thromboembolism, chemotherapeutic agents need not be discontinued if full anticoagulation can be pursued. With the exception of considering dose reduction or cessation of the offending chemotherapeutic agents, the management of cardiac toxicity does not differ very much from the management systolic or diastolic heart failure in other instances. The one exception is tachyarrhythmia, which requires therapy in patients with AL amyloidosis. Amiodarone is often better tolerated that beta-blockers or calcium channel blockers.

Immune Modulatory Drugs

There are three FDA approved drugs within the IMiD class: thalidomide, lenalidomide, and pomalidomide. These three drugs are known to have cardiovascular and vascular toxicity.

Thrombosis is an important complication for myeloma patients receiving IMiDs, especially when these drugs are administered with other therapies, such as corticosteroids or anthracyclines or even erythropoietin-stimulating agents, with venous thromboembolism (VTE) rates ranging from 11% to 26%.[21] The highest rates of thrombosis are seen in the first year after diagnosis.[22] Concomitant use of bortezomib with IMiD may abrogate that risk. In one randomized study of 659 patients receiving an induction regimen containing thalidomide and corticosteroids, the respective rates of VTE at 6 months were 5.9% in the low-dose aspirin, 3.2% in the enoxaparin arm, and 8.2% in the adjusted dose warfarin arm.[21] Patients who received concomitant bortezomib had the lowest rates of thromboembolism. Xa inhibitors are also an option to prevent VTE in patients with MM receiving IMiDs.[23]

Besides causing constipation, somnolence, and birth defects in unborn children, thalidomide is poorly tolerated in patients with AL amyloidosis, and it can cause bradycardia.[24,25] Lenalidomide[26] has been associated with an increased risk of thromboembolism, angina, atrial fibrillation, and bradycardia. Among patients with AL amyloidosis, hypotension and worsening heart failure has been observed.[27,28] Lenalidomide can also cause renal dysfunction in a minority of patients.[29] Pomalidomide may have the least cardiotoxicity in terms of hypotension.

Proteasome Inhibitors

The FDA approved proteasome inhibitors include bortezomib, carfilzomib, and ixazomib. Only carfilzomib, which is an irreversible proteasome inhibitor, has a clear cardiotoxicity signal, whereas the signal is less clear for bortezomib, a slowly reversible proteasome inhibitor, and is only anecdotal for ixazomib, a rapidly reversible oral proteasome inhibitor. The mechanism of action for this toxicity is poorly understood. Theories range from downregulation of the ubiquitin-proteasome system, endothelial nitric oxide synthase activity, and an adverse effect on vascular smooth muscle.

Carfilzomib

With carfilzomib, there is a clear signal for cardiovascular toxicity as further reviewed in Chapter 54. In the seminal ENDEAVOR trial (carfilzomib + dexamethasone vs. bortezomib + dexamethasone in the relapsed setting),[30] the following rates of adverse events were noted: dyspnea, 28% versus 13%; hypertension, 25% versus 9%; CHF 8% versus 2%; ischemic heart disease 3% versus 1%; and peripheral edema 21% versus 9%. In the ASPIRE trial (lenalidomide and dexamethasone with vs. without carfilzomib for patients with relapsed or refractory MM) the respective rates of AEs were dyspnea 19% versus 15%; hypertension, 14% versus 7%; CHF were 6% versus 4%; ischemic heart disease were 6% versus 5%l and VTE 10% versus 6%. Of note, these VTE rates occurred even in the presence of thromboprophylaxis, which is guideline mandated in this group of patients. Infusion schedule may not matter as much. For instance, a comparison of 30 minute infusion of 70 mg/m^2 once weekly versus 26 mg/m^2 over 10 minutes for two consecutive days each week did not appear to affect cardiovascular toxicity significantly: hypertension, 22% versus 20%; CHF, 4% versus 5%; ischemic heart disease, 2% versus 1%; and peripheral edema, 8% versus 11%.[31]

Bortezomib

The signal for cardiotoxicity for bortezomib is less clear. The labeling information for bortezomib was updated to include precautions regarding possible heart failure and QT prolongation, even though "causality has not been established."[26] In contrast to postmarking reports, two meta-analyses did not show a statistically significant increase in the rate of all-grade or high-grade cardiotoxicities with the use of bortezomib.[32,33] Finally, a retrospective, propensity matched analysis of administrative claims was performed to determine the relative risk of cardiac risk of bortezomib and lenalidomide.[26] The authors found no significant difference in cardiac hospitalization rates between the 895 bortezomib (B) treated patients and the 895 lenalidomide (L) treated patients, but interestingly, as compared with the general adult population (G), there were higher rates of myocardial infarction hospitalizations (B, 2.00/100 PY vs. L, 0.95/100 PY vs. G, 0.816/100 PY) and heart failure hospitalizations in bortezomib (B, 3.52/100 PY vs. L, 2.17/100 PY vs. G, 0.931/100 PY). The incidence of heart failure among patients with MM treated with these drugs was 12.7% compared with that of the general adult population at 2.1%.

High-Dose Chemotherapy Used as Conditioning for ASCT

High-dose cyclophosphamide-containing regimens have been associated with cardiotoxicity.[34] The mechanism is thought to be caused by toxic endothelial damage followed by extravasation of toxic metabolites with resultant myocyte damage and interstitial hemorrhage and edema. Pericardial effusion may also occur. This toxicity occurs during or within 3 weeks of administration. This toxicity is thought to be related to dose and schedule, rather than cumulative doses. These regimens may be used to mobilize stem cells or as conditioning chemotherapy.

High-dose melphalan is the most common conditioning therapy used for ASCT. The literature would suggest that it can induce arrhythmias in approximately 5% to 10% of patients.[34]

Fludarabine is another agent that may be used as part of the conditioning regimen for an allogeneic stem cell transplant. This drug has been associated with CHF in approximately 8% of patients.[34]

Anthracyclines

Anthracyclines (e.g., doxorubicin) are less commonly used in MM, but can cause cardiotoxicity (as detailed in Chapter 54).[18]

Immunotherapies

Therapeutic Monoclonal Antibodies

No cardiac toxicity signal was noted with either of the FDA approved antibodies targeting myeloma—elotuzumab or daratumumab.

Chimeric Antigen Receptor T-cell Therapy and Bispecific T-cell Receptor-Engaging Antibody

At the time of this writing, there are no approved chimeric antigen receptor T-cell therapy (CAR-T) or bispecific T-cell receptor-engaging antibody (BiTE) therapies for MM or AL amyloidosis, but a number of drugs are in trials for MM. Cytokine release syndrome (CRS) is the main, non-antigen-specific toxicity that occurs as a result of high-level immune activation.[35] In the case of CARTs and BiTEs, the symptom onset typically occurs days to occasionally weeks after the infusion, coinciding with maximal *in vivo* T-cell expansion. IL-6 is a central mediator of toxicity in CRS. Symptoms include high temperatures, often exceeding 40°C, cardiac dysfunction, hypotension, adult respiratory distress syndrome, neurologic toxicity, renal and/or hepatic failure, and disseminated intravascular coagulation. The cardiac dysfunction can be rapid in onset and severe, but it is typically reversible. It resembles the cardiomyopathy associated with seps and Takotsubo cardiomyopathy. Low-grade CRS is treated with fluids and vasopressors, but when oxygen requirement goes higher than 40% or multiple vasopressors are required, direct attempts at blunting the cytokine storm (i.e., tocilizumab ± corticosteroids) are required.

CONCLUSIONS

Significant advancements have been made in the treatment of MM and AL amyloidosis. Although these diseases are not considered to be curable, patients can survive for many years, in some instances, even decades. Many of the therapies are quite tolerable, but cardiac side effects are possible. Thromboembolism is a risk when thalidomide, lenalidomide, or pomalidomide are used in conjunction with corticosteroids or other chemotherapy. This risk can be reduced significantly with a daily aspirin, prophylactic low molecular weight heparin or full dose anticoagulants (Table 51.5). IMiDs are associated with high rates of cardiac intolerance among patients with AL amyloidosis. In those with MM, heart failure and hypertension are most common with carfilzomib, but following weights, blood pressure, and NT-proBNP can reduce morbidity. Excessive cardiac morbidity in a patient with MM should trigger an investigation for AL amyloidosis.

TABLE 51.5 Risk Assessment Model for the Preventive Management of Venous Thromboembolism in Multiple Myeloma Patients Treated with immunomodulatory drugs Drugs (IMiDs: Thalidomide, Lenalidomide, or Pomalidomide), in Agreement With the NCCN Guidelines

	ACTION
I. Individual Risk Factors	
Obesity[a]	If no risk factor or any one risk factor is present:
Previous venous thromboembolism	Aspirin 81–325 mg once daily
Central venous catheter or pacemaker	
A. Associated Disease	If two or more risk factors are present:
Cardiac disease	LMWH (equivalent of enoxaparin 40 mg once daily) or
Chronic renal disease	Full-dose warfarin (target INR 2–3) or
Diabetes	Factor Xa inhibitor
Acute infection	
Immobilization	
B. Surgery	
General surgery	
Any anesthesia	
Trauma	
C. Medications	
D. Erythropoietin	
E. Blood clotting disorders	
II. Myeloma-Related Risk Factors	
Diagnosis	
Hyperviscosity	
III. Myeloma Therapy	
High-dose dexamethasone[b]	LMWH (equivalent of enoxaparin 40 mg once daily) or
Doxorubicin	Full-dose warfarin (target INR 2–3) or
Multiagent chemotherapy	Factor Xa inhibitor

Obesity was defined as body mass index ≥30 kgm^{-2}.
≥480 mg per month.
INR, International normalized ratio; *LMWH*, low-molecular-weight heparin.
Adapted from Nature Publishing Group. Palumbo A, Rajkumar SV, Dimopolous MA, et al. Prevention of thalidomide and lenalidomide-associated thrombosis in myeloma. *Leukemia* 2008;22:414–423.

REFERENCES

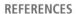

1. Siegel RL, Miller KD, Jemal A. Cancer statistics, 2018. *CA Cancer J Clin*. 2018;68:7–30.
2. Merlini G, Dispenzieri A, Sanchorawala V, et al. Systemic immunoglobulin light chain amyloidosis. *Nat Rev Dis Primers*. 2018;4:38.
3. Lousada I, Comenzo RL, Landau H, et al. Light chain amyloidosis: patient experience survey from the Amyloidosis Research Consortium. *Adv Ther*. 2015;32:920–928.
4. Gillmore JD, Maurer MS, Falk RH, et al. Nonbiopsy diagnosis of cardiac transthyretin amyloidosis. *Circulation*. 2016;133:2404–2412.
5. Palumbo A, Avet-Loiseau H, Oliva S, et al. Revised International Staging System for Multiple Myeloma: a report from International Myeloma Working Group. *J Clin Oncol*. 2015;33:2863–2869.
6. Muchtar E, Gertz MA, Kumar SK, et al. Improved outcomes for newly diagnosed AL amyloidosis between 2000 and 2014: cracking the glass ceiling of early death. *Blood*. 2017;129:2111–2119.
7. Muchtar E, Gertz MA, Kyle RA, et al. A modern primer on light chain amyloidosis in 592 patients with mass spectrometry-verified typing. *Mayo Clin Proc*. 2019;94:472–483.
8. Dispenzieri A, Gertz MA, Kyle RA, et al. Serum cardiac troponins and N-terminal pro-brain natriuretic peptide: a staging system for primary systemic amyloidosis. *J Clin Oncol*. 2004;22:3751–3757.
9. Kumar S, Dispenzieri A, Lacy MQ, et al. Revised prognostic staging system for light chain amyloidosis incorporating cardiac biomarkers and serum free light chain measurements. *J Clin Oncol*. 2012; 30:989–995.
10. Muchtar E, Kumar SK, Gertz MA, et al. Staging systems use for risk stratification of systemic amyloidosis in the era of high-sensitivity troponin T assay. *Blood*. 2019;133:763–766.
11. Lilleness B, Ruberg FL, Mussinelli R, et al. Development and validation of a survival staging system incorporating BNP in patients with light chain amyloidosis. *Blood*. 2019;133:215–223.
12. Dispenzieri A, Gertz MA, Kumar SK, et al. High sensitivity cardiac troponin T in patients with immunoglobulin light chain amyloidosis. *Heart*. 2014;100:383–388.
13. Kumar SK, Dispenzieri A, Lacy MQ, et al. Continued improvement in survival in multiple myeloma: changes in early mortality and outcomes in older patients. *Leukemia*. 2014;28:1122–1128.
14. Kumar SK, Rajkumar SV, Dispenzieri A, et al. Improved survival in multiple myeloma and the impact of novel therapies. *Blood*. 2008;111:2516–2520.
15. Kourelis TV, Kumar SK, Gertz MA, et al. Coexistent multiple myeloma or increased bone marrow plasma cells define equally high-risk populations in patients with immunoglobulin light chain amyloidosis. *J Clin Oncol*. 2013;31:4319–4324.
16. Hwa YL, Kumar SK, Gertz MA, et al. Induction therapy pre-autologous stem cell transplantation in immunoglobulin light chain amyloidosis: a retrospective evaluation. *Am J Hematol*. 2016;91:984–988.
17. Hwa YL, Shi Q, Kumar SK, et al. Beta-blockers improve survival outcomes in patients with multiple myeloma: a retrospective evaluation. *Am J Hematol*. 2017;92:50–55.
18. Wang Y, Bao L, Chu B, et al. Progressive elevation of NT-ProBNP during chemotherapy is related to asymptomatic cardiovascular events in patients with multiple myeloma. *Clin Lymphoma Myeloma Leuk*. 2019;19:167–176.e1.
19. Cornell RF, Ky B, Weiss BM, et al. Prospective study of cardiac events during proteasome inhibitor therapy for relapsed multiple myeloma. *J Clin Oncol*. 2019;37(22):1946–1955.
20. Thavendiranathan P, Poulin F, Lim KD, et al. Use of myocardial strain imaging by echocardiography for the early detection of cardiotoxicity in patients during and after cancer chemotherapy: a systematic review. *J Am Coll Cardiol*. 2014;63:2751–2768.
21. Palumbo A, Cavo M, Bringhen S, et al. Aspirin, warfarin, or enoxaparin thromboprophylaxis in patients with multiple myeloma treated with thalidomide: a phase III, open-label, randomized trial. *J Clin Oncol*. 2011;29:986–993.
22. Kristinsson SY. Thrombosis in multiple myeloma. *Hematology Am Soc Hematol Edu Program*. 2010;2010:437–444.
23. Cornell RF, Goldhaber SZ, Engelhardt BG, et al. Apixaban for primary prevention of venous thromboembolism in patients with multiple myeloma receiving immunomodulatory therapy. *Front Oncol*. 2019;9:45.
24. Dispenzieri A, Lacy MQ, Rajkumar SV, et al. Poor tolerance to high doses of thalidomide in patients with primary systemic amyloidosis. *Amyloid*. 2003;10:257–261.
25. Palladini G, Perfetti V, Perlini S, et al. The combination of thalidomide and intermediate-dose dexamethasone is an effective but toxic treatment for patients with primary amyloidosis (AL). *Blood*. 2005;105:2949–2951.
26. Reneau JC, Asante D, van Houten H, et al. Cardiotoxicity risk with bortezomib versus lenalidomide for treatment of multiple myeloma: a propensity matched study of 1,790 patients. *Am J Hematol*. 2017; 92:E15–E17.
27. Dispenzieri A, Dingli D, Kumar SK, et al. Discordance between serum cardiac biomarker and immunoglobulin-free light-chain response in patients with immunoglobulin light-chain amyloidosis treated with immune modulatory drugs. *Am J Hematol*. 2010;85: 757–759.
28. Tapan U, Seldin DC, Finn KT, et al. Increases in B-type natriuretic peptide (BNP) during treatment with lenalidomide in AL amyloidosis. *Blood*. 2010;116:5071–5072.
29. Specter R, Sanchorawala V, Seldin DC, et al. Kidney dysfunction during lenalidomide treatment for AL amyloidosis. *Nephrol Dial Transplant*. 2011;26:881–886.
30. Dimopoulos MA, Moreau P, Palumbo A, et al. Carfilzomib and dexamethasone versus bortezomib and dexamethasone for patients with relapsed or refractory multiple myeloma (ENDEAVOR): a randomised, phase 3, open-label, multicentre study. *Lancet Oncol*. 2016;17:27–38.
31. Moreau P, Mateos MV, Berenson JR, et al. Once weekly versus twice weekly carfilzomib dosing in patients with relapsed and refractory multiple myeloma (A.R.R.O.W.): interim analysis results of a randomised, phase 3 study. *Lancet Oncol*. 2018;19:953–964.
32. Xiao Y, Yin J, Wei J, Shang Z. Incidence and risk of cardiotoxicity associated with bortezomib in the treatment of cancer: a systematic review and meta-analysis. *PLoS One*. 2014;9:e87671.
33. Laubach JP, Moslehi JJ, Francis SA, et al. A retrospective analysis of 3954 patients in phase 2/3 trials of bortezomib for the treatment of multiple myeloma: towards providing a benchmark for the cardiac safety profile of proteasome inhibition in multiple myeloma. *Br J Haematol*. 2017;178:547–560.
34. Morandi P, Ruffini PA, Benvenuto GM, et al. Cardiac toxicity of high-dose chemotherapy. *Bone Marrow Transplant*. 2005;35:323–334.
35. Lee DW, Gardner R, Porter DL, et al. Current concepts in the diagnosis and management of cytokine release syndrome. *Blood*. 2014; 124:188–195.

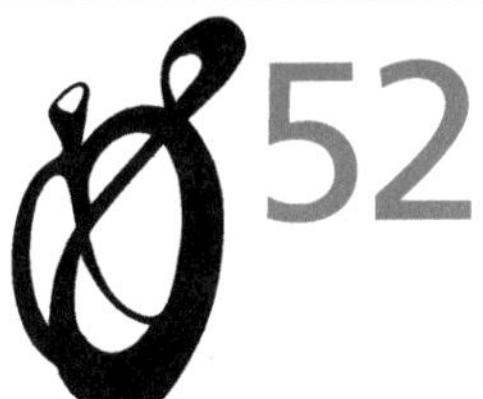

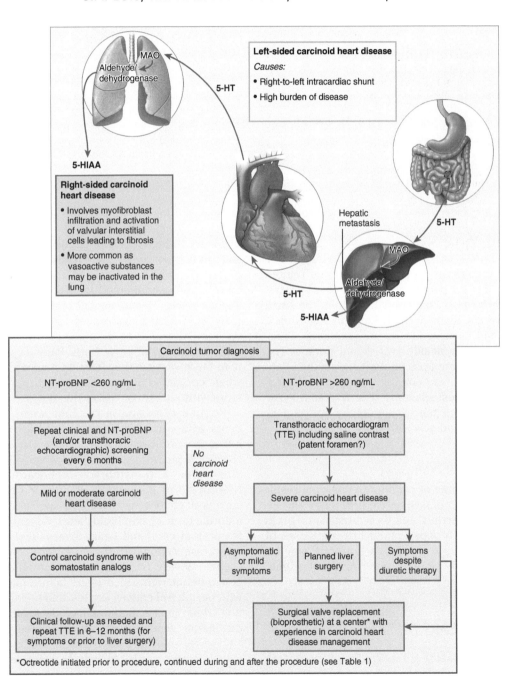

52 Carcinoid Tumors and Carcinoid Heart Disease

S.A. LUIS, T.R. HALFDANARSON, P.A. PELLIKKA, AND H.M. CONNOLLY

MAO
Aldehyde/dehydrogenase
5-HT
5-HIAA

Left-sided carcinoid heart disease

Causes:

- Right-to-left intracardiac shunt
- High burden of disease

Right-sided carcinoid heart disease

- Involves myofibroblast infiltration and activation of valvular interstitial cells leading to fibrosis
- More common as vasoactive substances may be inactivated in the lung

Hepatic metastasis
5-HT
MAO
Aldehyde/dehydrogenase
5-HT
5-HIAA

Carcinoid tumor diagnosis

NT-proBNP <260 ng/mL

Repeat clinical and NT-proBNP (and/or transthoracic echocardiographic) screening every 6 months

Mild or moderate carcinoid heart disease

Control carcinoid syndrome with somatostatin analogs

Clinical follow-up as needed and repeat TTE in 6–12 months (for symptoms or prior to liver surgery)

NT-proBNP >260 ng/mL

Transthoracic echocardiogram (TTE) including saline contrast (patent foramen?)

No carcinoid heart disease

Severe carcinoid heart disease

Asymptomatic or mild symptoms

Planned liver surgery

Symptoms despite diuretic therapy

Surgical valve replacement (bioprosthetic) at a center* with experience in carcinoid heart disease management

*Octreotide initiated prior to procedure, continued during and after the procedure (see Table 1)

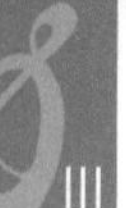

CHAPTER OUTLINE

KEY POINTS

- Carcinoid tumors are rare neuroendocrine tumors, arising from the small bowel (75% to 80%) or lung (20% to 30%).
- Carcinoid tumors secrete biologically active substances, including serotonin, histamine, tachykinins, kallikrein, and prostaglandins and they account for the presentation of carcinoid syndrome (flushing, diarrhea, and bronchospasm).
- Carcinoid syndrome typically occurs in patients with small-bowel primaries and hepatic metastases.
- Carcinoid syndrome therapy should be optimized prior to any cardiac or noncardiac procedure owing to the risk of intraprocedural carcinoid crisis. All patients with carcinoid syndrome should receive preprocedural octreotide, and intraprocedural hypotension should be treated with further doses of intravenous octreotide.
- Carcinoid heart disease occurs in approximately 20% of patients with carcinoid syndrome and has characteristic echocardiographic appearance, generally affecting the tricuspid and pulmonary valves.
- Cardiac surgical intervention is the only current effective treatment option for carcinoid heart disease, and surgical outcomes have improved over the past three decades.

INTRODUCTION

Carcinoid tumors are rare neuroendocrine tumors affecting 1.2 to 2.1 people per 100,000 people years. These tumors most commonly arise from the small bowel, typically ileum and appendix, in 75% to 80% of cases, and lungs in 20% to 30% of cases. Other less-common sites include ovaries and kidneys. The tumor secretes multiple biologically active substances, including serotonin, histamine, tachykinins, kallikrein, and prostaglandins. The overall 10-year survival with small bowel neuroendocrine tumors are 82% without and 42% with metastatic disease.[1]

Carcinoid Syndrome

Signs and symptoms of carcinoid syndrome result from the secretion of vasoactive hormones and include flushing, diarrhea, and bronchospasm. This is typically seen with hepatic metastases in cases of small-bowel primary tumors, as hormone may be cleared hepatically prior to entering the systemic circulation.

CARCINOID HEART DISEASE

Carcinoid heart disease is reported to affect at least 20% of patients suffering from carcinoid syndrome. Exposure to high levels of circulating serotonin results in fibrosis of the valve leaflets, without leaflet destruction. The right-sided cardiac valves are more commonly affected than the left (15%), with almost universal involvement of the tricuspid valve (~100%).[2] The disease process generally results in valvular regurgitation, less commonly valve stenosis, or a combination of both. Patients with carcinoid heart disease demonstrate a worse prognosis when compared with patients with carcinoid tumors without cardiac involvement.[3]

Routine screening is recommended for all patients with carcinoid syndrome at the time of the initial diagnosis using clinical assessment and an N-terminal pro-brain natriuretic peptide (NT-proBNP), plus/minus a transthoracic echocardiogram. A NT-proBNP of 260 μg/mL or greater (31 pmol/L) carries a good sensitivity and specificity for the identification of carcinoid heart disease.[4] Clinical features of carcinoid heart disease include symptoms of exertional dyspnea, fatigue, edema, and ascites. Severe tricuspid valve regurgitation with concomitant right-sided heart failure may present with peripheral edema, ascites, and hepatic congestion, thus clinical findings include jugular venous distension, generally with an associated prominent "V" wave, murmurs of tricuspid and pulmonary valve disease, a pulsitile liver, as well as edema and ascites. Clinically significant progression of valvula lesions can occur in as few as 6 months, especially among patients with elevated urinary 5-hydroxyindoleacetic acid (5-HIAA) levels (≥ 300 μmol/L) or active carcinoid symptoms (≥ 3 episodes of flushing/day).[5] Hence, repeat screening with clinical evaluation and NT-proBNP is recommended at 6 monthly intervals in patients without evidence of carcinoid heart disease. Further evaluation should be performed in all patients with an elevated NT-proBNP, or clinical features of carcinoid heart disease with follow up echocardiography recommended at 6 monthly intervals.[6]

Cardiac Imaging

Transthoracic echocardiography is the imaging test of choice for the assessment of patients with possible carcinoid heart disease (Fig. 52.1). It should include performance of agitated saline contrast injection to evaluate the interatrial septum, because an interatrial shunt is associated with an increased risk of left-sided valvular heart disease. Careful attention must be paid to the evaluation of all cardiac valves from multiple acoustic windows, including particularly the tricuspid and pulmonary valves. Particular attention should be paid to anatomic valvular leaflet motion, thickening and retraction, and resulting functional valvular regurgitation and/or stenosis. Valvular involvement seen in this disease is a progressive process with mild early leaflet thickening and restriction progressing eventually to the classic fixed and retracted leaflets seen late in this disease process.

Cardiac computed tomography and magnetic resonance imaging are used in select patients with known or suspected carcinoid heart disease. These imaging modalities may add incremental information in the clinical assessment, including images of the pulmonic valve which may be difficult to visualize by standard echocardiography, volumetric assessment of right heart size and function, and coronary artery assessment for preoperative purposes.

Management

Patients with carcinoid heart disease and associated edema may initially be treated with diuretic therapy, graduated compression stockings, and leg elevation. Combination diuretic therapy, including loop diuretics, thiazide diuretics, and aldosterone antagonists, may be required to maintain euvolemia. Where comorbid conditions and functional status allow, cardiac surgical valve replacement should be considered for ongoing symptoms (signs of right side of heart failure, shortness of breath, or fatigue related to low cardiac output) despite diuretic therapy.

Valve replacement surgery is associated with improvement in symptoms and survival, and should be performed at centers with experience in treating this high-risk patient group.[7] Preoperative evaluation should include a multidisciplinary approach incorporating oncologists, cardiologists, cardiac surgeons,

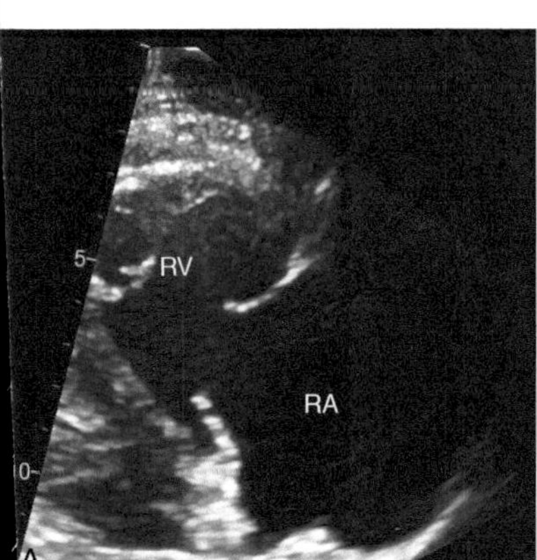

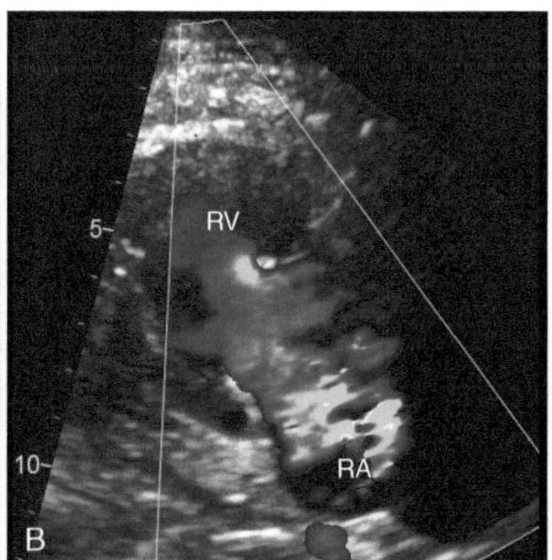

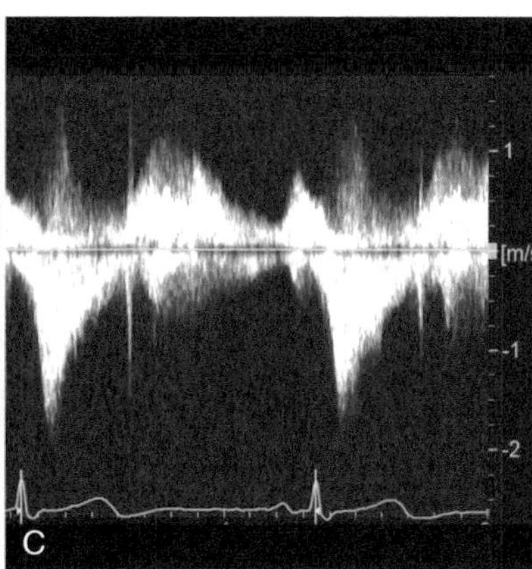

G. 52.1 Transthoracic echocardiogram demonstrating the classic features of carcinoid heart disease involving the tricuspid valve. (A) rasternal long axis right ventricular inflow view in mid systole demonstrating markedly thickened, retracted, and immobile tricuspid ve leaflets with leaflet noncoaptation. (B) Color Doppler in the parasternal long axis right ventricular inflow view demonstrating severe uspid regurgitation with laminar flow between the right ventricle and right atrium. (C) Continuous wave Doppler across the tricuspid ve demonstrating a dense, systolic, triangular-shaped regurgitant signal consistent with severe tricuspid regurgitation. *RA*, Right ium; *RV*, right ventricle.

and anesthetists with expertise in the treatment of carcinoid heart disease. It is imperative, as detailed in Tables 52.1 and 52.2, that management of carcinoid syndrome is optimized preoperatively, patients are premedicated with octreotide, and intraprocedural hypotension is treated with boluses of octreotide for carcinoid crises in order to minimize surgical morbidity and mortality. These measures have resulted in improved cardiac surgical outcomes.[8]

Although the choice of valve prosthesis remains somewhat contentious, the need for future noncardiac surgical intervention and risk of tricuspid mechanical valve prosthesis thrombosis make bioprosthetic valve replacement a reasonable choice. Long-term survival

TABLE 52.1 Suggested Periprocedural Management of Patients With Carcinoid Syndrome

PROCEDURE TYPE	PREPROCEDURAL RECOMMENDATIONS	MANAGEMENT OF INTRAPROCEDURAL HYPOTENSION
Minor procedures (e.g., colonoscopy, coronary angiography)	• 200 μg octreotide subcutaneously 1 hour prior to the procedure	• 50–100 μg octreotide intravenously as needed for flushing or hypotension
Major procedures (e.g., cardiac, liver, or bowel surgery)	• 200–500 μg octreotide subcutaneously in preoperative waiting area • Prior to anesthesia induction, commence 100–200 μg/h intravenous octreotide infusion • Continue octreotide infusion during and after surgery depending on symptoms, duration of surgery, and hemodynamic response, with a plan to taper infusion over 1–24 h	• 1000 μg intravenous octreotide bolus as needed with fluids • Repeated doses of octreotide may be necessary *Also consider:* • Intravenous fluids • Vasoactive medications (e.g., calcium, ephedrine, epinephrine) • Corticosteroids • H1 and H2 blockers—diphenhydramine and famotidine

TABLE 52.2 Management of Patients With Carcinoid Disease Before, During, and After Valve Surgery

PRESURGICAL ASSESSMENT
1. Assessment of coronary arteries with invasive CA or CT CA (depending on experience of the institution)
2. Assessment of all cardiac valves with TTE ± cardiac CT/CMR scanning
3. Assessment of right ventricular size and function (3D TTE/cardiac CT/CMR scanning)
4. Renal and liver function tests
5. Assessment of lung function tests
6. Carotid Doppler
7. Blood coagulation assessment
PERIOPERATIVE MANAGEMENT
1. Admission of a patient ≥ 48 h before surgery
2. Commencement of an octreotide infusion at the dosage of 50 mg/h administered 12 h before the procedure, throughout the operation, and 48 h after the operation, and increased to 100–200 mg/h, if necessary
3. Coordination of perioperative management by members of the multidisciplinary team
POSTOPERATIVE MANAGEMENT
1. Patients with a biological prosthesis should receive anticoagulation therapy with warfarin for 3–6 months.
2. Baseline postoperative echocardiogram should be performed early after operation.
3. First follow up echocardiogram at 3–6 months after cessation of anticoagulation and then at 6- to 12-month intervals
4. Intense control of carcinoid syndrome with an aim of 5-HIAA < 300 mmol/L

3D, Three-dimensional; *5-HIAA,* 5-hydroxyindoleacetic acid; *CA,* coronary angiogram; *CMR,* cardiac magnetic resonance; *CT,* computed tomography; *TT* transthoracic echocardiogram

From Davar J, Connolly HM, Caplin ME, et al. Diagnosing and managing carcinoid heart disease in patients with neuroendocrine tumors: an expert stat ment. *J Am Coll Cardiol.* 2017;69:1288–1304.

and freedom from cardiac surgical reoperation have been demonstrated to be similar in both prostheses types. Additionally, bioprosthetic valve dysfunction owing to carcinoid involvement is uncommon, with bioprosthetic dysfunction most commonly arising because of valve thrombosis.[8,9] Hence, oral anticoagulation using warfarin is recommended for a minimum of 3 to 6 months after bioprosthetic valve replacement, with regular cardiology follow up, including transthoracic echocardiography at 3 and 12 monthly intervals thereafter.[6] Development of bioprosthetic valve dysfunction, including a progressive increase in the transvalvular gradient compared with the baseline study, should raise concerns regarding possible bioprosthetic valve thrombosis.[10] A trial of therapeutic anticoagulation with warfarin should be considered in these instances, with a plan for lifelong anticoagulation if this is demonstrated to be the mechanism of bioprosthetic dysfunction.

TUMOR THERAPY

Somatostatin receptor analogs (octreotide or lanreotide) should be administered to all patients with carcinoid syndrome to achieve syndrome control prior to consideration of surgical intervention. Long-acting formulations of both agents are available and administered by four-weekly injection. Additional supplemental doses of short-acting octreotide and/or dose escalation of these long-acting preparations may be required to achieve carcinoid syndrome control in patients with ongoing symptoms. Somatostatin analogs can result in bradycardia and other conduction abnormalities that are rarely symptomatic. Telotristat, a tryptophan hydroxylase inhibitor, may be used in combination with these agents to achieve control of diarrhea, refractory to somatostatin receptor analogs and other standard medical therapies. Although the use of these agents has been demonstrated to control carcinoid syndrome symptoms effectively without cardiotoxicity, they unfortunately have not been demonstrated to decrease the risk and rate of progression of carcinoid heart disease or alter survival.

Carcinoid syndrome must be adequately controlled prior to planned interventions owing to the risk of carcinoid crisis. Despite prophylactic therapy with somatostatin analogs, carcinoid crisis may still occur and the pathophysiology is consistent with distributive shock.[11] Nonmetastatic carcinoid tumor should be excised surgically with the goal of achieving cure. However, given the gastrointestinal predominance of these tumors, patients are typically asymptomatic prior to the development of hepatic metastatic disease. Surgical resection of metastatic hepatic tumor or hepatic tumor embolization may improve control of carcinoid syndrome, reduce tumor burden, and prevent progression of carcinoid heart disease. Debulking of hepatic metastases, even if incomplete, likely improves overall survival. In patients undergoing surgical hepatic resection, transthoracic echocardiography should be performed prior to the procedure to assess for evidence of significant carcinoid heart disease. When carcinoid heart disease is present, attempt to assess the right atrial pressure, either noninvasively (by physical examination or through echocardiographic evaluation of inferior vena cava size and collapse) or invasively (by right-sided heart catheterization). The presence of severe right-sided carcinoid heart disease with elevated right atrial and hepatic venous pressure is associated with a reported increased risk of intraoperative bleeding. Cardiac surgical valve replacement for carcinoid heart disease prior to hepatic resection is associated with similar outcomes, when compared with patients without carcinoid heart disease undergoing hepatic resection for carcinoid syndrome.

Conventional cytotoxic chemotherapy is not typically used in carcinoid tumors due to low response rates. Everolimus, a mammalian target of rapamycin (mTOR) inhibitor, when used in combination with octreotide Long-acting repeatable (LAR) has been shown to prolong progression-free survival and reduce urinary 5-HIAA levels, but the efficacy is modest and the majority of patients will have progressive disease within 18 months. The use of everolimus is restricted to patients who have progressive disease while on somatostatin analog therapy or are intolerant of such therapy. Potential cardiac side effects of everolimus include hyperglycemia, hypertriglyceridemia, hypertension, congestive cardiac failure, peripheral edema, chest pain, and tachycardia. Interferon alpha has very modest activity and it is used rarely owing to troublesome side effects.

Peptide receptor radionuclide therapy (PRRT) utilizes a radiolabeled somatostatin analog to deliver targeted systemic radiotherapy to tumor cells while minimizing damage to normal tissues. Lutetium 177 is most commonly used and is the only radionuclide that has US Food and Drug Administration approval for therapy. Yttrium 90 is commonly used in Europe, but has not been compared with lutetium 177 in a randomized trial. PRRT is associated with a modest reduction in tumor size with an overall response rate of less than 20% and improved progression-free survival and likely overall survival.[12] PRRT is now widely considered the most effective and appropriate second-line therapy once progression is noted on somatostatin analog therapy. Patients need to abstain from long-acting octreotide or lanreotide for at least 4 weeks prior to each PRRT in order to allow binding of the radioligand to the somatostatin receptor. Short-acting octreotide can be used up to the day prior to PRRT and the long-acting preparations can be resumed after PRRT has been completed. This therapy is not known to be associated with cardiac side effects.

PERIPROCEDURAL CONSIDERATIONS

Procedural interventions carry a risk of precipitating carcinoid crisis in patients with poorly controlled carcinoid syndrome. Hence, carcinoid therapy must be optimized prior to undertaking any procedure. All patients with carcinoid syndrome must commence octreotide 2 to 4 weeks prior to any elective procedure, and a combination of long and short-acting octreotide may be required in patients with break-through symptoms. Ideally, major surgical procedures should be performed 14 to 21 days following the administration of octreotide LAR, in order to coincide with peak plasma concentrations. Despite receiving preoperative therapy, many patients may still have carcinoid crisis.[13,14] Timing of surgical intervention is less important with lanreotide, which achieves peak plasma concentration within 6 hours of administration followed by a very slow decrease in plasma concentration.

Preprocedural octreotide is recommended in all patients, with dosing based on procedure type (see Table 52.1).[6] Octreotide should be available in the procedure room during any procedure, because intraprocedural carcinoid crises are associated with high mortality and morbidity. Episodes of intraprocedural hypotension should be managed with additional doses of intravenous octreotide because these may be a manifestation of carcinoid crisis.[11] Octreotide may be administered liberally owing to the unlikely occurrence of octreotide toxicity.

CONCLUSIONS

All patients with carcinoid syndrome should receive preprocedural octreotide and intraprocedural hypotension should be treated with further doses of intravenous octreotide. Carcinoid heart disease occurs in over 20% of patients presenting with carcinoid syndrome and moderate or severe symptoms portend a poor prognosis. Routine screening of all patients with carcinoid syndrome using clinical evaluation, NT-proBNP and/or transthoracic echocardiography is recommended. Surgical valve replacement should be considered in patients with symptomatic tricuspid valve regurgitation and right-sided heart failure refractory to medical therapy, where comorbidities and functional status allow.

REFERENCES

1. Kim MK, Warner RR, Roayaie S, et al. Revised staging classification improves outcome prediction for small intestinal neuroendocrine tumors. *J Clin Oncol*. 2013;31:3776–3781.
2. Simula DV, Edwards WD, Tazelaar HD, Connolly HM, Schaff HV. Surgical pathology of carcinoid heart disease: a study of 139 valves from 75 patients spanning 20 years. *Mayo Clin Proc*. 2002;77:139–147.
3. Pellikka PA, Tajik AJ, Khandheria BK, et al. Carcinoid heart disease. Clinical and echocardiographic spectrum in 74 patients. *Circulation*. 1993;87:1188–1196.
4. Bhattacharyya S, Toumpanakis C, Caplin ME, Davar J. Usefulness of N-terminal pro-brain natriuretic peptide as a biomarker of the presence of carcinoid heart disease. *Am J Cardiol*. 2008;102:938–942.
5. Bhattacharyya S, Toumpanakis C, Chilkunda D, Caplin ME, Davar J. Risk factors for the development and progression of carcinoid heart disease. *Am J Cardiol*. 2011;107:1221–1226.
6. Davar J, Connolly HM, Caplin ME, et al. Diagnosing and managing carcinoid heart disease in patients with neuroendocrine tumors: an expert statement. *J Am Coll Cardiol*. 2017;69:1288–1304.
7. Connolly HM, Nishimura RA, Smith HC, et al. Outcome of cardiac surgery for carcinoid heart disease. *J Am Coll Cardiol*. 1995;25:410–416.
8. Nguyen A, Schaff HV, Abel MD, et al. Improving outcome of valve replacement for carcinoid heart disease. *J Thorac Cardiovasc Surg*. 2019;158:99–107.e2.
9. Connolly HM, Schaff HV, Abel MD, et al. Early and late outcomes of surgical treatment in carcinoid heart disease. *J Am Coll Cardiol*. 2015;66:2189–2196.
10. Egbe AC, Pislaru SV, Pellikka PA, et al. Bioprosthetic valve thrombosis versus structural failure: clinical and echocardiographic predictors. *J Am Coll Cardiol*. 2015;66:2285–2294.
11. Condron ME, Jameson NE, Limbach KE, et al. A prospective study of the pathophysiology of carcinoid crisis. *Surgery*. 2019;165:158–165.
12. Strosberg J, El-Haddad G, Wolin E, et al. Investigators N-T. Phase 3 trial of (177) Lu-dotatate for midgut neuroendocrine tumors. *N Engl J Med*. 2017;376:125–135.
13. Condron ME, Pommier SJ, Pommier RF. Continuous infusion of octreotide combined with perioperative octreotide bolus does not prevent intraoperative carcinoid crisis. *Surgery*. 2016;159:358–365.
14. Massimino K, Harrskog O, Pommier S, Pommier R. Octreotide LAR and bolus octreotide are insufficient for preventing intraoperative complications in carcinoid patients. *J Surg Oncol*. 2013;107:842–846.

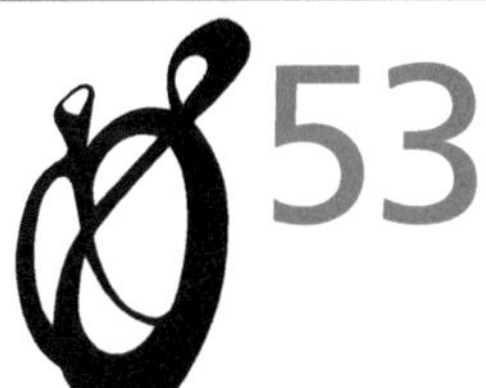

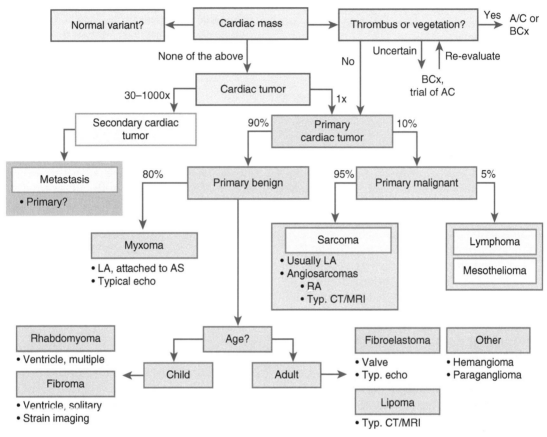

53 Neoplasms and the Heart

KYLE W. KLARICH AND JOSEPH J. MALESZEWSKIC

Cardiac mass
Normal variant?
Thrombus or vegetation?
Yes
A/C or BCx
Uncertain
Re-evaluate
BCx, trial of AC
No
None of the above
Cardiac tumor
30–1000x
1x
Secondary cardiac tumor
Primary cardiac tumor
90%
10%
Metastasis
• Primary?
80%
Primary benign
95%
Primary malignant
5%
Myxoma
• LA, attached to AS
• Typical echo
Sarcoma
• Usually LA
• Angiosarcomas
• RA
• Typ. CT/MRI
Lymphoma
Mesothelioma
Age?
Child
Adult
Rhabdomyoma
• Ventricle, multiple
Fibroma
• Ventricle, solitary
• Strain imaging
Fibroelastoma
• Valve
• Typ. echo
Lipoma
• Typ. CT/MRI
Other
• Hemangioma
• Paraganglioma

Cardiac mass algorithm. (Adapted from Bruce CJ. Cardiac tumours: diagnosis and management. *Heart*. 2011;97(2):151–60; with permission.)

CHAPTER OUTLINE

KEY POINTS

- Cardiac masses are uncommon, mostly encountered as an unexpected finding in clinical practice.
- The first step in the differential diagnosis is the question whether this mass could represent a normal variant.
- If not, the second step is to consider a vegetation (valvular lesions in particular) or thrombus (anywhere in the heart).
- If all of the above are negative, secondary cardiac masses (i.e., metastases) are more common than primary cardiac tumors.
- If no metastasis, benign cardiac tumors are more common than primary malignant cardiac tumors, and papillary fibroelastoma and sarcoma are the most common in these two categories, respectively.
- Local invasion, evidence of rapid growth, hemorrhagic pericardial effusion, precordial pain, right-sided location and presence of distant metastases are concerning for malignancy.
- The clinical context (age, extracardiac symptoms, and comorbidities) helps in providing an initial differential diagnosis; multimodality imaging is key and can be diagnostic, yet pathology, including biopsy, is often needed for the final diagnosis.

INTRODUCTION

This chapter will highlight the most common metastatic and primary neoplasms of the heart, accounting for more than 90% of the cardiac tumor practice. Clinical clues to narrowing the differential diagnosis of a cardiac mass include age, location, and syndromic characteristics (Table 53.1, Fig. 53.1).[1] Important imaging caveats also may be helpful to plan the diagnostic workup (Table 53.2). Echocardiography gives the best temporo-spatial resolution, especially for smaller, intracardiac, and highly mobile masses. Cardiac computed tomography (CT) has advantages over cardiac magnetic resonance imaging (CMR) for more rapid scanning and temporal resolution and, both CMR and cardiac CT are helpful in tissue characterization and evaluation of extracardiac extension of the mass.

MALIGNANT NEOPLASMS

Metastatic Neoplasms of the Heart

Metastatic disease is 20- to 30-fold more common than primary cardiac neoplastic disease and is typically associated with advanced disease; 9.1% of those with metastatic cancer, 14.2% of those with high-grade disease, and up to 18% of those with stage IV disease have metastases to the heart.[1,2]

Cancers that most frequently metastasize to the heart include breast and lung cancer, melanoma, and hematologic malignancies, such as lymphoma.[2] Cancers that have geographic proximity to the heart tend to metastasize to the heart by direct extension (breast, lung, and thymus). Hematogeneous spread is seen with melanoma and lymphoma, and lymphatic spread with carcinomas.[2,3] Some tumors may involve the heart by way of venous extension, such as hepatocellular and renal carcinomas, which have ready access to the large systemic veins (Fig. 53.2).

Clinically, metastatic disease often manifests as a nonspecific constellation of clinical signs and findings that are dictated by the tumor location and extent of cardiac involvement.[2] Pericardial effusions and clinical tamponade may be the first clinical clues to the presence of pericardial metastases. Over 60% of all cardiac metastases are pericardial in location.[2] The other third of cardiac metastases are myocardial in location and lead to any sinister symptoms, alone or in combination. Arrhythmias, chest pain, and even acute coronary syndrome can be the signs heralding the presence of the metastatic disease.[2,4] The extent of metastatic burden can be indicative of the consequences; myocardial invasion can lead to loss of contractility and even heart failure. Endocardial burden is rare, and may lead to embolism and possibly obstruction of a chamber or valve.[2]

Primary Cardiac Malignancies

Primary cardiac neoplasms are rare and much less common than metastatic disease to the heart. Their location makes their treatment problematic; yet, as with most malignancies, early detection is paramount for more successful treatment.

TABLE 53.1 **Primary Cardiac Neoplasms**

	AGE	LOCATION	GENETIC DRIVERS
Benign Neoplasms			
Papillary fibroelastoma	Adult	Valves	*KRAS*
Myxoma	Adult	Atria	*PRKAR1A*
Rhabdomyoma	Pediatric	Ventricles	*TSC1, TSC2*
Fibroma	Pediatric	Ventricles	*PTCH1*
Lipomatous hypertrophy of atrial septum	Adult	Atria	*HMGA2*
Lipoma	Adult	Pericardium	*HMGA2, TSC1, TSC2*
Hemangioma	Adult	Ventricles	—
Germ cell tumor	Pediatric	Pericardium	—
Histiocytoid cardiomyopathy	Pediatric	Ventricles	*MT-CYB*
Inflammatory myofibroblastic tumor	Pediatric	Ventricles, valves	—
Paraganglioma	Adult	Atria	*RET, VHL, SDH*
Granular cell tumor	Adult	Ventricles	—
Epithelioid hemangioendothelioma	Adult	Ventricles	*WWTR1-CAMTA1*
Hamartoma of mature cardiac myocytes	Adult	Ventricles	—
Schwannoma	Adult	Atria	—
Malignant Neoplasms			
Undifferentiated pleomorphic sarcoma	Adult	Atria	*MDM2*
Angiosarcoma	Adult	Atria	Complex cytogenetics
Mesothelioma	Adult	Pericardium	—
Lymphoma	Adult	Pericardium	—
Synovial sarcoma	Adult	Pericardium, valves	*SS18-SSX*
Rhabdomyosarcoma	Pediatric	Ventricles	—
Liposarcoma	Adult	Ventricles	—
Leiomyosarcoma	Adult	Vasculature	*TP53*[a]
Osteosarcoma	Adult	Atria	*TP53*[a]
Myxofibrosarcoma	Adult	Atria	*TP53*[a]
Solitary fibrous tumor	Adult	Pericardium	*STAT6*

[a]Association with Li Fraumeni syndrome.

Sarcomas

Undifferentiated High-Grade Pleomorphic Sarcoma (UHGPS)

The high-grade undifferentiated pleomorphic sarcoma, also previously called undifferentiated sarcoma or malignant fibrous histiocytoma,[5] is the most common primary cardiac malignancy (10%) with a slight female predominance and a mean age of presentation of 47 years. Anatomically, UHGPS tend to be in the left atrium and demonstrate tissue invasion.[5] The most common presenting signs and symptoms include chest pain, palpitations, and embolic phenomena.[6] Imaging by echocardiography, CT, or CMR will reveal a large and irregular intracavitary lesion with invasive features into the myocardium or pericardium. Imaging in this situation is often more important to distinguish nonmalignant from malignant and staging.[7]

Gross and tissue characteristics are required to make the diagnosis and treatment plans. UHGPS are endocardial neoplasms, often multiple, that project from the endocardium into the chambers

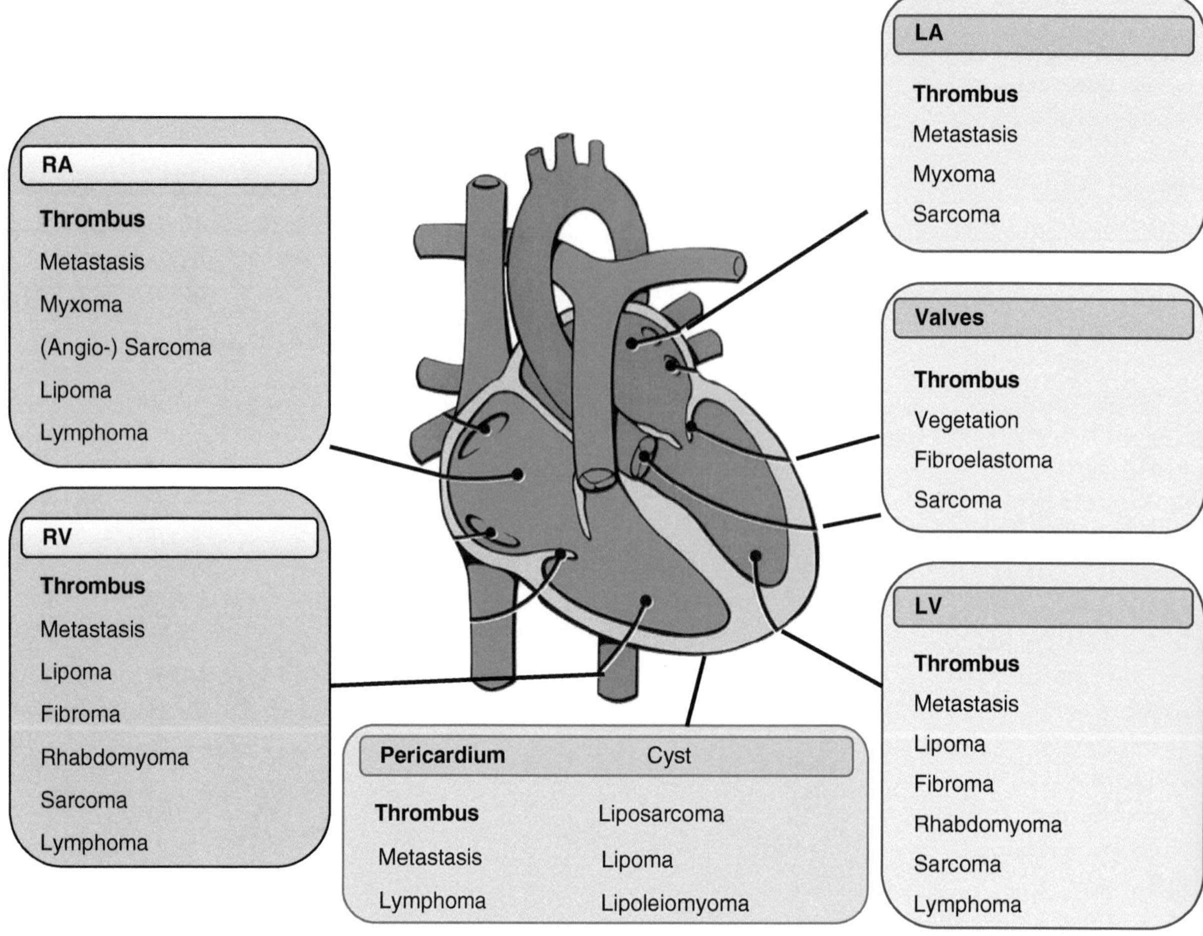

FIG. 53.1 Differential diagnoses of cardiac masses by location. (From Pieper MS, Araoz, PA. Cardiac tumors: imaging. In: Herrmann J, ed. *Clinical Cardio-Oncology*. Philadelphia: Elsevier; 2018: 77–90.)

TABLE 53.2 Imaging Characteristics for the Evaluation of Cardiac Tumors

	Echo	CMR	CT
Fat	++	++++	+++
Calcium	+++	+	++++
Thrombus	++	++++	+++
Mobility	++++	++	++
Foreign body	+++	+	+++
Extracardiac extension	+	+++	++++

of the heart. Histologically the cells are atypical, lack specific morphology. *MDM2* overexpression may support a primary cardiac etiology.[8]

Treatment requires a multidisciplinary team, and includes early detection, resection if possible, and adjuvant chemotherapy and/or radiation when the benefit is less certain. Outcomes are generally poor.[8–11] Although varying results for resection have been reported, in one study involving 95 patients, resection followed by chemotherapy suggested that removal of the primary tumor did not yield a survival advantage.[10] Another study did suggest an advantage for surgical resection: those who could undergo surgical resection had a 10-month survival advantage (15 months vs. 5 months).[11] The role of chemotherapy, either primary or adjuvant, radiation, or combined chemoradiotherapy has not been established. The rarity of cardiac sarcomas makes trials not feasible. In patients who had nonresectable cardiac sarcomas only 4 of 12 had any response to typical anthracycline-based therapies

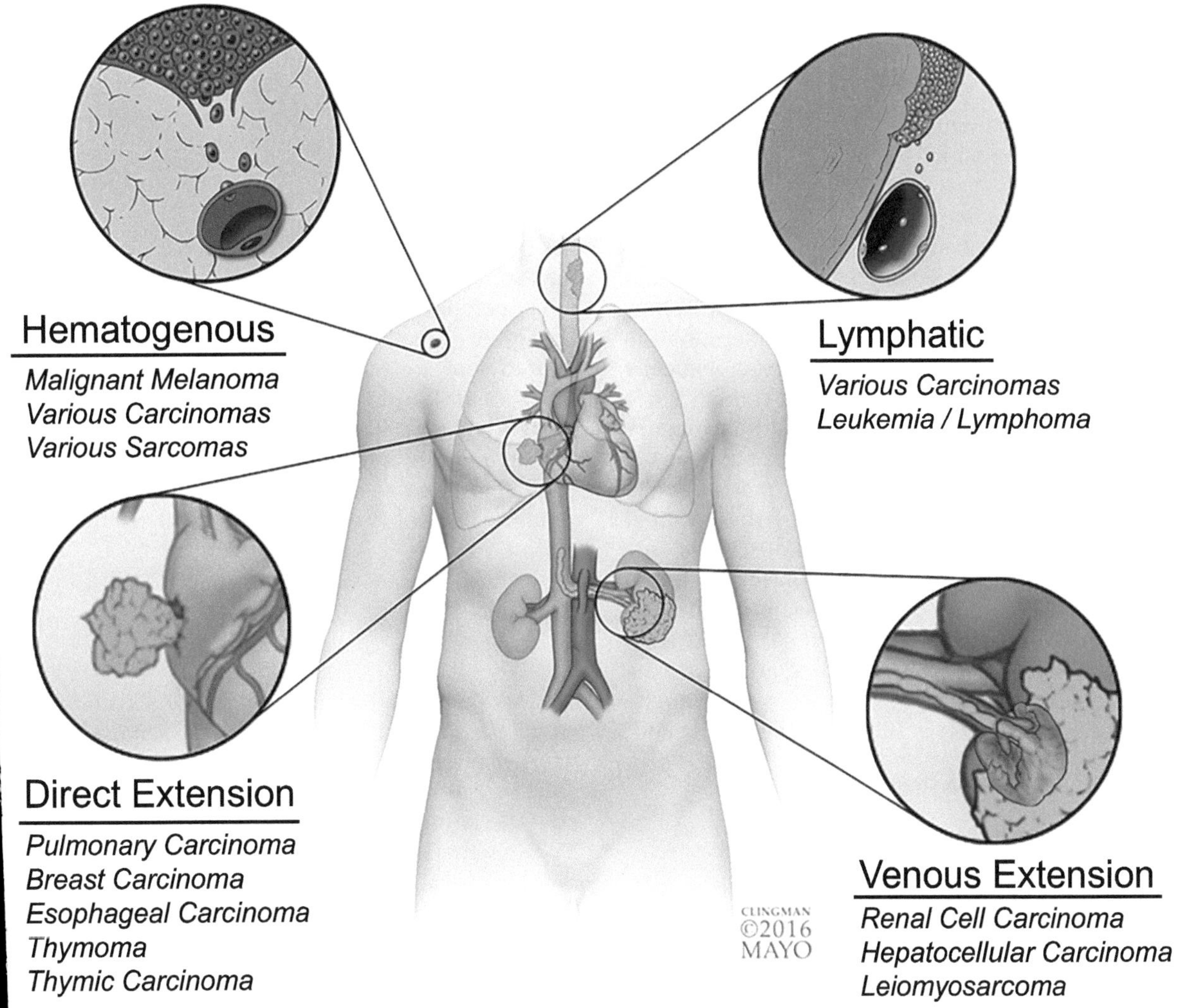

FIG. 53.2 Routes of metastatic involvement of the heart. (From Maleszewski JJ, Anavekar NS, Moynihan TJ, Klarich KW. Pathology, imaging, and treatment of cardiac tumours. Nat Rev Cardiol. 2017; 14(9): 536–549. Doi: 10.1038/nrcardio.2017.47, Used with permission of Mayo Foundation for Medical Education and Research. All rights reserved.)

all patients died within 2.5 years.[11] It is hoped for that advanced understanding of molecular markers and genetics of these aggressive tumors may lead to targeted therapies in the future.

Angiosarcoma

As opposed to UHGPS, angiosarcoma distinguishes itself by having differentiation and is most commonly situated along the right atrioventricular groove. Usually considered sporadic, familial cases have been described.[12,13] Like UHGPS they tend to affect middle-aged individuals (40 to 50 years) but, have been described in all age groups.[12,14]

Clinically it is very common that patients present with chest pain, dyspnea, weight loss, and malaise. Also, pericardial effusion, even tamponade, is not uncommon owing to the vascular nature of angiosarcomas. The effusion will often be bloody with negative cytology.[14] Such presentation may even precede the cancer diagnosis. Right atrial or atrioventricular groove location and the presence of a pericardial effusion (88%) is a strong clue to angiosarcoma as the culprit neoplasm. Echocardiography reveals a dense and irregular mass and associated pericardial involvement.[14] On CMR and CT scanning, the mass is often irregular, with myocardial infiltration, and pericardial effusion. CT scans show heterogeneous enhancement with contrast.[7] CMR shows T1 and T2 hyperintensity (tumor enhancement and necrosis) and superficial enhancement; however, the characteristics can be variable depending on the relative amounts of necrosis and hemorrhage.[15]

Angiosarcomas are usually red/brown, which is consistent with the hemorrhagic appearance. Histologically, these lesions have neoplastic cells that are spindle-shaped, rounded (epithelioid), or show a combination of both. Vascular differentiation needs to be demonstrated, either morphologically or based on the presence of antigen traits.[16] Once the diagnosis is established, a multidisciplinary treatment strategy can be planned, involving an experienced cardiac surgeon, cardiologist, oncologist, and radiation-oncology. Even with the most aggressive approaches, the median survival is only 5 months. A survival advantage, however, is noted with surgical debulking if the disease is confined to the heart (28- vs. 18-months survival).[11,14] Chemotherapy results for primary cardiac angiosarcoma have been disappointing as primary cardiac angiosarcoma are largely resistant to chemotherapy and/or radiation.

Primary Cardiac Lymphoma

Primary cardiac lymphomas are extra-nodal lymphomas that are believed to arise within the cardiac and pericardial lymphatics and by definition have limited extracardiac involvement. They account for approximately 1% to 2% of all cardiac neoplasms.[17] Primary cardiac lymphomas are seen in both immunocompetent (i.e., virus-associated) and immunocompromised hosts (i.e., transplant recipients). Like angiosarcoma, they have a predilection for the right side of the heart. Owning to its cardiac location it may typically cause chest pain, (bloody) pericardial effusion with or without tamponade and, unlike angiosarcoma, the cytology often is positive for lymphoma cells.[18] Occasionally malignant pulmonary emboli have been reported. B-symptoms, including fever and weight loss and night sweats, can be present as with lymphomas in general.

As in the case of other malignant cardiac tumors, imaging will reveal that the mass does not respect tissue boundaries.[11] Echocardiography, CT, and CMR are relatively nonspecific and can show any of the following: (1) pericardial effusion, (2) cardiac mass with right-sided location, and (3) myocardial infiltration.[7] Positron emission tomography imaging will reveal a hypermetabolic focus.

Pathologically, primary cardiac lymphomas appear as dense, infiltrating, homogeneous masses, trending along the right heart border in the pericardium and with invasion of the myocardium. A pericardial effusion can be present and is often bloody for this reason. Valves are spared. Histologically the most common form is diffuse B-cell lymphoma. Low-grade B-cell, T-cell lymphoma, Epstein–Barr related (particularly in patients after heart transplant) and Burkitt lymphoma have all been reported, often with extension by hematogenous spread and direct extension.[16,19]

Chemotherapy is the treatment of choice for primary cardiac lymphoma, directed by the lymphoma subtype.[17]

Indirect Cardiac Effects of Extracardiac Malignancies

Another important consequence of malignant disease entails the indirect effects of the tumors on the heart, such as nonbacterial thrombotic endocarditis (NBTE), carcinoid syndrome, and AL-type amyloidosis—the latter two covered in Chapters 51 and 52. NBTE (sometimes referred to as marantic endocarditis) is characterized by the deposition of thrombi secondary to a hypercoagulable state, such as that imparted by an underlying malignancy. Despite being the mimicker of "endocarditis," it is not associated with underlying infection. Because it typically affects the heart valves, it may cause systemic emboli, less commonly regurgitation, and even on rare occasion obstruction of the affected valve.

The pathology of NBTE is that of platelet/fibrin thrombi, without inflammation or underlying valvular injury.[20] A role for tumor-associated cytokines (tumor necrosis factor alpha, interleukin-1 beta, and vascular endothelial growth factor) as well as tumor genes (*MET* oncogene) have been implied.[21] NBTE deposits are typically seen in high flow areas and more on the left- than right-sided valves. The thrombi are typically attached to the atrial side of the atrioventricular valves and the ventricular side of the semilunar valves in descending order of frequency: aortic, mitral, combined aortic and mitral, tricuspid, and pulmonary.

Thromboembolism has been noted in approximately 40% of clinically recognized cases of NBTE,[22] manifesting as stroke, acute coronary syndrome, even sudden cardiac death, or valvular dysfunction. In autopsy series malignancies that are most frequently associated with NBTE are mucin-producing adenocarcinomas, such as those arising from the lung, pancreas, stomach, or ovary.[23]

Imaging studies should be carefully evaluated in patients with embolic signs or symptoms. A high level of clinical suspicion is required, followed by careful examination of the valves, which often requires high resolution transesophageal ultrasound. Although the nonbacterial vegetations can be large and even obstructive, they are usually subtle, presenting as small nodular masses attached to the valve at the closure margin.[24]

Treatment for NBTE is challenging and usually aimed at the underlying disease or malignancy. The most effective anticoagulant appears to be unfractionated heparin, which has been shown to be effective in reducing the incidence of recurrent episodes of thromboembolism.

PRIMARY BENIGN CARDIAC NEOPLASMS

Although masses arising primarily within the heart are regarded as histologically benign, they can still have devastating consequences because of their association with embolic phenomena (stroke and myocardial infarction), arrhythmia, and flow obstruction.

Papillary Fibroelastoma

Papillary fibroelastoma (PFE) is the commonly noted and the most frequently excised cardiac tumor.[25] PFEs are benign tumors of the heart, often an incidental finding at autopsy, at cardiac surgery, or during echocardiography. Although previously thought to be the second most common benign cardiac tumor (after cardiac myxoma) PFE is now known to be most common primary cardiac tumor, noted in 0.11% of echocardiograms performed.[25] Contrary to prior debates, PFEs are neoplastic, harboring a *KRAS* point mutation in 79% of cases.[26] Though predominantly valvular (80%) in location (aortic valve > mitral valve > tricuspid valve > pulmonary valve), PFEs have been described on every endocardial surface. They have been found in all age groups and show a notable increase after the fourth decade. PFEs are multiple in up to 20% of cases.[25]

Clinically the majority of patients are asymptomatic. When symptomatic, 30% of patients present with neurologic events owning to the embolic nature, followed by chest pain (20%).[25] Although embolism to nearly all vascular distributions has been reported, the most common locations are the cerebral, renal, mesenteric, retinal, lower extremity, and even pulmonary vasculature (owing to right-sided PFE).[25] Risk factors for PFE include prior cardiac surgery, chest radiation therapy exposing the heart, and hypertrophic cardiomyopathy.[27]

Echocardiography is the imaging of choice owing to its real-time spatial resolution. PFEs may be seen by CT and CMR and manifest as small (usually, <1 cm) masses with independent mobility. By tissue characteristics, PFEs are described as homogeneous speckled tumors with stippled, fluffy, shimmering edge that is best appreciated under high resolution.[28] Pathologically, these are small neoplastic masses (2 mm to 5 cm) in size. The papillary architecture is best appreciated in aqueous medium and so it may not be readily appreciated in an operative field, where the coalesced fronds can resemble myxoid tissue causing confusion with cardiac myxoma. Histologically they are avascular, with a single layer of endothelial cells, covering a core of elastin, collagen, myxoid tissue, smooth muscle cells.[29]

Owing to the risk of stroke, the recommended treatment is generally to remove the PFE by surgical excision irrespective of its size, location, and mobility (although some have reserved resection for highly mobile or large (≥1 cm) PFE).[25] This should be able to be accomplished with a valve-sparing procedure, simple shave excision in the vast majority of cases.[30] It should be recognized that PFEs are multiple in 20% of cases and an extensive and careful search for associated PFE should be carried out prior to surgery by transesophageal echocardiogram (TEE). Follow up should be considered, because there is a recurrence in 2% of patients.[25] In patients who are not deemed to be candidates or do not wish to proceed with surgery, we recommend antiplatelet therapy with aspirin; others have favored dual antiplatelet therapy or anticoagulation. No clinical trial data are available to guide treatment decisions at this point.

Hemangioma

Hemangiomas are benign vascular tumors that affect all age groups. They are very rare, yet account for 5% to 10% of all benign cardiac tumors. They have been reported in all cardiac chambers and have been seen on valves. Although hemangiomas are usually asymptomatic, they can cause chest pain, pericardial effusion, arrhythmias, and sudden cardiac death or dyspnea, depending on their location. The Kasabach-Merritt syndrome is a rare associated syndrome that consists of the presence of a giant hemangioma, leading to trapping and destruction of platelets and thereby thrombocytopenia and consumption coagulopathy.[31] The imaging characteristics of hemangioma include diffuse T2 hyperintensity on CMR, water attenuation on noncontrasted CT, and a gradual, nodular, discontinuous, peripheral to central enhancement pattern with administration of intravenous contrast agents on echocardiography.[29] Histologically, hemangioma are a mixture of blood vessels, cytologically consistent with endothelial cells.[32] Treatment is reserved for symptomatic patients. Surgical removal can be difficult due to their vascular and friable nature.[33]

Cardiac Myxoma

Cardiac myxoma (CM) is the second most common primary cardiac tumor in adults.[25] CM may be sporadic or as part of an underlying syndrome (i.e., Carney complex [CNC]), with the latter accounting for approximately 3% to 10% of cases.[32] Nonsyndromic CMs have a predilection for the left atrium, often attached to the atrial septum, with a slight female predominance (1.5:1) and can present at any age, but most commonly between the fourth and sixth decade.[34]

CNC is an autosomal-dominant disease characterized by endocrinopathy (Cushing syndrome, acromegaly, and so forth) and pigmented skin lesions (lentigines and blue nevus). It occurs as a result of underlying inactivating mutations in the genes encoding for the 1α regulatory subunit of the cAMP-dependent protein kinase type A. Myxomas occurring in this syndromic context are more likely than sporadic myxomas to occur in atypical locations within the heart and at extracardiac sites. They also demonstrate a higher recurrence rate throughout life.[35] Although clinical features are sufficient to establish a diagnosis of CNC, a combination of immune-histochemical staining and genetic testing is recommended to more completely understand the etiology of CNC in any given family.[35,36]

Even though many patients with CM are asymptomatic, some individuals with CM present with embolization, hemodynamic obstruction, heart failure, syncope, arrhythmias, chest pain, and stroke. Additional symptoms may include weight loss, malaise, fever, Raynaud's syndrome, and laboratory abnormalities, such as elevated inflammatory markers, specifically high sensitivity C-reactive protein, sedimentation rate, and interleukin-6.[35,37]

Diagnosis of CM hinges on multimodality imaging that emphasizes tissue characteristics and anatomic location. Echocardiographically, CMs are generally identified as a mass, typically in the left atrium. The tissue characteristics can be readily demonstrated by CMR and cardiac CT, owing to the relatively high water content which gives low attenuation on CT and high T2 hyperintensity and isointense T1 imaging on CMR. This is especially helpful for differentiation from an intracardiac thrombus. Two morphologic subtypes have been identified and can be appreciated on imaging—smooth (polypoid) with cysts, necrosis, and hemorrhage and villiform (papillary) with smooth fingerlike projections, often demonstrating a stalk attachment point. The villiform variety is more likely to embolize.[7,15,35]

Carney complexes can range in size from a few millimeters to 15 cm. Histologically, they consist of neoplastic "myxoma" cells set within a myxoid stroma. Immunohistochemical determination of *PRKAR1A* expression may serve as a potential screening tool to identify cases of potential CNC. Genetic screening may also be considered and is becoming more readily available.[36]

It is generally agreed that the treatment of CM is surgical excision. It is important to remove the entire base of attachment to avoid local recurrence. In the case of CNC, less noticeable tumors should be carefully searched for and also be removed for the same reason (to avoid or at least reduce the number of further surgeries).[38] Catheter ablation may also be used.[39] Surveillance is recommended at one and five years for the sporadic CM and more frequently in those with CNC.[35]

Rhabdomyoma

The most common benign primary cardiac tumor in infants and children is the cardiac rhabdomyoma. This hamartomatous tumor is usually associate with tuberous sclerosis (TS) and accounts for the vast majority of cardiac tumors identified prenatally (>90%).[40] TS is an autosomal-dominant condition, caused by underlying mutations in the *TSC1* or *TSC2* tumor suppressor genes which are involved in the control of the activity of the mammalian target of rapamycin signaling pathway.[41] Given the high frequency of TS in patients with cardiac rhabdomyomas and the high frequency of cardiac rhabdomyoma in those with TS, the finding of one should prompt evaluation for the other.[41]

Imaging by echocardiography will show an echodense, broad-based mass attached to the myocardium and protruding into the chamber or even completely within the myocardial wall of the chamber. Cardiac CT and CMR can be useful, but are employed less often in the pediatric populations. On CT scans rhabdomyomas will be hypodense on postcontrast myocardial images. CMR shows minimal delayed gadolinium enhancement.[7,42]

Pathologically, rhabdomyoma are firm, well-circumscribed, white-tan tumors, measuring upward of 9 cm. The histology reveals large, polygonal myocytes with sarcoplasmic clearing, and delicate sarcoplasmic strands that extend from the central nuclei to the sarcoplasmic membrane, causing the cells to look "spider-like."[43]

Fortunately, the vast majority of these tumors regress spontaneously. Surgical resection is considered only in extreme cases. Treatment with everolimus, a mammalian target of rapamycin pathway inhibitor, recently has been reported to hasten regression.[44]

Fibroma

Cardiac fibromas are uncommon benign tumors seen more frequently in children than in adults. Similar to rhabdomyoma, they represent hamartomatous proliferations that occur more frequently in the ventricles where they can be associated with arrhythmias or obstruction. Unlike rhabdomyoma, they are far more likely to arise as solitary lesions.

Cardiac fibromas may occur within the context of the nevoid basal cell carcinoma syndrome (NBCCS), also known as Gorlin syndrome, resulting from underlying mutations in the *PTCH1* gene. Imaging characteristics are similar to that seen in rhabdomyoma, with the exception that the fibromas are generally single and will have a particularly hyperdense core with homogeneous enhancement with gadolinium and microcalcifications that may be visible on CT, CMR, and echocardiography.[3,45]

Grossly, fibromas are solitary, whorled, white-tan masses that are sharply demarcated from the adjacent myocardium. Histologically, fibromas consist of a mix of spindle-shaped fibroblasts and collagen. Treatment is generally expectant. Surgical excision is reserved for symptomatic patients only and the "shelling" of the fibroma is usually incomplete owing to the microscopic extension of the tumor; however, this does not increase the likelihood of recurrence. Surgery may be challenging, depending on the tumor size and location. In some cases cardiac transplant is considered when excision risk is deemed too high.[45]

Lipoma

Cardiac lipoma is a benign proliferation of mature adipocytes, occurring sporadically without an age or sex predilection. Lipomas are encapsulated masses that may be located within the subendocardium (~50%), subpericardium (25%), or myocardium (25%). They most commonly arise in the left ventricle and right atrium, but are quite rare overall. They are usually asymptomatic and found incidentally on imaging or at the time of surgery for another reason (e.g., coronary artery bypass). When intramyocardial, they may be associated with arrhythmias.[46] There is also an association with TS, although it is highly likely that most of these tumors represent regressed rhabdomyomas.[47] Imaging also usually requires a multimodality approach, where echocardiographically lipoma will be hyperechoic masses. CT and CMR can be employed to define the tissue characteristics, and CMR can be very definitive in making the diagnosis (100% specific in the diagnosis of simple lipoma).[15]

Lipomatous hypertrophy of the atrial septum is an unencapsulated accumulation of fat within the atrial septum. It generally presents as a 1.5 cm or larger mass within the limbus of the fossa ovalis, making the atrial septum look a bit like a dumbbell. It occurs more commonly in older patients and is usually asymptomatic. When symptoms are present, they generally result from vena caval obstruction.[48,49] Atrial arrhythmias have been uncommonly reported.[50] CT and CMR are well equipped to determine the tissue characteristics of mature fat.[15]

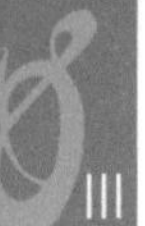

CONCLUSIONS

The treatment of cardiac neoplasms is entirely dependent on establishing a correct diagnosis. Although imaging and clinical examination provide important clues to the diagnosis, often tissue sampling is necessary for a definitive diagnosis. Thus, a multidisciplinary team is recommended for approaching these challenging lesions. A comprehensive overview of cardiac masses from pathology to imaging and management is provided in the book *Clinical Cardio-Oncology*.[51]

REFERENCES

1. Bruce CJ. Cardiac tumours: diagnosis and management. *Heart.* 2011;97(2):151–160.
2. Bussani R, De-Giorgio F, Abbate A, Silvestri F. Cardiac metastases. *J Clin Pathol.* 2007;60(1):27–34.
3. Maleszewski JJ, Anavekar NS, Moynihan TJ, Klarich KW. Pathology, imaging, and treatment of cardiac tumours. *Nat Rev Cardiol.* 2017;14(9):536–549.
4. Mankad R, Herrmann J. Cardiac tumors: echo assessment. *Echo Res Pract.* 2016;3(4):R65–R77.
5. Sebenik M, Ricci A Jr, DiPasquale B, et al. Undifferentiated intimal sarcoma of large systemic blood vessels: report of 14 cases with immunohistochemical profile and review of the literature. *Am J Surg Pathol.* 2005;29(9):1184–1193.
6. Okamoto K, Kato S, Katsuki S, et al. Malignant fibrous histiocytoma of the heart: case report and review of 46 cases in the literature. *Intern Med.* 2001;40(12):1222–1226.
7. Anavekar NS, Bonnichsen CR, Foley TA, et al. Computed tomography of cardiac pseudotumors and neoplasms. *Radiol Clin North Am.* 2010;48(4):799–816.
8. Neuville A, Collin F, Bruneval P, et al. Intimal sarcoma is the most frequent primary cardiac sarcoma: clinicopathologic and molecular retrospective analysis of 100 primary cardiac sarcomas. *Am J Surg Pathol.* 2014;38(4):461–469.
9. Agaimy A, Rosch J, Weyand M, Strecker T. Primary and metastatic cardiac sarcomas: a 12-year experience at a German heart center. *Int J Clin Exp Pathol.* 2012;5(9):928–938.
10. Ramlawi B, Leja MJ, Abu Saleh WK, et al. Surgical treatment of primary cardiac sarcomas: review of a single-institution experience. *Ann Thorac Surg.* 2016;101(2):698–702.
11. Simpson L, Kumar SK, Okuno SH, et al. Malignant primary cardiac tumors: review of a single institution experience. *Cancer.* 2008;112(11):2440–2446.
12. Leduc C, Jenkins SM, Sukov WR, Rustin JG, Maleszewski JJ. Cardiac angiosarcoma: histopathologic, immunohistochemical, and cytogenetic analysis of 10 cases. *Hum Pathol.* 2017;60:199–207.
13. Keeling IM, Ploner F, Rigler B. Familial cardiac angiosarcoma. *Ann Thorac Surg.* 2006;82(4):1576.
14. Kupsky DF, Newman DB, Kumar G, Maleszewski JJ, Edwards WD, Klarich KW. Echocardiographic features of cardiac angiosarcomas: the Mayo Clinic experience (1976–2013). *Echocardiography.* 2016;33(2):186–192.
15. Motwani M, Kidambi A, Herzog BA, Uddin A, Greenwood JP, Plein S. MR imaging of cardiac tumors and masses: a review of methods and clinical applications. *Radiology.* 2013;268(1):26–43.
16. Travis WD, Brambilla E, Burke AP, Marx A, Nicholson AG. *WHO Classification of Tumours of the Lung, Pleura, Thymus and Heart.* Lyon, France: World Health Organization, IARC; 2015.
17. Gowda RM, Khan IA. Clinical perspectives of primary cardiac lymphoma. *Angiology.* 2003;54(5):599–604.
18. Burling F, Devlin G, Heald S. Primary cardiac lymphoma diagnosed with transesophageal echocardiography-guided endomyocardial biopsy. *Circulation.* 2000;101(17):E179–E181.
19. Jeudy J, Burke AP, Frazier AA. Cardiac lymphoma. *Radiol Clin North Am.* 2016;54(4):689–710.
20. Eiken PW, Edwards WD, Tazelaar HD, McBane RD, Zehr KJ. Surgical pathology of nonbacterial thrombotic endocarditis in 30 patients, 1985–2000. *Mayo Clin Proc.* 2001;76(12):1204–1212.
21. Boccaccio C, Sabatino G, Medico E, et al. The MET oncogene drives a genetic programme linking cancer to haemostasis. *Nature.* 2005;434(7031):396–400.
22. Lopez JA, Ross RS, Fishbein MC, Siegel RJ. Nonbacterial thrombotic endocarditis: a review. *Am Heart J.* 1987;113(3):773–784.
23. Gonzalez Quintela A, Candela MJ, Vidal C, Roman J, Aramburo P. Non-bacterial thrombotic endocarditis in patients with cancer. *Acta Cardiol.* 1991;46(1):1–9.
24. Dutta T, Karas MG, Segal AZ, Kizer JR. Yield of transesophageal echocardiography for nonbacterial thrombotic endocarditis and other cardiac sources of embolism in patients with cancer with cerebral ischemia. *Am J Cardiol.* 2006;97(6):894–898.
25. Tamin SS, Maleszewski JJ, Scott CG, et al. Prognostic and bioepidemiologic implications of papillary fibroelastomas. *J Am Coll Cardiol.* 2015;65(22):2420–2429.
26. Wittersheim M, Heydt C, Hoffmann F, Buttner R. KRAS mutation in papillary fibroelastoma: a true cardiac neoplasm? *J Pathol Clin Res.* 2017;3(2):100–104.
27. Kumar G, Macdonald RJ, Sorajja P, et al. Papillary fibroelastomas in 19 patients with hypertrophic cardiomyopathy undergoing septal myectomy. *J Am Soc Echocardiogr.* 2010;23(6):595–598.
28. Klarich KW, EnriquezSarano M, Gura GM, Edwards WD, Tajik AJ, Seward JB. Papillary fibroelastoma: echocardiographic characteristics for diagnosis and pathologic correlation. *J Am Coll Cardiol.* 1997;30(3):784–790.
29. Maleszewski JJ, Bois MC, Bois JP, Young PM, Stulak JM, Klarich KW. Neoplasia and the heart: pathological review of effects with clinical and radiological correlation. *J Am Coll Cardiol.* 2018;72(2):202–227.
30. Ngaage DL, Mullany CJ, Daly RC, et al. Surgical treatment of cardiac papillary fibroelastoma: a single center experience with eighty-eight patients. *Ann Thorac Surg.* 2005;80(5):1712–1718.
31. Burke A, Johns JP, Virmani R. Hemangiomas of the heart. A clinicopathologic study of ten cases. *Am J Cardiovasc Pathol.* 1990;3(4):283–290.
32. Jain D, Maleszewski JJ, Halushka MK. Benign cardiac tumors and tumorlike conditions. *Ann Diagn Pathol.* 2010;14(3):215–230.
33. Li W, Teng P, Xu H, Ma L, Ni Y. Cardiac hemangioma: a comprehensive analysis of 200 Cases. *Ann Thorac Surg.* 2015;99(6):2246–2252.
34. Pinede L, Duhaut P, Loire R. Clinical presentation of left atrial cardiac myxoma. A series of 112 consecutive cases. *Medicine (Baltimore).* 2001;80(3):159–172.
35. Jain S, Maleszewski JJ, Stephenson CR, Klarich KW. Current diagnosis and management of cardiac myxomas. *Expert Rev Cardiovasc Ther.* 2015;13(4):369–375.
36. Maleszewski JJ, Larsen BT, Kip NS, et al. PRKAR1A in the development of cardiac myxoma: a study of 110 cases including isolated and syndromic tumors. *Am J Surg Pathol.* 2014;38(8):1079–1087.
37. Wang Z, Chen S, Zhu M, et al. Risk prediction for emboli and recurrence of primary cardiac myxomas after resection. *J Cardiothorac Surg.* 2016;11:22.
38. Garatti A, Nano G, Canziani A, et al. Surgical excision of cardiac myxomas: twenty years experience at a single institution. *An Thorac Surg.* 2012;93(3):825–831.
39. Konecny T, Reeder G, Noseworthy PA, Konecny D, Carney JA Asirvatham SJ. Percutaneous ablation and retrieval of a righ atrial myxoma. *Heart Lung Circ.* 2014;23(11):e244–e247.
40. Beghetti M, Gow RM, Haney I, Mawson J, Williams WG, Freedo RM. Pediatric primary benign cardiac tumors: a 15-year revie *Am Heart J.* 1997;134(6):1107–1114.
41. Tworetzky W, McElhinney DB, Margossian R, et al. Associatio between cardiac tumors and tuberous sclerosis in the fetus an neonate. *Am J Cardiol.* 2003;92(4):487–489.
42. Kiaffas MG, Powell AJ, Geva T. Magnetic resonance imaging eval ation of cardiac tumor characteristics in infants and children. *A J Cardiol.* 2002;89(10):1229–1233.
43. Burke AP, Virmani R. Cardiac rhabdomyoma: a clinicopatholog study. *Mod Pathol.* 1991;4(1):70–74.

44. Hoshal SG, Samuel BP, Schneider JR, Mammen L, Vettukattil JJ. Regression of massive cardiac rhabdomyoma on everolimus therapy. *Pediatr Int*. 2016;58(5):397–399.
45. ElBardissi AW, Dearani JA, Daly RC, et al. Analysis of benign ventricular tumors: long-term outcome after resection. *J Thorac Cardiovasc Surg*. 2008;135(5):1061–1068.
46. Hananouchi GI, Goff WB II. Cardiac lipoma: six-year follow-up with MRI characteristics, and a review of the literature. *Magn Reson Imaging*. 1990;8(6):825–828.
47. Winterkorn EB, Dodd JD, Inglessis I, Holmvang G, Thiele EA. Tuberous sclerosis complex and myocardial fat-containing lesions: a report of four cases. *Clin Genet*. 2007;71(4):371–373.
48. Kuester LB, Fischman AJ, Fan CM, Halpern EF, Aquino SL. Lipomatous hypertrophy of the interatrial septum: prevalence and features on fusion 18F fluorodeoxyglucose positron emission tomography/CT. *Chest*. 2005;128(6):3888–3893.
49. McNamara RF, Taylor AE, Panner BJ. Superior vena caval obstruction by lipomatous hypertrophy of the right atrium. *Clin Cardiol*. 1987;10(10):609–610.
50. Hutter AM Jr, Page DL. Atrial arrhythmias and lipomatous hypertrophy of the cardiac interatrial septum. *Am Heart J*. 1971;82(1):16–21.
51. Herrmann J, ed. *Clinical Cardio-Oncology*. Philadelphia: Elsevier; 2018.

PART IV

Cancer Drugs

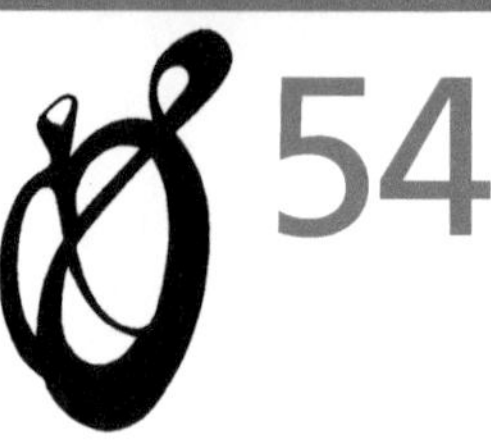

54 Cancer Therapeutic Drug Guide

JOERG HERRMANN, GAGAN SAHNI, ANDREA GALLARDO, AFERDITA SPAHILLARI, MATTHEW GALSKY, THOMAS ESCHENHAGEN, WENDY SCHAFFER, TOMAS G. NEILAN, GHOSH AK, TEODORA DONISAN, DINU VALENTIN BALANESCU, CEZAR ILIESCU, KEITH STEWART AND CAROLYN LARSEN

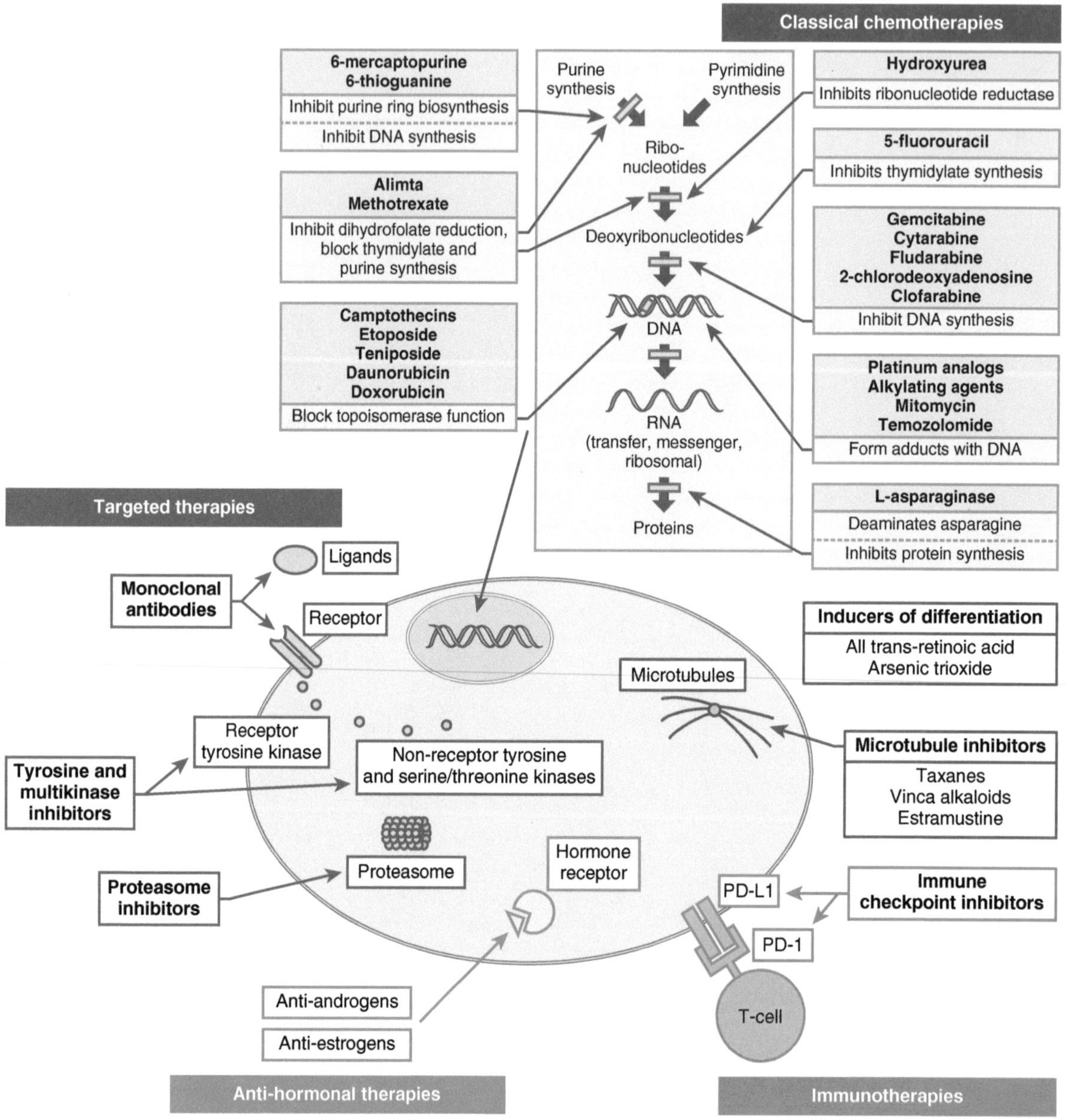

CHAPTER OUTLINE

Cancer drugs are a central part of cancer therapy and knowledge of their use, mode of action, and side effect profile is very important. This chapter is intended to provide an overview and to serve as a reference. With this intent, Table 54.1 lists the acronyms and components of a number of combination therapies and Tables 54.2 to 54.12 summarize the information for a number of cancer therapeutics organized by drug class.

ANTITUMOR ANTIBIOTICS AND TOPOISOMERASE INHIBITORS INCLUDING ANTHRACYCLINES

KEY POINTS

- Several of the antibiotic and plant alkaloids and their synthetic versions exert their antitumor action via several mechanisms, the most widely used and best example being anthracyclines.
- Anthracyclines, including doxorubicin and epirubicin, cause cancer cell death by inhibition of topoisomerase II, intercalation into the DNA, generation of oxidative stress, and induction of mitochondrial dysfunction.
- These mechanisms also account for cardiotoxicity, although topoisomerase II beta is the target in cardiomyocytes and topoisomerase II alpha in cancer cells.
- Traditionally acute cardiotoxicity (myocarditis-like presentation) and chronic cardiotoxicity (cardiomyopathy-like presentation) are differentiated.
- Recovery of cardiac function can be very protracted.
- Preventive measures include dexrazoxane, the beta-blockers carvedilol, nebivolol, and bisoprolol, angiotensin-converting enzyme (ACE) inhibitors/angiotensin receptor blockers (ARBs), and statins.

Antitumor antibiotics continue to take an important role in the treatment of malignancies (see Table 54.1). The anticancer effects of this class of drugs are broad and heavily directed toward the DNA. They include free radical formation with consequent induction of DNA damage or lipid peroxidation, DNA intercalation into the DNA leading to inhibition of macromolecular biosynthesis, and DNA binding, alkylation, and/or crosslinking or interference with DNA unwinding or DNA strand separation and helicase activity. Topoisomerases are

TABLE 54.1 **Acronyms of Chemotherapy Regimens**

NAME	COMPONENTS	EXAMPLE OF USES, AND OTHER NOTES
7+3, also known as DA or DAC in case of daunorubicin, or IA or IAC in case of idarubicin use	7 days of ara-C (cytarabine) plus 3 days of an anthracycline antibiotic, either daunorubicin [DA or DAC variant] or idarubicin [IA or IAC variant]	Acute myelogenous leukemia, excluding acute promyelocytic leukemia
ABVD	doxorubicin (Adriamycin), bleomycin, vinblastine, dacarbazine	Hodgkin lymphoma
AC	doxorubicin (Adriamycin), cyclophosphamide	Breast cancer
BACOD	bleomycin, doxorubicin (Adriamycin), cyclophosphamide, vincristine (Oncovin), dexamethasone	Non-Hodgkin lymphoma
BEACOPP	bleomycin, etoposide, doxorubicin (Adriamycin), cyclophosphamide, vincristine (Oncovin), procarbazine, prednisone bleomycin, etoposide, doxorubicin (Adriamycn), cyclophosphamide, vincristine (Oncovin), procarbazine, prednisone)	Hodgkin lymphoma
BEP	bleomycin, etoposide, platinum agent	Testicular cancer, germ cell tumors
CA	cyclophosphamide, doxorubicin (Adriamycin) (same as AC)	Breast cancer
CAF	cyclophosphamide, doxorubicin (Adriamycin), fluorouracil (5-FU)	Breast cancer
CAPOX or XELOX	capecitabine and oxaliplatin	Colorectal cancer
CAV	cyclophosphamide, doxorubicin (Adriamycin), vincristine	Lung cancer
CBV	cyclophosphamide, BCNU (carmustine), VP-16 (etoposide)	Lymphoma
CHOEP	cyclophosphamide, hydroxydaunorubicin (doxorubicin), etoposide, vincristine (Oncovin), prednisone	Non-Hodgkin lymphoma
CEPP	cyclophosphamide, etoposide, procarbazine, prednisone	Non-Hodgkin lymphoma
ChlVPP/EVA	chlorambucil, vincristine (Oncovin), procarbazine, prednisone, etoposide, vinblastine, doxorubicin (Adriamycin)	Hodgkin lymphoma
CHOP	cyclophosphamide, hydroxydaunorubicin (doxorubicin), vincristine (Oncovin), prednisone	Non-Hodgkin lymphoma
CHOP-R or R-CHOP	CHOP + rituximab	B-cell non-Hodgkin lymphoma
Clapped	clarithromycin, pomalidomide, dexamethasone	Multiple myeloma
CMF	cyclophosphamide, methotrexate, fluorouracil (5-FU)	Breast cancer
CMV	cisplatin, methotrexate, vinblastine	Transitional bladder carcinoma
CODOX-M	cyclophosphamide, vincristine, doxorubicin, high-dose methotrexate	Non-Hodgkin lymphoma
COP or CVP	cyclophosphamide, Oncovin or vincristine, prednisone	Non-Hodgkin lymphoma in patients with history of cardiovascular disease
COPP	cyclophosphamide, Oncovin (vincristine), procarbazine, prednisone	Hodgkin lymphoma
CT or TC	docetaxel (Taxotere), cyclophosphamide	Breast cancer
CTD	cyclophosphamide, thalidomide, dexamethasone	AL amyloidosis
CVAD and Hyper-CVAD	cyclophosphamide, vincristine, doxorubicin (Adriamycin), dexamethasone	Aggressive non-Hodgkin lymphoma, lymphoblastic lymphoma, some forms of leukemia
CVE	carboplatin, vincristin, etoposide	Retinoblastoma
CYBORD	cyclophosphamide, bortezomib, dexamethasone	Multiple myeloma, AL amyloidosi
DA or DAC	daunorubicin x 3 days plus ara-C (cytarabine) x 7 days, a variant of 7+3 regimen	Acute myeloid leukemia, excludin acute promyelocytic leukemia

TABLE 54.1 **Acronyms of Chemotherapy Regimens—cont'd**

NAME	COMPONENTS	EXAMPLE OF USES, AND OTHER NOTES
DAT	daunorubicin, cytarabine (ara-C), tioguanine	Acute myeloid leukemia
DCEP	dexamethasone, cyclophosphamide, etoposide, platinum agent	Relapsed or refractory multiple myeloma
DHAP	dexamethasone (a steroid hormone), cytarabine (ara-C), platinum agent	Non-Hodgkin lymphoma
DHAP-R or R-DHAP	dexamethasone (a steroid hormone), cytarabine (ara-C), platinum agent plus rituximab	Non-Hodgkin lymphoma
DICE	dexamethasone, ifosfamide, cisplatin, etoposide (VP-16)	Aggressive relapsed lymphomas, progressive neuroblastoma
DT-PACE	dexamethasone, thalidomide, platinum agent, doxorubicin (Adriamycin), cyclophosphamide, etoposide	Multiple myeloma
EC	epirubicin, cyclophosphamide	Breast cancer
ECF (MAGIC)	epirubicin, cisplatin, fluorouracil (5-FU)	Gastric cancer and cancer of the esophagogastric junction (Siewert classification III)
EOX	epirubicin, oxaliplatin, capecitabine	Esophageal cancer, gastric cancer
EP	etoposide, platinum agent	Testicular cancer, germ cell tumors
EPOCH	etoposide, prednisone, vincristine (Oncovin), cyclophosphamide, and hydroxydaunorubicin	Non-Hodgkin lymphoma
EPOCH-R or R-EPOCH	etoposide, prednisone, vincristine (Oncovin), cyclophosphamide, and hydroxydaunorubicin plus rituximab	B-cell non-Hodgkin lymphoma
ESHAP	etoposide, methylprednisolone (a steroid hormone), cytarabine (ara-C), platinum agent	Non-Hodgkin lymphoma
ESHAP-R or R-ESHAP	etoposide, methylprednisolone (a steroid hormone), cytarabine (ara-C), platinum agent plus rituximab	Non-Hodgkin lymphoma
FAM	fluorouracil, doxorubicin (Adriamycin), mitomycin	Gastric cancer
FAMTX	fluorouracil, doxorubicin (Adriamycin), methotrexate	Gastric cancer
FCM or FMC	fludarabine, cyclophosphamide, mitoxantrone	B-cell non-Hodgkin lymphoma
FCM-R or R-FCM or R-FMC or FMC-R	fludarabine, cyclophosphamide, mitoxantrone plus rituximab	B-cell non-Hodgkin lymphoma
FCR	fludarabine, cyclophosphamide, rituximab	B-cell non-Hodgkin lymphoma
FM	fludarabine, mitoxantrone	B-cell non-Hodgkin lymphoma
FM-R or R-FM or RFM or FMR	fludarabine, mitoxantrone, and rituximab	B-cell non-Hodgkin lymphoma
FEC	fluorouracil (5-FU), epirubicin, cyclophosphamide	Breast cancer
FEC-T	fluorouracil (5-FU), epirubicin, cyclophosphamide together, followed by docetaxel (Taxotere)	Breast cancer
FL (also known as Mayo)	fluorouracil (5-FU), leucovorin (folinic acid)	Colorectal cancer
FLAG	fludarabine, cytarabine, G-CSF	Relapsed or refractory acute myelogenous leukemia
FLAG-Ida or FLAG-IDA or IDA-FLAG or Ida-FLAG	fludarabine, cytarabine, idarubicin, G-CSF	Relapsed or refractory acute myelogenous leukemia
FLAG-Mito or FLAG-MITO or Mito-FLAG or MITO-FLAG or FLANG	mitoxantrone, fludarabine, cytarabine, G-CSF	Relapsed or refractory acute myelogenous leukemia
FLAMSA	fludarabine, cytarabine, amsacrine	Myelodysplastic syndrome, acute myeloid leukemia
FLAMSA-BU or FLAMSA-Bu	fludarabine, cytarabine, amsacrine, busulfan	Myelodysplastic syndrome, acute myeloid leukemia

Continued

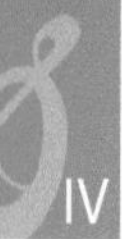

TABLE 54.1 Acronyms of Chemotherapy Regimens—cont'd

NAME	COMPONENTS	EXAMPLE OF USES, AND OTHER NOTES
FLAMSA-MEL or FLAMSA-Mel	fludarabine, cytarabine, amsacrine, melphalan	Myelodysplastic syndrome, acute myeloid leukemia
FLOT	fluorouracil (5-FU), leucovorin (folinic acid), oxaliplatin, docetaxel	Esophageal cancer, gastric cancer
FOLFIRI	fluorouracil (5-FU), leucovorin (folinic acid), irinotecan	Colorectal cancer
FOLFIRINOX	fluorouracil (5-FU), leucovorin (folinic acid), irinotecan, oxaliplatin	Pancreatic cancer
FOLFOX	fluorouracil (5-FU), leucovorin (folinic acid), oxaliplatin	Colorectal cancer
GC	gemcitabine, cisplatin gemcitabine, dexamethasone, and cisplatin	
GDP	gemcitabine, dexamethasone, cisplatin	Non-Hodgkin lymphoma and Hodgkin lymphoma
GemOx or GEMOX	gemcitabine, oxaliplatin	Non-Hodgkin lymphoma
GVD	gemcitabine, vinorelbine, pegylated liposomal doxorubicin	Hodgkin lymphoma
GemOx-R or GEMOX-R or R-GemOx or R-GEMOX	gemcitabine, oxaliplatin, rituximab	Non-Hodgkin lymphoma
IA or IAC	idarubicin × 3 days plus ara-C (cytarabine) × 7 days, a variant of classic 7+3 regimen	Acute myelogenous leukemia, excluding acute promyelocytic leukemia
ICE	ifosfamide, carboplatin, etoposide (VP-16)	Aggressive lymphomas, progressive neuroblastoma
ICE-R or R-ICE or RICE	ICE + rituximab	High-risk progressive or recurrent lymphomas
IFL	irinotecan, leucovorin (folinic acid), fluorouracil	Colorectal cancer
IVA	ifosfamide, vincristine, actinomycin D	Rhabdomyosarcoma
IVAC	ifosfamide, etoposide and high-dose cytarabine	Non-Hodgkin lymphoma
m-BACOD	methotrexate, bleomycin, doxorubicin (Adriamycin), cyclophosphamide, vincristine (Oncovin), dexamethasone	Non-Hodgkin lymphoma
MACOP-B	methotrexate, leucovorin (folinic acid), doxorubicin (Adriamycin), cyclophosphamide, vincristine (Oncovin), prednisone, bleomycin	Non-Hodgkin lymphoma
MAID	mesna, doxorubicin, ifosfamide, dacarbazine	Soft-tissue sarcoma
MINE	mesna, ifosfamide, novantrone, etoposide	Non-Hodgkin lymphoma and Hodgkin lymphoma in relapse or refractory cases
MINE-R or R-MINE	mesna, ifosfamide, novantrone, etoposide plus rituximab	Non-Hodgkin lymphoma and Hodgkin lymphoma in relapse or refractory cases
MMM	mitomycin, methotrexate, mitoxantrone	Breast cancer
MOPP	mechlorethamine, vincristine (Oncovin), procarbazine, prednisone	Hodgkin lymphoma
MVAC	methotrexate, vinblastine, doxorubicin (adriamycin), cisplatin	Advanced bladder cancer
MVP	mitomycin, vindesine, cisplatin	Lung cancer and mesothelioma
NP	cisplatin, vinorelbine	Non–small-cell lung carcinoma
PACE	platinum agent, doxorubicin (Adriamycin), cyclophosphamide, etoposide	
PCV	Procarbazine, CCNU (lomustine), vincristine	Brain tumors
PEB	cisplatin, etoposide, bleomycin	Non-seminomatous germ cell tumors
PEI	cisplatin, etoposide, ifosfamide	Small-cell lung carcinoma
platin + taxane	cisplatin/carboplatin, paclitaxel/docetaxel	Ovarian cancer
POMP	6-mercaptopurine (Purinethol), vincristine (Oncovin), methotrexate, and prednisone	Acute adult leukemia

TABLE 54.1 **Acronyms of Chemotherapy Regimens—cont'd**

NAME	COMPONENTS	EXAMPLE OF USES, AND OTHER NOTES
ProMACE-MOPP	methotrexate, doxorubicin (Adriamycin), cyclophosphamide, etoposide + MOPP	Non-Hodgkin lymphoma
ProMACE-CytaBOM	prednisone, doxorubicin (Adriamycin), cyclophosphamide, etoposide, cytarabine, bleomycin, vincristine (Oncovin), methotrexate, leucovorin	Non-Hodgkin lymphoma
RdC	lenalidomide (Revlimid), dexamethasone, cyclophosphamide	AL amyloidosis
R-Benda	rituximab + bendamustine	Follicular lymphoma and MALT lymphoma
R-DHAP or DHAP-R	rituximab + DHAP; that is, rituximab, dexamethasone (a steroid hormone), cytarabine (ara-C), platinum agent	Relapsed non-Hodgkin lymphoma and Hodgkin lymphoma
R-FCM or FCM-R	rituximab + FCM; that is, rituximab, fludarabine, cyclophosphamide, mitoxantrone	B-cell non-Hodgkin lymphoma
R-ICE or ICE-R or RICE	rituximab + ICE; that is, rituximab, ifosfamide, carboplatin, etoposide	High-risk progressive or recurrent lymphomas
RVD	lenalidomide (Revlimid), bortezomib, dexamethasone	
Stanford V	doxorubicin (Adriamycin), mechlorethamine, bleomycin, vinblastine, vincristine, etoposide, prednisone	Hodgkin lymphoma
TAC or ACT	docetaxel (Taxotere) or paclitaxel (Taxol), doxorubicin (Adriamycin), cyclophosphamide	Breast cancer ("TAC" can also refer to tetracaine-adrenaline-cocaine, used as local anesthetic)
TAD	tioguanine, cytarabine (ara-C), daunorubicin	Acute myeloid leukemia
TC or CT	docetaxel (Taxotere), cyclophosphamide	Breast cancer
TCH	docetaxel (Taxotere), carboplatin, trastuzumab (Herceptin)	Breast cancer with positive HER2/neu receptor
TCHP	docetaxel (Taxotere), carboplatin, trastuzumab (Herceptin), pertuzumab (Perjeta)	Breast cancer with positive HER2/neu receptor
Thal/Dex	thalidomide, dexamethasone	Multiple myeloma
TIP	paclitaxel (Taxol), ifosfamide, platinum agent cisplatin (Platinol)	Testicular cancer, germ cell tumors in salvage therapy
EE-4A	vincristine, actinomycin	Wilms' tumor
DD-4A	vincristine, actinomycin, doxorubicin (Adriamycin)	Wilms' tumor
VABCD	vinblastine, doxorubicin (Adriamycin), bleomycin, lomustine (CeeNU), dacarbazine	MOPP refractory Hodgkin lymphoma
VAC	vincristine, actinomycin, cyclophosphamide	Rhabdomyosarcoma
VAD	vincristine, doxorubicin (Adriamycin), dexamethasone	Multiple myeloma
VAMP	one of 3 combinations of vincristine and others	Hodgkin lymphoma, leukemia, multiple myeloma
Regimen I	vincristine, doxorubicin (Adriamycin), etoposide, cyclophosphamide	Wilms' tumor
VAPEC-B	vincristine, doxorubicin (Adriamycin), prednisone, etoposide, cyclophosphamide, bleomycin	Hodgkin lymphoma
VD-PACE	bortezomib, dexamethasone plus platinum agent, doxorubicin (Adriamycin), cyclophosphamide, etoposide	Multiple myeloma
VIFUP	vinorelbine, cisplatin, fluorouracil	Locally advanced/metastatic breast cancer
VIP	vinblastine, ifosfamide, platinum agent, (etoposide(VP-16) may substitute for vinblastine, making a regimen sometimes referred to as VIP-16)	Testicular cancer, germ cell tumors
VTD-PACE	bortezomib (Velcade), thalidomide, dexamethasone plus platinum agent, doxorubicin (Adriamycin), cyclophosphamide, etoposide	Multiple myeloma

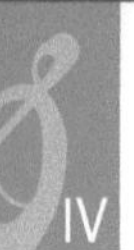

enzymes that facilitate the unwinding DNA that is required for normal replication or transcription. Topoisomerase I (TOP I) inhibition leads to single-stranded breaks in DNA, whereas topoisomerase II (TOP II) inhibition causes double-stranded breaks. Accordingly, a distinction of this diverse group of drugs can be made based on their ability to inhibit topoisomerase, and among topoisomerase inhibitors, one can furthermore differentiate between anthracyclines and nonanthracyclines (see Table 54.2).[1–3]

TABLE 54.2 Antitumor Antibiotics and Topoisomerase Inhibitors Including Anthracyclines

TREATMENTS/ DRUGS	THERAPEUTIC INDICATION	MECHANISMS OF CARDIOTOXICITY	RISK FACTORS	MANIFESTATIONS OF CARDIOTOXICITY	PREVENTION AND RISK REDUCTION STRATEGIES
Antitumor Antibiotics					
Mitomycin C Bleomycin	Gastric cancer Pancreatic cancer Bladder cancer Lung cancer Lymphomas Germ cell tumors Squamous cell CA	Unknown	• High cumulative dose > 30 mg/m^2 [Mitomycin C] • Concomitant with anthracycline or non-anthracycline-based chemotherapy • Prior coronary artery disease	CHF [Mitomycin C] Pericarditis [Bleomycin] Myocardial ischemia/ infarction [Bleomycin] Raynaud's [Bleomycin] Interstitial pneumonitis/ fibrosis/pulmonary hypertension [Bleomycin]	• Dose adjustment and limiting dose of other chemotherapies • Supportive care • Termination of treatment in case with pericarditis owing to Bleomycin
Topoisomerase Inhibitors					
Etoposide	Testicular cancer SCLC Hematologic cancer	Coronary artery vasospasm Direct injury to the myocardium Induction of an immune response	• Concurrent chemotherapy (esp., bleomycin, cisplatin, ifosfamide) • Preexisting CV disease	Myocardial ischemia/ infarction Vasospastic angina	• Unknown
Anthracyclines and Analogs					
TREATMENTS/ DRUGS (MAX. LIMITED DOSE, mg/m^2)	**THERAPEUTIC INDICATION**	**MECHANISMS OF CARDIOTOXICITY**	**RISK FACTORS**	**MANIFESTATIONS OF CARDIOTOXICITY**	**PREVENTION AND RISK REDUCTION STRATEGIES**
Doxorubicin (450–500) Daunorubicin (400–550) Epirubicin (800–900) Idarubicin (60)	Breast cancer Gastric tumor Leukemias Lymphomas Lung cancer Ovarian tumor Sarcomas	↑Toxic oxygen free radical ↑Oxidative stress Lipid peroxidation of membrane Replacement fibrous tissue ↓Endogenous antioxidant enzyme Iron accumulations complex Cellular apoptosis, DNA damage Topoisomerase IIb inhibition	• Concurrent chemotherapy • Prior/concurrent chest irradiation • High dose per cycle (>50 mg/m^2) • High cumulative dose (≥300 mg/m^2 of Doxorubicin, ≥600 mg/m^2 of Epirubicin) • IV bolus • Extreme age (Elderly >65, children <18) • Woman, pregnancy • Pre-existing CV disease (CAD, HT, LV dysfunction) • Hematopoietic cell transplantation	*Acute (Initial to several week after therapy)* • Arrhythmia (AF, SVT, VT, CHB, Mobitz II) • ST-T wave abnormalities • Anginal pain • LV dysfunction/CHF • Pericarditis/myocarditis • Myocardial ischemia/infarction *Chronic (early within 1 year and late onset beyond 1 year after therapy)* • Asymptomatic diastolic/systolic dysfunction, overt HF • Dilated cardiomyopathy Stroke	• Limiting lifetime cumulative dose • Structural modification (Liposome encapsulated molecule) and IV infusion schedule (>6 hours) • CV risk assessment before start chemotherapy • Intensive monitoring cardiac function during and after therapy • F/U ECG if QRS in limb leads ↓≥30% as associated with cardiomyopathy (Daunorubicin) • Adjunctive cardioprotective agent Dexrazoxane (Doxorubicin/ epirubicin) • Beta blocker (carvedilol, nebivolol) • ACE-I /ARB • Spironolactone • Statins

TABLE 54.2 Antitumor Antibiotics and Topoisomerase Inhibitors Including Anthracyclines—cont'd

TREATMENTS/ DRUGS (MAX. LIMITED DOSE, mg/m²)	THERAPEUTIC INDICATION	MECHANISMS OF CARDIOTOXICITY	RISK FACTORS	MANIFESTATIONS OF CARDIOTOXICITY	PREVENTION AND RISK REDUCTION STRATEGIES
Anthraquinolones					
Mitoxantrone (140 mg/m²)	Breast cancer, prostate cancer, NHL, AML Multiple sclerosis	↑Toxic oxygen-free radical ↑Oxidative stress	• Concurrent Chemotherapy • Prior/concurrent chest irradiation • High cumulative dose	Pericarditis-myocarditis syndrome CHF, arrhythmia Myocardial ischemia/ infarction	• Limiting lifetime cumulative dose • CV risk assessment before start chemotherapy • Intensive monitoring cardiac function during and after treatment

ALL, Acute lymphoblastic leukemia; *ACE-I*, angiotensin-converting-enzyme inhibitor; *AF*, atrial fibrillation; *AML*, acute myeloid leukemia; *CAD*, coronary artery disease; *CEL*, chronic eosinophilic leukemia; *CHB*, complete heart block; *CHF*, congestive heart failure; *CML*, chronic myelogenous leukemia; *CT*, computed tomography; *CV*, cardiovascular; *CYP3A4*, cytochrome p450 3a4 ; *DVT*, deep vein thrombosis; *ECG*, electrocardiogram; *GIST*, gastrointestinal stroma tumor; *GVHD*, graft versus host disease; *HF*, heart failure; *HR*, heart rate; *HT*, hormone therapy; *HTN*, hypertension; *ITP*, idiopathic thrombocytopenic purpura; *LBBB*, left bundle branch block; *LV*, left ventricular; *LVH*, left ventricular hypertrophy; *NHL*, non-Hodgkin lymphoma; *NCLC*, non–small-cell lung carcinoma; *PE*, pulmonary embolism; *RCC*, renal cell carcinoma; *ROS*, reactive oxygen species; *RT*, radiation therapy; *SCD*, sudden cardiac death; *SCLC*, small-cell lung carcinoma; *SPECT*, single photon emission computerized tomography; *SSS*, sick sinus syndrome; *SVT*, supraventricular tachycardia; *SVR*, stroke volume ratio; *TTP*, thrombotic thrombocytopenic purpura; *VT*, ventricular tachycardia; *WBC*, white blood cells.

Nontopoisomerase Inhibitors

The first antibiotic used as an antitumor agent and approved by the US Food and Drug Administration (FDA) in 1964 as such was **actinomycin D**, obtained from *Streptomyces griseus* in the mid 1950s. Actinomycin D inhibits the transcription of genes by interacting with a GC-rich duplex, a single-stranded or hairpin form of DNA, and interfering with the action of RNA polymerase.[1]

Mitomycin C was derived in the late 1950s as the second antitumor antibiotic from *Streptomyces caespitosus*. In tissues, mitomycin C is activated to an alkylating agent and is therefore covered in the following section.[1]

The third prominent antitumor antibiotic in the nontopoisomerase/nonanthracycline category is **bleomycin**.[1] It was isolated in 1966 from a strain of *Streptomyces verticillus*. Bleomycin acts by forming complexes with Fe^{2+} while binding to DNA. Oxidation of Fe^{2+} subsequently leads to the formation of free radicals, which results in DNA damage. Vascular side effects include flushing and Raynaud's phenomenon and the most concerning toxicity is pulmonary fibrosis (dose-dependent, commonly seen with cumulative doses greater than 300 units, pulmonary function testing with carbon monoxide diffusing capacity is to be obtained before initiation of therapy and with the onset of any symptoms).

Topoisomerase Inhibitors

Among the topoisomerase inhibitory antitumor antibiotics **anthracyclines** hold a special place for several reasons. They were the first group of cancer drugs that was discovered by a joint effort of a pharmaceutical company (Farmitalia) in collaboration with a research center (Istituto Nazionale dei Tumori in Milan).[2,3] This effort started in 1960 on a streptomyces strain, *Streptomyces peucetius*, found near Castel del Monte (Apulia). The new natural antitumor drug was called daunomycin (later daunorubicin), which showed higher efficacy compared with others antitumor drugs in patients with chronic lymphoproliferative diseases. In 1968, with expansion of the joint effort to include Memorial Sloan-Kettering Cancer Center in New York, a new molecule was extracted from a mutated strain of *S. peucetius* (obtained by treating the microorganism with N-Nitroso-N-methylurea): Adriamycin (later doxorubicin), which showed better activity against tumors in mouse and a greater therapeutic index. It has become the main anthracycline to be used, at least in the United States, for a variety of malignancies. Epirubicin, on the other hand, is used mainly for breast cancer, especially in Europe and idarubicin in the context of induction therapy for acute myeloid leukemia as part of the well-known 7+3 regimen (7 days cytarabine and 3 days idarubicin).

For all of these, a key mode of action is inhibition of topoisomerase II alpha, thereby prevention of the relaxation of supercoiled DNA and inhibition of DNA transcription and replication. Additional mechanisms include free radical formation with consequent induction of DNA damage or lipid peroxidation, DNA binding, and alkylation. These two mechanisms are also at play in the myocardium and account for cardiotoxicity. The same holds true for mitoxantrone, which is chemically related to the anthracyclines, an (amino-) anthraquinone that was synthesized in 1979. Unique is its use for metastatic hormone-refractory prostate cancer and in multiple sclerosis.

Currently, the other topoisomerase II inhibitors used clinically is **etoposide**. **Camptothecin**, isolated from the Chinese tree *Camptotheca acuminate*, was used for cancer treatment long before it was identified as a topoisomerase I inhibitor. Owing to its side effects, camptothecin is no longer used clinically. It was replaced by the more effective and safer derivates **irinotecan** and **topotecan**.[4]

Cardiovascular Toxicities

Anthracyclines are furthermore historically unique because of their unprecedented risk of cardiotoxicity in terms of potency and frequency.[5] In essence, it is only a matter of dose for cardiomyocytes to succumb to anthracyclines.[6] Clinically, two scenarios are differentiated: acute cardiotoxicity, which is a myocarditis-like presentation, and chronic cardiotoxicity, which is a dilated cardiomyopathy-like presentation.[7–9] Without testing, not many cases declare themselves acutely, even though injury may be present. The inflammation that can be seen in this setting may be classified best as toxic (reactive) myocariditis.[10] Cardiac function assessment (left ventricular ejection fraction [LVEF]) by imaging correlates poorly with cumulative dose and the histologic injury pattern.[11] Heart failure (HF), on the other hand, does seem to have a dose cutoff and follows a decline in cardiac function.[12] Two main mechanisms have prevailed over the years to explain the cardiotoxicity of anthracyclines. The first is the reactive oxygen species (ROS) or iron and free radical theory.[8] Anthracyclines have an affinity for cardiolipin, which brings them in close proximity to the respiratory chain in the mitochondria. In association with anthracyclines cardiolipin is reduced by nicotinamide adenine dinucleotide plus hydrogen (NADH), drawing an electron away from the mitochondrial respiratory chain and subsequently reducing oxygen to form a superoxide anion radical.[7] Further, the addition of an electron to the quinone moiety of anthracyclines leads to the formation of a semiquinone that reverts to the quinone state by reducing molecular oxygen to superoxide anion and its dismutation product hydrogen peroxide (the so called "redox cycling"). A surge in oxidative stress is generated when these products interact with low-molecular iron (Fenton reaction). Anthracyclines may also directly react with ferric iron ($Fe3+$) to form free radical and alcohol adducts. Collectively these processes lead to oxidative modification of proteins and lipids as well as genomic and mitochondrial DNA damage. Uncoupling of the electron transport chain with impairment of oxidative phosphorylation and adenosine triphosphate synthesis contributes further to mitochondrial dysfunction and damage. Oxidative stress activates a number of stress response pathways, including mitogen-activated protein kinase or extracellular signal-regulated kinase (MAPK/ERK). The phosphatidylinositol 3-kinase/protein kinase B (PI3K/AKT) pathway can take a protective role, activated, for instance by neuregulin-1 via human epidermal growth factor receptor-2 (HER2) signaling. This explains the syngergistic action in terms of cardiotoxicity when anthracyclines are combined with trastuzumab. An alternative or at least additional mechanism for anthracycline cardiotoxicity that emerged in recent years is the inhibition of topoisomerase II beta in cardiomyocytes.[13] Interfering with topoisomerase function anthracyclines may impair the repair of DNA as well, not only induce DNA damage, as described above.

Among the other antitumor antibiotics, mainly vascular toxicities have been seen. Mitomycin has been associated with thrombotic microangiopathy and HF on occasion (doses $> 30\ mg/m^2$). Bleomycin can cause abnormal vasoreactivity with Raynaud's phenomenon and chest pain syndromes as clinical presentations.[14–1 Bleomycin and cisplatin are the two drugs with the highest risk of drug-induced Raynaud's phenomenon.[1 Cases of acute ischemic events, including myocardia infarction, have been reported as well.

Patients with cardiovascular risk factors are a higher risk. Pericarditis is uncommon; pneumoniti and pulmonary fibrosis (with pulmonary hyperter sion) rank among the most concerning side effect (in up to 10% of patients).

Among the topoisomerase II inhibitors, irinoteca can cause vasodilation with hypotension and edem Cases of thromboembolism have been reported, b it is not one of the cancer drugs that have received consistent and widespread alerts in this regard. Etoposide is mainly known for causing hypotension; cases of myocardial ischemia and infarction have been reported as well.

Prevention and Treatment of Cardiotoxicity

The outlined mechanisms are important for the prevention and treatment of anthracycline cardiotoxicity. Reduction in the level of oxidative stress is a common denominator among agents that have been shown to be beneficial. These include beta blockers with antioxidant properties, ACE inhibitor and angiotensin receptor blockers (ARBs).[8,10] Furthermore, statins have been shown to be cardioprotective, possibly related to their antioxidant effects as well as reactivation of the PI3k/AKT kinase pathway. Dexrazoxane has become known as an iron chelator, but also as a strategy to modulate topoisomerase II beta to yield cardioprotective effects.[13]

ALKYLATING AGENTS

KEY POINTS

- Alkylating agents act by adding an alkyl group to the guanine base of the DNA molecule, causing structural damage to the DNA strands.
- Cardiomyopathy, pericarditis, and arrhythmias are the three main cardiovascular toxicities seen with alkylating agents.
- The risk of cardiovascular side effects is in part dose-related and also influenced by concomitant cardiotoxic chemotherapy.
- Older patients (age >50, females, those with known coronary artery disease, hypertension or heart failure (HF), prior or concomitant use of anthracycline, or mediastinal radiation are particularly susceptible to worsening HF and are at higher risk for arrhythmias; these patients should be monitored closely and treated for all cardiovascular risk factors.
- Emerging evidence suggests a role for acrolein in cyclophosphamide cardiotoxicity pointing toward acrolein inhibitors and scavengers as potential cardioprotective agents.
- No current guidelines exist for monitoring of cardiotoxicity with alkylating agents, but surveillance with echocardiograms and electrocardiograms is prudent, especially when higher doses are used.
- Early referral to cardiology/cardio-oncology is key in patients with suspected cardiotoxicity.

The recognition of the antitumor effects of alkylating agents dates back to the second decade of the 20th century and World War I as the vesicant properties of mustard gas were shown to induce suppression of lymphoid and hematologic functions.[1] The less-toxic, but closely related, nitrogen mustards of World War II, were selected for further trials in patients with lymphoma and they demonstrated regression of tumors with relief of symptoms. This led to the development of mechlorenthamine as the first alkylating agent used effectively in the treatment of human cancer.[2,3] An alternative route led to the approval of platinum drugs, which were discovered during studies on the influence of an electrical field on cell division, leading to the realization that the antiproliferative phenomenon had nothing to do with electricity, but rather with the release of a heavy metal, platinum, from the electrodes.

Although the alkylating agents react with cells in all phases of the cell cycle, their efficacy and toxicity result from interference with rapidly proliferating tissues (see Table 54.3).[4,5]

Mchanism of Action (see Fig. 54.1)

The cytotoxicity of alkylating agents can occur in two ways: conventional alkylation and unconventional methylation. Conventional alkylating agents form an aziridinium ion, which is an electrophilic cyclic ion that induces DNA alkylation either directly or through conversion to a carbonium ion. DNA structural change caused by alkylation blocks replication of new DNA (interstrand crosslink formation disrupts DNA separation) and inhibits transcription to mRNA for protein synthesis, impairing cell function, cell growth, and survival. These effects are amplified when alkylating agents form widespread interstrand crosslinks, inhibiting DNA repair and promoting apoptosis.[4]

These conventional alkylating reactions are generally classified through their kinetic properties as SN1 (nucleophilic substitution, first order) or SN2 (nucleophilic substitution, second order). The first-order kinetics of the SN1 reactions depends only on the concentration of the original alkylating agent (e.g., nitrogen mustards or nitrosoureas), which will decide the rate of formation of the reactive intermediate. The SN2 alkylation reaction (e.g., alkyl sulfonates) is a bimolecular nucleophilic displacement with second-order kinetics, where the rate

TABLE 54.3 **Alkylating Agents**

TREATMENTS/ DRUGS	THERAPEUTIC INDICATION	MECHANISMS OF CARDIOTOXICITY	RISK FACTORS	MANIFESTATIONS OF CARDIOTOXICITY	PREVENTION AND RISK REDUCTION STRATEGIES
Cyclophosphamide Ifosfamide	Leukemias Lymphomas Various solid tumors	Endothelial capillary damage	• High dose (not related to cumulative dose) • Elderly • Prior abnormal ejection fraction • Prior irradiation to chest wall • Prior anthracyclines	Hemorrhagic myocarditis/ pericarditis (common 1st week after high dose cyclophosphamide) Pericardial effusion/ tamponade LV dysfunction/CHF LVH	• Corticosteroid and analgesic with termination of treatment • Dose adjustment
Busulfan	Lymphomas Various solid tumors	Myocardial fiber fragmentation	• High-dose regimen • Use for lymphoma	Arrhythmias, ST-T wave change CHF	• Dose adjustment • ECG monitoring
Platinum drugs Cisplatin Carboplatin Oxaliplatin	CML	Unknown	• Unknown	Endocardial fibrosis/ pulmonary fibrosis HTN, arrhythmias Pericardial effusion	
	Germ cell tumors Ovarian cancer Lymphomas Head/neck tumors Lung cancer Sarcomas	Anaphylaxis and hypersensitivity reaction Endothelial injury/ apoptosis Arterial thrombosis Vascular fibrosis Electrolyte disturbance (hypokalemia, hypomagnesemia)	• Elderly • Prior mediastinal irradiation • Used for metastatic testicular cancer • Use with cyclophosphamide	*Early manifestation* • Venous and arterial thrombotic events • Myocardial ischemia/ infarction • Raynaud's phenomenon • HTN *Late manifestation* • Myocardial Ischemia/ infarction • HTN, stroke, LVH • Arrhythmia (SVT, bradycardia, LBBB) • (Ischemic) cardiomyopathy/CHF • Raynaud's phenomenon	• Adequate hydration and fluid balance • Electrolyte check-up and correction • Avoid concomitant renal toxic drug • Continuous infusion with infusion monitoring for hypersensitivity reaction

CHF, Congestive heart failure; *CML*, chronic myelogenous leukemia; *ECG*, electrocardiogram; *HTN*, hypertension; *LVH*, left ventricular hypertrophy.
Modified from Hermann J, ed. *Clinical Cardio-oncology.* Philadelphia: Elsevier; 2018.

depends on the concentration of both the alkylating agent and target nucleophile.[6]

In distinction, nonclassic or unconventional alkylating agents are synthetic inorganic nitrogen compounds that induce methylation of guanine bases, and therefore do not have the DNA crosslinking activity shown for classic alkylating agents.[4]

Nevertheless, the therapeutic and toxic effects of alkylating agents do not correlate directly with the subgroup to which they belong or with their chemical reactivity, because clinically useful agents include drugs with SN1 or SN2, and even some with both characteristics. The differences in their toxicity profiles and antitumor activity are more a consequence of their pharmacokinetics, membrane transport, metabolism and detoxification, lipid solubility, penetration of the central nervous system (CNS), and specific enzymatic reactions capable of repairing alkylation sites on DNA.[5]

Classic Alkylating Agents

Nitrogen Mustards

The nitrogen mustards are the most frequently used alkylating agents and the following have replaced mechlorethamine (the original "nitrogen mustard"): cyclophosphamide, ifosfamide, chlorambucil, and melphalan.

Cyclophosphamide is a prodrug that requires activation in the body to release active alkylating species. The initial activation reaction is carried out by cytochrome P450-mediated microsomal oxidation in the liver to produce 4-hydroxycyclophosphamide, after which it readily changes into its

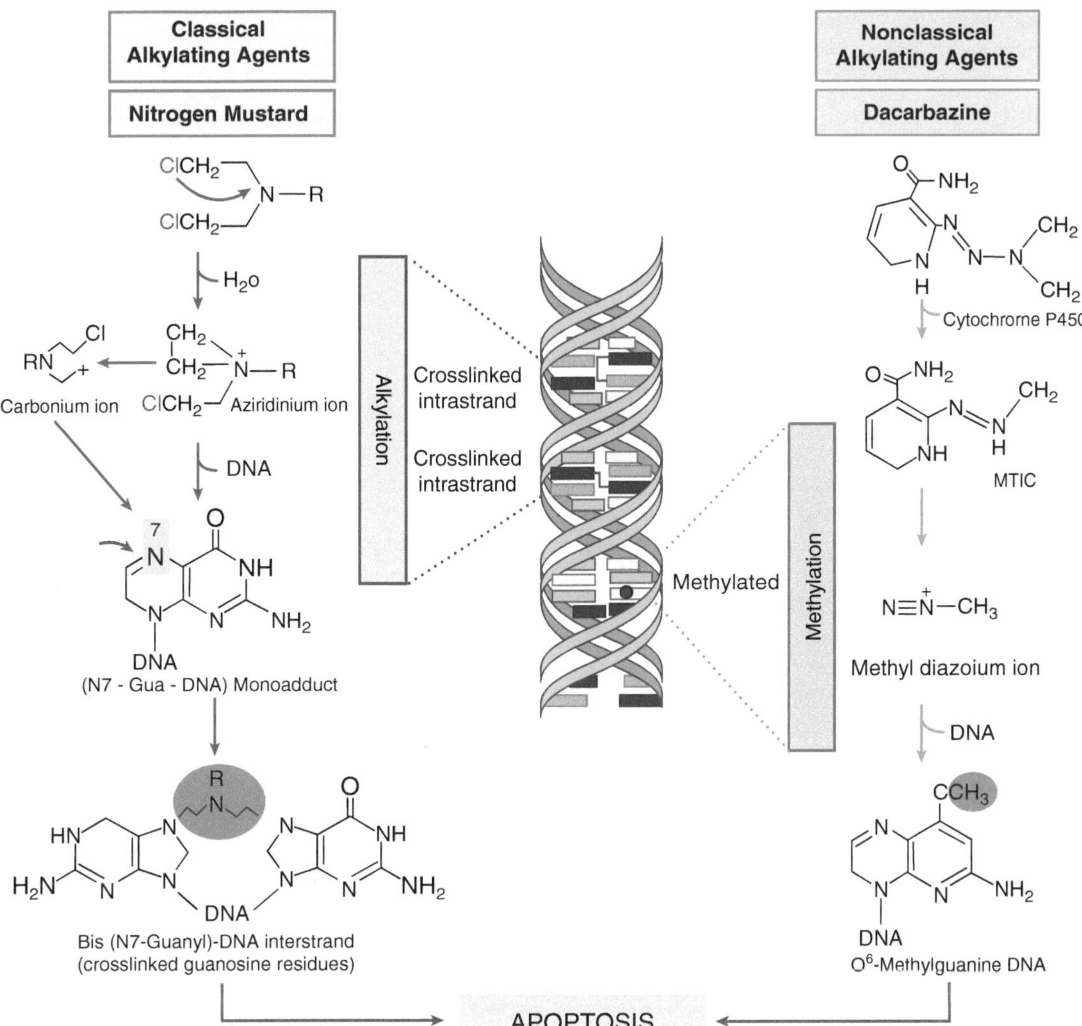

FIG 54.1 Alkylating agents mechanism of action. Classic alkylating anticancer agents (nitrogen mustard), undergo an intermolecular cyclization reaction to form the electrophilic aziridinium, which causes an alkylating reaction at the nucleophilic N7 of guanine, either directly or through a carbonium ion. This reaction can induce crosslinking when it occurs at two bases on complementary or identical strands. Alkylation of DNA impairs its function, affecting DNA replication and mRNA transcription for protein synthesis. This eventually leads to cellular apoptosis. Depending on the drug, such alkylation can occur only on one base, or on two bases within the same strand inducing crosslinking, or can occur on two bases from the complementary strands inducing interstrand crosslink. Unconventional or nonclassic alkylating agents (dacarbazine) form a methyldiazonium ion that induces methylation by reacting with O6 in guanine. Methylation occurring on a single strand leads to mismatched base pairing of the transformed guanine with thymine instead of cytosine during replication. This results in DNA truncation by DNA repair enzymes, leading to suppression of cell cycle progression or induction of apoptosis.

isomer aldophosphamide.[7,8] In cancer cells, aldophosphamide is broken down into the cytotoxic phosphoramide mustard and the byproduct acrolein. Phosphoramide mustard causes cytotoxicity by inducing DNA crosslinking between guanine molecules.[4,9] Cyclophosphamide was observed to have less toxicity in normal tissues, such as liver, bone marrow, and intestinal epidermal cells, compared with previous alkylating drugs. This is owing to the abundant amount of aldehyde-dehydrogenase in these tissues, converting 4-hydroxycyclophosphamide and aldophosphamide to carboxyphosphamide, which is not cytotoxic, is excreted in the urine and accounts for approximately 80% of an administered dose of cyclophosphamide.[10]

Ifosfamide is a structural isomer of cyclophosphamide, with subtle differences in the chemical properties of its reactive metabolite ifosfamide mustard, owing to the location of the chloroethyl group on the nitrogen ring. This makes it less reactive and hence less cytotoxic.[11,12] However, the oxidation of this chloroethyl side chain may produce either chloroataldehyde, which has been implicated in the neurotoxicity, or acrolein, which may contribute to the greater renal and bladder toxicity. Sodium-2-mercaptoethane sulfonate (mesna), can convert acrolein into a nontoxic compound and thereby prevent bladder toxicity (hemorrhagic cystitis). Mesna has been used until today to clinically prevent the side effects of ifosfamide, as approved by the FDA for testicular cancer and sarcoma.[13]

Chlorambucil's aromatic ring does not form a cyclic aziridinium ion, and therefore the drug exhibits lower toxicity than aliphatic nitrogen mustards. This low reactivity increases the chemical stability of chlorambucil and allows it to reach and stay in the DNA of target cancer cells for a longer time.[4]

Melphalan was developed by conjugating phenylalanine in place of the methyl group in mechlorethamine so that the drug could be delivered specifically to cancer cells through the L-phenylalanine active transport system. Reduced (bone marrow) toxicity and higher cancer cell specificity are the aspired consequences.[4]

Nitrosoureas

Nitrosoureas decompose to produce alkylating and carbamaylating compounds under physiologic conditions to induce DNA damage and to transform proteins, respectively. Representative drugs include **carmustine** (BCNU) and **lomustine** (CCNU). Their high lipophilicity allows them to easily penetrate the blood-brain barrier and to be used in CNS malignancies.[14]

Alkyl Sulfonates

Busulfan was one of the earliest alkylating agents. It has greater effect on myeloid cells than lymphoid cells (hence its main use in chronic myelogenous leukemia). It exhibits SN2 alkylation kinetics and shows nucleophilic selectivity for thiol groups, suggesting that it may exert cytotoxicity through protein alkylation rather than through DNA modification.[4,15]

Aziridines

Aziridines are analogs of ring-closed intermediates of nitrogen mustards and are less chemically reactive but therapeutically equally effective. These compounds are known to assault cancer cells by triggering DNA interstrand crosslinking.[4,5]

ThioTEPA acts through two mechanisms. The first is forming crosslinks through serial reactions. The second involves hydrolysis to produce an aziridine group, which then forms DNA monoadducts, separating the DNA strands and inducing apoptosis.[4,16]

Mitomycin C was approved by the FDA as a therapeutic agent for lung cancer and pancreatic cancer; however, owing to toxicities, such as hemolysis, and the introduction of other superior anticancer agents, its clinical use has largely declined.[17,18]

Platinum drugs

Platinum drugs remain of major use in the current treatment regimens of various cancers. Discovered by serendipity as mentioned above, **cisplatin** became the first platinum drug to be approved in 1978 for the treatment of testicular cancer. A variety of platinum complexes were tested thereafter with the collective knowledge of a structure–activity relationship, which was met by **carboplatin** and **oxaliplatin**. These platinum complexes, once aquated/activated, can react with nucleophilic centers on purine bases of the DNA (esp., the N7 positions of guanosine and adenosine residues). The two labile coordination sites on the platinum center permit crosslinking of adjacent guanine bases and, to a lesser extent, across different DNA strands to form interstrand crosslinks.[19]

Nonclassic Alkylating Agents

Hydrazine

Procarbazine was the first alkylating anticancer agent approved by the FDA among hydrazines. Its anticancer effect is by generating a methyldiazonium ion through spontaneous hydrolysis and inducing DNA methylation, which leads to truncation of chromatin threads and apoptosis.[20]

Triazenes

Dacarbazine acts as a prodrug. It becomes demeth ylated by cytochrome P450 (CYP3A4) and con verted into an activated monomethyl compound which methylates guanine in DNA, causing cytotox icity. It has the disadvantage of being extremel unstable in aqueous solution and needs to be directly injected into the blood vessels.[21]

Temozolomide is also a prodrug that undergoes spontaneous activation in solution to produce 5-(3-methyltriazen-1-yl) imidazole-4-carboxamide (MTIC), a triazine derivative. It crosses the blood–brain barrier with concentrations in the CNS approximating 30% of plasma concentrations with antitumor activity against gliomas and melanomas.[22]

Cardiovascular Toxicities

Alkylating agents can exert cytotoxic effects on the cardiovascular system, often magnified by the comorbid cardiovascular risk factors of an aging population, concomitant cardiotoxic chemotherapies, and radiation. Cardiotoxicity of these agents may range from asymptomatic pericardial effusion to myopericarditis, HF, and arrhythmias (see Table 54.3).

Left Ventricular Dysfunction

Asymptomatic reductions in LVEF as well as symptomatic HF has been reported with alkylating agents, especially with cyclophosphamide, ifosfamide, and mitomycin C.

Cyclophosphamide can cause structural damage, myocarditis, and HF.[23] This risk is dose-dependent, ranging from 7% to 28% with high-dose regimens and becoming evident within 1 to 10 days after administration. Animal studies have suggested that cyclophosphamide by itself is not directly cardiotoxic but acrolein, one of its metabolites, is 1000 times more toxic than doxorubicin.[24] It has been hypothesized that cyclophosphamide (via production of byproducts like acrolein) causes direct endothelial injury, followed by extravasation of toxic metabolites with cardiomyocyte injury, interstitial hemorrhage, and edema[25]; intracapillary microemboli may develop as well.[25] Myocardial ischemia caused from coronary vasospasm is another proposed mechanism of cardiotoxicity. Moreover, cyclophosphamide impairs cellular respiration and damages the inner mitochondrial membrane of cardiomyocytes, most likely through the induction of oxidative stress. Fulminant HF is seen most frequently in patients receiving a total dose of cyclophosphamide greater than 00 mg/kg prior to bone marrow transplantation. The clinical course is that of rapid onset of severe HF, which can be fatal within 10 to 14 days. The hearts of such patients are dilated, with patchy transmural hemorrhage and pericardial effusion. The microscopic findings consist of interstitial hemorrhage and edema, myocardial necrosis and vacuolar changes, and specific changes in the intramural small coronary vessels.[25,26] Cardiotoxicity could be seen in patients receiving lower doses of cyclophosphamide, if used in combination with other alkylating agents. Age above 50 years, previous adriamycin exposure, and concomitant radiation therapy to the left chest appear to increase the risk of cyclophosphamide cardiotoxicity.[27]

Given that **ifosfamide** and cyclophosphamide are structurally similar, it is possible that ifosfamide may induce HF through a similar mechanism. However, no histopathologic evidence of hemorrhagic myocarditis, which is the hallmark of cyclophosphamide toxicity, was found in patients treated with ifosfamide. Ifosfamide causes nephrotoxicity, which may delay the elimination of cardiotoxic metabolites and lead to acid-base and electrolyte disturbances and thereby cardiac function impairment and arrhythmias.[27]

Mitomycin C, particularly in combination with anthracyclines, may cause cardiomyopathy, probably owing to enhanced oxidative stress.[28] The risk seems to be related to cumulative drug dose (>30 mg/m^2).

Arrhythmias

Systemic use of alkylating agents has also been shown to cause a variety of atrial and ventricular tachyarrhythmias in 8% to 10% of patients within 72 hours of administration.[29,30] Marked symptomatic sinus bradycardia has also been described.[31] Alkylating agents may cause arrhythmias owing to direct damage of myocytes or through ischemia induced by coronary vasospasm and/or microthrombosis. Histopathologic studies have demonstrated that hypertrophy, fibrosis, and interstitial edema create a substrate vulnerable to arrhythmias.[29,30] However, **cyclophosphamide** and **ifosfamide** can cause arrhythmias even in the absence of left ventricular dysfunction. Other factors considered to increase the risk of bradyarrhythmias and atrioventricular block include excess vagal tone from severe nausea and emesis.[32–34] The nephrotoxic effects of ifosfamide with acid-base and electrolyte disturbances may contribute to arrhythmias. Ifosfamide specifically has been shown to cause ventricular tachycardias, atrial fibrillation, and reentry supraventricular tachycardia resistant to pharmacologic therapy.

Supraventricular tachycardia, especially atrial fibrillation (6.6% to 11%), is common after high-dose melphalan. Increased age (>60 years), higher baseline creatinine, larger left atrium size, and previous cardiac comorbidities are noted risk factors.

Pericarditis and Pericardial Effusion (Fig. 54.2)
Cyclophosphamide can cause pericarditis and pericardial effusion to the point of cardiac tamponade. The most feared complication is a hemorrhagic myocarditis/pericarditis, which occurs more commonly after 1 week of the administration of cyclophosphamide with doses greater than 40 mg/kg/day OR 1.4 g/m^2/day over a minimum of 2 consecutive days. This grave complication presents with HF symptoms, including new dyspnea at rest, elevated jugular venous pulsations, atypical chest pain, and peripheral edema. Tissue pathology demonstrates specific findings of intramyocardial extravasation of blood, fibrin, and fibrin-platelet microthrombi in capillaries. Fibrin strands in the interstitium is the most specific finding for the diagnosis of hemorrhagic myopericarditis. A decrease in QRS voltage can provide a clue. Pericardiocentesis should only be performed if necessary for tamponade.

Busulphan may occasionally cause pericardial and myocardial fibrosis, usually 4 to 9 years later and after a cumulative drug dose of more than 600 mg.[35] Intravenous busulphan may also induce tachycardia, hypertension, or hypotension and LV dysfunction; these complications are not observed after oral drug administration.[35]

Vascular Toxicities

Cisplatin (>carboplatin > oxaliplatin) has been associated with vascular events, primarily of two kinds: vasospasm, especially Raynaud's phenomenon, and thrombosis, including venous and arterial thrombosis. Coronary artery disease does not seem to be a prerequisite for acute coronary events to develop in patients undergoing platinum-based therapies. Intimal erosion secondary to induction of endothelial apoptosis has been suggested as the underlying mechanism (or thromboembolism from an alternate source). Of note, cisplatin levels can remain detectable over decades, indicating a potential long-term risk. Hypertension and renal toxicity are the other main side effects to be aware of for platinum drugs as it pertains to cardio-oncology.

Prevention and Treatment of Cardiotoxicity

Because most nitrogen mustards have dose-related cardiotoxicity, avoidance of higher doses of these drugs is a key preventative measure.

The relationship between acute toxicity and development of early and late cardiotoxicity is unclear. Clinical trials are required to determine if blocking acute toxicity (e.g., by the use of an ACE inhibitor or ARB) decreases the risk of subsequently developing later cardiotoxicity.[36] All patients who have already developed asymptomatic LV dysfunction or clinical HF, should be treated in keeping with HF guidelines.[37] Of the beta-blockers, carvedilol may have therapeutic advantages over the others, because it has been shown to possess antioxidant properties.[38] Its prophylactic use with alkylating agents is lacking.[38,39]

Management of arrhythmias should be individualized and decisions on the use of antiarrhythmic drugs or device therapy (implantable or external wearable cardioverter defibrillators) should consider the competing risks of cardiac and cancer-related life expectancy, quality of life, and complications. The diligent monitoring of electrolytes, QT interval on electrocardiogram and the use of QT prolonging agents, acid-base disturbances, and catabolic states are also key besides awareness of the direct arrhythmogenic effects of these drugs.

For complications, such as pericarditis, the use o standard therapy with nonsteroidal anti-inflammatory drugs and colchicine is recommended. Pericardiocentesis or pericardial window surgery should b considered in patients with refractory pericarditis o cardiac tamponade, provided they are not coagulo pathic or severely thrombocytopenic.

Hemorrhagic myopericarditis with cyclophospha mide and ifosfamide remains highly fatal and n standard treatment options have proven to reduc mortality. Use of corticosteroids, theophylline, no selective adenosine antagonist, ascorbic acid, or me chanical circulatory support have been anecdotall reported and must be guided by clinical judgemen No reports were found to demonstrate protectio with use of coadministration of mesna.[13]

Emerging Preventive Strategies

Animal studies have suggested that the cardiotox effects of cyclophosphamide are mediated throu

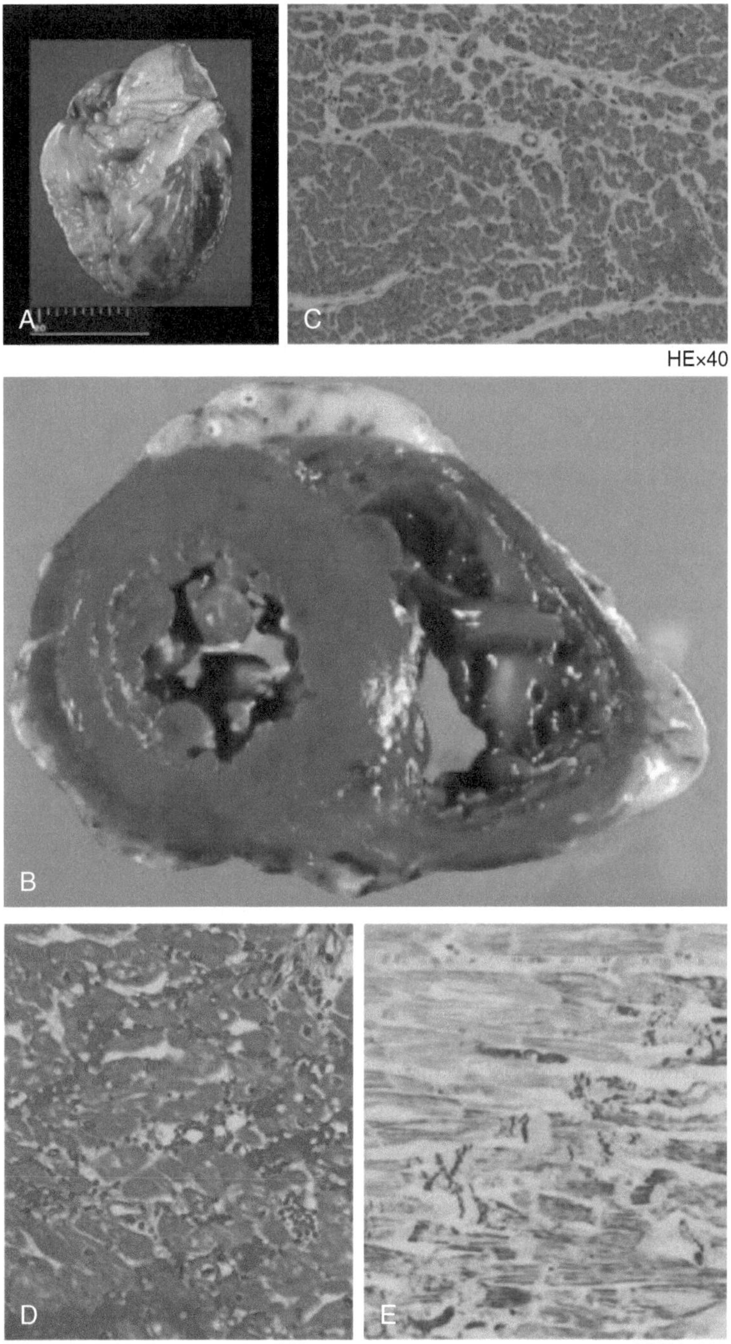

HE×40

HE×200

PTAH×200

IG 54.2 Postmortem examination in a lymphoma patient with fatal cyclophosphamide cardiotoxicity showing fibrinous pericarditis with potty pericardial hemorrhage (**A**). Cut surface of the myocardium showed diffusely hemorrhagic muscle and bulging appearance of yocardial tissue (**B**). Histologically, there were interstitial edema and extravasation of erythrocytes without infiltration of inflammatory ells or lymphoma cells (**C** and **D**). Although foci of contraction band necrosis were observed, most of the cardiac myocytes were histo-gically preserved. (From Katayama MI, Imai Y, Hashimoto H, et al. Fulminant fatal cardiotoxicity following cyclophosphamide therapy. *J Cardiol.* 09;54(2):330–334.)

the toxic reactive aldehyde acrolein, inducing extensive protein modifications and myocardial injury. Myocardial glutathione S-transferase P (GSTP), could prevent cyclophosphamide toxicity by detoxifying acrolein. Although this has only been seen in experimental studies in mice, humans with low cardiac GSTP levels or polymorphic forms of GSTP with low acrolein-metabolizing capacity may be more sensitive to cyclophosphamide toxicity.

Methyl palmitate may be of interest owing to its ability to suppress oxidative stress and to interrupt TLR4/NF-κB signaling pathway with reduction of apoptosis.[40] Similarly, by increasing carboxyethylphosphoramide mustard and decreasing acroline concentrations and ROS, N-acetylcysteine also has the potential to prevent cyclophosphamide cardiotoxicity.[24] Other agents that have shown promise as cardioprotectants include curcumine and piperine, oral glutamine, kolaviron, silymarin, blueberry anthocyanins-enriched extracts, green tea extract with hydrochlorothiazide, and many others still under clinical investigation.[41–46]

ANTIMETABOLITES

- Antimetabolites act by mimicking the structure of physiologic metabolites that are required for DNA synthesis or by interfering with their native synthesis; based on the metabolite, antifolates (e.g., methotrexate), antipurines (e.g., cytarabine), and antipyrimidines (e.g., 5-fluorouracil [5-FU]) are distinguished.
- From a cardiovascular perspective, 5-FU has received most attention with a broad spectrum of manifestations including chest pain, ischemia, ST segment elevation myocardial infarction (STEMI), non-STEMI (NSTEMI) arrhythmias, QT prolongation, HF, and stress cardiomyopathy, most of which has been related to altered vasoreactivity.
- The incidence of 5-FU cardiovascular toxicity is likely less than 1% overall, but 5% or more in patients with established coronary artery disease, most frequently occurring with first exposure.
- Dose-reduction, bolus infusion, and vasodilator therapy are recommendable management and prevention approaches.
- Risk/benefit of rechallenge in patients with prior cardiotoxicity should be carefully entertained.

Antimetabolites act by mimicking the structure of physiologic metabolites that are required for DNA synthesis or by interfering with their native synthesis. They most commonly affect cells in the S phase of the cell cycle (cell-cycle specific) when DNA replication is occurring. Based on the metabolite, antifolates, antipurines, and antipyrimidines are distinguished (see Table 54.4).

Antifolates

Antifolates were the first class of antimetabolites introduced in 1947 with aminopterin inducing complete remission of acute lymphoblastic leukemia. Amethopterin, better known as methotrexate, followed with conserved efficacy but less toxicity. It binds to and inhibits dihydrofolate reductase (DHFR), leading to inhibition of thymidylate and purine synthesis and, subsequently, to the induction of apoptosis.

Methotrexate was rationally designed nearly 60 years ago to potently block DHFR as an antimetabolite, thereby achieving temporary remissions in childhood acute leukemias. DHFR regenerates the reduced form of folate, a requirement for the biosynthesis of purines and thymidylate, which when missing leads to ineffective DNA synthesis and replication. When given in high doses, methotrexate is able to diffuse directly into cells leading to significant toxicity. Therapy is also toxic to nonmalignant cells, although leucovorin is able to bypass DHFR and rescue these cells. The strategy of high-dose therapy followed by leucovorin rescue is commonly used for the treatment of osteosarcoma and hematologic malignancies, especially when there is involvement of the CNS. As with all antimetabolites, methotrexate can cause myelosuppression and mucositis. It can also lead to renal dysfunction, which can be decreased with the use of urine alkalinization. Transaminitis can also be seen. The new generation antifolate pemetrexed is an antimetabolite with activity against certain lung cancers and mesothelioma. It is thought to affect many targets, including thymidylate synthetase, DHFR, and glycinamide ribonucleotide formyltransferase, which ultimately leads to a decreased production of purines and pyrimidines. Folic acid and vitamin B_{12} injections are given in conjunction to reduce side effects.

Antipurines and Anti(fluoro-) pyrimidines

Antipurines and anti(fluoro-)pyrimidines are ana logs to natural deoxynucleotides, competing for th

TABLE 54.4 **Antimetabolites**

TREATMENTS/ DRUGS	THERAPEUTIC INDICATION	MECHANISMS OF CARDIOTOXICITY	RISK FACTORS	MANIFESTATIONS OF CARDIOTOXICITY	PREVENTION AND RISK REDUCTION STRATEGIES
Fluorouracil (5-FU) Capecitabine	Breast cancer Colorectal cancer Pancreatic cancer	Endothelial cytotoxicity Vascular vasospasm (coronary) Exaggerated sympathetic stimulation Possible direct cytotoxic effect on cardiomyocytes	• Underlying CV disease • Infusion length and dose both in long-term and short-term • Previous treatment with 5-FU [Capecitabine] • Concomitant chemotherapy	Chest pain/angina (5-FU) Myocardial Ischemia/ infarction Myocarditis/pericarditis CHF, even cardiogenic shock Stress-induced cardiomyopathy (Takotsubo) (5-FU) Palpitations, arrhythmias, including ventricular tachycardia/fibrillation Sudden cardiac death	• Termination of treatment (reversible), retreatment after symptom improvement • IV bolus regimen, lower dose regimen • Antianginal treatment • Prophylactic coronary vasodilator therapy (limited efficacy)
Fludarabine Pentostatin Cladribine Cytarabine Methotrexate (MTX)	Leukemias Lymphomas Various solid tumors Autoimmune Disease	Unknown	• Unknown	Pericarditis (pericardial effusion/ tamponade) [cytarabine] Arrhythmia (bradycardia, supra/ventricular arrhythmia) [MTX] Hypotension/chest pain [fludarabine] Myocardial ischemia/ infarction CHF	• Termination of treatment (reversible), retreatment after symptom improvement • Steroid treatment in case of pericarditis from cytarabine • Antianginal treatment • Prophylactic coronary vasodilator (limited efficacy)

CHF, Congestive heart failure; *CV*, cardiovascular.
Modified from Herrmann J, ed. *Clinical Cardio-Oncology*. Philadelphia: Elsevier; 2018.

essential role in DNA synthesis, bases, and ribonucleosides. They can be divided into purine analogs (e.g., **fludarabine, cladribine**), pyrimidine analog (e.g., **cytarabine (ara-C), gemcitabine**), and the fluoropyrimidines (e.g., **5-FU, capecitabine**). 5-FU is readily incorporated into rapidly dividing malignant cells, especially those found within the gastrointestinal tract, explaining the widespread use of 5-FU in gastrointestinal malignancies. 5-FU has multiple mechanisms of action; its metabolite mediates inhibition of thymidylate synthase and 5-FU can also be incorporated into RNA and DNA. 5-FU is clinically administered with leucovorin to increase its antitumor activity. Capecitabine is a prodrug of 5-FU that is selectively activated in tumors overexpressing the activating enzyme thymidine phosphorylase.

5-Fluorouracil is one of the first and most successful designer chemotherapeutics, synthesized in 1957 by Heidelberger and colleagues, as a pyrimidine analog to slow a tumor's growth by interfering with DNA synthesis.[1] 5-FU-based chemotherapy is the standard of care for adjuvant treatment of stage II and III colorectal cancer (high-risk node-negative and node-positive disease) with a 20% to 30% reduction in mortality.[2] It is also a front-line agent for potentially curable, as well as metastatic, pancreatic cancer, metastatic esophageal and gastric cancer, early stage breast cancer with residual disease after anthracycline-based therapy, and metastatic breast, head, and neck cancers.[3–9]

Cardiovascular Toxicities

Most of the concerns have been residing with 5-FU and capecitabine in terms of cardio- and vascular toxicity and cytarabine for pericarditis and pericardial effusion (see Table 54.4). Coronary vasospasm during 5-FU infusion is well-documented, but 5-FU also causes cardiac hypertrophy, myocardial necrosis, apoptosis of myocardial and endothelial cells, vascular damage, and thrombus formation.[10–15] The complex pathophysiology of 5-FU results in a broad spectrum of cardiac toxicity including chest pain/angina, ischemia, NSTEMI and STEMI, silent ischemia noted on electrocardiogram (ECG) or ambulatory monitoring, bradyarrhythmias, ventricular arrhythmias, QT prolongation, HF and a stress cardiomyopathy.[1,16–20]

The risk of a cardiac event with 5-FU is 1.2% to 4.3% based on studies with over 400 patients, with the risk of treatment-related mortality of 0 to 0.5%.[21] It is reasonable to cite a risk of less than 1% for a life-threatening cardiac event in patients without known ischemic heart disease. For patients with ischemic heart disease, it is reasonable to cite a higher cardiac event risk (around 5%).[19,21,22] For patients with ischemic heart disease and a large ischemic burden despite guideline-directed therapy, inpatient cardiac monitoring for the first dose is not unreasonable. It is important when counseling patients to emphasize that, regardless of the risk, any chest pain with 5-FU or its oral prodrug, capecitabine, may represent a potentially life-threatening event and must be reported to health care providers immediately.

Cardiac events occur most frequently during the first cycle, (twice to eight times higher incidence than with later cycles).[22–27] Several studies report a median onset of symptoms within 72 hours of initiating 5-FU.[24,26,27] The effect of oral capecitabine is similar to a continuous low-dose infusion of 5-FU.[21] Though the incidence of cardiac events with capecitabine is higher during the first cycle (5.2% vs. 1.3% in later cycles) the onset of cardiac toxicity is even less predictable.[25]

Continuous infusion 5-FU may carry a higher risk of cardiac events than bolus alone.[21,23,28,29] The incidence of events with capecitabine appears similar to 5-FU continuous infusion over 5 days.[21,28–30] Dose reduction, bolus rather than continuous infusion, and prophylaxis with antianginal therapy (usually nitrates and/or calcium channel blockers) may be helpful.[27,28,31] Given the complex pathophysiology of 5-FU cardiotoxicity, prophylaxis to address coronary vasospasm is not sufficient to prevent all events.

Treatment of 5-FU cardiotoxicity includes nitrates and/or calcium channel blockers to address possible vasospasm. If underlying coronary artery disease cannot be definitively ruled out, acute management should include aspirin and statin. Emergent cardiac catheterization is recommended in the presence of significant ST segment elevation, depression, new left bundle branch block (LBBB) or hemodynamic instability. For patients with suggestive cardiac symptoms, but without diagnostic ECG changes, echocardiography for wall motion and ejection fraction, serial cardiac enzymes, and a focused cardiac care unit are indicated. In less urgent cases, CT angiogram or cardiac stress testing may also be helpful in evaluating whether ischemic heart disease is a contributing factor.

Whether to rechallenge a patient with a prior 5-FU cardiotoxicity is a complex decision that depends on the severity of the prior event, potential oncologic benefit of 5-FU, and availability of alternative treatments. For a patient who had chest pain and/or ECG changes without a troponin elevation, and for whom 5-FU promises the best oncologic outcome, one may consider inpatient admission with cardiac monitoring for the subsequent dose, and prophylaxis with nitrates and calcium-channel blockers. Dose reduction of 5-FU or bolus rather than continuous infusion is furthermore of consideration, although this may impact the efficacy. In case of exertional chest pain, exercise stress echo during 5-FU infusion can further risk stratify. For patients with more significant cardiotoxicity (troponin elevation, decline in ejection fraction, arrhythmias), rechallenging is generally advised, although there are individual cases where the potential for benefit is great and comparable treatment options are not available. In these cases, an appropriate consent process with the patient prior to proceeding and inpatient admission with cardiac monitoring are recommended.

MITOSIS INHIBITORS

KEY POINTS

- Mitosis inhibitors, also known as microtubule agents, are commonly used anticancer drugs, interfering with the segregation of chromosomes, an essential step to cell division and proliferation.
- Two subtypes are differentiated: microtubule stabilizers (esp., taxanes) and microtubule destabilizers (esp., vinca alkaloids).
- Acute side effects include nausea and vomiting and delayed toxicities myelosuppression and neurotoxicity.
- Cardiovascular side effects include mainly arrhythmias (bradycardia in particular) and vascular toxicities, including myocardial ischemia.
- Management is reactive.

Microtubules are required for the segregation o chromosomes during the M-phase of the cell cycl when the cell divides its DNA into two identical se of chromosomes (mitosis) as well as its cytoplasn (cytokinesis).[1] The mitotic spindles are fibrillar structures that are part of the cytoskeleton and composed of tubulin polymers. As one might expect, interference with the formation and function of microtubules can effectively disrupt mitosis and cell division, and even more, ultimately result in cell death.[2,3] Mitosis inhibitors are commonly classified as microtubule-destabilizing agents or microtubule-stabilizing agents based on their mode of action (i.e., either inhibiting the polymerization of microtubules via the interaction with the spindle assembly checkpoint [*Vinca* alkaloid and colchicine-binding sites] or stabilizing microtubules and preventing calcium- or cold-induced depolymerization, with subsequent blockage of mitotic fuse disassembly) (see Table 54.5).[2,4,5]

Microtubule Destabilizers

Microtubule destabilizers are mainly vinca alkaloids from the periwinkle plan (**vincristine** and **vinblastine**), first discovered in the late 1950s.[6] Initially used for the treatment of diabetes, their antitumor action was noticed in experimental models. In the 1960s their molecular mode of action was identified and several vinca derivates were synthesized (**vindesine, vinorelbine,** and **vinflunine**), all with depolymerizing action but greater therapeutic efficacy than the natural extract. Vinca alkaloids act by binding to the β-subunit near the guanosine triphosphate (GTP)-binding site on tubulin and thereby alter dimer conformation, inhibiting tubulin-dependent GTP hydrolysis and guanosine diphosphate (GDP)–GTP exchange.[7] At low concentrations, vinca alkaloids bind to the plus ends of microtubules, reducing the microtubule dynamics and contributing to mitotic arrest (so-called "end poisons" action).[7] At higher concentrations, the vinca alkaloids have affinity for free tubulin heterodimers, altering the geometry of the dimeric biological vector further into a curved shape, which favors the formation of paracrystals, spirals, and tubules.[8]

Microtubule Stabilizers

Microtubule stabilizers are mainly taxanes, plant alkaloids from the bark of the Pacific Yew tree, discovered in the 1970s. **Paclitaxel** was the first, **docetaxel** and **cabazitaxel** the second and third generation products. Taxanes target specific sites within the

TABLE 54.5 **Mitotic Inhibitors (Microtubule-Targeting Agents)**

TREATMENTS/ DRUGS	THERAPEUTIC INDICATION	MECHANISMS OF CARDIOTOXICITY	RISK FACTORS	MANIFESTATIONS OF CARDIOTOXICITY	PREVENTION AND RISK REDUCTION STRATEGIES
Vinca Alkaloids Vinblastine Vincristine Vinorelbine	Leukemias Lymphomas Nephroblastoma TTP/chronic ITP Brest cancer SCLC	Possible vasospasm Endothelial injury/ apoptosis	• Unknown	Hypertension Myocardial ischemia/infarction Vasoocclusive complication Raynaud's phenomenon	• Unknown
Taxane derivative Paclitaxel Docetaxel Eribulin Ixabepilone	Breast cancer Ovarian cancer NSCLC Kaposi's sarcoma Prostate cancer Gastric Adenocarcinoma	Anaphylaxis and Hypersensitivity reaction Possible vasospasm	• Congenital long QT syndrome • Concomitants chemotherapy • Concomitants with drug that prolonged QTc • Underlying CV disease	Conduction abnormalities (bradycardia, CHB) Arrhythmia (SVT), Angina Prolong QTc [Eribulin] Myocardial ischemia/ infarction Ventricular dysfunction Hypotension	• Pre-treatment with corticosteroid, H1 and H2 blocker agents • Dose adjustment and limiting dose of anthracycline • ECG monitoring [Paclitaxel, Eribulin] • Continuous infusion with infusion monitoring for hypersensitivity reaction

CHB, Complete heart block; *CV*, cardiovascular; *ECG*, electrocardiogram; *ITP*, idiopathic thrombocytopenic purpura; *NSCLC*, non–small-cell lung carcinoma; *SCLC*, small-cell lung carcinoma; *SVT*, supraventricular tachycardia; *TTP*, thrombotic thrombocytopenic purpura.
Modified from Herrmann J, ed. *Clinical Cardio-Oncology*. Philadelphia: Elsevier; 2018.

lumen of polymerized microtubules.[7] They bind to GDP-bound β-tubulin molecules changing their conformation to the more stable GTP-bound β-tubulin structure. This change aligns the dimer's biological vector with the vector of microtubule growth, increasing incorporation into the microtubule and its subsequent stabilization. This interaction between neighboring dimers results in an equilibrium shift from the soluble to the polymerized form of tubulin and a bundled phenotype of interphase microtubules. Microtubule over-polymerization ultimately leads to cell death by apoptosis.

Epothilones, like **ixabepilone**, are macrolide antibiotics and they represent a novel class of antimicrotubule agents, which by binding near the taxane-binding site cause microtubular stabilization and cellular arrest.

Eribulin mesylate is a nontaxane, completely synthetic microtubule inhibitor approved as third-line treatment of metastatic breast cancer refractory to anthracyclines and taxanes.[9] Eribulin is a synthetic analog of halichondrin B, a substance derived from a marine sponge. Unlike other antimicrotubule drugs, such as vinblastine and paclitaxel, which suppress the shortening and growth phases of microtubule dynamic instability, eribulin works through an end-poisoning mechanism, resulting in the inhibition of microtubule growth, but not of shortening. Tubulin is also sequestered into nonfunctional aggregates, resulting in irreversible G_2 to M-phase arrest and apoptosis.

Cardiovascular Toxicities

Vinca alkaloids, most commonly vinblastine, have been associated with vascular toxicity and most notably hypertension, although Raynaud's phenomenon, myocardial ischemia, and infarction have been reported as well.[10,11]

Paclitaxel has notoriously been associated with arrhythmias, mainly asymptomatic sinus bradycardia, which was recognized in 30% of patients monitored for hypersensitivity reactions with the Kolliphor EL (formerly known as Cremophor EL) formulation. Other, more worrisome types of arrhythmias, including atrioventricular and bundle branch blocks, and ventricular tachycardia have been reported in approximately 3% of patients. Most of these arrhythmias are noted within the first two cycles of paclitaxel therapy and tend to be self- imiting within 48 to 72 hours after discontinuation of therapy.[10] As mainly asymptomatic, routine monitoring is not recommended, at least not in those without risk factors.[12,13]

As blood pressure shifts can occur, frequent monitoring of vital signs is recommended, however, and those recognized to develop conduction abnormalities in this setting should have continuous monitoring during subsequent infusions. Important to know is that a scientific statement from the American Heart Association lists conventional paclitaxel as an agent that may either cause direct myocardial toxicity or exacerbate underlying myocardial dysfunction (magnitude: moderate).[14] This is supported by prospective data that up to 20% of patients on paclitaxel may experience a drop in LVEF and in 20% of these the drop will be by more than 20%.[15] Similar rates were reported in some but not all studies when paclitaxel was combined with doxorubicin. This being said, the impression has been that paclitaxel lowers the dose threshold for the development of HF in patients on doxorubicin. This effect has been attributed, in addition to the interference with the elimination of anthracyclines, to the stimulation of the conversion of doxorubicin to cardiotoxic metabolites (namely doxorubicin) inside cardiomyocytes.[16,17]

Nanoparticle albumin-bound paclitaxel (nab-paclitaxel, Abraxane) does not have a lower cardiovascular toxicity profile than the conventional formulation. Asymptomatic ECG abnormalities are seen in 35% of patients with a normal baseline, and in up to 60% otherwise. Hypertension and HF have been reported in 1% to 10% o patients, Chest pain, arterial and venous thrombolic events including acute myocardial infarction (AMI), even cardiac arrest can occur. The risk for severe events (grade 3 or higher) is ap proximately 3%.

Docetaxel can cause similar presentations a paclitaxel, although less frequently and with less o a causal link. Contrary to paclitaxel, docetaxel doe not affect doxorubicin's half-life elimination and it role in potentiating the cardiotoxicity of anthrac clines remains debated.[17]

With **Eribulin** the main concern is QTc prolonga tion, occurring late (or delayed), approximatel one week (but not on the first day) after the start o therapy. The FDA recommends ECG monitoring i patients who have HF, bradyarrhythmias, or are r ceiving drugs known to prolong the QTc interval. should be avoided in those with congenital long Q syndrome.

Ixabepilone seems to include the frequency of chest pain and cardiac dysfunction over what is seen with capecitabine alone, but maybe not in isolation. The labeling, however, suggests cautious use in patients with a history of cardiac disease and discontinuation of therapy in patients who develop cardiac ischemia or impaired cardiac function during therapy.

MONOCLONAL ANTIBODIES

KEY POINTS

- Monoclonal antibodies, which have revolutionized the treatment of malignancies, are widely used.
- Antigenicity is overcome by one of three designs: chimeric, humanized, and fully human.
- Affinity and efficacy are tailored further by point changes to the antibody in the antigen-binding and Fc regions.
- Interference with extracellular surface molecules is a key point of action of therapeutic antibodies.
- Induction of effector function, such as antibody-dependent cell-mediated or cellular cytotoxicity (ADCC), antibody-dependent cellular phagocytosis (ADCP), and complement-dependent cytotoxicity (CDC) add to it.
- Cardiovascular side effects relate to the signaling pathways and biological functions affected and include cardiomyopathy, myocarditis, vascular events, and arrhythmias to the point of sudden cardiac death.
- Management is reactive.

Currently 35 antibodies against 19 different antigen targets have FDA approval for the treatment of tumors (see Table 54.6). The most successful and important are the antibodies that target cluster differentiation 20 (CD20) and epidermal growth factor receptor (EGFR), including HER2, (VEGF), and programmed cell death protein 1 (PD-1) and its ligand (PD-L1). Based on the nature of the antibody generation, chimeric, humanized, and human antibodies can be differentiated.[1–4]

Chimeric Antibodies

Therapeutic monoclonal antibodies are typically IgGs composed of two heavy and two light chains. The two heavy chains form a "Y" structure and the two light chains run parallel to the open top portion of the heavy chain. The tips of the heavy-light chain pairs then form the antigen-binding sites with the primary antigen recognition regions. These are also known as the complementarity-determining regions (CDRs). The door to commercial monoclonal antibody production of predefined specificity was opened by César Milstein and Georges J. F. Köhler in 1975. Fusing and selectively growing cells from a myeloma cell line and spleen cells from a mouse immunized with sheep red blood cells, they generated a hybridoma cell line with the immortality of a myeloma cell and the ability to produce very large amounts of antibodies specific for sheep red blood cells. Several limitations to mouse monoclonal antibodies for the treatment of human cancers were noted, however. These included a broad range of target selections, that included those not critical for a specific malignancy, low overall potency, poor tumor penetration, and the development of human antimouse antibodies.

The availability of recombinant DNA technology allowed for a revised antibody design with reduced antigenicity of murine and other rodent-derived monoclonal antibodies in the early 1980s. Antigenicity and human antimouse antibodies responses could be further reduced by the development of chimeric antibodies, in which the constant domains of the human IgG were combined with the murine variable regions by transgenic fusion of the immunoglobulin genes. For instance, **cetuximab** was generated by immunizing mice with purified EGFR and replacing the mouse constant domains of the mouse antibody 225 with those of human IgG1. In addition to rendering less immunogenic molecules, chimerization allowed for the same or improved affinity than the parental mouse antibodies, but with enhanced effector functions.

Humanized Antibodies

In the mid to late 1980s, partially humanized antibodies were developed in which the CDRs of the heavy and light chains and a limited number of structural amino acids of the murine monoclonal antibody were grafted by recombinant technology to the CDR-depleted human IgG scaffold. Replacing human residues with the original mouse residues, especially those that guide antigen detection and interaction through a process of backmutation, improved affinity and efficacy. Prominent examples are **trastuzumab, pertuzumab, bevacizumab, and pembrolizumab**.

TABLE 54.6 **Monoclonal Antibodies**

TREATMENTS/ DRUGS	THERAPEUTIC INDICATION	MECHANISMS OF CARDIOTOXICITY	RISK FACTORS	MANIFESTATIONS OF CARDIOTOXICITY	PREVENTION AND RISK REDUCTION STRATEGIES
Trastuzumab	Breast cancer Gastric cancer Esophageal cancer	Direct blockage to HER2 effect to impair embryonic heart development and loss protective effect from cardiotoxin Anaphylaxis and hypersensitivity reaction	• Prior or concurrent anthracyclines > 300 mg/m² • Preexisting poor LV function • Age > 50 years • High BMI • Woman with underlying DM • Antihypertensive treatment	Cardiomyopathy and CHF (black box warning) Anaphylactic reaction Arrhythmias HTN Peripheral edema	• Dose adjustment and limiting dose of anthracycline, temporal separation • Termination of treatment, institution of beta-blocker and ACE inhibitor, may attempt retreatment after symptom improve (however, may not be reversible in all cases and/or may reoccur) • Continuous infusion with monitoring for hypersensitivity reaction • Weekly preferred over 3-weekly infusions
Rituximab	Lymphomas Leukemias Autoimmune diseases	Unknown Anaphylaxis and hypersensitivity reaction	• Preexisting CV disease • High number of circulating malignant cells ($\geq$ 25,000/mm³) with or without evidence of high tumor burden	Anginal pain Arrhythmia (ventricular fibrillation) Myocardial ischemia/ infarction Cardiomyopathy/ Takotsubo's Cardiogenic shock	• Cardiac function surveillance (baseline, 3, 6, 9, 12, months and at 18–24 months if sequential to anthracyclines) • Troponin I level can predict later cardiotoxicity and prognosis for trastuzumab-related cardiotoxicity • Termination of treatment (reversible) • Continuous Infusion with infusion monitoring for hypersensitivity reaction
Bevacizumab	Colorectal cancer Glioblastoma Breast cancer NSCLC RCC	Unknown Possible exacerbate of preexisting coronary and peripheral vessels owing to antibody of PIGF Infusion hypersensitivity reaction	• Preexisting CV disease, especially HTN and DM (possibly OSA) • Prior/concurrent anthracyclines • Age > 65 years • Previous arterial thromboembolic event	Anginal pain, dyspnea Myocardial ischemia/infarction Stroke, arterial and venous thromboembolic event Bleeding Severe hypertension Cardiomyopathy/Takotsubo's/HF	• Monitoring of BP on and off therapy • Optimal BP treatment • Assess and treat OSA • Infusion monitoring for hypersensitivity reaction • Aspirin in elderly with prior arterial thromboembolic event
Alemtuzumab	Lymphoma Leukemias Multiple sclerosis GVHD	Unknown Anaphylaxis and hypersensitivity reaction	• Unknown	Hypotension, cardiogenic shock Arrhythmia (AF, VT) CHF Myocardial ischemia/infarction	• Termination of treatment (reversible) • Continuous infusion with infusion monitoring for hypersensitivity reaction • Premedication with corticosteroid and H1 and H2 blockage agents
Cetuximab	Colorectal cancer Head/neck tumors	Unknown Anaphylaxis and hypersensitivity reaction Electrolyte imbalance (hypomagnesemia)	• Preexisting CV disease (previous CAD, HT, LV dysfunction or arrhythmia)	Arrhythmia, QTc prolongation Sudden cardiac arrest (black box warning) CHF Myocardial ischemia/infarction	• Termination of treatment (reversible) • Continuous infusion with infusion monitoring for hypersensitivity reaction • Monitor and correction of serum electrolyte and magnesium • Dose modification

ACE-I, Angiotensin-converting enzyme inhibitor; *AF*, atrial fibrillation; *ALL*, acute lymphoblastic leukemia; *AML*, acute myeloid leukemia; *CAD*, coronary artery disease; *CEL*, chronic eosinophilic leukemia; *CHB*, complete heart block; *CHF*, congestive heart failure; *CML*, chronic myelogenous leukemia; *CT*, computed tomography; *CV*, cardiovascular; *CYP3A4*, cytochrome p450 3a4; *DVT*, deep vein thrombosis; *ECG*, electrocardiogram; *GIST*, gastrointestinal stroma tumor; *GVHD*, graft versus host disease; *HF*, heart failure; *HR*, heart rate; *HT*, hormone therapy; *HTN*, hypertension; *ITP*, idiopathic thrombocytopenic purpura; *LBBB*, left bundle branch block; *LV*, left ventricular; *LVH*, left ventricular hypertrophy; *NCLC*, non–small-cell lung carcinoma; *NHL*, non-Hodgkin lymphoma; *PE*, pulmonary embolism; *RCC*, renal cell carcinoma; *ROS*, reactive oxygen species; *RT*, radiation therapy; *SCD*, sudden cardiac death; *SCLC*, small-cell lung carcinoma; *SPECT*, single photon emission computerized tomography; *SSS*, sick sinus syndrome; *SVR*, stroke volume ratio; *SVT*, supraventricular tachycardia; *TTP*, thrombotic thrombocytopenic purpura; *VT*, ventricular tachycardia; *WBC*, white blood cells.

[illegible] ed. *Clinical Cardio-Oncology*. Philadelphia: Elsevier; 2018.

Human Antibodies

Last but not least, fully human antibodies emerged in the 1990s with the development of two technology platforms: phage-display libraries and transgenic animals. The latter approach requires less optimization, carries less developability liability, and allows for shorter timelines to reach clinical development. This being said, this *in vivo* approach does not always lead to antibodies with the desired antibody affinity and specificity. On the other hand, phage display allows for designing and manipulating the repertoire of antibody genes to be used as a source of antibodies, and because conducted *in vitro*, optimal conditions for desired biophysical and biochemical properties can be selected; predefined epitopes can be targeted and locked in specific conformations; immunodominant epitopes can be avoided by masking them with other known antibodies; and/or focus the selection of rare or cross-reactive epitopes. In addition to the phage display system, ribosome, bacteria, yeast, and mammalian display platforms have been used, each with advantages and disadvantages. The yeast display is the most common and bears advantages over the phage display system in terms of efficiency in isolating with very high affinity and display of full IgG antibodies with glycosylation (whereas the phage system is limited to the display of antibody fragments such as scFvs or Fabs). Examples are **ramucirumab, ipilimumab, and nivolumab**.

Effector Functions

Most therapeutic antibodies are IgG1s, the most abundant subclass in humans, followed by IgG2s, IgG3s, and IgG4s. The half-life of all these is 21 days, with the exception of IgG3s (7 days). IgG3s show the highest complement activating capacity followed by IgG1s and IgG2s whereas IgG4s have none. IgG1 and IgG3 show high affinity to the Fc receptor on phagocytic cells. The Fc region has been recognized as being extremely important for the antitumor effect as it mediates effector functions such as ADCC, ADCP, and CDC.[5]

ADCC is triggered when an antibody simultaneously binds its cognate antigen on the surface of the target cell (via the Fab region) and Fc gamma receptors (FcγR) on the surface of an effector cell (via the Fc region). Effector cells include macrophages and neutrophils, which can express all low to high affinity FcγR subtypes as well as other immune cells: dendritic cells with high affinity FcγRI (CD64), Langerhans cells with intermediate affinity FcγRIIa (CD32a), and natural killer (NK) cells with low-affinity FcγRIIIa (CD16a). Upon FcγR activation the effector cells release cytotoxic granules that eliminate the antibody-coated cancer cell. This mechanism has been shown to contribute to the therapeutic efficacy of **rituximab**, **trastuzumab**, and **cetuximab**. **ADCP** is similar to ADCC, the difference being that phagocytosis is triggered by the binding surface antibody instead of the release of granules from the effector cell. **Trastuzumab** and **rituximab** are examples of therapeutic antibodies that trigger this response in the cancer tissue as well. Last, but not least, **CDC** is triggered when the antibody Fc region binds complement component 1q, which ultimately leads to the formation of transmembrane channels in the cell membrane of the target cancer cell with fatal consequences (membrane attack complex or terminal complement complex). Again, **rituximab**, **trastuzumab**, and **cetuximab** are prominent examples of therapeutic antibodies that trigger CDC.[6] Of note, even single point mutations can alter the potency of therapeutic antibodies to induce one or more of the effector functions as can glycosylation. In fact, the latter is critical for stabilization of the conformation and binding characteristics of the Fc region.

Based on the outlined effector functions, the affinity of the antibody for the target, and/or the biology of the target, the mode of action of the different therapeutic antibodies varies. In terms of biology, the target may be a component of a classic oncogenic pathways, such as HER2, or related to vessel formation (angiogenesis), such as VEGF, or the immune response/system, such as immune checkpoints.

Antibodies may thus lead to inhibition of malignant cell proliferation and/or induction of apoptosis, blockade of the formation of new blood vessels, and enhancement of the antitumor cytotoxic T cell (CTL) immune response to tumor cells.

Anti-CD20 Antibodies

Rituximab became the first therapeutic antibody to be approved for cancer therapy in 1997. It targets CD20, which is highly expressed on B cells (but not hematopoietic stem cells). The physiologic function of CD20 is not fully defined, but is assumed to play a role in calcium signaling of B-cell antigen receptor activation. CD20 remains on the surface upon antibody binding, allowing for the recruitment of immune cells and the broad range of effector functions, thereby effective elimination of malignant CD20-expression cells.

Anti-CD20 antibodies are classified as type I or type II according to their interaction with CD20 and the primary mode of action. Rituximab and ofatumumab are type I antibodies, which have full binding capacity, high CDC, and moderate direct cell death induction. Obinutuzumab, on the other hand, is a type II with half binding capacity, low CDC, and stronger direct cell death induction. In addition to specific epitopes binding, orientation of the antibodies once bound to CD20 seems to determine the therapeutic efficacy.

Anti-EGFR Antibodies Including HER2

The EGF receptors, including EGF receptor-2 or HER2 were among the first to be associated with human cancers and are prototypes for the dysregulation of growth factor pathways as a central mechanism to cancer. All three approved anti-EGFR therapeutic antibodies bind domain III (of four extracellular domains) and block the interaction with EGF. Cetuximab, necitumumab and panitumumab bind a very similar surface on EGFR, but have different functional epitopes and CDRs.

Although of similar structure and belonging to the class of EGF receptors, HER2 does not bind a ligand and functions primarily *via* heterodimerization with ligand-bound partners of the EGF receptor family, mostly HER3. Trastuzumab binds domain IV, interrupting HER2 dimerization and preventing cleavage of the extracellular domain, which leads to the active truncated receptor p95HER2. Interference with HER2-linked signaling furthermore interrupts intracellular signaling pathways that regulate, in particular, proliferation and survival.[7] Among these, the PI3K/AKT pathways takes a special role, last but not least, because it is also the main molecular link between HER2 targeting and cardiotoxicity.[8] Pertuzumab binds domain II and prevents heterodimerization of HER2 with HER3 and EGFR. Of note, the combination of pertuzumab and trastuzumab in breast cancer therapy has been shown to be more efficacious than the treatment with either drug alone.

VEGF and VEGF Receptor Antibodies

Bevacizumab is the first angiogenesis inhibitor to be approved for cancer therapy.[9,10] Bevacizumab is a recombinant humanized antibody that selectively binds to all isoforms of human VEGF with high affinity and thereby neutralizes the binding of VEGF to its receptors Flt-1 (VEGFR-1) and KDR (VEGFR-2) on the surface of endothelial cells and VEGF's biological activity. This activity is transmitted through the activation of the signaling pathway following receptor tyrosine phosphorylation and elicits mitogenic and prosurvival activity signals for the vascular endothelial cells. The thought has been that there is very low, if any expression of VEGF receptors in most normal tissues, but a significant upregulation in the tumor vasculature. Based on Judah Folkman's seminal work, tumor growth beyond a certain volume requires sufficient blood supply, in particular as most tumors are metabolically very active and in need of sufficient nutrient and oxygen supply. Interference with the development of the tumor vasculature and especially VEGF as the main angiogenic (growth) factor deemed very attractive. Experimental studies provided proof of concept and also outlined that anti-VEGF therapies have a relatively fast on-set and off-set.

Ramucirumab is fully human monoclonal antibody that binds the extracellular domain of the VEGFR-2 (KDR) and thereby blocks the interaction between VEGFR-2 (KDR) and its ligands.[11] VEGFR-2 is the main receptor to mediate the downstream actions of VEGF-A (but also binds VEGF-C, VEGF-D, and VEGF-E). Importantly, ramucirumab has approximately eight times more efficacy for binding this receptor than its natural ligand(s) and, once bound, it induces conformational changes as well as stearic hindrance for natural ligands to bind.[11]

Anti-PD-1/PD-L1 Antibodies

Programmed cell death protein 1 (PD-1) is expressed on T cells, its ligand (PD-L1) on antigen-presenting cells, such as macrophages, as well as in other tissues upon stimulation (e.g., in the setting of inflammation), avoiding autoimmune reactivity. Cancer cells can express PD-L1 as a mechanism o immune evasion, and targeting PD-1 and PD-L1 car reactivate immune activity and trigger an antitumo CTL response.

The epitopes for **pembrolizumab** and **nivolumal** overlap with part of the PD-L1 binding site, but th affinity of these anti-PD-1 antibodies is several o ders of magnitude stronger than the affinity of PD-L for PD-1. It has thus been assumed that the mai mode of action of pembrolizumab and nivolumab is through outcompeting PD-L1 for binding to PD-1. Of note, pembrolizumab and nivolumab are of the IgG4 isotypes, which lack effector functions such as ADCC and CDD, which could potentially be harmful to immune cells expressing PD-1 when targeting this ligand with antibodies.

Although atezolizumab, durvalumab, and avelumab bind distinct epitopes, all interfere with PD-1 binding and prevent PD-L1/PD-1 interaction. These three checkpoint inhibitors are of the IgG1 class, but the Fcs of atezolizumab and durvalumab have been modified to eliminate antibody effector functions. Atezolizumab is an aglycosylated antibody, whereas durvalumab is a Fc-modified triple mutant variant. Avelumab is reported to be a nonmodified IgG1. Therefore, as with the anti-PD-1 therapeutic antibodies, the mechanism of action of atezolizumab, durvalumab, and avelumab is an interplay between affinity, epitope, and Fc variants.

Cardiovascular Toxicities

Rituximab has been associated with a number of cardiovascular side effects, including myocardial ischemia and infarction, supraventricular and ventricular arrhythmias, HF and even cardiogenic shock (see Table 54.6). Takotsubo's cardiomyopathy has also been described. One caveat is that rituximab is often used in combination therapy, complicating adjudication of events and determination of the contributory role of the individual drug. Nevertheless, cardiac monitoring is recommended during and after the infusion for patients with a history of arrhythmias or ischemic heart disease or in those who develop clinically eminent or asymptomatic arrhythmias.

Ofatumumab can increase or decrease blood pressure and leads to peripheral edema. Tachycardia has been reported in 5% of patients. Last, but not least, obinutuzumab is one of the drugs that increase the risk of atrial fibrillation in a World Health Organization (WHO) pharmacovigilance study.[12]

Cetuximab carries a **black box warning for cardiopulmonary arrest or sudden cardiac death** based on the experience in patients with squamous cell carcinoma of the head and neck receiving cetuximab with radiation therapy or a cetuximab product with platinum-based therapy and fluorouracil (see Table 54.6). The recommendation is to monitor serum electrolytes, including serum magnesium, potassium, and calcium, during and after cetuximab administration and to use cetuximab with caution in patients with a history of coronary artery disease, HF, and arrhythmias.[13] In addition to ischemic heart disease, a two times higher risk of pulmonary embolism (4%) is noted.

Necitumumab has a high arterial (5%) and venous (9%) thromboembolic event rate. Fatal and nonfatal myocardial infarction, stroke, and pulmonary embolism have been noted (1% to 5%). Necitumumab likewise carries a **black box warning for cardiopulmonary arrest or sudden cardiac death**, which were noted in combination therapy with gemcitabine and cisplatin. Serum electrolytes, including serum magnesium, potassium, and calcium, need to be closely monitored and aggressively replaced during and after necitumumab administration. It is recommended to continue electrolyte monitoring for at least eight weeks after the last dose. Fatal cardiopulmonary events were more often seen in patients with a history of coronary artery disease, hypertension, and chronic obstructive pulmonary disease. The incidence of venous thromboembolism may be higher in patients over the age of 70.

Panitumumab carries a risk of thromboembolism, but much lower than the other two agents (1%), unless combined with fluorouracil (5-FU), leucovorin (folinic acid), oxaliplatin (FOLFOX; 5%).

Trastuzumab carries a **black box warning for cardiotoxicity** (see Table 54.6). The reported incidence of cardiac dysfunction varies greatly and depends on the study population and the thoroughness of cardiac function surveillance. Most patients developed some drop in LVEF and a decline by more than 10% is seen in up to 40% of patients. The diagnosis of cancer therapy-related cardiac dysfunction by American Society of Echocardiography (ASE) criteria is made in 15% to 20%. HF is less common, usually less than 5%, likely as a result of cardiac surveillance and early intervention. Hypertension has been reported in 4% of patients, arrhythmias and palpitations in 3% of patients. Peripheral edema can be noted in 5% to 10% of patients.

In agreement with the black box warning, LVEF should be evaluated in all patients prior to and during treatment (3-monthly during and 6-monthy for the first two years after). Caution has been advised in patients with preexisting cardiac disease or dysfunction, and additional risk factors proposed for trastuzumab cardiotoxicity include advanced age, high or low body mass index, smoking, diabetes, hypertension, and hyper-/hypothyroidism. However, in clinical practice it is noted that even patients with none of the listed factors develop trastuzumab cardiotoxicity. Although high afterload (hypertension, aortic stenosis, and so forth) and ischemia (coronary artery disease) can induce the reexpression of HER2 in the myocardium, anthracycline exposure is very potent and the highest incidence of cardiomyopathy and HF has been noted in those patients who received anthracycline treatment. It has been suggested that anthracyclines should be avoided for at least 7 months after the last trastuzumab dose, but this is not universally followed in clinical practice. The mantra that cardiac dysfunction in patients who receive trastuzumab therapy almost always recovers has been challenged. Patients noted to have a decline in cardiac function on trastuzumab should be seen in the cardio-oncology clinic for further evaluation and shared decision-making on continuation or hold of therapy. A temporary hold should be for at least three weeks followed by reassessment and decision on continuation of therapy. Those with a recurrent drop in LVEF will need permanent discontinuation. Initiation or intensification of beta-blocker therapy (especially carvedilol) and ACE inhibitors is recommended. These drugs are efficacious also in the primary preventive setting in patients exposed to anthracyclines.

Pertuzumab likewise carries a **black box warning for cardiotoxicity,** but the incidence of asymptomatic and symptomatic cardiac dysfunction is significantly lower (3% to 4% combined). The combination of pertuzumab and trastuzumab (plus docetaxel) does not increase the risk of cardiotoxicity. Studies have suggested that approximately half of the patients who experience symptomatic HF with pertuzumab therapy will recover. Baseline and three-monthly assessment of cardiac function while on treatment is recommended. Management recommendations are similar to those for trastuzumab.

The use of **bevacizumab** is confronted with a number of vascular side effects, most commonly hypertension (in up to 40%), peripheral edema (15%), venous thrombosis and thromboembolism (grades 3/4: 10%), and arterial thrombotic/thromboembolic events including angina, myocardial infarction, transient ischemic attacks, and strokes as well as mesenteric thrombosis (grades ≥ 3: 5%) (see Table 54.6). Among malignancies, the highest incidence of arterial thromboembolic events (ATE) has been seen in patients with glioblastoma. Other risk factors include a prior history of ATE, diabetes, and age 65 years or older. A decrease in LEVF/ left ventricular dysfunction can be seen as well (10%, grade 3 or 4 in 1%). The risk of HF and/or cardiac dysfunction is at least two times higher when bevacizumab is combined with chemotherapy and, most commonly, occurring within the first 6 months of therapy. The use of bevacizumab in combination with anthracycline-based chemotherapy is not indicated. Therapy with bevacizumab is to be discontinued in case of HF; reversibility is seen in nearly two thirds of patients.

Bevacizumab therapy should also be discontinued in patients with hypertensive crisis or hypertensive encephalopathy. Blood pressure monitoring should be conducted every week ideally, especially in the beginning, and every two to three weeks at a minimum thereafter. Blood pressure should be controlled as outlined in Chapters 11, 20, and 32.

Any patient with severe ATE or grade 4 VTE should discontinue bevacizumab therapy. In the context of decisions of antiplatelet and anticoagulation therapies it is important to consider the increase in bleeding risk with bevacizumab. Two distinct bleeding patterns are seen: minor or serious hemorrhage. Severe or fatal hemorrhage is up to five times more common in patients receiving bevacizumab, than in patients receiving chemotherapy alone. Serious or fatal pulmonary hemorrhage has been reported in nearly one third of patients with squamous non-small-cell lung cancer. Bevacizumab should not be administered to patients with a recent history of hemoptysis (≥ 2.5 mL red blood) and it should be discontinued in patients who develop grade 3 or 4 hemorrhage.

Ramucirumab has a cardiovascular toxicity pro-file similar to bevacizumab, but not as extensive frequent. Hypertension is seen in 25% of patients, o severe degree in 15%, Peripheral edema is noted i 25% of patients, Arterial thromboembolism occur in 2% of patients and includes myocardial infar tion, cardiac arrest, cerebrovascular accident, ar cerebral ischemia. These events constitute a re son to discontinue ramucirumab permanent Management of hypertension is similar to beva zumab.

The cardiovascular toxicity profile of **immu checkpoint inhibitors** is outlined in a separate se tion (see below).

MULTI-TYROSINE KINASE INHIBITORS

KEY POINTS

- Tyrosine kinases (TK), which are signaling nodes controlling cellular growth, survival, and metabolism and activating mutations in TK genes, are frequent causes of cancers by inducing growth that is independent of external signals such as growth factors (GFs).
- Small molecules that inhibit TK (tyrosine kinase inhibitors [TKIs]) can suppress the autonomous growth pathway activity and thereby reduce cancer cell proliferation.
- Multi-TKI can inhibit more than 10 kinase (including serine/threonine kinases) with on-target and off-target effects of significance for the cardiovascular system.
- The cardiovascular system needs GF/TK signaling to maintain its normal function, particularly under stress (beneficial actions include stimulation of cardiomyocyte and endothelial cell survival, growth, and adaptive metabolism).
- Contractile dysfunction, hypertension, arterial events, and arrhythmias are potential consequences of TKI use and the risk is increased in combination with other cardiotoxins and underlying cardiovascular risk factors and disease.
- Cardiotoxicity can be reduced by sequential administration and by determining and optimally treating the patient´s cardiovascular risk before initiating anticancer treatment.
- Monitoring for side effects is mandated, especially for drugs with the propensity for QTc prolongation, but also for atrial fibrillation, hypertension, and cardiac function.

Protein kinases (PK) are enzymes that catalyze the phosphorylation of other proteins. They form a arge, 518-member family and belong to the most mportant regulators of cell function. PK-mediated phosphorylation regulates both short-term responses (e.g., stimulation of cardiac contractility nd rate by PKA) and long-term functions, such as ell division, size, and metabolic adaptation. Depending on which amino acid is targeted, PK are ivided into serine/threonine and tyrosine kinases TK). Examples of the former are PKA, PKC, PKB AKT), mammalian target of rapamycin (mTOR), nd the mitogen-activated kinases raf-1, MEK1, nd MAPK (also known as ERK). TK encompass oth membrane-bound kinase domains of receprs (e.g., for insulin-, EGF, platelet-derived growth ctor-receptor [PDGF], HER2 [=ErbB2, receptor of neuregulin], c-Kit [receptor of stem cell factor SDF-1] and nonmembrane-bound cytosolic kinases, such as Abl [Abelson murine leukemia viral oncogene homolog 1], c-Src [cellular sarcoma kinase], and JNK [Janus kinases]). A shared characteristic of TK is that they transduce extracellular growth signals (e.g., by GFs or by cytokines) into cell proliferation, growth, and metabolic adaptation necessary for fast growth.

Somatic mutations (e.g., mutations not affecting the germline) that render TK autoactive (i.e., make them independent of GF) are a frequent cause of cancer. This fundamental observation underlies the protooncogene concept of cancer,[1,2] which was awarded with the Nobel Prize for Varmus and Bishop in 1989. It led to the development of the first "targeted cancer therapies" with the HER2 monoclonal antibody trastuzumab against HER2-overexpressing breast cancer,[3,4] followed by bevacizumab targeting the tumor vasculature.[5] Probably the most successful example of targeted cancer therapy is that directed to Philadelphia chromosome-positive chronic myeloid leukemia (CML) with the Abl-inhibitor imatinib, providing patients with an almost normal life expectancy under life-long therapy.[6]

Most PK inhibitors (both serine/threonine and tyrosine kinase inhibitors, TKI) target the ATP-binding pocket of the protein, which, by principle, shares homology among the vast PK family and beyond (e.g., adenosine phosphate [ATP]). Although imatinib relatively specifically inhibits the TK family and lapatinib appears quite specific for the EGFR, others such as sunitinib inhibit more than 50 kinases at therapeutic plasma concentrations, including many serine/threonine kinases.[7,8] Sunitinib and many newer compounds, such as vandetinib, axotinib, bosutinib, and erlotinib, are therefore termed multi-TKI. The advantage of targeting multiple pathways is two-fold: (1) It can be more effective by addressing one pathway on several levels and thus synergistically, similar to what is known from antibiotics (e.g., cotrimoxazole and combination therapy) and (2) it can overcome tumor resistance owing to *de novo* mutations in other growth factor pathways that often occur under therapy (e.g., in CML under imatinib) or are present early on (e.g., in typically heterogenous solid tumors). However, this broader MOA also causes more adverse effects in other, nonmalignant tissues (e.g., the heart).

Significance of TKs for the Cardiovascular System

It is important to realize that many pathways used by tumor cells to proliferate and adapt to the increased metabolic need are also critical for maintaining cardiac homeostasis, particularly under stress.[9] The most convincing evidence for the role of a certain kinase in the heart comes from genetic studies. This group of critical kinases include ErbB2, VEGFR, raf-1, and JAK1/STAT3 (reviewed by Chen et al.[10]

- Germline deletion of ErbB2 or ErbB4 or the ErbB4 ligand neuregulin (NRG) is embryonically lethal owing to impaired heart trabeculation. Mice with a partial conditional heart-specific deletion were born at normal Mendelian frequency, but later developed dilated cardiomyopathy, which was exaggerated by pressure overload.[11] The data substantiated critical roles of endothelial cell-derived NRG and its receptors ErbB4/ErbB2 for cardiac myocyte proliferation in the development and cardiac myocyte survival in adulthood. The latter involves the known prosurvival serine kinase ERK.
- Deletion of two VEGF isoforms led to ischemic cardiomyopathy[12] and tetracycline-inducible cardiac-specific overexpression of a VEGF-trap in adult mice quickly induced rarefication of cardiac vasculature and cardiac dysfunction.[13] Importantly for the cardiotoxicity of TKI targeting this pathway, the effects were fully reversible even after months. The data indicate that VEGF is necessary for maintenance of normal endothelial cell function and turnover and thereby normal function of the vasculature in the heart and circulation.
- Cardiac-specific deletion of raf-1 caused spontaneous cardiac dysfunction and dilation without lethality or hypertrophy.[14] Overexpression of a dominant-negative raf-1 isoform showed a blunted hypertrophic response to pressure overload, associated with dysfunction, increased apoptosis, and premature death,[15] substantiating the raf-1-ERK pathway to play a protective, growth-promoting and survival role in the heart.
- Cardiac-specific deletion of the imatinib-target Abl had no adverse effects, whereas global deletion was lethal and endothelial-specific deletion impaired vasculogenesis, suggesting a more important role of this kinase in the vasculature than in cardiomyocytes.[16]
- Another pathway shared between cancer and the heart is energy metabolism and one of the critical nodal points is AMP kinase (AMPK), which in response to a low energy state (high AMP/ATP ratio) activates several ATP-generating and inhibits ATP-consuming pathways. Inhibition or deletion of AMPK has been associated with cardiac dysfunction and implicated, for example, in cardiotoxicity of doxorubicin.[17]

Cardiovascular Toxicities

Although targeting of several of these pathways by multi-TKI is likely to bear a higher risk of cardiovascular toxicity than specific inhibition of a single pathway, no clear correlation has yet been established between a given kinase-inhibitory profile and the rate of cardiac side effects (see Table 54.7). Reasons are the lack of large systematic registries with long-term follow up, the complexity of cardiac biology, and the inhibition profile of TKI as well as the fact that many patients with cancer have cardiovascular comorbidities that obscure potential specific effects of compounds.

Four major forms of cardiovascular toxicities have been observed.

- **Cardiac (left ventricular, LV) dysfunction** is probably the most severe adverse effects of TKI and related compounds and also most commonly referred to when speaking of "cancer drug cardiotoxicity." Asymptomatic decreases of LVEF (mostly determined by echocardiography) can be differentiated from symptomatic LV dysfunction with HF. Cardiac dysfunction generally develops in several weeks to a few months after initiation of treatment[18] and is often (71%), but not always, reversible. Data on this question remain limited. Although the general concept as described above may explain cardiac side effects of multi-TKI, the specific mechanisms are still not known. Kinases with an established protective role in the heart are raf-1/ERK, PDGFR, and AMPK. Almost all TKI (likely exception imatinib) have been associated with cardiotoxicity. Large meta-analyses indicate that, as a group, TKI increase the risk of all-grade and high-grade HF 2.5- and 1.5-fold, respectively. Asymptomatic LV dysfunction is probably much more frequent. Although no clear differences were observed between different classes of TKI, inhibition of VEGFR may be associated with an earlier occurrence of HF and an increased risk of fatal adverse events (1.5- to 2-fold). Interestingly, this holds also in comparison with EGFR-active compounds.[18]

DRUGS	INDICATION	MECHANISMS OF CARDIOTOXICITY	RISK FACTORS	MANIFESTATIONS OF CARDIOTOXICITY	PREVENTION AND RISK REDUCTION STRATEGIES
Sorafenib Sunitinib	RCC/HCC/GIST Pancreatic neuroendocrine tumors Melanoma	Inhibition of ribosomal S6 kinase (RSK) Inhibition of RAF1 kinase activity Causes trigger and activation targeting apoptotic pathway result in increased apoptosis, myocyte loss and ATP depletion lead to left ventricular (LV) dysfunction	• History of HT and CAD	Arrhythmias Prolong of QTc/ST-T changes LV dysfunction/CHF ACS-myocardial ischemia/infarction HT	• Termination of treatment (reversible) • Monitoring ECG and LV function • Cardiac troponin and BNP show yield in early detection for cardiotoxicity
Regorafenib	Colorectal cancers	Unknown	• Preexisting CV disease	Myocardial ischemia/ infarction (rare)	• Unknown
Vandetanib	Medullary thyroid cancer Breast/lung cancers CML/CEL/ALL Mesothelioma	Unknown	• Congenital long QT syndrome • Electrolyte imbalance, hypocalcemia and hypomagnesemia • Concurrent drugs that prolong QTc interval	Prolong QTc/*Torsades de points*/SCD LV dysfunction/CHF HT	• Termination of treatment (reversible) • Monitoring ECG and QTc interval prior and during treatment • Correction of serum electrolyte, calcium, and magnesium before treatment • Avoiding for concurrent drugs that cause prolonged QTc or strong CYP3A4 inducers
Imatinib Nilotinib Dasatinib Bosutinib	GIST CML	Significant mitochondrial dysfunction Declines in ATP concentration ABL and/or ARG inhibition result in unrecognized function of cardiomyocytes	• Preexisting CV disease • Congenital long QT syndrome • Electrolyte imbalance, hypocalcemia, and hypomagnesemia • Concurrent drugs that prolong QTc interval	Prolong QTc Systolic and diastolic dysfunction Chest pain, HT Pericardial effusion Fatal myocardial ischemia/infarction LV dysfunction/CHF	• Termination of treatment (reversible) • Monitoring ECG and LV function • Correction of serum electrolyte calcium and magnesium before treatment • Avoiding for concurrent drugs that cause prolong QTc or strong CYP3A4 inhibitors
Lapatinib	Breast cancer Brain cancer	Unknown (rare cardiotoxicity, usually occurs when combine with other cardiotoxic agents)	• Concurrent systemic cardiotoxic agents	Prinzmetal's angina LV dysfunction/CHF	• Termination of treatment (reversible) • Dose adjustment and limiting dose of other chemotherapies
Crizotinib Vemurafenib	NSCLC Melanoma	Unknown	• Congenital long QT syndrome • Electrolyte imbalance and hypomagnesemia • Concurrent drugs that prolong QTc interval	Severe sinus bradycardia ($\leq$ 45 bpm) [Crizotinib] Arrhythmia, QTc prolongation, *Torsades de points* CHF, hypotension, syncope [Crizotinib]	• Termination of treatment (reversible) • QTc > 500 msec during treatment advice for termination of therapy • Monitoring ECG and correction of electrolyte and magnesium before therapy • Avoiding for concurrent drugs that cause prolong QTc or strong CYP3A4 inhibitors

ACE-I, Angiotensin-converting enzyme inhibitor; *AF*, atrial fibrillation; *ALL*, acute lymphoblastic leukemia; *AML*, acute myeloid leukemia; *CAD*, coronary artery disease; *CEL*, chronic eosinophilic leukemia; *CHB*, complete heart block; *CHF*, congestive heart failure; *CML*, chronic myelogenous leukemia; *CT*, computed tomography; *CV*, cardiovascular; *CYP3A4*, cytochrome p450 3a4; *DVT*, deep vein thrombosis; *ECG*, electrocardiogram; *GIST*, gastrointestinal stroma tumor; *GVHD*, graft versus host disease; *HF*, heart failure; *HR*, heart rate; *HT*, hormone therapy; *HTN*, hypertension; *ITP*, idiopathic thrombocytopenic purpura; *LBBB*, left bundle branch block; *LV*, left ventricular; *LVH*, left ventricular hypertrophy; *NCLC*, non–small-cell lung carcinoma; *NHL*, non-Hodgkin lymphoma; *PE*, pulmonary embolism; *RCC*, renal cell carcinoma; *ROS*, reactive oxygen species; *RT*, radiation therapy; *SCD*, sudden cardiac death; *SCLC*, small-cell lung carcinoma; *SPECT*, single photon emission computerized tomography; *SSS*, sick sinus syndrome; *SVR*, stroke volume ratio; *SVT*, supraventricular tachycardia; *TTP*, thrombotic thrombocytopenic purpura; *VT*, ventricular tachycardia; *WBC*, white blood cells.
Modified from Herrmann J, ed. *Clinical Cardio-Oncology*. Philadelphia: Elsevier; 2018.

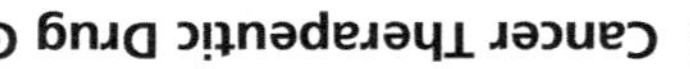

- **Hypertension** is a common adverse effect of many TKI, particularly those inhibiting VEGFR pathways. It is obvious that hypertension aggravates the direct cardiotoxicity, likely explaining the relatively strong cardiotoxicity of compounds such as sunitinib and sorafenib. Dasatinib has been specifically associated with an increased rate of **pulmonary arterial hypertension** and pleural edema (see Table 54.1).
- **ATEs** (e.g., myocardial infarction, stroke, peripheral occlusions) are increasingly recognized to be associated with many TKI, particularly with ponatinib, but also sunitinib, sorafenib, dasatinib, erlotinib, imatinib, and many newer TKI. The mechanism is not clear, but given the established protective role of VEGF, not only for angiogenesis, but endothelial cell integrity, inhibition of VEGFR may play a role. Indeed, a recent meta-analysis indicated a 3- and 1.5-fold increased risk of all-grade and high-grade ATE, respectively.[19]
- **QT prolongation**. Several TKI (as many other drugs) increase the QT interval, a surrogate of inhibition of repolarization reserve and a proarrhythmic state. Most often, this effect is due to inhibition of the main repolarizing K^+ current I_{Kr} (hERG channel), a typical off-target effect unrelated to the main MOA of the TKI. The most critical TKI (also carrying a black box warning in the prescription sheet) are ceritinib, crizotinib, dasatinib, nilotinib, sorafenib, sunitinib, vandetanib, and vemurafenib.[18,20] Erlotinib, nilotinib, sorafenib, and sunitinib have been associated with an increased rate of sudden death, but overall the clinical relevance of the TKI-induced QT prolongation has been judged as "remarkably low."[1]

Clinical Consequences

TKIs are associated with various forms of cardiovascular toxicity with cardiac dysfunction and with thromboembolic events being most critical. Whereas the mechanisms and the exact size of the problem are still insufficiently known, it is clear that it is relevant and growing, not at least because more and more patients are treated with these anticancer drugs, and the group of drugs is growing at fast a pace. Data suggest that less than 25% of rare but serious and potentially fatal adverse effects of anticancer drugs are reported in clinical trials, suggesting that the real problem is much greater than currently known.[21] The broad spectrum of pharmacologic actions, including (principally intended) on-target (e.g., VEGFR) and (unintended) off-target actions (e.g., inhibition of hERG channels), make it difficult to predict the risk-to-benefit ratio. Current data do not allow to single out specific drugs as "cardio-safe" or particularly "cardiotoxic," but VEGFR-active TKI may have a particularly high risk and EGFR-active drugs relatively little risk if not given in combination with anthracyclines.

The situation calls for increasing awareness and systematic efforts of cardio-oncology teams to (1) identify patients at risk, (2) closely monitor cardiovascular function under therapy and in the post-treatment phases, (3) systematically report these data, and (4) provide optimal treatment for patients at risk and for those who develop dysfunction. High blood pressure and HF can be managed with the usual combination therapy, and the available evidence suggests that this treatment is also effective and allows continuation of cancer treatment in the vast majority of cases.[22,23] The increased risk of ATE associated with TKI is a serious concern and may call for antiplatelet therapy, but no evidence exists supporting preemptive treatment. QT-prolonging actions of TKI need careful monitoring and the strict control of possible drug-drug-interactions (e.g., CYP3A4 inhibitors) and other QT-prolonging agents. In this respect, it is important to realize that TKI often induce vomiting and diarrhea, which can cause electrolyte imbalances (e.g., hypokalemia) that favor *Torsade de pointe* arrhythmias. Antiemetics, such as metoclopramide, droperidol, phenothiazines, and ondansetron, can increase the QT interval and further aggravate the proarrhythmic risk.

IMMUNE CHECKPOINT INHIBITORS

KEY POINTS

- Immune checkpoint inhibitors (ICIs) are approved for a broad range of advanced cancers (e.g., melanoma, non–small-cell lung cancer and urothelial carcinoma) and their use is being investigated even in earlier stage cancers.
- ICIs are either fully human or humanized antibodies that target immunomodulatory pathways (mainly CTLA-4 and PD-1/PD-L1) to activate primarily T cells in the immune response against cancer.
- Activation of the immune system via T cells, complement mediated inflammation, preformed antibodies, and inflammatory cytokines can lead to immune-related

adverse events (irAEs), most commonly dermatitis (rash), pneumonitis, colitis, hepatitis, and hypophysitis.

- Several adverse cardiovascular effects can be seen with ICI, including acute coronary syndromes, pericarditis, cardiomyopathy, and myocarditis.
- Although rare (< 1%), myocarditis is the most concerning entity as the most fatal of all ICI-related irAEs and often the most challenging to diagnose (cardiac fraction can be preserved even with evolving fulminant cases, and a myocardial biopsy may be necessary).
- Immunosuppressive therapy is the principal approach for all ICI irAEs; treatment of ICI myocarditis requires early initiation of high-dose steroid therapy and any additional measures as necessary (e.g., extracorporeal membrane oxygenation [ECMO]) in case of a fulminant course.

Immune checkpoint inhibitors (ICIs) are effective and approved against a broad range of advanced cancers and their use is being investigated in earlier stage cancers.

ICIs are a paradigm shift in the care of patients with cancer; currently they are approved for patients with several cancers, including melanoma, bladder cancer, lung and head, and neck cancer. The use of ICIs will expand because as over 1000 immune therapies are currently in development and several clinical trials expand the spectrum in cancer type and stage.[1,2] ICIs are used individually or as part of a combination therapy to augment the cellular immune response against cancer and treatment can be prescribed for months to years (see Table 54.8).

ICIs target immunomodulatory pathways to activate the immune response against cancer, which can also lead to immune-related adverse events.

ICIs are immunomodulatory antibodies that target T-cell surface molecules to activate the suppressed cellular immune response, allowing it to fight cancer. The most common immune-regulatory molecules targeted by ICIs include the cytotoxic T-lymphocyte–associated antigen 4 (CTLA-4) and programmed cell death-1 and its ligand (PD-1/PD-L1). These immune checkpoints have important roles in the maintenance of self-tolerance and reduction of inflammation.[3] In the tumor microenvironment, these pathways are exploited via upregulation of ligands that bind to CTLA-4 and PD-1 to prevent cytotoxic T-cell-mediated destruction of cancer cells and allow for immune evasion.[4] Antibodies that inhibit immune checkpoint pathways result in proliferation of cytotoxic T cells that effectively combat cancer. However, unintended inflammatory or autoimmune-like reactions (termed immune-related adverse events) can occur in most healthy organs, including the heart. The pathophysiology of immune-related events is not entirely clear, but it is postulated to be owing to unchecked immune activation involving T cells, antibodies, complement-mediated inflammation, and cytokines.[5,6]

Myocarditis, the main cardiovascular adverse effect of ICIs, is associated with a high mortality rate.

Myocarditis is the main cardiovascular adverse effect of ICIs with a high mortality rate of 46% in fulminant cases[7]; however, other presentations related to an unrestrained immune system, including pericarditis and acute coronary syndromes, have been noted. The incidence of myocarditis is wide and has ranged from 0.09% to 1%; the wide range likely relates to the difficulty of the diagnosis; the diagnostic tests used and the broad range of nomenclature applied in clinical trial reporting.[7,8] The frequency of myocarditis is greater in those undergoing combination therapy with multiple ICIs versus single therapy regimens and can be the first immune-related adverse effect noted in 50% of cases.[7,9] The median time to clinical presentation is 1 to 2 months with the majority of the cases occurring within 3 months of ICI initiation; however, cases presenting as late as 600 days after ICI initiation have been reported.[9] Presenting symptoms include chest pain, dyspnea, orthopnea, paroxysmal nocturnal dyspnea, and fatigue. Signs of HF, including jugular venous distention or pulmonary crackles, may or may not be present on examination. Ventricular arrhythmias or conduction system disease, such as complete heart block, can occur and indicate a poor prognosis if untreated.

Diagnosis of ICI myocarditis can be challenging and biopsy is often necessary.

Cardiac biomarkers, such as troponin and brain natriuretic peptide (BNP) or N-terminal pro-BNP (NT-proBNP), are often elevated. Troponin in acute presentations may be a marker of disease severity with greater elevation associated with a greater risk of a fulminant presentation.[9] LEVF is reduced in only half of the cases; however, major adverse events, including death and cardiogenic shock, can occur with a normal LVEF making LVEF a modest discriminator of outcomes.[9] Cardiac magnetic resonance imaging (MRI) may reveal findings typical of myocarditis, including edema, hyperemia, and late gadolinium enhancement,[10,11] as well as elevated values for native T_1, extracellular volume, and T_2 by novel

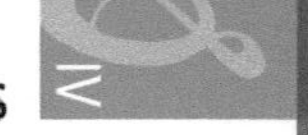

TABLE 54.8 **Immune Therapies**

TREATMENTS/ DRUGS	THERAPEUTIC INDICATION	MECHANISMS OF CARDIOTOXICITY	RISK FACTORS	MANIFESTATIONS OF CARDIOTOXICITY	PREVENTION AND RISK REDUCTION STRATEGIES
Immune Checkpoint Inhibitor					
CTLA-4 inhibitor Ipilimumab	Colorectal cancer Hepatocellular carcinoma Melanoma Non–small-cell lung cancer Renal cell carcinoma	Unknown	• Women • Age > 75 years • Preexisting cardiac disease • Diabetes • Autoimmune disease • (CTLA-4 plus) combination therapy	Myocarditis Pericarditis Vasculitis	• Serial cardiac troponin I and natriuretic peptide • ECG (new onset block patterns, ventricular ectopy, ventricular tachycardia, atrial fibrillation) • Cardiac MRI if the above are abnormal • Endomyocardial biopsy, as needed
PD-1 inhibitors Nivolumab	As above, plus esophageal cancer Head and neck Hodgkin lymphoma Small-cell lung cancer Urothelial carcinoma	Potential mechanisms include		Myocarditis Pericarditis Vasculitis Thromboembolism Hypertension Cardiomyopathy/ Takotsubo's	• Initiate high-dose steroids upon suspicion • Additional immunosuppressants, as needed • Circulatory support, as needed for fulminant myocarditis
Pembrolizumab,	As above, plus cervical cancer Cutaneous squamous cell carcinoma Endometrial carcinoma Gastric cancer Merkel cell carcinoma Primary mediastinal large B-cell lymphoma	• direct binding of ICIs to target molecules on nonlymphocytic cells, with downstream immune activation • formation of new T cells or reactivation of exhausted T cells against tumor antigens that crossreact with off-target tissues (shared antigen, molecular mimicry) • generation of autoantibodies and production of proinflammatory cytokines		Myocarditis Pericarditis Vasculitis Thromboembolism Hypertension Cardiomyopathy/ Takotsubo's Arrhythmias (may be an indicator of myocarditis)	
Cemiplimab	Cutaneous squamous cell carcinoma			Myocarditis Pericarditis Vasculitis Hypertension	

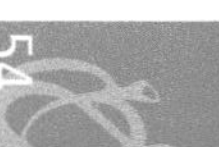

[illegible]	Hepatocellular carcinoma Melanoma Non–small-cell lung cancer Small-cell lung cancer Urothelial carcinoma			Myocarditis Pericarditis Vasculitis Thromboembolism	
Avelumab	Merkel cell carcinoma Renal cell carcinoma Urothelial carcinoma			Myocarditis Hypertension	
Durvalumab	Non–small-cell lung cancer Small-cell lung cancer Urothelial carcinoma			Myocarditis	
CAR T-Cell Therapy					
Tisagenlecleucel (CD19-directed)	Acute lymphoblastic leukemia Diffuse large B-cell lymphoma	Cytokine release	Cytokine release syndrome Neurotoxicity	Hypotension and shock Hypertension Arrhythmias (atrial fibrillation) Cardiac failure Thrombosis Capillary leak syndrome Cerebral infarction	Early treatment of cytokine release syndrome with interleukin-6 inhibitors
Bi-Specific T-Cell Engagers (BiTEs)					
Blinatumomab (CD19- directed, CD3-linked)	Acute lymphoblastic leukemia	Cytokine release	Unknown	Cardiac arrhythmias Hypotension and shock Hypertension Chest pain Capillary leak syndrome	Not defined

tissue characterization techniques.[12] However, several standard MRI features, LVEF, late gadolinium enhancement, and qualitative T2 sequences can be normal despite biopsy-confirmed myocarditis. If clinical suspicion for myocarditis is high, endomyocardial biopsy should be performed to confirm the diagnosis. Histologic features include T-cell–predominant lymphocytic infiltrate, which can be patchy or diffuse. In the absence of biopsy data, diagnosis can also be made by integrating clinical features with ECG, echocardiographic, biomarkers, and suggestive cardiac MRI findings.
Immunosuppressive agents are the principal approach for treatment of ICI myocarditis.

Once the diagnosis of ICI myocarditis is made, prompt institution of immunosuppressive therapy is necessary. No prospective trials have examined treatment of ICI myocarditis, therefore current treatment is based on expert opinion and institutional practices. Upfront therapy with high-dose intravenous corticosteroids is typically used and is associated with a lower adverse event rate and discharge troponin levels compared with smaller corticosteroid doses.[9] Other immunosuppressive agents have also been used, including intravenous immunoglobulin, mycophenolate, calcineurin inhibitors, antithymocyte globulin, and infliximab. The data are conflicting on the effect of immune-modulating therapies on cancer outcomes. Rechallenge with ICI is controversial and should be approached on a case-by-case basis after discussion with the oncology team and the patient. The pathophysiology, optimal diagnostic strategies, and therapeutic approaches are poorly defined and support the need for ongoing collaborations.[13]

CAR T-CELL THERAPY

KEY POINTS

- CD19-specific chimeric antigen receptor (CAR) T cells are effective and approved in the management of relapsing and refractory acute lymphoblastic leukemias in pediatric and young adult populations and B-cell lymphomas in adults.
- CD19-specific CAR T cells recognize the CD19 antigen expressed on all cells from the B-cell lineage, activating T cells and resulting in target cell lysis.
- The true extent of cardiotoxicity has yet to be defined, but includes profound hypotension, left ventricular systolic dysfunction, and rhythm disturbances.
- Cardiotoxicity associated with CAR T cells is managed supportively initially, and with tocilizumab, an IL-6 receptor antagonist, in more severe cases.

CD19-specific chimeric antigen receptor (CAR) T cells are novel therapies that have shown remarkable success in the treatment of pediatric and adult populations with refractory and relapsing hematological malignancies, including acute lymphoblastic leukemia (ALL) and large B-cell lymphoma. They have been associated with complete remission (CR) rates of 52% to 90%,[1–6] compared with a CR of 7% in patients treated with conventional therapies.[7] Two CD19-specific CAR T-cell products have received FDA approval (see Table 54.8).

CAR T cells are equipped with recombinant fusion proteins that enable T-cell activation upon recognition of a specific antigen, and this leads to target cell lysis. CD19 is expressed throughout B-cell lineage development and resultantly, it is frequently highly expressed on the surface of almost all B-cell malignancies. Furthermore, it is not found on other normal tissues. These factors render it an extremely effective target. The T cells are first harvested from the patient. Thereafter, *ex vivo* genetic modification with the help of lentiviral or retroviral vectors results in CARs on the T cells with the ability to recognize CD19 antigens. In order to further augment the CAR T-cell population and subsequently its anticancer activity, all patients receive lymphodepleting chemotherapy before the infusion of CAR T cells, usually with fludarabine and cyclophosphamide. The aim is to diminish the *in vivo* T-cell population, which subsequently stimulates the release of cytokines, such as interleukin (IL)-7 and IL-15, which promote T-cell expansion.[8]

The most frequent and well-described toxicity of CAR T-cell therapy is cytokine release syndrome (CRS), a multiorgan phenomenon that can have varied clinical manifestations. The consensus grading system from the American Society for Transplantation and Cellular Therapy[9] entails four grades. Fever (temperature ≥38°C, with or without constitutional symptoms, includes myalgia, arthralgia, and malaise) is require for all grades. Hypotension is part of grade 2 and higher; additional single or multiple agent va sopressor qualifies for grade 3 or 4 CRS, respectively Alternatively, or in conjunction, presence of hypoxia qualifies for grade 2 or higher with further modifica tion based on oxygen requirements: low-flow nasa cannula or blow-by (grade 2), low-flow nasal cannula facemask, nonrebreather, or Venturi mask (grade 3 or continuous positive airway pressure/bilevel pos tive airway pressure (CPAP/BiPAP) or mechanic ventilation (grade 4).

The extent of specific cardiovascular toxicities and complications remains incompletely defined. The most well-described cardiovascular complication is profound hypotension requiring vasopressor and intensive therapy unit support.[10,11] However, a much broader spectrum of cardiovascular toxicities has been observed. This ranges from ST segment changes and QT prolongation on ECG, to arrhythmias such as sinus tachycardia and atrial fibrillation, through to myocardial injury suggested by elevations in serum troponin and left ventricular systolic dysfunction.[10–12] Further, frequent abnormalities in NT-proBNP, lactate, and mixed venous saturations were evident in a small cohort of patients with serum cardiac biomarkers evaluations.[1]

Retrospective data suggest that a heavy burden of malignant disease, defined in one study as a pretreatment blast percentage greater than 25%, confers the greatest risk of cardiovascular complications. Other risk factors include left ventricular systolic and diastolic dysfunction prior to infusion of CAR T cells.[11]

The first-line management of cardiovascular complications, and in particular profound hypotension, is supportive care. This includes cessation or tapering of antihypertensives prior to T-cell infusion, frequent monitoring of vital signs, close cardiac surveillance with biomarkers (including troponin and NT-proBNP), ECG and transthoracic echocardiogram, fluid resuscitation, and Inotropes.[13]

In addition, tocilizumab should be considered in patients with profound hypotension requiring inotropic support. Tocilizumab is a monoclonal antibody directed against IL-6 receptor which has become an important strategy in managing severe grade 3 or 4 CRS, where IL-6 has been shown to be one of the main mediators of toxicity. It has been approved by the FDA for this indication and therefore has become standard therapy.[14] In two retrospective series by Fitzgerald and colleagues and Burstein and colleagues where 93% and 88% of their respective cohorts received tocilizumab, all of the patients experienced rapid clinical improvement within a number of hours.[10,11]

PROTEASOME INHIBITORS

KEY POINTS

- Proteasome inhibitors act as reversible and irreversible inhibitors primarily of the chymotrypsin-like proteolytic activity of the beta 5 subunit of the proteasome.
- Neutropenia, anemia, and thrombocytopenia are the most common side effects with all three proteasome inhibitors currently in clinical use.
- Peripheral edema, dyspnea, and fatigue are common nonhematologic side effects, which can raise concerns for heart failure.
- Cardiovascular side effects are most common with carfilzomib (incl., hypertension and heart failure).
- Older age and higher intensity (i.e., high dose and duration) are the main risk factors for proteasome inhibitor cardiotoxicity.
- Before and during proteasome inhibitor therapy patients should be followed for cardiovascular disease manifestations.
- Proteasome inhibitors should be held for grade 3 cardiovascular toxicities and thereafter resumed only very carefully, weighing risks and benefits and assuring appropriate management.

Proteasome inhibitors are used primarily in the treatment of multiple myeloma, amyloidosis, and less commonly low-grade lymphomas. The cardiovascular (CV) safety profile of multiple myeloma therapies is important to understand because patients with multiple myeloma tend to be older and have an increased burden of CV risk factors and CV disease at baseline.[1,2] Bortezomib, a first-generation proteasome inhibitor, is a component of many multiple myeloma directed therapies, both for initial therapy of newly diagnosed multiple myeloma and for relapsed/refractory multiple myeloma (RRMM). Carfilzomib and ixazomib are next-generation proteasome inhibitors currently approved for use in the treatment of RRMM, with ongoing studies investigating their use in frontline treatment.[3] This section will review the CV safety profile of the proteasome inhibitors, recognizing that hematologic side effects are most common and nonhematologic side effects, other than cardiovascular side effects, are sometimes more common (see Table 54.9). The multifactorial nature of peripheral edema, dyspnea, and fatigue should be taken into consideration and not automatically be equated with HF. Careful evaluation is required, including additional testing and the utilization of strict criteria, such as the Framingham criteria, for a diagnosis of HF.

Bortezomib

Congestive heart failure (CHF) and decreased LEVF have been reported in patients receiving bortezomib.

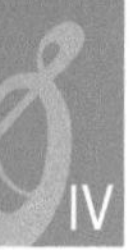

TABLE 54.9 **Proteasome Inhibitors**

TREATMENTS/ DRUGS	THERAPEUTIC INDICATION	MECHANISMS OF CARDIOTOXICITY	RISK FACTORS	MANIFESTATIONS OF CARDIOTOXICITY	PREVENTION AND RISK REDUCTION STRATEGIES
Proteasome inhibitors • Bortezomib • Carfilzomib • Ixazomib	Multiple myeloma Mantel cell lymphoma	Endoplasmatic reticulum stress Metabolic alterations Accumulation and crosslinking of ubiquitinated proteins Autophagy activation Oxidative stress Decreased cardiac myocyte contractility Abnormal vasoreactivity Endothelial dysfunction	Preexisting cardiovascular (CV) disease CV risk factor (e.g., poorly controlled hypertension and hypercholesterolemia) Prior and especially concurrent systemic cardiotoxic chemotherapies (esp., anthracyclines, possibly also cyclophosphamide) Age >70 years Higher dose (for carfilzomib) Short infusion time (for carfilzomib)	Orthostatic hypotension, syncope New onset/worsening preexisting heart failure (↓ left ventricular function can be seen, but less so for carfilzomib, incidence 8% with carfilzomib, 3% with bortezomib, 2% with ixazomib) Arrhythmia (bradycardia, heart block, atrial fibrillation) Cardiac arrest Myocardial ischemia/ infarction Systemic hypertension (9% with carfilzomib, 3% with bortezomib and ixazomib) Pulmonary arterial hypertension Dyspnea (5% with carfilzomib, 2% with bortezomib)	• Termination of treatment (potentially reversible) • Dose modification based on cardiac toxicity • Caution in patient with history of syncope • Avoid dehydration as well as overhydration (esp., for carfilzomib) • Blood pressure control • CV risk factor control in general

Modified from Herrmann J, ed. *Clinical Cardio-Oncology*. Philadelphia: Elsevier; 2018.

Case reports and case series of bortezomib use in real-world populations noted patients with reduced cardiac function and raised a general concern about an increased risk of CHF with bortezomib use.[4] This has been less so the case with randomized clinical trials (RCT). For examples, in a phase 3 clinical trial of bortezomib versus high-dose dexamethasone in RRMM, CHF was reported in 2% of patients in each treatment arm.[5] A retrospective analysis of phase 2 and 3 studies of bortezomib demonstrated no increase in cardiac risk (CHF, arrhythmias, ischemic heart disease, cardiac death) with bortezomib versus non-bortezomib-based treatment regimens for the treatment of newly diagnosed multiple myeloma or RRMM.[6] In this analysis, the incidence of all grade CHF was 2% to 7.6%, all grade ischemic heart disease 1.2% to 2.9%, and cardiac death 0 to 1.4%.[6] A separate meta-analysis that defined cardiotoxicity as left ventricular dysfunction, CHF, cardiomyopathy, cardiac arrest, or cardiac arrhythmia, reported a 3.8% incidence of all-grade cardiotoxicity with bortezomib. However, bortezomib use was not associated with a higher risk of cardiotoxicity compared with other treatment regimens.[7]

Similarly, a propensity matched analysis of more than 1600 real-world patients receiving bortezomib versus lenalidomide did not demonstrate a significantly increased risk of CHF, myocardial infarction, coronary revascularization, or arrhythmia with bortezomib.[2] Interestingly, rates of CHF hospitalization and myocardial infarction were higher in the multiple myeloma population than in the general population of the United States, suggesting a higher burden of CV disease in this population.[2]

Carfilzomib

Carfilzomib has significantly improved outcomes i RRMM as demonstrated in large phase 3 studies such as ASPIRE and ENDEAVOR.[8–10] However, CV ad verse events, including hypertension, dyspnea, an CHF, occurred with a higher frequency in patient treated with carfilzomib than in patients on noncarfi zomib regimens. Initial preclinical studies suggeste vascular toxicity as a potential mechanism. More r cently, experimental studies indicate that cardiotoxi ity with carfilzomib is an off-target effect, not relate to proteasome inhibition but alteration in autophag

A pooled analysis of over 2000 RRMM cases of patients treated with carfilzomib in phase 1 through 3 clinical trials found the incidence of grade 3 or greater CV adverse events to be as follows: hypertension (5.9%), dyspnea (4.5%), and CHF (4.4%).[11,12] In phase 3 clinical trials, grade 3 or greater cardiac failure occurred in 3.8% of patients treated with carfilzomib, lenalidomide, and dexamethasone versus 1.8% treated with lenalidomide and dexamethasone and in 4.8% of patients treated with carfilzomib and dexamethasone versus 1.8% treated with bortezomib and dexamethasone.[8,10] In the A.R.R.O.W. study, once weekly carfilzomib dosing (70 mg/m^2 once a week versus 27 mg/m^2 twice a week) improved progression-free survival in RRMM without an increased risk of CHF. However, there was in increased risk of treatment emergent grade 3 or greater hypertension in the once weekly group.[13] Higher dose (>36 to 45 mg/m^2), shorter infusion time (2 to 10 minutes), and older age (>70 years) appear to be the main risk factors for cardiac toxicity with carfilzomib.[9,14] Other risk factors include prior anthracycline and possibly even cyclophosphamide therapy, male gender, and the presence of cardiovascular risk factors/disease.

Interestingly, despite the increased risk for cardiac failure with carfilzomib, echocardiographic surveillance in a substudy of patients on a phase 3 clinical trial demonstrated no significant difference in the LVEF between treatment arms (carfilzomib and dexamethasone vs. bortezomib and dexamethasone) at any time during the study. Additionally, only three patients in each treatment arm had a significant decrease in their LVEF (defined as an absolute decrease of $\geq$ 10% for LVEF $<$ 55% at baseline or a decrease to $<$ 45% for LVEF $>$ 55% at baseline) at any time point and these decreases were largely reversible.[11] Single center data also support the largely reversible nature of LVEF declines in patients receiving carfilzomib.[15]

No increase in fatal CV failure or ischemic heart lisease adverse events was observed in patients eceiving carfilzomib versus noncarfilzomib regihens. Carfilzomib was not found to have a significant impact on cardiac repolarization as assessed y the QTc interval.[11]

It is important to emphasize that the benefits of arfilzomib in prolonging survival in multiple myoma outweigh the cardiac risk, especially with ppropriate safety measures.[11] In patients with rdiac risk factors, a baseline echocardiogram d NT-proBNP levels for monitoring have been suggested. Timely clinical management of treatment-emergent adverse effects, such as hypertension and peripheral edema, may play an important role in enabling patients to continue on carfilzomib containing regimens. Because dosing recommendations include significant fluid delivery before and after treatment, this may contribute to symptoms and recommendation to reduce or eliminate pre- and posttreatment fluids in susceptible or symptomatic patients. Cardio-oncology collaboration in the treatment of these patients is likely to be beneficial.

Ixazomib

Ixazomib is chemically similar to bortezomib, but orally delivered. As with bortezomib, adverse CV events can occur, but there is no uniform shift to increased risk compared with nonixazomib regimens. CHF, arrhythmias, hypertension, and myocardial infarction occurred at similar rates between the ixazomib, lenalidomide, dexamethasone, and the placebo, lenalidomide, and dexamethasone arms in a phase 3 trial in RRMM.[16]

Summary

Treatment regimens for multiple myeloma containing carfilzomib are associated with an increased risk of CHF, dyspnea, and hypertension versus non-carfilzomib-containing regimens. Reductions in LVEF with carfilzomib therapy, when observed, appear to be reversible based on available evidence. Collaboration with cardio-oncology providers is recommended for patients with multiple myeloma with cardiac risk factors who are going to be receiving carfilzomib. Patients with baseline cardiac risk or cardiac amyloidosis may be particularly susceptible.

In contrast, bortezomib- and ixazomib-containing regimens do not appear to lead to a generally increased overall CV risk compared with other treatment regimens, although individual case reports linking bortezomib to reduced cardiac function have been reported. However, regardless of the therapy they are receiving, patients with multiple myeloma may benefit from aggressive CV risk factor modification and careful monitoring for signs or symptoms of CV disease owing to their age and baseline burden of CV risk factors. Early recognition and treatment of CV events are important to minimize morbidity and mortality in this population.

mTOR/PHOSPHATIDYLINOSITOL-3-KINASE (PI3K) INHIBITORS

KEY POINTS

- The phosphatidylinositol-3-kinase (PI3K)/AKT/mammalian target of rapamycin (mTOR) signaling pathway is important for cell metabolism, proliferation, growth, and survival.
- Aberrant activation of the pathway is commonly observed in many human cancers, especially breast, lung, endometrial, gastrointestinal tract, and brain (glioblastoma).
- Despite the strong evidence that mTORC1 and mTORC2 control events that are important for cell growth and survival, which are processes of key importance in cancer cells, progress in successfully applying rapamycin and rapalogs as anticancer agents has been limited and the same holds true for PI3K inhibitors.
- Temsirolimus was approved by the FDA for advanced renal cell carcinoma in 2007 and since then everolimus has been passed for use in certain other cancers, including neuroendocrine tumors and, as a combination therapy, for HER2-positive breast cancer, as well as for certain tuberous sclerosis complex (TSC)-related tumors.
- Cardiovascular side effects relate to the signaling pathways and biological functions affected, but hypertension stands out as the most consistent class effect.
- Management of hypertension should follow the outline provided in Chapters 11, 20, and 32.

The phosphatidylinositol-3-kinase (PI3K)/AKT/mammalian target of rapamycin (mTOR) pathway is one of the most important intracellular signaling pathways and an attractive target for cancer therapy.[1–6]

It regulates cell metabolism, proliferation, and survival. Of the three classes of PI3Ks, class I has been most implicated in cancer.[4] Class I PI3Ks are activated by receptor tyrosine kinases (RTKs) or G protein–coupled receptors (GPCRs) and convert phosphatidylinositol 4,5-bisphosphate (PI4,5P2) to phosphatidylinositol 3,4,5-trisphosphate (PIP3). PIP3 activates AKT by recruitment to the plasma membrane. AKT, also known as protein kinase B (PKB), operates as a serine/threonine protein kinase on multiple targets, one key target being mTOR. mTOR acts both upstream and downstream of AKT in two different multiprotein complexes, target of rapamycin complex (TORC) 1 and TORC2.

TORC1 assumes a role in activation of multiple anabolic pathways, including protein synthesis, ribosome production, lipogenesis, and nucleotide synthesis, as well as in the suppression of key catabolic processes such as autophagy. It is estimated that TORC1 is hyperactivated in up to 70% of all human tumors. Similar information is not available for TORC2, but it phosphorylates AKT/PKB and thereby serves an important positive feedback role. mTOR and PI3K are the two drug targets in this pathway with the following options: mTOR inhibitors, dual PI3K/mTOR inhibitors, pan-PI3K inhibitors, and isoform-specific PI3K inhibitors (see Table 54.10).

mTOR Inhibitors

Rapamycin is the best known prototype mTOR inhibitor, originally approved in 1997 as an immunosuppressant to prevent allograft rejection. Though recognized a decade earlier, rapamycin's application in cancer therapy emerged around the same time in conjunction with the development of several analogs, often termed as rapalogs. Several downsides to rapamycin explain this conundrum. First, rapamycin does not directly inhibit the catalytic activity of mTOR; instead it binds, togethe with FKBP12, to a domain adjacent to the active kinase site of mTORC1, but not mTORC2. This bein said, by binding to mTORC1, rapamycin prevent mTOR from associating with the mTORC2-specifi partner protein Rictor, therefore causing a gradua decline in mTORC2 levels. Indeed, inhibition o mTORC2 is evident upon prolonged treatment, bu only some types of cancer cells. With mTORC1 rapamycin inhibits mainly its weaker substrate such as the PK termed ribosomal protein rpS6 ki nase, and showed very limited, if any, effect o stronger substrates, such as the eIF4E-binding pr tein 4E-BP1. 4E-BP1 is the substrate through whic mTORC1 controls cell proliferation, which likel explains the poor efficiency of rapamycin as an a tihyperplastic agent. Furthermore, by impairi mTORC1, rapamycin can promote growth fact signaling via various feedback loops (e.g., interfe ing with the S6K-dependent negative feedback lo of PI3K/AKT signaling), resulting in enhanced PI3 AKT activity. The inhibition of mTORC1 induc stress responses and leads to a reduction in prot synthesis and induction of autophagy, protecti cancer cells.

TABLE 54.10 **mTOR and PI3K Inhibitors**

TREATMENTS/ DRUGS	THERAPEUTIC INDICATION	MECHANISMS OF CARDIOTOXICITY	RISK FACTORS	MANIFESTATIONS OF CARDIOTOXICITY	PREVENTION AND RISK REDUCTION STRATEGIES
mTOR Inhibitors					
Everolimus	Breast cancer Neuroendocrine tumors Renal cell carcinoma	• mTOR (mechanistic target of rapamycin) is a master regulator of several crucial cellular processes, including protein synthesis, cellular growth, proliferation, autophagy, lysosomal function, and cell metabolism	• Preexisting CV disease • History of CAD disease	Hypertension Hyperlipidemia Insulin resistance Chest pain Arrhythmias Heart failure	• Optimal blood pressure control • Consideration for statin therapy • Consideration of metformin
Temsirolimus	Renal cell cancer	• Complete genetic disruption of mTORC1 or mTORC2 in the heart impairs the development of compensatory cardiac hypertrophy in response to stress and abrogates the ability of the heart to adapt to mechanical and ischemic injury, but applicability to mTOR inhibitors is unknown	• Unknown	Chest pain DVT/PE Hypertension	
PI3K Inhibitors					
Idelalisib	• Chronic lymphocytic leukemia • Follicular B-cell non-Hodgkin lymphoma • Small lymphocytic lymphoma	• Overexpression of AKT/PKB in the heart causes resistance to apoptosis, whereas knockout enhances apoptosis in response to myocardial ischemia • Loss or gain of PTEN activity leads to reduced or enhanced apoptosis		Peripheral edema	
Copanlisib	Follicular lymphoma	No fully defined		Hypertension Hyperglycemia	As above • Optimal blood pressure control • Consideration of metformin
Duvelisib	Follicular lymphoma Chronic lymphocytic leukemia				

AKT/PKB, Protein kinase B; *CAD*, coronary artery disease; *CV*, cardiovascular; *DVT*, deep vein thrombosis; *PE*, pulmonary embolism; *PTEN* phosphatase and tensin homolog.
Modified from Herrmann J, ed. *Clinical Cardio-Oncology*. Philadelphia: Elsevier; 2018.

The pharmacologic properties of rapamycin itself are also not ideal for clinical purposes. For instance, rapamycin is poorly water soluble, reducing bioavailability. Addressing these shortcomings has been the focus of the development of rapalogs (temsirolimus, everolimus, and ridaforolimus), accomplished by replacing the hydrogen at C-40-O position with different moieties. Temsirolimus became the first rapalog approved by the FDA for advanced renal cell carcinoma in 2007 and thereafter for endometrial cancer. Everolimus is approved for renal cell carcinoma, neuroendocrine tumors, and, in combination with exemestane, for hormone receptor-positive, HER2 receptor-negative breast cancer. This limited list speaks of limited success in the majority of cancer, possibly due to genetic variations conferring rapalog resistance to cancer cells. Likely a more important reason is the fact that rapamycin and its analogs are generally not cytotoxic (rather cytostatic) in their effect.

Bypassing these limitations, two strategies have been used: (1) pairing with cytotoxic agents (e.g., paclitaxel and carboplatin for advanced ovarian cancer and metastatic melanoma or in conjunction with hormonal therapy in endocrine cancers for sensitization), and (2) developing inhibitors that target both PI3K and mTOR or, selectively, mTOR. In the latter case, because mTOR serves as the catalytic subunits for both mTORC1 and mTORC2, drugs inhibiting the kinase activity as ATP competitive inhibitors are expected to affect both complexes, and consequently, also the mTORC2-dependent activation of AKT. Because of sequence similarities of mTOR and PI3K, many ATP competitive mTOR inhibitors also block PI3K and vice versa, which can increase anticancer potency but also toxicity. As such, selective inhibitors for either mTOR or PI3k are considered to be better tolerated and clinically preferred. Second-generation mTOR inhibitors emerged toward the end of the first decade of the new millennium. None of them has yet been approved.

PI3K Inhibitors

The PI3K family is divided into three different classes (I, II, and III), based on protein domains and interactions with regulatory subunits. The PI3K class I (p110 catalytic and p85 regulatory unit) is further subdivided into class 1A (activated by receptor tyrosine kinases) and class 1B (activated by G protein–coupled receptors). Class 1A is the subfamily most implicated in human cancer, and tissue-specific isoforms determine the distribution and the activity and toxicity of PI3K inhibitors. There are five variants of the p85 regulatory subunit, and three of the catalytic p110 subunit. The first two p110 isoforms (alpha and beta) are expressed in all cells, but p110δ is expressed primarily in leukocytes, which explains both its use in lymphoid malignancies as well as its inflammatory toxicities.

Indeed, idelalisib, targeting PI3K delta (class 1A) was the first PI3K inhibitor approved by the FDA in 2014 for the use in relapsed/refractory chronic lymphocytic leukemia, follicular lymphoma, and small lymphocytic lymphoma. Although efficacious, unexpected autoimmune and infectious toxicities were demonstrated even to the point of requiring intensive care. Autoimmune toxicities included pneumonitis, hepatitis, noninfectious colitis, and infections *Pneumocystis jirovecii* pneumonia, cytomegalovirus infection, and fungal infections. Idelalisib carries a black box warning for hepatotoxicity, diarrhea/colitis, pneumonitis, and intestinal perforation. Other FDA-approved PI3K inhibitors include the dual PI3k alpha and delta (class 1) inhibitor copanlisib and the dual PI3K delta (class 1A) and gamma (class 1B) inhibitor duvelisib.

Cardiovascular Toxicities

mTOR Inhibitors

The most common cardiovascular side effects with **everolimus** are peripheral edema (up to nearly 40%) and hypertension (up to nearly 15%). Chest pain can be seen in 5% of patients, arrhythmias in 3%, and HF in 1%. With **temsirolimus**, peripheral edema is equally common, but chest pain is more common (~ 15%). Deep vein thrombosis or pulmonary embolism is seen in 2%. Hypertension is seen in 7%. Additional CV risk factor dyscontrol includes hyperglycemia and hyperlipidemia.

PI3K Inhibitors

The most important cardiovascular side effect of **copanlisib** is hypertension in up to 70% of individuals (49% grade 3 and higher).[7] The reasons for this phenomenon are not known, especially as idealisib is not associated with hypertension and the difference in molecular targets, additional inhibition of PI3K alpha by copanlisib does not seem to explain it. However, the fact that copanlisib is also associated with a much higher rate of hyperglycemia (70%, 30% grade 3 and higher) points into the direction of a much stronger inhibition of insulin-receptor-related signaling. A differential effect on the autonomic nervous system is another consideration. For **idealisib** peripheral edema is the most common CV side effec in 10% of patients.

Based on the fact that the mTOR signaling pathway is so important and links to AMPK as a maste regulator of cell metabolism, the impact of PI3 and mTOR inhibition on cardiomyocyte functio and survival has been debated. Arguments for and against a detrimental role of these drugs for cardiac function, especially under situations of stress such as doxorubicin, have been published. As a general rule, if in doubt, more frequent cardiac surveillance should be implemented until the clinical trajectory is defined.[7–13]

BIOLOGICAL RESPONSE MODIFIERS AND DIFFERENTIATION AGENTS

KEY POINTS

- Biological response modifiers and differentiation agents are a heterogeneous group of agents that are used to treat cancer by modulating naturally occurring processes, especially the immune response, or by inciting the maturation (differentiation) of immature cancer cells, thereby slowing growth and spread.
- All-trans retinoid acid (ATRA) and arsenic trioxide (ATO) are examples of differentiation agents.
- Differentiation syndrome is a potentially life-threatening complication of therapy with ATRA and ATO, characterized by dyspnea, fever, peripheral edema, hypotension, weight gain, pleuro-pericardial effusions, acute kidney injury, musculoskeletal pain, and hyperbilirubinemia.
- Interferon-α (IFN-α) and interleukin-2 (Il-2) are examples of biological response modifier. Cardiovascular complications are rare, but include cardiomyopathy, arrhythmias, ischemic events, and pericarditis.

The concept of targeted therapy emerged from the need to minimize the adverse events associated with conventional anticancer therapies. Biological therapy involves the use of agents that engage the immune system into "treating" the underlying condition rather than using chemical drugs or invasive herapies.[1] These agents are collectively termed 'biological response modifiers" and are increasngly used as anticancer therapies. Differentiation herapy is an alternative approach to cancer therpy compared with both biological and convenional treatments. Differentiation agents work by ltering malignant phenotypes and reverting maligant cells to normal.[2] Although immunomodulating nd differentiation treatments exert less direct toxcity compared with conventional chemotherapies, ne nonspecific engagement of the immune system ay still lead to significant side effects, including ardiovascular events (see Table 54.11).

DIFFERENTIATION AGENTS AND DIFFERENTIATION SYNDROME

All-trans retinoic acid (ATRA) and arsenic trioxide (ATO) are associated with complete clinical remission in a high proportion of patients with acute promyelocytic leukemia (APL) by inducing the differentiation of malignant cells into phenotypically mature myeloid cells.[3] Differentiation syndrome (DS), formerly known as retinoic acid syndrome, is a relatively frequent (20% to 25% incidence) and severe complication in APL patients treated with ATRA and/or ATO. DS does not appear when ATRA and/or ATO are used as consolidation or maintenance therapies in APL or for other malignancies.[4]

The proposed mechanism for DS is the activation of various pathophysiologic pathways[5]:

- Interleukin (IL)-1, IL-β, IL-6, IL-8, and tumor necrosis factor-α release, leading to a systemic inflammatory response syndrome.[6]
- Cathepsin G release, enhancing capillary permeability and damaging the endothelium.
- Changes in adhesion molecule interaction, promoting promyelocyte aggregation, leukostasis, and leukocyte tissue infiltration, leading to vessel occlusion and multiorgan failure.[7]

Clinical manifestations include dyspnea with interstitial infiltrates and unexplained fever (most commonly), weight gain, peripheral edema, pleuropericardial effusions (owing to serositis), hypotension, renal and hepatic dysfunction, and rash.[6] Myocarditis, pulmonary hemorrhage and Sweet syndrome (acute febrile neutrophilic dermatosis) have been reported in DS, but the incidence is unclear.[8]

A diagnosis of DS can be made in the presence of two or more of the following signs and symptoms: fever, weight gain, dyspnea, radiologic opacities on chest X-ray, pleural or pericardial effusions, hypotension, or renal failure. The major limitation of these diagnostic criteria is that they are highly nonspecific. Rapid improvement with glucocorticoids supports a diagnosis of DS. DS can have a bimodal time distribution, occurring more commonly in the first or third week of induction treatment with ATRA and/or ATO. Earlier occurrence is associated with worse outcomes. DS is not dose-dependent, nor is the risk proportional to white blood cell count.

Steroid use (prednisone, methylprednisolone, dexamethasone) has been proposed as a preventive

TABLE 54.11 **Biological Response Modifiers and Differentiation Agents**

TREATMENTS/ DRUGS	THERAPEUTIC INDICATION	MECHANISMS OF CARDIOTOXICITY	RISK FACTORS	MANIFESTATIONS OF CARDIOTOXICITY	PREVENTION AND RISK REDUCTION STRATEGIES
Biological Response Modifiers					
Interferon-alpha	Leukemia Lymphomas Melanoma Various solid tumors	Unknown Complex of interferon and cardiac tissue stimulating an auto-immune or inflammatory reaction (unclear mechanism)	• Pre-existing CV disease • History of CAD disease	*Early manifestation* • Arrhythmias (supraventricular/ ventricular) and heart block • Sudden cardiac death (Case report) • Hypertension • Acute pericarditis (effusion/ tamponade, high dose related case report) *Late manifestation* • LV dysfunction/CHF • Dilated cardiomyopathy	• Termination of treatment (reversible)
Interleukin-2	Melanoma RCC	Capillary leakage syndrome with increased vascular permeability (high dose) Direct myocardial toxicity (Unclear mechanism)	• Unknown	*Early manifestation* • Hypotension (↓SVR, ↑HR)-peak at 4 hours after therapy • Arrhythmias (SVT/VT) • Myocarditis • Thrombotic events *Late Manifestation* • Dilated cardiomyopathy	• Termination of treatment (reversible) • Response well with fluid replacement • Vasopressors as indicated
Denileukin difitox	Lymphomas Leukemias	Fatal capillary leakage syndrome Hypersensitivity reaction	• Preexisting CV disease	Hypotension, tachycardia Chest pain Myocardial ischemia/infarction Arrhythmias CHF	• Termination of treatment (reversible) • Continuous infusion with monitoring for hypersensitivity reaction
Differentiation Agents					
All-trans retinoic acid (ATRA) Arsenic trioxide (ATO)	Leukemias (AML esp., in acute promyeloblastic leukemia)	Direct myocyte injury and damage ↑oxidative stress and DNA fragmentation ↑Apoptosis of myocardial cells Capillary leakage syndrome	• WBC $\geq$ 10,000/mm^3 • Rapidly increasing WBC count • Presence of CD 13 expression on leukemic cells • Hypokalemia, Hypomagnesemia [ATO]	Differentiation syndrome (Both) • Hypotension • CHF/pulmonary edema • Pericardial effusion/tamponade • Myocardial ischemia/infarction QTc Prolongation/*Torsades de points/* SCD [ATO]	• Prompt IV corticosteroid • Continue chemotherapy (termination recommended only in case severe differentiation syndrome) • Generalize supportive care (oxygen, diuretic) • Monitoring ECG and correction of serum electrolyte and magnesium [ATO] • Resveratrol treatment [ATO-case report]

AML, Acute myeloid leukemia; *CAD*, coronary artery disease; *CHF*, congestive heart failure; *CV*, cardiovascular; *ECG*, electrocardiogram; *HR*, heart rate; *LV*, left ventricular; *RCC*, renal cell carcinoma; *SCD*, sudden cardiac death; *SVR*, stroke volume ratio; *SVT*, supraventricular tachycardia; *VT*, ventricular tachycardia; *WBC*, white blood cell.
Modified from Herrmann J, ed. *Clinical Cardio-Oncology*. Philadelphia: Elsevier; 2018.

strategy, but uniform evidence for this approach regarding timing, duration, preferred agent, or dose is lacking.[9] The ongoing preferred strategy is that of selective prophylaxis with dexamethasone (2.5 mg/m^2 per 12 hours intravenously for 15 days) for patients with leukocytosis or increased serum creatinine levels.[10]

Full-blown DS can be life-threatening, so treatment with corticosteroids (dexamethasone 10 mg twice daily intravenously) should be initiated as soon as the first signs or symptoms appear.[11] Although other severe complications, such as bacteremia, sepsis, pulmonary hemorrhage, pneumonia, renal failure, or CHF, can present similarly, they can occur at the same time with DS, making the differential diagnosis challenging. Empiric treatment to cover all suspected complications, including DS, is recommended.[10] ATRA or ATO can be safely continued except in the case of severe DS (e.g., renal failure, respiratory distress requiring intensive care unit admission) or if DS is unresponsive to dexamethasone. ATRA and/or ATO can be resumed after the disappearance of all DS signs and symptoms. DS can recur, albeit rarely, and is similarly treated with dexamethasone. Fortunately, early dexamethasone treatment with additional supportive measures, as needed, can lead to a dramatic and rapid resolution of DS within 12 to 24 hours.

Cardioprotective Effects of ATRA

All-trans retinoic acid has been studied for its cardioprotective effects against doxorubicin cardiotoxicity in experimental models. ATRA appears to counteract doxorubicin-induced cardiomyopathy through antioxidative and anti-inflammatory properties and by suppressing mitochondrial apoptosis activation, without compromising antitumoral efficacy[12]

ATO Cardiotoxicity

Although ATO has been proven as an efficient and safe agent in the treatment of APL, the clinical efficacy of ATO is limited by its poor tissue selectivity, damaging both malignant and normal cells. The very mechanisms through which ATO exerts its antitumoral effects are the ones that generate cardiotoxicity:

- Free radical-mediated oxidative damage.
- Apoptosis induction through direct mitochondrial membrane effects leading to release of cytochrome C intracellularly and caspase activation.
- Cardiac ion channel dysfunction by inhibiting potassium currents and stimulating L-type calcium currents.
- Endothelial function changes through induction of growth factors and inflammatory cytokines.
- Enzymatic activation and gene expression induction contributing to its carcinogenic effects.

Arsenic trioxide cardiotoxicity is dose-dependent and can manifest in various ways, either acutely (e.g., arrhythmias, stroke, myocardial infarction, pericarditis, sudden cardiac death) or chronically (e.g., atherosclerosis, peripheral vascular disease, hypertension, type 2 diabetes). Arrhythmias are among the most common side effects associated with ATO, including prolongation of the QT interval, *Torsades de pointes* and, more rarely, bradycardias and heart blocks. Treatment of these arrhythmias is challenging, because responses to treatment may be impaired.

Acute ATO toxicity can be severe or fatal, even at therapeutic doses, in susceptible patients. Supportive care and urgent chelation therapy with unithiol (3 to 5 mg/kg every 4 to 6 hours intravenously) or dimercaprol (3 to 5 mg/kg every 4 to 6 hours intramuscularly) are warranted. Chronic exposure to ATO has been proven to increase the risk of mortality caused by myocardial injury, arrhythmias, and cardiomyopathy. Chelation therapy has not proven to be useful for chronic ATO toxicity, the only useful strategy being to limit ATO exposure as much as possible. Attempts to limit the cardiotoxicity associated with ATO without compromising its anticancer effects have been made. Various agents (e.g., herbal extracts, omega-3 fatty acids, resveratrol) have been studied for their potential to limit the cardiotoxicity associated with ATO, but they are not currently used in clinical practice.

BIOLOGICAL RESPONSE MODIFIERS

Interferon-α

Interferon-α (IFN-α) is a cytokine with complex antiproliferative, antiviral, and immunoregulatory activities. It is also involved in cell differentiation and antitumor defense processes, making tumor cells more vulnerable to chemo- and radiotherapy. These results are achieved through:

- Apoptosis induction via death receptor activation, mitochondrial pathways, or stress kinase cascade activation.[13]
- Cell cycle mitotic arrest in various phases.[13]

- Angiogenesis inhibition by the downregulation of proangiogenic factors (VEGF, basic fibroblast growth factor, IL-8, matrix metalloproteinase 9 expression).[14]
- Immune effector cell activation (cytotoxic T-lymphocyte, natural killer-cells, and monocyte activation).[15]

Interferon-α has been used in the treatment of various hematologic and solid malignancies, but its use has been limited by its significant side effect profile.[16] The interest in IFN-α has been renewed by the appearance of the better-tolerated pegylated form and by its complementary action to TKIs.[14]

Acute manifestations of IFN-α toxicity are caused by cytokine release and include flu-like symptoms, such as fever, chills, headache, and myalgia. These occur in almost all patients, shortly after starting IFN-α administration and lasting for several hours. If necessary, the symptoms can be managed by pretreatment with acetaminophen, antiemetics, or cyclooxygenase inhibitors, adequate hydration during treatment, or by decreasing the INF-α dose.[17] If the symptoms are severe or persistent, patients should be evaluated for rhabdomyolysis, systemic infection, pneumonitis, or pneumonia.

Delayed manifestations include effects on all organ systems: hematologic (e.g., anemia, leukopenia, thrombocytopenia), hepatic (e.g., increased transaminase levels, cytochrome p450 inhibition), gastrointestinal (e.g., nausea, vomiting, diarrhea), psychiatric (e.g., depression, cognitive dysfunction, delirium), neurologic (e.g., seizures, neuropathies, myasthenia gravis, multiple-sclerosis-like disease), renal (e.g., proteinuria), pulmonary (e.g., pneumonitis), endocrine (e.g., thyroid disorders, diabetes mellitus, hypopituitarism), dermatologic (e.g., alopecia, injection site reactions, rash, pruritus, vitiligo, lichen planus, psoriasis), and general fatigue.[16]

Cardiovascular complications are rare, encountered in less than 5% of patients,[18] but they can be life-threatening and include:

- Dilated cardiomyopathy, presumably caused by mitochondrial dysfunction.[19] The occurrence of cardiomyopathy could be underestimated, as its symptoms (e.g., fatigue and poor exercise tolerance) can be confounded by the typical side effects of IFN-α.[20]
- Arrhythmias, caused by inflammatory infiltrates in or around nerves, leading to conduction abnormalities[19]
- Ischemic events through various mechanisms: coronary vasospasm at the time of administration, capillary wall thickening leading to luminal size decreases, and triglyceride and very low density lipoprotein (VLDL) increases with concomitant high-density lipoprotein decreases.[21]
- Pericarditis and pericardial effusions, which are caused by inflammatory infiltrates within the pericardial space or by autoimmune processes.[22]

Cardiotoxicity does not appear to be closely correlated with IFN-α dose and the cardiovascular effects (including cardiomyopathy) appear to be reversible upon discontinuation.[17] Pegylated IFN-α-induced cardiotoxicity, however, seems to have a poor prognosis.[23] IFN-α can also cause vascular adverse events: hypotension (related to administration pathway and dose), Raynaud-like phenomena, thrombotic thrombocytopenic purpura, pulmonary hypertension, and retinopathy.[16] The mechanisms for these appear to be capillary wall thickening, endothelial dysfunction, vasospasm, and autoimmunity.

Recommendations regarding prevention or treatment of IFN-α toxicity are limited to supportive treatment and IFN-α interruption. Cardiac assessment is recommended monthly for the first four months, then every three months.[17] Thyroid function should be assessed, because it can be concomitantly affected by INF-α and can predispose to cardiac complications. An important objective of IFN therapy is to maintain the dose intensity to achieve maximum therapeutic benefits. In light of this objective, all means to maintain patient comfort and to avoid dose reductions should be pursued.[17]

Interleukin-2

Interleukin-2, either as a single-agent or in combina tion with other antineoplastic agents, has bee shown to induce durable remission in a small sub set of patients with metastatic melanoma and meta static renal carcinoma. It works by:

- Upregulating proinflammatory cytokines
- Expanding CD4+ cells
- Augmenting natural killer cell activity[24]

Because of the widespread effects of cytokin on the body, the toxicities of IL-2 affect all orga systems,[25] but they are usually predictable, manag able, and resolve quickly with treatment.[26] The terruption or discontinuation of IL-2 treatment, ne ertheless, is often required owing to the severity the side effects. Careful patient selection and treatment at experienced centers can limit and control toxicities.[27]

Before IL-2 treatment initiation, cardiac evaluation with a careful personal and family history, physical evaluation, ECG, and a cardiac stress test are important to assess adequate cardiac function and to exclude patients at risk for cardiotoxicity.[27] Reversible ischemia is a contraindication to IL-2 treatment, because it makes patients who experience hypotension during treatment vulnerable to myocardial infarction. The initial evaluation includes a thoracic computed tomography, on which the presence of pericardial fluid should be carefully assessed. Effusions can worsen owing to capillary leak syndrome, making them a contraindication to IL-2 treatment.

During treatment, patients should be placed on continuous telemetry monitoring, to rapidly diagnose arrhythmias and to monitor heart rate and blood pressure. Hypotension with reflexive tachycardia is the most frequent cardiac side effect (50% to 70%). It is caused by nitric oxide release from endothelial cells giving rise to decreased systemic vascular resistance and third spacing of fluid, comprising capillary leak syndrome.[28] Antihypertensive agents should be discontinued 24 to 48 hours before IL-2 treatment and can be resumed 24 to 48 hours after blood pressure has stabilized following each cycle. Beta-blockers should not be discontinued abruptly, but rather tapered; smaller doses can be kept if beta-blockers are used for tachyarrhythmia control.

Hypotension can be observed within 2 hours after he first dose, is cyclic, and peaks 4 to 6 hours after ach dose. It can be managed with saline boluses for goal systolic blood pressure below 80 to 90 mm Hg. luid resuscitation should be reduced to 1.5 L/day to imit the exacerbation of capillary leak syndrome. If ypotension persists despite fluid resuscitation, doamine (preferred) or phenylephrine (in case of chyarrhythmias) can be used. If maximized vasoressor support is inefficient in controlling blood ressure, IL-2 treatment should be discontinued and ypotension should resolve within 24 to 48 hours.

Cardiac dysrhythmias are usually asymptomatic d severe arrhythmias are uncommon. If arrhythias occur, they are usually brief, responsive to meditiom, and cease upon IL-2 treatment interruption. us tachycardia is expected during therapy and of- responds to fluids. Although supraventricular or nonsustained ventricular tachycardia can be present, atrial fibrillation is more common.[29] If premature ventricular contractions are frequent or occur in patterns (e.g., quadrigeminy, couplets), it may be necessary to hold IL-2 until recovery. Serum electrolytes should be checked and monitored throughout treatment to minimize arrhythmias.

Myocardial infarction and myocarditis have been reported in patients with IL-2 treatment.[28] Myocarditis is rare and difficult to diagnose, usually leading to elevated cardiac enzymes with a normal ECG, in the context of low-grade fever and mild chest pain.[27] Owing to the similar presentation between myocarditis and myocardial infarction, it is presumed that the true incidence of myocarditis has been underestimated. It can present days after IL-2 treatment. It is thought to occur because of cytokine-induced migration of activated lymphocytes and other inflammatory cells into the myocardium, leading to microcirculation disruption, cytotoxic damage, and myocyte necrosis.[30] If myocarditis or ischemia is suspected, cardiac enzymes should be monitored daily and, if confirmed, IL-2 should be discontinued. Transthoracic echocardiogram is currently used to guide the decision regarding IL-2 treatment continuation after an adverse cardiac event, but this is an imperfect assessment for myocarditis.[28] Cardiac magnetic resonance has been successfully used to diagnose IL-2-induced myocarditis and to avoid unnecessary invasive procedures.[31]

Fluid administration and capillary leak syndrome can lead to peripheral edema, with patients gaining 10% to 15% of their body weight. Careful physical examination for fluid overload and daily weights to monitor weight gain should be performed. After IL-2 treatment completion, patients return to their baseline weight within 2 to 3 days. If not and the edema causes significant discomfort, diuretics can be used.

Judicious patient selection, vigilant monitoring for acute and delayed toxicities, and prompt intervention are essential to ensure safe and successful IL-2 treatments.

CONCLUSIONS

Biological therapy is associated with significant cardiovascular effects. IFN-α is used in various hematologic and solid malignancies and chronic use may lead to cardiomyopathy, arrhythmias, ischemic events, or pericardial disease. Patients requiring IL-2 treatment should be evaluated with an ECG and a cardiac stress test and may experience hypotension, myocardial infarction, arrhythmias, or myocarditis. Physicians administering ICIs should exert vigilance regarding cardiac side effects, of which myocarditis appears to be the most severe. Differentiation therapies associated with cardiovascular side effects are ATRA and ATO, because patients may experience differentiation syndrome or a broad range of cardiotoxic events.

MISCELLANEOUS

A few cancer therapeutics were not covered in detail because their use is very confined, or relates to specific disease entities, such as hormonal therapies for breast and prostate cancer, covered in Chapters 35 and 37. A summary, however, is provided in Table 54.12.

TABLE 54.12 **Miscellaneous**

TREATMENTS/ DRUGS	THERAPEUTIC INDICATION	MECHANISMS OF CARDIOTOXICITY	RISK FACTORS	MANIFESTATIONS OF CARDIOTOXICITY	PREVENTION AND RISK REDUCTION STRATEGIES
Anti-Hormonal Therapy					
Diethylstilbestrol Estramustine	Breast cancer Prostate cancer	Unknown • Estrogen related CV side effect	• Pre-existing CV disease	• Arterial thrombosis • Myocardial ischemia/ infarction/stroke • Venous thrombosis-DVT, PE • HTN • ↑CV death for overall	• Use with caution in patients with CV risk factors • Diethylstilbestrol: now no longer available in the United States due to teratogenic effect.
Selective Estrogen Receptor Modulators					
Tamoxifen Raloxifen	Breast cancer	• Changes in coagulation factors, esp. decrease in antithrombin III and protein C levels	• VTE risk factors • CV risk factors	• Venous (and arterial) thromboembolism	• Ambulation for VTE prophylaxis • Optimization of CV risk factors
Aromatase Inhibitors					
Anastrozole Letrozole Exemestane	Breast cancer	• Increase in LDL cholesterol • Exemestane decreases antithrombin III and protein C levels	• CV risk factors and CV disease	Increased CV risk, including heart failure and CV mortality (compared with tamoxifen but not confirmed against placebo)	• Optimize CV risk factors, possibly even aspirin in view of increased arterial risk
Antiandrogens					
Enzalutamide, Darolutamide, Apalutamide *CPY17 inhibitor* Abiraterone	Prostate cancer	• Induction of a metabolic syndrome state (dyslipidemia, adiposity, and insulin resistance) • Promotion of atherosclerosis	• CV risk factors • ASCVD • MI history	• Myocardial ischemia and infarction • Hypertension • Heart failure • Arrhythmias • QTc prolongation	• Cautious use in patients with CV disease, especially MI, heart failure and arrhythmias; close follow-up • Monitor and optimize blood pressure control • Monitor QTc interval, avoid any factors contributing to QTc prolongation

TABLE 54.12 **Miscellaneous—cont'd**

TREATMENTS/ DRUGS	THERAPEUTIC INDICATION	MECHANISMS OF CARDIOTOXICITY	RISK FACTORS	MANIFESTATIONS OF CARDIOTOXICITY	PREVENTION AND RISK REDUCTION STRATEGIES
Gonadotropin-Releasing Hormone [GnRH] Agonist					
Leuprolide Goserelin Triptorelin Buserelin Histrelin	Prostate cancer	As above	• CV risk factors • ASCVD • MI history	• Hypertension • Myocardial ischemia and infarction • Venous thromboembolism • Arrhythmias including atrial fibrillation • QTc prolongation • Syncope • Heart failure	• Cautious use in and follow closely patients with CV disease, especially MI, heart failure and arrhythmias • Monitor and optimize CV risk factors and vascular health (optimal lipid and glucose control) • Monitor QTc interval and avoid concomitant QTc prolonging drugs • Aspirin in those at thrombotic risk
GnRH Antagonist					
Degarelix Relugolix	Prostate cancer	As above	• CV risk factors • ASCVD • MI history	• Hypertension • QTc prolongation	• Lower risk than above listed androgen depreviation therapies, but caution advised
Immuno-Modulatory Drugs (IMDs)					
Thalidomide Lenalidomide	MM, amyloidosis, Waldenstrom's CLL, diffuse large B-cell lymphoma, mantel cell lymphoma, MM, MDS	• Not clearly defined (alternation in coagulation factors and vWF)	• Combination with chemotherapy (doxorubicin) or dexamethasone • Advanced age • Previous thromboembolism • Indwelling central venous catheter • Comorbidities (e.g. infections, diabetes, CV disease, obesity) • Immobilization, recent surgery • Inherited thrombophilia	• Venous > arterial thromboembolic events **[Black box warning for both]** • Arrhythmia	• Appropriate prophylaxis based on risk factor stratification (MM patients: SAVED score or IMPEDE DVT score) with LMWH or warfarin (high risk) or aspirin (low risk) • Optimize vascular health
CDK 4/6 Inhibitors					
Ribociclib Palbociclib Abemaciclib	Breast cancer	• Down-regulation of *KCNH2* expression (encoding for potassium channel hERG) and up-regulation of SCN5A and SNTA1 (encoding for sodium channels Nav1.5 and syntrophin-α1)	Ribociclib: • Long QT syndrome uncontrolled or significant cardiac disease (e.g., recent MI, unstable angina, CHF, bradyarrhythmias) • Electrolyte abnormalities • Tamoxifen use	Ribociclib: • QTc prolongation (dose-dependent) • Torsades de pointes • SCD • Syncope	• Evaluate ECG prior to treatment, and proceed only if QTcF <450 msec • Repeat ECG on day 14 of cycle 1, at the beginning of cycle 2, and as clinically indicated • Monitor and correct electrolyte and magnesium before the start medication • Avoid use in patients with risk factors or in combination with medications known to prolong the QTc interval and/or strong CYP3A inhibitors • Avoid concomitant tamoxifen use

Continued

TABLE 54.12 **Miscellaneous—cont'd**

TREATMENTS/ DRUGS	THERAPEUTIC INDICATION	MECHANISMS OF CARDIOTOXICITY	RISK FACTORS	MANIFESTATIONS OF CARDIOTOXICITY	PREVENTION AND RISK REDUCTION STRATEGIES
Histone Deacetylase Inhibitors [HDAC-I]					
Vorinostat Romidepsin	T-cell lymphoma NSCLC	Unknown	• Pre-existing CV disease • Congenital long QT syndrome • Concurrent drugs that prolong QTc interval or inhibit CYP3A4 • Electrolyte disturbance or hypomagnesemia	• Prolongation of QTc, ST-T changes (transients) • Arrhythmias (supraventricular/ ventricular) • Hypotension, syncope • DVT	• No routine ECG monitoring, recommendation only in high risk • Monitor and correct electrolyte and magnesium before start medication • Avoid concurrent drugs that prolong the QTc or inhibit CYP3A4

AF, Atrial fibrillation; *ASCVD*, atherosclerotic cardiovascular disease; *CV*, cardiovascular; *DVT*, deep vein thrombosis; *ECG*, electrocardiogram; *HTN*, hypertension; *LDL*, low density lipoprotein; *LMWH*, low molecular weight heparin; *MM*, multiple myeloma; *MDS*, myelodysplatic syndrome; *MI*, myocardial infarction; *PE*, pulmonary embolism; *SCD*, sudden cardiac death; *VTE*, venous thromboembolism; *vWF*, von Willebrand factor.
Modified from Herrmann J, ed. *Clinical Cardio-Oncology*. Philadelphia: Elsevier; 2018.

REFERENCES

Antitumor Antibiotics and Topoisomerase Inhibitors Including Anthracyclines

1. Szucs Z, Jones RL. Introduction to systemic antineoplastic treatments for cardiologists. *Clin Cardio-Oncol.* 2017;1:15–38.
2. Falzone L, Salomone S, Libra M. Evolution of cancer pharmacological treatments at the turn of the third millennium. *Front Pharmacol.* 2018;9:1300.
3. Cassinelli G. The roots of modern oncology: from discovery of new antitumor anthracyclines to their clinical use. *Tumori.* 2016;2016:226–235.
4. Delgado JL, Hsieh CM, Chan NL, Hiasa H. Topoisomerases as anticancer targets. *Biochem J.* 2018;475:373–398.
5. Gianni L, Herman EH, Lipshultz SE, Minotti G, Sarvazyan N, Sawyer DB. Anthracycline cardiotoxicity: from bench to bedside. *J Clin Oncol.* 2008;26:3777–3784.
6. Chen B, Peng X, Pentassuglia L, Lim CC, Sawyer DB. Molecular and cellular mechanisms of anthracycline cardiotoxicity. *Cardiovasc Toxicol.* 2007;7:114–121.
7. Geisberg C, Pentassuglia L, Sawyer DB. Cardiac side effects of anticancer treatments: new mechanistic insights. *Curr Heart Fail Rep.* 2012;9:211–218.
8. Herrmann J, Lerman A, Sandhu NP, Villarraga HR, Mulvagh SL, Kohli M. Evaluation and management of patients with heart disease and cancer: cardio-oncology. *Mayo Clin Proc.* 2014;89:1287–1306.
9. Henriksen PA. Anthracycline cardiotoxicity: an update on mechanisms, monitoring and prevention. *Heart.* 2018;104:971–977.
10. Herrmann J. Adverse cardiac effects of cancer therapies: cardiotoxicity and arrhythmia. *Nat Rev Cardiol.* 2020;17:474–502.
11. Ewer MS, Ali MK, Mackay B, et al. A comparison of cardiac biopsy grades and ejection fraction estimations in patients receiving adriamycin. *J Clin Oncol.* 1984;2:112–117.
12. Mitani I, Jain D, Joska TM, Burtness B, Zaret BL. Doxorubicin cardiotoxicity: prevention of congestive heart failure with serial cardiac function monitoring with equilibrium radionuclide angiocardiography in the current era. *J Nucl Cardiol.* 2003;10:132–139.
13. Zhang S, Liu X, Bawa-Khalfe T, et al. Identification of the molecular basis of doxorubicin-induced cardiotoxicity. *Nat Med.* 2012;18: 1639–1642.
14. Doll DC, Ringenberg QS, Yarbro JW. Vascular toxicity associated with antineoplastic agents, *J Clin Oncol.* 1986;4:1405–1417.
15. Herrmann J, Yang EH, Iliescu CA, et al. Vascular toxicities of cancer therapies: the old and the new—an evolving avenue. *Circulation.* 2016;133:1272–1289.
16. McGrath SE, Webb A, Walker-Bone K. Bleomycin-induced Raynaud's phenomenon after single-dose exposure: risk factors and treatment with intravenous iloprost infusion. *J Clin Oncol.* 2013;31:e51–e52.
17. Khouri C, Blaise S, Carpentier P, Villier C, Cracowski JL, Roustit M. Drug-induced Raynaud's phenomenon: beyond beta-adrenoceptor blockers. *Br J Clin Pharmacol.* 2016;82:6–16.

Alkylating Agents

1. Adair FE, Bagg HJ. Experimental and clinical studies on the treatment of cancer by dichlorethylsulphide (mustard gas). *Ann Surg.* 1931;93(1):190199.
2. Rhoads C. Nitrogen mustards in treatment of neoplastic disease. *JAMA.* 1946;131:656658.
3. Jacobson LP, Spurr CL, Barron ESG, et al. Studies on the effect of methyl-bis(beta-chloroethyl) amine hydrochloride on neoplastic diseases and allied disorders of the hematopoietic system. *JAMA.* 1946;132:263.
4. Kim K. Roh JK, Wee H, Kim C. *Cancer Drug Discovery: Science and History*. Springer; 2016.
5. DeVita VT Jr, Lawrence TS, Rosenberg SA. *Cancer: Principles & Practice of Oncology*, ed 10. Philadelphia, PA: Wolters Kluwer Health; 2015.
6. Coles B. Effects of modifying structure on electrophilic reactions with biological nucleophiles. *Drug Metab Rev.* 1985;15:1307–1334.
7. Ross W. Alkylating agents. In: *Biological Alkylating Agents*. London Butterworth; 1962.
8. Fenselau C, Kan MN, Rao SS, et al. Identification of aldophospha mide as a metabolite of cyclophosphamide in vitro and in vivo i humans. *Cancer Res.* 1977;37:2538–2543.
9. Zon G, Ludeman SM, Brandt JA, et al. NMR spectroscopic studie of intermediary metabolites of cyclophosphamide. A compreher sive kinetic analysis of the interconversion of cis- and trans- hydroxycyclophosphamide with aldophosphamide and the co comitant partitioning of aldophosphamide between irreversib fragmentation and reversible conjugation pathways. *J Med Che* 1984;27:466.
10. Chabner BA. Alkylating agents. In: Chabner BA, Collins JM, ed *Cancer Chemotherapy: Principles and Practice*. Lippincott Willia & Wilkins; 1990: 276–313.
11. Boddy AV, Cole M, Pearson ADJ, Idle JR. The kinetics of the au induction ifosfamide metabolism during continuous infusion. *C cer Chemother Pharmacol.* 1995;36:53.
12. Colvin M. The comparative pharmacology of cyclophosphami and ifosfamide. *Semin Oncol.* 1982;9:2.

13. Brock N, Pohl J, Stekar J. Studies on the urotoxicity of oxazaphosphorine cytostatics and its prevention. 2. Comparative study on the uroprotective efficacy of thiols and other sulfur compounds. *Eur J Cancer Clin Oncol.* 1981;17:1155–1163.
14. Colvin M, Brundrett RB, Cowens W, et al. A chemical basis for the antitumor activity of chloroethylnitrosoureas. *Biochem Pharmacol.* 1976;25:695.
15. Galton DAG, Till M, Wiltshaw E. Busulfan (1, 4-dimethyl-sulfonoxybutane, myleran): summary of clinical results. *Ann N Y Acad Sci.* 1958;68:967.
16. Sykes MP, Karnofsky DA, Philips FS, Burchenal JH. Clinical studies on triethylene-phosphoramide and diethylenephosphoramide, compounds with nitrogen-mustard-like activity. *Cancer.* 1953;61:—142–148.
17. Hata T, Sano Y, Sugawara R, et al. Mitomycin, a new antibiotic from Streptomyces. *J Antibiot.* 1956;9:141–146.
18. Szybalski W, Iyer VN. Cross-linking of DNA by enzymatically or chemically activated mitomycins and porfiromycins, bifunctionally "alkylating" antibiotics. *Fed Proc.* 1964;23:946–957.
19. Johnstone JC, Young Park G, Lippard SJ. Understanding and improving platinum anticancer drugs—phenanthriplatin. *Anticancer Res.* 2014;34:471–476.
20. Zeller P, Gutmann H, Hegedus B, et al. Methylhydrazine derivatives, a new class of cytotoxic agents. *Experientia.* 1963;19:129.
21. Shealy YF, Struck RF, Holum LB, Montgomery JA. Synthesis of potential anticancer agents. XXIX. 5-Diazoimidazole-4-carbox amide and 5-Diazo-c-triazole-4-carboxamide. *J Org Chem.* 1961;26:2396–2401.
22. Newlands ES, Blackledge GRP, Slack JA, et al. Phase I trial of temozolomide (CCRG 81045: M&B 39831: NSC 362856). *Br J Cancer.* 1992;65:287–291.
23. Herrmann J, Lerman A, Sandhu NP, Villarraga HR, Mulvagh SL, Kohli M. Evaluation and management of patients with heart disease and cancer: cardio-oncology. *Mayo Clin Proc.* 2014;89:1287–1306.
24. Kurauchi K, Nishikawa T, Miyahara E, Okamoto Y, Kawano Y. Role of metabolites of cyclophosphamide in cardiotoxicity. *BMC.* 2017;10(1):406.
25. Morandi P, Ruffini PA, Benvenuto GM, Raimondi R, Fosser V. Cardiac toxicity of high-dose chemotherapy. *Bone Marrow Transplant.* 2005;35:323–334.
26. Quezado ZM, Wilson WH, Cunnion RE, et al. High-dose ifosfamide is associated with severe, reversible cardiac dysfunction. *Ann Intern Med.* 1993;118:31–36.
27. Yeh ET, Bickford CL. Cardiovascular complications of cancer therapy: incidence, pathogenesis, diagnosis, and management. *J Am Coll Cardiol.* 2009;53:-2231–2247.
28. Schimmel K, Richel D, van den Brink R, Guchelaar HJ. Cardiotoxicity of cytotoxic drugs. *Cancer Treat Rev.* 2004;30:181–191.
29. Tamargo J, Caballero R, Delpon E. Cancer chemotherapy and cardiac arrhythmias: a review. *Drug Saf.* 2015;38:129–152.
30. Kupari M, Volin L, Suokas A, Hekali P, Ruutu T. Cardiac involvement in bone marrow transplantation: serial changes in left ventricular size, mass and performance. *J Intern Med.* 1990;227:259–266.
31. Cil T, Kaplan MA, Altintas A, Pasa S, Isikdogan A. Cytosine-arabinoside induced bradycardia in patient with non-Hodgkin lymphoma: a case report. *Leuk Lymphoma.* 2007;2007;48:1247–1249.
32. Agarwal N, Burkart TA. Transient, high-grade atrioventricular block from high-dose cyclophosphamide. *Tex Heart Inst J.* 2013; 40(5):626–627.
33. Sculier JP, Coune A, Klastersky J. Transient heart block. An unreported toxicity of high dose chemotherapy with cyclophosphamide and etoposide. *Acta Clin Belg.* 1985;40(2):112–114.
34. Ramireddy K, Kane KM, Adhar GC. Acquired episodic complete heart block after high-dose chemotherapy with cyclophosphamide and thiotepa. *Am Heart J.* 1994;127(3):701–704.
35. Yeh ET. Cardiotoxicity induced by chemotherapy and antibody therapy. *Annu Rev Med.* 2006;57:485–498.
36. Nakamae H, Tsumura K, Terada Y, et al. Notable effects of angiotensin II receptor blocker, valsartan, on acute cardiotoxic changes after standard chemotherapy with cyclophosphamide, doxorubicin, vincristine, and prednisolone. *Cancer.* 2005;104:2492–2498.
37. Hunt SA; American College of Cardiology, American Heart Association Task Force on Practice Guidelines (Writing Committee to Update the 2001 Guidelines for the Evaluation and Management of Heart Failure). ACC/AHA 2005 guideline update for the diagnosis and management of chronic heart failure in the adult: a report of the American College of Cardiology/American Heart Association Task Force on Practice Guidelines (Writing Committee to Update the 2001 Guidelines for the Evaluation and Management of Heart Failure). *J Am Coll Cardiol.* 2005;46:e1–e82.
38. Kalay N, Basar E, Ozdogru I, et al. Protective effects of carvedilol against anthracycline-induced cardiomyopathy. *J Am Coll Cardiol.* 2006;48:2258–2262.
39. Ewer MS, Vooletich MT, Durand JB, et al. Reversibility of trastuzumab-related cardiotoxicity: new insights based on clinical course and response to medical treatment. *J Clin Oncol.* 2005;23:7820–7826.
40. El-Agamy DS, Elkablawy MA, Abo-Haded HM. Modulation of cyclophosphamide-induced cardiotoxicity by methyl palmitate. *Cancer Chemother Pharmacol.* 2017;79:399–409.
41. Chakraborty M, Bhattacharjee A, Kamath JV. Pharmacodynamic interaction of green tea extract with hydrochlorothiazide against cyclophosphamide-induced myocardial damage. *Indian J Pharmacol.* 2017;49(1):65–70.
42. Chakraborty M, Bhattacharjee A, Kamath JV. Cardioprotective effect of curcumin and piperine combination against cyclophosphamide-induced cardiotoxicity. *Indian J Pharmacol.* 2009;25(7–8): 812–817.
43. Todorova V, Vanderpool D, Blossom S, et al. Oral glutamine protects against cyclophosphamide-induced cardiotoxicity in experimental rats through increase of cardiac glutathione. *Nutrition.* 2019;25:812–817.
44. Omole JG, Ayoka OA, Alabi QK, et al. Protective effect of kolaviron on cyclophosphamide-induced cardiac toxicity in rats. *J Evid Based Integr Med.* 2018;23:2156587218757649.
45. Avci H, Epikmen ET, Ipek E, et al. Protective effects of silymarin and curcumin on cyclophosphamide-induced cardiotoxicity. *Exp Toxicol Pathol.* 2017;69(5):317–327.
46. Liu Y, Tan D, Shi L, et al. Blueberry anthocyanins-enriched extracts attenuate cyclophosphamide-induced cardiac injury. *PLoS One.* 2015;10(7):e0127813. doi:10.1371/journal.pone.0127813.

Antimetabolites

1. Heidelberger C, Chaudhuri NK, Danneberg P, et al. Fluorinated pyrimidines, a new class of tumour-inhibitory compounds. *Nature.* 1957;179(4561):663–666.
2. Benson AB III, Venook AP, Al-Hawary MM, et al. NCCN Guidelines Insights: Colon Cancer, Version 2.2018. *J Natl Compr Canc Netw.* 2018;16(4):359–369.
3. Khorana AA, Mangu PB, Berlin J, et al. Potentiallyc curable pancreatic cancer: American Society of Clinical Oncology Clinical Practice Guideline Update. *J Clin Oncol.* 2017;35(20):2324–2328.
4. Sohal DP, Mangu PB, Khorana AA, et al. Metastatic pancreatic cancer: American Society of Clinical Oncology Clinical Practice Guideline. *J Clin Oncol.* 2016;34(23):2784–2796.
5. Oshaughnessy JA, Blum J, Moiseyenko V, et al. Randomized, open-label, phase II trial of oral capecitabine (Xeloda) vs. a reference arm of intravenous CMF (cyclophosphamide, methotrexate and 5-fluorouracil) as first-line therapy for advanced/metastatic breast cancer. *Ann Oncol.* 2001;12(9):1247–1254.
6. Fumoleau P, Largillier R, Clippe C, et al. Multicentre, phase II study evaluating capecitabine monotherapy in patients with anthracycline- and taxane-pretreated metastatic breast cancer. *Eur J Cancer.* 2004;40(4):536–542.
7. Masuda N, Lee SJ, Ohtani S, et al. Adjuvant capecitabine for breast cancer after preoperative chemotherapy. *N Engl J Med.* 2017; 376(22):2147–2159.
8. Colevas AD, Yom SS, Pfister DG, et al. NCCN Guidelines Insights: Head and Neck Cancers, Version 1.2018. *J Natl Compr Canc Netw.* 2018;16(5):479–490.
9. Enzinger PC, Burtness BA, Niedzwiecki D, et al. CALGB 80403 (Alliance)/E1206: A randomized phase II study of three chemotherapy regimens plus cetuximab in metastatic esophageal and gastroesophageal junction cancers. *J Clin Oncol.* 2016;34(23):2736–2742.
10. Tsibiribi P, Bui-Xuan C, Bui-Xuan B, et al. Cardiac lesions induced by 5-fluorouracil in the rabbit. *Hum Exp Toxicol.* 2006;25(6):305–309.

11. Cwikiel M, Zhang B, Eskilsson J, Wieslander JB, Albertsson M. The influence of 5-fluorouracil on the endothelium in small arteries. An electron microscopic study in rabbits. *Scanning Microsc.* 1995; 9(2):561–576.
12. Cwikiel M, Eskilsson J, Wieslander JB, Stjernquist U, Albertsson M. The appearance of endothelium in small arteries after treatment with 5-fluorouracil. An electron microscopic study of late effects in rabbits. *Scanning Microsc.* 1996;10(3):805–818; discussion 819.
13. Cwikiel M, Eskilsson J, Albertsson M, Stavenow L. The influence of 5-fluorouracil and methotrexate on vascular endothelium. An experimental study using endothelial cells in the culture. *Ann Oncol.* 1996;7(7):731–737.
14. Luwaert RJ, Descamps O, Majois F, Chaudron JM, Beauduin M. Coronary artery spasm induced by 5-fluorouracil. *Eur Heart J.* 1991;12(3):468–470.
15. Sudhoff T, Enderle MD, Pahlke M, et al. 5-Fluorouracil induces arterial vasocontractions. *Ann Oncol.* 2004;15(4):661–664.
16. Stewart T, Pavlakis N, Ward M. Cardiotoxicity with 5-fluorouracil and capecitabine: more than just vasospastic angina. *Intern Med J.* 2010;40(4):303–307.
17. Talapatra K, Rajesh I, Rajesh B, Selvamani B, Subhashini J. Transient asymptomatic bradycardia in patients on infusional 5-fluorouracil. *J Cancer Res Ther.* 2007;3(3):169–171.
18. Wacker A, Lersch C, Scherpinski U, Reindl L, Seyfarth M. High incidence of angina pectoris in patients treated with 5-fluorouracil. A planned surveillance study with 102 patients. *Oncology.* 2003;65(2):108–112.
19. Labianca R, Beretta G, Clerici M, Fraschini P, Luporini G. Cardiac toxicity of 5-fluorouracil: a study on 1083 patients. *Tumori.* 1982;68(6):505–510.
20. Schober C, Papageorgiou E, Harstrick A, et al. Cardiotoxicity of 5-fluorouracil in combination with folinic acid in patients with gastrointestinal cancer. *Cancer.* 1993;72(7):2242–2247.
21. Polk A, Vaage-Nilsen M, Vistisen K, Nielsen DL. Cardiotoxicity in patients with cancer treated with 5-fluorouracil or capecitabine: a systematic review of incidence, manifestations and predisposing factors. *Cancer Treat Rev.* 2013;39(8):974–984.
22. Meyer CC, Calis KA, Burke LB, Walawander CA, Grasela TH. Symptomatic cardiotoxicity associated with 5-fluorouracil. *Pharmacotherapy.* 1997;17(4):729–736.
23. Kelly C, Bhuva N, Harrison M, Buckley A, Saunders M. Use of raltitrexed as an alternative to 5-fluorouracil and capecitabine in patients with cancer with cardiac history. *Eur J Cancer.* 2013;49(10):2303–2310.
24. Meydan N, Kundak I, Yavuzsen T, et al. Cardiotoxicity of de Gramont's regimen: incidence, clinical characteristics and long-term follow-up. *Jpn J Clin Oncol.* 2005;35(5):265–270.
25. Ng M, Cunningham D, Norman AR. The frequency and pattern of cardiotoxicity observed with capecitabine used in conjunction with oxaliplatin in patients treated for advanced colorectal cancer (CRC). *Eur J Cancer.* 2005;41(11):1542–1546.
26. Akhtar SS, Salim KP, Bano ZA. Symptomatic cardiotoxicity with high-dose 5-fluorouracil infusion: a prospective study. *Oncology.* 1993;50(6):441–444.
27. Jensen SA, Sorensen JB. Risk factors and prevention of cardiotoxicity induced by 5-fluorouracil or capecitabine. *Cancer Chemother Pharmacol.* 2006;58(4):487–493.
28. Kosmas C, Kallistratos MS, Kopterides P, et al. Cardiotoxicity of fluoropyrimidines in different schedules of administration: a prospective study. *J Cancer Res Clin Oncol.* 2008;134(1):75–82.
29. Tsavaris N, Kosmas C, Vadiaka M, et al. 5-fluorouracil cardiotoxicity is a rare, dose and schedule-dependent adverse event: a prospective study. *J BUON.* 2005;10(2):205–211.
30. Van Cutsem E, Hoff PM, Blum JL, Abt M, Osterwalder B. Incidence of cardiotoxicity with the oral fluoropyrimidine capecitabine is typical of that reported with 5-fluorouracil. *Ann Oncol.* 2002; 13(3):484–485.
31. Cianci G, Morelli MF, Cannita K, et al. Prophylactic options in patients with 5-fluorouracil-associated cardiotoxicity. *Br J Cancer.* 2003;88(10):1507–1509.

Mitotic Inibitors

1. Szucs Z, Jones RL. Introduction to systemic antineoplastic treatments for cardiologists. *Clin Cardiol.* 2017;1:15–38.
2. Jordan MA, Wilson L. Microtubules as a target for anticancer drugs. *Nat Rev Cancer.* 2004;4:253–265.
3. Morris PG, Fornier MN. Microtubule active agents: beyond the taxane frontier. *Clin Cancer Res.* 2008;14:7167–7172.
4. Dumontet C, Jordan MA. Microtubule-binding agents: a dynamic field of cancer therapeutics. *Nat Rev Drug Discov.* 2010;9:790–803.
5. Perez EA. Microtubule inhibitors: differentiating tubulin-inhibiting agents based on mechanisms of action, clinical activity, and resistance. *Mol Cancer Ther.* 2009;8:2086–2095.
6. Falzone L, Salomone S, Libra M. Evolution of cancer pharmacological treatments at the turn of the third millennium. *Front Pharmacol.* 2018;9:1300.
7. Stanton RA, Gernert KM, Nettles JH, Aneja R. Drugs that target dynamic microtubules: a new molecular perspective. *Med Res Rev.* 2011;31:443–481.
8. Risinger AL, Giles FJ, Mooberry SL. Microtubule dynamics as a target in oncology. *Cancer Treat Rev.* 2009;35:255–261.
9. Jain S, Vahdat LT. Eribulin mesylate. *Clin Cancer Res.* 2011;17:6615–6622.
10. Herrmann J. Vascular toxic effects of cancer therapies. *Nat Rev Cardiol.* 2020.
11. Herrmann J, Yang EH, Iliescu CA, et al. Vascular toxicities of cancer therapies: the old and the new—an evolving avenue. *Circulation.* 2016;133:1272–1289.
12. Arbuck SG, Strauss H, Rowinsky E, et al. A reassessment of cardiac toxicity associated with Taxol. *J Natl Cancer Inst Monogr.* 1993:117–130.
13. Rowinsky EK, Eisenhauer EA, Chaudhry V, Arbuck SG, Donehower RC. Clinical toxicities encountered with paclitaxel (Taxol). *Semin Oncol.* 1993;20:1–15.
14. Page RL II, O'Bryant CL, Cheng D, et al.; American Heart Association Clinical Pharmacology and Heart Failure and Transplantation Committees of the Council on Clinical Cardiology; Council on Cardiovascular Surgery and Anesthesia; Council on Cardiovascular and Stroke Nursing; and Council on Quality of Care and Outcomes Research Drugs that may cause or exacerbate heart failure: a scientific statement from the American Heart Association. *Circulation.* 2016;134:e32–69.
15. Osman M, Elkady M. A prospective study to evaluate the effect o paclitaxel on cardiac ejection fraction. *Breast Care (Basel)* 2017;12:255–259.
16. Gianni L, Herman EH, Lipshultz SE, Minotti G, Sarvazyan N, Sawye DB. Anthracycline cardiotoxicity: from bench to bedside. *J Cli Oncol.* 2008;26:3777–3784.
17. Perotti A, Cresta S, Grasselli G, Capri G, Minotti G, Gianni L. Ca diotoxic effects of anthracycline-taxane combinations. *Expe Opin Drug Saf.* 2003;2:59–71.

Monoclonal Antibodies

1. Ross JS, Gray K, Gray GS, Worland PJ, Rolfe M. Anticancer antibo ies. *Am J Clin Pathol.* 2003;119:472–485.
2. Sun Z, Fu YX, Peng H. Targeting tumor cells with antibodies e hances anti-tumor immunity. *Biophys Rep.* 2018;4:243–253.
3. Zafir-Lavie I, Michaeli Y, Reiter Y. Novel antibodies as anticanc agents. *Oncogene.* 2007;26:3714–3733.
4. Adler MJ, Dimitrov DS. Therapeutic antibodies against canc *Hematol Oncol Clin North Am.* 2012;26:447–481, vii.
5. Weiner LM, Surana R, Wang S. Monoclonal antibodies: versat platforms for cancer immunotherapy. *Nat Rev Immunol.* 2010; 317–327.
6. Rogers LM, Veeramani S, Weiner GJ. Complement in monoclo antibody therapy of cancer. *Immunol Res.* 2014;59:203–210.
7. Moasser MM. The oncogene HER2: its signaling and transformi functions and its role in human cancer pathogenesis. *Oncoge* 2007;26:6469–6487.
8. De Keulenaer GW, Doggen K, Lemmens K. The vulnerability of heart as a pluricellular paracrine organ: lessons from unexpec triggers of heart failure in targeted ErbB2 anticancer therapy. *Res.* 2010;106:35–46.
9. Ignoffo RJ. Overview of bevacizumab: a new cancer therape strategy targeting vascular endothelial growth factor. *Am J He Syst Pharm.* 2004;61:S21–S26.
10. Kazazi-Hyseni F, Beijnen JH, Schellens JH. Bevacizumab. *Onc gist.* 2010;15:819–825.

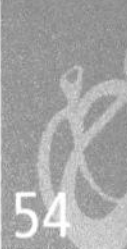

11. Tiwari P. Ramucirumab: boon or bane. *J Egypt Natl Canc Inst.* 2016;28:133–140.
12. Alexandre J, Salem JE, Moslehi J, et al. Identification of anticancer drugs associated with atrial fibrillation—analysis of the WHO pharmacovigilance database. *Eur Heart J Cardiovasc Pharmacother.* 2021;7(4):312–320. doi:10.1093/ehjcvp/pvaa037. PMID: 32353110.
13. Tang XM, Chen H, Liu Y, et al. The cardiotoxicity of cetuximab as single therapy in Chinese chemotherapy-refractory metastatic colorectal patients with cancer. *Medicine (Baltimore).* 2017;96:e5946.

Multi-Tyrosine Kinase Inhibitors

1. Bishop JM. Clues to the puzzle of purpose. *Nature.* 1985;316:483–484.
2. Varmus HE. The molecular genetics of cellular oncogenes. *Annu Rev Genet.* 1984;18:553–612.
3. Slamon DJ, Leyland-Jones B, Shak S, et al. Use of chemotherapy plus a monoclonal antibody against HER2 for metastatic breast cancer that overexpresses HER2. *N Engl J Med.* 2001;344:783–792.
4. Romond EH, Perez EA, Bryant J, et al. Trastuzumab plus adjuvant chemotherapy for operable HER2-positive breast cancer. *N Engl J Med.* 2005;353:1673–1684.
5. Folkman J. Tumor angiogenesis: therapeutic implications. *N Engl J Med.* 1971;285:1182–1186.
6. Hochhaus A, Larson RA, Guilhot F, et al. Long-term outcomes of imatinib treatment for chronic myeloid leukemia. *N Engl J Med.* 2017;376:917–927.
7. Bantscheff M, Eberhard D, Abraham Y, et al. Quantitative chemical proteomics reveals mechanisms of action of clinical ABL kinase inhibitors. *Nat Biotechnol.* 2007;25:1035–1044.
8. Karaman MW, Herrgard S, Treiber DK, et al. A quantitative analysis of kinase inhibitor selectivity. *Nat Biotechnol.* 2008;26:127–132.
9. Hoshijima M, Chien KR. Mixed signals in heart failure: cancer rules. *J Clin Invest.* 2002;109:849–855.
10. Chen MH, Kerkela R, Force T. Mechanisms of cardiac dysfunction associated with tyrosine kinase inhibitor cancer therapeutics. *Circulation.* 2008;118:84–95.
11. Ozcelik C, Erdmann B, Pilz B, et al. Conditional mutation of the ErbB2 (HER2) receptor in cardiomyocytes leads to dilated cardiomyopathy. *Proc Natl Acad Sci U S A.* 2002;99:8880–8885.
12. Carmeliet P, Ng YS, Nuyens D, et al. Impaired myocardial angiogenesis and ischemic cardiomyopathy in mice lacking the vascular endothelial growth factor isoforms VEGF164 and VEGF188. *Nat Med.* 1999;5:495–502.
13. May D, Gilon D, Djonov V, et al. Transgenic system for conditional induction and rescue of chronic myocardial hibernation provides insights into genomic programs of hibernation. *Proc Natl Acad Sci U S A.* 2008;105:282–287.
14. Yamaguchi O, Watanabe T, Nishida K, et al. Cardiac-specific disruption of the c-raf-1 gene induces cardiac dysfunction and apoptosis. *J Clin Invest.* 2004;114:937–943.
15. Harris IS, Zhang S, Treskov I, Kovacs A, Weinheimer C, Muslin AJ. Raf-1 kinase is required for cardiac hypertrophy and cardiomyocyte survival in response to pressure overload. *Circulation.* 2004;110:718–723.
16. Chislock EM, Ring C, Pendergast AM. Abl kinases are required for vascular function, Tie2 expression, and angiopoietin-1-mediated survival. *Proc Natl Acad Sci U S A.* 2013;110:12432–12437.
17. Wang S, Song P, Zou MH. Inhibition of AMP-activated protein kinase alpha (AMPKalpha) by doxorubicin accentuates genotoxic stress and cell death in mouse embryonic fibroblasts and cardiomyocytes: role of p53 and SIRT1. *J Biol Chem.* 2012;287:8001–8012.
18. Shah RR, Morganroth J. Update on cardiovascular safety of tyrosine kinase inhibitors: with a special focus on QT interval, left ventricular dysfunction and overall risk/benefit. *Drug Saf.* 2015;38:693–710.
19. Liu B, Ding F, Zhang D, Wei GH. Risk of venous and arterial thromboembolic events associated with VEGFR-TKIs: a meta-analysis. *Cancer Chemother Pharmacol.* 2017;80:487–495.
20. Shah RR, Morganroth J, Shah DR. Cardiovascular safety of tyrosine kinase inhibitors: with a special focus on cardiac repolarisation (QT interval). *Drug Saf.* 2013;36:295–316.
21. Seruga B, Sterling L, Wang L, Tannock IF. Reporting of serious adverse drug reactions of targeted anticancer agents in pivotal phase III clinical trials. *J Clin Oncol.* 2011;29:174–185.
22. Eschenhagen T, Force T, Ewer MS, et al. Cardiovascular side effects of cancer therapies: a position statement from the Heart Failure Association of the European Society of Cardiology. *Eur J Heart Fail.* 2011;13:1–10.
23. Pareek N, Cevallos J, Moliner P, et al. Activity and outcomes of a cardio-oncology service in the United Kingdom-a five-year experience. *Eur J Heart Fail.* 2018;20:1721–1731.

Immune Checkpoint Inhibitors

1. Reck M, Rodriguez-Abreu D, Robinson AG, et al. Pembrolizumab versus chemotherapy for PD-L1-positive non-small-cell lung cancer. *N Engl J Med.* 2016;375:1823–1833.
2. Hodi FS, O'Day SJ, McDermott DF, et al. Improved survival with ipilimumab in patients with metastatic melanoma. *N Engl J Med.* 2010;363:711–723.
3. Boussiotis VA. Molecular and biochemical aspects of the PD-1 checkpoint pathway. *N Engl J Med.* 2016;375:1767–1778.
4. Melero I, Hervas-Stubbs S, Glennie M, Pardoll DM, Chen L. Immunostimulatory monoclonal antibodies for cancer therapy. *Nat Rev Cancer.* 2007;7:95–106.
5. Naidoo J, Page DB, Li BT, et al. Toxicities of the anti-PD-1 and anti-PD-L1 immune checkpoint antibodies. *Ann Oncol.* 2015;26:2375–2391.
6. Postow MA, Sidlow R, Hellmann MD. Immune-related adverse events associated with immune checkpoint blockade. *N Engl J Med.* 2018;378:158–168.
7. Moslehi JJ, Salem JE, Sosman JA, Lebrun-Vignes B, Johnson DB. Increased reporting of fatal immune checkpoint inhibitor-associated myocarditis. *Lancet.* 2018;391:933.
8. Johnson DB, Balko JM, Compton ML, et al. Fulminant myocarditis with combination immune checkpoint blockade. *N Engl J Med.* 2016;375:1749–1755.
9. Mahmood SS, Fradley MG, Cohen JV, et al. Myocarditis in patients treated with immune checkpoint inhibitors. *J Am Coll Cardiol.* 2018;71:1755–1764.
10. Friedrich MG, Sechtem U, Schulz-Menger J, et al. International Consensus Group on Cardiovascular Magnetic Resonance in Myocarditis. Cardiovascular magnetic resonance in myocarditis: a JACC White Paper. *J Am Coll Cardiol.* 2009;53:1475–1487.
11. Ganatra S, Neilan TG. Immune checkpoint inhibitor-associated myocarditis. *Oncologist.* 2018;23:879–886.
12. Lurz P, Luecke C, Eitel I, et al. Comprehensive cardiac magnetic resonance imaging in patients with suspected myocarditis: The MyoRacer-Trial. *J Am Coll Cardiol.* 2016;67:1800–1811.
13. Neilan TG, Rothenberg ML, Amiri-Kordestani L, et al., Checkpoint inhibitor safety working group. Myocarditis associated with immune checkpoint inhibitors: an expert consensus on data gaps and a call to action. *Oncologist.* 2018;23:874–878.

Chimeric Antigen Receptor (CAR) T Cell Therapy

1. Maude SL, Laetsch TW, Buechner J, et al. Tisagenlecleucel in children and young adults with B-cell lymphoblastic leukemia. *N Engl J Med.* 2018;378:439–448.
2. Maude SL, Frey N, Shaw PA, et al. Chimeric antigen receptor T cells for sustained remissions in leukemia. *N Engl J Med.* 2014;371:1507–1517.
3. Schuster SJ, Bishop MR, Tam C, et al. Sustained disease control for adult patients with relapsed or refractory diffuse large B-cell lymphoma: an updated analysis of Juliet, a global pivotal phase 2 trial of tisagenlecleucel. *Blood.* 2018;132:1684–1684.
4. Schuster SJ, Bishop MR, Tam CS, et al. Tisagenlecleucel in adult relapsed or refractory diffuse large B-cell lymphoma. *N Engl J Med.* 2019;380:45–56.
5. Locke FL, Ghobadi A, Jacobson CA, et al. Long-term safety and activity of axicabtagene ciloleucel in refractory large B-cell lymphoma (ZUMA-1): a single-arm, multicentre, phase 1–2 trial. *Lancet Oncol.* 2019;20:31–42.
6. Neelapu SS, Locke FL, Bartlett NL, et al. Axicabtagene ciloleucel CAR T-cell therapy in refractory large B-cell lymphoma. *N Engl J Med.* 2017;377:2531–2544.
7. Crump M, Neelapu SS, Farooq U, et al. Outcomes in refractory diffuse large B-cell lymphoma: results from the international SCHOLAR-1 study. *Blood.* 2017:blood-2017-03-769620.

8. Brudno JN, Kochenderfer JN. Chimeric antigen receptor T-cell therapies for lymphoma. *Nat Rev Clin Oncol*. 2017;15:31.
9. Lee DW, Santomasso BD, Locke FL, et al. ASTCT Consensus grading for cytokine release syndrome and neurologic toxicity associated with immune effector cells. *Biol Blood Marrow Transplant*. 2019;25:625–638.
10. Burstein DS, Maude S, Grupp S, Griffis H, Rossano J, Lin K. Cardiac profile of chimeric antigen receptor T cell therapy in children: a single-institution experience. *Biol Blood Marrow Transplant*. 2018;24:1590–1595.
11. Fitzgerald JCMDP, Weiss SLMDM, Maude SLMDP, et al. Cytokine release syndrome after chimeric antigen receptor T cell therapy for acute lymphoblastic leukemia. *Crit Care Med*. 2017;45:e124–e131.
12. Asnani A. Cardiotoxicity of immunotherapy: incidence, diagnosis, and management. *Curr Oncol Rep*. 2018;20:44.
13. Brudno JN, Kochenderfer JN. Toxicities of chimeric antigen receptor T cells: recognition and management. *Blood*. 2016;127:3321.
14. Subklewe M, von Bergwelt-Baildon M, Humpe A. Chimeric antigen receptor T cells: a race to revolutionize cancer therapy. *Transfus Med Hemother*. 2019;46:15–24.

Proteasome Inhibitors

1. Chari A, Mezzi K, Zhu S, et al. Incidence and risk of hypertension in patients newly treated for multiple myeloma: a retrospective cohort study. *BMC Cancer*. 2016;16(1):912.
2. Reneau JC, Asante D, van Houten H, et al. Cardiotoxicity risk with bortezomib versus lenalidomide for treatment of multiple myeloma: a propensity matched study of 1,790 patients. *Am J Hematol*. 2017;92(2):E15–E17.
3. Kumar SK, Callander NS, Alsina M, et al. Multiple myeloma, version 3. 2017, NCCN Clinical Practice Guidelines in Oncology. *J Natl Compr Canc Netw*. 2017;15(2):230–269.
4. Enrico O, Gabriele B, Nadia C, et al. Unexpected cardiotoxicity in haematological bortezomib treated patients. *Br J Haematol*. 2007;138(3):396–397.
5. Richardson PG, Sonneveld P, Schuster MW, et al. Bortezomib or high-dose dexamethasone for relapsed multiple myeloma. *N Engl J Med*. 2005;352(24):2487–2498.
6. Laubach JP, Moslehi JJ, Francis SA, et al. A retrospective analysis of 3954 patients in phase 2/3 trials of bortezomib for the treatment of multiple myeloma: towards providing a benchmark for the cardiac safety profile of proteasome inhibition in multiple myeloma. *Br J Haematol*. 2017;178(4):547–560.
7. Xiao Y, Yin J, Wei J, Shang Z. Incidence and risk of cardiotoxicity associated with bortezomib in the treatment of cancer: a systematic review and meta-analysis. *PLoS One*. 2014;9(1):e87671.
8. Dimopoulos MA, Moreau P, Palumbo A, et al. Carfilzomib and dexamethasone versus bortezomib and dexamethasone for patients with relapsed or refractory multiple myeloma (ENDEAVOR): a randomised, phase 3, open-label, multicentre study. *Lancet Oncol*. 2016;17(1):27–38.
9. Dimopoulos MA, Stewart AK, Masszi T, et al. Carfilzomib, lenalidomide, and dexamethasone in patients with relapsed multiple myeloma categorised by age: secondary analysis from the phase 3 ASPIRE study. *Br J Haematol*. 2017;177(3):404–413.
10. Stewart AK, Rajkumar SV, Dimopoulos MA, et al. Carfilzomib, lenalidomide, and dexamethasone for relapsed multiple myeloma. *N Engl J Med*. 2015;372(2):142–152.
11. Chari A, Stewart AK, Russell SD, et al. Analysis of carfilzomib cardiovascular safety profile across relapsed and/or refractory multiple myeloma clinical trials. *Blood Adv*. 2018;2(13):1633–1644.
12. *Common Terminology Criteria for Adverse Events (CTCAE). Version 4.03*. 2010, National Cancer Institute. NIH Publication no. 09-5410: Bethesda, MD.
13. Moreau P, Mateos MV, Berenson JR, et al. Once weekly versus twice weekly carfilzomib dosing in patients with relapsed and refractory multiple myeloma (A.R.R.O.W.): interim analysis results of a randomised, phase 3 study. *Lancet Oncol*. 2018;19(7):953–964.
14. Ludwig H, Dimopoulos MA, Moreau P, et al. Carfilzomib and dexamethasone vs bortezomib and dexamethasone in patients with relapsed multiple myeloma: results of the phase 3 study ENDEAVOR (NCT01568866) according to age subgroup. *Leuk Lymphoma*. 2017;58(10):2501–2504.
15. Jain T, Narayanasamy H, Mikhael J, et al. Systolic dysfunction associated with carfilzomib use in patients with multiple myeloma. *Blood Cancer J*. 2017;7(12):642.
16. Moreau P, Masszi T, Grzasko N, et al. Oral Ixazomib, lenalidomide, and dexamethasone for multiple myeloma. *N Engl J Med*. 2016;374(17):1621–1634.

mTOR and PI3K Inhibitors

1. Tian T, Li X, Zhang J. mTOR signaling in cancer and mTOR inhibitors in solid tumor targeting therapy. *Int J Mol Sci*. 2019;20.
2. Pons-Tostivint E, Thibault B, Guillermet-Guibert J. Targeting PI3K signaling in combination cancer therapy. *Trends Cancer*. 2017;3:454–469.
3. Janku F. Phosphoinositide 3-kinase (PI3K) pathway inhibitors in solid tumors: from laboratory to patients. *Cancer Treat Rev*. 2017;59:93–101.
4. Greenwell IB, Ip A, Cohen JB. PI3K inhibitors: understanding toxicity mechanisms and management. *Oncology (Williston Park)*. 2017;31:821–828.
5. Yang J, Nie J, Ma X, Wei Y, Peng Y, Wei X. Targeting PI3K in cancer: mechanisms and advances in clinical trials. *Mol Cancer*. 2019;18:26.
6. Janku F, Yap TA, Meric-Bernstam F. Targeting the PI3K pathway in cancer: are we making headway? *Nat Rev Clin Oncol*. 2018;15:273–291.
7. Gratia S, Kay L, Potenza L, et al. Inhibition of AMPK signalling by doxorubicin: at the crossroads of the cardiac responses to energetic, oxidative, and genotoxic stress. *Cardiovasc Res*. 2012;95:290–299.
8. Yang Y, Li N, Chen T, et al. Trimetazidine ameliorates sunitinib-induced cardiotoxicity in mice via the AMPK/mTOR/autophagy pathway. *Pharm Biol*. 2019;57:625–631.
9. Timm KN, Tyler DJ. The role of AMPK activation for cardioprotection in doxorubicin-induced cardiotoxicity. *Cardiovasc Drugs Ther*. 2020;34:255–269.
10. Lv X, Zhu Y, Deng Y, et al. Glycyrrhizin improved autophagy flux via HMGB1-dependent AKT/mTOR signaling pathway to prevent doxorubicin-induced cardiotoxicity. *Toxicology*. 2020;441:152508.
11. Li M, Sala V, De Santis MC, et al. Phosphoinositide 3-kinase gamma inhibition protects from anthracycline cardiotoxicity and reduces tumor growth. *Circulation*. 2018;138:696–711.
12. Hullin R, Metrich M, Sarre A, et al. Diverging effects of enalapril or eplerenone in primary prevention against doxorubicin-induced cardiotoxicity. *Cardiovasc Res*. 2018;114:272–281.
13. Elmadani M, Khan S, Tenhunen O, et al. Novel screening method identifies PI3Kalpha, mTOR, and IGF1R as key kinases regulating cardiomyocyte survival. *J Am Heart Assoc*. 2019;8:e013018.

Biological Response Modifiers and Differentiation Agents

1. Kuroki M, Miyamoto S, Morisaki T, et al. Biological response modifiers used in cancer biotherapy. *Anticancer Res*. 2012;32:2229–2233.
2. Warrell RP Jr, Frankel SR, Miller WH Jr, et al. Differentiation ther-
apy of acute promyelocytic leukemia with tretinoin (all-trans-retinoic acid). *N Engl J Med*. 1991;324:1385–1393.
3. Shen ZX, Shi ZZ, Fang J, et al. All-trans retinoic acid/As2O3 combi
nation yields a high quality remission and survival in newly diag
nosed acute promyelocytic leukemia. *Proc Natl Acad Sci U S A*
2004;101:5328–5335.
4. Kuley-Bagheri Y, Kreuzer KA, Monsef I, Lubbert M, Skoetz N. Ef
fects of all-trans retinoic acid (ATRA) in addition to chemotherap
for adults with acute myeloid leukaemia (AML) (non-acute promy
elocytic leukaemia [non-APL]). *Cochrane Database Syst Re*
2018;8:CD011960.
5. Luesink M, Jansen JH. Advances in understanding the pulmonar
infiltration in acute promyelocytic leukaemia. *Br J Haemato*
2010;151:209–220.
6. Dubois C, Schlageter MH, DE Gentile A, et al. Hematopoiet
growth factor expression and ATRA sensitivity in acute promyel
cytic blast cells. *Blood*. 1994;83:3264–3270.
7. Larson RS, Brown DC, Sklar LA. Retinoic acid induces aggregati
of the acute promyelocytic leukemia cell line NB-4 by utilization
LFA-1 and ICAM-2. *Blood*. 1997;90:2747–2756.
8. Manna A, Cadenotti L, Motto A, Ballo P. Reversible cardiac dy
function without myocytolysis related to all-trans retinoic ac

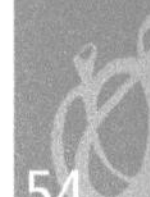

administration during induction therapy of acute promyelocytic leukemia. *Ann Hematol.* 2009;88:91–92.

9. Burnett AK, Hills RK, Grimwade D, et al. Inclusion of chemotherapy in addition to anthracycline in the treatment of acute promyelocytic leukaemia does not improve outcomes: results of the MRC AML15 trial. *Leukemia.* 2013;27:843–851.
10. Sanz MA, Montesinos P. How we prevent and treat differentiation syndrome in patients with acute promyelocytic leukemia. *Blood.* 2014;123:2777–2782.
11. Sanz MA, Grimwade D, Tallman MS, et al. Management of acute promyelocytic leukemia: recommendations from an expert panel on behalf of the European LeukemiaNet. *Blood.* 2009;113:1875–1891.
12. Khafaga AF, EL-Sayed YS. All-trans-retinoic acid ameliorates doxorubicin-induced cardiotoxicity: in vivo potential involvement of oxidative stress, inflammation, and apoptosis via caspase-3 and p53 down-expression. *Naunyn Schmiedebergs Arch Pharmacol.* 2018;391:59–70.
13. Vitale G, Van Eijck CH, Van Koetsveld Ing PM, et al. Type I interferons in the treatment of pancreatic cancer: mechanisms of action and role of related receptors. *Ann Surg.* 2007;246:259–268.
14. Talpaz M, Mercer J, Hehlmann R. The interferon-alpha revival in CML. *Ann Hematol.* 2015;94(suppl 2):S195–207.
15. Rizza P, Moretti F, Belardelli F. Recent advances on the immunomodulatory effects of IFN-alpha: implications for cancer immunotherapy and autoimmunity. *Autoimmunity.* 2010;43:204–209.
16. Sleijfer S, Bannink M, Van Gool AR, Kruit WH, Stoter G. Side effects of interferon-alpha therapy. *Pharm World Sci.* 2005;27:423–431.
17. Hauschild A, Gogas H, Tarhini A, et al. Practical guidelines for the management of interferon-alpha-2b side effects in patients receiving adjuvant treatment for melanoma: expert opinion. *Cancer.* 2008;112:982–994.
18. Motzer RJ, Murphy BA, Bacik J, et al. Phase III trial of interferon alfa-2a with or without 13-cis-retinoic acid for patients with advanced renal cell carcinoma. *J Clin Oncol.* 2000;18:2972–2980.
19. Kondo Y, Yukinaka M, Nomura M, Nakaya Y, ITO S. Early diagnosis of interferon-induced myocardial disorder in patients with chronic hepatitis C: evaluation by myocardial imaging with 123I-BMIPP. *J Gastroenterol.* 2000;35:127–135.
20. Choy-Shan A, Berezovskaya S, Zinn A, Sedlis SP, Bini EJ. Nonischemic cardiomyopathy related to pegylated interferon and ribavirin. *Eur J Gastroenterol Hepatol.* 2009;21:1438–1440.
21. Fernandez-Miranda C, Castellano G, Guijarro C, et al. Lipoprotein changes in patients with chronic hepatitis C treated with interferon-alpha. *Am J Gastroenterol.* 1998;93:1901–1904.
22. Rauw J, Ahmed S, Petrella T. Pericardial effusion and tamponade following interferon alpha treatment for locally advanced melanoma. *Med Oncol.* 2012;29:1304–1307.
23. Condat B, Asselah T, Zanditenas D, et al. Fatal cardiomyopathy associated with pegylated interferon/ribavirin in a patient with chronic hepatitis C. *Eur J Gastroenterol Hepatol.* 2006;18:287–289.
24. Henney CS, Kuribayashi K, Kern DE, Gillis S. Interleukin-2 augments natural killer cell activity. *Nature.* 1981;291:335–338.
25. Kim-Schulze S, Taback B, Kaufman HL. Cytokine therapy for cancer. *Surg Oncol Clin N Am.* 2007;16:793–818, viii.
26. Hamm C, Verma S, Petrella T, Bak K, Charette M. Biochemotherapy for the treatment of metastatic malignant melanoma: a systematic review. *Cancer Treat Rev.* 2008;34:145–156.
27. Marabondo S, Kaufman HL. High-dose interleukin-2 (IL-2) for the treatment of melanoma: safety considerations and future directions. *Expert Opin Drug Saf.* 2017;16:1347–1357.
28. Schwartzentruber DJ. Guidelines for the safe administration of high-dose interleukin-2. *J Immunother.* 2001;24:287–293.
29. White RL Jr, Schwartzentruber DJ, Guleria A, et al. Cardiopulmonary toxicity of treatment with high dose interleukin-2 in 199 consecutive patients with metastatic melanoma or renal cell carcinoma. *Cancer.* 1994;74:3212–3222.
30. Zhang J, Yu ZX, Hilbert SL, et al. Cardiotoxicity of human recombinant interleukin-2 in rats. A morphological study. *Circulation.* 1993;87:1340–1353.
31. Tan MCC, Ortega-Legaspi JM, Cheng SF, Patton KK. Acute myocarditis following high-dose interleukin-2 treatment. *J Cardiol Cases.* 2017;15:28–31.

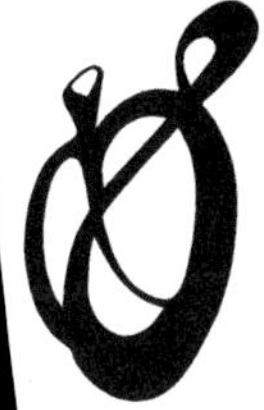

Index

Page numbers followed by 'f' indicate figures, 't' indicate tables, and 'b' indicate boxes.

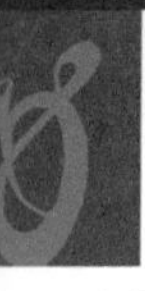

C

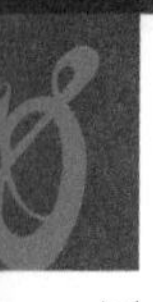

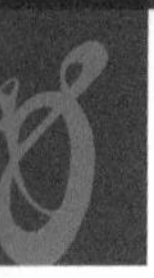

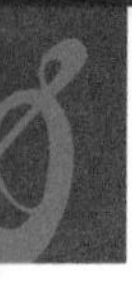